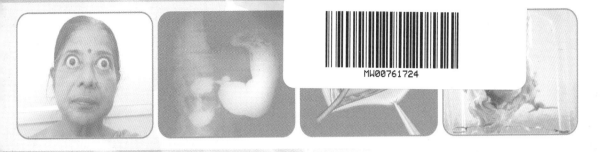

SURGERY

Bedside Clinics in Surgery

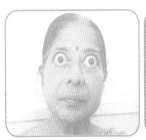
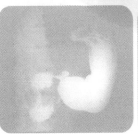
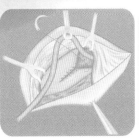
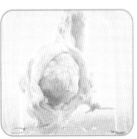

SURGERY

Bedside Clinics in Surgery

Long and Short Cases, Surgical Problems, X-rays
Surgical Pathology, Preoperative Preparations
Minor Surgical Procedures, Instruments
Operative Surgery and Surgical Anatomy

Makhan Lal Saha

MBBS MS (Surgery) FMAS FAIS

Professor
Department of General Surgery
IPGME & R/SSKM Hospital, Kolkata, West Bengal, India
Formerly, Associate Professor
Department of General Surgery, Calcutta Medical College
North Bengal Medical College

Forewords
**Bhabatosh Biswas
N Chintamani
Manoj Kumar Bhattacharya**

The Health Sciences Publisher
New Delhi | London | Panama

Jaypee Brothers Medical Publishers (P) Ltd

Headquarters

Jaypee Brothers Medical Publishers (P) Ltd
4838/24, Ansari Road, Daryaganj
New Delhi 110 002, India
Phone: +91-11-43574357
Fax: +91-11-43574314
Email: jaypee@jaypeebrothers.com

Overseas Offices

J.P. Medical Ltd
83 Victoria Street, London
SW1H 0HW (UK)
Phone: +44 20 3170 8910
Fax: +44 (0)20 3008 6180
Email: info@jpmedpub.com

Jaypee Brothers Medical Publishers (P) Ltd
17/1-B Babar Road, Block-B, Shaymali
Mohammadpur, Dhaka-1207
Bangladesh
Mobile: +08801912003485
Email: jaypeedhaka@gmail.com

Jaypee-Highlights Medical Publishers Inc
City of Knowledge, Bld. 235, 2nd Floor, Clayton
Panama City, Panama
Phone: +1 507-301-0496
Fax: +1 507-301-0499
Email: cservice@jphmedical.com

Jaypee Brothers Medical Publishers (P) Ltd
Bhotahity, Kathmandu
Nepal
Phone: +977-9741283608
Email: kathmandu@jaypeebrothers.com

Website: www.jaypeebrothers.com
Website: www.jaypeedigital.com

© 2018, Author

Bedside Clinics in Surgery

First Edition: 2004
Second Edition: 2013
Reprint: 2014
Third Edition: 2018
ISBN 978-93-5270-314-2
Printed at Replika Press Pvt. Ltd.

Dedicated to

My late parents Madhusudan Saha and Pushpa Rani Saha,
my revered uncle Shri Jadulal Saha
and my teachers
for whom what I am today.

Foreword to the Third Edition

It is a matter of great pleasure and honor for me to write the 'Foreword' for the third edition of the *Bedside Clinics in Surgery* authored by Professor Makhan Lal Saha.

In this context, I have no hesitation to declare this "Volume" as a perfect blend of hard core clinical practice along with profound knowledge and vast experience of the author.

Translation of knowledge to clinical practice has always been a great challenge, and Professor Saha has been successful in showing the perfect roadmap to face the challenge for the surgical trainees.

Professor Makhan Lal Saha is known to me since his student days, as serious learner, committed surgeon and passionate teacher. His vast teaching experience has been clearly reflected in selection of "Contents" of this book with 23 chapters of great surgical importance.

I am sure, this volume would prove immensely beneficial for the surgical students and trainees of all the programs including MBBS, MS, Nursing, AYUSH as well as other health science courses.

Here I would like to recommend this edition, not only for undergraduate and postgraduate medical students but also for surgical teachers and trainers.

Prof (Dr) Bhabatosh Biswas
MS DNB MCh (Cardiothoracic Surgery) FRCS
LLB LLM MBA MSW MA (Education)
Formerly Vice-Chancellor, The West Bengal University of Health Sciences, Kolkata
Formerly Vice-President, National Board of Examinations (NBE), New Delhi
Past President, Indian Association of Cardiothoracic Surgeons
Editor (Thoracic Surgery), Asian Cardiovascular and Thoracic Annals
Member of Academic Council of NIMHANS, Bengaluru
Visiting Professor, Indira Gandhi Institute of Medical Science, Patna
Formerly Head, Department of Cardiothoracic and Vascular Surgery, RG Kar Medical College, Kolkata

Foreword to the Second Edition

"He who loves his work never labors."
—**Jim Stovall**

It gives me great pleasure and joy to write a foreword for this extra-ordinary book on *Bedside Clinics in Surgery* the second edition by Dr Makhan Lal Saha published by M/s Jaypee Brothers Medical Publishers (P) Ltd, New Delhi, India. The book is a classic example of how to make reading exhaustive yet lucid and enjoyable.

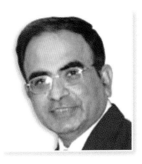

I have known the author for more than a decade and I can vouch for his dedication and keen interest in the teaching of the science and art of surgery. Having authored a few books myself, I am sure that any book is a true reflection of the author's love for the subject, his readers and students and it is clearly palpable in this book. Dr Saha's exceptional way of narrating the text makes this book a masterpiece for bedside learning of surgery.

Like in the first edition, the very simple way of teaching even the complex aspects of surgery has its impact on the reader. The litmus test for any book on bedside clinics is the utility during various undergraduate and postgraduate examinations. The book is surely going to pass that test with flying colors as it is a wonderful blend of all the essential aspects of performance in the examinations and in real-life scenario as a doctor.

The mandatory aspect of learning of surgery involves a thorough understanding of the surgical anatomy. The addition of various essential aspects of surgical anatomy with very easily discernible pictures adds tremendous value to this book. There are very limited texts available that address the issue of surgical anatomy of relevant regions.

A picture is worth a thousand words and the presentation of various clinical scenarios with real-life clinical pictures is truly remarkable. The demonstration of bedside physical signs and performance of certain important procedures have been addressed using a very simple and understandable method. The book is strongly recommended for all undergraduates, postgraduate trainees and trainers alike.

N Chintamani
MS FRCS (Ed) FRCS (Glas) FRCS (Irel)
FACS FICS (Surg Oncol) FIMSA
Vardhman Mahavir Medical College and Safdarjung Hospital, New Delhi, India
Honorary Secretary, Association of Surgeons of India-2012
Governing Council Member, Association of Surgeons of India
President (Elect), Association of Breast Surgeons of India
Editorial Secretary, Indian Association of Surgical Oncology
Controller of Examinations, College of Surgeons of India
Past President, Indian Society of Wound Management
Chief Editor, Surgical Clinics of India
Joint Editor, Indian Journal of Surgical Oncology
Associate Editor, Indian Journal of Surgery

Foreword to the First Edition

It is my pleasure to write a Foreword for Dr Makhan Lal Saha's book, *Bedside Clinics in Surgery*. I know him for more than a decade and though he being a general surgeon worked under me in my neurosurgery department for two years with keen interest and proved his worth.

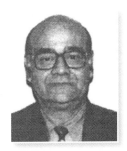

I have gone through the proofs of his venture and I am sure his efforts will prove results both to the undergraduate and postgraduate students in surgery.

I am confident that his dedication to author this book for last five years and practical experience will be very much useful to them for whom he has written. I am sure his book will be highly appreciated, amply rewarded and accepted by the entire medical students community.

HB 267 Salt Lake, Sector-3
26th January, 2004

Manoj Kumar Bhattacharya
MS MCh (Neurosurgery)
Formerly, Dean
Faculty of Medicine
University of Calcutta
Kolkata, West Bengal, India

Preface to the Third Edition

Keeping in mind the acceptance of the second edition of the book by both undergraduate and postgraduate students of surgery, the basic format of the book is being retained. Almost all the sections have been revised. The concept of exact measurement of a swelling by using a Vernier caliper instead of a tape measurement has been incorporated. A new long case on management of diabetic foot has been added in the long case section. The TNM classification of all the malignant tumors has been updated as per 7th Edition of American Joint Committee on Cancer (AJCC). In X-ray section, interpretation of mammography has been added. In surgical anatomy section, discussions on lower leg compartments and cervical fascia have been added.

Makhan Lal Saha
E-mail: drmlsaha@yahoo.com

Preface to the First Edition

Practical examination in surgery is exhaustive, encompassing long cases, short cases, surgical problems, surgical pathology, radiology, surgical instruments, minor surgical procedures, preoperative preparation and operative surgery. At present, there is no book available, which covers all these aspects in a comprehensive manner, suitable for preparation in final MBBS examination. The impetus for writing a book was primarily initiated by one of my favorite students, Dr Shamik Nandy of Calcutta Medical College. This book, very different in its approach, content and design, provides students of MBBS the basic and accurate knowledge of the practical problems, which can be assimilated in a reasonable but short time. With six years of extensive hard work, I have been able to present this book to the students of surgery.

This book covers discussions on almost all aspects of practical examinations. In long and short cases, a sample summary is given and management is discussed based on that particular case. The detailed discussion about that particular disease is presented afterward. The summary described may not be reproducible in examination, but provides a valuable guideline as to how to write a good summary of a particular case. Demonstration of physical signs with photographs and schematic diagrams are also included in each section of the long and short cases. In long and short case discussions, the students have to plan relevant management of the particular clinical situation presented by him in the said examination. The section on surgical problems covers both emergency and non-emergency conditions. A general outline for answer in such a situation is presented. In X-rays section, representative plates are presented and discussion is based on the findings of the particular X-rays. Discussions on the relevant clinical situation are also covered. In surgical pathology section, a representative specimen is described and this section mainly deals with the pathological aspects of the particular disease. For better clarity and understanding, the surgical pathology specimens are printed in color. Preoperative preparations for elective major surgery as well as those associated with common coexisting medical diseases are discussed. The section on minor surgical procedures is not exhaustive and only covers the important procedures commonly asked in examinations. Operative surgery is not discussed in a separate section but important operations are discussed with long and short cases and in other sections of the book. In instrument section, relevant points for identification of the instrument are mentioned. While discussing the use of instruments, emphasis has been given to mention the particular operations where the instrument is used. Sterilization of instruments are discussed in detail. Every attempt has been made to create a condensation of information by pointwise framing that will fulfil the students' need during examination. Throughout the text, emphasis has been given for methods of demonstration of clinical signs. An attempt has been made to maximize the number of illustrations to complement the general text materials. Photographs and schematic diagrams have been used for demonstration of clinical signs and operative procedures. The book contains 485 illustrations, numerous photographs and X-ray plates.

This book, however, is not a textbook of surgery. I would recommend all the students to go through standard textbooks of surgery for acquiring basic concepts. This book provides a very simple, comprehensive, updated, and well-illustrated account, which may be used as a revision book for preparation for practical examination in surgery. At places, the discussions are exhaustive and may not be required for undergraduate students. These are indicated by *italic fonts*. I would like to thank Dr Shamik Nandy, who has gone through the whole manuscript and suggested important modifications to make the book suitable for undergraduate students. I would like to thank Prof Biswanath Mukhopadhyay, Professor of Pediatric Surgery, Dr Anadinath Acharya, Assistant Professor of Surgery, Dr Sasanka Sekhar Chatterji, Associate Professor of Plastic Surgery and Dr Sukumar Maiti, Associate Professor of Surgery who have provided majority of the clinical photographs included in the long and short case sections of the book. I would like to thank all the faculty members of the Department of Surgery IPGME & R/SSKM Hospital, Kolkata, West Bengal, India, namely Prof PK Gupta, Dr Sushma Banerji, Dr QM Rahaman, Dr PK Sarkar, Dr Abhimanyu Basu, Dr PS Paul, Dr DK Sarkar, Dr S Das Chowdhury, and Dr SK Halder for their constant help and encouragement while I was preparing this book. They have also gone through the proof of the book. One of my postgraduate students, Dr Srinjoy Saha spent lots of his time in taking different photographs included in this book. Dr Krishnendu Maity, postgraduate student at Calcutta Medical College has also taken some photographs included in this book. Dr Ranjit Das, Dr Kaushik Ghosh, Dr Budhadeb Saha for help in preparation of some sections of this book. I thank my friend and well wisher Prof Sekhar Mukhopadhaya for his constant encouragement while I was writing this book. He has also helped in designing the cover page of this book. I would like to thank Dr Bansari Goswami, Professor and Head, Department of Surgery, NRS Medical College, and Dr Mrityunjoy Mukherji, Professor and Head, Department of Surgery, Calcutta National Medical College for allowing me to take the photographs of surgical pathology specimens included in this book. Dr Sudip Chakraborty, Professor and Head, Department of Urology, and Dr AG Ghosal, Professor and Head, Department of Chest Medicine, IPGME & R, provided some X-ray plates for inclusion in this book. Dr Satinath Mukherji, Associate Professor, Department of Endocrinology for help in writing the section on diabetes and surgery.

I would like to thank Mr Bimal Dhur and Sri Dipankar Dhur of Academic Publishers who were always after me over these years and for their sincere efforts to publish this book in time. Other members of staff of Academic Publishers Sri Abhijit Chakraborty, Sri Biswajit Seal and Sri Swapan Dutta also worked hard for making this publication successful. I thank Mr Narayan Sur and Mr Dilip Das who have drawn the different diagrams included in this book.

I am indebted to my wife Smt Priti Saha and my daughters Priyanka and Monica for their wholehearted support in this endeavor. I will never forget their sacrifice of long hours of family associations over these years while I was busy in preparing this book.

My sincere thanks are due to my enthusiastic young students, friends, relatives and well-wishers for their constant support, encouragement and help.

In spite of all precautions, a good number of printing errors might have gone unnoticed. I would request all the students to go through the corrigendum and correct the text to avoid confusion.

I hope this book will be beneficial to students of surgery and my efforts will be amply rewarded only if this book is accepted by the students and teachers of surgery. I apologise for any inadvertent mistakes, which might have been overlooked. I will be happy to receive comments, criticisms and suggestions for the improvement of this book in future from my readers, which I shall duly incorporate in the next edition of the book. The comments and the suggestions may please be sent to me at my residential address or to my E-mail address.

Makhan Lal Saha

E-mail: drmlsaha@yahoo.com

Acknowledgments

Prof Susanta Banerjee (Director of Medical Education), Prof Indrajit Saha (Joint Secretary, Department of Health and Family Welfare), Swasthya Bhavan (Salt Lake City, Kolkata), for giving me necessary permission for publishing this book.

My sincere thanks and gratitude to the following persons for their constant help and encouragement during preparation of this book:

- Prof Pradip Kumar Mitra (Director, IPGME & R), Prof Tamal Kanti Ghosh (Vice-Principal and Medical Superintendent), Dr Ajit Kumar Maity (Former Director), Dr DD Chattopadhyay (Former Surgeon and Superintendent), Dr Arabinda Narayan Chowdhury (Ex-Professor of Psychiatry and Superintendent, Institute of Psychiatry), Dr Nanda Dulal Chatterjee (Ex-Professor and Head, Department of Orthopedics), Dr Anup Majumder (Professor and Head, Department of Radiotherapy), Prof Rajen Pandey (Head, Department of Nephrology), Dr Abhijit Tarafdar (Ex-Professor and Head, Department of Nephrology), Prof Pradip Kumar Saha (Superintendent, Institute of Psychiatry), Dr Subhankar Chowdhury (Professor and Head, Department of Endocrinology), Dr Parimal Tripathy (Professor and Head, Department of Neurosurgery), Prof PK Ghosh (Ex-Professor and Head, Department of Forensic and State Medicine), Dr Bijay Kumar Majumdar (Professor and Head, Department of Plastic Surgery), Dr Alakendu Ghosh (Professor, Department of Medicine), Dr PK Mishra (Professor, Department of Pediatric Surgery), Dr D Kar (Medical Officer, Department of Surgery), Dr Abhijit Chowdhury (Professor, Department of Gastroenterology), Prof GK Dhali (IPGME & R and SSKM Hospital), Prof Samarendranath Ghosh (Head, Department of Neurosurgery), and all my postgraduate students, to name particularly—Dr Sarvesh Gupta, Dr Asif Ayaz, Dr Sidhartha Bhattacharya, Dr Subhamitra Chowdhury, Dr Vivek Sharma, Dr Subhendu Majhi, Dr Kamal Singh Kanwar, Dr Albinus Lakra, Dr Sanghamitra Sarkar, Dr Kallol Ray, Dr Gopal Singh Yadav, Dr Suddha Swatya Sen, Dr Sohabrata Das, Dr Harbans Bansal, Dr Puneet Goel, Dr Sushil Pandey, Dr Mala Mistry, Samir Saha, and Dr Rajan Tondon [MS MCh (PDT)], Department of Plastic Surgery, Institute of Postgraduate Medical Education and Research (IPGME & R), Kolkata, West Bengal, India.
- My teacher and well-wisher Dr Satyabrata Dasgupta, Ex-Professor and Head, Department of Surgery, Calcutta Medical College, Kolkata, West Bengal, India.
- Prof Bitan Kumar Chattopadhyay, Prof Amitava Sarkar, Prof Prasanta Bhattacharya, Prof Diptendra Kumar Sarkar, Dr Shyamal Kumar Halder, Dr Anadi Nath Acharya, Dr Rajat Subhra Moral, Dr Susnata De, Dr Subhra Ganguly, Dr Subhasis Saha, Dr Soumya Mondal, Dr Saurav Das, Dr Partha Bhar, Dr Soumen Das, Dr Prakash Bhagat, Dr Mainak Pal, Dr Barun Kumar Saha, Dr Partha Sarathi Dutta, Institute of Postgraduate Medical Education and Research, Kolkata, West Bengal, India.
- Prof Kashinath Das, Prof Sukumar Maity, Prof Utpal De, Prof Debabrata Kundu, Prof Shibajyoti Ghosh, Prof Gargi Banerjee, Prof Udipta Roy, Dr Shantanu Sinha, Dr Arijit Mukherjee and other faculty members, Calcutta Medical College, Kolkata, West Bengal, India.
- Prof Nemai Nath, Prof Sushil Ranjan Ghosal, Prof Sudev Saha, Prof Subodh Ranjan Saha, Prof Nirjhar Bhattacharya, Prof Saugata Samanta, Prof TD Chattopadhyay and other faculty members, Department of Surgery, Nil Ratan Sarkar Medical College and Hospital, Kolkata, West Bengal, India.

- Prof Saibal Mukherjee, Prof Manju Banerjee, Prof Subhabrata Das, Dr Ambar Ganguly, Dr Subhasis Karmakar, Dr Nilanjan Panda, Dr Shamik Bandhopadhyay, Dr Ramanuj Mukherjee and other faculty members, Department of Surgery, RG Kar Medical College and Hospital, Kolkata, West Bengal, India.
- Prof Debabrata Roy, Prof Hiranmoy Bhattacharya, Prof Ujjwal Bhattacharya, Dr Abhiram Majhi, Dr Madhumita Mukhopadhyay and other faculty members, Department of Surgery, Calcutta National Medical College, Kolkata, West Bengal, India.
- Prof Mrityunjoy Mukherjee, Prof Manas Kumar Gumta and other faculty members, Department of Surgery, Sagar Dutta Medical College, Kolkata, West Bengal, India
- Prof Anil Kumar Saha, Dr Saugata Roy, Dr Amit Kumar Roy, Dr Mrityunjay Pal, Dr Mala Mistri and other faculty members, Medinipur Medical College and Hospital, Medinipur, West Bengal, India.
- Prof Gautam Ghosh, Dr Ramkrishna Mondal, Dr Sukhendu Bikash Saha, Dr Sudangshu Sarkar and other faculty members, Department of Surgery, Bankura Sammilani Medical College, Bankura, West Bengal, India.
- Prof Tomanosh Chowdhury, Prof RN Majumder, Prof Rabishankar Biswas, Dr Shamita Chatterji and other faculty members, Department of Surgery, Burdwan Medical College, Burdwan, West Bengal, India.
- Prof Narendrananth Mukherjee, Prof Gautam Das, Prof SS Bhej, Prof Sudangshu Sekhar Bhoj, Dr AN Sarkar, Dr JS Basunia and other faculty members, Department of Surgery, North Bengal Medical College, Darjeeling, West Bengal, India.
- Prof Abhimanyu Basu, Prof Manoranjan Kar, Dr Dushmanta Burman and other faculty members, Department of Surgery, Malda Medical College, Malda, West Bengal, India.
- Dr Tandra Mukherjee (Registrar), Dr G Dasgupta (Registrar), Dr S Das, Dr S Banerjee, Dr KL Dey, Dr B Mukherjee (Medical Officer), PG Polyclinic, Kolkata, West Bengal, India.
- My teachers and senior colleagues—Prof Manoj Kumar Bhattacharya (Former Dean of Medical Faculty, University of Calcutta), Prof AP Majumder (Ex-President, AS1, WB Chapter), Prof Urmila Khanna, Prof Sushila Sripad, Prof Purnima Mukherji, Prof Samar Pal, Prof D Sarbapally, Prof Rita Sarkar, Dr RN Ghosh, Dr Gayatri Roy, Dr Chandreyi Gupta, Dr Collin Roy.
- My friends and well-wishers—Pradip Kumar Gupta (MGM Medical College, Kishanganj, Bihar, India), Dr Aniruddha Dasgupta, Dr SP Saha, Dr Samiran Saha, Dr KG Saha, Dr JN Kabiraj, Dr S Babu Thakur, Dr SN Bhowmik, Dr PK Paul, Dr L Naha Biswas, Dr TK Paul, Dr TN Sen, Dr SK Das, Dr Debjani Roy, Dr S Paul, Dr S Roy, Dr Tanusree Roy, Dr GD Mitra, Dr S Purakayastha, Dr Manish Bose, Dr Om Tantia, Dr Shomnath Ghosh, Dr Aloke Kumar Roy, Dr Manab Sarkar, Dr Sikha Adhikary, Dr Rama Das, Dr Sutapa Mondal, Dr Bhaswati Basu, Dr Debashis Basu, Dr Dipak Pal, Dr Diptendu Bikash Sengupta, Miss Sikha Das, Sister Moni Mandi, Sister Pronita Chakraborty, Sister Sumana and Sister Subhra.
- Dr N Chintamani, Dr Manoj Kumar Bhattacharya and Dr Bhabatosh Biswas for their remarks in the Foreword.
- Shri Jitendar P Vij (Group Chairman), Mr Ankit Vij (Group President), Ms Ritu Sharma (Director–Content Strategy), Ms Sunita Katla (PA to Group Chairman and Publishing Manager), Mr Rajesh Sharma (Production Coordinator), Ms Seema Dogra (Cover Visualizer), Ms Geeta Srivastava (Proofreader), Mr Kulwant Singh (DTP Operator) and Mr Gopal Singh Kirola (Graphic Designer) of M/s Jaypee Brothers Medical Publishers (P) Ltd, New Delhi, India.
- My all relatives who have always stood beside me.

Contents

Section 1 Surgical Long Cases

1. Introduction 1

Outline for Writing a Surgical Long
Case 1
- Physical Examination 5
- Clinical Questions on General Survey 9

Outline for Writing a Case of Swelling 25
- Clinical Questions 27

Outline for Writing a Case of Ulcer 35

Outline for Writing a Case of Sinus or
Fistula 36

2 Hernias 38

Outline for Writing a Case of Hernia 38
- History 38
- Physical Examination 39
- Summary of the Case 41
- Provisional Diagnosis 41
- Investigations Suggested 42
- Differential Diagnosis 42
- Indirect Reducible Inguinal Hernia in an
  Adult 42
- Inguinal Hernia with Features of
  Prostatism 68
- Recurrent Inguinal Hernia 70

Incisional Hernia: Outline for Writing a
Long Case of Incisional Hernia 71
- History 71
- Physical Examination 72
- Summary of the Case 72
- Provisional Diagnosis 72
- Investigations Suggested 72

3. Abdomen 85

Outline for Writing an Abdominal Case 85
- History 85
- Physical Examination 87
- Summary of the Case 90
- Provisional Diagnosis 90
- Investigations Suggested 90
- Differential Diagnosis 90

Cases Presenting with Gastric Outlet
Obstruction 103
- Gastric Outlet Obstruction due to
  Carcinoma of Stomach 103
- Discussion on Gastric Lymphoma 117
- Discussion on Gastrointestinal Stromal
  Tumor 120
- Gastric Outlet Obstruction due to
  Complication of Chronic Duodenal
  Ulcer 124

Peptic-Ulcer Disease 126
- Chronic Gastric Ulcer and Chronic
  Duodenal Ulcer 126

Case of Chronic Cholecystitis 138

Cases Presenting with Obstructive
Jaundice 147
- Obstructive Jaundice due to
  Periampullary Carcinoma or Carcinoma
  of Head of Pancreas 147
- Obstructive Jaundice due to
  Choledocholithiasis 166
- Carcinoma of Gallbladder (Presenting with
  or without Obstructive Jaundice) 171
- Discussion on Cholangiocarcinoma 177
- Obstructive Jaundice due to Choledochal
  Cyst 181

Cases Presenting with Abdominal
Lump 185
- Abdominal Lump due to Hydatid Cyst of
  Liver 185
- Pseudocyst of Pancreas 193
- Carcinoma of Colon 199

4. Urinary Cases 210

Outline for Writing Urinary Cases 210
- History 210
- Physical Examination 211
- Summary of the Case 214
- Provisional Diagnosis 214
- Differential Diagnosis 214

Clinical Questions   214
- Hydronephrosis   216
- Carcinoma of Kidney   220

5. **Breast**   226

Writing a Long Case of Carcinoma of Breast   226
- History   226
- Physical Examination   227
- Summary of the Case   229
- Provisional Diagnosis   229
- Differential Diagnosis   229
- Investigations Suggested   229

Early Carcinoma of Breast in a Premenopausal Woman   238

Locally Advanced Carcinoma of Breast   251

Management of Carcinoma of Breast with Distant Metastasis   255

6. **Thyroid**   272

Writing a Long Case of Thyroid Disease   272
- History   272
- Physical Examination   274
- Summary of the Case   276
- Provisional Diagnosis   276
- Investigations Suggested   277
- Differential Diagnosis   277

Nontoxic Multinodular Goiter or Colloid Goiter   284

Solitary Thyroid Nodule   291

Primary Thyrotoxicosis (Graves' Disease)   295

Carcinoma of Thyroid Gland   305
- Discussion on Anaplastic Thyroid Carcinoma   315
- Discussion on Medullary Carcinoma of Thyroid   316

7. **Varicose Veins**   321

Outline for Writing a Long Case of Varicose Veins   321
- History   321
- Physical Examination   322
- Varicose Veins   323

8. **Peripheral Vascular Disease**   345

Outline for Writing a Long Case of Buerger's Disease and Atherosclerotic Peripheral Vascular Disease   345
- History   345
- Physical Examination   346
- Summary of the Case   349
- Provisional Diagnosis   349
- Differential Diagnosis   349
- Investigations Suggested   349
- Buerger's Disease   349
- Atherosclerotic Peripheral Vascular Disease   365
- Diabetic Foot   365
- Local Examination—Examination of Both Lower Limbs   366

Section 2   Surgical Short Cases

9. **Skin and Subcutaneous Tissue 381**

Skin and Subcutaneous Tissue   382
- Dermoid Cyst   382
- Implantation Dermoid   387
- Submental Dermoid   388
- Sebaceous Cyst   389
- Lipoma   392
- Keloid   395
- Postburn Contracture   397

- Questions about Burns   399
- Malignant Melanoma   400
- Malignant Melanoma with Lymph Node Metastasis   404
- Benign Pigmented Nevus   413
- Squamous Cell Carcinoma   416
- Basal Cell Carcinoma   422
- Marjolin's Ulcer   426
- Soft Tissue Sarcoma   428

10. Blood Vessels and Nerves 439

- Hemangioma 439
- Plexiform Hemangioma (Cirsoid Aneurysm) 442
- Glomus Tumor 444
- Raynaud's Disease/Raynaud's Syndrome 445
- Arteriovenous Fistula 449
- Neurofibroma 452
- Plexiform Neurofibromatosis (Pachydermatocele) 454
- Generalized Neurofibromatosis (von Recklinghausen's Disease) 456
- Meningocele/Meningomyelocele 458
- Meningomyelocele 461

Nerve Injuries 462
- Radial Nerve Injury 463
- Ulnar Nerve Injury 473
- Median Nerve Injury 477

11. Neck Swellings 484

- Cystic Hygroma 484
- Ranula 487
- Thyroglossal Cyst 490
- Thyroglossal Fistula 493
- Branchial Cyst 494
- Branchial Sinus (Fistula) 499
- Tubercular Cervical Lymphadenitis 501

Metastatic Cervical Lymph Node Swelling with Unknown Primary 507
- Malignant Lymphoma 513
- Cervical Rib 518
- Carotid Body Tumor 522
- Pharyngeal Pouch 525

12. Salivary Gland 530

- Mixed Parotid Tumor 531
- Adenolymphoma 539
- Carcinoma Parotid Gland 540
- Chronic Sialadenitis of Left Submandibular Salivary Gland due to Calculus in Submandibular Duct 546
- Carcinoma of Submandibular Salivary Gland 549
- Parotid Fistula 551

13. Mouth and Oral Cavity 553

- Clinical Examination 553
- Cleft Lip 554

- Bilateral Cleft Lip 561
- Cleft Palate 563
- Oral Leukoplakia 568
- Carcinoma of Tongue 570
- Carcinoma of Lip 579
- Carcinoma of Cheek 582
- Carcinoma of the Floor of Mouth 584
- Carcinoma of Hard Palate and the Upper Alveolus 586
- Dental Cyst 587
- Dentigerous Cyst 588
- Ameloblastoma or Adamantinoma 589
- Osteomyelitis of Jaw 591
- Epulis 592

14. Breast, Hernias and Abdominal Wall 594

- Carcinoma in Male Breast 594
- Bilateral Gynecomastia 596
- Fibroadenoma Breast 598
- Cystosarcoma Phyllodes or Phyllodes Tumor in Breast 599
- Congenital Hernia 600
- Umbilical Hernia 602
- Paraumbilical Hernia in Adults 605
- Epigastric Hernia 608
- Femoral Hernia 609
- Lumbar Hernia 613
- Persistent Vitellointestinal Duct 614
- Umbilical Adenoma or Raspberry Tumor 616
- Urachal Fistula 617
- Desmoid Tumor in the Lower Abdominal Wall 618

15. Genitalia and Urethra 620

- Vaginal Hydrocele 620
- Encysted Hydrocele of the Cord 626
- Cyst of Epididymis 627
- Varicocele 628
- Undescended Testis 634
- Filarial Scrotum and Ramhorn Penis 643
- Phimosis 646
- Peyronie's Diseases 650
- Carcinoma Penis 651
- Hypospadias 660
- Ectopia Vesicae 666
- Testicular Tumor 669

Section 3   Surgical Problems

16. Surgical Problems   677

- Road Traffic Accident   677
- Head Injury   685
- Chest Injury   689
- Abdominal Injury   695
- Splenic Injury   699
- Liver Injury   703
- Pancreatic Injury   708
- Renal Injury   713
- Ruptured Urethra   717
- Burn Injury   719
- Acute Pain in Right Upper Quadrant of Abdomen   726
- Acute Pain in Right Lower Quadrant of Abdomen   729
- Lump in Right Iliac Fossa   731

- Acute Pancreatitis   735
- Peptic Perforation   742
- Intestinal Obstruction   744
- Brust Abdomen   747
- Postoperative Pyrexia   749
- Acute Retention of Urine   751
- Hematuria   754
- Solitary Thyroid Nodule   756
- Respiratory Distress Following Thyroidectomy   758
- Gangrene of Foot   759
- Abnormal Nipple Discharge   462
- Breast Lump   763
- Deep Vein Thrombosis   765
- Wound Infection   768

Section 4   X-rays

17. X-rays   775

- Straight X-ray of Chest/Abdomen with Free Gas Under Both Domes of Diaphragm   776
- Plain X-ray of Abdomen, Multiple Air Fluid Levels   781
- Sigmoid Volvulus   788
- Radiopaque Gallstone and Kidney Stone   794
- Radiopaque Kidney Stones and Bladder Stone   796
- Cannonball Metastasis   799
- Subphrenic Abscess   803
- Endoscopic Retrograde Cholangiopancreatography   806
- Worm in Common Bile Duct   808
- Endoscopic Retrograde Cholangiopancreatography—Chronic Pancreatitis   810
- T-tube Cholangiogram   813
- Barium Swallow X-ray of Esophagus— Achalasia Cardia   816

- Barium Swallow—Carcinoma of Esophagus   818
- Barium Meal X-ray—Chronic Duodenal Ulcer   822
- Barium Meal X-ray—Benign Gastric Ulcer   822
- Barium Meal X-ray—Carcinoma Stomach   824
- Barium Meal X-ray—Gastric Outlet Obstruction and Duodenal Obstruction   826
- Barium Meal Follow-through—Ileocecal Tuberculosis/Jejunal Stricture   829
- Barium Meal Follow-through— Recurrent Appendicitis   833
- Barium Enema—Carcinoma Colon   836
- Intravenous Urography— Hydronephrosis   842
- Intravenous Urography—Carcinoma Kidney   844
- X-ray Skull—Skull Bone Fracture   845
- Chest X-ray– Chest Injury   847
- Mammography   851

Section 5 Surgical Pathology

18. Surgical Pathology 855

- Benign Gastric Ulcer 855
- Perforated Benign Gastric Ulcer 859
- Carcinoma of Stomach 860
- Acute Appendicitis 865
- Small Cut Stricture 869
- Intussusception 871
- Meckel's Diverticulum 874
- Polyposis of Colon 876
- Carcinoma of Colon 879
- Carcinoma of Rectum 883
- Ulcerative Colitis 886
- Hydatid Cyst 889

- Gallstone Disease 894
- Cholesterolosis of Gallbladder 901
- Carcinoma of Gallbladder 902
- Polycystic Kidney 904
- Hydronephrosis 906
- Carcinoma of Kidney (Hypernephroma) 909
- Tuberculosis of Kidney 912
- Papillary Carcinoma of Urinary Bladder 914
- Benign Enlargement of Prostate 919
- Testicular Tumors 922
- Carcinoma of Penis 926
- Carcinoma of Breast 928

Section 6 Preoperative Preparations

19. Preoperative Preparations 933

Preoperative Preparation for an Elective Major Surgery 933

Preoperative Preparation in a Case of Toxic Goiter 937

Preoperative Bowel Preparation for Colorectal Surgery 937

Preoperative Preparation in a Case of Gastric Outlet Obstruction 938

Preoperative Preparation in a Case with Obstructive Jaundice 939

Preoperative Preparation of a Patient with Diabetes Mellitus 940

Preparation of Patient with Associated Heart Disease for Surgery 944

Preparation of Patient with Chronic Respiratory Disease for Elective Major Surgery 946

Preoperative Preparation of Patient with Chronic Renal Disease 947

Section 7 Minor Surgical Procedures

20. Minor Surgical Procedures 949

Insertion of a Nasogastric Tube 949

Starting an Intravenous Line 950

Arterial Blood Gas 951

Establishing a Central Venous Line by Subclavian Vein Puncture 952

Internal Jugular Vein Cannulation 953

Catheterization for Retention of Urine 954

Abscesses 955
- Drainage of Peritonsillar Abscess 956
- Ludwig's Angina 956
- Parotid Abscess 957
- Axillary Abscess 957
- Perinephric Abscess 958
- Anorectal Abscesses 959
- Breast Abscess 960
- Hand Infections 961
- Drainage of Pulp Space Infection of Finger 962

- Volar Space Infection   963
- Web Space Infection   963
- Infection of Middle Palmar Space   964
- Thenar Space Infection   964
- Infection of Ulnar Bursa of the Hand   965
- Drainage of Infection in Space of Parona   966
- Infection of Flexor Tendon Sheaths   966

Aspiration of Pleural Fluid (Thoracocentesis)   966

Insertion of a Chest Drain   967

Pericardiocentesis   968
- Peritoneal Fluid Tap   969

Cricothyrotomy   970

Sclerotherapy for Piles   971

Sclerotherapy for Ganglion   972

Lymph Node Biopsy   972

Excision of Sebaceous Cyst   972

Excision of Lipoma   973

Management of Ingrowing Toe Nail   973

Dorsal Slit of Prepuce   974

Sclerotherapy for Varicose Veins   974

Exposure and Ligature of External Carotid Artery   975

Exposure of Subclavian Artery in the Neck   976

Exposure of the Third Part of the Subclavian Artery   976

Exposure and Ligature of the Internal Iliac Artery   977

Exposure of the External Iliac Artery   979

Exposure of the Femoral Artery in the Thigh (in Adductor Canal)   980

Exposure of the Popliteal Artery   981

Peripheral Nerve Blocks   982
- Digital Nerve Block   982
- Median Nerve Block   982
- Ulnar Nerve Block   982
- Posterior Tibial Nerve Block   983

Section 8   Instruments

21. Instruments   985
- Sterilization of Instruments   986
- Rampley's Swab Holding Forceps   987
- Towel Clips   989
- Bard-Parker's Handles   990
- Surgical Blades   990
- Hemostatic Forceps   993
- Kocher's Hemostatic Forceps   997
- Mosquito Hemostatic Forceps   998
- Mayo's Pedicle Clamp   999
- Lister's Sinus Forceps   999
- Allis Tissue Forceps   1000
- Babcock's Tissue Forceps   1001
- Lanes' Tissue Forceps   1001
- Plain Dissecting Forceps   1002
- Toothed Dissecting Forceps   1003
- Needle Holders   1004
- Needles   1005
- Skin Closure Clips and Accessories   1009
- Skin Staplers   1010
- Mayo's Scissors   1010
- McIndoe Scissors   1011

- Metzenbaum Scissors   1012
- Heath's Suture Cutting Scissors   1012
- Langenbach's Retractor   1013
- Czerny's Retractor   1013
- Morris' Retractor   1013
- Hook Retractors   1014
- Cat's Paw or Volkman's Retractor   1015
- Fisch Nerve Hook   1015
- Deaver's Retractor   1015
- Self-retaining Abdominal Retractor (Balfour's Type) with Provision for Attachment for Third Blade   1016
- Millin's Self-retaining Bladder Retractor with a Provision for Attachment of Third Blade   1017
- Joll's Thyroid Retractor   1018
- Kocher's Thyroid Dissector   1018
- Cord Holding Forceps   1019
- Malleable Olive Pointed Probe   1020
- Olive Pointed Fistula Director with Frenum Slit   1023
- Piles Holding Forceps   1023
- Right Angled Forceps (Lahey's Forceps)   1026

❑ Cholecystectomy Forceps   1027
❑ Desjardin's Choledocholithotomy
Forceps   1028
❑ Kehr's T-Tube   1029
❑ Gastric Occlusion Clamps   1030
❑ Lane's Paired Gastrojejunostomy
Clamps   1032
❑ Intestinal Occlusion Clamps   1033
❑ Payrs' Crushing Clamps   1036
❑ Pyelolithotomy Forceps   1038
❑ Suprapubic Cystolithotomy
Forceps   1039
❑ Simple Rubber Catheter No. 10   1039
❑ Foley's Balloon Catheter   1040
❑ Malecot's Catheter No. 30 Fr   1041
❑ De Pezzer's Catheter No. 24 Fr   1042
❑ Catheter Introducer   1042
❑ Metallic Bougie   1043
❑ Female Metallic Catheter   1045
❑ Male Metallic Catheter   1046
❑ Volkman's Spoon or Scoop   1047
❑ Kelly's Rectal Speculum
(Proctoscope)   1047
❑ Flatus Tube   1048
❑ Doyen's Mouth Gag   1049

❑ Airway Tubes   1050
❑ Fuller's Bivalved Metallic Tracheostomy
Tube   1051
❑ Single-Bladed Blunt Hook   1053
❑ Single-Bladed Sharp Hook   1053
❑ Tracheal Dilator   1054
❑ Corrugated Rubber Sheet Drain   1054
❑ Aneurysm Needle   1055
❑ Suture Materials   1058
❑ Natural Absorbable Suture:
Catgut   1060

Synthetic Absorbable Sutures   1063
❑ Common Features   1063
❑ Polyglycolic Acid Suture (Dexon)   1063
❑ Polyglactin Sutures (Vicryl)   1063
❑ Polyglactin Rapide (Vicryl Rapide)
Suture   1065
❑ Polydioxanone Suture (PDS-II)   1066
❑ Natural Nonabsorbable Sutures:
Silk   1067
❑ Synthetic Nonabsorbable Sutures   1069
❑ Stainless Steel Wire   1071
❑ Instruments for Laparoscopic
Surgery   1071
❑ Laparoscopic Instruments   1071

Section 9   Operative Surgery

22. Operative Surgery   1083
❑ Steps of Lichtenstein Hernioplasty   1083
❑ Steps of Herniotomy for Congenital
Hernia   1084
❑ Steps of Transabdominal Preperitoneal
Operation   1085
❑ Steps of Total Extraperitoneal Operation
for Inguinal Hernia   1088
❑ Anatomy of Abdominal Incisions   1089
❑ Steps of D2 Gastrectomy for Gastric
Cancer   1092
❑ Steps of Total Gastrectomy   1094
❑ Steps of Truncal Vagotomy and
Gastrojejunostomy   1097
❑ Steps of Repair of Peptic
Perforation   1099
❑ Steps of Laparoscopic
Cholecystectomy   1100
❑ Open Cholecystectomy   1103
❑ Steps of Choledocholithotomy   1104

❑ Steps of Choledochoduodenostomy   1107
❑ Steps of Whipple's
Pancreaticoduodenectomy   1107
❑ Steps of Lateral
Pancreaticojejunostomy   1110
❑ Steps of Right Hemicolectomy   1112
❑ Steps of Low Anterior Resection   1114
❑ Steps of Abdominoperineal
Resection   1116
❑ Steps of Transverse Colostomy   1119
❑ Steps of Closure of Colostomy   1120
❑ Step of Appendiccctomy   1121
❑ Splenectomy   1123
❑ Nephrectomy   1125
❑ Steps of Modified Radical
Mastectomy   1126
❑ Steps of Lumbar Sympathectomy   1128
❑ Steps of Total Thyroidectomy   1129
❑ Steps of Left Hemithyroidectomy   1131
❑ Steps of Superficial
Parotidectomy   1133

❏ Steps of Submandibular
    Sialoadenectomy   1134
❏ Steps of Type I Modified Radical Neck
    Dissection   1135
❏ Venous Cut Down (Venesection)   1137

❏ Tracheostomy   1139
❏ Gastrostomy   1140
❏ Steps of Eversion of Sac   1142
❏ Circumcision   1142

Section 10   Surgical Anatomy

23. Surgical Anatomy   **1145**

❏ Inguinal Canal   1145
❏ Anatomical Concept in View of
    Laparoscopic Repair of Hernia   1151
❏ Anterior Abdominal Wall   1152
❏ Esophagus   1156
❏ Stomach   1158
❏ Anatomy of Liver and Extrahepatic
    Biliary System   1166
❏ Appendix   1176
❏ Autonomic Nervous System   1184
❏ Breast   1187

❏ Cervical Fascia   1197
❏ Thyroid Gland   1199
❏ Subclavian Artery   1203
❏ Anatomy of Common Carotid Artery in
    the Neck   1204
❏ Cervical Lymph Nodes   1208
❏ Salivary Glands   1209
❏ Anatomy of Testis, Blood Supply and
    Lymphatic Drainage   1209
❏ Fascial Compartments of the
    Thigh   1214
❏ Fascial Compartments in the Leg   1218

Index   *1221*

Surgery Curriculum for MBBS Students

Clinical Classes in Surgery: Total 26 weeks

3rd Semester : 6 weeks

4th Semester : Nil

5th Semester : 4 weeks

6th Semester : Nil

7th Semester : 4 weeks

8th Semester : 6 weeks

9th Semester : 6 weeks

Final MBBS Surgery Examination: Marks Distribution for Surgery

- **Theory:** 2 Papers: 120 (60+ 60) 2½ hours duration in each paper
  - *Paper I:*
    - Section 1: General surgery
    - Section 2: Orthopedic surgery
  - *Paper II:*
    - General surgery
    - Anesthesiology
    - Dentistry
    - Radiotherapy
    - Radiology

- **Oral:** 20 marks

- **Practical:** 100 marks
  - **Internal assessment:** 60 (Theory 30 + Practical 30)
  - **Total marks:** 300 marks
  - **Pass criteria:** 50% in aggregate.
    - Practical minimum 50%
    - Theory and oral minimum 50%.

Honours: 75% marks in the subject provided other subjects are cleared in one chance.

Surgery Theory Examination

- *Paper I:* 60 marks

  Section I:

  1. Long question type (compulsory) 10 + 5 = 15
     - » General principle/Basic science.
  2. Long question (1 out of 2) – 15
     - » Gastrointestinal tract.

3. Short answer type (5 out of 6) $2 \times 5 = 10$
   » General surgery.

Section II:

4. Short notes (5 out of 7) $4 \times 5 = 20$
   » Orthopedics.

- *Paper II:*   60 marks
  1. Long question (Compulsory) – 15
     » Endocrine and breast:
       Thyroid
       Parathyroid
       Adrenal
       Breast.
  2. Long question ($1 \times 15 = 15$) or Short notes (3 out of 5) $3 \times 5 = 15$
     » Genitourinary.
  3. Short answer type (2 out of 3) $2 \times 5 = 10$
     » Pediatric
     » Plastic
     » Neurosurgery
     » Cardiothoracic and vascular surgery.
  4. Short notes (4 out of 5) $4 \times 5 = 20$
     » Anesthesiology
     » Radiology
     » Dental
     » Radiotherapy, etc.

Surgery Practical Examination

One long case (30 minutes)   40 marks
• History: 15 marks
• Clinical examination: 10 marks
• Discussion: 15 marks

Two short cases ($5 \times 2 = 10$ minutes) – $20 \times 2 = 40$ marks
• Discussion on clinical findings
• Clinical demonstration
• Management

Operative: 20 marks
• Operative steps: 10
• Surgical anatomy/Preoperative/Postoperative: 10

Oral : 20 marks
• X-ray/other imaging: 5 marks
• Instrument: 5
• Specimen: 5
• Problems and recent advances: 5

Introduction

Long case is an important part of practical examination. Separate marks are earmarked for writing good history and recording the physical examination. There should be no spelling mistakes while writing history and it should be written neatly and should include all the points.

There are two important parts for writing a surgical long case:

1. History
2. Physical examination.

OUTLINE FOR WRITING A SURGICAL LONG CASE

History

1. Particulars of the Patient

* Name
* Age
* Sex
* Religion
* Occupation
* Address
* Date of admission
* Date of examination
* Bed No. (bed number allotted in the examination hall).

2. Chief Complaint

If there are more than one chief complaint write as *chief complaints*

* Write the presenting complaint in chronological order with duration
* Do not write two symptoms in one sentence in chief complaint, e.g. pain in abdomen and jaundice for 2 years.

Better write as

◆ Pain in right upper half of abdomen for 2 years
◆ Yellowish discoloration of eyes and urine for 2 years

Do not write a long list of symptoms in chief complaint. Write up to 3–4 symptoms in chief complaint.

3. History of Present Illness

◆ Start with a comment that the patient was apparently well before this episode of illness which started (months/years) back. Avoid writing that patient was absolutely well or perfectly well—as patient may have some minor complaints earlier.
◆ Elaborate each chief complaint in one paragraph in history of present illness.
◆ If patient's chief complaints are pain, jaundice and vomiting, write details about pain, jaundice and vomiting in three different paragraphs maintaining the chronological order.
◆ Once the chief complaints are elaborated then write about other relevant symptoms.
◆ Symptoms pertaining to different systems should be asked and relevant symptoms are to be written.

Gastrointestinal symptoms:

◆ Appetite
◆ Weight loss
◆ Pain abdomen
◆ Heartburn
◆ Acidity
◆ Flatulence
◆ Sensation of fullness after meals
◆ Vomiting
◆ Hematemesis
◆ Any sensation of rolling mass in abdomen
◆ Jaundice
◆ Fever
◆ Details of bowel habit—number of motions per day, consistency of stool, any change in bowel habit, any history of passage of mucus with stool, melena, bleeding per rectum.

Urinary symptoms:

◆ Any renal or ureteric colic
◆ Pain in loin
◆ Details of urinary habit
◆ Frequency, both diurnal and nocturnal
◆ Hematuria
◆ Pyuria
◆ Difficulty in passing urine
  – Any burning sensation during micturition
◆ Hesitancy and urgency
◆ Any history of incontinence (involuntary passage of urine).

Respiratory symptoms:

* Chest pain
* Cough
* Hemoptysis
* Breathlessness
* Fever

Cardiovascular symptoms:

* Palpitation
* Exertional chest pain
* Breathlessness on exertion
* Swelling of the face or feet (may occur in congestive cardiac failure)
* Any history of paroxysmal nocturnal breathlessness associated with expectoration of pink frothy sputum (suggestive of acute left ventricular failure).

Neurological symptoms:

* Headache
* History of loss of consciousness
* History of convulsion
* Any symptom pertaining to cranial nerve palsy
* Any history of loss of smell sensation (olfactory nerve palsy)
* Any difficulty in vision (optic nerve palsy)
* Any difficulty in eye movement (3rd, 4th and 6th nerve palsy)
* Presence of squint
* Double vision
* Any difficulty in chewing (trigeminal nerve palsy)
* Any loss of sensation in face
* Any loss of hearing (vestibulocochlear nerve palsy)
* Any difficulty in speech (vagus nerve palsy)
* Any history of nasal regurgitation of food
* Any alteration of voice
* Any loss of taste sensation (hypoglossal nerve palsy)
* Any drooping of shoulder/difficulty in turning the head to either side (spinal root of accessory nerve)
* Any difficulty in tongue movement and wasting of tongue (hypoglossal nerve)
* Any weakness in upper and lower limbs
* Any sensory loss.

4. Past History

* Do not write or say "nothing significant"
* Mention about any major medical ailment in the past
* Any history of operations. If so, the type of operation, any postoperative complications. Any complications of anesthesia
* Any history of pulmonary tuberculosis (Koch's) in the past

- Any history of diabetes or hypertension which may be present earlier to this period
- If disease characterized by relapse and remission enquire about similar illness in the past.

5. Personal History

Write about the following points:
- Marital status: Married or unmarried
- Number of children
- Status of health of spouse and children
- Dietary habit
- Any addiction: Cigarette, alcohol, betel, tobacco chewing (addiction implies physical and mental dependence on a particular substance or drug and if denied that particular substance patient will have withdrawal symptoms. Otherwise mention these as habit of smoking or alcohol
- Sleep
- Bowel habit/bladder habit (to be mentioned here if not mentioned in the history of present illness). In an abdominal case, usually bowel and bladder habits are mentioned in history of present illness
- Socioeconomic status: Poor/average income/high income group.

In female patients:
- Menstrual history
  - Age of menarche
  - Cycle
  - Duration of period
  - Amount of blood loss (assessed by number of pads used or if there is history of passage of clots)
  - Last menstrual period (mention the date)
  - In postmenopausal woman mention the time (months/years) of menopause
- Obstetrical history
  - Number of pregnancies (Mention as P_{*+*})
  - Number of abortions
  - Number of live births:
    - Male
    - Female
  - Mode of delivery
  - Last childbirth
  - Any complications following childbirth.

6. Family History

Do not write as "family history nothing significant", instead write as:
- *Parents:* If parents are alive, write their status of health. If parents are not alive, write when they had died and what was the disease he/she died of.
- *Siblings:* Number of brothers and sisters, and their status of health.
- In some hereditary diseases, e.g. carcinoma of breast, polyposis coli. Take history of 2–3 generations for similar disease or related diseases.

7. Treatment History
* Treatment received so far for the present disease
* Any other medications for other diseases.

8. Any History of Allergy to Drug or Food and immunization history.

■ PHYSICAL EXAMINATION

In surgical long case, physical examination will be done under three headings:
1. General survey: Quick overview of patient from head to foot.
2. Local examination
3. Systemic examination.

1. General Survey
* Mental state: Conscious, alert, cooperative
* Performance status: mention either in Karnofsky scale or Eastern Cooperative Oncology Group (ECOG) scale, particularly in patient with malignant disease
* Built
* Facies
* Gait
* Decubitus
* Hydration status
* Nutrition
* Anemia
* Jaundice
* Cyanosis
* Clubbing
* Edema
* Neck veins
* Cervical lymph node
* Pulse
* Blood pressure
* Respiration
* Temperature
* Any obvious deformity
* Any pigmentation.

2. Local Examination

Mention the region that is to be examined in local examination, e. g.
* Local examination of abdomen
* Local examination of breasts
* Local examination of inguinoscrotal region, etc.
* Write details of local examination, which will vary according to region being examined.

Examination headings are:

* Inspection
* Palpation
* Percussion (wherever applicable)
* Auscultation (wherever applicable).

3. Systemic Examination

This examination includes system other than that mentioned in local examination:

* Do not write systemic examination as "no abnormality detected"
* Better write in brief about each system.

Examination of abdomen:

* Inspection:
  - Shape of abdomen: Normal/obese/scaphoid/distended
  - Position of umbilicus: Central/deviated/pushed up/pushed down
  - Movements of abdomen: Respiratory/peristaltic/pulsatile
  - Skin over the abdomen: Any scar/pigmentation/venous engorgements
  - Any obvious swelling: Brief description of the swelling
  - Hernial sites: Any expansile impulse on cough
  - External genitalia
* Palpation:
  - Superficial palpation
    - Temperature
    - Tenderness
    - Any muscle guard
    - Any swelling
  - Deep palpation
    - Any tenderness in any of the deep tender spots
    - Any other sites of tenderness
    - Palpation of liver/spleen/kidneys
    - Deep palpation of any swelling
    - Fluid thrill
* Percussion:
  - General note over abdomen
  - Shifting dullness
  - Upper border of liver dullness
  - Upper border of splenic dullness
  - Percuss over the renal angle area
* Auscultation:
  - Bowel sounds
  - Any added sound
* Perrectal examination:
* Pervaginal examination (if applicable).

Examination of respiratory system:
- Inspection:
  - Respiratory rate
  - Shape of chest
  - Movement of chest
- Palpation:
  - Position of trachea
  - Tenderness over the chest
  - Movement of chest
  - Vocal fremitus
- Percussion:
  - Note over chest
- Auscultation:
  - Breath sound
  - Any added sound: Crepitation/rhonchi
  - Vocal resonance.

Examination of cardiovascular system:
- Inspection:
  - Shape of precordium
  - Apex beat
  - Any pulsation
- Palpation:
  - Apex beat
  - Left parasternal heave
  - Any thrill
- Auscultation:
  - 1st/2nd heart sound
  - Any murmur
  - Any gallop.

Examination of nervous system:
- Higher functions:
  - Conscious, alert, cooperative
  - Speech: Normal/any special character
  - Cranial nerve: I to XII. Any palsy
- Motor system:
  - Tone, power, coordination of upper limb
  - Tone, power, coordination of lower limb
- Sensory system:
  - Superficial sensation: Pain, touch, temperature
    - Face, neck
    - Upper limbs
    - Trunk
    - Lower limbs

     – Deep sensation
       - Joint sensation
       - Vibration sense
     – Deep reflexes: Jerks
     – Superficial reflexes
       - Abdominal reflex
       - Plantar response
     – Cerebellar sign: Absent
     – Gait: Normal.

Examination of cranium and spine:

- Normal

Summary of the Case

Write summary of the case of the patient in two paragraphs. In first paragraph, write in brief about the history of the patient.

In second paragraph, write briefly about the examination, such as important points from general survey and local examination, including points from inspection, palpation, percussion, auscultation, and positive findings on systemic examination.

Provisional Diagnosis

Try to give a complete diagnosis, such as:

- This is a case of carcinoma of the left breast T2N1M0 (stage II) in a premenopausal woman
- This is a case of obstructive jaundice probably due to carcinoma of head of the pancreas.

Investigations Suggested

Investigations may be mentioned under the following headings:

- Investigations for confirmation of diagnosis
- Investigations to stage the disease (in case of a malignant disease)
- Investigations to assess fitness of patient for anesthesia and surgery.

Investigations may also be mentioned under the following headings:

- Baseline investigations
  - Blood for hemoglobin, total leukocyte count (TLC), differential leukocyte count (DLC) and erythrocyte sedimentation rate (ESR)
  - Blood for sugar, urea and creatinine
  - Urine for routine examination
  - Stool for routine examination for ova/parasite/cyst
  - Chest X-ray (posteroanterior view)
  - 12-lead electrocardiogram.
- Special investigations
  - Depends on the provisional diagnosis.

Differential Diagnosis

♦ Write few relevant differential diagnoses. In list of differential diagnosis the more probable diagnosis should be written before the rare diagnosis.

In a long case examination: Examiner usually asks *what is your case?* Then you should mention the summary of the patient and end up by giving the provisional diagnosis.

♦ If the examiner asks you what is your diagnosis. Then straightway give a complete diagnosis.

■ CLINICAL QUESTIONS ON GENERAL SURVEY

Q. What are symptoms and signs?

Ans. Symptom is what the patient complains of and the sign is what the clinician elicits. Patient complains of pain at one site. When the clinician presses the area and patient experiences pain, this is tenderness. Pain is the symptom and tenderness is the sign.

Q. How will you assess mental state?

Ans. While taking history try to make some initial assessment of the patient's intelligence, mental and emotional state. If the patient has been able to narrate the history well, cooperated with the clinician for the clinical examination patient may be considered conscious, alert, cooperative and oriented.

Q. How will you assess performance status of the patient?

Ans. Originally performance status was assessed for consideration of patient fitness for administration of chemotherapy. This assessment of performance status may also be applied to surgical patient for assessing fitness for surgery and also to assess the surgical outcome.

There are two different ways for assessing the performance status.

The Eastern Cooperative oncology group (ECOG) performance status is as follows:

♦ Performance scale:
  – 0: Fully active and is able to carry out normal activities without any restriction.
  – 1: Symptoms restrict strenuous activity but is able to carry out light sedentary activities.
  – 2: Ambulatory but unable to carryout normal activities. Up and about >50% waking hours.
  – 3: Only limited self-care. Confined to bed for >50% of waking hours.
  – 4: Completely confined to bed, disabled, need assistance.
  – 5: Dead.
  So, ECOG performance status is written as score of 0, 1, 2, 3, 4 or 5.

Karnofsky scale for performance status is as follows:

♦ Able to carry on normal activity and to work; no special care needed (100–80).
  – 100: Normal, no complaints; no evidence of disease.
  – 90: Able to carry on normal activity; minor signs or symptoms of disease.
  – 80: Normal activity with effort; some signs or symptoms of disease.
♦ Unable to work; able to live at home and care for most personal needs; varying amount of assistance needed (70–50).

    – 70: Cares for self; unable to carry on normal activity or to do active work.
    – 60: Requires occasional assistance, but is able to care for most of his personal needs.
    – 50: Requires considerable assistance and frequent medical care.

◆ Unable to care for self; requires equivalent of institutional or hospital care; disease may be progressing rapidly (40–0).

    – 40: Disabled; requires special care and assistance.
    – 30: Severely disabled; hospital admission is indicated although death not imminent.
    – 20: Very sick; hospital admission necessary; active supportive treatment necessary.
    – 10: Moribund; fatal processes progressing rapidly.
    – 0: Dead.

Karnofsky performance status expressed as score of 100, 90.............

Q. How will you assess built or physique?

Ans. Built is the skeletal structure of an individual in relation to age and sex. Built may be described as short (Fig. 1.1), average or gigantism in comparison to a normal individual of the same age and sex.

Q. What is Facies?

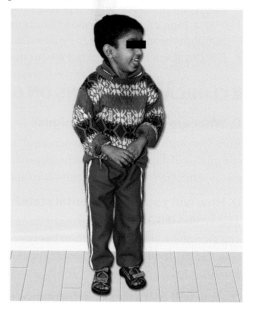

Fig. 1.1: Short stature 20 years male patient (height: 3ft 8 inches).
Source: Prof Subhankar Chowdhury, IPGME & R, Kolkata.

Ans. Observe the patient's face. The facial expression particularly the eyes indicate the facies of the patient. Some typical facies are thyrotoxic facies (Fig. 1.2A), facies of myxedema, moon facies of Cushing's syndrome (Fig. 1.2B), acromegaly (Fig. 1.2C), facies Hippocratica, anxious facies, etc.

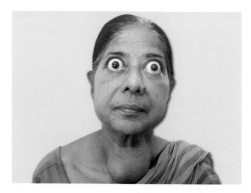

Fig. 1.2A: Facies of thyrotoxicosis (Note the stare look, exophthalmos, visibility of both upper and lower sclera)

Sources: Prof Satinath Mukhopadhyay, IPGME & R, Kolkata

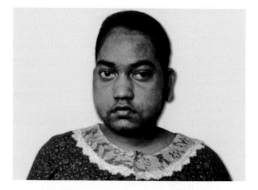

Fig. 1.2B: Facies of Cushing syndrome (Note the rounded face, hirsutism and facial acne)

Sources: Prof Abhimanyu Basu, IPGME & R, Kolkata

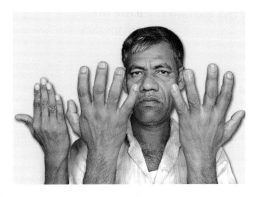

Fig. 1.2C: Facies of acromegaly (Note the enlarged face, thick and enlarged lips, nose, pinna and forehead. Note the enlarged hand and fingers—compare with normal hand).

Sources: Prof Subhankar Chowdhury, IPGME & R, Kolkata.

Q. How will you assess gait?

Gait is observed while the patient walks. Patient examined in the bed is asked to sit, stand and then walk.

Decubitus or the Physical Attitude

Attitude of the patient in bed is called decubitus. Patient with abdominal pain due to peritonitis may lie still, while patient with colic may be restless and even roll with an attempt to get relief. Various neurological diseases may have characteristics posture. When the patient is comfortable in any position then the decubitus may be described as "decubitus of choice".

Q. How will you assess hydration status of the patient?

Ans. Assessment of the hydration status is important in surgical patient. Some diseases may cause chronic dehydration either due to failure of intake (dysphagia due to carcinoma esophagus) or excessive fluid loss due to vomiting (gastric outlet obstruction) or diarrhea (ulcerative colitis or Crohn's disease). There may be evidence of fluid overload in patient with renal failure.

Hydration status is assessed by:
- Look at tongue and oral mucosa—normally moist. In case of dehydration will appear dry.
- Pull the skin and release. Normal skin is elastic. In case of dehydration, the skin turgor will get lost (Figs 1.3A and B).
- Patient will feel thirsty and urine output will also diminish.

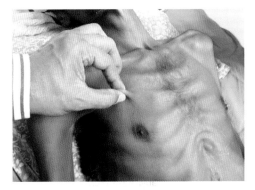

Fig. 1.3A: Pinch the skin up in between fingers and then release

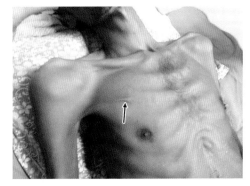

Fig. 1.3B: Release the fingers-observe—in dehydration the skin turgor will be lost

Q. How will you assess nutritional status of the patient?

Ans. Nutritional status is assessed by:
* Calculating the body mass index.
* Assessing the thickness of the subcutaneous fat in the arm, forearm or the back (Fig. 1.4A)
* Assessing the bulk of the muscle by measuring the mid upper arm circumference (Figs 1.4B and C**).**
* Look for any evidence of vitamin deficiency: Night blindness, xerophthalmia, Bitots spot (vitamin A deficiency), skin changes (dermatitis), stomatitis, glossitis cheilitis (vitamin B complex deficiency), bleeding and swollen gums (vitamin C deficiency) (Fig. 1.4D), etc.

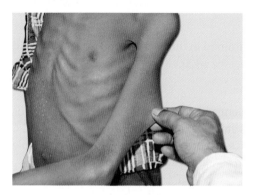

Fig. 1.4A: Assessment of subcutaneous fat by skinfold thickness

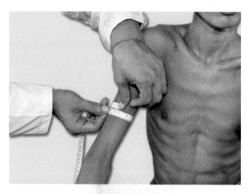

Fig. 1.4B: Assessment of midarm circumference. Note the midarm circumference of a malnourished patient (18 cm)

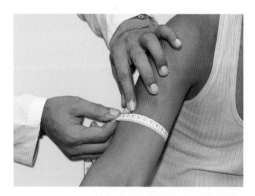

Fig. 1.4C: Assessment of midarm circumference. Note the midarm circumference of a normal person (25 cm)

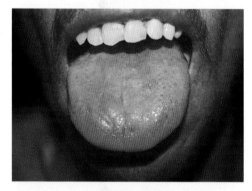

Fig. 1.4D: Look at the tongue for evidence of glossitis. Note the red and smooth tongue

Q. What is body mass index?

Ans. Body mass index (BMI) is calculated by:
* Body mass index = Weight in kg/height in meter^2.

- Body weight—60 kg, height—1.5 meter
- BMI = 60/2.25 = 26.6
- Depending on the BMI patient may be classified as:
  - Underweight   : BMI <18.5
  - Normal   : BMI 18.5–24.9
  - Overweight   : BMI 25–29.9
  - Obese   : BMI 30–35
  - Morbid obesity   : BMI >35
  - Supermorbid obesity   : BMI >55
- Nutritional state is described as poor, average or overnutrition.
- In practical examination, it may not be possible to measure BMI, unless you have a weighing machine and a height scale.

Q. How will you assess anemia?

Ans. Anemia is quantitative or qualitative reduction of hemoglobin or red blood cell (RBC) or both in relation to standard age and sex.

Anemia is assessed by presence of pallor at the lower palpebral conjunctiva, tip and dorsum of the tongue, soft palate, nail beds and the skin on the palm and sole and the general body skin (Figs 1.5A to D).

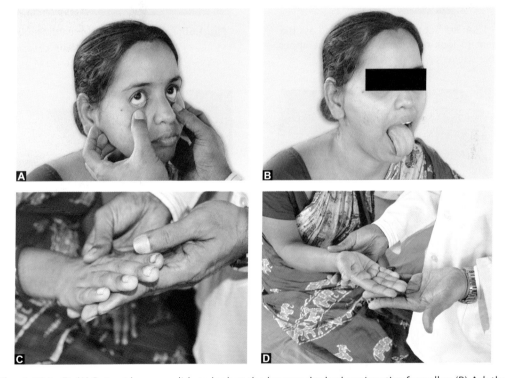

Figs 1.5A to D: (A) Retract lower eyelids to look at the lower palpebral conjunctiva for pallor; (B) Ask the patient to show the tongue and look for pallor; (C) Look at the nail bed for pallor; (D) Look at the palm for pallor

Depending on the degree of pallor anemia is described as mild, moderate and severe anemia:
- Mild anemia: When the hemoglobin is 50–60% of the normal
- Moderate anemia: When the hemoglobin is 40–50% of normal
- Severe anemia: When the hemoglobin is less than 40% of normal.

Q. How will you assess jaundice?

Jaundice is defined as yellowish discoloration of skin, eyes and mucous membrane due to excessive bilirubin in blood. Jaundice is looked for in upper bulbar sclera, soft palate, undersurface of tongue, palms, soles and general body skin (Figs 1.6A to D).

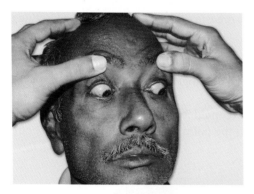

Fig. 1.6A: Retract the upper eyelid and ask the patient to look downward and look at upper bulbar sclera

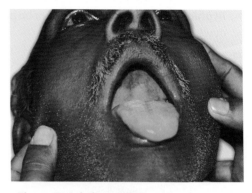

Fig. 1.6B: Ask the patient to open the mouth and look at the soft palate

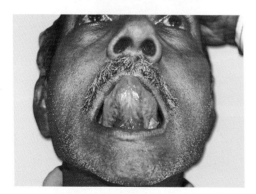

Fig. 1.6C: Ask the patient to show the undersurface of the tongue. Ask the patient to lift the tongue and touch the roof of the mouth with the tip of the tongue so that the under surface of the tongue is visible

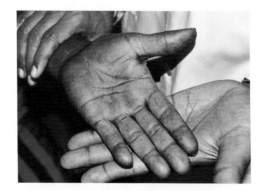

Fig. 1.6D: Look at the palm and soles

- In deep jaundice there is yellowish hue of general body skin surface. Jaundice is also looked in general body skin surface, palms and soles
- Normal bilirubin: Serum bilirubin value of 0.2–0.8 mg%

• Latent jaundice: Serum bilirubin between 1 mg% and 1.9 mg%
• Clinical jaundice is seen when the bilirubin level is more than 2 mg%.

Q. What is cyanosis?

Ans. Bluish discoloration of the skin and mucous membrane due to excessive amount of reduced hemoglobin in circulation, i.e. more than 5 g% of reduced hemoglobin in circulation. The cyanosis may be:

• *Peripheral cyanosis:* Arterial oxygen saturation is normal but there is more oxygen desaturation at the venocapillary bed. This may be due to peripheral vasoconstriction or sluggish circulation.
• *Central cyanosis:* This is due to excessive oxygen desaturation of the arterial blood.

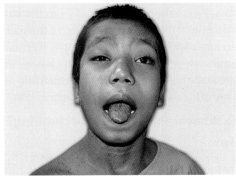

Q. Where will you look for cyanosis?

Ans. Peripheral cyanosis is looked for at the tip of nose, ear lobule, tips of fingers and toes, and palms and soles. Central cyanosis is looked for in the tongue, inner surface of the lips in addition to the sites of peripheral cyanosis (Fig. 1.7).

Fig. 1.7: Central cyanosis. Note bluish discoloration of tongue, lips and tip of the nose
Source: Prof Shankar Mondal, IPGME & R, Kolkata.

Q. How will you assess for presence of clubbing?

Ans.
• Look at the nail from the side to look for increased curvature of the nail (Fig. 1.8A) and assessment of angle between the nail and nail bed.
• Look for fluctuation at the base of the nail with two index fingers (Fig. 1.8B).
• Look for Schamroth sign (Fig. 1.8C).

Clubbing is characterized by increase in transverse and longitudinal curvature of the nail with increase of the angle between the nail and the nail bed (Lovibond's angle) (Fig. 1.8D). This is also associated with bulbous changes and diffuse enlargement of the terminal phalanges. These changes are due to proliferation of subungual connective tissues.

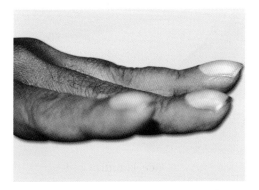

Fig. 1.8A: Look at the nail from the side

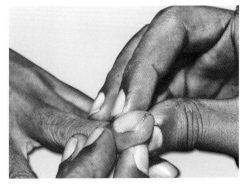

Fig. 1.8B: Fluctuation at the base of the nail with two index fingers

Q. What is Schamroth's sign?

Ans. When the nails of two normal fingers are apposed, there is a diamond-shaped gap. In clubbing this diamond-shaped gap disappears. This is known as Schamroth sign (Fig. 1.8C).

Q. What is Lovibond angle?

Ans. When the nail is viewed from the side, the skin fold of the nail and the base of the nail make an angle known as Lovibond angle. Normally this angle is less than 165 degrees. In case of clubbing the angle between the skin of the nail fold and the base of the nail is more than 180 degrees (Fig. 1.8D).

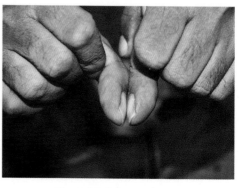

Fig. 1.8C: Schamroth sign

Q. What are the degrees of clubbing?

Ans.

- *1st degree:* There is only increased fluctuation of the nail bed.
- *2nd degree:* In addition to fluctuation, there is increased anteroposterior and transverse diameter of the nail.
- *3rd degree:* Above changes with increased pulp tissue in the terminal phalanges.
- *4th degree:* Combination of above changes with subperiosteal thickening of bones of wrist and ankle (hypertrophic osteoarthropathy).

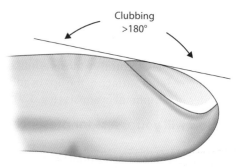

Fig. 1.8D: Lovibond angle

Q. Where will you look for presence of edema?

Ans. Edema is defined as excessive accumulation of fluid in the extravascular compartment.

In ambulant patient, edema is looked for by pressing on the medial surface of the tibia about 2.5 cm above the medial malleolus for about 5–10 seconds. If edema is present, a dimple will appear in the skin (Figs 1.9A and B).

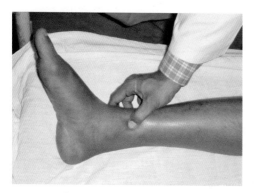

Fig. 1.9A: Press on the medial aspect of the leg 2.5 cm above the medial malleolus

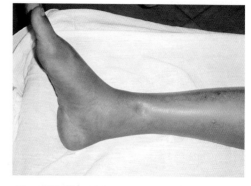

Fig. 1.9B: Note the pitting edema on release of finger pressure

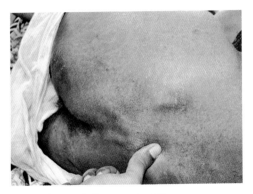

Fig. 1.9C: Press against the sacrum

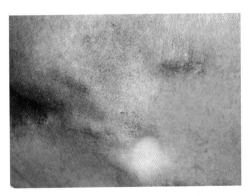

Fig. 1.9D: Note the edema at the sacral region

In nonambulant patient, you should look for edema at the sacral region by pressing over the sacrum for 5–10 seconds, a dimple appears if there is edema (Figs 1.9C and D).

Q. How will you assess jugular venous pressure?

Ans. The jugular venous pressure reflects the hemodynamics of the right atrium. Patient is made to lie supine with head end propped up to about 45° and the upper level of the jugular venous pulsation is localized by the clinician looking from the side (Fig. 1.10). The height of the upper point of jugular venous pulsation measured from the level of the sternal angle in centimeter is the jugular venous pressure (Fig. 1.11).

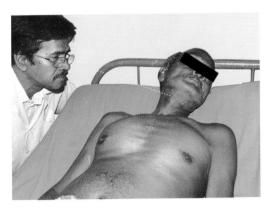

Fig. 1.10: Assessment of the upper level of jugular venous pulsation. Look tangentially from the side, keeping eye at the same level

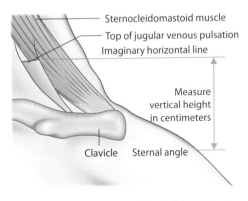

Fig. 1.11: Measurement of the height of jugular venous pressure

In normal individuals, the jugular venous pressure does not exceed 2 cm vertically above the sternal angle. The jugular venous pressure is elevated in patients with congestive heart failure and in superior mediastinal syndrome.

Q. What are the characteristics of jugular venous pulsation wave?

Ans. Normal jugular venous pulse wave is characterized by both positive and negative waves. a, c, and v are positive waves and x and y are negative waves (Fig. 1.12).

* *a wave*: Due to right atrial contraction.
* *c wave*: Due to right ventricular contraction when the tricuspid valve bulges into the right atrium.
* *x wave*: Due to atrial diastole—there is filling of right atrium and the tricuspid valve moves down.
* *v wave*: Due to right atrial filling.
* *y wave*: Due to opening of tricuspid valve resulting in emptying of right atrium.

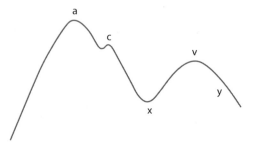

Fig. 1.12: Jugular venous pulse wave

Q. What are the different lymph node groups in the neck?

Ans. Depending on the location of the lymph nodes in relation to the investing layer of deep cervical fascia the cervical lymph nodes may be:

* *Superficial:* Lymph nodes lying superficial to the investing layer of the deep cervical fascia
* *Deep:* Lymph nodes lying deep to the investing layer of deep cervical fascia.
  These lymph nodes may further be subdivided into horizontal chain and vertical chain.

Q. What are the different levels of lymph nodes in the neck?

Ans. There are six levels of lymph nodes in the neck (Fig. 1.13).

* Level I: Submental lymph nodes lying in the submental triangle (IA) and submandibular lymph nodes situated in the submandibular triangle (IB).
* Level II (Upper jugular group): Lymph nodes located around the upper third of the internal jugular vein from the level of carotid bifurcation to the base of the skull.
* Level III (Middle jugular group): Lymph nodes located around the middle third of the internal jugular vein extending from the carotid bifurcation above to the cricothyroid membrane below.

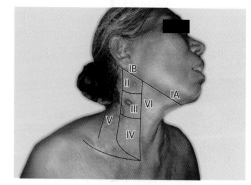

Fig. 1.13: Levels of lymph nodes in the neck

* Level IV (Lower jugular group): Lymph nodes located around the lower third of the internal jugular vein lying between the cricothyroid membrane above and the clavicle below.
* Level V (Posterior Triangle Group): Lymph nodes located in the posterior triangle extending laterally up to the anterior border of the trapezius and medially up to the lateral border of sternomastoid. The supraclavicular nodes are also included in this group.
* Level VI (Anterior compartment group): This includes the perilaryngeal, pericricoid and peritracheal nodes lying above up to the hyoid bone, below up to the suprasternal notch, and laterally extend up to the medial border of sternomastoid.
  (Lymph nodes in the anterior mediastinum are included as level VII nodes).

Q. What is Virchow's gland?

Ans. The left supraclavicular lymph node lying between the two heads of sternocleidomastoid is called the Virchow's lymph node. This lymph node may be involved by metastasis from carcinoma of stomach, testicular tumor, carcinoma of esophagus and bronchogenic carcinoma (Fig. 1.14).

Q. How will you palpate the cervical lymph nodes?

Ans. The cervical lymph nodes may be palpated both from front and the back.

The clinician stands behind the patient. The neck is slightly flexed and turned to the side of examination. The different groups of lymph nodes levels I to VI are then palpated systematically with one hand.

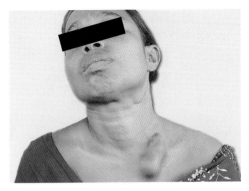

Fig. 1.14: Enlarged Virchow's lymph node

- Level IA lymph nodes are palpated at the submental triangle with the pulp of the fingers directed upwards with the neck slightly flexed and turned to the same side (Fig. 1.15A)
- Similarly level IB nodes are palpated at the submandibular triangle (Fig. 1.15B)
- Level II, III and IV nodes are palpated along the line of internal jugular vein with the pulp of the fingers (Figs 1.15C to E).

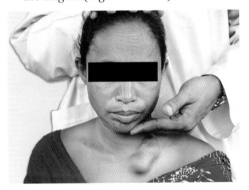

Fig. 1.15A: Palpation of level IA (submental group) lymph node

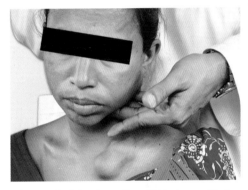

Fig. 1.15B: Palpation of level IB (submandibular group) lymph nodes

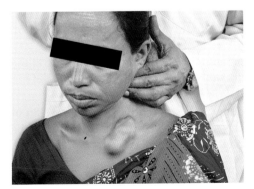

Fig. 1.15C: Palpation of level II lymph nodes (along the upper third of internal jugular vein)

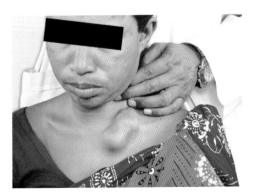

Fig. 1.15D: Palpation of level III lymph nodes (along the middle third of internal jugular vein)

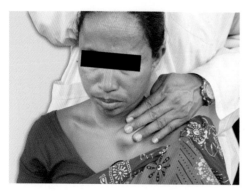

Fig. 1.15E: Palpation of level IV lymph nodes (along the lower third of internal jugular vein)

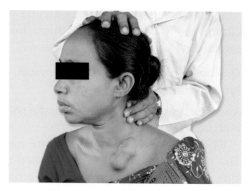

Fig. 1.15F: Palpation of level V lymph nodes: palpate along the posterior border of sterno-cleido-mastoid muscle

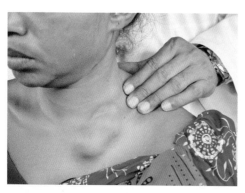

Fig. 1.15G: Palpation of level V lymph nodes (palpate along the anterior border of trapezius muscle)

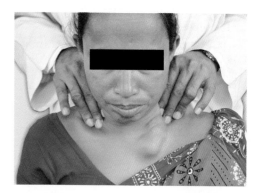

Fig. 1.15H: Palpation of level V lymph nodes. Palpate the supraclavicular fossa for supraclavicular lymph nodes

- Level V nodes are palpated at the posterior triangle with the pulp of the fingers (Figs 1.15F and G)
- The supraclavicular nodes (Level V) are palpated with the pulp of the fingers kept at the supraclavicular fossa and asking the patient to shrug the shoulder up (Fig. 1.15H)
- Level VI nodes are palpated at the pre- and paralaryngeal and tracheal region.
- The number of lymph nodes, size, surface, margins, consistency and fixity to the skin or underlying structures are noted. If the lymph nodes are enlarged the drainage area is to be examined for any evidence of infection or any malignant tumor.

Q. How will you examine pulse?

Ans. Pulse is the lateral expansion of the arterial wall due to a column of arterial blood forced into the arteries by the contraction of the heart.

Palpate the radial pulse just above the wrist on the anterior aspect of the lower end of the radius lateral to the tendon of the flexor carpi radialis (Fig. 1.16).

Look for rate, rhythm, volume, tension, condition of arterial wall, equality of pulse with the opposite radial and femoral pulses, any special character of the pulse.

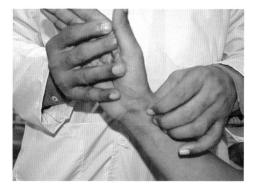

Fig. 1.16: Palpation of radial pulse

Regarding rate:

* *Normal heart rate:* It is 60–100 beats per minute, average 72 beats per minute
* *Bradycardia:* Heart rate less than 60 beats per minute
* *Tachycardia:* Heart rate more than 100 beats per minute
* *Relative bradycardia:* When there is fever, there is rise of pulse rate. for each degree rise of temperature and there is rise of 10 beats per minute. When with per degree rise of temperature, the pulse rate increase is less than 10 beats per minute then it is called relative bradycardia, e. g. enteric fever (1st week)
* *Relative tachycardia:* With per degree rise of temperature, the pulse rate rise is more than 10 beats per minute, e. g. rheumatic carditis.

Regarding rhythm: Appearance of successive pulse waves with time—

* *Normal rhythm:* The successive pulse beats are appearing at definite intervals
* *Irregular rhythm:* The successive pulse beats are not appearing at definite interval. This may be
  – Irregularly irregular
  – Successive beats are appearing at irregular intervals or the rhythm may be occasionally interrupted by a slight irregularity coming at definite interval
  – Regularly irregular.

Q. How would you assess volume of pulse?

Ans. The amplitude of the pulse is defined as the pulse volume and is palpated with the fingers. This may be normal, low volume or high volume depending on the amplitude of the pulse wave.

Q. How will you assess tension of the pulse wave?

Ans. Tension of pulse is defined as the pressure required to obliterate the pulse wave.

Q. How will you assess the condition of the arterial wall?

Ans. Empty the segment of the artery by using two middle fingers and then palpate with the two fingers and try to roll the artery against the bone. The arterial wall may be thickened in atherosclerosis (Figs 1.17A to C).

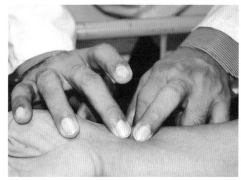

Fig. 1.17A: Empty the artery by milking with the middle finger of both hands

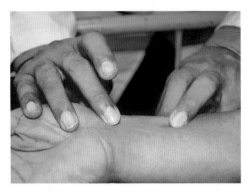

Fig. 1.17B: The segment of radial artery is emptied

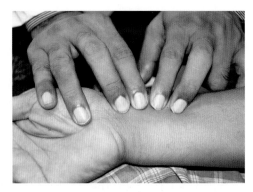

Fig. 1.17C: The arterial wall is palpated with the index finger of both hands

Q. How will you measure blood pressure?

Ans. Blood pressure is measured by sphygmoma-nometer (Fig. 1.18).

The patient lies supine in the bed. The blood pressure cuff is wrapped around the arm firmly and evenly around the arm one inch above the elbow joint, with the middle of the rubber bag lying over the brachial artery. The blood pressure cuff is then inflated till the radial pulse disappears. The diaphragm of the stethoscope is placed over the brachial artery under the edge of the sphygmomanometer cuff taking care not to press the diaphragm too heavily over the brachial artery.

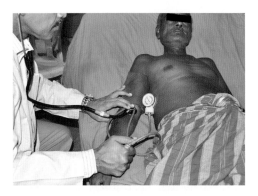

Fig. 1.18: Measurement of blood pressure

The blood pressure cuff is then deflated gradually and listen with the stethoscope when clear tapping sound becomes first audible. This is the point which indicates systolic blood pressure. The cuff is continually deflated. The character of the audible sounds changes and the sound becomes muffled and then disappears. This is the point which indicates diastolic blood pressure.

The blood pressure may also be measured by *palpatory method*. The blood pressure cuff is inflated till the radial pulse disappears. The cuff is then deflated slowly. The point at which the radial pulse reappears is the systolic blood pressure. The cuff is then continually deflated and the radial pulse assumes a water hammer character and then suddenly resumes the normal character. The point at which pulse resumes normal character indicates diastolic blood pressure.

Q. What is hypertension?

Ans. Persistent systolic blood pressure above 140 mm Hg and diastolic blood pressure above 90 mm Hg is defined as hypertension.

Q. What is hypotension?

Ans. Persistent systolic blood pressure below 90 mm Hg is defined as hypotension.

Q. How will you assess respiration?

Ans. Normal respiration is abdominothoracic and the normal rate is 18–20 breaths per minute. Allow the patient to take normal breathing and observe the rate of respiration by noting the movement of chest and abdomen in one minute. Look for rhythm of respiration and any special type of respiration. Note whether the respiration is thoracic, abdominal or abdominothoracic.

Q. What is Cheyne–Stokes breathing?

This is a special type of respiration, when there is a period of hyperpnea followed by apnea. The respiration becomes deeper and deeper until a peak is reached when there is apnea followed by hyperpnea. The period of hyperpnea lasts for 1–3 minutes, whereas the period of apnea lasts for 10–30 seconds.

This type of respiration is usually found in patients with increased intracranial pressure, renal failure and morphine poisoning.

Q. How will you measure temperature?

Ans. Temperature is measured by clinical thermometer and is expressed in either Fahrenheit or Centigrade scale. In surgical case, temperature is not recorded routinely.
* *Normal body temperature:* 98–99°F
* *Subnormal temperature:* Below 98°F
* *Pyrexia:* Above 99°F
* *Hyperpyrexia:* Above 106°F
* *Hypothermia:* Below 95°F.

Types of fever (Fig. 1.19):
* *Continuous fever:* The daily fluctuation of temperature is less than 1.5°F, and the temperature does not touch the baseline. It is found in pneumococcal pneumonia, in second week of enteric fever and rheumatic fever.
* *Remittent fever:* The daily fluctuation is more than 2°F and the temperature does not touch the baseline. This is found in urinary tract infection and pulmonary tuberculosis.
* *Intermittent fever:* Fever continues for several hours and returns to normal during the day. This may be:
  - *Quotidian:* The paroxysm of intermittent fever occurs daily.
  - *Tertian:* The paroxysm of intermittent fever occurs on alternate days.
  - *Quartan:* The paroxysm of intermittent fever occurs every 3 days.
  - *Relapsing fever:* There cyclic periods of fever and periods of apyrexia.

Q. What is Pel-Ebstein fever?

Ans. This is a type of relapsing fever when there is fever for a period of 14 days and there is apyrexial period of 14 days. Found in brucellosis and Hodgkin's lymphoma.

Q. What do you mean by pyrexia of unknown origin (PUO)?

Ans. When a fever of more than 101°F persists for more than 2 weeks with the cause remaining obscure in spite of intensive investigations is called pyrexia of unknown origin.

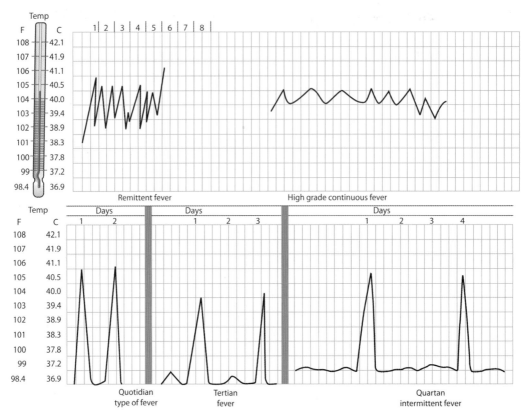

Fig. 1.19: Types of fever

Q. Where do you look for pigmentation?

Ans. The usual sites to be looked for pigmentation are face, oral cavity, tongue, creases of palms and soles and general body skin. Pigmentation may be seen in Cushing's syndrome, Addison's disease, Peutz–Jegher's syndrome (Figs 1.20A and B) and other dermatological diseases.

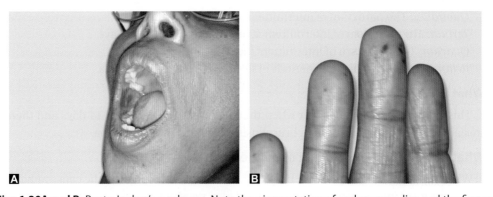

Figs 1.20A and B: Peutz-Jegher's syndrome. Note the pigmentation of oral mucosa, lips and the fingers

OUTLINE FOR WRITING A CASE OF SWELLING

History

- Duration: How long is the swelling present?
- Site: Where was the swelling first noticed?
- Mode of onset: Whether swelling appeared following trauma, or developed spontaneously.
- Progress of swelling:
  - Static: Same as onset, no increase in size
  - Slowly increasing in size since beginning (usually benign swelling)
  - Rapidly increasing in size since beginning (usually malignant)
  - Initially slowly increasing in size, later (after a variable period) started rapidly increasing in size (benign swelling showing malignant change)
  - Initially increasing size. Later the swelling regressed with time or treatment (inflammatory)
  - Ask the patient what was the size of the swelling when he first noticed it. Earlier this was described as either pea, marble, lemon or orange shaped. It is better to describe the approximate size of the swelling in centimeter at the onset. From patient description try to assess the approximate size of the swelling at onset and describe as the swelling was about 2 cm/3 cm/4 cm in size at the onset and then describe the progress of the swelling.
- Pain over the swelling:
  - Duration of pain
  - Site of pain
  - Character of pain
  - Any radiation of pain
  - Periodicity of pain
  - Relation of pain with the swelling
- Any other swelling in the body
- Any history of fever, loss of appetite, loss of weight
- Any subsequent changes over the swelling, e. g. ulceration, satellite nodules. Ask when these changes were first noticed
- In a suspected malignant disease enquire about symptoms which will suggest metastasis, chest pain, cough, hemoptysis, bone pain, headache, vomiting, loss of consciousness, convulsion, pain abdomen, abdominal distension and jaundice
- Any history of previous excision of the swelling and recurrence
- History of similar swelling in the past
- Any history of tuberculosis: Past history/personal history/family history/treatment history/ history of allergy.

Physical Examination

- General survey
- Local examination

1. Inspection (Fig. 1.21)

- Number
- Site
- Extent
- Shape
- Size
- Surface
- Margin
- Skin over the swelling
  - Scar
  - Venous prominence
  - Pigmentation
  - Ulcer, any discharge
  - Peau D'orange
  - Satellite nodule
- Impulse on cough (for hernias and meningocele)
- Any pressure effect
  - Swelling of limbs
  - Muscle wasting.

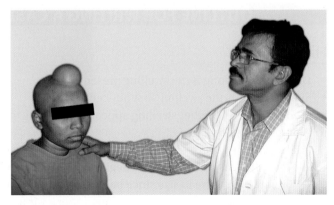

Fig. 1.21: Inspection of the swelling. Note the site and extent, size and shape, surface and margin and skin over the swelling

2. Palpation

- Temperature
- Tenderness
- Site
- Extent
- Shape
- Size
- Surface
- Margin
- Consistency
- Fluctuation, if the swelling is cystic
- Transillumination, if swelling is cystic
- Reducibility:
  - Reducible or not
- Compressible or not
- Palpable impulse on cough
- Fixity of the swelling to skin
- Fixity of the swelling to deeper structure
  - Muscle: Test mobility with muscle relaxed and contracted
  - Tendon: Test mobility with tendon relaxed and after tendon is made taut with contraction of muscle
  - Bones: Swelling is fixed as such
  - Vessel compression effect: Absence of pulse distal to the swelling
  - Nerve compression effect: Test for muscle power and sensation
- Pulsation: If present, transmitted or expansile pulsation
- Any thrill on palpation.

3. Percussion

4. Auscultation

5. Movement of adjacent joint

6. Examination of regional lymph nodes.

■ CLINICAL QUESTIONS

Q. How will you examine temperature over the swelling?

Ans. The temperature of the swelling is ascertained by palpation with the dorsum of the fingers. Compare the temperature over the swelling with the temperature of the adjacent area or corresponding area of the body (Fig. 1.22).

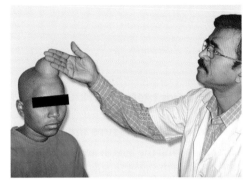

Fig. 1.22: Ascertaining temperature over the swelling

Q. How to ascertain tenderness over the swelling?

Ans. Press the swelling with the pulp of the fingers and look at the patient face. If the patient experiences pain on pressure, tenderness is said to be present.

Q. How will you measure the size of the swelling?

Ans. Conventionally, we used to measure the size of the swelling by using a measuring tape in inches/cm (Figs 1.23A and B). But measurement with a tape is faulty in many situations. If the swelling bulging outward and tape is placed over the swelling, this in fact gives a measurement of half of the circumference of the swelling rather than length/breadth of the swelling.

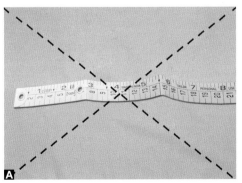

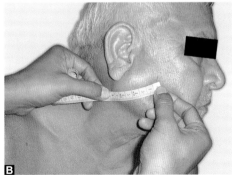

Figs 1.23A and B: Picture of a measuring tape

The better way of measuring the size of the swelling would be by using a Vernier caliper which can measure the exact length and breadth of the swelling in mm (Fig. 1.24). All students should carry a Vernier caliper for clinical examination of a swelling.

If the swelling is spherical mentioning the diameter of the swelling is enough. For elongated swelling, measure the length and breadth of the swelling.

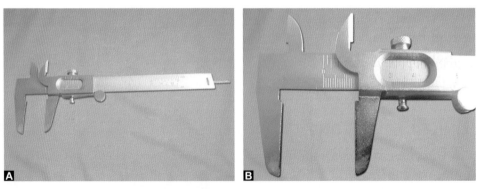

Figs 1.24A and B: Pictures of a Vernier caliper (Give exact measurement in mm)

Q. How will you measure the size of the swelling with the help of Vernier caliper?

Ans. Measuring the length and breadth of a swelling with a Vernier caliper.

The size of the swelling on inspection is assessed approximately and expressed in centimeter.

Palpate the swelling and place markers at the periphery of the swelling. Place the Vernier caliper on the marked point and measure the distance. If the swelling is spherical the measurement of diameter is sufficient. In other swelling measure the length and breadth of the swelling and express in centimeter (Figs 1.25 and 1.26).

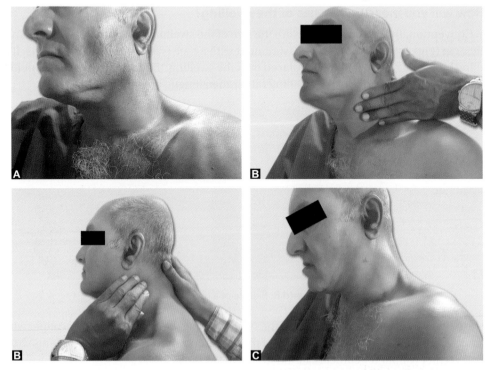

Figs 1.25A to D: Measurement of length and breadth of the swelling. (A) Patient showing swelling in the neck; (B and C) Palpate the swelling and mark the extent of the swelling horizontally and vertically; (D) Palpate the swelling and mark the margin of the swelling horizontally and vertically

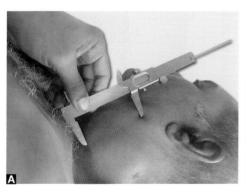
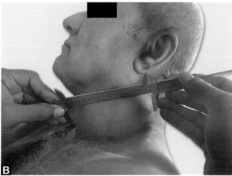

Figs 1.26A and B: (A) Place the Vernier caliper vertically and measure the distance; (B) Place the Vernier caliper horizontally and measure the distance

How will you measure the diameter of a globular swelling?

Ans. Palpate the swelling and mark the peripheral limit of the swelling. Place the Vernier caliper on these two points and measure the diameter of the swelling in mm (Fig. 1.27).

Q. How will you examine the surface of the swelling?

Ans. Palpate with the pulp of the finger over the surface of the swelling. The surface of the swelling may be smooth, irregular (the irregular surface may be granular, nodular or lobulated) (Fig. 1.28).

Q. How will you assess the margin of the swelling?

Ans. Palpate the periphery of the swelling with the pulp of the finger (Figs 1.29A and B).

The margin of the swelling may be well-defined (when it can be palpated well) or ill-defined when the margins are not delineated well on palpation.

The margin of the swelling may be regular (when it is uniform throughout) or irregular (when the periphery of the swelling is not uniform).

Q. How will you assess underlying bony indentation?

Ans. Some swelling like long-standing dermoid cyst may show bony indentation.

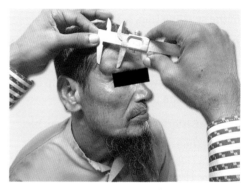

Fig. 1.27: Measurement of the diameter of a globular swelling

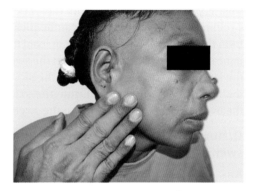

Fig. 1.28: Palpation of the surface of the swelling

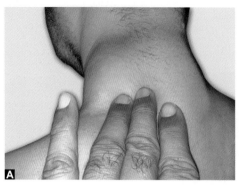 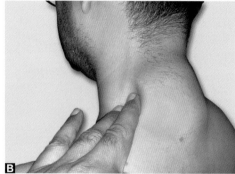

Figs 1.29A and B: Ascertaining the margin of the swelling

Palpate at the periphery deep to the margin of the swelling. If there is bony indentation the raised bony margin can be felt deep to the margin of the swelling (Fig. 1.30).

Q. How will you assess consistency of the swelling?

Ans. Press the swelling with the pulp of the finger and assess the feel (see Fig. 1.28).

The consistency of the swelling may be:

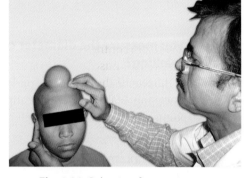

Fig. 1.30: Palpation for ascertaining underlying bony indentation

* Soft (feel of a relaxed muscle) or
* Firm (feel of a contracted muscle)
* Hard (feel of bone)
* The consistency of a swelling may be described as variegated when the swelling has a variable feel soft, firm or hard at different parts of the swelling.

Q. How will you demonstrate fixity of the swelling to skin?

Ans. Try to pick up the skin from the underlying swelling (Fig. 1.31). If the skin can be picked up from the swelling, the swelling is not fixed to skin. If the skin cannot be picked up from the swelling, the swelling is said to be fixed to the skin. The malignant swelling may infiltrate the skin and the overlying skin may be fixed to the swelling.

Q. How will you ascertain relation of the swelling with the underlying muscle?

Ans. A swelling may lie either superficial or deep to the muscle or it may arise from the muscle itself.

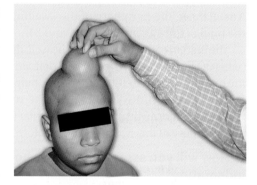

Fig. 1.31: Demonstration of skin fixity. The skin can be picked up from the swelling

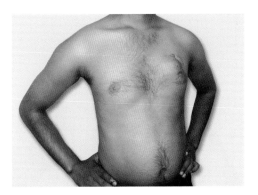

Fig. 1.32A: Ascertaining relation of a chest wall swelling to the underlying pectoralis major muscle. The swelling is first examined with the muscle relaxed

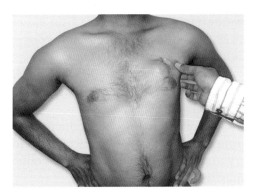

Fig. 1.32B: Patient is then asked to contract the pectoralis major muscle—the swelling becomes more prominent with the muscle contracted—suggesting that the swelling lies superficial to the pectoralis major muscle

Ask the patient to contract the muscle. If the swelling becomes more prominent, the swelling lies superficial to the muscle (Figs 1.32A and B). If the swelling becomes less prominent, it lies deep to the muscle. If the swelling remains same or becomes less prominent and becomes immobile, it may arise from the muscle.

Q. How will you ascertain fixity of the swelling to the underlying muscle?

Ans. A swelling may become fixed to the underlying muscle or bone. Before testing for fixity of the swelling to the muscle it is necessary to exclude whether swelling is fixed to the underlying bone or not.

Hold the swelling and try to move it with the underlying muscle relaxed both along and across the axis of the muscle (Figs 1.33A and B).

If the swelling is immobile with the muscle being relaxed, this indicates that the swelling is fixed to the underlying bone. It is not necessary now to ask the patient to contract the muscle

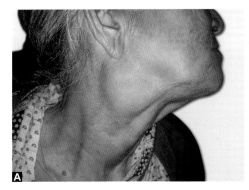

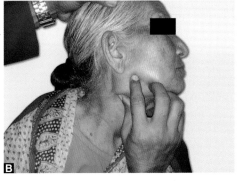

Figs 1.33A and B: Ascertaining fixity of the swelling with the underlying muscle. The swelling is moved with the muscle relaxed. The swelling is mobile—suggesting that the swelling is not fixed to the underlying bones and prevertebral fascia

and test for fixity of the swelling to the muscle. The swelling has to be fixed to the underlying muscle as it fixed to the underlying bone.

If the swelling is mobile with the muscle relaxed, this indicates the swelling is not fixed to the underlying bone.

Ask the patient to contract the muscle (confirmed by palpating the contracted muscle), and try to move the swelling over the contracting muscle in both axes (Fig. 1.33C).

If the swelling is freely mobile, this indicates that the swelling is not fixed to the underlying muscle.

Restriction of mobility of the swelling over the contracted muscle indicates fixity of the swelling to the underlying muscle.

Q. How will you demonstrate fluctuation?

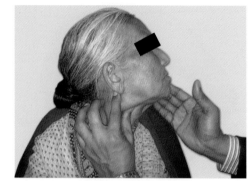

Fig. 1.33C: The right sternocleidomastoid muscle is contracted by asking the patient to look to the opposite side against resistance and the mobility is tested again. if the mobility remains same, then the swelling is not fixed to the underlying sternocleidomastoid muscle, if the mobility becomes restricted—the swelling is fixed to the underlying muscle

Ans. Fluctuation means transmitted impulse in two planes at right angles to each other.

Depending on the size of the swelling one finger or two fingers of each hand is used to demonstrate fluctuation. The finger which presses the swelling is called the displacing finger while the static fingers, which appreciate the displacement is called the watching finger.

Usually index and middle fingers straight with slight flexion at metacarpophalangeal joint are placed over the swelling. The tip of the pulp of the left index middle finger is placed halfway between the center and the periphery of the swelling. This is the watching finger and is kept static throughout the procedure. The tip of the pulp of the right index and middle finger is placed at similar point diagonally opposite the right index and middle finger. This is the displacing finger.

The displacing fingers are pressed inward, if the watching fingers are displaced by this pressure in both axes of the swelling then fluctuation is said to be positive (Figs 1.34A and B).

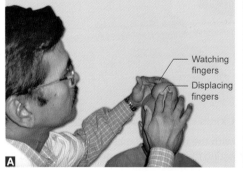
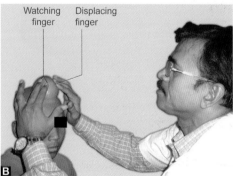

Figs 1.34A and B: Demonstration of fluctuation

In small swelling, the two fingers of the left hand are placed apart over the swelling and this acts as the watching finger. The right index finger acting as the displacing finger exerts pressure at the center of the swelling. If the watching finger is displaced in both axes of the swelling then fluctuation is said to be positive (Fig. 1.34C).

In small swelling the fluctuation may be demonstrated by Paget's test. The swelling is fixed at the periphery with two fingers and feel the swelling from center to the periphery. The swelling feels softer at the center than at the periphery.

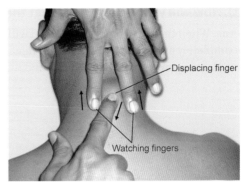

Fig. 1.34C: Demonstration of fluctuation in small swelling

In case of a mobile swelling, the swelling should be fixed by an assistant and the fluctuation demonstrated by the above method.

If the swelling is very small (< 2 cm), it is difficult to demonstrate fluctuation.

Q. How will you differentiate transmitted and expansile pulsation?

Ans. Place the index and middle finger over the swelling. If the pulsation is transmitted, the fingers move up parallel to each other with each pulsation. If the pulsation is expansile, the fingers are lifted up and also move apart with each pulsation (Figs 1.35A to C).

The transmitted pulsation is present when there is a swelling in front of an artery. Expansile pulsation is present in cases of an aneurysm.

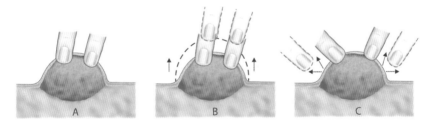

Figs 1.35A to C: (A) Demonstration of transmitted and expansile pulsation; (B) Both the fingers are lifted up; (C) The fingers are both lifted up and moved apart

Q. How will you demonstrate transillumination?

Ans. The transillumination is usually demonstrated by placing a torch over the swelling and usually under the shade of a screen. The normal skin transillumination should be taken into account before commenting that the swelling is transilluminant.

The important brilliantly transilluminant swelling includes:

* Vaginal hydrocele
* Cystic hygroma
* Encysted hydrocele of the cord
* Hydrocele in the canal nuck
* Congenital hernia in infants may show positive transillumination.

Q. How will you demonstrate that the swelling is compressible?

Ans. When the swelling is compressed with the fingers it diminishes in size and may disappear completely and when the pressure is released, it reappears slowly (Figs 1.36 and 1.37).

Hemangiomas, lymphangiomas and meningocele or meningomyelocele are compressible.

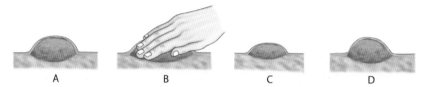

A   B   C   D

Figs 1.36A to D: (A) Demonstration of compressibility of a swelling; (B) The swelling is pressed with the fingers; (C) The swelling diminishes in size; (D) On release of compression the swelling reappeared

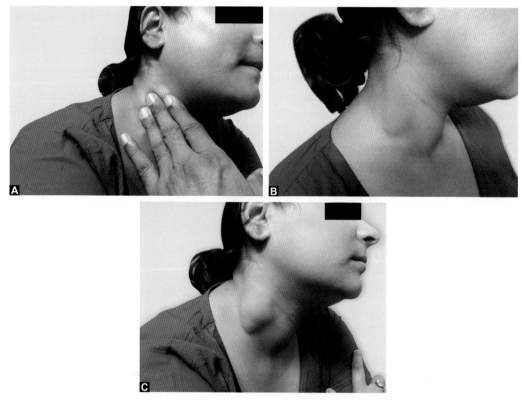

Figs 1.37A to C: Demonstration of compressibility. (A) Swelling is compressed with the fingers; (B) Swelling diminished in size; (C) On release of compression, the swelling reappeared

Q. What do you mean by indentation of a swelling?

Ans. Press the swelling for 15–30 seconds. if a dimple appears over the swelling then the swelling is said to have shown the sign of indentation (Figs 1.38A to D).

Cysts containing pultaceous materials as in dermoid cyst or sebaceous cyst are said to be indentable.

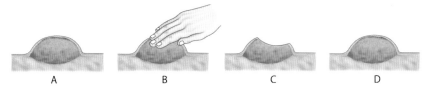

Figs 1.38A to D: (A) Demonstration of indentation. (B) Swelling is pressed with the fingers. (C) An indentation appears on the surface of the swelling. (D) On release of compression, the swelling refilled

OUTLINE FOR WRITING A CASE OF ULCER

History

- Duration: For how long ulcer is present?
- Mode of onset: Following trauma or spontaneously or following a swelling
- Site: Where first noticed?
- Progress of the ulcer: Change in size and shape
- Any pain over the ulcer: Site of pain, any radiation, character of pain and severity
- Any discharge: serous/purulent/hemorrhagic
- Any associated disease: Diabetes/sickle cell anemia/pulmonary tuberculosis/varicose vein/ systemic malignancy/AIDS
- Past history of similar ulcer, any history of tuberculosis in the past
- Personal history: Enquire about smoking, alcohol intake.

Physical Examination

General survey: A detail general survey.

1. Local Examination of Ulcer

Inspection:

- Number
- Site: Describe in relation to the region or bony landmark
- Extent
- Shape: Circular, oval, irregular or serpiginous
- Size
- Margin (Fig. 1.39): This is the junction of normal skin and the periphery of the edge of the ulcer
- Edge of the ulcer: Area of the ulcer between the floor and the margin. The edge may be (Fig. 1.40):

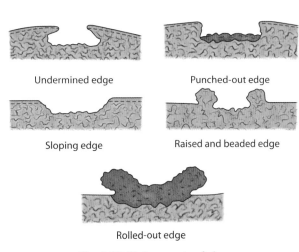

Undermined edge   Punched-out edge

Sloping edge   Raised and beaded edge

Rolled-out edge

Fig. 1.39: Various parts of ulcer

- Sloping
- Undermined
- Punched out
- Sloping
- Raised and rolled out
- Raised and beaded
- Floor of ulcer: Exposed portion of the ulcer. Floor may be covered by red granulation tissue/ pale granulation tissue/slough
- Discharge character, amount, smell
- Adjacent area:
  - Any swelling
  - Any skin change
  - Any secondary changes, pigmentation, pallor
  - Any associated venous diseases.

Palpation:

- Temperature: Palpate the area adjacent to the ulcer for any rise of local temperature
- Tenderness: Over the ulcer and adjacent area
- Size of the ulcer: Measure with a tape from one margin to the other
- Margin and edge of ulcer: Type, any induration
- Base: The area on which ulcer rests (Fig. 1.40) (Feel the base by picking up the ulcer in between the thumb, index and middle finger)
- Test mobility of ulcer over the deeper structure
- Any discharge during palpation: Bleeding or mucus discharge

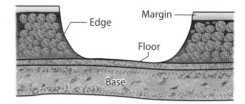

Fig. 1.40: Different types of edge of ulcers

2. Examination of regional lymph nodes

3. Examination of adjacent joints: Both active and passive movements

4. Examination for vascular disease

5. Examination for any nerve lesion

6. Examination of chest (in cases of tuberculous ulcer).

OUTLINE FOR WRITING A CASE OF SINUS OR FISTULA

Sinus is a blind tract having an opening on one side. Sinus is usually lined by granulation tissue or sometimes may be epithelialized, e.g. preauricular sinus, submental sinus, pilonidal sinus, etc.

A fistula is a tract having opening at both ends of the tract. The fistula tract may communicate a viscus to the external surface (enterocutaneous fistula, urethrocutaneous fistula), may communicate two viscera (colovesical fistula communication between the colon and urinary bladder. Vesicovaginal fistula, communication between the vagina and urinary bladder).

History

Duration and onset: Mode of onset. Some sinuses or fistula may be congenital and may be present since birth (branchial fistula).

Some sinus or fistula may develop following incision and drainage of an abscess (perianal fistula).

Some sinus or fistula may develop following incomplete excision of a congenital swelling (thyroglossal fistula may develop following incomplete excision of a thyroglossal cyst).

* Preceding history of swelling, pain and fever.
* History of discharge:
  – Type of discharge (purulent, mucous, bilious, feculent or urine), any discharge of bony spicules (may suggest underlying osteomyelitis)
  – Quantity of discharge, color and odor
  – Progress: sometimes discharge may stop and opening may be blocked. Recollection occurs in the tract and discharge comes out through the same or a different opening
* Any history of pain
* History of fever.

Past history: Any history of tuberculosis, actinomycosis or inflammatory bowel disease and any history of operation. Thyroglossal fistula may result following incomplete removal of thyroglossal cyst. Incision and drainage of perianal abscess may result in perianal fistula.

Physical Examination

* General survey
* Local examination

Inspection

* Site of fistula
* How many external openings: Single or multiple?
* Appearance of external opening: Any presence of granulation tissue, margin of the opening.
* Any discharge from the opening: Character of discharge and the odor of discharge.
* Appearance of the area adjacent to the external opening: any swelling, any scar, pigmentation.

Palpation

* Temperature of the local area.
* Tenderness around the site of external opening
* Palpate the wall of the tract: Any thickening
* Palpate for any swelling adjacent to the sinus/fistula
* Palpate for any bone thickening adjacent to the external opening (Bone thickening found in osteomyelitis)
* In case of perianal fistula—Rectal examination to assess the presence of internal opening
* In case of vesicovaginal or rectovaginal fistula: per vaginal examination.

Examination of Regional Lymph Nodes

* Systemic examination.

Hernias

■ HISTORY

1. **Particulars of the Patient** (Same as mentioned in general scheme of case taking)
2. **Chief Complaints**
   Usual chief complaints are:
   – Swelling in (right/left) groin for .... months/years
   – Swelling in (right/left) groin and scrotum for .... months/years
   – Pain over the swelling for .... months/years
3. **History of Present Illness**
   – Write in details about the swelling in first paragraph, details about the pain in the second paragraph and in the next paragraph write about any straining factor and any systemic symptoms
   – Patient was apparently well before he had noticed the swelling in groin..........months/ year back
   – Mode of onset—gradual or acute
   – How did the swelling appear first—following straining or spontaneously
   – Where did the swelling appear first—in the groin or in the scrotum
   – Progress of the swelling—size and extent of the swelling at onset—whether the swelling descended from groin to the scrotum or from scrotum to the groin
   – What happens to the swelling when the patient stands up, walks about and strains?
   – What happens to the swelling when the patient lies down?
   – Any period of irreducibility of the swelling
   – Any inguinoscrotal swelling on the opposite side
   – In the next paragraph write about the history of pain
   – Site of pain in the groin or over the swelling
   – Any radiation of pain
   – Character of pain—usually dull aching. In case of obstructed hernia the pain may be colicky
   – Relation of pain with straining: usually pain increases with straining
   – How is the pain relieved—usually relieved on lying down
   – In third paragraph write about any straining factor
   – History of chronic cough, breathlessness, any history of chronic bronchial asthma

- Bowel habits: Whether normal or there is any history of constipation or straining at stools. Write in details the usual bowel habit
- Bladder habit: Write in details about bladder habit to exclude any prostatic enlargement or urethral stricture
  - Any dysuria
  - Hesitancy/urgency/precipitancy
  - Narrowing of stream
  - Frequency of micturition, during daytime and nocturnal (ask whether patient has to wake up at night to micturate)
  - Any history of acute retention of urine
- Mention about any other important systemic symptom.
4. **Past History:** Any history of similar swelling in the same or opposite side. Any history of operation.
5. **Personal History**
6. **Family History**
7. **Treatment History**
   Whether using truss or not.
8. **Any History of Allergy**

■ PHYSICAL EXAMINATION

1. **General Survey:** Same as general scheme of case taking (See page 5, Chapter 1).
2. **Local Examination:** Examination of both inguinoscrotal regions:
   (In majority of hernia cases the swelling gets reduced partly or completely on lying down. So description of details of the swelling in lying down position will be fallacious. Main part of hernia examination will be in standing position and patient will lie down while doing some special tests only.)

In standing position:
- *Inspection* (Fig. 2.1):
  - Side where the swelling is present—right/ left
  - Position and extent of the swelling:
    » The swelling is seen in the inguinal region
    » A swelling is seen in (right/left) inguinoscrotal region
    » The swelling extends above up to the inguinal canal and below up to the bottom of scrotum
  - Size: Mention approximate size of the swelling—longitudinal and transverse dimension
  - Shape: Pyriform or globular
  - Surface: Smooth/irregular
  - Margin: Rounded/ill-defined

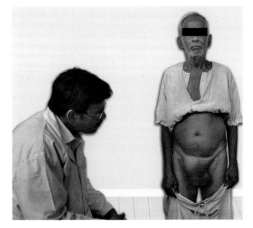

Fig. 2.1: Inspection of both inguinoscrotal regions in standing position

- Expansile impulse on cough over the swelling
- Skin over the swelling: Any scar/engorged vein/pigmentation
- Any visible peristalsis over the swelling
- Position of penis: Any deviation
- Testis: Whether testis could be seen separately from the swelling or swelling is seen all around the testis.
– *Palpation*
  - Temperature over the swelling
  - Tenderness over the swelling
  - Whether it is possible to get above the swelling (For an inguinoscrotal swelling it is not possible to get above swelling)
  - Position and extent of the swelling
  - Size: Longitudinal and transverse dimension, to be measured and mentioned, e.g. 5 cm × 4 cm
  - Shape: A complete hernia is usually pyriform in shape. A direct hernia is globular in shape
  - Surface
  - Margin
  - Consistency
    - » Soft and elastic (when content is intestine)
    - » Doughy (when content is omentum)
    - » Tense and tender (obstructed hernia)
  - Relation of the swelling to pubic tubercle:
    - » If the swelling is situated above and medial to pubic tubercle—inguinal hernia.
    - » If the swelling is situated below and lateral to pubic tubercle—femoral hernia
  - Relation of swelling to testis: Whether testis can be felt separately from the swelling or not.
    - » Testis not felt separately and hernia is reaching up to the bottom of the scrotum— complete hernia
    - » Testis felt separately from the hernia swelling and swelling stops at the upper pole of testis—incomplete hernia
  - Reducibility (to test for reducibility patient has to *lie down*):
    - » Whether swelling reduces *spontaneously* on lying down, partially or completely
      - ▷ If not reduced spontaneously—whether swelling can be reduced by *manipulation*
      - ▷ Which part of the swelling is easy to reduce—first part or last part
    - » In omentocele, first part reduces easily, but last part is difficult to reduce
    - » In enterocele, first part is difficult to reduce, but last part reduces easily
  - Invagination test:
    - » The invagination test is usually not done nowadays. The demonstration of this test is painful. This is no longer necessary to mention about this test in routine examination of hernia, unless examiner is specifically interested to know about the test
    - » On invagination test, comment about the size of the superficial inguinal ring. Normally the superficial ring does not admit the tip of index finger. When the hernia has reached the scrotum, superficial inguinal ring becomes patulous
    - » Ask patient to cough and assess where the impulse is felt—pulp or tip

- Deep ring occlusion test:
  - » Hernia is <u>reduced</u> and the <u>deep inguinal ring is occluded</u> by the <u>thumb</u> and patient is asked to <u>cough.</u> Test is positive when no impulse or hernia bulge is seen medial to the deep inguinal ring on coughing after the deep ring is occluded, suggesting this to be an indirect inguinal hernia
  - » Test is negative, i.e. an expansile impulse or hernia bulge is seen in inguinal canal medial to the occluded deep ring suggesting this to be a direct inguinal hernia
  - Palpation of testis epididymis and spermatic cord.
- *Percussion:*
  - Percuss over the hernial swelling keeping the content out in the hernial sac (patient in standing posture)
    - » <u>Resonant note</u> over the swelling suggests <u>enterocele</u>
    - » <u>Dull note</u> over the swelling suggests <u>omentocele</u>
- *Auscultation (Patient in standing posture):*
  - <u>Bowel sound</u> over the swelling suggests <u>enterocele</u>
- Mention about normal side of inguinoscrotal region:
  - No swelling in the opposite inguinoscrotal region
  - No expansile impulse on cough
  - Testis/epididymis and spermatic cord—normal
- Examination of tone of abdominal muscles—good or poor with bulge in the flanks
- <u>Per-rectal examinations</u>: It is important in a male patient with symptoms of <u>prostatism.</u>

3. **Systemic Examination**
   - Examination of abdomen
   - Examination of respiratory system (emphasize, if there is history of respiratory symptoms)
   - Examination of cardiovascular system
   - Examination of nervous system
   - Examination of spine and cranium.

▌SUMMARY OF THE CASE

▌PROVISIONAL DIAGNOSIS

Give a complete diagnosis mentioning:
- Side: Right or left
- Inguinal or femoral
- Direct or indirect
- Complete or incomplete
- Reducible or irreducible
- Content: Intestine or omentum
- Complicated or uncomplicated.

For example: This is a case of right-sided reducible complete indirect inguinal hernia containing intestine without any features of complication at present.

■ INVESTIGATIONS SUGGESTED

- Baseline investigation to assess fitness of patient for surgery:
  - Chest X-ray (posteroanterior view)
  - Electrocardiography (ECG)
  - Blood for Hb%, TLC, DLC and ESR
  - Blood for sugar, urea and creatinine
  - Urine for routine examination
- If patient has urinary symptom:
  - Ultrasonography (USG) of kidney, ureter and bladder (KUB) region
- If patient has chronic obstructive pulmonary disease—a pulmonary function test
- If the patient has cardiac disease—echocardiography/coronary angiography.

■ DIFFERENTIAL DIAGNOSIS

To be mentioned.

■ INDIRECT REDUCIBLE INGUINAL HERNIA IN AN ADULT

Q. What is your case? (Summary of a case of inguinal hernia)

Ans. A 40-year-old gentleman, a manual laborer by occupation, presented with a swelling in his right groin and scrotum for last 2 years and pain over the swelling for last 6 months. The swelling appeared insidiously, initially in the right groin and gradually increased in size for last 2 years and descended to the bottom of the right scrotum. The swelling disappears completely when the patient lies down, but the swelling reappears on standing and increases in size as the patient walks, coughs and strains at defecation. Patient complains of a dull aching pain over the swelling for last 6 months. The pain increases with straining as the

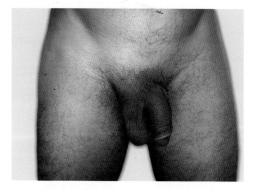

Fig. 2.2: Right-sided inguinal hernia

swelling increases, but the pain subsides with rest when the swelling gets reduced. Bladder and bowel habits are normal. No history of chronic constipation, or difficulty in micturition. Patient complains of chronic cough and breathlessness for last 3 years, which particularly aggravates during the winter season (Fig. 2.2).

On physical examination general survey is essentially normal. On local examination of inguinoscrotal regions, on inspection, there is a swelling in right inguinoscrotal region extending from the right inguinal canal to the bottom of the scrotum. The swelling is pyriform in shape. Skin over the swelling is normal and there is visible peristalsis and expansile impulse over the swelling. On palpation temperature is normal and there is no tenderness over the swelling. It is not possible to get above the swelling and there is palpable expansile impulse over the swelling. The swelling extends above up to the deep inguinal ring and below upt o the upper pole of right testis. The swelling is soft and elastic in feel. The swelling lies above and medial to the pubic tubercle. On lying down the swelling is easily reducible. The content of the swelling reduces with a gurgling sound. The deep ring occlusion test is positive and on percussion the swelling is resonant and bowel sounds are audible over the swelling on auscultation. The left inguinoscrotal region is normal and the systemic examination is also normal.

Q. What is your diagnosis?

Ans. This is a case of right sided, incomplete, reducible, indirect inguinal hernia containing intestine without any complication at present.

Q. Why do you say this is a case of hernia?

Ans. This 40 years male patient presented with a swelling which started in right groin and subsequently increased in size and descended to the scrotum. The swelling increased in size after walking and following strenuous activities. The swelling disappears (or reduces partially) on lying down.

On examination of inguinoscrotal region there is a right sided inguinoscrotal swelling as it is not possible to get above the swelling. There is expansile impulse on cough over the swelling.

On lying down swelling is reducible. So this is a hernia.

Q. What is hernia?

Ans. Hernia is abnormal protrusion of a part or whole of a viscus through the wall of its containing cavity.

Q. Why do you say this is an inguinal hernia?

Ans. This patient presented with a swelling in the groin which subsequently descended to the scrotum. This hernial swelling lies above and medial to the pubic tubercle. So this is an inguinal hernia. In case of femoral hernia, the hernia swelling lies below and lateral to the pubic tubercle.

Q. Why do you say this is an indirect and not a direct hernia?

Ans. Indirect hernia is usually unilateral, more commonly complete and more commonly found in young adults.

On inspection the swelling extends downward and forward from the inguinal canal up to the bottom of the scrotum.

During reduction the hernial contents go upward and backward. The deep ring occlusion test is positive. So this is an indirect inguinal hernia.

Q. Why do you say this is a reducible hernia?

Ans. The content of the hernia can be reduced into the abdominal cavity, so this is a reducible hernia.

Q. Why do you say this is an incomplete hernia?

The hernia has extended up to upper pole of the right testis. The testis and epididymis can be palpated separately from the hernial swelling, so this is an incomplete hernia (Fig. 2.3C).

Q. What do you mean by bubonocele?

Ans. Bubonocele is an incomplete inguinal hernia where the hernial sac is confined to the inguinal canal (Fig. 2.3B).

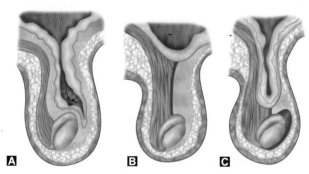

Figs 2.3A to C: Types of inguinal hernia: (A) Complete; (B) Bubonocele (incomplete); (C) Funicular (incomplete)

Q. What is funicular type of inguinal hernia?

Ans. In this type, the hernial sac goes beyond the superficial inguinal ring and reaches up to the upper pole of testis. The testis and epididymis can be felt separately from the hernial contents (Fig. 2.3C).

Q. What do you mean by complete hernia?

Ans. In complete hernia, the hernial contents reach up to the bottom of scrotum (Fig. 2.3A). Testis and epididymis could not be felt separately from the hernial swelling.

Q. Why do you say this is an enterocele?

Ans. By definition, enterocele is one which contains intestine.

From history, patient says that while he lies down the hernial content reduces with a gurgling sound.
- On inspection there is visible peristalsis over the swelling.
- On palpation the swelling is soft and elastic in feel. While attempting reduction, the first part was difficult to reduce, but the last part reduces easily with a gurgling sound.
- On percussion the swelling is resonant.
- On auscultation bowel sounds are audible over the swelling.
- So this is an enterocele.

Q. What are the differential diagnoses in this patient?

Ans. The important causes of inguinal or inguinoscrotal swellings are:
- Indirect inguinal hernia
- Direct inguinal hernia
- Femoral hernia
- Congenital hydrocele
- Funicular type of hydrocele
- Encysted hydrocele of the cord
- Lipoma of the cord
- Epididymal cyst
- Varicocele.

Q. Why hernia examination should be done in standing position?

Ans. In majority of patients with hernia the swelling reduces on lying down position. So in lying down position the description of the swelling will be fallacious.

Q. How will you demonstrate the sign "to get above the swelling"?

Ans. Start palpating the swelling from the bottom of the scrotum between the thumb in front and index and middle fingers behind and gradually palpate upward toward the root of the scrotum.

In case of the inguinoscrotal swelling the thumb and other two fingers do not meet at the root of the scrotum as the swelling continues in the groin. So it is not possible to get above the swelling in case of inguinoscrotal swelling (Figs 2.4A and B).

In case of a scrotal swelling the thumb and other two fingers meet each other at the root of the scrotum and only the spermatic cord is palpable in between the fingers; suggesting this to be a scrotal swelling (Figs 2.5A and B).

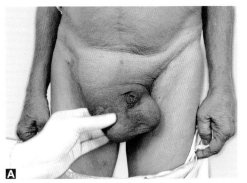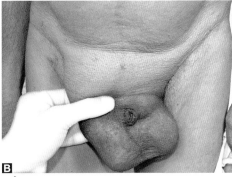

Figs 2.4A and B: (A) Start palpation at the scrotum; (B) Palpation at root of scrotum—the swelling is still palpable—so it is not possible to get above the swelling—inguinoscrotal swelling

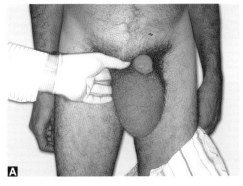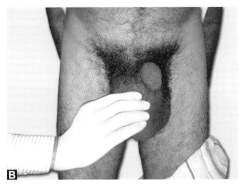

Figs 2.5A and B: In scrotal swelling it is possible to get above the swelling. (A) Start palpation at the scrotum; (B) At the root of scrotum swelling is not palpable—spermatic cord may be felt. It is possible to get above the swelling—scrotal swelling

Q. How will you demonstrate expansile impulse on coughing?

Ans. On inspection patient is asked to cough—the expansile impulse on cough may be seen over the swelling. This is visible expansile impulse on cough.

On palpation: Keep thumb in front and index and middle fingers behind the swelling at the root of the scrotum and ask the patient to cough. The expansile impulse can be appreciated by the palpating finger as the thumb and other fingers get separated (Figs 2.6A and B).

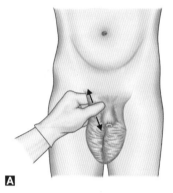 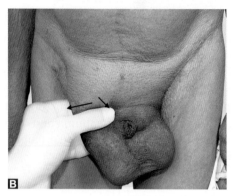

Figs 2.6A and B: Palpate with the thumb in front and the index and middle finger behind and ask the patient to cough. Expansile impulse may be appreciated by the palpating fingers

Q. What other swellings show expansile impulse on cough?

Ans. Apart from hernia the following swellings may show expansile impulse on cough:
* Meningocele
* Encephalocele
* Laryngocele.
* Empyema necessitates.

Q. How will you measure the dimension of a hernial swelling?

Ans. Patient should be in standing posture so that the whole hernial swelling is visible. Patient may be asked to cough for the full bulge to appear. Mark the proximal and distal point of the swelling. Use a Vernier Caliper to measure the vertical extent of the swelling. Similarly measure the horizontal extent of the swelling.

Q. How will you do invagination test?

Ans. As discussed earlier the invagination test is no longer routinely done in hernia examination. The method for demonstration invagination is however described. Patient is asked to lie down and the hernial content is reduced. The scrotal skin is invaginated with the tip of the index finger from the upper pole of the testis and the finger reaches up to the superficial inguinal ring (Figs 2.7A to C).

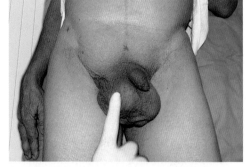

Fig. 2.7A: Start invaginating the scrotal skin with the index finger from the upper pole of testis (do not take the testis up)

The finger first assesses the size of the superficial inguinal ring. Normally the superficial inguinal ring does not admit the tip of index finger.

Once the size of the superficial inguinal ring is assessed and when it is patulous, the finger is pushed further. The finger may go directly back into the inguinal canal suggesting this to be a

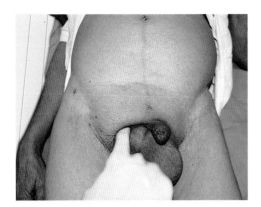

Fig. 2.7B: Push the index finger up to reach the superficial inguinal ring

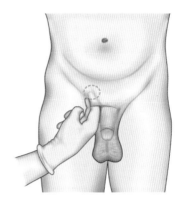

Fig. 2.7C: Invagination test: The index finger assess the superficial inguinal ring

direct inguinal hernia or the finger may go upward and laterally suggesting this to be an indirect inguinal hernia.

• The finger is kept in the inguinal canal with the nail pointing towards the roof and patient is asked to cough.
  – If the impulse touches the pulp of the finger, it is likely to be a direct inguinal hernia.
  – If the impulse touches the tip or dorsum of the index finger, it is likely to be an indirect inguinal hernia.

Q. How will you test for reducibility?

Ans. In some cases hernia gets reduced once the patient lies down. In majority of cases patient can reduce the hernia better. Some cases require taxis for reduction of the hernia. However, forcible taxis should not be done for reduction of hernia.

Patient lies down supine, leg flexed at the hip and knee, keep the thigh adducted. The fingers of one hand surround the swelling near the superficial inguinal ring and guide the content through the superficial inguinal ring into the inguinal canal. The other hand grasps the swelling near the fundus. Gentle squeezing is carried out with one hand alternating with the other till the hernia is reduced (Figs 2.8A and B).

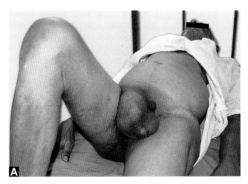

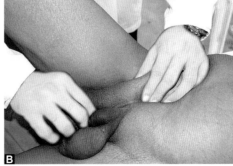

Figs 2.8A and B: (A) Method for reduction of hernia: Patient lies down and flex the hip and knee; (B) Keep fingers of one hand at the superficial inguinal ring and the other hand at the fundus of hernia—hernia sac and the hernial contents are then pushed upward from the scrotum. The fingers in the superficial ring guide the contents into the inguinal canal

Q. How will you do deep ring occlusion test?

Ans. Patient is asked to lie down and the hernia is reduced. The position of deep inguinal ring is marked out. The deep ring lies 1.25 cm above the midinguinal point, which is situated at the midpoint between anterior superior iliac spine and symphysis pubis.

The anterior superior iliac spine is marked by following the groin crease towards the lateral side. The first bony point at the lateral end is the anterior superior iliac spine. If you follow the iliac crest from back, the last bony point is the anterior superior iliac spine (Figs 2.9A and B).

To find the pubic symphysis follow the midline from below the umbilicus. The first bony point in the midline is the symphysis pubis (Figs 2.10A and B).

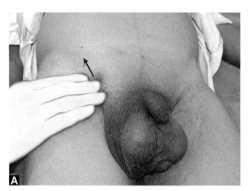 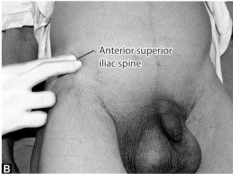

Figs 2.9A and B: (A) Finding the anterior superior iliac spine—pass the finger along the groin crease laterally. (B) The first bony point felt at the lateral end of the groin crease is anterior superior iliac spine

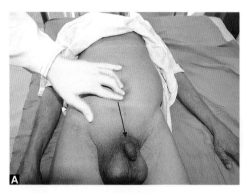 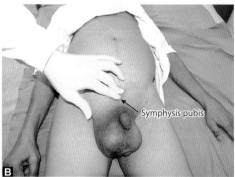

Figs 2.10A and B: (A) Follow the midline below the umbilicus; (B) The first bony point in the midline is the symphysis pubis

Measure the distance between the anterior superior iliac spine and the symphysis pubis using a tape and take the midpoint at the inguinal ligament. This is midinguinal point which lies over the inguinal ligament. The deep ring is located 1.25 cm above this point (Figs 2.11A to C).

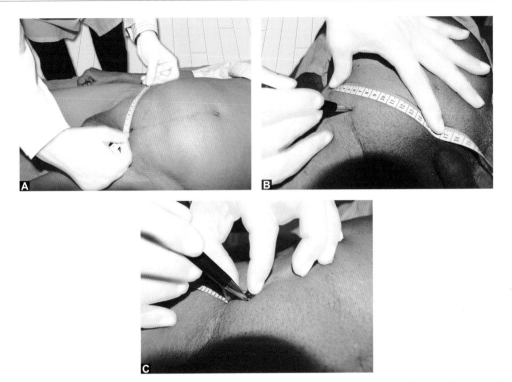

Figs 2.11A to C: (A and B) The midinguinal point is found out by measuring the distance between the anterior superior iliac spine and the symphysis pubis; (C) The deep inguinal ring is marked 1.25 cm above the midinguinal point

The thumb is placed over the deep ring and patient is asked to cough. Look whether any cough impulse is seen medial to the deep ring. If no expansile impulse is seen in lying down position patient is asked to stand with the deep ring occluded and is asked to cough again. Again look for any expansile impulse on cough medial to deep ring (Fig. 2.12).

Q. How to interpret deep ring-occlusion test?

Ans. On occlusion of deep ring and asking patient to cough—no expansile impulse on cough is seen medial to deep ring, suggesting this to be an indirect inguinal hernia (Fig. 2.13). This is described as deep ring occlusion test is positive.

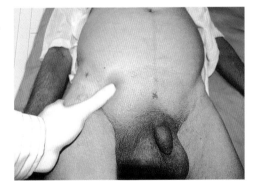

Fig. 2.12: Occlude the deep inguinal ring by pressing with the thumb

On occlusion of the deep ring and asking patient to cough—expansile impulse on cough is seen medial to the deep ring suggesting this to be direct inguinal hernia (Fig. 2.14). This is described as deep ring occlusion test is negative.

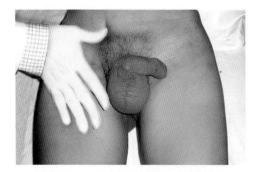

Fig. 2.13: On asking the patient to cough, there is no expansile cough impulse medial to the deep ring, suggesting this to be an indirect inguinal hernia

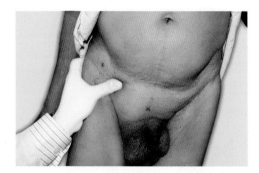

Fig. 2.14: On asking the patient to cough with the deep ring occluded, there is expansile cough impulse medial to the occluded deep ring, suggesting this to be a direct inguinal hernia

Q. What is Zieman's test?

Ans.

* Hernia is reduced. Three fingers are placed—index finger over the deep ring, middle finger over the superficial ring and ring finger over the femoral ring and the patient is asked to cough
* If impulse touches the index finger—indirect inguinal hernia
* If impulse touches the middle finger—direct hernia
* If impulse touches the ring finger—femoral hernia.

However, it is difficult to appreciate the impulse with three fingers placed apart at three sites. So, Zieman's test is not favored by many at present (Figs 2.15A to C).

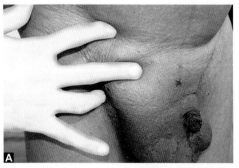

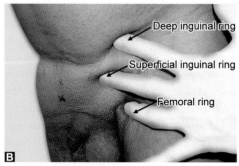

Deep inguinal ring

Superficial inguinal ring

Femoral ring

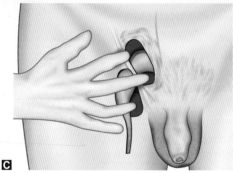

Figs 2.15A to C: Zieman's test

Q. How will you assess tone of abdominal muscles?

Ans. This is tested by rising test. Patient lies supine on the bed. He is asked either to lift the head and chest or both the legs above the bed. If there is weakness of abdominal muscles, the flank will bulge out. This is called Malgaigne's bulging. The contracting muscle may be palpated with the hand placed on the abdominal wall (Figs 2.16A to C).

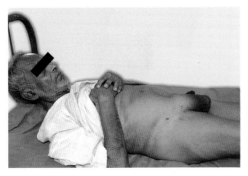

Fig. 2.16A: Ask the patient to keep his hands over the chest and lift the head above the level of bed and look at the flanks for appearance of any bulging. Appearance of bulging in the flanks suggest poor abdominal muscle tone

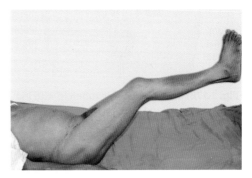

Fig. 2.16B: Abdominal muscle tone and appearance of bulging in the flanks may also be observed by leg rising test

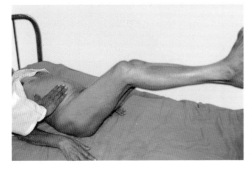

Fig. 2.16C: Patient is asked to lift the leg above the bed (leg rising) and the tone of the abdominal muscles are assessed with the palpating fingers

Q. How will you differentiate inguinal and femoral hernia?

Ans.

* *Relation with pubic tubercle:* Inguinal hernia lies above and medial, and the femoral hernia lies below and lateral to the pubic tubercle (Figs 2.17A to C).

Q. How would you find the pubic tubercle?

Ans. The patient is asked to adduct the thigh against resistance. The tendon of the adductor longus is palpated at the upper medial aspect

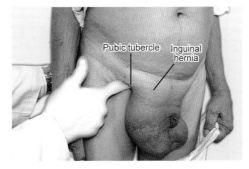

Fig. 2.17A: The finger is placed in the pubic tubercle. The hernial sac lies above and medial to the pubic tubercle, suggesting this to be an inguinal hernia

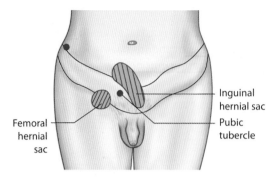

Fig. 2.17B: Relation of pubic tubercle with inguinal and femoral hernia

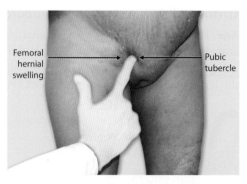

Fig. 2.17C: Femoral hernia, the hernia sac lies below and lateral to the pubic tubercle

of the thigh. Trace the adductor longus tendon upward, it reaches up to a bony point that is pubic tubercle (Fig. 2.18). Alternatively follow the groin crease medially the first bony point reached is pubic tubercle. It may also be reached by marking the symphysis pubis and going laterally along the pubic crest to reach the bony eminence which is pubic tubercle.

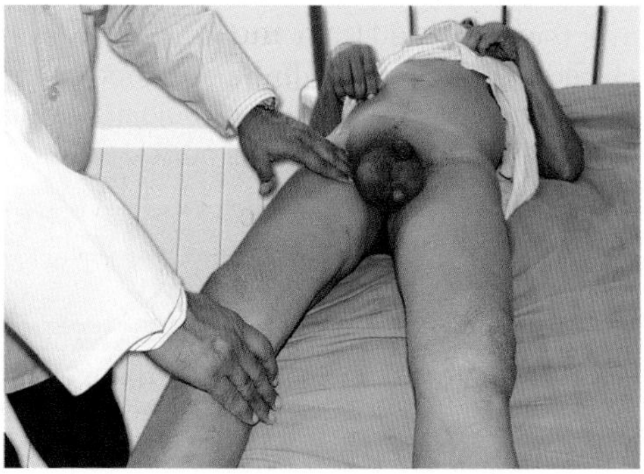

Q. How will you differentiate direct and indirect inguinal hernia?

Ans.

Fig. 2.18: Leg adducted against resistance, follow adductor longus tendon. The bony point reached is the pubic tubercle

* Direct hernia comes out through the Hesselbach's triangle, whereas the indirect inguinal hernia comes out through the deep inguinal ring
* Alternatively follow the groin crease medially along the inguinal ligament, the bony point reached in the pubic tubercle
* The pubic tubercle may also be reached by passing laterally from the symphysis pubis along the pubic crest
* Direct hernia is more commonly incomplete whereas indirect hernias are commonly complete
* Direct hernias are commonly bilateral whereas indirect hernias are commonly unilateral
* On cough the direct hernia appears as a direct forward bulge, whereas the indirect hernia comes out downward and forward
* On invagination test, the palpating finger goes directly backward in direct hernia, whereas in indirect hernia the finger goes upward and backward. The cough impulse will touch the tip or dorsum of the finger in indirect hernia and pulp of the finger in direct hernia
* Deep ring occlusion test is positive in indirect inguinal hernia.

Q. How will you do percussion of hernia swelling?

Ans. This is to be done with the patient in standing position, as the swelling may get reduced on lying down (Fig. 2.19).

- Dull percussion note—suggest content is omentum (omentocele).
- Resonant percussion note—suggest content is intestine (enterocele).

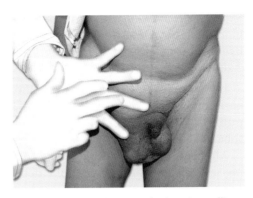

Fig. 2.19: Percussion over the hernia swelling in standing position

Q. How will you manage this patient?

This adult male patient presented with indirect, incomplete, uncomplicated reducible inguinal hernia. I will plan for surgical treatment after some routine investigations.

I will suggest following investigations:

- Blood for Hb%. Total count and differential count (TLC–DC)
- Blood for sugar, urea and creatinine
- Urine for routine examination
- Chest X-ray (posteroanterior view)
- 12-lead-ECG.
    This patient complains of chronic cough and breathlessness. I will do a pulmonary function test to exclude any obstructive or restrictive pulmonary disease.

Q. What operation will you do in this patient?

Ans. I will consider Lichtenstein tension free mesh hernioplasty in this patient under regional anesthesia.

Q. What anesthesia will you prefer for hernia surgery in adult?

Ans.

- Spinal and epidural anesthesia is excellent for hernia operation. Less postoperative pain following regional anesthesia. In adult local infiltration anesthesia may be used for hernia repair
- General anesthesia is also used
- Both surgeon and anesthetist should be flexible with regard to type of anesthesia to be used, suiting to the general condition and preference of the patient.

Q. Can this operation be done under local anesthesia?

Ans. Hernia operation can also be done under local anesthesia. In day-care surgery units often the hernia operations are done under local anesthesia and patient is discharged on the same day.

Q. What is the technique of local infiltration for inguinal hernia surgery?

Ans. A large volume of local anesthetic is required so either lignocaine 0.5% with adrenaline or without adrenaline is to be used. If used with adrenaline larger volume may be used. There are two technique of local anesthetic block.

Shouldice technique: This is a type of field block with local anesthetic. 1% lignocaine hydrochloride is used as anesthetic (Fig. 2.20).

Here 4 cm wide area is infiltrated from anterior superior iliac spine to symphysis pubis. The first layer of infiltration is subcutaneous tissue.

After skin and subcutaneous tissue are incised similar infiltration is done deep to external oblique aponeurosis.

After external oblique aponeurosis is incised the inguinal canal is exposed. The hernial sac is then infiltrated.

Point Block (Fig. 2.21):

* The midinguinal point area is infiltrated with 10 mL of 0.5% lignocaine (1)
* The pubic tubercle area is infiltrated with 10 mL of 0.5% of lignocaine (2)
* A point below the inguinal ligament lateral to femoral artery is infiltrated with 10 mL to 0.5% lignocaine (blocks genital branch of genitofemoral nerve) (3)
* A point 2 cm above and medial to anterior superior iliac spine is infiltrated with 10 mL of 0.5% lignocaine (blocks iliohypogastric nerve) (4)
* The line of skin incision is infiltrated with 10 mL of 0.5% of lignocaine (5)
* During dissection of the hernial sac inject 10 mL of 0.5% of lignocaine into the neck of the hernial sac.

Q. What is Lichtenstein tension-free repair?

Ans. In 1993, Lichtenstein described a technique of repair of both direct and indirect hernia by a tension-free technique without closing the defect by direct suturing and by placement of a mesh in the defect of inguinal canal (Fig. 2.22).

Procedure may be done under local anesthesia. The hernial sac is dealt with by dissecting the sac and invaginating it into the

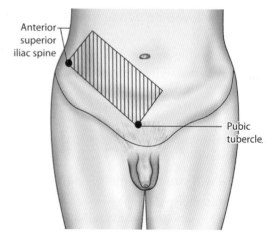

Fig. 2.20: Shouldice technique for local anesthetic block

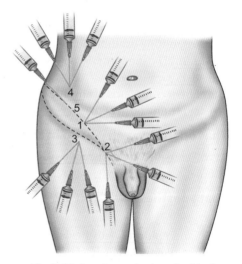

Fig. 2.21: Local anesthetic point block for hernia repair

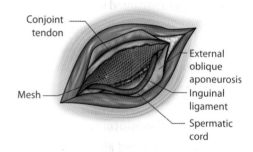

Fig. 2.22: Lichtenstein mesh repair

abdomen. In case of large direct hernia this sac may be invaginated by imbricating suture using an absorbable suture to allow proper placement of the mesh.

A mesh of size 11 cm × 6 cm is sutured along the lower edge to pubic tubercle, the lacunar ligament and the inguinal ligament to beyond the deep ring with a continuous suture of 3-0 polypropylene. The medial edge of the mesh is sutured to the rectus sheath. The superior edge is sutured to the conjoint tendon. The lateral edge of the mesh is split around the cord at the deep inguinal ring. The two split arch of the mesh are then crossed over each other and sutured down to the inguinal ligament to create a new deep ring. The external oblique aponeurosis is sutured in front of the spermatic cord.

Q. Describe the steps of Lichtenstein mesh hernioplasty.

Ans. *See* Operative Surgery Section, Page No, 1083 Chapter 22.

Q. What is modified Bassini's repair?

Ans.

* There are various modifications of Bassini's repair.
* Lichtenstein modification of Bassini's repair is as follows (Fig. 2.23):
  – Herniotomy is done first. The lower edge of the transversus abdominis aponeurosis and the conjoint tendon with fascia transversalis attached to it is apposed to inguinal ligament with interrupted nonabsorbable suture. Tension may be relieved by Tanner's slide.
  – The internal oblique muscle is bulky here and does not hold suture well so it is not included in suture in modified Bassini's repair.

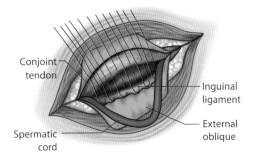

Fig. 2.23: Modified Bassini's repair: Conjoint tendon apposed to inguinal ligament

Q. What was original Bassini's operation?

Ans. In 1884, Bassini first performed herniorrhaphy. He dissected the hernial sac up to the deep inguinal ring and ligated the neck of the sac high up near the deep inguinal ring.

He reinforced the posterior wall of the inguinal canal by apposing internal oblique, transversus abdominis and upper leaf of fascia transversalis to lower leaf of fascia transversalis, and inguinal ligament using interrupted silk suture. The rectus sheath comes in the medial end of the repair. The external oblique aponeurosis is sutured in front of the cord.

Q. What is herniotomy?

Ans. Herniotomy involves dissection of the hernial sac and once the sac is dissected it is opened at the fundus. The content of the sac is reduced and a sliding component is excluded. The hernial sac is twisted and ligated at the neck and redundant part of the sac is excised.

Q. While doing herniotomy where do you ligate the sac?

Ans. The sac is dissected all around the deep inguinal ring twisted and ligated in the neck of the sac.

However, the proximal end of the sac may not be ligated and simply inverted into the peritoneal cavity. The defect closes rapidly within hours or days.

The pain in postoperative period is less when hernial sac is not ligated proximally.

Q. How will you identify the neck of an indirect hernia sac?

Ans. The indirect hernial sac is dissected up to the neck of the sac. The neck of the indirect hernial sac is identified by:

* This is the most constricted part of the sac.
* There is a collar of fat pad around the neck of the sac.
* The inferior epigastric vessels cross the neck of the sac from the medial side.

Q. What is the standard skin incision for inguinal hernia repair?

Ans. For herniorrhaphy/hernioplasty in adult, the incision should be long, starting from the pubic tubercle at the medial end and taken laterally along the inguinal canal beyond the deep inguinal ring.

An adequate incision provides good exposure for dissection of the sac and repair of posterior wall can be done easily.

Q. Why absorbable sutures are not used for hernia repair?

Ans. Following hernia repair, process of healing takes about 1 year. 80% wound tensile strength is achieved in 6 months. Absorbable suture like catgut loses 50% of their tensile strength within 1 week and gets absorbed within 6 weeks. So it is not an ideal suture for hernia repair.

Q. Why braided silk is not preferred for hernia repair?

Ans. Silk sutures lose 40% of their tensile strength within 6 weeks. These sutures being braided polyfilament suture causes more tissue reaction, may perpetuate infection once there is infection.

Q. Which suture is ideal for hernia repair?

Ans.

* Monofilament nonabsorbable synthetic suture like polypropylene and polyamide sutures are ideal for hernia repair
* Even if there is infection these sutures need not be removed
* Monofilament stainless steel sutures may also be used for hernia repair.

Q. When can a patient return to normal activities after operation?

Ans.

* There is no advantage in limiting postoperative activities. Patient can return to normal activities as soon as postoperative discomfort is over. There is no evidence that lengthy rest reduces the chance of recurrence
* Recurrence rate depends on the technique used for hernia repair and does not depend on postoperative activity of the patient.

Q. What is Shouldice repair for inguinal hernia?

Ans. This is a multilayered repair of hernia first practiced at Shouldice clinic in Toronto.

* Usually done under local anesthesia. Using stainless steel wire or polypropylene as suture material

- Skin incision in the groin from anterior superior iliac spine to the pubic tubercle. Cremaster muscle is excised
- Hernial sac is dissected and ligated at neck at the deep inguinal ring
- Redundant transversalis fascia is excised from deep ring to pubic tubercle
- The lower flap of fascia transversalis is sutured behind the upper flap of fascia transversalis
- The upper flap of fascia transversalis is sutured to inguinal ligament from deep inguinal ring to the pubic tubercle
- This double breasting of fascia transversalis forms a new strong posterior wall of the inguinal canal
- The posterior wall is further strengthened by double layer of suture apposing conjoint tendon to the inguinal ligament starting from pubic tubercle and carrying laterally to deep ring and back from deep inguinal ring to the pubic tubercle
- The cut margins of the external oblique aponeurosis are sutured in front of the cord in two layers
- Skin closure with interrupted 2-0 monofilament polyamide suture
- Recurrence rate following this type of repair is less than 1%.

Q. What is modified Shouldice repair for inguinal hernia?

Ans. Berliner modified six layers repair of inguinal hernia. He initially started repair of posterior wall in three layers and later modified it with repair in two layers. The fascia transversalis is split from pubic tubercle to the deep inguinal ring. The upper leaf of fascia transversalis and transversus abdominis aponeurosis is apposed to lower leaf of fascia transversalis. The second layer of continuous suture approximates the superior margin of fascia transversalis and transversus abdominis aponeurosis to the inguinal ligament. The external oblique aponeurosis is sutured in front of the spermatic cord in single layer.

Q. What is McVay repair for inguinal hernia?

Ans.
- It is also known as Lothiessan's repair or Cooper's ligament repair
- Herniotomy is done. The Cooper's ligament is dissected by dividing the iliopubic tract. Beginning at pubic tubercle a series of sutures are placed between the upper edge of the fascia transversalis and aponeurosis of transversus abdominis and the Cooper's ligament up to the medial margin of femoral vein
- Femoral ring is closed by interrupted suture apposing the Cooper's ligament to anterior femoral fascia and inguinal ligament
- In the lateral part the transversus aponeurosis and fascia transversalis is apposed to the inguinal ligament with interrupted sutures
- The external oblique aponeurosis is sutured in front of the spermatic cord.

Q. What is the role of laparoscopic repair of groin hernia?

Ans. The laparoscopic repair of inguinal hernia, a relatively newer modality in the armamentarium of the surgeon and has established its rightful place in the surgical practice.

In this type of repair, a sheet of mesh is placed in the preperitoneal space to cover the myopectineal orifice of Fruchaud and is fixed with sutures/tacker to prevent its migration.

The placement of the mesh may be accomplished either via:

◆ TAPP technique (transabdominal preperitoneal repair)
◆ TEP technique (totally extraperitoneal repair).

Q. What is TAPP repair?

Ans. In this technique the approach is through the transperitoneal route. 10 mm subumbilical port for camera and two 5 mm port in right and left iliac fossae. Induction of pneumoperitoneum. The peritoneal flap is raised medial to anterior superior iliac spine and hernia sac dissected. The preperitoneal space is dissected delineating the Fruchaud myopectineal orifice and medially dissecting the space of Retzius. A 15 cm × 12 cm polypropylene mesh is placed in the preperitoneal space and fixed medially to Cooper ligament. No fixation to be done laterally (Triangle of pain).

Q. Describe the steps of TAPP operation.

Ans. *See* Operative Surgery Section, Page No. 1085, Chapter 22.

Q. What is TEP repair?

Ans. In this technique approach is through the extraperitoneal space. Entry to extraperitoneal space is through a subumbilical 10 mm incision. Anterior rectus sheath is incised and rectus muscle is retracted laterally. A balloon is inserted into the preperitoneal space and inflated thus creating a prepritoneal space. Alternatively this space may be created by telescopic dissection. Two more 5 mm ports are made in the midline one just above the symphysis pubis and another midway between the subumbilical port and suprapubic port. The preperitoneal space is dissected and the hernia sac is dissected and placed in the preperitoneal space. The lateralization of the cord structures are done. A 15 cm × 12 cm polypropylene mesh is placed in the preperitoneal space covering the Fruchaud myopectineal orifice and space of Retzius. The mesh is fixed medially to Cooper ligament by suture/tacker.

Q. Describe the steps of TEP operation.

Ans. *See* Operative Surgery Section, Page No. 1088, Chapter 22.

Q. What are the indications of Laparoscopic hernia repair?

Ans. Laparoscopic repairs provide very good results where surgeons have expertise in the technique. It results in very low postoperative pain, fewer wound infection, and quick return to daily activity and working. This is suitable for unilateral, bilateral and recurrent groin hernias.

Q. What are the current recommendations for groin hernia repair?

Ans. At present strong recommendations exist in favor of Lichtenstein repair. American College of Surgeons choose this technique as "gold standard" for repair of groin hernia. The National Institute of Clinical Excellence (NICE) from UK and The National Agency for Accreditation and Evaluation in Health (ANAES) from France recommended Lichtenstein mesh repair as the standard technique for inguinal hernia repair.

Laparoscopic repairs also provide very good results where surgeons have expertise in the technique. It results in very low postoperative pain, fewer wound infection, and quick return to daily activity and working.

There is great competition between open and laparoscopic mesh repairs. Majority of hernia repairs are still done with open technique throughout the world. However, the rate of laparoscopic repair are increasing.

The prime indications for laparoscopic repair at present are bilateral hernias and recurrent hernias after open repair. But some center with surgical expertise unilateral hernias are also being managed laparoscopically with comparable results.

Q. How will you treat asymptomatic hernia?

Ans. There were different studies with regard to natural history of asymptomatic hernias. In one study 364 men assigned to watchful waiting and 356 were assigned routine operations. Only two patients in the watchful waiting group developed strangulation over a period of 2–4.5 years and required emergency operation. About one-third of the waiting group required operation due to symptom progression. There were no untoward complications for delay in surgery.

The current recommendation is, there is a role for watchful waiting in asymptomatic hernias.

Q. What is the current recommendation for unilateral inguinal hernia?

Ans. There has been excellent result with both open and laparoscopic repair of groin hernias. The experience of the surgeon is one of the most important factors for choosing the type of procedure.

In infants and children with indirect inguinal hernia herniotomy by anterior approach is adequate.

In adults with inguinal hernia prosthetic repair by an open approach is the standard of care at present.

Laparoscopic repair is not suitable in following circumstances:

- Obstructed and strangulated hernia
- Previous lower abdominal surgery
- Previous pelvic irradiation—fibrosis may hamper laparoscopic dissection.

Q. What are the evidences in favor of laparoscopic and open hernia operation?

Ans. A recent meta-analysis of open versus laparoscopic hernia repair compared the recurrence and surgery related morbidity. TEP repair was associated with a higher recurrence rate in comparison to open hernia repair. However, in TAPP repair recurrence was not higher. TAPP repair was associated with higher perioperative complications. Overall laparoscopic hernia repair was associated with less chronic groin pain and numbness.

Q. What are the strategies for recurrent groin hernia?

Ans. If previous surgery was an open anterior repair, preferred approach will be laparoscopic approach or open posterior approach for repair of recurrent inguinal hernia.

If previous repair was done laparoscopically, the preferred technique will be open anterior approach.

Q. What are the strategies for bilateral hernia?

Ans. For bilateral hernia laparoscopic repair is preferred over the open approach. Bilateral operation may be done with the same ports. Although operating time in laparoscopic repair is greater, the recovery time, risk of wound infection and chronic groin pain is much less in laparoscopic repair.

Q. What are the important complications of herniorrhaphy/hernioplasty?

Ans.

General Complications

* *Pulmonary:* Atelectasis, pneumonia and pulmonary embolism
* *Cardiac:* Particularly in patient with overt cardiac diseases
* *Urinary retention:* Usually caused by overzealous fluid administration leading to diuresis and atony of the overfilled bladder.

Local Complications

* Hemorrhage
* Urinary bladder or bowel injury during dissection and ligation of the sac
* Injury to testicular vessels during dissection, leading to:
  – Testicular swelling
  – Testicular atrophy
* Closing the superficial inguinal ring tightly may cause testicular swelling and subsequent atrophy
* Injury to vas deferens
* Injury to nerve like iliohypogastric, ilioinguinal and genital branch of genitofemoral nerve
* Wound infection
  – Incidence 1–5%. Minor or major wound infection
* Recurrence of hernia
* Hydrocele or lymphocele
* Edema of the penis due to injury to superficial external pudendal vein.

Q. What are the parts of a hernia?

Ans. A hernia consists of:
* Hernial sac
* Contents in the sac
* Coverings of the sac.

Q. What are the parts of hernial sac?

Ans. The hernial sac is the prolongation of the parietal peritoneum. The hernial sac has following parts (Fig. 2.24):
* Mouth of the sac: The opening into the peritoneal cavity (1)
* Neck of the sac: The constricted part of the sac beyond the mouth (2)
* Body of the sac (3)
* Fundus of the sac: The most distal closed part of the sac (4).

Q. What may be the different contents of a hernia?

Ans. The hernia may contain different intra-abdominal structures which include:

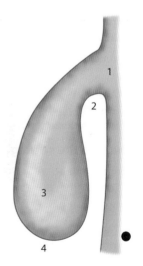

Fig. 2.24: Parts of a hernial sac

- Omentum: Omentocoele
- Intestine: Enterocoele
- A portion of the circumference of the bowel: Richter's hernia
- A portion of the urinary bladder
- Appendix
- Meckel's diverticulum: Littre's hernia
- Fallopian tubes
- Fluid: Secondary to ascites.

Q. What are the coverings of complete inguinal hernia?

Ans. Apart from skin, subcutaneous tissue and dartos, the coverings of hernia are:
- External spermatic fascia derived from external oblique aponeurosis
- Cremasteric muscle and fascia derived from internal oblique
- Internal spermatic fascia derived from the fascia transversalis
- Deep to this is hernial sac derived from the parietal peritoneum.

When the hernia sac is exposed at the inguinal canal, the coverings include the cremasteric muscle and fascia, and the internal spermatic fascia.

Q. What is Richter's hernia?

Ans. When the hernial sac contains a portion of the circumference of the bowel then it is called Richter's hernia (Fig. 2.25).

Q. What is sliding hernia?

When the wall of the hernial sac (usually the posterior wall) is formed by a viscus then it is called a sliding hernia. On the right side cecum or urinary bladder may form the posterior wall of the sac and on the left side sigmoid or urinary bladder may form the posterior wall of the hernial sac (Figs 2.26A and B).

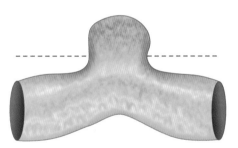

Fig. 2.25: Richter's hernia (circumference of the colon lying in the hernial sac)

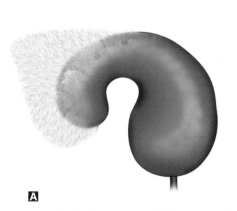

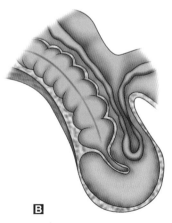

A **B**

Figs 2.26A and B: Sliding hernias. (A) Posterior wall of hernia sac formed by urinary bladder; (B) Posterior wall of hernia sac formed by cecum

Q. What is Littre's hernia?

Ans. Hernial sac containing Meckel's diverticulum as the content and is called Littre's hernia.

Q. What do you mean by pantaloon (or saddle bag) hernia?

Ans. A pantaloon hernia is described as having both a direct and indirect inguinal hernial sac lying on either side of inferior epigastric vessels. It is also known as dual hernia.

Q. What is Cooper's ligament?

Ans. It is the extension of the inguinal ligament, which is attached to the pecten pubis from pubic tubercle and laterally extends up to the femoral ring. It is quite strong and forms the lower boundary of the Fruchaud's myopectineal orifice.

Q. What are the different types of inguinal hernia depending on the distal extent of the hernia?

Ans. The hernia may be:
* Complete: When the hernial sac reaches up to the bottom of scrotum and the testis cannot be felt separately (*see* Fig. 2.3A).
* Incomplete hernia: When the hernial sac does not descend up to the bottom of the scrotum. This can be:
  - Bubonocele: When the hernial sac is confined to the inguinal canal and does not reach beyond the superficial inguinal ring (*see* Fig. 2.3B).
  - Funicular: When hernial sac goes beyond the superficial inguinal ring and reaches up to the upper pole of the testis (*see* Fig. 2.3C).

Q. What do you mean by hernioplasty?

Ans. When the repair of hernia is done by reinforcing the gap by placement of some prosthetic materials like mesh or natural tissues like fascia lata.

Q. What are the different techniques of hernioplasty?

Ans. *Abrahamson nylon darn repair:* The principle of this operation is to reinforce the posterior wall of the inguinal canal with the muscle of the musculoaponeurotic arch along with a simple lattice of monofilament suture under no tension on which fibrous tissue develops. The hernial sac is dealt with. The repair begins by suturing the medial edge of rectus sheath and the musculoaponeurotic arch (conjoint tendon) to the posterior portion of the inguinal ligament and to the iliopubic tract with a continuous suture of 2-0 polypropylene. If the conjoined tendon and inguinal ligament cannot be apposed without tension then approximation is not forced and a gap is left between the inguinal ligament or the upper elements of repair. The gap is bridged by a number of layers of the polypropylene suture.

    The first bite is to take over the most medial fiber of inguinal ligament over the pubic tubercle and then through the medial edge of the rectus sheath. The suture is then taken laterally taking bites below to the inguinal ligament and above to rectus sheath medially and laterally to the conjoint tendon and more laterally muscular part of transversus abdominis and internal oblique, up to the deep inguinal ring. The suture is not tied tightly, but kept loose and the suture is then continued medially taking bites of the same structures and ending up at the most medial end of inguinal ligament and rectus sheath. A third layer of suture may be applied from lateral to medial end thus providing a lattice of nylon suture in posterior wall of inguinal canal. External oblique aponeurosis is sutured in front of the cord.

Q. What is Rives prosthetic repair of inguinal hernia?

Ans.
* Rives recommended placement of mesh in the preperitoneal space
* The hernial sac is dealt with:
  - The fascia transversalis is slit open and is dissected all around widely to create a preperitoneal space.
  - The lower margin of the mesh is folded over and stitched to the Cooper's ligament and fascia iliaca. The mesh is passed upward behind the cord, transversalis fascia, transversus abdominis aponeurosis and rectus sheath into the preperitoneal space. The mesh is fixed above by interrupted suture to the combined thickness of internal oblique, transversus abdominis muscle and the edge of rectus sheath.
  - The superolateral edge of the mesh is split to accommodate the cord and the tails of the mesh are also fixed to the full thickness of internal oblique and transversus abdominis muscle.
  - The mesh is covered by suturing the musculoaponeurotic arch of the transversus abdominis and internal oblique muscle and fascia transversalis above to the fascia transversalis and inguinal ligament below. The external oblique is closed in front of the cord.
  - Rives also uses a midline subumbilical abdominal approach with a preperitoneal dissection to place a large sheet of mesh over the inguinal defect between the peritoneum and the abdominal wall. This technique is recommended for difficult recurrent hernia where Cooper's ligament is already destroyed.

Q. What is GPRVS (Stoppa procedure)?

Ans. This is called giant prosthetic reinforcement of visceral sac devised by Stoppa.

Q. Where is the mesh placed in GPRVS?

Ans. A large sheet of mesh (mersilene, dacron or polypropylene) is placed between the peritoneum and anterior, inferior, and lateral abdominal wall. The mesh stretches in the lower abdomen and pelvis from one end to the other enveloping the lower half of the parietal peritoneum with which it gets incorporated by scar tissue.

Q. What is the approach for placement of the mesh?

Ans. The mesh may be placed in the preperitoneal space by either a midline abdominal incision or Pfannenstiel incision. Unilateral mesh placement may also be done by an inguinal incision.

Q. How do you measure the size of the mesh required for a bilateral giant mesh placement?

Ans. The mesh is chevron-shaped and the width of the mesh is 2 cm less than the distance between the two anterior superior iliac spines. The vertical dimension equals the distance between the umbilicus and the symphysis pubis.

Q. How is the mesh anchored in place?

Ans. When correctly placed, this large prosthesis does not require any anchoring suture. The prosthesis may be fixed by a single suture to umbilical fascia only.

Q. In which hernia repair GPRVS is more suitable?

Ans. This technique is particularly useful for:
* Elderly patient with bilateral hernias
* Large hernias
* Recurrent hernias
* Patient with collagen disease, Ehlers–Danlos syndrome or Marfan syndrome.

Q. What is Lytle's repair?

Ans. When the deep ring is patulous, the fascia transversalis is plicated by suture narrowing the deep ring. This is called Lytle's repair (Fig. 2.27).

Q. What is Nyhus classification for groin hernia?

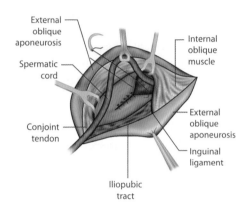

Fig. 2.27: Lytle's repair—narrowing the deep inguinal ring

Ans. Depending on the anatomical defects in the groin, Nyhus has classified groin hernias into four types:
* *Type I:* No defects in the deep inguinal ring or the inguinal canal. There is presence of persistent processus vaginalis, e.g. hernias in newborn and infants.
* *Type II:* Deep ring is patulous, but the inguinal canal is intact. Small indirect inguinal hernias.
* *Type III:* Variable defect in the deep inguinal ring or the inguinal canal. This includes large indirect inguinal hernias, sliding hernias, direct hernias and pantaloon hernias.
* *Type IV:* All recurrent hernias.

Q. What is Gilbert's classification for groin hernia?

Ans. Gilbert, in 1987, described an anatomical classification for hernia. However, it is not universally accepted.
* *Type I:* Patent processus vaginalis—Snug internal inguinal ring. Inguinal canal intact.
* *Type II:*
  - Moderately splayed deep inguinal ring
  - Admits one finger
  - Inguinal canal is otherwise intact
* *Type III:*
  - Large internal inguinal ring
  - Admit two or more fingers
  - Inguinal canal is weak
* *Type IV:*
  - Typical direct hernia
  - Full blow out of the posterior wall of the inguinal canal
  - Internal ring is intact

- *Type V:*
  - A type of direct hernia through a punched out hole in fascia transversalis
  - Internal inguinal ring is intact.

Q. What is European Hernia Society (EHS) classification for groin hernia?

Ans. The European Hernia Society (EHS) Board recently agreed on a new classification based on Aachen system and asked all surgeons practicing hernia surgery to report the class of the hernia in the operative reports.

EHS classification defines the location of hernia with ((Table 20.1):

- L: Lateral (Indirect inguinal hernia)
- M: Medial (Direct inguinal hernia)
- F: Femoral.

The size of hernia is indicated with:

- 1: ≤ one finger.
- 2: one-two fingers
- 3: ≥ three fingers.

Table 2.1: The European Hernia Society (EHS) groin hernia classification

EHS Groin Hernia Classification	Primary		Recurrent	
	0	1	2	3	x
L					
M					
F					

If the patient has two types of hernia together (e.g. direct + indirect, direct + femoral, indirect + femoral) appropriate boxes in the table are ticked.

In addition, P or R letter is encircled for a primary or recurrent hernia.

No matter which classification system is used the type of hernia should be recorded according to intraoperative findings.

For bilateral hernia each side should be described separately and clearly.

Q. What are the different options for inguinal hernia repair?

Ans. There are various techniques for repair of groin hernia:

- Tissue-suture repair:
  - Modified Bassini repair
  - Shouldice repair
  - Modified Shouldice repair
- Tension-free repair:
  - Anterior repair:
    - Lichtenstein tension-free repair
    - Plug repair
    - Plug and patch repair
    - Double layer devices.
  - Posterior repair (Preperitoneal repair)
    - Open preperitoneal mesh repair via an inguinal approach
    - Stoppa reapir
    - Laparoscopic mesh repair
      » TAPP (Transabdominal preperitoneal repair)
      » TEP (Total extraperitoneal repair).

Q. What do you mean by groin hernia?

Ans. All the hernias occurring through the myopectineal orifice of Fruchaud at the groin are grouped as groin hernias. These include the indirect inguinal hernia, direct inguinal hernia and the femoral hernia.

Q. What is the boundary of Fruchaud myopectineal orifice?

Ans. Fruchaud myopectineal orifice is an osseo-myo-aponeurotic tunnel through which all the groin hernia comes out (Fig. 2.28). This orifice is bounded by:

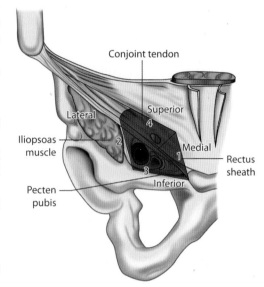

- Medially by the lateral border of the rectus sheath (1)
- Laterally by the iliopsoas muscle (2)
- Below by the pecten pubis and fascia covering it and the Cooper's ligament (3)
- Above by the arched fibers of internal oblique, transversus abdominis muscle and the conjoint tendon (4).

Anatomy of inguinal canal (*See* Surgical Anatomy Section, Page No. 1145, Chapter 23).

Fig. 2.28: Schematic diagram of Fruchaud myopectineal orifice

Q. What are the complications of hernia?

Ans. Untreated the hernias may lead to a number of complications. These include:

- Irreducible hernia
- Obstructed hernia
- Incarcerated hernia
- Strangulated hernia
- Inflamed hernia due to inflammation of the contents of hernia
- Hydrocele of the hernial sac.

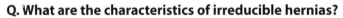

Q. What are the characteristics of irreducible hernias?

Ans. The contents of the hernial sac cannot be reduced inside the abdomen on lying down or after manipulation. This is usually due to adhesion of the hernial contents. Apart from irreducibility there are no symptoms and signs. However, irreducibility may lead to obstruction or strangulation. So, irreducible hernia should be operated early.

Q. What do you mean by obstructed hernia?

Ans. Hernia containing intestine may lead to acute intestinal obstruction due to obstruction of the lumen of the gut inside the hernia.

In addition to irreducibility patient complains of colicky pain initially over the hernia and later on colicky abdominal pain. The hernia becomes tense and tender and there may be visible peristalsis over the hernia. Unrelieved the patient may present with cardinal features of acute intestinal obstruction—pain abdomen, vomiting, abdominal distension and absolute constipation.

Unrelieved the obstruction may lead to impairment of blood supply to the gut causing strangulation of the hernial contents.

Q. What are the characteristics of strangulated hernia?

Ans. Due to impairment of blood supply there is ischemic necrosis of the hernial contents.

The hernial swelling becomes irreducible, no cough impulse, tense, tender and there may be rebound tenderness.

In strangulated omentocele, the symptoms and signs may be mild and if not relieved ischemic necrosis of omentum may lead to bacterial invasion leading to a localized abscess.

In strangulated enterocele, symptoms and signs are more severe with features of acute intestinal obstruction and if not treated patient condition will deteriorate rapidly. The ischemic gut may perorate leading to initially localized and then generalized peritonitis and septicemia.

Q. What do you mean by inflamed hernia?

Ans. When the contents of the hernial sac get inflamed, this is known as inflamed hernia. Patient complains of pain over the swelling and may be febrile. the hernia may become irreducible, there may be localized tenderness over the hernia.

Q. What do you mean by incarcerated hernia?

Ans. This is a type of obstructed hernia where the lumen of the colon is blocked with fecal matter. The hernial contents may be indented with the finger.

The term incarcerated hernia is often used as an alternative to obstructed or strangulated hernia.

Q. What are the etiological factors for development of hernia?

Ans.

* *Chronic straining factors:* Any chronic straining factors like chronic cough, lower urinary tract obstruction, straining at defecation may increase the intra-abdominal pressure which may be one of the important precipitating factors for development of hernia.
* Increased intra-abdominal pressure due to an underlying intra-abdominal malignancy or ascites may result in a hernia.
* *Obesity:* May cause stretching of muscles due to interposition of fat in between muscles which makes the muscles weak. Fat may also weakens the fascia and aponeurosis and may lead to hernias.
* *Smoking:* Smoking may result in an acquired collagen deficiency and may result in hernia.
* Chronic peritoneal dialysis may result in hernia either due to weakness of the abdominal wall or enlargement of a persistent processus vaginalis.

Q. What is herniography?

Ans. Radiographic contrast material is injected into peritoneal cavity and patient is turned to different position. X-ray of local area will demonstrate contrast in the hernial sac, if hernia is present.

■ INGUINAL HERNIA WITH FEATURES OF PROSTATISM

Q. What is your diagnosis?

Ans. This is a case of right sided incomplete, direct, reducible inguinal hernia containing intestine with features of benign prostatic enlargement in a gentleman aged 60 years.

(In this case a detailed history of bladder habit needs to be taken along with mention of P/R examination and comment on prostatic status) (Fig. 2.29).

Q. How will you manage this patient?

Ans. As this patient has chronic urinary obstruction due to prostatic enlargement, I will do the following special investigations in addition to routine investigation.

* USG of kidney, ureter and bladder (KUB) region to assess the size of the prostate, amount of residual urine and back pressure changes in the urinary tract
* Uroflowmetry study to decide about the necessity of operation for prostatic enlargement
* Serum PSA level.

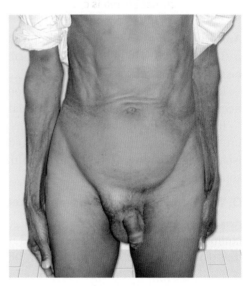

Fig. 2.29: Direct inguinal hernia

Q. If the patient has significant prostatic enlargement, how will you treat this patient?

Ans. As the patient has significant prostatic enlargement, the patient should be treated by prostatectomy and hernia repair in same sitting.

I will do transurethral resection of prostate and right-sided inguinal hernioplasty in same sitting.

Q. What is the role of medical treatment in benign prostatic hyperplasia?

Ans. *See* Page No. 922, Chapter 18.

Q. Can you do open prostatectomy and hernia repair in same sitting?

Ans. Yes. This can also be done. A Pfannenstiel incision extending slightly to the side of hernia is suitable. A transvesical or retropubic prostatectomy and repair of hernia may be done in same sitting.

Q. What is direct inguinal hernia?

Ans. When the hernia occurs through Hesselbach's triangle, it is called direct inguinal hernia.

Q. What are the characteristics of direct inguinal hernia?

Ans.
- Direct inguinal hernia is common in elderly male patient
- The neck of the direct hernial sac is wide so the chance of strangulation is less
- The direct hernia is usually incomplete
- A direct hernia is always acquired. Smoking, strenuous activities, damage to ilioinguinal nerve are predisposing factors.

Q. What is funicular direct inguinal hernia?

Ans. This is a variety of direct inguinal hernia where a narrow necked sac descend through a small defect in the most medial part of the Hesselbach's triangle just above the pubic tubercle.

The chance of strangulation is high in this variety of direct inguinal hernia.

Q. How will you tackle a direct hernial sac?

Ans. The neck of the sac is wide and hernia is usually incomplete. After dissection of the hernial sac it may just be inverted into the peritoneal cavity. Excision of the sac is usually not required. In case of a large hernial sac the fascia transversalis may be plicated to keep the sac reduced.

Only when direct hernial sac is like a diverticulum with a narrow neck, the sac is dissected, ligated at neck and redundant sac is excised.

Q. How will you differentiate a direct and indirect inguinal hernia at operation?

Ans.
- The direct hernia is a bulge through the Hesselbach's triangle, an indirect inguinal hernia descends through the deep inguinal ring
- The direct hernial sac lies posteromedial to the spermatic cord whereas an indirect hernial sac lies anterolateral to the cord
- The neck of direct hernial sac is wide and lies medial to inferior epigastric artery, whereas the neck of indirect inguinal hernia is narrow and lies lateral to inferior epigastric artery.

Q. How will you repair a direct inguinal hernia?

Ans. In direct hernia there is usually a wide gap in the posterior wall of the inguinal canal, so I will consider Lichtenstein tension-free mesh hernioplasty in this patient.

Q. What are other techniques for repair of direct inguinal hernia?

Ans.
- Shouldice repair
- Cooper's ligament repair
- Rives preperitoneal mesh repair
- Stoppa's GPRVS
- Laparoscopic mesh repair (TAPP and TEP).

■ RECURRENT INGUINAL HERNIA

Q. What is your diagnosis?

Ans. This is a case of recurrent right sided complete, reducible indirect inguinal hernia containing omentum in a gentleman aged 45 years (Fig. 2.30).

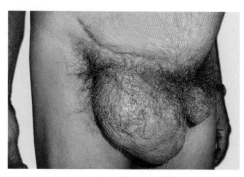

Q. What is the most important factor for development of recurrence after operation?

Ans.

+ The most important cause of *early recurrence* of hernia is due to technical reasons
+ *Late recurrences* are due to tissue failure.

Fig. 2.30: Right-sided recurrent inguinal hernia

Q. What are the important causes of recurrence of hernia?

Ans.

+ Repair under tension
+ Wound infection
    – 50% of recurrences are due to infection following repair
    – Wound hematoma contribute to increased chance of infection
+ Use of absorbable suture
+ Size of the hernia:
    – Larger the hernia, greater the chance of recurrence
+ Failure to identify and leaving behind a part of the sac
+ Missed hernial sac while repairing direct inguinal hernia, an indirect hernial sac may be overlooked
+ Smoking
+ Ascites and other causes of increased intra-abdominal pressure
+ Surgeons *expertise*
+ Multiple recurrences of repeated repair may be due to disorder of *collagen* production, maintenance and absorption.

Q. What is the incidence of recurrence of hernia after repair?

Ans. Varies between 1% and 3%.

Q. What are the problems of surgery in recurrent hernia?

Ans. Because of previous repair, the anatomy of the inguinal canal is distorted. There is scarring of tissues. The inguinal and Cooper's ligaments are usually attenuated.

The hernia usually descends through a large defect in the inguinal canal.

Q. What investigations will you do in this patient?

Ans. I will do a routine workup to assess his fitness for surgery.

Other special investigations depending on any underlying disease:

+ If patient have urinary symptoms: USG of KUB region, uroflowmetry
+ If patient has obstructive airway disease: Chest X-ray/pulmonary function test.

Q. What operation will you do in this patient?

Ans. As the patient has undergone an open operation earlier, it will be difficult to dissect the different layers in the inguinal canal. It is preferable to do a laparoscopic mesh repair of hernia in this patient.

Q. What other operation may be suitable to this patient?

Ans.

* An open preperitoneal approach for repair of this hernia may be undertaken and a mesh may be placed in preperitoneal space to overlap the myopectineal orifice
* Stoppa's GPRVS for large multiple recurrent hernia
* If anatomy is not distorted too much, then either Cooper's ligament repair or Shouldice repair may be attempted.

Q. What is the indication of orchiectomy?

Ans. When in a recurrent hernia cord cannot be dissected free from the scar tissue then excision of the cord and orchiectomy may be considered. Orchiectomy may also be required when cord has been damaged during dissection or in repair of complicated recurrent hernia. Informed consent is to be taken for orchiectomy.

INCISIONAL HERNIA: OUTLINE FOR WRITING A LONG CASE OF INCISIONAL HERNIA

■ A. HISTORY

1. **Particulars of the Patient**
2. **Chief Complaints**
   - Swelling in the abdomen for last....................months/years
   - Pain over the swelling/abdomen for.......................................
3. **History of Present Illness**
   - If the swelling started shortly after the operation then start writing history of present illness with history of operation including details of postoperative course
   - If hernia developed after a long duration following operation then the operation history may be described in past history
   - Detailed history about the swelling—mode of onset, progress of the swelling—size at the onset and approximate present dimension. What happens to the swelling on standing, walking, straining and lying down
   - Detail history about pain—onset, duration, site, character, radiation. Relation of pain with the swelling, any aggravating or relieving factor
   - If operative history and appearance of the swelling is not a long gap (less than a year), then details of the operation may be included in the history of present illness, otherwise the history of operation may be written in past history. The operative history includes—type of operation, emergency or elective, nature of operation, postoperative recovery, any history of cough or abdominal distension in the postoperative period any wound infection, any wound gaping or burst abdomen, whether required secondary suture, duration of hospital stay. Time gap between the operation and appearance of swelling

- Any straining factors like chronic cough, constipation or difficulty in micturition
- Details of bowel and bladder habits
- Any other systemic symptoms—ask details about systemic symptoms.
4. **Past History**
   - Detail history about the operation, if not included in history of present illness.
5. **Personal History**
6. **Family History**
7. **Treatment History: Whether using abdominal belt.**
8. **Any History of Allergy.**

■ B. PHYSICAL EXAMINATION

1. General Survey
2. Local Examination: Examination of abdomen
   Detail abdomen examination: inspection, Palpation, Percussion and Auscultation
   - To comment about the hernial swelling site, extent, size, shape, surface, margin the patient should be examined in standing as with lying down the swelling may disappear or may reduce in size
   - For testing reducibility the patient should lie down and the clinician pushes the swelling through the gap in the abdominal wall
   - The gap in the abdominal wall should be assessed.
3. **Systemic Examination.**

■ C. SUMMARY OF THE CASE

■ D. PROVISIONAL DIAGNOSIS

■ E. INVESTIGATIONS SUGGESTED

Q. What is your case?

Ans. A 40-year-old lady presented with gradual onset of a swelling in lower abdomen since last 1 year. She underwent abdominal hysterectomy through a midline incision for uterine-fibroid 1.5 years back. Patient also underwent LUCS 5 years back. Following hysterectomy patient developed wound infection and the wound required dressings for about 2 months for healing.

1 year back the swelling appeared at the site of abdominal wound, starting at the lower end of the wound, gradually increased in size over the last 1 year with occasional episodes of pain, dull-aching in nature, which aggravated when the swelling increases in size and gets relieved on rest when the swelling reduces in size. The swelling appears on standing and walking and gets aggravated on coughing and other strenuous activities and disappears fully on lying down and manipulation by the patient. There is no period of irreducibility. She is not a known diabetic and hypertensive (Fig. 2.31).

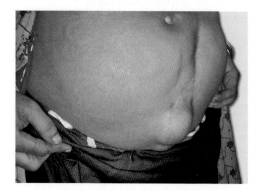

Fig. 2.31: Incisional hernia

On examination patient is obese. There is a wide-scar of lower-midline incision in right abdomen. A swelling appears on coughing in lower-abdomen 8 cm × 7 cm in dimension, reducing completely on lying down. The skin over the swelling is tense, thinned out with evident visible-peristalsis. The gap in the abdomen is about 6 cm vertically and 4 cm horizontally in diameter. No other organomegaly or lump abdomen detected. Chest is clear. Cardiovascular system appears within normal limit.

Q. What is your diagnosis?

Ans. This is a case of incisional hernia through lower midline incision following hysterectomy, content of hernia being intestine and it is reducible.

Q. What operative history is relevant in a case of incisional hernia?

Ans.
◆ Type of operation
◆ Elective or emergency
  – Postoperative complications more with emergency surgery
◆ Incision, suture material used, surgeon's expertise, any intraoperative complication (if information is available from the OT-note)
◆ Postoperative period
  – Wound infection/wound hematoma
  – Gaping of wound/burst-abdomen
  – Duration of postoperative stay
  – Any history of postoperative cough, straining, abdominal distension
◆ History of previous abdominal operations
◆ Patient factors
  – Systemic illness, e.g. hypertension, diabetes mellitus
  – Malnutrition
  – Anemia
  – Smoking
  – Any straining factors—constipation, any history of chronic cough, any urinary problems
  – Prostatism.

Q. How will you assess the gap in the abdominal wall?

Ans. The hernial content is reduced and the gap in the anterior abdominal wall may be felt with the fingers. Patient is asked to lift both the legs with knee extended and with both arms folded over chest. This causes contraction of muscle of abdominal wall and hernial gap may be felt distinctly. In an irreducible hernia the gap cannot be felt properly.

Q. What are the important causes for development of incisional hernias?

Ans. Many factors singly or in combination are responsible for development of incisional hernia.
◆ *Poor surgical technique*
  – Nonanatomic incision:
    - Battle's pararectal incision damaging number of nerves has high incidence of incisional hernia
    - Vertical incision (midline or paramedian) has high chance of developing hernia than the transverse incision

- Method of closure: Layered closure has higher incidence of developing incisional hernia than wound closed in single layer.
- Inappropriate suture material: The wound gains about 85% of normal strength in 6 months. Maximum strength is gained in 1 year. Sutures are responsible for maintaining wound strength for 6 months. Wound closed with nonabsorbable suture material are followed by a far lesser incidence of postoperative hernia than wound closed with absorbable suture.
- Suturing technique: Closing abdominal incision with suturing under tension causes pressure necrosis of intervening tissues and is an important cause for development of incisional hernia.
- Drainage tube: When drain tubes are brought out through the main wound the chance of developing incisional hernia is increased.

◆ *Preoperative straining factors:* Chronic cough, chronic constipation and urinary obstruction.

◆ *Postoperative complications:* Abdominal distension, cough, respiratory distress due to pneumonia or lung collapse, and postoperative wound infection.

◆ *General factors:* Age (elderly patients), malnutrition, hypoproteinemia, jaundice, malignancy, diabetes, chronic renal failure, steroid or immunosuppressive therapy and alcoholism.

◆ *Tissue failure:* Late development of hernia after 5, 10 or more years after operation is usually associated with tissue failure. Abnormal collagen production and maintenance has been shown to be associated with increased incidence of incisional hernia.

Q. When does majority of incisional hernia start?

Ans. Majority of incisional hernia starts in the immediate postoperative period due to partial disruption of deep layers of the wound. As the skin remains intact the event may pass unnoticed in immediate postoperative period.

Q. What are the types of defects in incision line?

Ans. The hernial opening may vary in size. The whole of the incision line may have a long and wide gap. A small area may have gap or there may be multiple gaps ("Swiss cheese" defect) along the incision line.

Q. What is the role of rectus abdominis muscle in midline incisional hernia?

Ans. Due to gap in midline the rectus muscle is stretched and pushed laterally. Contraction of rectus muscle now expels the abdominal contents out into the hernial sac rather than retaining them into the abdominal cavity.

Q. What are the problems with large incisional hernias?

Ans.

◆ In large incisional hernia, large amount of omentum small gut and large gut may remain outside the abdominal cavity into the hernial sac. If this continues for a long time the intra-abdominal capacity is reduced. During operation, if such contents are reduced into abdominal cavity forcibly under tension, it may cause compression of inferior vena cava and may also cause splinting of diaphragm leading to respiratory distress (abdominal compartment syndrome).

◆ Large incisional hernia may cause reduction of intra-abdominal pressure and may cause edema of the mesentery and stasis in IVC and splanchnic vascular bed. It may be difficult to raise the intra-abdominal pressure leading to problems of micturition and defecation.

◆ Lordosis may occur and back pain is a common complain.
◆ The skin and subcutaneous tissue overlying a large incisional hernia are stretched and damaged. Skin becomes atrophic devoid of subcutaneous fat and spontaneous ulceration may develop in the skin.

Q. Does all incisional hernia need operation?

Ans.
◆ If the neck of the incisional hernia is wide, shows no signs of increase in size and patient has no symptom, it may be observed
◆ Symptomatic hernia, which is showing sign of increase needs repair
◆ Large hernia with a small opening has high incidence of strangulation and need to be repaired early. Attacks of subacute intestinal obstruction, irreducibility and strangulation are definite indications for repair of incisional hernias.

Q. How will you manage this patient?

Ans.
◆ The patient has incisional hernia through lower midline incision. Patient does not have any medical disease and there are no straining factors, I will prepare this patient for surgery
◆ Associated cardiovascular disease, if any or hypertension needs to be treated
◆ Associated respiratory disease, if any, needs treatment
◆ If diabetic, needs good control before surgery
◆ If obese, weight reduction before surgery is helpful
◆ Intertrigo or any infected skin lesion overlying the hernia needs attention
◆ Investigation for any intra-abdominal pathology: USG/upper gastrointestinal (GI) endoscopy.

Q. What operation is preferable for this patient?

Ans. In this patient the hernial gap is about 6 cm × 4 cm, so I will consider mesh repair in this patient.

Q. Why do you like to do mesh repair?

Ans. In case of incisional hernia with a small gap (<2 cm) the tissue can be apposed without tension. In those cases anatomical repair may be done. In this patient the gap is 6 cm × 4 cm so an anatomical repair may cause tension in the suture line. So a mesh repair is preferable in this patient.

Q. In case of midline incisional hernia, what do you mean by anatomical repair?

Ans.
◆ Anatomical repair involves apposition of the different layers of the abdomen to repair the defect.
◆ Either transverse or vertical elliptical incision. The skin flaps are raised.
◆ The hernial sac is dissected up to the lateral edge of the gap and redundant sac excised.
◆ The linea alba is apposed in the midline by continuous or interrupted polypropylene suture taking heavy bite.
◆ Skin apposed by interrupted suture using monofilament polyamide sutures.

Q. What do you mean by anatomical repair in case of hernias through paramedian incision?

Ans.

* The hernial sac is dissected and the redundant sac is excised up to the lateral edge of the gap.
* The medial edge of the defect will be the intact linea alba and remains of the rectus sheath along it. The lateral edge will be composed of anterior and posterior rectus sheath and rectus muscle in between, with all three layers fused by scar tissue.
* The medial leaf is dissected separating the peritoneum with the posterior rectus sheath and the anterior rectus sheath. The lateral edge is incised and the anterior and posterior rectus sheath is dissected free.
* The peritoneum with the posterior rectus sheath is approximated by continuous polypropylene suture.
* The anterior rectus sheath is apposed by continuous or interrupted polypropylene suture.
* Alternatively: Mass approximation of the medial and lateral edge by continuous or interrupted polypropylene suture taking good bite of tissue from the edge.

Q. What is Shoelace darn technique for repair of incisional hernia?

Ans.

This technique of repair restores the normal anatomy and function of abdominal wall. A new strong linea alba is reconstructed and the new midline anchor allows the rectus muscle to straighten and return to lie alongside the midline and also reconstruct the anterior rectus sheath and fix them to the new linea alba (Figs 2.32A to D).

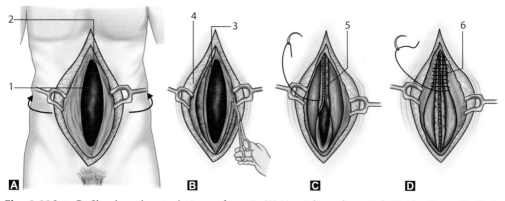

Figs 2.32A to D: Shoelace darn technique of repair: (A) Hernial sac dissected; (B) The linea alba incised 1 cm from the margin; (C) The medial cut edge sutured by a running polypropylene suture; (D) A neo linea alba created by running suture apposing the lateral cut edge and taking bites from the apposed medial cut edge [(1) Margin of linea alba; (2) Hernial sac; (3) Medial cut margin of linea alba; (4) Lateral cut margin of linea alba; (5) Medial cut margin suture; (6) Lateral cut margin suture]

There are two steps of this operation:

* The first step is to reconstitute a strong new midline by suturing a strip of fascia from the medial edge of each anterior rectus sheath. The second step is to restore the recti muscle to their normal position by drawing together the lateral cut edges of the anterior rectus sheath.

- Either a vertical or transverse abdominal skin incision is made, and the redundant skin and subcutaneous fat is excised.
- The skin flaps are dissected off the sac of the hernia and from anterior rectus sheath on either side. The anterior rectus sheath is sufficiently exposed to allow for splitting of the anterior rectus sheath. The sac is not opened and inverted into the abdominal cavity. The sac is opened only when the operation is done for obstruction or strangulation. The anterior rectus sheath around the hernial opening is defined. An incision is made over the anterior rectus sheath 1–1.5 cm from the medial edge of the rectus sheath on either side. The incision is extended up and down 2 cm beyond the gap on either side.
- The medial edge of the rectus sheath is sutured from above downward by a continuous suture of polypropylene. This creates a new linea alba and return the unopened sac into the peritoneal cavity.
- The lateral edge of the anterior rectus sheath is situated at a gap from the newly constructed linea alba. This gap is closed by a second suture running between the lateral edges of the rectus sheath and while passing the midline it takes a bite through the newly constructed linea alba. The sutures should be applied 5 mm apart and each suture passes through the new midline. The second layer of suture begins at the top end of the incision in the rectus sheath. In cases with large gap the to and fro shoelace suture across the fascial defect helps in functionally substituting for the missing anterior rectus sheath.

Q. How will you prepare an obese patient with incisional hernia for surgery?

- Obesity is associated with higher rate of recurrence following repair.
- Obese patient should lose weight.

Q. What is the role of mesh repair in incisional hernia?

Ans. The mesh repair is an excellent method for repair of incisional hernia. It may be used for all types of incisional hernias, for large incisional hernias with a wide gap, or when the aponeurotic gap cannot be properly apposed or tissue is thinned out.

Q. What is an ideal mesh?

Ans. Ideal mesh should be:

- Easy to handle
- Can be cut to a desired shape
- Flexible
- Rapidly incorporated in tissues
- Inert and should excite minimal tissue reaction
- Should not be rejected in presence of infection
- Noncarcinogenic
- Cheap.

Q. What are the different types of mesh used for hernial repair?

Ans.

- Polypropylene mesh
- Vypro mesh (Polypropylene + Polyglycolic acid)
- Dacron mesh
- Polytetrafluoroethylene (PTFE) mesh
- Polyglycolic acid mesh (Vicryl mesh).

Q. What are the different ways of mesh placement for repair of incisional hernia?

Ans.

- *Inlay graft:* A sheet of mesh of the size of the defect is sutured to the margin of the defect, the mesh bridging the hernial gap.
- *Onlay mesh:* The hernial gap is apposed and a mesh is placed to reinforce the repaired defect. The onlay mesh may be placed as:
  - Underlay: The mesh is placed in the preperitoneal space after closure of the peritoneum and the anterior sheath sutured in front of the mesh. The mesh is placed deep to the rectus muscle.
  - Overlay: The mesh may be placed as an onlay on the anterior surface of the rectus sheath deep to the subcutaneous tissue after apposing the gap in the rectus sheath.

Q. What is Rive Stoppa's technique of mesh repair of incisional hernia?

Ans. The important steps in this technique of repair are:

- The operation is done under general anesthesia
- Old scar excised: Hernial sac dissected up to the margin of the myoaponeurotic edges of the hernial opening
- The sac is opened and its contents inspected. All bowel loops and omentum freed and returned to the abdomen
- The redundant sac is excised
- The margin of the sac along with the peritoneum is closed with a running vicryl suture
- A preperitoneal space is created between the rectus muscle anteriorly and the hernial sac blended with the posterior rectus sheath posteriorly
- A large mesh is placed in the preperitoneal space created extending 4–5 cm beyond the hernial defect above, below and laterally up to the lateral edge of the rectus sheath
- The prolene mesh is then fixed by polypropylene suture passing through full thickness of abdominal wall and a stab wound is made in the skin and sutures are brought out and tied. The mesh is thus fixed all around
- The medial edge of the cut rectus sheath is sutured together by polypropylene suture
- Excess skin is excised and skin closed by interrupted skin sutures keeping a suction drain in preperitoneal space.

Q. Can the mesh be placed in the preperitoneal space without fixation?

Ans. Yes. The mesh when placed in the preperitoneal space may be held in place by normal intra-abdominal pressure and suture fixation may not be necessary.

Q. What is Mayo's repair?

Ans. Mayo's repair involves tackling of hernial sac in the usual way. The repair is done by double breasting of rectus sheath whereby one flap of rectus sheath overlaps the other.

Q. What is the drawback of Mayo's repair?

Ans. Mayo's repair with double breasting usually causes tension on the suture line and there is 50% chance of recurrence following Mayo's repair.

Q. What are problems with intraperitoneal inlay mesh placement?

Ans. When mesh is placed intraperitoneally, there is chance of adhesion and fistula formation.

Q. How will you manage postoperatively?

Ans.
- Nasogastric (NG) aspiration to prevent gastric distension
- IV fluid till patient passes flatus
- Urinary catheterization if there is difficulty in passing urine
- Prophylactic antibiotics
- Early ambulation is advisable.

Q. What is the incidence of recurrence following repair of incisional hernia?

Ans. Most series incidence of recurrence following incisional hernia repair is 30–40%. With mesh repair incidence of recurrence is less—about 10%.

Q. What is the role of laparoscopic repair of incisional hernia?

Ans. Repair of incisional hernia has been tried laparoscopically. However, this is suitable only for small reducible incisional hernias. The mesh is placed either in the preperitoneal space or placed in the gap of hernia inside peritoneum. Intraperitoneal mesh placement (IPOM) is associated with increased incidence of adhesion particularly if a polypropylene mesh is used. Placement of polytetrafluoroethylene (PTFE) mesh cause least chance of adhesion.

Q. What do you mean by complex ventral hernia?

Ans. A ventral hernia that:
- Involves a compromised surgical field in which GI, biliary or genitourinary procedures are performed or frank infection is present
- Includes enterocutaneous or enteroatmospheric fistulas
- Includes an infected prosthetic mesh
- Hernial defect is large (>10 cm in any dimension) ± loss of domain
- Has recurred.

Q. What is component separation technique for repair of giant incisional hernia?

Ans. The component separation technique (CST), first described by Ramirez et al., provides tensionless closure of large, full thickness anterior abdominal wall defects with autologous tissue. This technique was described without the use of prosthetic material and there were high recurrence rates ranging from 0% to 30%. Subsequent modifications of the CST have incorporated the use of prosthetic materials, with consequent reductions in hernia recurrence rates.

Bilateral components separation is a preferred technique, as synthetic mesh may be placed as underlay or bridging fascial defects.

Two of the three abdominal oblique muscles must be intact or a flank hernia will result.

Q. What are the anatomical disposition of abdominal wall?

Ans. A clear understanding of the anatomy of the abdominal wall is essential when performing ventral herniorrhaphy with component separation. Such knowledge results in the best clinical outcomes by providing a well-vascularized, innervated, and correctly oriented abdominal wall reconstruction.
- The vertically oriented rectus abdominis muscles originate at the pubic symphysis and insert on the costal cartilage of 5th to 7th ribs. These muscles lie on either side of the intact, midline linea alba.

- On each side of the rectus, three flat semihorizontally oriented muscles are found layered on one another: From superficial to deep these are—the external oblique muscle, the internal oblique muscle, and the transversus abdominis muscle.
- Disruption of the linea alba permits unopposed lateral pull on the recti by the lateral musculature and contributes to increase in size of incisional midline hernias.
- External oblique muscle and the aponeurosis. At the lateral border of the rectus the aponeurosis of the external oblique alongwith the anterior lamella of internal oblique aponeurois forms the anterior rectus sheath which forms the linea alba by joining the sheath from the opposite side.
- Internal oblique muscle and the aponeurosis: The aponeurosis of the internal oblique splits at the lateral border of the rectus abdominis muscle. The posterior lamella of the aponeurosis alongwith the transversus abdominis forms the posterior rectus sheath.
- Below the arcuate line the internal oblique aponeuroris does not split and alongwith transversus aponeurosis and external oblique aponeurosis forms the anterior rectus sheath.
- Linea semilunaris: At the lateral border of the rectus abdominis the aponeurosis of external oblique and internal oblique blends to form the linea semilunaris. The transverses abdominis muscle and the aponeurosis is not densely adherent at the linea semilunaris.
- The transversus abdominis muscle and the aponeurosis: The innermost flat muscle of the abdominal wall. The aponeurosis joins the posterior lamella of the internal oblique and forms the posterior rectus sheath. Below the arcuate line the posterior rectus sheath is deficient.
- For retrorectus repair, it is important to note that the transversus abdominis does not contribute to the linea semilunaris. Its muscle belly extends medial to the linea semilunaris, behind the rectus muscle, in the upper one-third of the abdomen.
- Each rectus muscle receives blood supply from the inferior and superior epigastric arteries as well as intercostal arterial branches that enter the muscle belly laterally.
- The intercostal branches are also the main blood supply to the lateral musculature. The intercostal vessels and the nerves and the thoracoabdominal nerves and vessels (T7–T12) runs in the "neurovascular plane" located between the internal oblique and transversus abdominis muscles.
- In addition to supplying the lateral abdominal musculature and skin, these branches innervate the rectus muscle posteriorly and slightly medial to the linea semilunaris.
- Both anterior and posterior component separations are able to preserve these intercostal neurovascular bundles due to their location deep to the internal oblique.
- For anterior component separation, where lipocutaneous flaps are created, knowledge of the skin vascularity is also critical.
- For a classic component separation (external oblique release), transection of the deep epigastric perforating vessels leaves the central abdominal wall without its major blood supply. PUPS component separation preserves these vessels to reduce the risk of ischemia-related wound complications.

Q. What is posterior component separation technique for repair of ventral hernia?

Ans.

Posterior Component Separation Technique

- The patient is positioned in a supine position with arms abducted. A Foley catheter and an nasogastric (NG) tube are placed.

- A full midline elliptical skin incision is made, removing the old scar, thin skin over the hernia, or ulcerated wounds. The incision is stopped at the level of the pubis and above up to the xiphoid process. Safe access to the abdominal cavity is critical to avoid bowel injury and is best achieved by traversing fascia in an area remote from the hernia (above or below the old incision).
- Adhesiolysis and foreign body excision and visceral adhesions to the anterior abdominal wall and pelvis are fully lysed. This is critical to allow full medial mobility of the posterior abdominal wall components.
- Care must be taken to avoid excess injury to the posterior layers of the abdominal wall (peritoneum and transversalis fascia) during this portion of the procedure.
- Interloop adhesions are typically ignored unless the patient has a history of adhesive related small bowel obstruction.
- Any foreign bodies (tacks, suture material, old mesh) are fully removed.
- A sterile towel is packed over the viscera to protect them during the component separation.
- Retrorectus dissection using electrocautery: An incision is made in the posterior rectus sheath within 0.5 cm of its medial boarder. This incision is extended superiorly and inferiorly, spanning the entire length of the rectus muscle. Working medial to lateral, the plane is continued using blunt and electrocautery dissection. Care must be taken to avoid injury to the epigastric vessels, which should remain with the muscle, not the posterior sheath, during the dissection. The lateral limit of this dissection is the linea semilunaris at the lateral boarder of the rectus muscle, where the anterior and posterior rectus sheaths fuse. Identification and preservation of the intercostal neurovascular structures as they enter the posterior aspect of the rectus muscle is crucial. Superiorly, this plane is extended into the retroxiphoid/retrosternal space. Inferiorly, the plane extends into the space of Retzius. Blunt dissection in this avascular plane permits exposure to the midline symphysis pubis and Cooper's ligaments bilaterally. Care must be exercised here to avoid injury to the inferior epigastric vessels at their origin on the iliac vessels.
- Transversus abdominis release (TAR): In patients with large gap dissection in the retrorectus space just up to the linea semilunaris is insufficient to permit adequate abdominal wall reconstruction because of the insufficient retrorectus space to permit adequate prosthetic reinforcement of the hernia. Methods to extend the retrorectus dissection lateral to the linea semilunaris is by dividing the transversus abdominis muscle.
- Approximately 0.5 cm medial to the linea semilunaris, electrocautery is used to incise the posterior sheath, exposing the transversus muscle. This is most easily accomplished in the upper half of the abdomen, where the muscle belly is well defined. Using a right-angled clamp to assist dissection, electrocautery is used to hemostatically transect the transversus abdominis muscle. Care must be taken to avoid injury to the transversalis fascia/peritoneal layer that lies deep to this.
- Once divided, the muscle can be retracted anteriorly and the avascular retromuscular plane developed bluntly. Superiorly, this plane extends beyond the costal margin to the diaphragm, inferiorly to the myopectineal orifice, and laterally to the psoas muscle.
- The TAR is then completed on the contralateral side.
- Reconstruction of posterior layer: The posterior rectus sheath is reapproximated in the midline using running 2-0 polyglycolic acid (vicryl) suture. Any holes created in the posterior

layer during dissection must be closed; this prevents bowel from contacting the unprotected mesh and prevents bowel from slipping in between the posterior layer and the mesh, which can result in a bowel obstruction from internal herniation.

- Fenestrations in the posterior layer are common in areas where the abdominal wall has been traversed (laparoscopic port sites, drain sites, old incisions) and below the arcuate line (where there is no transversus abdominis muscle within the posterior layer). Small holes that cannot be repaired primarily with suture can be closed with native tissue (omentum, colon epiploicae, hernia sac). Larger holes are best closed by patching the defect with absorbable mesh (vicryl) secured with a running absorbable suture. The newly created visceral sac and abdominal wall are irrigated with 3 L of antibiotic lavage solution.
- Mesh placement: For patients with clean wounds a large (30.5 × 30.5-cm) lightweight, macroporous, polypropylene mesh is used in the space created. There is emerging evidence that use of this mesh is also acceptable in patients with multiple comorbidities (diabetes, obesity, prior mesh infection) or in clean-contaminated circumstances (fistula takedown, enterotomy closure, small bowel resection, stoma formation or relocation). The mesh is turned into a diamond configuration and is anchored inferiorly using a single transfascial stitch just above the pubic ramus or bilateral sutures placed into Cooper's ligaments. The mesh is fixed by using 0 monofilament absorbable suture (polyglyconate or polydioxanone) to secure the mesh. For inferior midline defects, the mesh can be positioned deep in the space of Retzius and the anchoring stitch(es) backed off the edge to permit adequate overlap (at least 4 cm). For concurrent inguinal or femoral hernias, the mesh can be positioned to cover the myopectineal orifice. For superior midline defects, the mesh is positioned well beyond the costal margin (at least 4 cm to allow adequate overlap of the defect) and is anchored with transfascial sutures placed around the xiphoid process.
- Fixation of mesh: The mesh is fixed on either side by using full-thickness transfascial sutures in 3 cardinal points. A Reverdin needle facilitate transfascial suture placement.
- Kocher clamps are placed on the medial edge of the rectus muscle on the ipsilateral side and the abdominal wall is pulled toward the midline as the transfascial sutures are placed. This not only permits primary fascial closure over the mesh, but also reduces the tension on the midline closure. The mesh will not buckle or wrinkle when the linea alba is recreated, reducing the space for seroma to accumulate.
- Reconstruction of the anterior layers: With the mesh circumferentially secured, the linea alba is recreated by suturing the anterior rectus sheaths to each other in the midline using multiple figure of eight stitches using 0 monofilament absorbable suture.
- Placement of drain: Closed suction drains are positioned anterior to the mesh and in the dependent (inferior and lateral) portions of the repair. Because of the substantial rectus medialization afforded by TAR and by physiologically tensioning the mesh, it is uncommon to not complete the anterior fascial closure over the mesh.
- The subcutaneous tissues can be closed in layers with absorbable suture. Subcutaneous drains are placed only in circumstances in which there is a large dead space not effectively closed with sutures
- The skin is stapled.

Q. What is anterior component separation for repair of giant ventral hernia?

Ans.

Surgical Technique: Anterior Component Separation

* Incision, adhesiolysis, and foreign body (mesh) excision proceed identical to posterior component separation as described earlier.
* *Formation of subcutaneous flaps:* Once the fascia medial to the rectus has been identified, lipocutaneous flaps are created by dissecting the subcutaneous tissues off the anterior rectus sheath. These flaps extend superiorly to the costal margin, inferiorly to inguinal ligament, and laterally to just beyond the linea semilunaris (lateral border of rectus muscles).
* *External oblique release:* With electrocautery, the external oblique aponeurosis and muscle fibers are divided 1–2 cm lateral to the linea semilunaris from just above the costal margin to just above the inguinal ligament.
* An assessment is then made as to whether the linea alba can be recreated at the midline without undue tension. If no tension is found, mesh placement and fascial closure can begin. If the midline fascia will not reapproximate, retrorectus dissection (as described for posterior component separation) can be performed to permit greater medialization of the rectus muscle.
* *Mesh placement:* Mesh can be placed as an underlay (within the peritoneal cavity), sublay (within the retrorectus space), or as an onlay (over anterior rectus sheath), depending on the types of release performed.
* Underlay mesh is secured via transabdominal sutures passed through the lateral cut edge of the external oblique fascia. If synthetic mesh is used here, it must have an antiadhesive barrier.
* Sublay mesh is placed within the retrorectus space after the posterior layer has been closed. Transabdominal sutures are passed through the medial cut edge of the external oblique at the level of the linea semilunaris.
* Onlay mesh is placed over the closed midline repair, and is secured to the lateral cut edges of the external oblique bilaterally.
* *Placement of drains:* Drains are generally placed above the Multiple closed suction drains (2–4) are placed to evacuate fluid from the dead space.
* *Closure of subcutaneous tissue and skin:* The subcutaneous tissues can be closed in layers with absorbable suture. The skin is stapled.

Q. What are the procedures of the postoperative care?

Ans.

Postoperative Care

* *Airway management:* In cases with prolonged operative times, patients with underlying pulmonary disease, patient may be kept intubated overnight. If the plateau airway pressure increases more than 6 cm H_2O following approximation of the linea alba, the patient is also kept intubated for 24 hours.
* *Pain management:* Epidural catheters are recommended in all patients and are maintained for 3–4 days postoperatively. For patients in whom an epidural cannot be placed (or is contraindicated) or who have delayed bowel function at the time of epidural removal, an IV patient-controlled analgesia device is used. Patients are transitioned to oral narcotic analgesia when they tolerate a diet.

- Diet retching and emesis can jeopardize the repair. Patients are kept nil per mouth until flatus is passed, at which time clear liquids are begun. When bowel function has returned, patients are advanced to an appropriate diet.
- Nasogastric tube decompression is used only in patients with extensive adhesiolysis or in whom small bowel resection has been performed.
- *Drains (anterior component separation):* Subfascial drains are typically removed before hospital discharge (within 7 days). Subcutaneous drains are left until output is less than 30 mL per day for two consecutive days. This can result in drains that are in place for several weeks postoperatively.
- *Drains (posterior component separation):* When synthetic mesh is used, drains are removed when then the output is less than 30 mL per day or on the day of discharge (whichever is first). This typically occurs on day 4–7. When biologic mesh is used, drains are kept in place for 2 weeks irrespective of the output volume.
- *Abdominal binder:* An abdominal binder is usually used in the immediate postoperative period. Following discharge, the patient may wear the binder as desired. If there is concern for the viability of lipocutaneous skin flaps, most will not place a binder.
- *Prophylaxis against deep vein thrombosis:* Mechanical and pharmacologic venous thromboembolism prophylaxis is instituted in all patients beginning in the operating room.
- *Prophylactic antibiotics:* Given within 1 hour of skin incision and are discontinued within 24 hours. For patients with active mesh or soft tissue infections, antibiotics are given until resolution of the infection.

Q. What are the postoperative complications?

Ans.

- *Wound complications:* Surgical site infections (SSIs) are a major source of morbidity following open ventral hernia repair. In the highest-risk populations, the SSI rate has been reported to be as high as 27–41%. Wound complications are more common and more severe in anterior component separation than posterior component separation techniques.
- Infected collections (including seromas and hematomas) are drained percutaneously or operatively. Asymptomatic fluid collections are generally followed conservatively.
- *Skin flap necrosis:* Necrosis of skin or subcutaneous tissues is addressed with early operative debridement.
- *Pulmonary complications:* Diaphragm function and pulmonary toilet are both negatively affected by abdominal wall reconstruction, leaving patients vulnerable to pulmonary complications. As many as 20% of patients will experience a postoperative respiratory complication following component separation hernia repair. Aggressive pulmonary toilet, including incentive spirometer use, chest physiotherapy, adequate analgesia, and upright posture, are all critical to minimizing these complications.
- *Gastrointestinal complications:* Paralytic ileus is common following ventral hernia repair, although the exact rate is not reported. Prolonged ileus, or symptoms suggestive of an early small bowel obstruction, should prompt further investigation. A CT scan of the abdomen and pelvis will demonstrate an internal hernia (bowel is seen protruding through a rent in the posterior layer). Prompt surgical re-exploration in this case is mandatory.
- Intra-abdominal hypertension: Except in the smallest ventral hernia repairs, some degree of intra-abdominal hypertension (IAH) is likely created in the course of reapproximating the linea alba.

Abdomen

OUTLINE FOR WRITING AN ABDOMINAL CASE

▮ HISTORY

1. **Particulars of the Patient**
2. **Chief Complaints (with duration)**
   - The usual chief complaints are:
     - Pain abdomen
     - Vomiting
     - Sensation of fullness after meals
     - Vomiting of blood
     - Passage of black tarry stool
     - Yellowish discoloration of eyes and urine
     - Loss of appetite
     - Weight loss
     - Alteration of bowel habit
     - Fever
     - Swelling in abdomen.
3. **History of Present Illness**
   - Detailed history about pain:
     - Onset: Sudden/insidious
     - Duration: Short-lived/persistent
     - Initial site of pain
     - Radiation/shifting/referral
     - Character of pain: Dull-aching (chronic cholecystitis)/stabbing (pancreatitis)/colicky (renal colic)
     - Periodicity of pain: Appearance after a definite period of days/months
     - Relation with food intake: Before/after, i.e. on empty stomach or full stomach
     - Relation with vomiting: Relief/aggravation
     - Aggravating and relieving factors: Food/vomiting/medicines
     - Relation with defecation and micturition

- Details of vomiting:
  - Duration
  - Frequency: The exact number
  - Relationship with food intake
  - Character of the act: Projectile or effortless
  - Character of the vomitus
  - Amount
  - Color
  - Taste
  - Smell
  - Contains any food taken more than 12 hours earlier
  - Any blood in vomiting: Suggestive of upper gastrointestinal bleeding
  - Any relation with pain.
- Details of blood vomiting (Hematemesis):
  - Duration
  - Number of bouts of blood vomiting
  - Color
  - Amount
  - Whether associated with black tarry stool or not.
- Details of jaundice:
  - Duration
  - Onset
  - Any prodromal symptom before onset of jaundice: Fever/arthralgia/generalized weakness/loss of appetite/skin rash suggestive of viral-hepatitis
  - Any history of biliary colic preceding the onset of jaundice
  - Progress of jaundice
    » Progressively increasing
    » Diminishing after an initial deepening
    » Waxing and waning
    » Static
  - Associated symptoms with jaundice:
    » Pruritis: Obstructive jaundice
    » Clay colored stool (obstructive jaundice)
  - History of fever with chill and rigor—cholangitis
  - History of biliary colic
  - History of black tarry stool with waxing and waning of jaundice
- Bowel habit
  - What was the usual bowel habit before the illness started?
  - What is the present bowel habit?
  - What is the change in bowel habit?
  - Any history of bleeding P/R or black tarry stool, passage of mucus in stool
  - Any history of sensation of incomplete defecation
  - Any history of tenesmus
- Details of loss of weight and appetite: To mention exact figure of weight loss in kilogram and the duration.

- Details of swelling in the abdomen
  - Duration
  - Site where first noticed
  - Size of the swelling when first noticed
  - Progress of the swelling
- Details of urinary symptoms: Loin pain/mass in loin/frequency of micturition (diurnal and nocturnal)/difficulty in passing urine/any burning during micturition/any urgency or hesitancy/any history of passage of blood or pus in urine.

4. **Past History**
5. **Personal History**
6. **Family History**
7. **Treatment History**
8. **Any History of Allergy**

∎ PHYSICAL EXAMINATION

1. **General Survey**
2. **Local Examination of Abdomen**
   - *Inspection*
     (Patient supine with arms kept on sides and exposed from mid-chest to mid-thigh)
     - Shape and contour of abdomen
       - » Normal/scaphoid/distended
     - Umbilicus
       - » Position (normal position lies midway between the xiphisternum and the symphysis pubis)
       - » Normally inverted/deeply inverted/flushed/everted.
     - Skin over the abdomen
       - » Scar (If operative scar describe as upper midline/lower midline/upper paramedian/right or left subcostal incision scar) (Fig. 3.1)
       - » Pigmentation
       - » Striae (white striae found in multiparous women is to be described as striae albicans)
       - » Engorged vein (if engorged veins are present ascertain the direction of blood flow in the engorged veins)

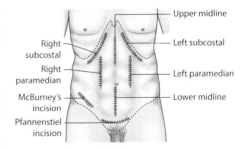

Fig. 3.1: Scars of different incision

     - Movements
       - » Respiratory movements whether all region are moving normally with respiration
       - » Visible peristalsis
       - » Pulsatile movements
     - Visible swelling
       - » Site and extent
       - » Size

» Shape
» Surface
» Margin
» Moving with respiration or not
» Rising test—whether swelling is parietal or intra-abdominal
- Hernial sites
  » Any swelling
  » Any expansile impulse on cough
- External genitalia.
– *Palpation*
  - Superficial palpation:
    » Temperature: Examine all the regions of the abdomen (compare temperature of abdomen with temperature of chest with the dorsum of finger)
    » Any superficial tenderness.
    » Feel of the abdomen:
      ▷ Soft and elastic feel is normal
      ▷ Muscle guard
      ▷ Rigidity
    » Lump palpable: details of the lump are to be described under deep palpation
  - Deep palpation:
  - Deep tender spots: Any tenderness over the following sites (Fig. 3.2):
    1. Gastric point: A point in the midepigastrium
    2. Duodenal point: A point in the transpyloric plane 2.5 cm to the right of midline
    3. Gallbladder point: A point at the junction of lateral border of right rectus abdominis and the tip of right 9th costal cartilage
    4. McBurney's point: A point in the right spinoumbilical line at the junction of medial two-thirds and lateral one-third
    5. Amebic point: Point on left spinoumbilical line corresponding to McBurney's point on right side
    6. Renal point: A point at the junction of lateral border of erector spinae and the 12th rib (*See* Figs 4.2A and B, Page No. 212).

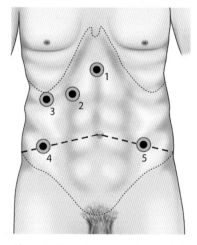

Fig. 3.2: Deep tender spots (For 1, 2, 3, 4, 5 see text)

  - Murphy's sign
    » Found positive in patient with acute cholecystitis
    » Usually not demonstrable in chronic cholecystitis
  - Palpation of organs:
    » Liver
    » Spleen
    » Kidneys
    » Gallbladder is not normally palpable

- If gallbladder is distended or there is a mass in relation to gallbladder, the gallbladder may be palpable—the detail of gallbladder examination is to be recorded
- Stomach is normally not palpable. In cases with gastric outlet obstruction, the distended stomach may be palpable in epigastrium, which disappears with passage of peristaltic waves from left to right
- Normal pancreas is also not palpable
- Palpation of any other lump:
  » Position and extent in relation to abdominal regions
  » Shape
  » Size
  » Surface
  » Margin
  » Consistency
  » Mobility: with respiration
  » Mobility from side to side, up and down
  » Fixity to skin or underlying structure
  » Rising test to confirm intra-abdominal or parietal swelling
  » Knee elbow position and examine the swelling again to decide whether swelling is intraperitoneal or retroperitoneal
- However, this position is very inconvenient for the patient, now this test is usually avoided.
- Hernial sites
- External genitalia.
– *Percussion*
  - Normal percussion note over the abdomen
  - Shifting dullness
  - Fluid thrill
  - Succusion splash over stomach
  - Upper border of liver dullness
  - Upper border of splenic dullness
  - Percussion over any abdominal lump palpable.
– *Auscultation*
  - Peristaltic sound
  - Bruit
  - Venous hum
  - Any added sound.
– *Ausculto-percussion*
  - In case of gastric outlet obstruction to delineate the greater curvature of the stomach.
– Per rectal examination
– Per vaginal examination.
3. **Systemic Examination**
   Describe all system.

■ SUMMARY OF THE CASE

■ PROVISIONAL DIAGNOSIS

■ INVESTIGATIONS SUGGESTED

■ DIFFERENTIAL DIAGNOSIS

Q. How far you should expose for an abdominal examination?

Ans. Patient lying supine in bed with exposure from the mid-thigh to just above the xiphisternal junction.

Q. How do you divide the abdomen into different quadrants?

Ans. For clinical examination abdomen may be divided into four quadrants by drawing a vertical line in the midline and a horizontal line at right angle to the vertical line crossing at the umbilicus (Fig. 3.3).

- Right upper quadrant
- Right lower quadrant
- Left upper quadrant
- Left lower quadrant.

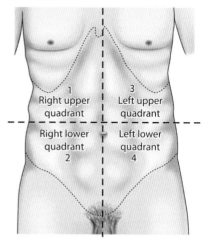

Fig. 3.3: Quadrants of abdomen

Q. How do you divide abdomen into different regions?

Ans. For clinical examination abdomen may be divided into nine regions. Two horizontal planes and two vertical planes divide the abdomen into nine regions.

The upper horizontal plane is the transpyloric plane (TPP), which is drawn midway between the suprasternal notch and the symphysis pubis. This also corresponds to a plane drawn one hands breadth (of patient) below the xiphisternal junction and passes through the tip of ninth costal cartilages on either side.

The lower horizontal plane is the transtubercular plane (TTP), which is drawn by joining the tubercle of the iliac crest on either side. The tubercle of the iliac crest is found out by palpating backward from the anterior superior iliac spine where the tubercle is palpated in the iliac crest and usually lies 5 cm behind the anterior superior iliac spine.

The vertical planes are drawn on either side by joining the midclavicular point and the midinguinal point (Fig. 3.4).

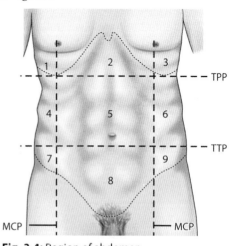

Fig. 3.4: Region of abdomen

Abbreviations: TPP: transpyloric plane; TTP: transtubercular plane; MCP: midclavicular plane

The nine regions are:

1. Right hypochondrium
2. Epigastrium
3. Left hypochondrium
4. Right lumbar
5. Umbilical
6. Left lumbar
7. Right iliac fossa
8. Hypogastrium
9. Left iliac fossa.

Q. How will you ascertain position of the umbilicus?

Ans. The normal umbilicus is situated in the midline midway between the xiphisternal junction and the symphysis pubis.

Q. How will you look for peristaltic movements in the abdomen?

Ans. Gross peristaltic waves may be seen on simple inspection.

Sit by the side of the patient and look tangentially. Ask the patient to take a deep breath and hold the breath at the end of expiration so long he can. Observe for any visible peristaltic wave. If peristaltic waves are seen describe the character of the peristaltic wave (Fig. 3.5).

Gastric peristaltic waves are large peristaltic waves seen in the epigastrium, umbilical or as low as hypogastrium moving from left to right (Figs 3.6A and B).

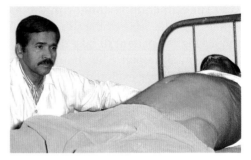

Fig. 3.5: Sit by the side of the patient and look tangentially. Ask the patient to take a deep breath and hold the breath at the end of expiration so long he can. This should be observed for about 30 secondss to 1 minute

Small intestinal peristaltic waves are seen in central abdomen showing in step ladder pattern.

Peristaltic waves in transverse colon may be seen in the right hypochondrium, epigastrium, umbilical and left hypochondriac region moving from right to left.

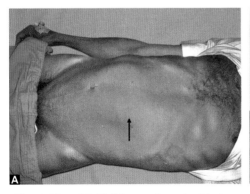
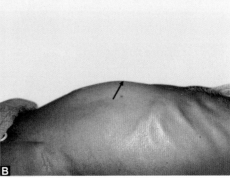

Figs 3.6A and B: Visible gastric peristalsis: Large peristaltic waves seen moving from left to right

Q. How will you look for pulsation in abdomen?

Ans. Patient lies supine. The examiner looks tangentially from the side to look for any pulsation in the abdomen (Fig. 3.5). The patient is asked to hold the breath at the end of expiration to obscure the respiratory movement so that pulsation, if present, is seen well.

Q. How will you ascertain whether the pulsation is transmitted or expansile?

Ans. This is done by palpation. The index and the middle fingers of both hands are placed close to each other on the epigastrium on either side of the midline.

In case of transmitted pulsation all the fingers are simply lifted up.

In case of expansile pulsation the fingers of two hands are lifted up and are also separated (*See* Figs 1.35A to C, Page No. 33).

Q. How will you palpate the abdomen?

Ans. The palpation is done with the patient supine, with the arms by the side of the patient and asking the patient to take deep breathing with the mouth open. The abdominal muscle gets relaxed during expiration and in the pause between inspiration and expiration. The forearm of the clinician should be kept horizontally at the same level of the abdomen. Palpate with a warm hand particularly during winter. If hands are cooler rub two hands together to make the hand warm before palpating the abdomen (Fig. 3.7).

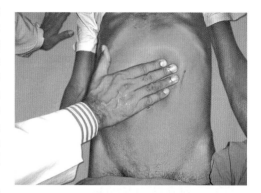

Fig. 3.7: Palpation of abdomen

The palpation is best done with the flexor surfaces of the fingers and not with the tip of the fingers.

Q. How will you ascertain temperature in abdomen?

Ans. This is done by palpating with the back of the fingers in all the quadrants of the abdomen. The temperature of the abdomen is compared with the temperature of the chest or the other covered parts of the body (Figs 3.8A to C).

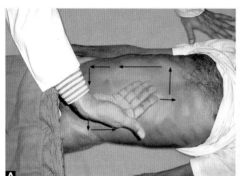 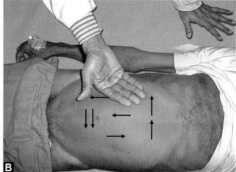

Figs 3.8A and B: Ascertaining the temperature of the abdomen with dorsal aspect of the fingers

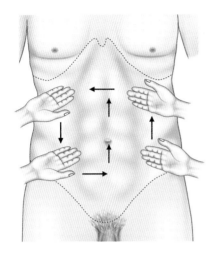

Fig. 3.8C: Ascertaining the temperature of the abdomen

Q. When you find engorged veins in the abdominal wall, how will you ascertain the flow?

Ans. In normal person, the flow in the veins in abdominal wall is away from the umbilicus both above and below the umbilicus (Fig. 3.9A).

Engorged veins in the abdominal wall may be due to:

* Portal hypertension
* Inferior vena cava obstruction
* Superior vena cava obstruction.

The direction of flow may be ascertained by palpation. Empty a segment of vein above the umbilicus by milking with index finger of both hands (Figs 3.9B and C).

Remove the lower finger: If the vein remains collapsed, the flow is from above downward. The veins fill quickly, if the flow is from below upward (Fig. 3.9D).

Empty the vein segment in the same way. Remove the upper finger: the vein remains collapsed if the flow is from below upward. The vein fills quickly, if the flow is from above downward.

The same procedure is repeated by emptying a segment of vein below the umbilicus.

* In portal hypertension, the flow will be away from the umbilicus in both segments of the vein below and above the umbilicus.

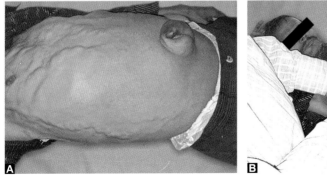
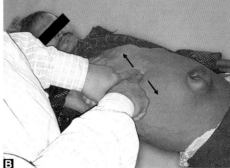

Figs 3.9A and B:

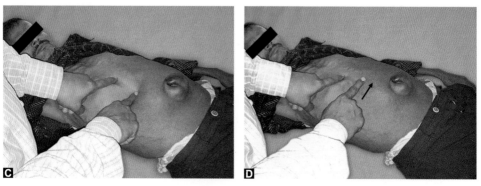

Figs 3.9C and D:

Figs 3.9A to D: Ascertaining the direction of flow in engorged veins in abdominal wall

* In inferior vena cava obstruction, the flow will be from below to up in both segments of the vein
* In superior vena cava obstruction, the flow will be from above to down in both segments of the vein.

Q. How will you assess feel of the abdomen?

Ans. The feel of the abdomen is assessed during superficial palpation. The normal feel of the abdomen is soft and elastic. As the abdomen is pressed it yields and on release the abdomen recoils back to original position.

In perforative peritonitis there may be muscle guard or rigidity. In presence of muscle guard, there is resistance when trying to yield the abdomen. In case of rigidity the abdomen cannot be yielded at all.

This can be better appreciated by palpating with two hands one placed over the other. The lower hand is pressed by the upper hand gently and the feel of the abdomen is assessed (Figs 3.10A and B).

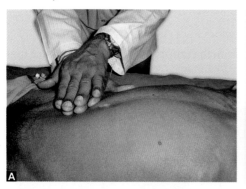
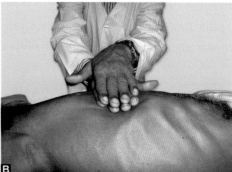

Figs 3.10A and B: Superficial palpation with two hands

Q. How will you palpate liver?

Ans. Patient supine with legs flexed at the hips and knees.

Place the hand flat on the abdomen parallel to the right costal margin with the fingers pointing upward and placed lateral to the rectus muscle and the fingertips are placed to lie parallel to the edge of the liver. Start palpating from the right iliac fossa and move upward. Ask the patient to take deep breaths with open mouth. With each expiration the hand is moved nearer to the right costal margin. If the liver is enlarged the margin of the liver will ride over the tip of the fingers. Palpate the margin of the liver—sharp, rounded, firm, smooth or irregular. Using the palmar aspect of the fingertips the margin and the surface of the liver is palpated by changing the position of the fingertips along the surface and margin of the liver (Figs 3.11A and B).

Alternatively the enlarged liver border may be palpated with the radial border of the index finger. Start palpating from right iliac fossa toward the right costal margin keeping the radial border of index finger parallel to the right costal margin. Describe the enlargement as.....cm. below the right costal margin (Figs 3.11C and D).

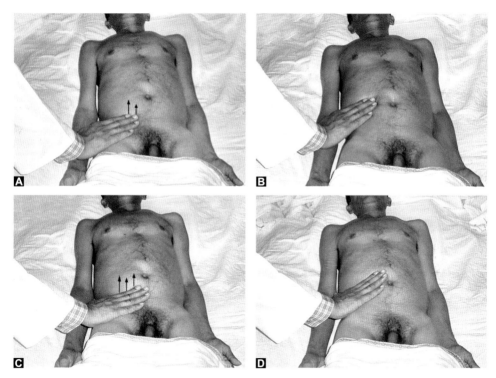

Figs 3.11A to D: (A) Start palpation at right iliac fossa using the tip of the fingers; (B) Palpate upward toward the costal margin using the tip of fingers; (C) Start palpation at right iliac fossa using the radial border of index finger; (D) Palpate upward toward the right costal margin using the radial border of the index finger

Q. How will you delineate the upper border of liver?

Ans. Start percussing in the right midclavicular line at second intercostal space, and if, clear resonant note is obtained percuss downward until a dull note is obtained. This marks the upper border of liver dullness (Fig. 3.12).

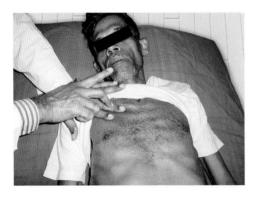

Fig. 3.12: Percussion from second intercostal space to delineate the upper border of liver

Q. When normal liver is palpable?

Ans. In infants below 3 years of age liver may be palpable 2–3 fingers breadth below the right costal margin.

In healthy thin adult liver may be palpable just below the costal margin.

Q. How will you palpate liver in presence of ascites?

Ans. This is done by dipping method. The pulp of the fingers is placed on the abdominal wall. By a quick push the fingers are dipped into the abdominal wall. The enlarged liver may be felt by the dipping fingers (Fig. 3.13).

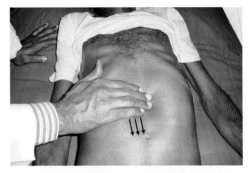

Fig. 3.13: Palpation by dipping method

Q. How will you palpate the gallbladder?

Ans. The normal gallbladder is not palpable. The method for palpation of gallbladder is same as for liver. If the gallbladder is enlarged, it is palpated in the right lumbar or even in right iliac fossa. Its lower margin, lateral and medial margins are palpable and the upper margin either becomes continuous with the enlarged liver or passes under the right costal margin (Fig. 3.14).

Q. What are the important causes of palpable gallbladder?

- Acute cholecystitis
- Mucocele
- Empyema
- Carcinoma gallbladder
- Carcinoma of head of pancreas (Courvoisier's law).

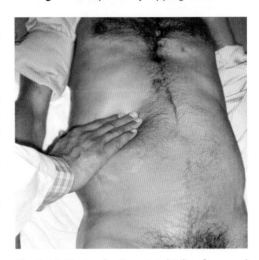

Fig. 3.14: Start palpation at right iliac fossa and go upward to the right costal margin to palpate the gallbladder. If gallbladder is palpable feel the medial border, lower border and the lateral border. The upper border is not palpable and passes deep to the costal margin or the enlarged liver. Feel the surface of the gallbladder

Q. How will you elicit Murphy's sign?

Ans. In Moynihan's method for elicitation of Murphy's sign, the patient lies supine. Place the left hand on the right costal margin so that the thumb lies over the region of the fundus of gallbladder (area just lateral to the junction of the lateral border of right rectus abdominis and the tip of the right 9th costal cartilage). Exert moderate pressure with the thumb and ask the patient to take deep breaths.

At the height of inspiration when the inflamed gallbladder impinges on the thumb there will be a catch in breath and patient will wince with pain. The Murphy's sign is said to be positive (Fig. 3.15A).

This sign may also be elicited with the patient in sitting position keeping hand in the right costal margin as described above (Fig. 3.15B).

This is found in acute cholecystitis. Not found in chronic cholecystitis or uncomplicated gallstone disease.

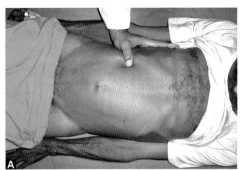 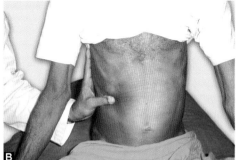

Figs 3.15A and B: (A) Eliciting Murphy's sign in supine position; (B) Eliciting Murphy's sign in sitting posture

Q. How to palpate the spleen?

Ans. The normal spleen is not palpable and becomes palpable only when enlarged 1.5 times or 2 times the normal size. The spleen enlarges toward the right iliac fossa after emerging from below the left costal margin.

Patient supine with the arms by the side of the patient: the left hand is placed over the left lateral chest wall exerting some amount of compression. Start palpating from the right iliac fossa with the fingertips pointing toward the left costal margin. Ask the patient to take deep breathing. At the zenith of inspiration, if the spleen is enlarged the edge of the spleen will ride over the tip of the fingers (Figs 3.16A to C).

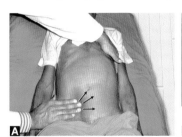 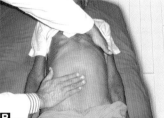 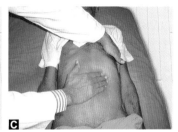

Figs 3.16A to C: Palpation of spleen: Start palpation at right iliac fossa and palpate upward toward the left costal margin using the tip of the fingers

Spleen may also be palpated with the radial border of the index finger starting from the right iliac fossa and moving upwards towards the left costal margin (Figs 3.16D and E).

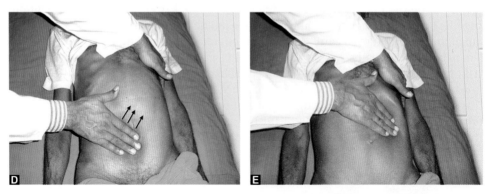

Figs 3.16D and E: Palpation in the same way by using the radial border of the index finger

If the spleen is not palpable by this method turn the patient to the right lateral position and palpate with the tip of the fingers below the right costal margin (Fig. 3.16F).

* *Palpation by hooking for minor enlargement:*

Patient supine with the arms by the side of the patient and knees flexed. Patient's left fist is placed behind the left side of chest pushing forward. The clinician stands on the left side of the patient and places the fingers of the hand below the left costal margin. Patient is asked to take deep breathing, if the spleen is enlarged this can be palpated with the fingers (Fig. 3.16G).

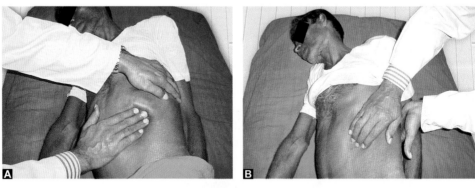

Figs 3.16F and G: (F) For minor enlargement: Patient is turned to right side and palpate near the left costal margin; (G) Palpation of spleen by hooking method

Q. How will you palpate the kidneys?

Ans. Kidney is palpated by bimanual method.

For palpation of the right kidney, place the left hand posteriorly in the right loin between the 12th rib and the right iliac crest and lateral to erector spinal muscle. Place the right hand horizontally anteriorly in the right lumbar region. Ask the patient to take deep breath and press the right hand backward and press the left hand forward. Kidney is normally not palpable. If kidney is enlarged it may be palpated between the two hands (bimanually palpable). The palpable kidney may be pushed from one hand to the other, as kidney is ballotable (Figs 3.17A and B).

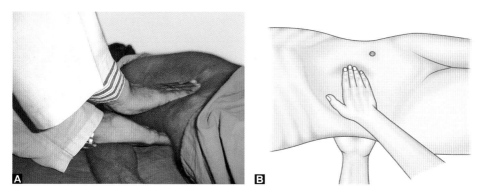

Figs 3.17A and B: Palpation of right kidney

Palpation of the left kidney is done in the same way by placing the left hand posteriorly in the loin and placing the right hand horizontally anteriorly in the left lumbar region and is palpated as above (Figs 3.18A and B).

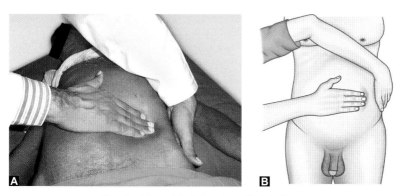

Figs 3.18A and B: Palpation of left kidney

Q. How will you elicit rebound tenderness?

Ans. Pressure of palpation may elicit a painful response in the region of the abdomen suggesting an inflammatory lesion underneath. Sudden withdrawal of the palpating finger may aggravate the painful response, which is called rebound tenderness. This is due to sudden movement of deeply placed inflamed or ischemic organ resulting in pain (Figs 3.19A and B).

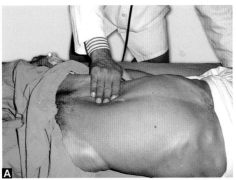
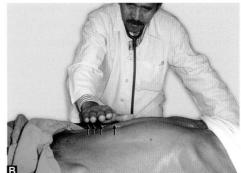

Figs 3.19A and B: (A) Right iliac fossa pressed firmly; (B) The hand is lifted suddenly. Eliciting rebound tenderness

Q. How will you elicit fluid thrill?

Ans. Patient is laid supine. Place one hand flat over the lumbar region of one side. Ask the patient to keep the side of his hand firmly in the midline of the abdomen. Tap the opposite lumbar region. A fluid thrill is felt as wave in the palpating hand laid flat in the lumbar region (Fig. 3.20).

Fluid thrill is demonstrable in presence of huge ascites.

Q. How will you demonstrate shifting dullness?

Ans. Patient is asked to empty the bladder and is laid supine in the bed. Palpate for any swelling in the abdomen. If a swelling is present avoid percussing over the swelling.

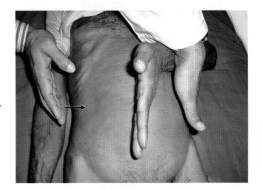

Fig. 3.20: Eliciting fluid thrill

Start percussion from below the xiphoid to the symphysis pubis (Fig. 3.21A). Then percuss from the center of the abdomen toward the flank on one side and mark the point from where the note is dull (Figs 3.21B and C). Percuss from the center of the abdomen to the other flank and mark the point from where it is dull (Figs 3.21D and E). The area of dullness on both flanks is marked out (Fig. 3.21F).

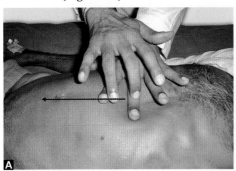
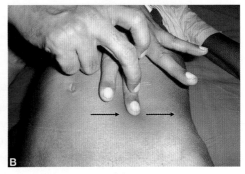

Figs 3.21A and B: (A) Percussion in midline from below xiphoid to the hypogastrium; (B) Percussion towards left flank

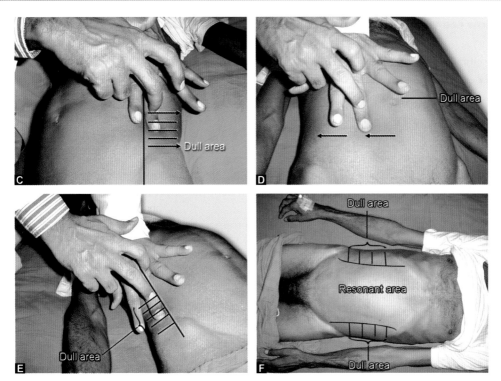

Figs 3.21C to F: (C) Percussion continued till the lateral end and the dull area on the left side marked out; (D) Percussion toward right flank; (E) Percussion till the lateral end of right flank to mark the dull area; (F) Mark out the dull and resonant area

Turn the patient to right side and wait for a few seconds. Now start percussing from the left flank toward the right flank. The dull area in the left flank now becomes resonant and dullness on the right flank is pushed more medially (Figs 3.21G and H). The percussion is repeated by turning the patient to the opposite side. Positive shifting dullness is found when at least 1 liter of free fluid is present in the abdomen.

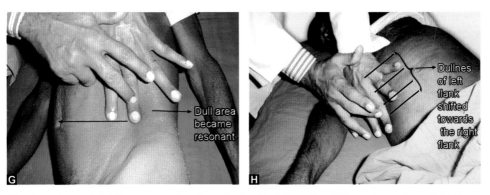

Figs 3.21G and H: (G) Start percussion from the left flank from the dull area toward the right flank; (H) Percuss toward the right flank and mark the dull area

Q. How can you demonstrate minimal free fluid in abdomen?

Ans. This can be demonstrated by Puddle sign. Percuss around the umbilicus with the patient in knee elbow position. About 100 mL of free fluid should be present for Puddle sign to be positive.

This is a very inconvenient position for the patient and is no longer practiced.

Q. When an abdominal mass is palpable how to decide that the lump is parietal or intra-abdominal?

Ans. This can be done by head rising or leg rising test (Carnett's test).

Ask the patient to keep his hands over his chest and ask him to lift his head and shoulder off the pillow. If the swelling disappears or becomes less prominent then the swelling is intra-abdominal. If the swelling becomes more prominent or remains the same then the swelling is parietal (Fig. 3.22).

For lower abdominal swelling this can be ascertained by leg rising test. Patient lies supine and is asked to lift both the legs from the bed. The interpretation is same as for head rising test (Fig. 3.23).

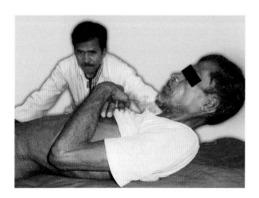

Fig. 3.22: Head rising test

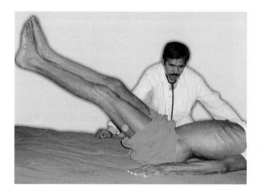

Fig. 3.23: Leg rising test

Q. How to ascertain that the swelling is intraperitoneal or retroperitoneal?

Ans. The intra-abdominal swelling may be intraperitoneal or retroperitoneal. Examine the lump in knee elbow position. If the lump disappears or becomes less prominent then it is a retroperitoneal swelling. If the lump becomes more prominent or remains the same then it is intraperitoneal (Fig. 3.24).

This is a very inconvenient position for the patient and is usually avoided.

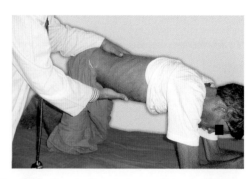

Fig. 3.24: Examination in knee elbow position to ascertain intraperitoneal or retroperitoneal lump. (Not a favored test, uncomfortable for the patient, better avoided)

CASES PRESENTING WITH GASTRIC OUTLET OBSTRUCTION

■ GASTRIC OUTLET OBSTRUCTION DUE TO CARCINOMA OF STOMACH

Q. What is your case? (Summary of a case of gastric outlet obstruction)

Ans. A gentleman aged 60 years presented with sensation of fullness after meals and vomiting for last 6 months and anorexia and weight loss for last 4 months. The sensation of fullness after meal is more toward the evening. He complains of a rolling mass in the abdomen moving from left to right. Complains of vomiting for last 6 months occurring almost daily for last 4 months, but for last 2 months vomiting has become less as he is taking less food. Vomiting is projectile in nature. Vomitus contains food material taken more than 12 hours earlier. No history of hematemesis or melena. Complains of loss of appetite and significant weight loss for last 4 months. No history of peptic ulcer disease in the past (Fig. 3.6A).

On physical examination, on general survey patient's nutrition is poor, pallor is present, no cervical lymphadenopathy, pulse 90 beats per minute. There is evidence of dehydration.

On local examination of abdomen, abdomen is normal in shape with fullness in upper abdomen and umbilicus is present at normal site and is normally inverted. Visible peristalsis is seen in upper abdomen and peristaltic waves are seen moving from left hypochondriac region to the epigastrium, umbilical and right hypochondriac region. Distended stomach is palpable in the left hypochondriac, epigastric and the umbilical region, which disappears under the examining finger. A firm intra-abdominal lump is palpable in the epigastric region, globular in shape, 3 cm in diameter, surface irregular, margin well-defined, moving up and down with respiration, mobile from side to side. No other lump is palpable. Liver/spleen is not palpable. No free fluid in abdomen. Normal bowel sounds are audible. Succussion splash is present. Ausculto-percussion revealed a distended stomach with greater curvature lying below the umbilicus. Per rectal examination is normal. Systemic examination is normal.

Q. What is your diagnosis?

Ans. This is a case of gastric outlet obstruction due to carcinoma of stomach.

Q. Why do you say this is a case of gastric outlet obstruction?

Ans.

* This elderly male patient presented with history of sensation of fullness after meals for last 6 months
* Patient complains of vomiting for last 6 months
* He is having vomiting almost daily for last 6 months
* Patient has vomiting mainly toward the evening
* The vomitus is sour in taste sometimes contains food materials taken more than 12 hours earlier
* Patient complains of a rolling mass in abdomen moving from left to right
* On examination of abdomen there is fullness in the upper abdomen

- There is visible peristalsis moving from left hypochondriac region to the epigastric, umbilical and the right hypochondriac region
- The distended stomach is palpable in the epigastric and the umbilical region, which disappears under the palpating fingers
- Succussion splash is present suggesting dilated stomach with retained food residue
- On ausculto-percussion the greater curvature of the stomach is lying below the umbilicus suggesting a distended stomach.

Q. Why do you say gastric outlet obstruction is due to carcinoma stomach in this patient?

Ans. History:
- Elderly male patient presented with short history of about 6 months
- Patient complains of anorexia, generalized weakness and weight loss for last 4 months
- Patient has features suggestive of gastric outlet obstruction
- No history of peptic ulcer disease in the past.

On Examination

- In addition to features of gastric outlet obstruction a firm intra-abdominal lump is palpable in the epigastric region, which is likely to be arising from the stomach.
- So I think this is a case of carcinoma of stomach causing gastric outlet obstruction.

Q. How to demonstrate succussion splash?

Ans.
- Patient should not eat or drink within last 3 hours
- Place stethoscope in the midepigastrium and fix it with two thumbs and shake the patient's abdomen side-to-side with other fingers of the two hands holding the lower end of the rib cage. A splashing sound will be heard, if the test is positive (Fig. 3.25)

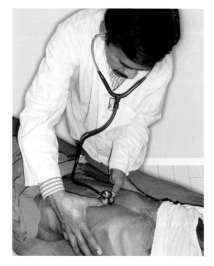

Fig. 3.25: Demonstration of succussion splash

In gross dilatation of stomach the splashing sound may be heard directly by keeping the ears close to the abdomen.

This may also be demonstrated by dipping method. The hand is laid over the epigastrium and short, sudden dipping movements are made audible gurgle indicates a positive succussion splash (Fig. 3.26).

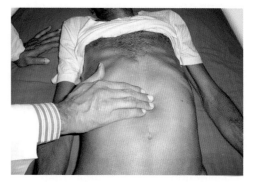

Fig. 3.26: Demonstration of succussion splash by dipping method

Q. How to do ausculto-percussion?

Ans.

- Ausculto-percussion outlines the greater curvature of the stomach
- The bell of the stethoscope is placed in the midepigastrium
- With the back of a pencil, abdominal wall is scratched radially from the edge of the bell of stethoscope starting from below the left costal margin up to the right hypochondriac region. When the scratch is made over the stomach region, scratch sound is easily audible. When scratch goes out of stomach outline no sound is audible. A point is marked at the junction of sound being audible and not audible. The line joining these points marks the greater curvature of stomach. In gastric outlet obstruction the greater curvature usually lies below the level of umbilicus (Figs 3.27A to C).

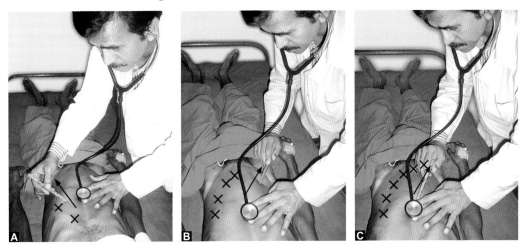

Figs 3.27A to C: Delineation of greater curvature of stomach by ausculto-percussion.

Q. What are the other possibilities?

Ans.

- Gastric outlet obstruction due to chronic duodenal ulcer
- Extrinsic compression near the pylorus due to enlarged lymph node mass either due to lymphoma or tuberculous lymph node
- Lymphoma of stomach
- Gastric outlet obstruction due to a bezoar
- Gastrointestinal stromal tumor involving the stomach (leiomyoma and leiomyosarcomas)
- Carcinoma head of the pancreas causing gastric outlet obstruction
- Adult hypertrophic pyloric stenosis.

Q. What are the consequences of gastric outlet obstruction?

Ans.

- Anatomical effect: Because of obstruction there is hyperperistalsis of the stomach leading to *hypertrophy* of the musculature of the stomach and later on there is huge *dilatation* of the stomach

* Metabolic effect: Because of vomiting there is chronic dehydration, prerenal azotemia and there is loss of H^+, Cl^- and K^+ ion leading to hypochloremic, hypokalemic metabolic alkalosis
* In early stage: Loss of H^+ and Cl^- ion leading to hypochloremic alkalosis. Sodium may be normal and hypokalemia may not be obvious
* Kidney tries to compensate metabolic alkalosis by excreting low chloride and more bicarbonate. While excreting bicarbonate sodium is also lost in urine
* If vomiting continues patient becomes more dehydrated and hyponatremia develops
* To conserve circulatory volume kidney reabsorbs water and sodium due to aldosterone effect. Sodium is retained by the distal renal tubule in exchange of H^+, K^+ ions. To conserve Na^+ ions H^+ and K^+ ions are excreted in urine
* At this late stage of metabolic alkalosis, the kidney passes acidic urine due to passage of H^+ ion in urine in exchange of sodium ion. This is called paradoxical aciduria as on the background of metabolic alkalosis kidney should have excreted alkaline urine.

Q. Why there is paradoxical aciduria in metabolic alkalosis due to gastric outlet obstruction?

Ans. Due to vomiting there is hypochloremic metabolic alkalosis. As a compensatory mechanism to metabolic alkalosis kidney excretes low chloride with bicarbonate. Sodium is lost along with bicarbonate. With time patient becomes progressively dehydrated and hyponatremic. Because of dehydration and hyponatremia the aldosterone response occurs in the body. Aldosterone effect tries to conserve sodium. In distal renal tubule sodium is conserved in exchange of H^+ ion and K^+ ion leading to paradoxical aciduria and hypokalemia.

Q. How will you correct these metabolic abnormalities?

Ans. These metabolic abnormalities may be corrected by infusing normal saline solution. Once the urine output is optimal add potassium chloride with normal saline infusion.

Q. How will you treat refractory metabolic alkalosis?

Ans.
* Earlier ammonium chloride or arginine hydrochloride infusion was used, but ammonium chloride infusion may cause ammonia toxicity
* Use of 0.1–0 2 N HCl is a safe and effective therapy for correction of severe resistant metabolic alkalosis. 1–2 liters of solution infused over a period of 24 hours. Monitor pH, $PaCO_2$ and serum electrolyte every 4 hours
* Underlying cause should be corrected.

Q. What is the cause of tetany in patient with gastric outlet obstruction?

Ans. Due to alkalosis plasma ionized calcium level may fall, and this may lead to mental confusion and tetany due to hypocalcemia.

Q. How will you manage this patient?

Ans. I would like to confirm my diagnosis by doing an upper gastrointestinal (GI) endoscopy.

Q. What information can be obtained by upper GI endoscopy?

Ans.
* The lesion can be seen, photographed and biopsy may be taken
* Gastric juice may be aspirated, centrifuged and examined for malignant cells by Papanicolaou stain

* If facility is available endoscopic ultrasonography (USG) may be done, which may clearly show the depth of invasion of the tumor in the stomach wall.

Q. How endoscopic USG may help in diagnosis of carcinoma of stomach?

Ans. Endoscopic USG can clearly show the different layers of stomach as alternating hypoechoic and hyperechoic layers. This can show the relative depth of tumor invasion in stomach wall (T staging). The overall accuracy varies between 57% and 85% for tumor staging.

This is also helpful for assessing the lymph node status (N staging). The overall accuracy for N staging varies between 50% and 80%.

Q. What is the role of barium-meal study?

Ans. With a good video-endoscopic study a barium-meal study is not essential.

However, barium meal study is helpful in linitis plastica when barium meal study will clearly show the contracted stomach.

Barium meal study is also helpful when the endoscope cannot be negotiated properly beyond the growth or if there is no facilities for endoscopy.

Q. What other investigations are indicated?

Ans. To assess the stage of the disease the following investigations are advised:
* Liver function test
  - USG of abdomen to assess any liver enlargement, lymph node enlargement and any pelvic deposit
  - Contrast enhanced computed tomography (CECT) scan of abdomen
* Chest X-ray (posteroanterior view).

Q. How does the CECT scan help in evaluation of carcinoma stomach?

Ans. The CECT scan is useful for assessment of locoregional disease for tumor and nodal status. The depth of invasion of the primary tumor may be assessed. However, the accuracy is less than endoscopic USG.

The more important point for CECT scan is to detect the intra-abdominal metastatic disease in liver, pelvis. The diagnostic accuracy for detection of metastatic disease is around 85%. However, the detection of peritoneal metastasis is around 50%.

Q. What is CT scan staging of carcinoma of stomach?

Ans.
* Stage I: Intraluminal growth without wall thickening
* Stage II: Wall thickening greater than 1 cm
* Stage III: Direct invasion to adjacent structures
* Stage IV: Metastatic lesion to liver, lymph node or other distant site.

Q. What other investigations are required?

Ans. Some other investigations are to be undertaken to assess any biochemical abnormalities and to assess patient's fitness for anesthesia.
* Complete hemogram: May reveal anemia and high erythrocyte sedimentation rate (ESR)
* Stool for occult blood: May be positive
* Blood for sugar, urea and creatinine
* Serum electrolytes—sodium, potassium and chloride.

Q. What do you expect in hemogram of patients with carcinoma of stomach?

Ans. Low Hb% and high ESR.

Q. What do you expect in LFT?

Ans.

* Low serum albumin, high serum enzymes
* Increased alkaline phosphatase is an important marker for metastasis to liver
* Until metastasis impairs at least 75% of liver function, liver function test (LFT) is not altered.

Q. How USG of abdomen helps in evaluation of patient of carcinoma of stomach?

Ans.

* Stomach cancer may spread to liver or to adjacent lymph node
* USG may detect liver deposits and also pre- and para-aortic lymph node enlargement. However, it is very difficult to evaluate the stomach growth by USG.

Q. What is the role of endoscopic USG in evaluation of carcinoma stomach?

Ans. Endoscopic USG may detect the wall invasion by the growth and also can pick up liver and lymph node metastasis. The overall accuracy for T staging is 65–92%.

Q. When you find a suspicious lesion in stomach on endoscopy how many biopsies will you take?

Ans. At least 10 biopsy bits from different sites covering all the quadrants.

Q. What is the role of PET-CT scan in evaluation of carcinoma stomach?

Ans. Only 50% of gastric cancer patients are PET avid. Hence, PET-CT scan is not very helpful for primary evaluation of carcinoma stomach.

In advanced disease where neoadjuvant chemotherapy is contemplated PET-CT scan is useful for evaluation of response to neoadjuvant chemotherapy.

Q. What is the role of diagnostic laparoscopy in carcinoma stomach?

Ans. Even with advanced imaging the peritoneal and small liver metastasis may be missed, laparoscopy may detect these small metastases. Staging laparoscopy with peritoneal lavage cytology is now considered as part of the work-up for majority of gastric carcinoma patients to avoid unnecessary laparotomy in patient with advanced disease. The overall sensitivity of detecting metastasis is around 95%.

Q. How will you prepare the patient for surgery?

Ans. This patient has multiple problems, which need correction before surgery. He is:

* Chronically dehydrated
* Electrolyte imbalance—hypokalemia, hyponatremia, hypochloremia and metabolic alkalosis
* Anemia and hypoproteinemia
* Stomach is dilated and contains lots of food residue.

The preparation includes:

* Correction of dehydration either by oral fluid or by intravenous (IV) normal saline infusion. Adequate urine output suggests proper hydration

◆ Correction of electrolyte imbalance by IV infusion of normal saline. Once urine output is adequate potassium should be supplemented to correct hypokalemia
◆ Correction of anemia by blood transfusion
◆ Correction of hypoproteinemia by oral high protein diet, amino acid or human albumin infusion
◆ Gastric lavage before each feed 4–5 days prior to surgery.
  Gastric lavage removes the food residue, decreases the mucosal edema and also brings back the gastric tonicity.

Q. How will you do gastric lavage?

Ans. Gastric lavage is done before each feed 4–5 days before surgery. A 16 or 18 Fr Ryles tube is inserted into the stomach and the gastric juice is aspirated. Normal saline is allowed to run through the Ryles tube and then aspirated back. This is repeated till the return is clear. This requires lavage with about 1–2 liters of normal saline.

Q. How will you treat this patient?

Ans. After adequate preoperative preparation I will plan for an exploratory laparotomy with intent for curative resection.
◆ On exploration of abdomen, assess for:
  – Presence of ascites
  – Any evidence of distant spread to liver
  – Any pelvic deposits
  – Any omental deposit
  – Any peritoneal deposits
◆ Assessment of the local growth:
  – The site and extent of the growth is assessed
  – Whether the growth invaded into the adjacent structures like, liver, pancreas, spleen, major vessels and the retroperitoneum
◆ Any lymph node involvement number of lymph node involvement, mobile or fixed.

If localized and resectable: I will plan to do a lower radical gastrectomy. Only the proximal stomach is preserved. The lesser curvature side is closed by suture or stapler and the greater curvature side is anastomosed to a Roux-en-Y loop of jejunum.

Q. What will you remove in a lower radical gastrectomy?

Ans.
◆ Entire greater and lesser omentum and the superior layer of transverse mesocolon
◆ Distal stomach along with the growth. Proximal clearance of 6 cm proximal to the growth and distal line of resection taking up to 2 cm of proximal duodenum
◆ Appropriate lymph node dissection D1, D2 or D3, depending on the lymph node involvement
◆ Distal pancreas and spleen was routinely removed in lower radical gastrectomy earlier. But presently pancreas and spleen are not included in the resection in view of increased morbidity and mortality due to pancreatic and splenic resection
◆ Continuity is maintained by either a loop or Roux-en-Y gastrojejunostomy.

Q. Describe the steps of lower radical gastrectomy (D2 gastrectomy).

Ans. *See* Operative Surgery Section, Page No. 1092, Chapter 22.

Q. What are the lymph node stations in lymphatic drainage of stomach?

Ans. There are 18 lymph node stations described by Japanese classification (Fig. 3.28).

1. *Right cardiac node*
2. *Left cardiac node*
3. *Lymph nodes along the lesser curvature*
4. *Lymph nodes along greater curvature*
   4sa—lymph nodes along short gastric vessels
   4sb—lymph nodes along left gastroepiploic vessels
   4d—lymph nodes along right gastroepiploic vessels
5. *Suprapyloric lymph nodes*
6. *Subpyloric lymph nodes*
7. *Lymph nodes along left gastric artery*
8. *Lymph nodes along common hepatic artery*
9. *Lymph nodes along the celiac axis*
10. *Lymph nodes at the splenic hilum*
11. *Lymph nodes along the splenic artery*
12. *Lymph nodes at hepatoduodenal ligament*
13. *Retroperitoneal duodenal lymph nodes*
14. *Lymph nodes at root of mesentery*
15. *Lymph nodes around middle colic artery*
16. *Lymph nodes around aorta—para-aortic lymph nodes*
17. *Around lower esophagus*
18. *Supradiaphragmatic nodes.*

In addition lymph nodes around the lower esophagus, lymph nodes at the esophageal hiatus, supradiaphragmatic and infradiaphragmatic nodes also receive lymphatics from the cardiac end of the stomach.

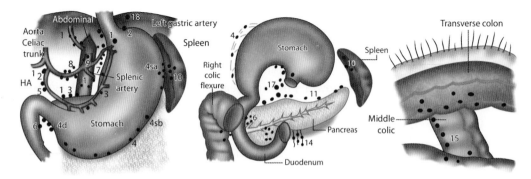

Fig. 3.28: Lymph node stations of stomach according to the Japanese classification (*See* text)

Abbreviation: HA: hepatic artery

Q. What is TNM classification for gastric cancer?

Ans. The tumor-node-metastasis (TNM) classification for gastric cancer is described in Table 3.1 and anatomic stage is given in Table 3.2.

Table 3.1: TNM classification for gastric cancer	
Primary tumor	
TX	Primary tumor cannot be assessed
T0	No evidence of primary tumor
Tis	Carcinoma in situ: Intraepithelial tumor without invasion of the lamina propria
T1	Tumor invades lamina propria, muscularis mucosae, or submucosa
T1a	Tumor invades lamina propria or muscularis mucosae
T1b	Tumor invades submucosa
T2	Tumor invades muscularis propria
T3	Tumor penetrates subserosal connective tissue without invasion of visceral peritoneum or adjacent structures
T4	Tumor invades serosa (visceral peritoneum) or adjacent structures
T4a	Tumor invades serosa (visceral peritoneum)
T4b	Tumor invades adjacent structures
Regional lymph nodes (N)	
NX	Regional lymph node(s) cannot be assessed
N0	No regional lymph node metastasis
N1	Metastasis in 1–2 regional lymph nodes
N2	Metastasis in 3–6 regional lymph nodes
N3	Metastasis in seven or more regional lymph nodes
N3a	Metastasis in 7–15 regional lymph nodes
N3b	Metastasis in 16 or more regional lymph nodes
Distant metastasis (M)	
M0	No distant metastasis
M1	Distant metastasis

Table 3.2: Anatomic stage/prognostic groups			
Stage	*T*	*N*	*M*
0	Tis	N0	M0
IA	T1	N0	M0
IB	T2	N0	M0
	T1	N1	M0
IIA	T3	N0	M0
	T2	N1	M0
	T1	N2	M0

Contd...

Contd...

Stage	T	N	M
IIB	T4a	N0	M0
	T3	N1	M0
	T2	N2	M0
	T1	N3	M0
IIIA	T4a	N1	M0
	T3	N2	M0
	T2	N3	M0
IIIB	T4b	N0	M0
	T4b	N1	M0
	T4a	N2	M0
	T3	N3	M0
IIIC	T4b	N2	M0
	T4b	N3	M0
	T4a	N3	M0
IV	Any T	Any N	M1

Q. What is the extent of lymph node dissection (D1, D2 and D3) in carcinoma stomach?

Ans. The extent of lymph node dissection in carcinoma stomach is a debatable issue. Depending on the extent of lymph node dissection the operation is classified as D1, D2 and D3 resection.

The extent of lymph node dissection for a growth in the body of the stomach:

D1 resection:
- Removal of perigastric lymph node within 3 cm of stomach serosa (N1 node)
- 1 and 2—right and left cardiac nodes
- 3 and 4—lymph nodes along lesser and greater curvature
- 5 and 6—supra and subpyloric lymph nodes.

D2 resection:
- D1 resection + removal of second tier of lymph node along main arterial trunk (N2 nodes)
- 7—lymph nodes along left gastric artery
- 8—lymph nodes along common hepatic artery
- 9—lymph nodes along celiac trunk
- 10—lymph nodes at splenic hilum
- 11—lymph nodes along splenic artery.

D3 resection:
- D2 resection + lymph nodes resection of:
    - 12—lymph nodes at hepatoduodenal ligament
    - 13—retroperitoneal duodenal lymph nodes
    - 14—lymph nodes at root of mesentery
    - 15—lymph nodes around middle colic artery
    - 16—lymph nodes around aorta—para-aortic lymph nodes.

Q. What is the recent concept of lymph node dissection in carcinoma stomach?

Ans. The N staging in American Joint Committee on Cancer (AJCC) system of TNM staging (1997) is not defined by the location of the lymph nodes but by the number of positive nodes. Consequent to this change there has been a recommendation that at least 15 lymph nodes should be removed for adequate staging. To achieve 15 lymph nodes dissection a formal D2 dissection should be the standard of care.

Q. What do you mean by R0, R1 and R2 resection?

Ans.
- *R0 resection:* In R0 resection, the growth has been resected with both macroscopic and microscopic free margin
- *R1 resection:* There is macroscopic free margin of resection but there is microscopic positive invasion at the margin
- *R2 resection* of growth with a macroscopic positive margin.

Q. Is distal pancreatectomy and splenectomy mandatory in radical gastrectomy?

Ans. In traditional radical gastrectomy distal pancreas and spleen was removed routinely enbloc with the stomach. However, this is associated with increased mortality and morbidity and splenectomy related complication.

Now a radical gastrectomy preserves spleen and pancreas. Proximal gastric cancer with extension to spleen or pancreas will require splenectomy with distal pancreatectomy.

Q. What are the signs of incurability?

Ans. Unequivocal signs of incurability are:
- Hematogenous distant metastasis
- Involvement of distant peritoneum
- N4 nodal diseases
- Fixation to structures that cannot be removed. Involvement of another organ does not imply incurability provided that it can be removed.

Q. What are the indications of total gastrectomy in carcinoma of stomach?

Ans.
- Proximal gastric cancer involving the cardia
- Diffuse gastric cancer (Borrmann's type 4)
- Growth involving two or all three sectors of the stomach
- Generalized linitis plastica.

Q. How will you establish continuity following total gastrectomy?

Ans. By a Roux-en-Y esophagojejunostomy. Roux loop should be at least 50 cm long to avoid bile reflux. It may be placed either antecolic or retrocolic. Jejunojejunostomy is done at a distance of 50 cm from esophagojejunal anastomosis (Fig. 3.29).

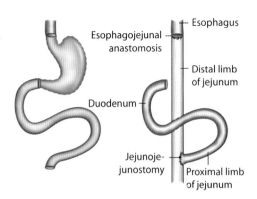

Fig. 3.29: Roux-en-Y anastomosis of the jejunum to the esophagus

Q. What should be the extent of gastric resection?

Ans.

+ In early gastric cancer, a 2 cm margin is acceptable
+ In advanced gastric cancer, a proximal 6 cm margin is essential, as lateral spread may occur up to 5 cm
+ Distal margin is usually 2 cm beyond the pylorus.

Q. What is omentectomy?

Ans. Omentectomy involves excision of both greater and lesser omentum along with radical gastrectomy. The lesser omentum should be detached from the liver. The whole of the greater omentum including the superior layer of transverse mesocolon needs to be removed to bare the colic arteries and veins to remove the lymph nodes around these vessels.

Q. What is the role of radiotherapy?

Ans.

+ Radiotherapy is not helpful in carcinoma of stomach
+ There are a number of radiosensitive tissues in the gastric bed and this limits the use of radiotherapy in gastric cancer
+ Indicated only when there is painful bony metastasis.

Q. What is the role of chemotherapy in gastric cancer?

Ans. Following R0 resection, there has been high incidence of recurrence (up to 30%) in 2 years.

+ Gastric cancer responds well to combination chemotherapy and there have been claims of improved survival with use of chemotherapy
+ A combination of epirubicin, cisplatin and 5FU is very effective
+ In Japan, intraperitoneal mitomycin-C impregnated with charcoal has been tried. This is taken up by intraperitoneal lymphatic and may target the site of local recurrence, such as the gastric bed
+ However, the benefits of adjuvant chemotherapy have not been well-established.

Q. What is MAGIC trial for chemotherapy in gastric carcinoma?

Ans. In view of poor outcome of postoperative adjuvant chemotherapy perioperative chemotherapy has been tried in carcinoma stomach. MAGIC trial is a randomized controlled trial comparing perioperative chemotherapy with surgery alone in patient with Stage II or higher gastric cancer in 503 patients.

The treatment group receives preoperative three cycles of combination chemotherapy with epirubicin, cisplatin and continuous infusion of 5 FU. Three postoperative cycles with the same regime. This trial has shown encouraging results. The rates of local recurrence (14.4% vs 20.6%), distant metastasis (24.4% vs 36.8%) and 5 year survival (36.3% vs 23%) were significantly improved in chemotherapy group than compared with the surgery only group.

Based on MAGIC trial and French trial FF CD9703, carcinoma stomach patient should be evaluated for preoperative systemic chemotherapy.

Q. What is the role of neoadjuvant chemotherapy in advanced gastric cancer?

Ans. In advanced gastric cancer preoperative combination chemotherapy with epirubicin, cisplatin and 5FU has been tried with a view to down stage the tumor and it has been observed that inoperable cancers may be rendered operable. This is still under trial.

Q. What is the treatment for stage IV carcinoma stomach?

Ans.
*   The treatment of stage IV carcinoma stomach is palliative
*   The median survival of patient with distant metastatic disease is 3–5 months with best supportive therapy
*   Combination chemotherapy with epirubicin, cisplatin and 5FU has been tried. The results are better than supportive care alone. However, overall survival is not altered
*   The main treatment is supportive
*   Palliative surgery: Some patients with significant symptom may require surgery even in the setting of metastatic disease
*   If there are signs of incurability what palliative surgery may be done?
*   In patients with bleeding or obstruction
*   A palliative resection is appropriate
*   If growth is not resectable palliative gastrojejunostomy is to be done for relief of gastric outlet obstruction.
*   For inoperable gastroesophageal junction growth:
    –   Stenting or recanalization with laser may be helpful
    –   Alternatively esophagojejunostomy and gastric exclusion may be done.

Q. How will you manage acute bleeding in patient with advanced carcinoma stomach?

Ans.
*   Resuscitation with IV fluid/blood transfusion
*   Endoscopic treatment: Electrocautery, clipping or injection of adrenaline
*   Angiography and coil embolization
*   If other methods failed: Surgery—limited resection with a negative margin.

Q. What is the strategy for surgery in locally advanced gastric cancer?

Ans. The objective of multiorgan resection in locally advanced gastric cancer is to achieve a R0 resection. Recent reports have demonstrated promising results following multiorgan resection for locally advanced gastric cancer. In patient where a R0 resection is possible with multiorgan resection, an aggressive surgical approach is justified.

In patients with a clear evidence of nonresectable disease, palliative resection is not justified.

Q. What is the role of biological therapy in gastric cancer?

Ans. *Biological or targeted therapy for advanced gastric cancer has been described. The agents tried are:*
*   *Cetuximab: Epidermal growth factor receptor inhibitor (EGFR)*
*   *Trastuzumab (Herceptin): Human epidermal growth factor receptor 2 inhibitor (HER2)*
*   *Bevacizumab: Monoclonal antibody of VEGFR family*
*   *Combination of herceptin with 5Fu and cisplatin has shown better results with no increase in adverse events*
*   *Cetuximab has been evaluated as monotherapy and combined with 5FU.*

Q. What do you mean by early gastric cancer?

Ans. Gastric cancer confined to mucosa and submucosa is called early gastric cancer.

Q. What are the strategies for treatment of early gastric cancer?

Ans. *Minimal surgery in the form of endoscopic submucosal resection (EMR) is being tried in early gastric cancer confined to the mucosa. This is widely practiced in Japan. The indications of EMR include:*
- *Tumor smaller than 2 cm*
- *Tumor confined to the mucosa*
- *No lymphovascular invasion*
- *No surface ulceration.*
- *Tumor larger than 2 cm, submucosal invasion, surface ulceration or with lymphovascular invasion should undergo gastrectomy with appropriate lymph node dissection.*

Q. What is the technique of endoscopic submucosal resection?

Ans. *This is done under endoscopic guidance. Indigo carmine is sprayed around the lesion. Submucosal injection of saline with epinephrine is done deep to the lesion to elevate the mucosa with the lesion. The line of resection is marked with electrocautery. The tumor with the mucosa is resected using a snare or electrosurgical knife.*

Q. What are the patterns of recurrence in carcinoma of stomach?

Ans. Recurrence after gastrectomy is high and varies between 40% and 80%. Most of the recurrences occur within first 2 years.
- Most common site of recurrence is the gastric bed
  - Most common site is the gastric remnant at the site of anastomosis
- Nodal metastasis
- Intraperitoneal metastasis
- Systemic spread to liver, lungs and bones.

Q. How would you evaluate in follow-up?

Ans.
- Frequency of follow-up: Every 4 months for 1 year, every 6 months for next 2 years and then annually
- History and physical examination
- Routine hemogram and liver function test
- Chest X-ray and CT scan if indicated
- Annual endoscopy.

Q. What are the premalignant lesions in stomach?

Q. What is the relation between H. pylori and carcinoma of stomach?

Q. What is Lauren's classification for gastric cancer?

Q. Which genes have been related to development of carcinoma of stomach?

Q. What do you mean by early gastric cancer?

Q. What is Japanese classification for early gastric cancer?

Q. What is Borrmann's classification for advanced gastric cancer?

Q. What is the most important histological marker for development of gastric cancer?

Q. How nitrates are related to development of gastric cancer?

Q. What are the different types of intestinal metaplasia?

Q. What are common tumor markers in gastric cancers?

Q. How does carcinoma of stomach spread?

For answer to these questions, *See* Surgical Pathology, Section, Page No. 855–865, Chapter 18.

■ DISCUSSION ON GASTRIC LYMPHOMA

Q. What are the types of gastric lymphoma?

Ans. Gastric lymphoma may be:
- *Primary: When localized to stomach. Constitute 5% of gastric neoplasm*
- *Secondary: Stomach is involved secondary to generalized lymph node disease. This is more common than the primary lymphoma of stomach.*

Q. What is the cell of origin of primary gastric lymphoma?

Ans. Primary gastric lymphoma arises from B cell and from mucosa associated lymphoid tissue (MAL Toma).

Q. What is the pattern of involvement in primary gastric lymphoma?

Ans.
- *In early stage there is diffuse mucosal thickening which ulcerate later on*
- *Lymph node involvement is late.*

Q. What is the correlation between H. pylori infection and lymphoma?

Ans.
- *Lymphocytes are usually not found in normal gastric mucosa but have been found in association with H. pylori infection*
- *In some cases of early gastric lymphoma treatment for H. pylori eradication has caused regression of lymphomatous process thereby suggesting a strong correlation between H. pylori infection and primary gastric lymphoma.*

Q. How will you diagnose gastric lymphoma?

Ans.
- *May present with signs and symptoms suggestive of gastric cancer—anemia, anorexia, asthenia (3As)*

- *May present with features of gastric outlet obstruction, i.e. sensation of fullness after meals and vomiting*
- *May present with lump in the abdomen*
- *May present with bleeding—hematemesis or melena*
- *Endoscopy and biopsy usually confirm the diagnosis*
  - *Mucosal thickening or ulceration on endoscopy.*

Q. How to ascertain whether it is primary or secondary gastric lymphoma?

Ans.

- *History and clinical examination*
- *Full blood count*
- *Bone marrow examination*
- *USG and CT scan of abdomen and CT scan of chest*
- *Criteria for diagnosis of primary gastric lymphoma*
  - *Disease localized to the stomach*
  - *No superficial or mediastinal lymphadenopathy*
  - *White cell count is normal*
  - *Liver and spleen are normal*
  - *Normal bone marrow.*

  In secondary gastric lymphoma there may be lymphocytosis in the peripheral blood count, bone marrow may be involved, USG and CT scan may show lymphadenopathy in other sites.

Q. What is Ann Arbor staging of gastric lymphoma?

Ans.

- *Stage IE: Tumor confined to the stomach*
- *Stage IIE: Tumor with spread to the regional lymph nodes*
- *Stage IIIE: Tumor with spread beyond the regional lymph nodes (para-aortic, iliac)*
- *Stage IVE: Tumor with spread to other intra-abdominal organs (liver, spleen) or beyond abdomen (chest, bone marrow).*

Q. What is Paris staging system for primary gastrointestinal lymphomas?

Ans. The Paris staging system is as follows:

TX	Lymphoma extent not specified
T0	No evidence of lymphoma
T1	Lymphoma confined to the mucosa/submucosa
T1m	Lymphoma confined to mucosa
T1sm	Lymphoma confined to submucosa
T2	Lymphoma infiltrates muscularis propria or subserosa
T3	Lymphoma penetrates serosa (visceral peritoneum) without invasion of adjacent structures
T4	Lymphoma invades adjacent structures or organs

Contd...

Contd...

N-Lymph node involvement NX	Involvement of lymph nodes not assessed
N0	No evidence of lymph node involvement
N1‡	Involvement of regional lymph nodes
N2	Involvement of intra-abdominal lymph nodes beyond the regional area
N3	Spread to extra-abdominal lymph nodes
MX	Dissemination of lymphoma not assessed
M0	No evidence of extranodal dissemination
M1	Noncontinuous involvement of separate site in gastrointestinal tract (e.g. stomach and rectum)
M2	Noncontinuous involvement of other tissues (e.g. peritoneum, pleura) or organs (e.g. tonsils, parotid gland, ocular adnexa, lung, liver, spleen, kidney, breast, etc.)
B-Bone marrow involvement BX	Involvement of bone marrow not assessed
B0	No evidence of bone marrow involvement
B1	Lymphomatous infiltration of bone marrow

Depending on the T, N, and M scores, the tumor is then designated a stage:

TNM stage I	$T_1 N_0 M_0$ $T_2 N_0 M_0$ $T_3 N_0 M_0$
TNM stage II	$T_{1-3} N_1 M_0$ $T_{1-3} N_2 M_0$
TNM stage IIE	$T_4 N_0 M_0$
TNM stage IV	$T_{1-4} N_3 M_0$ $T_{1-4} N_{0-3} M_1$

Q. How will you treat primary gastric lymphoma?

Ans. *Earlier surgery was treatment of choice for primary gastric lymphomas. Most patients are now treated with combination chemotherapy.*

A prospective study comparing surgery alone, chemotherapy alone, surgery plus radiation and surgery plus chemotherapy has concluded better results in patients with chemotherapy alone and in patients with surgery plus chemotherapy.

Extent of surgery involves:

* *Lesion in the antrum—distal subtotal radical gastrectomy*
* *Lesion in the fundus or proximal stomach total gastrectomy.*

Q. What is the treatment for secondary gastric lymphoma?

Ans. *Systemic chemotherapy.*

Q. What are the regimes of chemotherapy in gastric lymphoma?

Ans. *Chemotherapy regime is same for other lymphomas. There are four effective regimes for treatment of lymphomas:*
* *MOPP: Mechlorethamine, oncovin (vincristine), procarbazine and prednisone*
* *COMLA: Cyclophosphamide, oncovin, methotrexate, leucovorin, ara-cytosine (cytarabine)*
* *BACOP: Bleomycin, adriamycin, cyclophosphamide, oncovin and prednisone*
* *CHOP: Cyclophosphamide, hydroxydaunomycin, oncovin and prednisone.*

Q. What are the indications of surgery in secondary gastric lymphoma?

Ans.
* *Bleeding and perforation*
    – *This may occur following initiation of chemotherapy*
    – *Usually requires total gastrectomy*
    – *Gastric outlet obstruction.*

■ DISCUSSION ON GASTROINTESTINAL STROMAL TUMOR

Q. What is gastrointestinal stromal tumor (GIST)?

Ans. *Gastrointestinal stromal tumor (GIST) is the most common mesenchymal tumor of the GI tract arising from the cells of Cajal (intestinal pacemaker cell). Originally GIST is believed to be arising from the smooth muscle of the GI tract (leiomyoma and leiomyosarcomas). GIST has now been recognized as a unique tumor based on KIT (CD117) expression which is found in 95% of patients. Platelet derived growth factor alpha (PDGFR alfa) mutations has been found in 5% of patients who lacks KIT expression.*

Q. What are sporadic and familial GIST?

Ans. *GIST is usually sporadic. In this only one family member is affected and there is no affection of other family members. Familial GIST may occur. In these families there is germline KIT mutation in exon 11.*

Q. What is Carney's triad?

Ans. *This is a variety of familial GIST. Young women are usually affected and include:*
* *Functioning extra-adrenal paragangliomas*
* *Pulmonary chondromas*
* *Gastric GIST.*

Q. What is the association of GIST with neurofibromatosis type 1 (NF-1)?

Ans. *GIST can occur in patients with NF-1. GIST is usually found in small intestine. However, it is different from other forms as it lacks KIT or PDGFR alfa mutation.*

Q. What is the behavior of GIST?

Ans. *GIST has a wide spectrum from benign to malignant. GIST may occur from esophagus to the anus. Small intestinal GIST has highest chance of malignancy (40%) and stomach has the lowest chance of malignancy (20%).*

Q. What are the different ways of presentation of GIST?

Ans. There are various modes of presentation:
- Asymptomatic—GISTs are often diagnosed incidentally during a physical examination or in course of some investigations for other disease (smaller size GIST: <2.5 cm)
- Microcytic anemia due to slow hemorrhage
- Nonspecific symptoms like—anorexia, weight loss and anemia
- Significant GI hemorrhage (hematemesis and melena) may occur in 25% of patients
- Symptoms due to mass effect—nausea, vomiting, early satiety or abdominal distension.

Q. What are the diagnostic investigations?

Ans.
- *Upper GI endoscopy: For gastroduodenal GIST. Appear as a submucosal mass*
- *CECT scan of abdomen: Can assess the local extent of the tumor. Smaller tumors may appear as gut wall thickening*
- *MRI abdomen: Appear as low intensity signal in T1-weighted image and high intensity signal in T2-weighted image with enhancement on administration of gadolinium contrast*
- *FDG-PET scan: Uptake is sensitive but not specific. This is generally not necessary in most patients. Useful as an early test for treatment response*
- *Endoscopic USG: May assess the actual depth of the tumor.*

Q. What is the role of FNAC in GIST?

Ans. *Fine needle aspiration cytology (FNAC) is not indicated in routine evaluation of GIST. GISTs are usually fragile and may rupture if biopsied. These tumors are hypervascular and FNAC may cause intratumoral hemorrhage. The pathologist cannot diagnose GIST in fine needle aspirate.*

Q. What is the role of endoscopic biopsy?

Ans. *Endoscopic biopsy is less likely to cause hemorrhage. May differentiate the lesion from lymphoma, which is similar in appearance. In nonresectable disease endoscopic biopsy may be useful for consideration of neoadjuvant imatinib therapy. Endoscopic biopsy may be inconclusive as the tumor is in submucosa and a proper biopsy may not be possible.*

Q. What are the immunohistochemical characteristics of GIST?

Ans.
- KIT receptor positivity (present in 95%)
- CD 34 a hematopoietic progenitor cell antigen (60–70% of GIST)
- Desmin similar to smooth muscle tumors
- Protein kinase C theta in KIT negative tumor.

Q. How will you assess malignant potential in GIST?

Ans.
- Benign: Size <2 cm no more than 5 mitoses/50 HPF
- Probably benign: >2 cm ≤5 cm, no more than 5 mitoses/50 HPF
- Malignant:
  - >5 cm but ≤10 cm, >5 mitoses/HPF.
  - >10 cm, > 5 mitoses /HPF

Q. What is TNM classification for gastrointestinal stromal tumors?

Ans. The TNM classification for gastrointestinal stromal tumors is given in Table 3.3 and anatomic stage is dissected in Table 3.4.

Table 3.3: TNM classification for gastrointestinal stromal tumors	
Primary tumor (T)	
TX	Primary tumor cannot be assessed
T0	No evidence of primary tumor
T1	Tumor ≤ 2 cm
T2	Tumor > 2 cm but ≤ 5 cm
T3	Tumor > 5 cm but ≤ 10 cm
T4	Tumor > 10 cm in greatest dimension
Regional lymph nodes (N)	
N0	No regional lymph node metastasis
N1	Regional lymph node metastasis
Distant metastasis (M)	
M0	No distant metastasis
M1	Distant metastasis
Histologic grade (G)	
GX	Grade cannot be assessed
G1	Low grade; mitotic rate 5/50 per high-power field (HPF) or less
G2	High grade; mitotic rate > 5/50 HPF

Table 3.4: Anatomic stage/prognostic groups				
Gastric GIST				
Stage	*T*	*N*	*M*	*Mitotic rate*
IA	T1 or T2	N0	M0	Low mitotic rate
IB	T3	N0	M0	Low mitotic rate
II	T1	N0	M0	High mitotic rate
	T2	N0	M0	High mitotic rate
	T4	N0	M0	Low mitotic rate
IIIA	T3	N0	M0	High mitotic rate
IIIB	T4	N0	M0	High mitotic rate
IV	Any T	N1	M0	Any rate
	Any T	Any N	M1	Any rate

Contd...

Contd...

Small intestinal GIST				
Stage	T	N	M	Mitotic rate
I	T1 or T2	N0	M0	Low mitotic rate
II	T3	N0	M0	Low mitotic rate
IIIA	T1	N0	M0	High mitotic rate
	T4	N0	M0	Low mitotic rate
IIIB	T2	N0	M0	High mitotic rate
	T3	N0	M0	High mitotic rate
	T4	N0	M0	High mitotic rate
IV	Any T	N1	M0	Any rate
	Any T	Any N	M1	Any rate

Q. What is the treatment for resectable GIST?

Ans. *Surgery is the mainstay of treatment for resectable GIST. Complete resection provides a chance for cure. GISTs are normally surrounded by a pseudocapsule. Due to exophytic growth of GIST a wedge or segmental resection is adequate. A 1 cm margin around the tumor and an excision outside the pseudocapsule is adequate for complete resection.*

If the tumor is adherent to the adjacent organ, additional resection of the adjacent organ may be required for curative resection.

Q. What is the role of adjuvant therapy in GIST?

Ans. Patient with larger lesion has higher incidence of local recurrence and surgery alone is inadequate.

Imatinib is the drug of choice as adjuvant treatment.

Q. What is the role of imatinib in GIST?

Ans. Imatinib may be used as:
* Adjuvant therapy: In resectable disease, if the tumor is low-risk of malignancy no adjuvant therapy is required
* In tumor with high chance of recurrence (>3 cm, >5 mitoses/HPF) adjuvant imatinib is indicated
* Neoadjuvant therapy: In nonresectable disease, imatinib may be given as neoadjuvant, if the tumor responds and become resectable; surgery may be done followed by imatinib therapy
* As main modality of treatment in metastatic disease
* In nonresectable metastatic disease imatinib may be the sole mode of treatment.

Q. How will you treat imatinib resistant disease?

Ans. In some cases of imatinib therapy KIT mutation may develop in some part of the tumor, which may continue to grow. In such cases surgical resection of the resistant nodule may be considered and the treatment continued with imatinib.

In some cases, the tumor may continue to grow with imatinib therapy at a dose of 400 mg/day. The dose can be escalated to 800 mg/day. There is 5% chance of response with dose escalation to 800 mg/day.

Some patients who have continued growth of GIST with imatinib therapy or who do not tolerate imatinib may be treated with sunitinib. Sunitinib is a multitargeted tyrosine kinase inhibitor that has both antitumor and antiangiogenic properties. Sunitinib inhibits vascular endothelial growth factor receptor 1, 2, 3, KIT, PDGFR alfa, PDGFR beta, FMs such as tyrosine kinase 3 receptor and the RET proto-oncogene receptor.

Q. What are the other tyrosine kinase inhibitors?

Ans.
- *Vatalanib (PTK787/ZK222584)*
- *Dasatinib (BMS354825)*
- *Everolimus.*

Q. What is the role of radiotherapy in GIST?

Ans. GISTs are radioresistant tumors and there are no prospective trials of effect of radiation in GIST.

Q. What is the role of conventional chemotherapy?

Ans.
- *The result of treatment with conventional chemotherapy in GIST is not promising*
- *Treatment with Gemcitabine and Doxorubicin only 10% response rate*
- *There is no response also with ifosfamide and etoposide.*

Q. How does GIST spread?

Ans.
- *They usually spread by bloodstream to liver, lungs and bone*
- *Lymphatic metastasis is uncommon.*

■ GASTRIC OUTLET OBSTRUCTION DUE TO COMPLICATION OF CHRONIC DUODENAL ULCER

Q. What is your case? (Summary of a case of gastric outlet obstruction due to chronic duodenal ulcer)

Ans. A 45-year-old gentleman presented with pain in central part of abdomen for last 4 years. Pain was dull aching, in nature, felt in the central part of the upper abdomen. Pain was more in empty stomach and relieved with intake of food. Pain was periodic, in nature, initially occurring for 2–3 months with a pain free interval of 3–4 months. But for last 5 months patient is having dull aching constant pain in the central abdomen. Complains of vomiting for last 6 months. Vomiting occurs after almost every feed, but more toward evening. Vomiting is projectile in nature and contains food materials taken more than 12 hours or earlier. Vomiting is sour in taste and is colorless (does not contain bile). Complains of heart burn and acidity for last 5 years. Patient complains of sensation of a rolling mass in the abdomen moving from left to right more so after taking meals.

On general survey, patient is emaciated with poor nutrition. Pallor is present. Abdominal examination revealed scaphoid abdomen with fullness in upper abdomen. Visible peristalsis is seen in the upper abdomen moving from left to right. Distended stomach is palpable in the left hypochondriac, epigastrium and right hypochondriac region. The palpable stomach disappears under the palpating fingers. Succussion splash is present over the epigastrium and ausculto-percussion revealed dilated stomach. Other systemic examination is normal.

Q. What is your diagnosis?

Ans. This is a case of gastric outlet obstruction due to chronic complication of chronic duodenal ulcer.

Q. What are the other possible causes for gastric outlet obstruction in this patient?

Ans. *See* Gastric Outlet Obstruction, Page No. 103.

Q. If it is a complication of duodenal ulcer where is the stenosis located?

Ans.
* The stenosis is actually at the first part of duodenum and not in the pylorus as this is the complication of chronic duodenal ulcer
* True pyloric stenosis occurs as a complication of pyloric channel ulcer.

Q. How will you manage this patient?

Ans.
* To confirm diagnosis an upper GI endoscopy is to be undertaken. There may be lots of food residue in the stomach. The stomach is dilated and usually it is not possible to pass the endoscope beyond the pylorus in severe pyloric stenosis
* Apart from upper GI endoscopy—following investigations are also suggested:
  - Complete hemogram, Hb%, total leukocyte count (TLC), differential leukocyte count (DLC) and erythrocyte sedimentation rate (ESR)
  - Blood for sugar, urea and creatinine
  - Blood for serum electrolyte Na, K and Cl
  - Chest X-ray (PA view)
  - Urine for routine examination (RE)
  - Stool for occult-blood
  - Liver function test (LFT). Serum protein may be low.

Q. Is a barium-meal study mandatory?

Ans. As upper GI endoscopy is readily available and can give a reasonable diagnosis of gastric outlet obstruction and its possible cause, a barium-meal study is not essential.

Q. How will you prepare the patient for surgery?

Ans. *See* Carcinoma of Stomach, Page No. 108.

Q. What operation you will do in this patient?

Ans. Truncal vagotomy and gastrojejunostomy.

Q. Describe the steps of truncal vagotomy and gastrojejunostomy.

Ans. *See* Operative Surgery Section, Page No. 1097, Chapter 22.

Q. What are other options for surgical treatment?

Ans.
- Highly selective vagotomy with gastrojejunostomy
- Partial gastrectomy, but this operation is associated with increased morbidity and mortality
- Highly selective vagotomy with pyloric dilatation
- In elderly frail patient with poor general condition only gastrojejunostmy may be helpful.

Q. Is it possible to do a pyloroplasty?

Ans. In gastric outlet obstruction due to complication of chronic duodenal ulcer there is gross scarring of pyloric region so pyloroplasty is not feasible.

Q. Is there any nonoperative means of correcting pyloric stenosis?

Ans. Pyloric stenosis is a manifestation of burnt out duodenal ulcer disease. A nonoperative treatment has been tried particularly in elderly patient unfit for surgery. Balloon dilatation of stenosed area via an endoscope may be helpful and may need repeated dilatation at an interval of few weeks. Patient also needs treatment with proton pump inhibitors (PPIs).

PEPTIC-ULCER DISEASE

▄ CHRONIC GASTRIC ULCER AND CHRONIC DUODENAL ULCER

Q. What is your case? (Summary of a case of chronic duodenal ulcer)

Ans. A 35-year-old gentleman presented with history of pain in upper central part of abdomen for last 6 years. The pain was insidious in onset and started 6 years back. The pain used to occur at an interval of about 4–6 months and used to persist for 2–3 months. The pain is burning in character, occurs after 3–4 hours of intake of meals and in empty stomach. The patient has relief of pain with intake of food and some antacids. But for last 1 year patient is having pain at more frequent intervals and he has partial relief of pain with antacids. He complains of heartburn and acidity for same duration. He has a history of passage of black tarry stool 6 months back, which lasted for 2 days and was relieved with medicines. No history of vomiting and no hematemesis. Bowel and bladder habits are normal. No other systemic symptoms. There is no major ailment in the past.

Personal history: He is from a low socioeconomic status and he used to smoke 10–20 *bidis* a day for last 10 years. He has given up smoking 1 year back.

On examination, general survey is essentially normal. Abdominal examination is also normal except deep tenderness over the duodenal point. No visible peristalsis. Liver and spleen are not palpable. No free fluid in abdomen and normal bowel sounds are audible.

Q. What is your diagnosis?

Ans. This is a case of chronic duodenal ulcer.

Q. What are the other possibilities?

Ans.
- Chronic gastric ulcer
- Chronic cholecystitis
- Chronic pancreatitis
- Hiatus hernia with reflux esophagitis.

Q. What are the characteristics of pain in chronic duodenal ulcer?

Ans. The pain is epigastric, burning in character, usually occurs 3–4 hours after meals and in empty stomach, has relief with intake of food, periodicity of pain is present-symptoms occurs for few weeks to months and then relieved spontaneously and recurs after weeks or months.

Q. Where is the duodenal point?

Ans. Duodenal point is situated in the transpyloric plane 2.5 cm to the right of midline. Tenderness is elicited over the duodenal point in chronic duodenal ulcer (*see* Fig. 3.2, Page No. 88).

Q. Where is the gastric point?

Ans. Gastric point is situated in the midepigastrium and tenderness is elicited at the gastric point in chronic gastric ulcer (*see* Fig. 3.2, Page No. 88).

Q. What investigations are suggested in this patient?

Ans. To confirm diagnosis an esophagogastroduodenoscopy is to be done, which may show the ulcer and exclude any other lesion in the esophagus and stomach. If a gastric ulcer is found multiple biopsies should be taken from different quadrants to rule out malignancy.

Aspirated gastric juice may be used for a rapid urease test to detect *Helicobacter pylori* infection.

Aspirated gastric juice may be centrifuged and Papanicolaou stain done to exclude malignant lesion in the stomach.

Q. How to treat this patient?

Ans. As the patient has received adequate medical treatment and he has history of melena I will consider surgical treatment in this patient. However, a course of intensive medical therapy may be tried for a period of 4–6 weeks.

If the rapid urease test shows evidence of *H. pylori* infection, then *H. pylori* eradication therapy is to be started. Effective eradication therapy may help in healing of the ulcer and may reduce the incidence of relapse of ulceration.

Q. What are the regimes for medical treatment of chronic duodenal ulcer or chronic gastric ulcer?

Ans. The aim of medical treatment is to reduce the acid secretion thereby helping the ulcer to heal.

Components of medical treatment are:
* Lifestyle changes: Stop smoking, avoid alcohol
* Bland diet at frequent intervals. Avoid remaining in empty stomach for long time
* If there is a component of anxiety, tranquillizer drugs, like alprazolam or diazepam
* Stop NSAIDs
* Antisecretory drugs: Proton-pump inhibitor (PPI) like omeprazole 20 mg daily for 4 weeks followed by omeprazole 10 mg daily for 3–6 months as maintenance therapy.

Q. How will you treat associated H. pylori infection?

Ans.
* A combination of amoxicillin, clarithromycin and a PPI omeprazole is very effective and is given for 7–14 days

- Amoxicillin at a daily dose of 1,500 mg in two divided doses
- Clarithromycin at a daily dose of 500 mg in two divided doses
- Omeprazole in a dose of 40 mg daily in two divided doses
- Omeprazole is continued at a daily dose of 20 mg daily for 4–6 weeks.

Q. What other drugs regime are effective against H. pylori infection?

Ans.
- A combination of colloidal bismuth with amoxicillin and metronidazole
- A combination of omeprazole, amoxicillin and metronidazole
- Pantoprazole may be used instead of omeprazole.

Q. What other drugs are effective for peptic ulcer treatment?

Ans. Three groups of drugs are effective for treatment of peptic ulcer:
1. Drugs acting against *H. pylori*: effective treatment of *H. pylori* allows ulcer healing.
   - A combination clarithromycin, amoxicillin and omeprazole
2. Drugs that reduces acid secretion or causes chemical neutralization of acids. These include:
   - *Antacids:* It can neutralize the gastric acid. Most effective when given 1 hour after a meal. Dosage of 200–1,000 mmol/day may allow ulcer healing in a month. But the large dosage required is a limiting factor of adequate treatment with antacids
   - H_2 *receptor antagonist: Ulcer* healing occurs after 4–6 weeks of therapy
     - Ranitidine: 300 mg BD × 4–6 weeks
     - Famotidine: 40 mg OD × 4–6 weeks
   - Proton-pump inhibitors: PPI are most potent antisecretory drugs. PPI requires an acid environment for its activation. So, PPI should not be used in combination with H_2 receptor antagonists and antacids.
     - Pantoprazole: 40 mg daily
     - Omeprazole: 40 mg daily
     - Esomeprazole: 40 mg daily
     - Rabeprazole: 20 mg daily
     - Dexrabeprazole: 10 mg daily.
   Proton-pump inhibitors are more effective and the ulcer may heal in 2–4 weeks' time
3. Drugs increasing the mucosal protective barrier: Sucralfate—an aluminum salt of sulfated sucrose dissociates in the acidic environment of the stomach and the sucrose polymerizes and binds to the protein in the ulcer crater to produce a protective coating and allow ulcer healing in 4–6 weeks' time.

Q. What are the problems with the drug therapy?

Ans. The antisecretory drugs such as H_2 receptor antagonist and the proton-pump inhibitors reduce acid secretion and causes healing of the ulcer. Proton-pump inhibitors are more effective and provide relief of symptoms in few days and healing of ulcer in 2 weeks' time. But there is high chance of relapse following cessation of therapy.

So, maintenance therapy with these drugs is required to prevent the relapse of the ulcer. The maintenance therapy may be continued for 6 months to 1 year.

Q. When will you consider surgical treatment in this patient?

Ans. In *H. pylori* positive cases anti-*H. pylori* treatment is to be given. PPIs are continued for 6 weeks along with the general measures. If this intensive medical treatment fails surgical treatment is to be contemplated.

If the patient has already received adequate medical treatment and the ulcer is there for long duration (> 5 years) then surgical treatment is indicated.

Q. What surgery is appropriate in this patient?

Ans. As this patient does not have a gastric outlet obstruction, the idea of operation in this case is to reduce the gastric acid secretion. Highly selective vagotomy will be appropriate.

Q. What is highly selective vagotomy?

Ans. In highly selective vagotomy the vagal branches from anterior and posterior vagus to the fundus and body of stomach are divided keeping the *nerve of Latarjet* supplying the antrum intact. The nerve branches to the lower 5 cm of esophagus are also divided for complete denervation of the parietal cells of the stomach (Fig. 3.30).

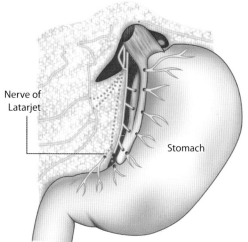

Fig. 3.30: Highly selective vagotomy

Q. What is nerve of Latarjet?

Ans. The anterior and posterior nerves of Latarjet are terminal branches of anterior and posterior vagal nerve trunk. This nerve branches like a crow's feet and supplies the pyloric antrum region of the stomach. The supply of nerve of Latarjet ends approximately 7 cm proximal to the pylorus. So all nerve branches 7 cm proximal to the pylorus is divided for completeness of highly selective vagotomy (Fig. 3.30).

Q. What is criminal nerve of Grassi?

Ans. This is a branch of posterior vagus nerve, which passes posteriorly to the fundus of the stomach. For completeness of highly selective vagotomy this criminal nerve of Grassi has to be divided (Fig. 3.31).

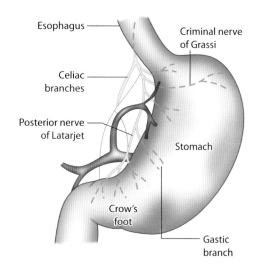

Fig. 3.31: Criminal nerve of Grassi

Q. Why a drainage operation is not required with highly selective vagotomy?

Ans. The main advantage of highly selective vagotomy is that a drainage procedure is not required as the nerve supply to the pyloric antrum part of the stomach is retained, which is mainly responsible for the propulsion of the food material from stomach to the duodenum.

Q. What are the problems with highly selective vagotomy?

Ans. It is a technically difficult operation. The chance of recurrent ulceration is 2–10%, little higher as compared to truncal vagotomy and drainage where chance of recurrent ulceration is 2–7%.

However, slight epigastric fullness and mild dumping may occur following highly selective vagotomy.

Q. What are the other options for surgery for chronic duodenal ulcer?

Ans.

- *Truncal vagotomy and a drainage procedure (gastrojejunostomy or pyloroplasty):* This is a standard operation for chronic duodenal ulcer. Both anterior and posterior vagal trunks are divided above the celiac and hepatic branches. The nerve branches to the lower 7 cm of esophagus are to be divided for completeness of vagotomy. As it denervates the whole stomach a drainage procedure is required to avoid gastric retention. The drainage procedure is either a gastrojejunostomy or pyloroplasty.
- *Vagotomy and antrectomy:* In addition to vagotomy the antrum of the stomach is removed to remove the source of gastrin. The incidence of recurrent ulceration is very low 1%. In view of increased mortality and morbidity due to antrectomy this is not a very effective procedure for chronic duodenal ulcer.
- *Billroth II gastrectomy:* It was done earlier for chronic duodenal ulcer. Although the chance of recurrent ulceration is much less 1–4%, in view of increased mortality and morbidity (postgastrectomy syndrome) of the procedure, it is not a good acceptable procedure for chronic duodenal ulcer.
- *Only gastrojejunostomy:* Performance of simple gastrojejunostomy may allow the ulcer to heal. As the acid secretion is not suppressed there is high chance of recurrent ulceration (50%). There is increased incidence of stomal ulceration. So, only gastrojejunostomy is also not a very effective procedure for chronic duodenal ulcer.

Q. What are the drainage operations following truncal vagotomy?

Ans. It may be either pyloroplasty or gastrojejunostomy.

Q. What is Heineke-Mikulicz pyloroplasty?

Ans. This is a form of drainage procedure following truncal vagotomy. It involves a longitudinal incision of the pyloric ring extending both to the duodenum (1") and the pyloric antrum (2"). The incision is then closed transversely with a single layer of interrupted polyglactin (vicryl) sutures (Fig. 3.32).

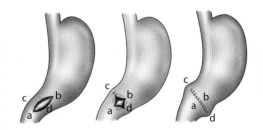

Fig. 3.32: Heineke-Mikulicz pyloroplasty

Q. What is an ideal gastrojejunostomy?

Ans. A posterior *(Retrocolic), short or no loop, isoperistaltic* gastrojejunostomy is an ideal gastrojejunostomy.

Q. How to treat a patient with chronic gastric ulcer?

Ans.

♦ The medical treatment for gastric and duodenal ulcer is same
♦ The options for surgical treatment of gastric ulcer are:
  – *Highly selective vagotomy with excision of the gastric ulcer.* Side effects of surgery is less, but there is slight increased incidence of recurrent ulceration
  – *Truncal vagotomy,* or *drainage (pyloroplasty or gastrojejunostomy) and excision of the ulcer* is very effective and avoids the side effects associated with gastrectomy
  – *Partial gastrectomy with the excision of the ulcer bearing area*—Billroth I or Billroth II type. This is very effective procedure but the side effects associated with gastrectomy limits its application for treatment of gastric ulcer.

Q. What are the factors for development of chronic peptic ulcer?

Ans. *Gastric acidity:* Gastric acidity is one of the prime factors for development of peptic ulceration. In chronic duodenal ulcer there is hypersecretion of acid. In Zollinger-Ellison syndrome there is very high secretion of acid, which may lead to extensive peptic ulceration. Acid pepsin digestion of the mucosa leads to development of chronic peptic ulcer. In chronic gastric ulcer, however, the acid levels may be normal or even low. However, all ulcers heal in absence of acid. So, acid is the most important factor for development of peptic ulcer.

Genetic factors: Patients with blood group "O" has increased incidence of chronic duodenal ulcer.

Smoking: Predisposes to increased incidence of peptic ulceration and also increases the relapse rate.

Nonsteroidal anti-inflammatory drugs and steroid: Prolonged treatment with NSAIDs and steroid predisposes to increased incidence of peptic ulceration.

H. pylori infection: There is increasing evidence that infection with *H. pylori* is one of the very important factors for development of peptic ulceration. *H. pylori* hydrolyze urea resulting in formation of ammonia, which is a strong alkali. This released ammonia causes stimulation of antral G cells leading to hypergastrinemia, which in turn leads to gastric hypersecretion and leads to formation of peptic ulceration. The infection with *H. pylori* may lead to disruption of gastric mucous membrane due to some enzymes secreted by the organism. The organism also secretes cytotoxin, which can damage the gastric epithelial cells and lead to peptic ulceration.

H. pylori do not colonize the duodenum normally. *H. pylori* induced gastric hypersecretion leads to gastric metaplasia of the duodenum due to the excess acidity. Following gastric metaplasia, the duodenum may be colonized by the *H. pylori* and leads to same inflammatory process as it causes in the gastric epithelium leading to formation of peptic ulceration.

Q. What lesions may be caused by H. pylori infection?

Ans. *H. pylori* infection may lead to:

♦ Chronic gastritis
♦ Peptic ulceration
♦ Carcinoma of stomach
♦ Gastric lymphoma.

Q. How do the H. pylori look like and what is the route of infection?

Ans. *H. pylori* is a spiral-shaped flagellate organism, which normally colonizes the gastric epithelium (Fig. 3.33).

* The fecal oral spread is the most likely route of infection
* The infection is more prevalent in low socioeconomic groups.

Q. How to detect H. pylori infection?

Ans. *Rapid urease test:* The organism's obligate urease activity may be utilized in a slide test which will show the color change suggesting a positive test.

C13 and C14 breath test.

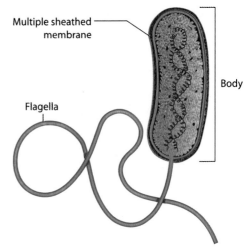

Fig. 3.33: Schematic diagram of the *Helicobacter pylori*

Gastric biopsy: The organism may be detected histologically by Giemsa's stain. The organism may also be cultured using appropriate media.

Serological test: Previous or current infection with *H. pylori* may be detected by enzyme-linked immunosorbent assay (ELISA) test for *H. pylori* antibody.

Q. How will you treat H. pylori infection?

Ans. Discussed under *H. pylori* infection.

Q. What are the sites of peptic ulcers?

Ans. The peptic ulcer is caused by acid peptic digestion and may occur in sites exposed to acid pepsin exposure.

Stomach: Common site is the body of stomach near the lesser curvature. Pyloric channel and prepyloric ulcers behaves like duodenal ulcers.

Duodenum: Most common in the first part of duodenum.

Lower end of esophagus due to reflux of gastric juice.

Meckel's diverticulum due to presence of heterotopic gastric mucosa in the Meckel's diverticulum.

In the stoma of gastrojejunostomy, the recurrent ulcer usually forms near the jejunal side of the stoma.

Q. What are the characteristic features of chronic duodenal ulcer and chronic gastric ulcer?

Ans. The characteristic features of chronic duodenal ulcer and chronic gastric ulcer are given in Table 3.5.

Table 3.5: Characteristic features of chronic duodenal ulcer and chronic gastric ulcer

	Chronic duodenal ulcer	Chronic gastric ulcer
Site of pain	Epigastric	Epigastric
Timing of pain	Occurs in empty stomach 3–4 hours after meals. Often pain in early hours of morning	Occurs after intake of food
Periodicity of pain	Marked periodicity of pain. Relief of symptoms for weeks/months	Periodicity present
Relieving factors	Food or antacids	Vomiting
Vomiting	Usually absent unless developed gastric outlet destruction	Marked vomiting
Bleeding	Hematemesis: Melena—60:40	Hematemesis: Melena—40:60
Tenderness	Tenderness 2.5 cm to the right of midline in transpyloric plane	Tenderness in the center of epigastrium

Q. What are the different types of gastric ulcer?

Ans. *Gastric ulcer may occur at any location in the stomach.*
* *Type I—gastric ulcer: Usually located at the lesser curvature. Not associated with excessive acid secretion. Acid secretion is low or normal.*
* *Type II: Usually occurs in the body of the stomach. Associated with excessive acid secretion. There may be associated duodenal ulcer.*
* *Type III: These are prepyloric ulcers. These ulcers behave like duodenal ulcer and are associated with excessive acid secretion.*
* *Type IV: These ulcers occurs high in the lesser curvature near GE junction. Not associated with high acid secretion.*
* *Type V: May occur at any site in the stomach. Associated with chronic NSAID intake.*

Q. What are the complications of peptic ulcer?

Ans. The complications of peptic ulcer are given in Table 3.6.

Table 3.6: Complications of peptic ulcer

Acute	Subacute	Chronic

1. Bleeding
  – Hematemesis
  – Melena
	1. Residual abscess	1. Stenosis
		  – Pyloric
		  – Duodenal

2. Perforation – Peritonitis		2. Hour glass stomach 3. Penetration into the pancreas or liver 4. Malignant change

Q. What are the complications of peptic ulcer surgery?

Ans. Immediate complications

* *General complications:* Pulmonary, cardiac and thromboembolic
* *Specific complications* of peptic ulcer surgery:
  – Bleeding
  – Paralytic ileus
  – Stomal obstruction
  – Duodenal fistula
  – Acute postoperative pancreatitis.

Late Complications

* Recurrent ulcer
* Gastrojejunocolic fistula
* Early and late dumping syndromes
* Bilious vomiting
* Anemia
* Nutritional deficit
* Intestinal obstruction
* Diarrhea
* Decalcifying bone diseases
* Gallstones
* Carcinoma in the gastric remnant.

Q. Following gastrojejunostomy there is bleeding in the postoperative period, how to manage?

Ans. *Conservative:* The initial treatment is conservative.

* Sedative.
* Injection pethidine (50 mg) intravenously
* Blood transfusion
* Gastric lavage with normal saline
* Monitoring of the patient's vitals: Pulse, blood pressure, urine output.

Surgical: If the bleeding is persistent and continuous, the patient needs re-exploration. The anterior layer is opened up and often the bleeding is found in the posterior anastomotic line. The bleeding points are under-run.

Q. Following gastrojejunostomy patient has very high nasogastric aspirate even on 9th postoperative day. What may be the likely cause and how to manage such a situation?

Ans. This may be due to:

* *Stomal obstruction* caused by edema of the stoma and technical factors causing a small stoma
* *Kinking of efferent loop*
* *Prolonged gastric atony* due to vagotomy
* *Rarely due to jejunogastric* intussusception.

If obstruction is due to stomal edema or gastric atony the treatment is to persist with nasogastric aspiration and IV fluid with correction of fluid and electrolyte imbalance.

If there is mechanical obstruction due to stomal narrowing, kinking of efferent loop and jejunogastric intussusception revision surgery may be required.

Q. How will you diagnose duodenal stump blow out?

Ans. Duodenal stump blow out is a serious complication following Billroth II gastrectomy. If a drain is kept during surgery, patient will have excessive bilious drainage through the drain. Patient may complain of intense thoracoabdominal pain, and if untreated will develop symptoms and signs of diffuse peritonitis.

Q. When does blow out occur?

Ans. Duodenal stump blow out usually occurs on the 4th to 5th postoperative day.

Q. How can you take care to prevent development of duodenal stump blow out?

Ans. Avoid suturing the duodenum when there is active inflammation in the duodenum. An alternative operation like gastrojejunostomy may be done or a controlled fistula is created by introducing a tube inside the duodenum. Ensure that there is no obstruction in the afferent loop which is a predisposing factor for development of duodenal stump blow out.

Q. How a duodenal stump blows out is managed?

Ans. If a drain is already in situ and draining well and there is no evidence of peritonitis, conservative treatment with:
* Total parenteral nutrition
* Correction of fluid and electrolyte balance
* Care of the local part.

It may allow spontaneous closure of the duodenal fistula.

If the drain is not in situ, a tube or sump suction drain is placed in the hepatorenal pouch of Morrison and total parenteral nutrition is continued.

If there is no distal obstruction almost all fistulas heal with conservative treatment and it may need long time even up to 4–6 weeks.

Q. What do you mean by recurrent peptic ulcer?

Ans. Recurrence of peptic ulcer following effective surgical treatment is called recurrent peptic ulcer. The usual sites of recurrent ulcer are:
* Anastomotic ulcer at the gastrojejunostomy
* Anastomotic ulcer at the gastroduodenal stoma
* Ulcer in the stomach remnant
* Ulcer in the duodenum.

Q. What are the causes of recurrent peptic ulcer?

Ans.
* Incomplete surgery: Vagotomy was not complete or the stomach resection was inadequate
* Cigarette smoking
* Endocrine disorder like gastrinoma.

Q. How will you diagnose recurrent peptic ulcer?

* Severe, persistent pain aggravated after intake of food

- Bleeding may be slow leading to anemia or there may be hematemesis or melena
- Rarely perforation may occur
- Diagnosis may be confirmed by endoscopy.

Q. How will you treat recurrent peptic ulcer?

Ans. *Medical treatment:*

- H_2 blockers or PPIs are effective, but long-term therapy is required
- Investigate for hypergastrinemia or hypercalcemia. If present, treatment of the primary condition.

Surgical treatment: Indicated in situation, if there is failure of medical treatment.

Q. What are the options for surgical treatment for recurrent peptic ulceration?

Ans. If vagotomy was done earlier completeness of vagotomy is to be ascertained by doing spit and chew test.

If this is positive, it suggests incomplete vagotomy and surgical treatment in such situation involves a thorough search for intact vagal nerve fibers during surgery. If intact vagal fibers are found the operation should be revagotomy. If the stoma is inadequate it should be revised. Alternatively partial gastrectomy is to be considered.

If Billroth II gastrectomy is done earlier, if hypersecretion is present and the stoma is adequate a vagotomy will be a suitable procedure.

If Billroth I gastrectomy has been done earlier, vagotomy or revision gastrectomy will cure the ulcer.

Q. What are postcibal syndromes?

Ans. The postcibal syndromes are important complications following gastrectomy or vagotomy and drainage. Depending on relation to timing of meals these are further subdivided into early and late postcibal syndromes.

Q. What are the characteristics of early postcibal syndrome?

Ans. Immediately after intake of food patient complains of some vasomotor symptoms like sweating, sensation of warmth, tachycardia and abdominal symptoms like colicky abdominal pain and diarrhea. The attack usually lasts for 30–40 minutes and is usually relieved by lying down.

Q. Why does the patient develop these symptoms?

Ans. Following gastrectomy there is rapid emptying of stomach leading to distension of afferent loop. The small bowel is filled with food from the stomach which has a high osmotic load. There is sequestration of fluid from the circulation into the small intestine also. This results in a net fall in blood volume leading to the vasomotor symptoms.

The alternative explanation is, after intake of a carbohydrate meal there is initial transient hyperglycemia. This leads to suppression of absorption of further glucose from the intestine and the intestinal content becomes hyperosmotic and there is shift of fluid from blood into the intestinal lumen leading to hypovolemia and the resultant vasomotor symptoms.

Q. How will you treat early postcibal syndrome?

Ans. With passage of time there may be spontaneous regression of these symptoms.

Others measures include:

- Small meals preferably dry and with less carbohydrate
- Somatostatin analog, i.e. octreotide administered before meals is beneficial for some patients
- Codeine phosphate may reduce the intestinal hurry
  Persistent symptoms may need revisional surgery
- If Billroth II operation has been done a conversion to a Billroth I may help
- The intestinal hurry may be avoided by interposition of a 10 cm antiperistaltic jejunal loop between the stomach and duodenum.

Q. What are characteristics of late postcibal syndrome?

Ans. This usually occurs about 2 hours after meals and patient complains of tremor, faintness and nausea, and is usually relieved by glucose intake and aggravated by exercise.

Q. How late postcibal syndromes develop?

Ans. With rapid gastric emptying there is transient hyperglycemia. This leads to increased secretion of insulin, which results in hypoglycemia and blood sugar may be as low as 50 mg%. This explains relief of symptoms with administration of glucose.

Q. How late dumping is treated?

Ans. Conservative measures are same as early dumping syndrome. Octreotide is very effective.

Q. What are the nutritional problems following gastrectomy?

Ans.
- *Weight loss* due to less food intake and less absorption
- *Steatorrhea* due to poor pancreatic function or inactivation of pancreatic enzyme in the afferent loop
- *Diarrhea:* Due to intestinal hurry or steatorrhea
- *Iron deficiency anemia* due to reduced absorption or blood loss from the gastric mucosa. Iron deficiency is more pronounced when the duodenum is bypassed. Megaloblastic anemia is due to gastric mucosal atrophy or following total gastrectomy. This may be due to a combination of reduced intrinsic factor or bacterial colonization of gut which results in destruction of the B_{12} in the gut.
- *Calcium deficiency:* Due to reduced absorption of calcium in the small intestine or due to reduced acidity in the proximal small intestine. This may lead to osteoporosis.

Q. How will you treat megaloblastic anemia following gastrectomy?

Ans. There is very large store of vitamin B_{12} in the body and it takes long time for B_{12} deficiency to develop. However, following gastrectomy B12 supplementation is desirable.

Intramuscular injection of cyanocobalamin: 100 μg weekly till the blood picture is normal. Thereafter maintenance dose of cyanocobalamin every month.

Q. What are the effects of vagotomy on the GI tract?

Ans.

* *Acid secretion:* Complete vagotomy leads to anacidity of the gastric juice.
* *Loss of motility of the stomach* leads to delayed emptying, retention of food particle, nausea and vomiting and foul eructations.
* *Effect on rest of bowel:* Variable. 30% patient may have increased bowel activity leading to diarrhea.
* *Gallbladder:* Motility function may be disturbed leading to increased incidence of gallstone disease.

Q. What is the relation between peptic ulcer surgery and carcinoma of stomach?

Ans. Following partial gastrectomy, the stomach remnant is slightly more prone to develop carcinoma of stomach. Also following vagotomy and drainage there is slightly increased risk of carcinoma of stomach. This is related to anacidity (absence acid secretion due to vagotomy), atrophic gastritis and bile reflux gastritis following peptic ulcer surgery. The lag period between the ulcer surgery and development of carcinoma is usually 10–15 years. However, highly selective vagotomy has not been found to be associated with increased incidence of carcinoma of stomach.

Q. What are the causes of postvagotomy diarrhea?

Ans. About 5% patients following peptic ulcer surgery (except highly selective vagotomy) may suffer from intractable diarrhea.

The exact mechanism of diarrhea is uncertain. This may be related to rapid gastric emptying, denervation of small and large gut and exaggerated peptide response.

Q. How will you treat postvagotomy diarrhea?

Ans.

* Some authors regard diarrhea and dumping syndrome as being essentially the same problem. It is difficult to treat postvagotomy diarrhea
* Antidiarrheal like codeine phosphate may help
* Octreotide is not very effective in postvagotomy diarrhea
* Revisional surgery is also not very helpful.

CASE OF CHRONIC CHOLECYSTITIS

Q. What is your case? (Summary of a case of chronic cholecystitis)

Ans. A 35-year-old lady presented with history of recurrent attack of pain in right upper half of abdomen for last 1 year. The pain started in the right upper half of the abdomen 1 year back, which was sudden in onset. The pain was colicky in nature, severe in intensity and was relieved by analgesics. The pain radiated to the back of the right side of the chest and right shoulder region. Patient has similar attacks of pain for last 1year initially at an interval of 3–4 months, but for last 1 month patient is having dull aching constant pain in right upper half of abdomen. Patient complains of heart burn, acidity, flatulence and sensation of fullness after meals for the same duration. Bowel and bladder habits are normal. There are no significant symptoms suggestive of any systemic disease. There are no significant past family or personal history.

On examination: On general survey patient is conscious and cooperative, no jaundice, anemia, pulse 86 beats/min. On abdominal examination, on inspection, the shape and contour of the abdomen is normal. Umbilicus is normal. Abdomen is moving normally with respiration, no visible peristalsis, no pulsatile movement and skin of the abdomen is normal. On palpation the abdomen has a normal soft elastic feel. There is no superficial or deep tenderness in abdomen. Liver and spleen are not palpable. No other mass is palpable. On percussion the abdomen is normally tympanitic and there is no free fluid in abdomen. On auscultation normal bowel sounds are heard. External genitalia are normal. Per rectal and per vaginal, examination is not done. Systemic examination is normal.

Q. What is your diagnosis?

Ans. This is a case of chronic cholecystitis.

(In case of mucocele of gallbladder, the history and examination part is the same as chronic cholecystitis, except on abdominal examination on inspection there is a globular intra-abdominal lump in the right hypochondriac and right lumbar region moving up and down with respiration. On palpation a lump is palpable in the said region, which is intra-abdominal, moving up and down with respiration, nontender, surface is smooth, lower margin, medial and lateral margins are palpable, but the upper margin is passing deep to the costal margin, it is tense cystic in feel. Liver and spleen are not palpable.

Q. How will you demonstrate Murphy's sign?

Ans. *See* abdomen examination (Figs 3.15A and B, Page No. 97).

Q. When do you find Murphy's sign is positive?

Ans. Murphy's sign is positive in acute cholecystitis. In chronic cholecystitis Murphy's sign is not positive.

Q. What are the other possibilities in this patient?

Ans.
* Chronic duodenal ulcer
* Chronic gastric ulcer
* Chronic pancreatitis
* Recurrent appendicitis
* Hiatus hernia
* Right-sided renal calculus
* Chronic pyelonephritis.

Q. How will you manage this patient?

Ans. I would like to confirm my diagnosis by doing a USG of upper abdomen.

Q. How ultrasonography helps in diagnosis of biliary tract disease?

Ans. Ultrasonography is a reliable investigation for evaluation of biliary tract disease.
* *Gallbladder:*
  – Size of the gallbladder whether gallbladder is normal sized, contracted or distended
  – Walls of the gallbladder—normal wall thickness or any thickening of wall

- Intraluminal calculi—intraluminal calculi may be seen as a echogenic shadow in the gallbladder lumen with both anterior and posterior acoustic shadow. Any associated mass in gallbladder may be seen.
- *Common bile duct:* The upper end of common bile duct may be seen and its diameter may be measured. Any intraluminal calculi in the bile duct lumen may be seen. However, stone at lower end of bile duct may sometimes be missed on USG.
- *Liver:* Liver may be seen well and any solid or cystic lesion in the liver may be ascertained. Any dilatation of the intrahepatic biliary radicles may be seen well.
- *Pancreas:* The pancreas may be seen and any mass in relation to the pancreas may be seen well. The diameter of the pancreatic duct may be measured. Any calculus in the pancreatic duct or parenchymal calcification may be seen. The parenchymal echotexture may be seen clearly and chronic or acute pancreatitis may be diagnosed.

Q. If USG shows stone in gallbladder what else would you like to do?

Ans. If USG shows stone in gallbladder and common bile duct is normal and there is no history of jaundice or cholangitis then no further investigation is required to confirm diagnosis of gallstone disease.

We would like to do some more investigation to assess fitness of the patient for general anesthesia.
- Complete hemogram: Hb%, TLC, DLC and ESR
- Blood for sugar, urea and creatinine
- Liver function test
- Urine for routine examination
- Chest X-ray (posteroanterior view)
- ECG.

Q. When will you consider doing an ERCP on MRCP in patient with gallstone disease?

Ans. Ultrasonography is not always reliable for evaluation of bile duct as it is difficult to study the lower part of the bile duct due to overlapping bowel gas shadow. So evaluation of CBD may need to be done in following situations:
- If there is suspicion of stone in the common bile duct on USG examination
- If there is history of jaundice or the patient is having jaundice
- If LFT shows elevation of serum enzymes—ALT, AST and alkaline phosphatase
- USG shows dilatation of common bile duct.

Q. What are the advantages and disadvantages of MRCP for evaluation of bile duct?

Ans. Magnetic resonance cholangiopancreatography (MRCP) is a newer modality of investigation and it provides virtual reconstruction of the whole biliary tree from the slices of MRI of the hepatobiliary tree and can give very good picture of the entire biliary tree. It is a non-invasive investigation, no radiation exposure, no dye is required. The biliary tract dilatation, any obstruction due to stone or growth may be ascertained.

The limitation of MRCP is that it has only diagnostic value as no intervention is possible.

Q. What are the advantages and disadvantages of ERCP?

Ans. The advantage of ERCP is therapeutic intervention like sphincterotomy and stone extraction or biliary stenting is possible. Bile aspirated may be used for exfoliative cytology. Biopsy from periampullary lesion or brush cytology from the bile duct may be taken.

This is an invasive investigation. It requires introduction of a gastroduodenoscope, cannulation of bile and pancreatic duct and injection of a dye. There is chance of postprocedure cholangitis or pancreatitis, which may be life-threatening.

Q. How will you treat this patient?

Ans. I will treat this patient by cholecystectomy. I would prefer to do laparoscopic cholecystectomy.

Q. Why do you prefer laparoscopic cholecystectomy?

Ans.

* Laparoscopic cholecystectomy has been established as gold standard for the treatment of gallstone diseases
    – Surgery is safe in the hands of a trained surgeon
    – Less pain, less hospital stays
    – Cosmetic
    – Early return to work is possible
    – More acceptance by the patient.

Q. While you take consent for laparoscopic cholecystectomy what consent should be taken?

Ans. Informed consent is to be taken. Patient should be explained that if laparoscopic procedure is not safe it may need conversion to open cholecystectomy.

Q. Describe the steps of laparoscopic cholecystectomy?

Ans. *See* Operative Surgery Section, Page No. 1100–1102, Chapter 22.

Q. What are the incisions for open cholecystectomy?

Ans.

1. Right subcostal incision (Kocher's incision)
2. Right upper paramedian incision
3. Midline incision
4. Mayo Robson's incision. Right paramedian with extension to midline
5. Upper abdominal transverse incision (Fig. 3.34).

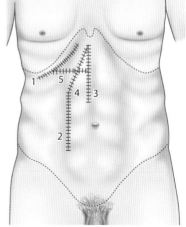

Fig. 3.34: Incisions for open cholecystectomy (See text for 1, 2, 3, 4, 5)

Q. Where do you place mops during open cholecystectomy?

Ans. During open cholecystectomy after opening the peritoneum and confirmation of diagnosis, three mops are placed properly to expose the gallbladder area. One mop is placed in the hepatorenal pouch of Morrison to retract the hepatic flexure of the colon downward. (1) Another mop is inserted to retract the transverse colon and the duodenum. (2) The third mop is placed medially to retract the stomach. (3) The Calot's triangle area is exposed by retracting these structures with the left hand of the assistant and by retracting the liver upwards by placement of a Deaver's retractor (Fig. 3.35).

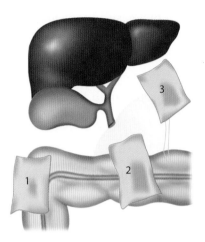

Fig. 3.35: Placement of mops during cholecystectomy (See text for 1, 2, 3)

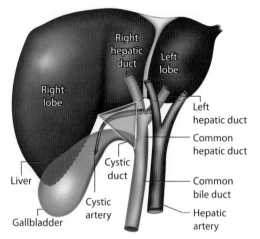

Fig. 3.36: Boundary of Calot's triangle

Q. What is the boundary of Calot's triangle?

Ans. Calot's triangle is bounded below by the cystic duct, medially by the common hepatic duct and above by the inferior surface of the liver. The triangle is crossed by the cystic artery (Fig. 3.36).

Q. What is cystic pedicle?

Ans. It is the two layers of peritoneum covering the cystic duct and the cystic artery and extends from the neck of the gallbladder to the lesser omentum.

Q. Sometime during cholecystectomy Calot's triangle area is found densely adherent and the structures in the Calot's triangle area cannot be identified properly what do you do then?

Ans. In such situation there is risk of injury to the bile duct by blind dissection so it is better to do a fundus first cholecystectomy. The fundus of the gallbladder is dissected first from the gallbladder bed and the gallbladder is dissected off up to the neck of the gallbladder. Thus cystic duct may be identified and ligated and divided avoiding injury to the bile duct. If there is bleeding it should be controlled by pressure and packing rather than by blind clamping.

Q. What is mini-cholecystectomy?

Ans. Open cholecystectomy done through a small right subcostal incision of about 5 cm is called mini-cholecystectomy. This is a good technique with very little postoperative pain, shorter hospital stay and it has been claimed to be comparable to laparoscopic cholecystectomy.

Q. If the cystic duct is found densely adherent to the common bile duct what will you do?

Ans. In such situation there is risk of injury to the bile duct while dissecting the cystic duct. It is better to open the gallbladder and the stones are removed. Gallbladder removed leaving behind a sleeve of neck and the neck of the gallbladder is oversewn with silk suture.

Q. While doing cholecystectomy when will you decide to explore the common bile duct?

Ans. This decision will depend on:

* *Preoperative criteria:*
  - Patient is icteric or there is history of jaundice or cholangitis
  - LFT is abnormal with elevation of ALT/AST and alkaline phosphatase
  - Preoperative USG/ERCP/MRCP has shown stone in common bile duct or the common bile duct is dilated.
* *Intraoperative criteria:*
  - Palpable stone in common bile duct is the absolute indication for opening the common bile duct
  - Common bile duct is dilated more than 1 cm
  - Gallbladder contains a single facetted stone with cystic duct dilatation
  - Intraoperative cholangiogram shows a stone in common bile duct.

Q. What is postcholecystectomy syndrome?

Ans. In 15% cases cholecystectomy fails to relieve the symptoms for which the operation was done. This is called postcholecystectomy syndrome.

The important causes of postcholecystectomy syndrome are:

* Missed stone in common bile duct
* A stone in cystic duct stump
* Operative damage to biliary tree
* Peptic ulcer
* Hiatus hernia
* Gastroesophageal reflux disease.

Q. How will you manage a patient with postcholecystectomy syndrome?

Ans.

* Clinical evaluation by detailed history and physical examination and relevant examination
* Liver function test
* USG of upper abdomen
* Upper GI endoscopy
* Barium meal X-ray of esophagus, stomach and duodenum
* Appropriate treatment depending on the cause.

Q. What are the different types of gallstone?

Ans.

* Cholesterol stone
* Pigment stone
* Mixed stone.

Q. What are the characteristics of cholesterol gallstones?

Q. What are the characteristics of pigment gallstones?

Q. What are the characteristics of mixed gallstones?

Q. How cholesterol stones are formed in the gallbladder?

Q. Which factors determine solubility of cholesterol in bile?

Q. When bile becomes supersaturated with cholesterol?

Q. In which form cholesterol remains in solution in bile?

Q. What is nucleation?

Q. Which factors initiate cholesterol precipitation?

Q. Which factors increase cholesterol secretion in bile?

Q. What are the conditions causing reduced bile salts concentration in bile?

Q. Why infection is important for development of gallstones?

Q. What are the compositions of mixed stones?

Q. How chenodeoxycholic acid (CDCA) and ursodeoxycholic acid (UDCA) may prevent stone formation?

For answer to these question. *See* Surgical Pathology Section, Gallstones Diseases, Page No. 894–901, Chapter 18.

Q. What may be the presentation of patients with gallstones?

Ans. Patients with gallstones may have varied presentations:
* Stones remaining in the gallbladder
    – Silent stones: Patient is asymptomatic and gallstone detected in routine check-up
    – Biliary colic
    – Acute cholecystitis and its sequelae: Gangrene/perforation/local abscess/biliary peritonitis
    – Chronic cholecystitis
    – Mucocele of gallbladder
    – Empyema of gallbladder
    – Carcinoma of gallbladder
* Stones migrated into the bile duct
    – Obstructive jaundice
    – Recurrent cholangitis
    – Acute pancreatitis
* Stones migrated into the intestine
    – Gallstone ileus.

Q. Describe a classical attack of biliary colic?

Ans. Acute onset of pain in right upper quadrant of abdomen, severe spasmodic in nature, may radiate to back of chest or shoulder. Pain may last for few minutes to several hours. Pain is often precipitated by a fatty meal. Attacks of pain are usually self-limiting, but recur in an unpredictable manner. Fever and leukocytosis are uncommon. Pain may occur in the epigastrium or rarely in the left upper quadrant of the abdomen (in 4% cases).

Q. What are the features of acute cholecystitis?

Ans.

* History
  - Acute onset pain in right upper quadrant of abdomen. Severe spasmodic in nature with radiation to back or the right shoulder. Later on pain becomes dull aching and constant and usually lasts longer than 24 hours
  - Marked nausea and vomiting
  - Fever
* Examination
  - Tachycardia and jaundice may be present
  - Abdominal examination may reveal marked tenderness in right upper quadrant of abdomen
  - Murphy's sign will be positive
  - A vague mass may be palpable
* Investigation
  - Leukocytosis is usually a feature
  - Liver function test: There may be mild rise of serum bilirubin
  - USG examination may diagnose acute cholecystitis, wall thickening, pericholecystic fluid collection.

Q. What are the sequelae of acute cholecystitis?

Ans.

* *Resolution:* Inflammation subsides and patient recovers
* *Gangrene:* Infection may lead to gangrenous change in gallbladder manifested by increasing pain, toxemia and appearance of rebound tenderness
* *Perforation of gallbladder:* Perforation may be
  - *Localized:* Localized abscess formation manifested by severe pain, fever with chill and rigors, and extreme tenderness in right upper quadrant of abdomen
  - *Generalized perforation:* Leading to generalized biliary peritonitis manifested by generalized pain abdomen, muscle guard or rigidity and extreme tenderness all over abdomen
  - *Perforation into a neighboring* viscus most commonly duodenum, stomach or colon.

Q. What is mucocele of gallbladder?

Ans. When there is obstruction to the cystic duct or the neck of the gallbladder by a stone or a growth then the contained bile in the gallbladder is absorbed by the gallbladder epithelium and is replaced by mucus secreted by the gallbladder epithelium. The content is usually a clear sterile fluid.

Q. What is empyema of gallbladder?

Ans. Gallbladder is filled with pus and may follow as a consequence of acute cholecystitis or as result of infection of a mucocele. In 50% cases the contained pus is sterile.

Q. What is acalculous cholecystitis?

Ans. Acute or chronic inflammation of the gallbladder in absence of gallstone is known as acalculous cholecystitis.

Q. What are the predisposing factors for development of acalculous cholecystitis?

Ans.
- Critically ill patients in intensive therapy unit
- Following major surgery, trauma or burns.

Q. What is strawberry gallbladder?

Ans. There is deposition of cholesterol crystals in the submucosa and they may appear as yellow specks and the interior of the gallbladder looks like a strawberry. This may be associated with cholesterol stones in gallbladder.

Q. What is lithogenic bile?

Ans. In normal bile the cholesterol, phospholipids and bile salts remain in optimum concentration. This keeps the cholesterol in solution. Bile supersaturated with cholesterol is known as lithogenic bile as this predisposes to gallstone formation (Fig. 3.37).

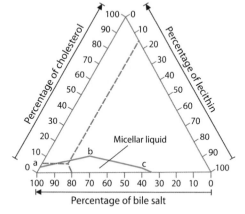

Fig. 3.37: Cholesterol solubility in bile salt. (a, b, c denote normal solubility range of cholesterol in percentage of bile salts and lecithin)

Q. What do you mean by silent gallstone?

Ans. Incidentally found gallstones during examination for other pathology or in routine health check-up that does not produce symptoms are called silent gallstones.

Q. What is the incidence of silent gallstones?

Ans. In western population, 10% of men and 20% of women have silent gallstones.

Q. What is the natural history of silent gallstones?

Ans. There is high incidence of silent gallstones in the community. However, all the patients do not develop symptoms. In long follow-up it is established that the chance of developing symptoms is approximately 1% per year. So, only 20% patients have the chance of developing symptoms over 20 years.

Q. When do you consider prophylactic cholecystectomy in silent gallstones?

Ans. Prophylactic cholecystectomy is not indicated in all patients with silent gallstones. Prophylactic cholecystectomy is indicated in population at high risk of developing complications. This includes:
- Diabetic patients
- Patients on immunosuppressive therapy
- Candidates for renal transplant
- Large gallstones (>2.5 cm)
- Multiple small gallstones
- Patients living in high-risk areas where there is increased incidence of gallbladder carcinoma
- Porcelain gallbladder in view of increased risk of carcinoma of gallbladder.

Q. What is incidental cholecystectomy?

Ans. Different series has reported high incidence of biliary symptoms following abdominal surgery with incidental finding of gallstones. Increased incidence of cholecystitis in the postoperative period is due to bile stasis, dehydration, fasting, use of narcotics and associated gallstones.

Simple cholecystectomy is now widely recommended as a concomitant procedure during the course of laparotomy for unrelated condition, provided the exposure is adequate and there are no associated hepatobiliary risk factors, e.g. abnormal LFT, cirrhosis, shrunken gallbladder and dilated common bile duct.

CASES PRESENTING WITH OBSTRUCTIVE JAUNDICE

There are a number of long cases, which presents with obstructive jaundice
1. Obstructive jaundice due to periampullary carcinoma or carcinoma head of pancreas
2. Obstructive jaundice due to cholangiocarcinoma involving the bile duct
3. Carcinoma of gallbladder with obstructive jaundice due to metastasis in the porta hepatis or invasion to the bile duct
4. Obstructive jaundice due to choledocholithiasis
5. Gastrointestinal malignancy with metastasis in the porta hepatis or liver metastasis.

■ OBSTRUCTIVE JAUNDICE DUE TO PERIAMPULLARY CARCINOMA OR CARCINOMA OF HEAD OF PANCREAS

Q. What is your case? (Summary of a case of obstructive jaundice due to periampullary carcinoma)

Ans. A 65-year-old gentleman presented with yellowish discoloration of eyes and urine for last 6 months and anorexia and weight loss for the same duration. Patient noticed gradual onset of yellowish discoloration of eyes and urine for last 6 months. The yellowish discoloration was gradually deepening for about 4 months and afterward there was diminution of yellowish discoloration for about 1 month. But for last 1 month the yellowish discoloration is again increasing in intensity. Patient complains of itching all over the body. Patient is passing clay colored stool since the onset of yellowish discoloration of eyes and urine. Patient complains of anorexia and significant loss of weight over last 6 months. Complains of sensation of fullness after meals for last 3 months. No history of vomiting or hematemesis. History of passage of black tarry stool 2 months back, which lasted for about 7 days. Passing stool twice a day, no history of alteration of bowel habit. No urinary complaint. Patient complains of a mass in right upper half of abdomen for last 5 months. Patient has no other systemic symptoms.

On examination on general survey, nutrition is poor, pallor is present and the patient is deeply jaundiced. No cervical lymphadenopathy. Abdominal examination—shape and contour of abdomen normal. Umbilicus is normal. Liver and spleen are not palpable. A lump is palpable in the right hypochondriac region extending to the epigastric and right lumbar region. The lower, medial and the lateral margins are palpable and the upper margin passes deep to the right costal margin. The palpable swelling appears to be the palpable gallbladder. There is no free fluid in the abdomen. Bowel sounds are audible. Per rectal (in female both per rectal and per vaginal) examination not done.

So, this is a case of obstructive jaundice probably due to periampullary carcinoma.

(If the jaundice is progressively increasing and there is no history of melena with associated diminution of jaundice—the provisional diagnosis may be given as: obstructive jaundice due to carcinoma head of pancreas).

Q. What is your diagnosis?

Ans. This is a case of obstructive jaundice due to periampullary carcinoma (or carcinoma head of pancreas).

Q. Why do you say this is a case of obstructive jaundice?

Ans. Patient complains of gradually progressive increase in yellowish discoloration of eyes and urine. Patient is having itching all over the body and he is passing clay colored stool since the onset of jaundice. So, this is a case of obstructive jaundice.

Q. Why do you say obstructive jaundice due to periampullary carcinoma in this patient?

Ans. Patient is elderly and presented with history of painless progressive jaundice for last 6 months. Jaundice is associated with itching all over the body and passage of clay colored stool. Patient had melena 2 months back which was followed by diminution in intensity of jaundice. Patient also complains of anorexia and weight loss for last 6 months. Patient also complained of a lump in his right side of upper abdomen for last 3 months. No history of biliary colic.

On examination, patient is deeply jaundiced, malnourished and abdominal examination gallbladder is palpable, which is tense cystic in feel and is nontender. Liver and spleen is not palpable.

So, obstructive jaundice in this patient is likely to be due to periampullary carcinoma in this patient.

Q. What are the other possibilities?

- Cholangiocarcinoma involving the bile duct
- Carcinoma of gallbladder
- Choledocholithiasis
- Lymph node mass in the porta causing biliary obstruction (metastatic lymphoma, tuberculosis)
- Bile duct stricture
- Sclerosing cholangitis
- Chronic pancreatitis.

Q. How will you palpate the gallbladder?

Ans. *See* Palpation of Gallbladder (*see* Fig. 3.14, Page No. 96).

Q. How will you palpate the liver?

Ans. *See* Palpation of Liver (*see* Figs 3.11A to D, Page No. 94-95).

Q. How will you palpate the spleen?

Ans. *See* Palpation of Spleen (see Figs 3.16A to G, Page No. 97-98).

Q. Why spleen palpation is important in patient with obstructive jaundice?

Ans. Associated splenomegaly may suggest associated portal hypertension. Portal hypertension may be due to extrahepatic portal venous obstruction due to splenic vein thrombosis or secondary biliary cirrhosis.

Q. What are the causes of pain in carcinoma of pancreas?

Ans.
* The pain in carcinoma of pancreas may be due to:
    – Involvement of retropancreatic nerve by the malignant growth
    – Pancreatic duct obstruction causing stasis within the gland.

Q. What may be the cause of hepatomegaly in carcinoma of pancreas?

Ans. Hepatomegaly in carcinoma pancreas may be either due to:
* Metastasis in the liver
* Biliary stasis causing hepatomegaly due to hydrohepatosis.

Q. What is Courvoisier's law?

Ans. If in a jaundice patient, the gallbladder is palpable, then it is not due to choledocholithiasis as the gallbladder would have been fibrosed by previous cholecystitis (Figs 3.38A and B).

Q. What are the exceptions to Courvoisier's law?

Ans.
* Double impaction of stone—one at common bile duct and another at cystic duct
* Primary CBD stone
* Distended gallbladder due to large stone load.

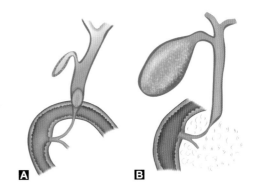

Figs 3.38A and B: Courvoisier's Law. (A) Choledocholithiasis gallbladder fibrosed and contracted. (B) Carcinoma of head pancreas gallbladder distended

Q. In what percentage of cases of carcinoma of pancreas gallbladder is found palpable?

Ans. Gallbladder is palpable in 30% of cases of carcinoma of head of pancreas and in 50% cases of periampullary carcinoma.

Q. What do you mean by periampullary carcinoma?

Ans. This includes a group of malignant tumors arising at or near the ampulla
* Adenocarcinoma from head of pancreas adjacent to the ampulla (within 2 cm): 40–60%
* Ampullary tumor arising from ampulla of Vater: 20–40%
* Distal bile duct carcinoma:10%
* Duodenal carcinoma adjacent to the ampulla: 10%.

Q. What investigation will you suggest in this patient?

Ans. I will do some investigations for confirmation of diagnosis.
* Liver function test
    – Serum bilirubin:
        - Total
        - Conjugated
        - Unconjugated

  – Alkaline phosphatase
  – Serum enzymes ALT/AST
  – Serum protein: Total/albumin/globulin
  – Prothrombin time.
+ USG of hepatobiliary system.
Further investigations will be guided by the USG report.

Q. What changes do you expect in liver function test?

Ans. In obstructive jaundice conjugated bilirubin will be high, serum alkaline phosphatase will be high, ALT and AST may show some increase. Serum proteins may be low. Prothrombin time may be prolonged.

Q. Why prothrombin time is prolonged in obstructive jaundice?

Ans. In obstructive jaundice there is defect in absorption of fat soluble vitamins like vitamin A, D, E and K from the gut. Vitamin K is required for synthesis of prothrombin in the liver. Deficiency of vitamin K dependent coagulation factors may cause prolongation of prothrombin time.

Q. How can you correct prolonged prothrombin time in obstructive jaundice?

Ans. Parenteral administration of vitamin K (deep intramuscular) for 5–7 days will correct prothrombin time in patients with obstructive jaundice.

A patient of obstructive jaundice received vitamin K for 5 days for prolonged prothrombin time but there is no improvement. What does it indicate?

If there is associated hepatocellular dysfunction then prolonged prothrombin time will not be corrected by administration of vitamin K.

Q. How will you correct prothrombin time in such situation?

Ans. Prolonged prothrombin time in such situation may be corrected by fresh frozen plasma and fresh blood transfusion.

Q. How ultrasonography helps in evaluation of patients with obstructive jaundice?

Ans.
+ It can delineate the anatomy and any lesion in liver, gallbladder, common bile duct, pancreas and any associated lymphadenopathy
+ Can detect any stone in gallbladder and common bile duct
+ In case of periampullary or carcinoma head pancreas USG may show the lesion. However, in small ampullary tumor USG may not show the lesion
+ In periampullary carcinoma (or carcinoma head pancreas) the bile duct may appear dilated. The pancreatic duct may also be dilated (double duct sign).

Q. What other investigations will you do in this patient?

Ans. If USG showed a mass in the pancreas and there is dilatation of biliary and pancreatic tree (double duct sign), I will do a pancreatic protocol CECT scan.

Q. What do you mean by pancreatic protocol CECT scan?

Ans. Pancreatic protocol CECT scan is required for evaluation of focal pancreatic lesion. This involves taking images in number of phases with axial thickness of 1–4 mm. In this study a negative oral contrast (either water or mannitol) is given to differentiate distended duodenum from pancreas.

- Precontrast scan is done from diaphragm to the third part of duodenum.
- After unenhanced scanning administer 1.5 mL/kg of iopromide intravenously for 30 seconds using a power injector at a rate of 3–5 mL/sec.
- Triple-phase, dynamic CT scans were then obtained. The scanning delay for the arterial, pancreatic, and portal-venous phases was approximately 25s, 40s, and 70s, respectively, after the initiation of the contrast injection
- Multiple postcontrast images are obtained:
  - Arterial phase: 25 seconds after contrast injection. The hypervascular neuroendocrine tumors are better seen in arterial phase
  - Pancreatic parenchymal phase: 40 seconds after contrast injection. Hypovascular pancreatic adenocarcinomas are better seen in pancreatic parenchymal phase. The hypovascular tumor is seen in contrast to the normally enhancing pancreatic parenchyma.
  - Portal venous phase: 70 seconds after injection of contrast. Vascular invasion by the tumor and liver metastases are better seen in the portal venous phase. Some endocrine tumors are also better seen in portal venous phase.

Q. How does CT scan help in evaluation of pancreatic head lesion?

Ans. Contrast-enhanced computed tomography (CECT) is helpful for:
Delineation of the pancreatic mass
- Relationship of the mass to the portal vein and superior mesenteric vessels
- Level of bile duct obstruction
- Any dilatation of the pancreatic duct
- Any regional lymph node enlargement
- Any liver deposits or pelvic deposits
- Presence of ascites.

Q. When will you consider ERCP?

Ans. Routine endoscopic retrograde cholangiopancreatography (ERCP) is not indicated in patient with obstructive jaundice due to carcinoma head pancreas or periampullary carcinoma.
- In suspected periampullary carcinoma a side viewing endoscopy may show the ampullary region, if any growth is found it can be biopsied
- Both bile duct and pancreatic duct may be cannulated and dye injected to visualize both the bile duct and the pancreatic duct
- May show site of obstruction in the common bile duct with proximal dilatation
- Bile may be collected during ERCP and exfoliative cytology from the bile aspirated may help in diagnosis of cholangiocarcinoma
- Brush cytology during ERCP may be helpful for diagnosis of cholangiocarcinoma
- Endoscopic biliary stenting may be done for palliation of jaundice or relief of jaundice in preoperative period to improve liver function.

Q. What is the role of preoperative biliary stenting?

Ans. Preoperative biliary stenting is not routinely recommended in patient with obstructive jaundice due to a periampullary or head lesion. The usefulness of preoperative stenting is questionable in patients who are candidates for surgical resection. Preoperative biliary stenting may increase the chance of wound infection.

So, ERCP is reserved for cases in whom palliation of jaundice is required in advance cases. Also indicated when neoadjuvant chemotherapy is indicated before surgical treatment is considered.

Q. What is the role of angiography in evaluation of carcinoma of pancreas?

Ans.
- With good quality contrast CT scan which may show any invasion of vessels by the pancreatic growth, an angiography is not routinely required
- Angiographic appearance of occlusion of celiac, superior mesenteric vessels or portal vein suggests nonresectability
- Distortion of the vessels is commonly seen.

Q. How can a barium meal X-ray help in diagnosis of periampullary carcinoma?

Ans.
- Although not done routinely some finding in barium meal X-ray helps in diagnosis of periampullary carcinoma or carcinoma head of pancreas
- In ampullary growth:
  - Mucosal irregularity, *rose thorn appearance* of medial border of duodenum
  - Filling defect in the region of ampulla giving an *inverted 3 appearance*
- Carcinoma of head of pancreas
  - Widening of C-loop
  - Gastric distension due to gastric outlet obstruction.

Q. Do you like to do a percutaneous transhepatic cholangiography (PTC) in this case?

Ans. With advancement in imaging CECT scan can delineate the whole biliary tree.

With advent of MRCP, which can delineate the whole biliary tree nicely the role of PTC has become very limited as it is an invasive procedure.
- If patient is deeply jaundiced and a percutaneous transhepatic biliary drainage is contemplated then a PTC followed by PTBD may be done.

Q. What is double duct sign?

Ans. In ERCP or MRCP or other imaging if both the bile duct and the pancreatic duct show dilatation with constriction of both the ducts in the region of head of pancreas it is called double duct sign.

This is found in periampullary carcinoma (or carcinoma of head of pancreas).

This may also be found in chronic pancreatitis.

Q. What other investigations would you like to do in this patient?

Ans. I would like to do some more investigations to assess the patient for fitness for GA.
- Complete hemogram—Hb% TLC, DLC and ESR
- Chest X-ray (posteroanterior view)
- ECG
- Blood for sugar/urea and creatinine
- Blood for serum electrolytes—Na, K and Cl
- Urine for routine examination.

Q. What is the role of endoscopic ultrasonography (EUSG) in evaluation of carcinoma pancreas?

Ans. Endoscopic ultrasonography (EUSG) has an important role in evaluation of pancreatic tumors. Small tumors (<2 cm) can be well-demonstrated in EUSG. The relationship of the tumor to the vasculature may be well seen. The regional lymph nodes may also be seen well. If required an EUSG-guided FNAC may be done.

However, a good quality CT scan may provide these informations. So EUSG is not routinely indicated.

Q. What is the role of FDG-PET scan?

Ans. Fluorodeoxyglucose positron emission tomography (FDG-PET) scan combined with a CT scan has been advocated for evaluation of carcinoma pancreas. FDG-PET scan combined with CT scan is able to differentiate between benign and malignant pancreatic lesion. However, inflammatory lesion in pancreas may show false positive results. Further studies are required to recommend FDG-PET scan as a routine for evaluation of pancreatic cancer.

Q. What is the role of laparoscopy in evaluation of carcinoma of pancreas?

Ans.
- Not very much helpful for diagnosis
- Staging laparoscopy has a role in management of pancreatic cancer
- Staging laparoscopy identifies about additional 30% of patient to have advanced disease (small liver and peritoneal metastasis) who appear resectable on imaging and a laparotomy may be avoided
- However, current imaging interpreted properly may identify these small metastases
- Staging laparoscopy is however indicated in some high-risk cases where chance of occult metastasis is high:
  – Large tumors> 3 cm
  – Significant elevation of tumor marker CA 19-9 (>100 U/mL)
  – Body and tail tumors
- Experienced laparoscopists are also trying biliary and gastric bypass laparoscopically.

Q. What operation will you plan for this patient?

Ans.
- Clinically, there are no symptoms and signs of disseminated disease and if CT scan also reveals no signs of local spread, I will go for curative surgery
- I would like to do an exploratory laparotomy to confirm my diagnosis and if operable I will proceed to do Whipple's pancreaticoduodenectomy.

Q. What preoperative preparation will you do for this patient?

Ans.
- Patient is usually anemic. If Hb level is less than 10 g%—correction of anemia by preoperative blood transfusion.
- Because of associated hepatocellular dysfunction glycogen reserve is reduced in these patients. Glycogen store may be replenished by administration of plenty of glucose by mouth
- Patients with obstructive jaundice usually have chronic dehydration and impaired renal function. Correct dehydration by oral and IV fluid before operation. Adequate rehydration is indicated by good urinary output.

- Prothrombin time may be prolonged due to decreased synthesis of prothrombin consequent to vitamin K deficiency—may be corrected with injection of vitamin K for 5–7 days before operation.
- Renal function may be impaired in obstructive jaundice and may be complicated by postoperative renal failure. One mechanism for postoperative renal failure has been said to be due to blockage of renal tubules by deposition of bile salts. Gram-negative septicemia has been said to be the other mechanism for development of renal failure in patients with obstructive jaundice. Needs treatment with adequate IV fluid and IV furosemide or mannitol to ensure adequate diuresis.
- There is increased chance of infection in patients with obstructive jaundice and are prone to develop Gram-negative septicemia. Patient is started on a broad spectrum antibiotic like second generation cephalosporin and aminoglycoside combination 1–2 days before surgery.
- If patient is malnourished enteral or parenteral nutrition may be given preoperatively.
- Evaluation of pulmonary function by chest X-ray and pulmonary function test. Pulmonary physiotherapy is to be started from the preoperative period.

Q. What are the criteria of a resectable tumor on clinical assessment?

Ans. Resectable tumor is defined as:
- Tumor localized to the pancreas
- No evidence of SMV or portal vein involvement
- Preserved fat plane between the tumor and the SMA and celiac trunk branches
- No evidence of distant metastasis.

Q. What are the signs of advance disease (inoperability) in a case of periampullary carcinoma?

Ans. Obvious signs of inoperability are:
- Ascites
- Peritoneal metastasis
- Multiple liver metastasis
- Extensive lymph node metastasis
- Invasion of growth to IVC
- Invasion of growth to superior mesenteric vessels, portal vein or celiac axis.

Q. What do you mean by borderline resectable disease?

Ans. National comprehensive cancer network (NCCN) guidelines defines following criteria as borderline resectable disease:
- Unilateral or bilateral superior mesenteric vein-portal vein (SMV-PV) impingement
- Less than 180° tumor abutment on SMA
- Abutment or encasement of hepatic artery, if reconstructible
- Short segment occlusion of SMV, if reconstructible.

These tumors were earlier considered as non-resectable tumors. The resection of these tumors should be undertaken only by an experienced surgeon working in a high volume center.

Q. How will you diagnose carcinoma of periampullary region on exploration?

Ans.
- Nodular growth in the ampulla or lower end of bile duct or the head of pancreas
- Lymph node, if enlarged is hard in feel
- Liver metastasis may be present
- Wide dilatation of biliary tree may be seen.

Q. How will you suspect chronic pancreatitis rather than malignancy?

Ans. It is at times very difficult to differentiate even on exploration.

◆ Pancreas as a whole is hard and nodular and may be shrunken
◆ Nodes, if enlarged will be soft
◆ Gallbladder is often fibrosed and may contain calculi.

Q. What structures will you remove in Whipple's operation?

Ans. Whipple's pancreaticoduodenectomy involves excision of following structures (Figs 3.39 and 3.40):

◆ Whole of duodenum up to 10 cm of proximal jejunum
◆ Head and neck of pancreas including uncinate process
◆ Distal 40–50% of stomach
◆ Lower end of common bile duct (CBD)
◆ Gallbladder
◆ Pericholedochal, periduodenal and peripancreatic lymph nodes.

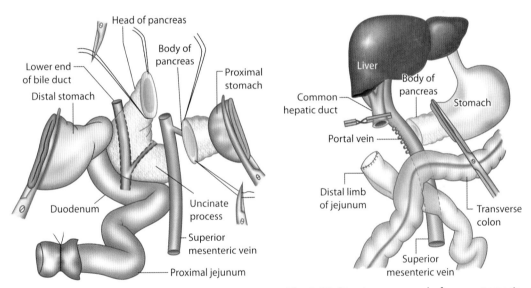

Fig. 3.39: Structures that are to be removed in Whipple's operation are shown to the right of superior mesenteric artery

Fig. 3.40: Structures as seen before anastomosis

Q. How will you maintain continuity following resection for Whipple's operation?

Ans.
1. Pancreaticojejunostomy (end-to-side)
2. Hepaticojejunostomy (end-to-side) 10–15 cm beyond the pancreaticojejunostomy
3. Beyond 10–15 cm of hepaticojejunostomy gastrojejunostomy (Fig. 3.41).

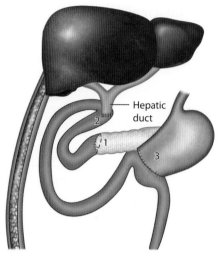

Fig. 3.41: Reconstruction after pancreaticoduodenecto-my. (1: Pancreaticojejunostomy; 2: Hepaticojejunostomy; 3: Gastrojejunostomy)

Q. What do you mean by pylorus conserving pancreaticoduodenectomy?

Ans. In further modification of Whipple's operation the distal third of the stomach is not removed to avoid the complications related to gastrectomy. The line of resection is 2 cm distal to the pylorus and other structures described above are removed. In 1978, Traverso and Longmire described this modification.

Q. What is the rationality of total pancreatectomy in carcinoma of pancreas?

Ans.
* Growth involving head and body need total pancreatectomy for curative surgery
* Pancreatic growth may be multicentric, hence, total pancreatectomy remove the other foci of carcinoma
* Resection lines may be positive after Whipple operation and there is increased chance of local recurrence
* Viable malignant cells may be present in pancreatic duct
* Pancreaticojejunal anastomosis has chance of leakage and fistula formation and is an important cause of morbidity and mortality. Total pancreatectomy avoids a pancreaticojejunal anastomosis
* No risk of postoperative pancreatitis.

Q. What are the problems with total pancreatectomy?

Ans.
* *Surgery is more extensive and there is little more incidence of mortality due to surgery*
* *Permanent diabetes mellitus needs insulin for lifelong*
* *Permanent pancreatic enzyme deficiency needs pancreatic enzyme replacement therapy.*

Q. What is extended Whipple's operation?

Ans. When growth has involved superior mesenteric vessels and adjacent lymph nodes—a wider clearance is possible by resecting a segment of superior mesenteric vessels with bypass graft and dissection of adjacent lymph nodes.

Q. If on exploration you find the growth is inoperable what will you do?

Ans. In that case palliative surgery is to be undertaken, including:
* Relief of jaundice by
  - Roux-en-Y choledochojejunostomy or
  - Roux-en-Y cholecystojejunostomy or
  - Choledochoduodenostomy, if no duodenal obstruction is present
* If patient has gastric outlet obstruction
  - A gastrojejunostomy is to be done
* Relief of pain by celiac plexus blockade with absolute alcohol.

Q. If there is no gastric outlet obstruction will you do a gastrojejunostomy?

Ans.
* If there is impending gastric outlet obstruction a gastrojejunostomy should be done
* About 30% of patient may develop gastric outlet obstruction subsequently, if there is no evidence of distant metastasis. If there is possibility of longer survival (when distant metastasis is absent) a prophylactic gastrojejunostomy should be added.

Q. What are the drawbacks of adding a gastrojejunostomy routinely?

* Prolongs the operation
* Morbidity increased to some extent
* In some cases it may not be necessary at all if there is no duodenal obstruction.

Q. How will you manage a postoperative patient following Whipple's operation?

Ans.
* Patient should be treated in an intensive therapy unit
* Patient may require respiratory assistance for 12–24 hours
* Surgery is usually prolonged and particularly elderly patient may have respiratory depression and poor respiratory effort in immediate postoperative period
* Nasogastric decompression by a Ryle's tube to prevent gastric distension due to paralytic ileus
* IV fluid till bowel sounds return
* Maintenance fluid with 5% dextrose and normal saline. Monitoring of serum electrolyte and replacement of potassium
* Patient with carcinoma pancreas may be diabetic
* Strict diabetic control is required in postoperative period. Blood sugar is to be checked 4 hourly and administer appropriate dose of insulin. This may be done by making a sliding-scale of insulin-dosage. This is followed by checking CBG (capillary blood glucose) and administering insulin according to the scale
* Postoperative hemorrhage is a problem
* Bleeding may occur from the anastomotic lines or there may be bleeding from the raw areas into the peritoneal cavity. Observe for any signs of bleeding—needs treatment with blood transfusion
* Prophylactic antibiotics is to be continued for 5–7 days
* Maintain intake output chart
* Monitor pulse/blood pressure/jugular venous pressure/urine output hourly.

Q. If patient is inoperable clinically and on investigation how will you manage this patient?

Ans.

- Patient may be having advanced disease with signs of inoperability on clinical ground. In that case only palliative treatment is advisable
- *Relief of jaundice:*
  - Relief of jaundice may be achieved by endoscopic stenting of the bile duct. A metal stent is better in malignant obstructive jaundice
  - Surgical relief of obstructive jaundice is done by either choledochojejunostomy, cholecystojejunostomy or choledochoduodenostomy (Provided there is no duodenal obstruction).
- *Relief of gastric outlet obstruction:*
  - Endoscopic stenting may provide short-term relief of gastric outlet obstruction
  - Surgical relief of gastric outlet obstruction—by gastrojejunostomy
  - If patient is found to have advanced disease on exploratory laparotomy both choledochojejunostomy and gastrojejunostomy is to be done for relief of jaundice and gastric outlet obstruction.
- *Relief of pain:*
  - Analgesics—NSAIDs, opioids
  - Celiac plexus block—by injecting bupivacaine and absolute alcohol into the celiac plexus
  - Celiac plexus block may be done either during laparotomy or by percutaneous approach (EUSG or CT guided)
  - Adjuvant chemotherapy may be tried.

Q. What is the role of adjuvant therapy in periampullary carcinoma?

Ans. Role of radiotherapy is very limited in terms of long-term survival and quality of life.

- Cytotoxic chemotherapy
- Combination chemotherapy with:
  - 5 Fluorouracil + Cyclophosphamide + Methotrexate or vincristine
  - 5 Fluorouracil + Mitomycin
  - Gemcitabine.
  Results of chemotherapy are not encouraging.

Q. How will you provide relief of pain in carcinoma of pancreas?

Ans.

- Analgesics: NSAIDs and opioids
- Relief of pain may be achieved with celiac plexus blockade with absolute alcohol or glycerol either during surgery or by percutaneous block
- Pancreatic duct decompression by pancreaticojejunostomy or pancreaticogastrostomy.

Q. What is average age of presentation of carcinoma of head of pancreas?

Ans. It affects elderly patients—50% in more than 75 years of age.

Q. What are the important etiological factors for development of carcinoma head of pancreas?

Ans. Etiological factors for development of carcinoma pancreas:

- *Smoking:* The risk is proportional to both the duration and intensity of smoking. Smoking roughly doubles the risk of pancreatic cancer. Smoking is calculated to have caused about 25% of burden of pancreatic cancer.
- *Alcohol:* Alcohol is a leading cause of chronic pancreatitis. Chronic pancreatitis increases the risk of pancreatic cancer 10–20 fold.
- *Diet:* Diet high in protein and fats has been incriminated for causation of pancreatic cancer. Diet rich in fruits and vegetables would lower the risk of pancreatic cancer. However, the dietary factors have not been well-established in different studies.
- *Chronic pancreatitis:* There is 10–20 fold higher risk of pancreatic cancer for patients with chronic pancreatitis. This includes all types of chronic pancreatitis including tropical pancreatitis found in south India.
- *Diabetes:* The overall risk of pancreatic cancer is 60% greater in patients with diabetes mellitus than in general population. This risk is limited to patients with type II diabetes. In some cases diabetes may be the presenting symptom of pancreatic cancer.
- *Infectious disease: H. pylori* infection has been associated with higher risk of pancreatic cancer. This, however, needs further study.
- *Genetic:* Some inherited disorder has been linked to pancreatic cancer. *BRCA2 gene* has been associated with 7–10% of sporadic pancreatic cancer and 10–20% of patients with family history of cancer.

Q. What are the usual presentations of patient with pancreatic cancer?

Ans.
- *Painless progressive jaundice* is described as the classic presentation. Jaundice is found in 65–90% of patient with mass in head of pancreas. In patient having carcinoma involving the body and tail less than 20% may present with jaundice
- *Epigastric pain*: Dull aching epigastric pain, radiating to the back, worse at night and in supine position with some relief in leaning forward may be the presenting symptom in about 70% patient with mass in head and in about 90% patients with carcinoma in body and tail of pancreas. The pain is explained to be due to:
  - Perineural and splanchnic neuronal compression
  - Invasion to adjacent organ
  - Adjacent organ compression
- *Nonspecific symptoms:* Malaise, weight loss, nausea and vomiting
- *Diarrhea or steatorrhea*
- *New onset diabetes mellitus* is found in 6–8% patients with carcinoma pancreas
- *Rarely patient may present* with signs and symptoms of acute pancreatitis
- *Migratory thrombophlebitis* (Trousseau sign) may be found in about 10% of patients.

Q. Carcinoma is common in which part of the pancreas?

Ans. It commonly involves the head and neck of the pancreas. The relative incidence is: Head and neck: Body and tail = 8:1.

Q. What is TNM classification for pancreatic cancer?

Ans. The TNM classification for pancreatic cancer is given in Table 3.7 and anatomic stages are given in Table 3.8.

Table 3.7: TNM classification for pancreatic cancer

Primary tumor (T)

TX	Primary tumor cannot be assessed
T0	No evidence of primary tumor
Tis	Carcinoma in situ
T1	Tumor limited to the pancreas, ≤2 cm in greatest dimension
T2	Tumor limited to the pancreas, >2 cm in greatest dimension
T3	Tumor extends beyond the pancreas but without involvement of the celiac axis or the superior mesenteric artery
T4	Tumor involves the celiac axis or the superior mesenteric artery (unresectable primary tumor)

Regional lymph nodes (N)

NX	Regional lymph nodes cannot be assessed
N0	No regional lymph node metastasis
N1	Regional lymph node metastasis

Distant metastasis (M)

M0	No distant metastasis
M1	Distant metastasis

Table 3.8: Anatomic stage/prognostic groups

Stage	T	N	M
0	Tis	N0	M0
IA	T1	N0	M0
IB	T2	N0	M0
IIA	T3	N0	M0
IIB	T1	N1	M0
	T2	N1	M0
	T3	N1	M0
III	T4	Any N	M0
IV	Any T	Any N	M1

Q. What are the features of cystadenocarcinoma?

Ans.

* Incidence is 1%
* They may attain very large size
* Usually slow growing
* Have both cystic and solid component.

Q. Does carcinoma of pancreas always present with painless progressive jaundice?

Ans.

* No. In 65–90% of cases painless jaundice is the presenting symptom in carcinoma head pancreas
* Patient may present with other features.

Q. What is the prognosis of carcinoma of pancreas?

* Median survival is 6 months
* 5 years survival after curative resection of carcinoma head of pancreas is 3% while that for periampullary carcinoma is 30%.

Q. What is the operative mortality rate for Whipple's operation?

Ans. Earlier it was quoted as 8%. With improvement in technique and intensive postoperative care the acceptable mortality following Whipple's operation is 1–2%.

Q. What is the usual extent of disease in carcinoma of pancreas at presentation?

Ans.

* Only 10% are confined to the pancreas at diagnosis
* About 40% has locally advanced disease
* About 50% has evidence of distant spread.

Q. What is the peculiarity of presentation in carcinoma of body and tail of pancreas?

Ans.

* Symptoms appear usually late
* Disease is usually advanced at diagnosis
* Usually presents with vague symptoms like anorexia, weight loss and pain. Jaundice is usually not the presenting symptom. Prognosis is usually worse.

Q. What are different tumor markers helpful in diagnosis of carcinoma of pancreas?

Ans. CEA, CA 19-9 and CA 494 are the different tumor markers which may be elevated in carcinoma of pancreas.

CA 19-9 level is most encouraging having 80% sensitivity. However, colorectal and gastric carcinoma may also have elevated CA 19-9 level.

Q. Is it rational to do pancreaticoduodenectomy when there is confusion in diagnosis between carcinoma of head of pancreas and chronic pancreatitis?

Ans. Sometimes it is very difficult to differentiate carcinoma of pancreas from chronic pancreatitis even on exploration. Pancreaticoduodenectomy may be considered in such situation. Frozen section biopsy is unreliable. Treatment of chronic pancreatitis with jaundice and pancreatic ductal obstruction may be done by Whipple's procedure.

Q. What is the relationship between diabetes and pancreatic cancer?

Ans. Hereditary type of diabetes mellitus which may be already present poses an increased risk of development of pancreatic cancer.

In another group hyperglycemia develops subsequent to the development of pancreatic cancer.

Q. What is the relation between pancreatic cancer and chronic pancreatitis?

Ans. Pancreatitis has been found to be associated with pancreatic cancer.

In one group histological pancreatitis may be found in patient with pancreatic cancer presumably due to ductal obstruction and/or direct destruction of parenchymatous tissue.

The hereditary type of pancreatitis seen to have higher predisposition to pancreatic cancer than the general population.

The acquired variety of chronic pancreatitis does not seem to be related to pancreatic cancer.

Q. What may be the cause of upper GI hemorrhage in carcinoma of pancreas?

Ans. Growth invading into the duodenal wall may cause hemorrhage.

Growth may obstruct the portal vein causing portal hypertension and bleeding may be due to rupture of esophageal varices.

Q. What is Trousseau's sign?

Ans. Migratory thrombophlebitis in patients with an underlying abdominal malignancy is known as Trousseau's sign. This may be found in pancreatic malignancy and in other gastrointestinal malignancy.

Q. What is Troisier's sign?

Ans. Left supraclavicular lymph node enlargement due to metastasis from an intra-abdominal malignancy is known as Troisier's sign.

Q. What are the causes of delay in diagnosis of carcinoma of pancreas?

Ans. The factors responsible for late diagnosis are:
- *Tumor is asymptomatic in early stage:* Preclinical stage of the tumor may be present for months or years before the tumor becomes apparent.
- *Patient's delay:* Early symptoms are vague and nonspecific. Patient often tolerates these symptoms and does not report to a physician.
- *Physician's delay:* As symptoms are vague and physical signs are sparse at the early stage, if the physician does not have a high index of suspicion and fail to properly evaluate the patient the diagnosis may be delayed.
- *Difficulty of the patient to reach a proper place for diagnosis.*

Q. When do you suspect that the lesion is advanced?

Ans. Presence of physical signs, such as a palpable mass in abdomen, liver metastasis and presence of Trousseau's sign or Troisier's sign usually indicate advanced disease.

Q. What are the indications of adjuvant therapy in patients with carcinoma of pancreas?

Ans.
- Patient with regional disease—tumors with capsular invasion and or regional lymph node spread may benefit from adjuvant therapy
- A combination of radiotherapy and chemotherapy may help.

Q. What was the original Whipple's operation?

Ans. In 1935, Whipple reported a two stage enbloc resection of head of pancreas and duodenum.
In the first stage cholecystogastrostomy and gastrojejunostomy were done. After the jaundice has subsided and the nutrition has improved the second stage operation was done.

The second stage involves enbloc resection of duodenum and a small wedge of pancreas. Pancreatic stump was closed without a pancreaticoenteric anastomosis.

Q. Who first performed one stage pancreaticoduodenectomy?

Ans. Trimble in 1941 performed first one stage pancreaticoduodenectomy.

Q. What is the role of endoscopic ultrasonography in evaluation of carcinoma of pancreas?

Ans.

◆ In this technique, a high frequency transducer is placed in the gastric and duodenal lumen in close proximity to the pancreas
◆ Detect small lesion less than 2 cm in pancreas
◆ Detect lymph node and vascular involvement
◆ Invasion of ampullary tumors into duodenal wall and pancreas
◆ This modality of investigation is superior to USG/CT/and angiography.

The option for treatment of carcinoma of pancreas is given in Table 3.9.

Table 3.9: Option for treatment of carcinoma of pancreas		
Mass in pancreatic head without metastasis	**Mass in head with metastasis**	**Mass in body and tail usually advanced at diagnosis**
Resectable—Whipple's operation Nonresectable—Biliary and/or gastric bypass	Biliary and/or gastric bypass	FNAC positive Avoid surgery and endoscopic stenting

Q. What are the criteria to define borderline resectable pancreatic cancer?

Ans. Borderline resectable pancreatic cancer are a group of patient of pancreatic cancer which were earlier considered as nonresectable in view of their critical relationship to local vascular structures—superior mesenteric vein, portal vein, hepatic artery and the celiac trunk. Several studies now established these patients may undergo safe resection following neoadjuvant chemoradiation therapy.

The consensus definition for borderline resectable pancreatic ductal adenocarcinoma (PDAC) includes tumors with following characteristics:

◆ *Tumor abutment, encasement, or short segment venous occlusion of superior mesenteric vein/ portal vein, but with suitable vessel proximal and distal to the area of vessel involvement, allowing for safe resection and reconstruction*
◆ *Tumor encasement of gastroduodenal artery extending up to the hepatic artery*
◆ *Tumor involving a short segment encasement/direct tumor abutment of the hepatic artery with no extension to the celiac axis*
◆ *Tumor abutment of superior mesenteric artery less than 180°.*

Q. What are Ishikawa radiographic criteria for assessment of vascular involvement?

Ans. *The Ishikawa classifications based on radiographic findings that demonstrate the relationship of the tumor to the PV-SMV (Fig. 3.42).*

- *Normal*
- *Smooth shift without narrowing*
- *Unilateral narrowing*
- *Bilateral narrowing*
- *Bilateral narrowing and the presence of collateral.*

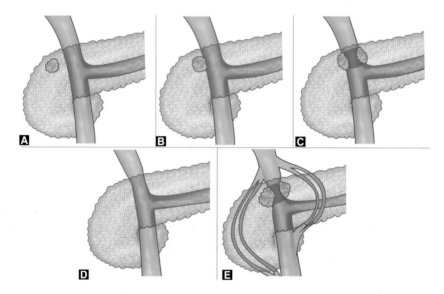

Figs 3.42A to E: Ishikawa classification of portal and/or superior mesenteric vein involvement. (A) Normal; (B) Smooth shift without narrowing; (C) Unilateral narrowing; (D) Bilateral narrowing; (E) Bilateral narrowing with collateral veins

Q. What do you mean by tumor vein interface (TVI)?

Ans. *Tran Cao described a simplified radiographic classification system with regard to circumferential tumor-vein interface. The TVI system was found to be predictive of the need for venous resection and survival.*

Tumor vein interface grouping includes:

- *No TVI*
- *≤ 180° of vessel circumference*
- *TVI > 180° of vessel circumference, or occlusion requiring for venous resection.*

Q. What are the preoperative investigations required for borderline resectable PDAC?

Ans. *Preoperative imaging*

CECT scan: A pancreatic protocol triphasic contrast (noncontrast, arterial, pancreatic parenchymal, portal venous) with 2–3 mm slices. CT performed in this manner has an excellent negative predictive value for unresectability, but it is not as accurate at predicting resectability. This is due to its lack of sensitivity for identifying small hepatic and peritoneal metastases.

MRI pancreas: Recently, some studies have suggested an MRI pancreas protocol is valuable due to more sensitive visualization of subcentimeter tumors/liver metastases, peritoneal carcinomatosis, and minimal signs of vascular infiltration.

PET-CT scan: The role of PET-CT in the evaluation of potentially resectable pancreatic cancer remains unclear. PET-CT may detect metastases in high-risk patients and is useful for assessment of response to chemoradiation.

PET-CT may be useful in certain circumstances but routine use is not recommended.

Q. What is the role of tissue diagnosis?

Ans. *Although histologic diagnosis is not required for patients with pancreatic cancer who are undergoing upfront surgery, biopsy is required prior to initiation of neoadjuvant therapy in patients with borderline resectable pancreatic cancer.*

Fine needle aspiration (FNA) is the preferred method for obtaining a tissue diagnosis. While this can be performed percutaneously, under ultrasound (US) or CT guidance endoscopic ultrasound (EUS) with FNA is favored. EUS-FNA offers decreased potential for peritoneal seeding compared to percutaneous biopsy.

Q. What is role of ERCP in borderline resectable pancreatic cancer?

Ans. *Borderline resectable pancreatic cancer patients with obstructive jaundice should be stented prior to starting neoadjuvant therapy. Stenting, these patients, provides symptomatic relief, reduces risk of cholangitis, and prevents coagulopathy. Some chemotherapeutic drugs cannot be given in presence of abnormal liver function.*

Q. What is the role of tumor marker study?

Ans. *CA 19-9 (Sialylated Lewis antigen) is the best validated in pancreatic cancer. Although relatively sensitive, its specificity is suboptimal as CA19-9 levels are often elevated in association with other pancreatic and hepatobiliary pathology.*

Q. What is the optimal treatment planning for borderline resectable PDAC?

Ans. *Neoadjuvant therapy is currently the preferred initial treatment for PDAC. Reevaluation and surgical treatment is the definitive treatment.*

Q. How neoadjuvant therapy helps in borderline resectable PDAC?

Ans.
+ *Provide early treatment of micrometastasis*
+ *Potential to achieve some degree of downstaging*
+ *Increase likelihood of R0 resection*
+ *Lymph node metastasis may regress*
+ *Most of the patients need postoperative chemotherapy. Postoperative complications may delay the initiation of postoperative chemotherapy. Preoperative chemotherapy avoids delay in adjuvant treatment.*

Q. What are the different regimes of neoadjuvant therapy?

Ans.
* *5-FU and radiation followed by re-evaluation for resection*
* *Gemcitabine based chemoradiation*
* *Induction chemotherapy using gemcitabine/cisplatin/5-FU followed by chemoradiation with 5-FU*
* *Modified FOLFIRINOX regime (oxaliplatin, irinotecan, leucovorin 400 mg/m^2) followed by external beam radiation therapy (50.4 Gy) with capecitabine (825 mg/m^2).*
  After restaging, patients who are deemed candidates for resection proceed with surgery followed by postoperative gemcitabine.

Q. What are the outcomes of neoadjuvant treatment in borderline resectable PDAC?

Ans. *There are large number of reports in literature establishing the benefits of neoadjuvnat chemoradiation in borderline resectable PDAC. The largest series of case report is from MD Anderson Cancer Center. Out of 160 patients 84 had borderline resectable PDAC. Neoadjuvnat chemoradiation with different regimes were administered in all 84 patients.*

Following neoadjuvant treatment 38% underwent resection of which 97% were R0. The median survival of all patients was 21 months. 40 months for resected patients and 15 months for patients who did not undergo resection. Afterwards multiple smaller and few similarly sized retrospective reviews have reported similar findings.

More recently, Katz reported on 129 patients with borderline resectable tumors who underwent neoadjuvant treatment at MD Anderson. On post-treatment re-evaluation of 122 patients, only 15 (12%) showed partial response by RECIST criteria. Despite this, 85 (69%) underwent resection, of which R0 resection was 81 (95%). Median overall survival of those who underwent resection was 33 months, which did not correlate with RECIST response indicating that a lack of radiographic evidence of tumor response in PDAC is of little clinical value as prognostic or predictive marker. So, the recommendation is aggressive surgical resection in patients with adequate performance status and absence of disease progression.

■ OBSTRUCTIVE JAUNDICE DUE TO CHOLEDOCHOLITHIASIS

Q. What is your case? (Summary of a case of obstructive jaundice due to choledocholithiasis)

Ans. A 45-year-old lady presented with pain in right upper quadrant of abdomen for last 1 year and yellowish discoloration of eyes and urine for last 2 months. Patient had recurrent attacks of severe colicky pain in right upper quadrant of abdomen for last 1 year. Pain used to radiate to the back of the right side of the chest and to the right shoulder. Initially patient had recurrent attacks of similar pain at an interval of 2–3 months. For the last 2 months patient has a constant dull aching pain in the right upper quadrant of abdomen. Patient complains of yellowish discoloration of eyes and urine for last 2 months. The onset of jaundice was preceded by an attack of severe colicky pain 2 months back. The yellowish discoloration was increasing in intensity for last 6 weeks, but during last 2 weeks the intensity of yellowish discoloration is diminishing. Patient complains of itching all over the body for last 2 months and from last week the itching has also diminished. Patient is passing clay colored stool for last 2 months. There is history of fever with chill and rigor with the attack of pain for last 2 months, which subsided with treatment. Bowel and bladder habits are normal and there are no other systemic symptoms.

On examination patient is conscious and cooperative. Mild pallor and moderate jaundice is present. There are scratch marks in the skin due to itching. On abdominal examination, inspection is normal. On palpation there is no tenderness. Liver is palpable 2 cm below the right costal margin firm, nontender, smooth surface. Spleen not palpable, gallbladder is not palpable. No other mass is palpable in abdomen. Hernial sites and external genitalia are normal.

Q. What is your diagnosis?

Ans. This is a case of obstructive jaundice due to choledocholithiasis.

Q. What are the other possibilities?

Ans. *See* Page No. 148.

Q. How will you palpate the gallbladder?

Ans. *See* Palpation of Gallbladder (*see* Fig. 3.14, Page No. 96).

Q. What is Courvoisier's law?

Ans. *See* Courvoisier's Law (*see* Page No. 149).

Q. What are the exceptions to Courvoisier's law?

Ans. *See* Courvoisier's Law (see Page No. 149).

Q. What investigations will you suggest in this patient?

Ans. I will do some investigations to confirm my diagnosis.
* Liver function test:
    - Bilirubin: Total, conjugated and unconjugated
    - Serum proteins: Total, albumin and globulin
    - Liver-enzymes: AST, ALT and alkaline-phosphatase
    - Prothrombin time.
* USG of upper abdomen will demonstrate gallstones and the bile duct diameter and any stone in the bile duct.
* I would suggest an endoscopic retrograde cholangiopancreatography (ERCP) along with endoscopic sphincterotomy and stone retrieval by Dormia basket catheter through the endoscope, if choledocholithiasis is found on USG.

Q. How else can you evaluate common bile duct?

Ans. Magnetic resonance cholangiopancreatography (MRCP) is a newer imaging investigation, which helps in very good delineation of both bile duct and the pancreatic duct. This is a noninvasive investigation and does not entail radiation exposure. But therapeutic intervention is not possible.

Endoscopic ultrasound has been emerged as a reliable method for demonstrating common bile duct stones. The probe which is placed in duodenum is also helpful for detecting any lesion in the pancreas, distal bile duct or the ampulla of Vater which may be the cause of jaundice.

Q. Which serum enzymes are important?

Ans. The serum alkaline phosphatase and gamma glutamyl transpeptidase (GGT) are sensitive indicators of bile duct obstruction, i. e. obstructive jaundice.

ALT and AST may be elevated in long-standing biliary obstruction.

Q. Would you like to do a CT scan in this patient?

Ans. If USG and the cholangiography have shown stone disease then CT scan is not helpful as an additional mode of investigation.

Q. What other investigations will you do in this patient?

Ans. Routine investigations to assess patient's fitness for general anesthesia:
* Hemogram
* Blood for sugar, urea and creatinine
* Chest X-ray
* ECG.

Q. How will you treat this patient?

Ans. If facilities are available, I will advise endoscopic sphincterotomy and bile duct stone extraction by a Dormia basket catheter introduced through the endoscope followed by laparoscopic cholecystectomy.

In absence of such facilities conventional open cholecystectomy with bile duct exploration is the standard operation.

Q. What is the role of laparoscopy in choledocholithiasis?

Ans. With advancement in laparoscopic technique it is now possible to do both laparoscopic cholecystectomy and laparoscopic choledocholithotomy in patients with cholelithiasis and choledocholithiasis.

Q. What are the problems with ERCP stone extraction?

Ans.
* In 5–10% the procedure may not be possible
* Stones larger than 1.5 cm is not suitable for extraction endoscopically unless there is facility for contact lithotripsy
* There is 1–5% mortality and 5–10% morbidity following the procedure
* Risk of postprocedure cholangitis, pancreatitis, bleeding or rarely duodenal perforation remains. Usual success rate is 86–96% in expert hand.

Q. What is transcystic exploration of bile duct?

Ans. The common duct stones may be approached via the transcystic route. The cystic duct may be dilated and a choledochoscope introduced through the cystic duct may visualize the interior of the bile duct and the stones retrieved by a Dormia basket catheter. Once the bile duct is cleared off all stones the cystic duct stump may be ligated.

Q. What are the limitations of transcystic bile duct stone extraction?

Ans.
* Stones more than 1 cm in diameter cannot be retrieved in this approach

- Stones in the proximal hepatic and right and left hepatic cannot be retrieved transcystically as it is difficult to pass the choledochoscope proximally by bending it in a cephalad direction
- If the cystic duct is friable transcystic approach is not suitable.

Q. What is Charcot's triad?

Ans.
- Intermittent pain
- Intermittent jaundice
- Intermittent fever.
  This triad of symptoms suggests cholangitis.

Q. What is Reynold's pentad?

Ans.
- Charcoat's triad (intermittent pain, intermittent jaundice, intermittent fever)
- Along with mental status changes and evidence of shock (hypotension).
  This is found in severe cholangitis with septicemia.

Q. What are primary bile duct stones?

Ans. The stones that form in bile duct itself are called primary bile duct stones. Primary bile duct stones are usually brown pigment stones.

Brown stones are usually associated with biliary tract infection. The bacterial enzyme hydrolyzes bilirubin diglucuronide into free bilirubin which then precipitates and forms a complex with cholesterol.

Q. What are secondary bile duct stones?

Ans. The stones that form in gallbladder and then migrate into the bile duct are called secondary bile duct stones.

Q. What are retained or residual bile duct stones?

Ans. Stones in the bile duct detected within two years following cholecystectomy are defined as retained stones. Stones missed during cholecystectomy with or without bile duct exploration are called residual or retained bile duct stones and the stones have the characteristics of secondary bile duct stones.

Q. What are recurrent bile duct stones?

Ans. Stones which form within the bile duct 2 years after initial operation are grouped as recurrent bile duct stones. This has the characteristics of primary bile duct stones.

Q. What are the characteristics of primary bile duct stones?

Ans. About 99% of primary bile duct stones are pigment type. The principal composition of the pigment stone is calcium bilirubinate. The pigment stones are either brown or black. The brown stones are associated with infection in the biliary tree. The black stones are associated with chronic hemolytic diseases.

Q. What are the usual presentations of patients with bile duct stones?

Ans.
- *Charcot's triad:* Intermittent pain, intermittent fever, intermittent jaundice

♦ *Obstructive jaundice:* Itching, clay colored stool
♦ *Associated pancreatitis* may cause pain in the back
♦ *Abdominal examination* may be normal in between attacks
♦ *Abdominal tenderness* may be present in right upper quadrant during an attack of cholangitis
♦ *Gallbladder is usually* not palpable.

Q. What is the role of intraoperative cholangiography in evaluation of bile duct stones?

Ans. Operative cholangiography is an important diagnostic tool for detection of bile duct stones. There has been debate regarding routine use of operative cholangiography.

The routine operative cholangiography is justified because:

♦ About 5–7% of patients who are found to have stones during operative cholangiogram have no preoperative indication of bile duct stones
♦ Ductal abnormalities may be identified thereby reducing the incidence of bile duct injury.
  However, newer diagnostic modalities like MRCP has increased the diagnostic accuracy of bile duct stones.

Q. How will you do intraoperative cholangiography?

Ans. The cystic pedicle is dissected and cystic duct isolated and a ligature passed around the cystic duct. An opening is made in the anterior wall of the cystic duct. A fine cannula is introduced through the cystic duct into the bile duct. About 2 mL of urografin 60% is injected through the cannula and X-ray exposure taken or seen under a fluoroscope. This is called transcystic intraoperative cholangiogram (Fig. 3.43).

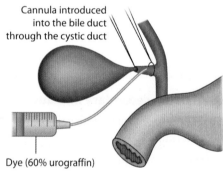

Cannula introduced into the bile duct through the cystic duct

Dye (60% urograffin)

Fig. 3.43: Intraoperative cholangiography

Q. Cholecystectomy and choledocholithotomy has been done and the postoperative T-tube cholangiography has shown a residual stone in the bile duct—how will you manage?

Ans. This situation may be avoided by doing a completion T-tube cholangiogram on table to detect any residual stone.

There are a number of ways of tackling such stones:

♦ *Mechanical flushing with heparinized saline:* If small (<1 cm) the stones may be flushed off by irrigating the bile duct with heparinized saline (250 mL of normal saline) mixed with 25,000 IU of heparin is irrigated through the T-tube tract for 3 days.
♦ *Contact dissolution:* If the stone is a cholesterol one, contact dissolution by infusing monooctanoin or methyl tert-butyl ether via the T-tube tract may be helpful.
♦ *Burrhene technique:* Patient is discharged home with the T-tube in situ, and waiting period of 4–6 weeks allow the T-tube tract to get matured. The retained stone is extracted through the matured T-tube tract. The T-tube is removed and the T-tube tract is dilated under fluoroscopic

control. A Dormia basket catheter is introduced through the T-tube tract into the bile duct and the stones may be removed.

- Alternatively a choledoscope may be passed through the matured T-tube tract and the stones from the bile duct may be removed under vision.
- *ERCP and endoscopic sphincterotomy* and stone extraction by a Dormia basket catheter introduced through the endoscope.
- *Extracorporeal shock wave lithotripsy (ECSWL):* If there is a single stone ECSWL may be applied.
- *Laparoscopic choledocholithotomy.*
- *Open choledocholithotomy:* If the above measures fail, open surgery is to be done.

Q. If the retained stone is detected after the removal of T-tube. How will you manage?

Ans.
- *Endoscopic sphincterotomy and stone* extraction by a Dormia basket catheter introduced through the endoscope.
- *Extracorporeal shock wave lithotripsy:* If the stone is large it may not be suitable for ECSWL. 50% patients need adjunctive procedure like endoscopic extraction, biliary lavage and stenting.
- *Percutaneous transhepatic route* may be used to pass a cholangioscope to visualize the bile duct stones and removal by using Dormia basket catheter introduced through the cholangioscope.
- *Laparoscopic or open choledocholithotmy.*

■ CARCINOMA OF GALLBLADDER (PRESENTING WITH OR WITHOUT OBSTRUCTIVE JAUNDICE)

Q. What is your case? (Summary of a case of carcinoma of gallbladder)

Ans. A 55-year-old lady presented with history of pain in right upper quadrant of abdomen for last 3 years. Patient has recurrent attacks of colicky pain in right upper quadrant of abdomen for last 3 years. Initially patient had colicky pain in right upper quadrant of abdomen but for last 3 months patient is having dull aching continuous pain in the same region. The pain radiates to the back of the chest and the central part of the abdomen. Patient complains of anorexia and marked weight loss for last 6 months.

On examination on general survey patient has moderate pallor, jaundice is absent, no lymphadenopathy. Abdominal examination revealed tenderness in right hypochondriac region. Gallbladder is palpable, firm in consistency moving up and down with respiration, tender. Liver and spleen is not palpable. No other mass is palpable. No free fluid in abdomen. Normal bowel sounds are heard.

Q. What is your diagnosis?

Ans. This is a case of carcinoma of gallbladder.

Q. What are the other possibilities?

Ans. If patient has jaundice give the differential diagnosis of obstructive jaundice.
- Periampullary carcinoma
- Cholangiocarcinoma involving the bile duct
- Choledocholithiasis

* Lymph node mass in the porta causing biliary obstruction (metastatic, lymphoma, tuberculosis)
* Bile duct stricture
* Sclerosing cholangitis
* Chronic pancreatitis.

Differential diagnosis of a patient presenting with a gallbladder mass:

* Mucocele of gallbladder
* Empyema of gallbladder
* Carcinoma of gallbladder
* Periampullary carcinoma
* Cholangiocarcinoma involving the distal bile duct
* Distal bile duct obstruction due to lymph node metastasis.

Q. What investigations will you suggest in this patient?

Ans. I would like to do some investigations to confirm my diagnosis.

* Liver function test
* USG of abdomen to assess the lesion in relation to the gallbladder. If a mass is found in gallbladder whether it has spread into the liver and the involvement of lymph nodes. The status of the common bile duct is to be assessed. Any lesion in pancreas is to be looked for
* USG may reveal a heterogeneous mass in gallbladder, asymmetrical thickening of gallbladder wall
* CECT scan of abdomen: If USG shows a neoplastic lesion in the gallbladder, a CECT scan is essential for further evaluation to assess the operability and to stage the disease.

Q. In carcinoma gallbladder when you will not plan further investigation after doing an ultrasonography?

Ans. Most cases of gallbladder carcinoma are advanced at presentation. If USG revealed advanced disease—ascites, multiple liver metastasis, extensive lymphadenopathy and infiltration of the gallbladder mass to the porta hepatis, then further investigations like CECT scan will not be very much helpful for planning palliative treatment.

Q. Will you do a preoperative FNAC?

Ans. In patient with early stage disease a preoperative FNAC is not required for diagnosis. While doing curative resection a frozen biopsy may be done in selected cases.

In patients with advanced disease who are considered for palliative treatment a USG or CT-guided FNAC may be done for confirmation of diagnosis.

Q. What other investigations will you do in this patient?

Ans. Further investigations will depend on the CECT scan report of the patient. If the CECT scan revealed the gallbladder mass and there is no metastasis to the liver and no lymph node spread I will plan for surgical treatment.

I will do baseline investigations to assess the patient's fitness for general anesthesia.

* Complete hemogram
* Blood for sugar, urea and creatinine
* Chest X-ray PA view
* ECG.

Q. What is the role of MRCP in evaluation of carcinoma gallbladder?

Ans. As this patient does not have jaundice, MRCP is not required. In patient with obstructive jaundice MRCP can give a very good delineation of biliary tree and the site of obstruction may be localized.

Q. What is the role of ERCP in carcinoma gallbladder?

Ans. In advanced carcinoma gallbladder presenting with jaundice when surgery is not indicated, palliation of jaundice may be done by ERCP and stenting.

Q. How will you treat this patient?

Ans. I will review the clinical findings and the investigations report. If the disease is localized and there is no distant spread then I will plan for curative surgery. I will do an exploratory laparotomy and assess the operability and if it is operable I will do radical cholecystectomy.

Q. What is the role of diagnostic laparoscopy?

Ans. CECT scan can miss small liver and peritoneal metastasis. A diagnostic laparoscopy may detect these lesions in an otherwise operable case and a laparotomy is avoided.

Q. Under which circumstances a curative resection is not feasible?

Both the patient factors and tumor factors should be taken into consideration for assessing resectability. Following factors preclude a curative resection:
- *Patient factors:*
  - Age: Elderly patient tolerate radical surgery poorly
  - Poor general condition
  - Comorbid condition
  - Sepsis
- *Tumor factors:*
  - Distant metastasis: Intraperitoneal or extra-abdominal is an absolute contraindication for curative resection
  - Extensive metastasis in both lobes of the liver
  - Invasion of growth into the portal vascular structures
  - Invasion of growth into the duodenum, pancreas or colon.

   Metastasis confined to one lobe of liver or invasion to duodenum or pancreas or colon without liver metastasis may be amenable to extended resection.

Q. What structures will you remove in radical cholecystectomy?

Ans.
- Cholecystectomy with a 2 cm wedge of liver tissue at the gallbladder bed to ensure a tumor free margin. Some advocates resection of segments V and IVb.
- Lymph node dissection removing pericholedochal, periportal, hepatoduodenal, nodes along the hepatic artery, portal vein, lymph nodes behind 2nd part of duodenum, peripancreatic nodes around the head of pancreas and lymph nodes around the celiac plexus.

Q. On exploration you found that a curative resection is not feasible in view of local or distant spread, what will you do then?

- *Simple cholecystectomy*, if it is possible, provides tissue diagnosis and prevents development of acute cholecystitis. Palliative procedures may be undertaken if indicated.
- *Relief of jaundice:* Surgical bilioenteric bypass. A choledochojejunostomy with a Roux-en-Y limb of jejunum. If the hilum is invaded by the tumor a segment III anastomosis with a Roux en Y limb of jejunum may be done.
- *If there is impending gastric outlet obstruction* either due to lymph node metastasis or invasion of growth to the pylorus a gastrojejunostomy is to be done to relieve gastric outlet obstruction.
- *Relief of pain*: Celiac ganglion blockade with alcohol will provide relief of pain reduce the dose of analgesics.

Q. After cholecystectomy, histopathology report shows carcinoma gallbladder, how will you manage the patient?

Ans. Further treatment depends on tumor staging. Histopathology report is to be reviewed.

Further treatment will depend on the depth of invasion.

- If the histology of the gallbladder shows that the tumor is confined to the mucosa and submucosa (TIa) simple cholecystectomy is adequate. No further surgery is required.
- If the tumor involves the muscular layer (TIb) and tumor extending beyond the muscularis (T2) the likelihood of lymph node metastasis is high and revision surgery (radical cholecystectomy) is to be considered.

    A 2 cm wedge of liver in the gallbladder bed or segment IVb and V along with the lymph nodes at the porta, hepatoduodenal ligament and peripancreatic lymph nodes are removed.

Q. Why only right lobectomy is not adequate in gallbladder carcinoma?

Ans. Gallbladder fossa is the anatomical demarcating line between the right and left lobes and may spread to both lobes so a right lobectomy is not enough to resect the disease.

Q. How will you manage patient presenting with advanced gallbladder cancer?

Ans. These patients need palliative treatment only:

- *Palliation of jaundice:* ERCP and stenting with a self-expanding metallic stent provides relief of jaundice with less need for repeated change of stent.
- *Palliation of gastric outlet obstruction:* Gastric outlet obstruction may also be relieved by endoscopic duodenal stenting or by open operation of gastrojejunostomy.
- *Palliation of pain:* NSAID → Opioids → percutaneous neurolysis of celiac plexus by injecting alcohol.

Q. What is the role of chemotherapy in carcinoma of gallbladder?

Ans. Chemotherapy is not very effective in carcinoma gallbladder. Most frequently 5-fluorouracil and mitomycin have been used. Cisplatin has shown better results.

Q. What is the role of radiotherapy in carcinoma of gallbladder?

Ans. Radiation therapy has been used after resectional surgery as an adjuvant. No survival advantage has been reported. Radiation sensitizer 5-fluorouracil along with radiation provides some benefit.

Advanced unresectable disease radiotherapy is not useful.

Q. What are the etiological risk factors for carcinoma of gallbladder?

Ans. The etiological risk factors are:
1. Gallstone disease
2. Choledochal cyst
3. Anomalous pancreaticobiliary duct junction
4. Gallbladder polyp >1 cm
5. Adenomyomatosis of gallbladder
6. Chronic typhoid carriers
7. Carcinogens, e.g. nitrosamines
8. Occupational exposure—persons working in rubber and textile industries
9. Genetic—mutation of p53 and *k ras* gene
10. Chronic *H. pylori* infection.

Q. What is the relation between gallstone disease and carcinoma of gallbladder?

Ans. *See* Surgical Pathology Section, Page No. 902–904, Chapter 18

Q. What is the correlation between stone size and carcinoma of gallbladder?

Ans. *See* Surgical Pathology Section, Page No. 903–904, Chapter 18

Q. How anomalous pancreaticobiliary duct junction can cause carcinoma of gallbladder?

Ans. *See* Surgical Pathology Section, Page No. 903–904, Chapter 18

Q. What are the sequences of changes in development of carcinoma gallbladder?

Ans. *See* Surgical Pathology Section, Page No. 903, Chapter 18

Q. What are the macroscopic types of carcinoma of gallbladder?

Ans. *See* Surgical Pathology Section, Page No. 903, Chapter 18

Q. What are the histological types of carcinoma of gallbladder?

Ans. *See* Surgical Pathology Section, Page No. 903, Chapter 18

Q. How does carcinoma gallbladder spread?

Ans. *See* Surgical Pathology Section, Page No. 903, Chapter 18

Q. What is Nevin's staging for carcinoma of gallbladder?

Ans. Nevin's stages:
* Stage I: Intramucosal only
* Stage II: Extends to the muscularis propria
* Stage III: Extends through the liver
* Stage IV:- Transmural involvement
* Stage V: Direct extension.

Q. What are TNM definitions for carcinoma of gallbladder?

Ans. T groups for gallbladder cancer
* TX: The primary tumor's extent cannot be assessed.
* T0: There is no evidence of primary tumor.

- Tis (carcinoma in situ): Tumor confined to the epithelium and have not grown into deeper layers of the gallbladder.
- T1: The tumor has grown into the lamina propria or the muscle layer (muscularis propria).
  - T1a: Tumor has grown into lamina propria.
  - T1b: Tumor has grown into the muscularis propria.
- T2: Tumor penetrating into perimuscular fibrous tissue.
- T3: Tumor extending through the serosa and/or it has grown from the gallbladder directly into the liver and/or one nearby structures such as the stomach, duodenum, colon, pancreas, or extrahepatic biliary tree.
- T4: Tumor invading the portal vein or hepatic artery or it has grown into two or more structures outside of the liver.

N Groups for Gallbladder Cancer

- NX: Nearby (regional) lymph nodes cannot be assessed.
- N0: The cancer has not spread to nearby lymph nodes.
- N1: Cancer spread to lymph nodes near the gallbladder, cystic lymph node, pericholedochal lymph node, nodes along hepatic artery, and portal vein.
- N2: Cancer has spread to lymph nodes farther away from the gallbladder, such as the lymph nodes along the aorta (periaortic), the vena cava (pericaval), the superior mesenteric artery, and the celiac artery.

M Groups for Gallbladder Cancer

- M0: No distant metastasis.
- M1: Distant metastasis present.

Stage Grouping

- Stage 0: Tis, N0, M0: Tumor confined to the epithelial layer of the gallbladder'
- Stage I: T1 (a or b), N0, M0: Tumor confined to the lamina propria (T1a) or the muscle layer (T1b)
- Stage II: T2, N0, M0: Tumor invading the perimuscular fibrous tissue (T2)
- Stage IIIA: T3, N0, M0: The tumor extends through the serosa (outer layer of the gallbladder) and/or directly grows into the liver and/or one other nearby structure (T3). No lymph nodes (N0) or no distant metastasis (M0)
- Stage IIIB: T1 to T3, N1, M0: Tumor confined to gallbladder wall or invading the liver or invading one adjacent structure (T1 to T3), but involved the nearby lymph nodes (N1). No distant metastasis (M0)
- Stage IVA: T4, N0 or N1, M0: Tumor invading portal vein or hepatic artery or invaded to more than one nearby organ other than the liver (T4). Lymph node spread may or may not be there (N0 or N1). No distant metastasis (M0)
- Stage IVB: Either of the following:
  - Any T, N2, M0: **Primary** tumor of any T. Lymph node involvement beyond the peri-gallbladder area (N2). No distant metastasis. (M0).
    OR
  - Any T, any N, M1: Primary tumor of any T. Any lymph node status. But distant metastasis present (M1).

Q. How the patients with carcinoma of gallbladder present?

Ans.

* Patient may present in different ways:
    - Symptoms and signs suggestive of acute cholecystitis
    - Symptoms and signs of chronic biliary tract disease—right upper quadrant pain, jaundice
    - General symptoms and signs suggestive of a malignant disease—anorexia, weight loss, generalized weakness
    - Symptoms and signs suggestive of disease outside the biliary tract—gastric outlet obstruction and gastrointestinal bleeding
    - Symptoms and signs suggestive of advanced malignant disease   palpable gallbladder mass, hard nodular liver and ascites.
* Carcinoma of gallbladder is suspected in a patient who has long-standing history of gallstone disease in which a recent change in symptomatology and pain has occurred.

Q. Laparotomy has been done for gallstone disease and found to have carcinoma of gallbladder, what will you do in that situation?

Ans.

* Occult gallbladder carcinoma diagnosed by opening the gallbladder before closure of abdomen. Frozen section biopsy is to be done
* If the tumor has not invaded beyond submucosa (pT1a) simple cholecystectomy is enough
* If the tumor has invaded beyond the submucosa and the muscle layer (pT1b and pT2)—radical cholecystectomy is to be done straightway
* If the gallbladder carcinoma is diagnosed on histological examination afterwards the management strategy is same
* Gallbladder carcinoma obvious on exploratory laparotomy—cancer confined to the gallbladder, but no evidence of distant spread—the optimum procedure is radical cholecystectomy
* Gallbladder carcinoma with evidence of local invasion but no distant spread (T3/T4 tumors) extended or radical cholecystectomy may be done but the survival is poor as compared to early disease
* Gallbladder carcinoma with both local invasion and evidence of distant spread—no role of curative resection. Biopsy to confirm the diagnosis.
    - For jaundice, bilioenteric bypass, a segment III bypass with a Roux-en-Y limb of jejunum. Alternatively endoscopic stenting may be considered later
    - For gastric outlet obstruction—gastrojejunostomy
    - For pain relief—celiac plexus blockade with alcohol.

Q. Which tumor markers are important in carcinoma of gallbladder?

Ans. CEA and CA 19-9 may be elevated in carcinoma gallbladder. But these markers may be elevated in other GI malignancy.

▮ DISCUSSION ON CHOLANGIOCARCINOMA

It is difficult to give a diagnosis of obstructive jaundice due to cholangiocarcinoma depending on history and examination. This will come up as a differential diagnosis for obstructive jaundice.

Q. What are the important etiological factors for development of cholangiocarcinoma?

Ans. The important etiological factors are:
* Stone disease: 20–50% patients of cholangiocarcinoma have associated bile duct stones. The association between bile duct stone and cholangiocarcinoma is however not clear
* Bacterial induced endogenous carcinogens in the bile may cause increased incidence of cholangiocarcinoma
* Sclerosing cholangitis and ulcerative colitis predisposes to increased incidence of cholangiocarcinoma
* Choledochal cyst also predisposes to increased incidence of cholangiocarcinoma in the whole biliary tree
* Parasitic infestation of bile duct. Clonorchis sinensis is an important etiological factor.

Q. What are the different types of cholangiocarcinoma?

Ans.
* Depending on the sites of involvement of the biliary tree the cholangiocarcinoma may be:
  - Intrahepatic: Involves the minor intrahepatic duct. May be multicentric difficult to differentiate from hepatocellular carcinoma.
  - Extrahepatic
    - Proximal: Arises either from right or left hepatic ducts or the confluence or the proximal common hepatic duct (Klatskin's tumor)
    - Middle: Involves the common hepatic duct and the proximal common bile duct
    - Distal: From distal common bile duct and the periampullary region.
* Depending on the gross appearance cholangiocarcinomas may be divided into:
  - Scirrhous type: Causes diffuse thickening of wall of the bile duct. Intensely fibrotic lesion and is difficult to differentiate from sclerosing cholangitis
  - Nodular variety: Form extraductal nodule in addition to intraluminal projection
  - Papillary variety: Mainly involves the distal bile duct and the periampullary region. Friable vascular growth may fill the bile duct lumen and bleeds easily leading to hemobilia.

Q. What are the histological types of cholangiocarcinoma?

Ans.
* Majority are adenocarcinoma.
* Rare types may include squamous cell carcinoma, adenosquamous cell carcinoma, lymphoma, carcinoid, melanoma and very rarely APUDomas.

Q. How does the cholangiocarcinoma spreads?

Ans.
* It may spread directly to invade the portal vein or liver
* Perineural spread and lymphatic spread may occur.

Q. What are the usual presentations of patients with cholangiocarcinoma?

Ans.
* Obstructive jaundice in 90% cases
* Dull upper abdominal pain
* Anorexia, weight loss
* May present with acute cholangitis
* Gallbladder may be palpable in distal bile duct lesion.

Q. What is silvery stool?

Ans. Silvery stool is combination of steatorrhea and altered blood giving a bright silvery appearance of the stool. This may be found in periampullary carcinoma associated with upper gastrointestinal hemorrhage.

Q. How will you evaluate a patient of cholangiocarcinoma?

Ans.
* Liver function test
* USG can show dilatation of biliary tree but cannot localize the tumor
* CECT scan
* ERCP or MRCP
* Celiac axis angiography: Vascular encasement signifies inoperability.

Q. What is TNM classification for cholangiocarcinoma?

Ans. The TNM classification for cholangiocarcinoma is given in Table 3.10 and anatomic stage is discussed in Table 3.11

Table 3.10: TNM classification for cholangiocarcinoma	
Primary tumor (T)	
TX	Primary tumor cannot be assessed
T0	No evidence of primary tumor
Tis	Carcinoma in situ (intraductal tumor)
T1	Solitary tumor without vascular invasion
T2a	Solitary tumor with vascular invasion
T2b	Multiple tumors, with or without vascular invasion
T3	Tumor perforating the visceral peritoneum or involving the local extrahepatic structures by direct invasion
T4	Tumor with periductal invasion (the pathologic definition of periductal invasion is the finding of a longitudinal growth pattern along the intrahepatic bile ducts on both gross and microscopic examination)
Regional lymph nodes (N)	
NX	Regional lymph nodes cannot be assessed
N0	No regional lymph node metastasis
N1	Regional lymph node metastasis present
Distant metastasis (M)	
M0	No distant metastasis
M1	Distant metastasis present
Histologic grading	
G1	Well-differentiated
G2	Moderately differentiated
G3	Poorly differentiated
G4	Undifferentiated

Table 3.11: Anatomic stage			
Stage	*T*	*N*	*M*
0	Tis	N0	M0
I	T1	N0	M0
II	T2	N0	M0
III	T3	N0	M0
IVA	T4	N0	M0
	Any T	N1	M0
IVB	Any T	Any N	M1
	Any T	Any N	M1

Q. How will you treat patient with cholangiocarcinoma showing signs of advanced disease?

Ans. Palliative treatment for relief of jaundice either by surgical bilioenteric bypass or endoscopic stenting or percutaneous transhepatic biliary drainage (PTBD).

Q. In inoperable hilar lesion how will you do a surgical bilioenteric bypass?

Ans. Anastomosis of a Roux-en-Y loop of jejunum to segment III duct using the round ligament approach.

Q. How will you treat an operable middle cholangiocarcinoma?

Ans. The best treatment is excision extending from below the confluence of the hepatic duct down up to the duodenum along with pericholedochal lymph nodes.

Q. What will be the treatment for a distal or periampullary cholangiocarcinoma?

Ans. Whipple pancreaticoduodenectomy is the ideal procedure in such situation.

Q. How will you treat Klatskin's tumor?

Ans. Klatskin tumor is cholangiocarcinoma involving the confluence of the hepatic ducts.

If there are no signs of spread, excision of the tumor with both right and left hepatic duct anastomosis with a Roux-en-Y loop of jejunum.

Tumor involving either of the hepatic duct may be treated with hepatic lobectomy and reconstruction of the biliary tree.

Q. What is the role of radiotherapy in cholangiocarcinoma?

Ans. Some reports say that postoperative adjuvant radiotherapy may reduce the incidence of local recurrence.

Q. What is the role of chemotherapy in cholangiocarcinoma?

Ans.
- Not much helpful.
- Some success has been claimed with combination chemotherapy with 5-fluorouracil plus mitomycin and doxorubicin.

■ OBSTRUCTIVE JAUNDICE DUE TO CHOLEDOCHAL CYST

It is difficult to give a diagnosis of choledochal cyst clinically. It may come as differential diagnosis of patient with obstructive jaundice particularly in young adults.

Q. What is your case? (Summary of a case of obstructive jaundice due to choledochal cyst)

Ans. A 15-year-old girl presented with recurrent attacks of pain in right upper-half of abdomen for last 3 years. Pain is acute in onset, severe colicky in nature and often there is radiation of pain to the back of the chest and the central part of the abdomen and patient gets relief only with medicines. At the beginning patient had history of pain at an interval of 3–4 months, but for last 1 month patient has history of dull aching continuous pain in the right upper-half of abdomen. Associated with history of pain patient has history of yellowish discoloration of eyes and urine which persists for about 2 weeks and gradually disappears. Patient has recurrent attacks of such yellowish discoloration for last 3 years. Patient has occasional history of mild fever along with pain and jaundice. No other systemic symptoms. Bowel and bladder habits are normal.

On examination, general survey is essentially normal except mild jaundice. Abdominal examination is normal. Systemic examination is also normal.

In view of the patient's age and the history of recurrent cholangitis I think this to be a case of choledochal cyst.

Q. What are the other possibilities?

Ans.
* Cholelithiasis with choledocholithiasis
* Cholangiohepatitis due to worm infestation
* Chronic pancreatitis
* Obstructive jaundice due to bile duct obstruction due to lymph node mass in the porta due to tuberculosis or lymphoma.

Q. What investigation will you suggest for the diagnosis?

Ans. The primary investigation will be a liver function test and USG of hepatobiliary tree.

Q. What further investigation you will do in this patient?

Ans. Further investigations will depend on the ultrasonographic findings.
* If the USG shows there is choledochal cyst, I will prefer to do MRCP
* If USG shows that there is gallstone disease with choledocholithiasis I will suggest ERCP with endoscopic sphincterotomy and endoscopic extraction of CBD stone using a Dormia basket catheter.

Q. How MRCP helps in diagnosis?

Ans. With advent of MRCP the role of diagnostic ERCP has become very limited. MRCP can give a very good delineation of biliary tree and a diagnosis of choledochal cyst may be done with confidence.

Q. Does CT scan has any role in this case?

Ans. For evaluation of a suspected choledochal cyst a CT scan is not essential. However, CECT scan may also demonstrate the dilated biliary tree.

Q. What other investigation you will do in this patient?

Ans. I will do routine work-up to assess the patient's fitness for general anesthesia.

Q. How will you treat this patient?

Ans. I will plan for operative treatment. The optimum surgical treatment is total excision of the choledochal cyst and hepaticojejunostomy with a Roux-en-Y limb of jejunum.

Q. What is the distal and proximal extent of resection of the cyst?

Ans. Initially the gallbladder is mobilized and the cyst is then dissected distally to the point of entry into the pancreatic parenchyma where it is divided. The cyst is then dissected proximally and usually the dilatation ends just below the confluence where it is divided and a hepaticojejunostomy with a Roux-en-Y limb of jejunum is done.

If the cystic dilatation involves the confluence then the confluence may be excised and right and left hepatic duct may be anastomosed separately to a Roux-en-Y limb of jejunum. The anastomosis may be stented by a transhepatic tube.

Q. While excising the lower limit of the cyst what precaution you should take?

Ans. By doing preoperative investigation or intraoperative cholangiography the pancreatic duct opening should be localized. If there is anomalous pancreaticobiliary duct junction while excising the lower limit of the cyst the injury to the anomalous opening of the pancreatic duct should be avoided.

Q. Why a cystoenterostomy is not an ideal surgical procedure?

Ans. The mucus lining of the choledochal cyst shows inflammation and fibrosis—so there is chance of anastomotic obstruction from scarring at the site of anastomosis.

The fibrous thick walled cyst does not contract after drainage and acts as a receptacle for stagnant bile and the risk of cholangitis remains.

Choledochal cyst is a premalignant lesion and the chance of developing malignancy remains there. So, cystoenterostomy is not an ideal procedure.

Q. How will you manage if there is gross pericholecystic adhesion and the cyst is adherent to the hepatic artery or the portal vein?

Ans. Recurrent attacks of cholangitis can lead to such situation and an attempt to do a complete excision may lead to injury to the important structures.

A modified approach is required to remove such cyst. The anterior and lateral wall of the cyst is excised. An arbitrary plane is created within the posterior wall of the cyst and the inner lining of the cyst is dissected and excised leaving behind the outer layer of the cyst that lies adherent to the portal structures. Thus, the anterior, lateral and the inner lining of the posterior wall of the cyst are excised. This is called Lily's modification for excision of choledochal cyst.

Q. What is choledochal cyst?

Ans. Choledochal cyst is congenital dilatation of extrahepatic or intrahepatic biliary tree or both.

Q. What are the different types of choledochal cyst?

Ans. Choledochal cyst is classified into different types by Alonso Lej. Subsequently Todani et al. proposes a modification which is as follows (Fig. 3.44).

- Type I: Dilatation of extrahepatic biliary tree—Ia-Cystic, Ib-Focal, Ic-Fusiform
- Type II: Saccular diverticulum of extrahepatic bile duct
- Type III: Dilatation of intraduodenal part of bile duct—choledochocoele
- Type Iva: Dilatation of both intrahepatic and extrahepatic biliary tree
- Type IVb: Multiple extrahepatic cysts
- Type V: Dilatation of intrahepatic ducts only (Caroli's disease).

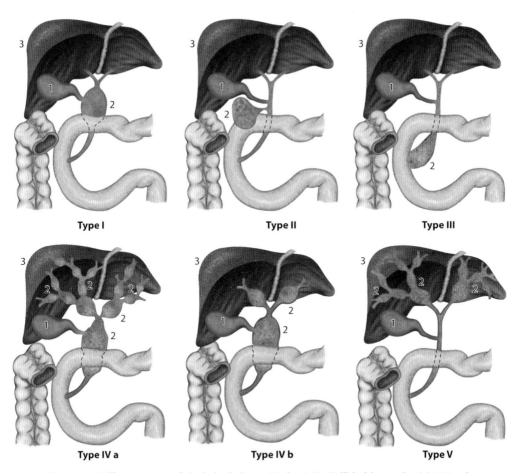

Fig. 3.44: Different types of choledochal cyst (Todani). [1: Gallbladder; 2: Cyst(s); 3:Liver]

Q. What are the histological types of choledochal cyst?

Ans. Histologically, the choledochal cyst may be of two types:

1. *Glandular type:* Normal cuboidal epithelium present along with glandular cavities in the mucosal layer.
2. *Fibrotic type:* Bile duct is thickened with plenty of fibrous tissues in the wall of the cyst.

Q. How does the choledochal cyst develop?

Ans. There are three theories to explain the development of choledochal cyst:

- *First theory—Babbit hypothesis:* There is anomalous pancreaticobiliary duct junction. There is reflux of pancreatic juice into the bile duct. This causes increase in pressure in the bile duct and also there is enzymatic destruction of bile duct wall leading to ductal weakening and dilatation.
- *Second theory:* Abnormal canalization of bile duct during embryogenesis with distal obstruction. The distal obstruction causes increased proximal pressure leading to ductal dilatation.
- *Third theory:* Pathogenesis of choledochal cyst involves abnormalities of autonomic innervation of the extrahepatic biliary tree. There is reduction of postganglionic neurons in the narrow distal portion of the cyst in comparison to the dilated part of the cyst.

Q. How the patient with choledochal cyst does usually present?

Ans. It may present in infancy or in adult.

Classic triad of choledochal cyst:

- Jaundice
- Right upper quadrant mass and
- Right upper quadrant abdominal pain.
  This triad is present in only minority of patients (5–30% of cases). Majority presents with one or two symptoms of the triad. pancreatic ductal adenocarcinoma
- Other symptoms are: Nausea, pruritus and weight loss
- Adults may present with: Features of acute pancreatitis or acute cholangitis
- May rarely present with acute rupture of the cyst with S/S of acute biliary peritonitis.

Q. What are the complications of choledochal cyst?

Ans.

- Jaundice
- Recurrent cholangitis
- Pancreatitis
- Gallstones and stones in the cyst, cholecystitis and cholangitis
- Carcinoma of gallbladder and bile duct
- Cirrhosis and portal hypertension
- Rupture of cyst.

Q. What is the treatment of type III choledochal cyst?

Ans. Choledochocele is treated either by transduodenal sphincteroplasty or sphincterotomy.

Q. What is the treatment for Caroli's disease? (Type V)

Ans.

- Confined to one lobe or segment—lobectomy or segmental resection
- Diffuse disease involving both lobe—liver transplantation.

CASES PRESENTING WITH ABDOMINAL LUMP

■ ABDOMINAL LUMP DUE TO HYDATID CYST OF LIVER

Q. What is your case? (Summary of a case of abdominal lump due to hydatid cyst of liver)

Ans. A 35-year-old lady presented with a swelling in right side of upper abdomen for last 5 years, which is gradually increasing in size for last 5 years. There is no history of rapid increase in size of the swelling. Patient complains of occasional dull aching pain over the right upper of abdomen for last 2 years. No history of fever and no other systemic symptoms. There is no history of major ailment in the past. Patient used to keep pet dogs at home for long time.

On examination, general survey is essentially normal. On local examination of abdomen, liver is enlarged 9 cm below the right costal margin in the right midclavicular line and a cystic swelling is palpable in relation to the liver 7 cm × 5 cm in dimension, nontender. No other mass is palpable. No free fluid in the abdomen and normal bowel sounds are audible. Systemic examination is normal.

Q. What is your diagnosis?

Ans. This is a case of a cystic lesion in right lobe of liver probably hydatid cyst.

Q. Why do you say this is a cystic swelling arising from the liver?

Ans. Patient complained of the swelling in the right upper half of the abdomen and on examination the liver is found to be enlarged and the cystic swelling, which is palpable in the epigastrium and the right hypochondriac region is found to be continuous with the enlarged liver and the liver dullness is continuous the dull note over the swelling and it is not possible to insinuate the finger between the swelling and the costal margin. So this is a cystic swelling in relation to the liver.

Q. What is the differential diagnosis for such a cystic lesion in liver?

- Simple or congenital cyst in liver
- Polycystic liver: A few cysts may be larger which are palpable
- Lymphatic cyst in liver
- Pseudocyst of pancreas
- Proliferative cyst: Cystadenoma
- Traumatic cyst in liver: Usually filled with bile, no cyst lining
- Hepatic adenoma
- Hepatoma with cystic degeneration
- Metastatic liver with cystic degeneration.

Q. What investigation will you suggest in this patient?

Ans. To confirm diagnosis following investigations are suggested:

- USG of abdomen, which will show the cyst in the liver. It can show laminated membrane or hydatid sand which is detached from daughter cyst
- Enzyme-linked immunosorbent assay (ELISA) test for *Echinococcus* antigen.

Q. How ultrasonography will help?

Ans. Ultrasonography will show:
* Extent of liver enlargement
* Nature of palpable swelling—solid or cystic
* Dimension of the swelling
* Any other cyst in liver or kidney (to exclude polycystic disease).

In case of hydatid cyst it will show:
* Size of the cyst
* Number of cyst
* Location of the cyst in relation to liver segment
* Vascular and biliary relationship of the cyst
* The laminated membrane and hydatid sand may be demonstrated.

Q. How the cysts are classified according to USG findings?

Ans. Depending on the appearance in USG the cysts are classified as:
* CL type (Univesicular cyst): Well-circumscribed, round cyst. Well-defined wall with anechogenic image
* CE 1 type: There is a concentric hyperechogenic halo around the cyst and the cyst contains free floating hyperechogenic foci (hydatid sand)
* CE 2 type: multivesicular cyst. The characteristic appearance of daughter cyst identified by honeycomb, rosette or spoke wheel appearance
* CE 3 type: Characterized by partial or total detachment of the chitinous layer showing dual wall, water lily and water snake sign
* CE 4 type: Cysts containing cystic and solid components
* CE 5 type: Cyst with a matrix or amorphous mass with soild appearance. Calcification at the periphery is common.

Q. What is water lily sign?

Ans. It is the ultrasonographic appearance of hydatid cyst. Separation of laminated membrane produces a "split wall" appearance and its complete collapse results in water lily sign.

Q. What is cart wheel appearance?

Ans. This is an ultrasonographic finding showing multiple cyst like the wheel of a cart and is suggestive of a multivesiculated cysts.

Q. Is CT scan indicated in this patient?

Ans. If on USG a single unilocular cyst is found and the rest of the liver is normal then a CT scan of abdomen is not essential. In case of multiple hydatid cysts on USG, a CT scan is indicated to delineate different cysts, more in relation to the liver segments, which will help to plan operative management. CECT is invaluable for recurrent cyst. Spiral CT scan is now the gold standard investigation.

Q. What is the role of MRI in hydatid cyst diagnosis?

Ans. MRI can demonstrate the cystic lesion in liver. MRCP can give a good delineation of intrahepatic and extrahepatic biliary tree and its relationship to the cyst and any evidence of cystobiliary communication.

Q. What is the role of ERCP in hydatid cyst?

Ans. Routine ERCP is not required in hydatid cyst. In patient presenting with obstructive jaundice due to cystobiliary communication. Endoscopic sphincterotomy can allow removal of daughter cyst from the biliary tree.

Q. What other investigations are to be done in this patient?

Ans. Apart from above investigation following are suggested:
- Chest X-ray to exclude pulmonary hydatid
- Complete hemogram Hb%, TLC, DLC and ESR. May show eosinophilia
- Blood for sugar, urea and creatinine
- Liver function test
- ECG
- Serological test—ELISA test for detection of hydatid antigen. Immunoelectrophoresis for detection of antibody to hydatid antigen (diagnostic value: 91–94%).

Q. How will you treat this patient?

Ans. Surgical treatment is to be considered in this patient. As this is a single cyst simple excision of the cyst with partial excision of the pericyst (partial cystopericystectomy) is sufficient. Before surgery a course of albendazole for 3 weeks is to be undertaken.

Q. Why surgical treatment is indicated?

Ans. The cyst is larger than 5 cm and the large cysts are unlikely to resolve with drug treatment.

Q. What is the role of albendazole before surgery?

Ans. Preoperative albendazole therapy has some advantages.
- Some of the cyst may regress to some extent
- The albendazole has scolicidal activity
- In case of accidental spillage of hydatid cyst fluid during operation, due to the scolicidal effect, peritoneal seedling will be prevented.

Q. What is the technique of cystectomy?

Ans.
- Abdomen explored cyst localized
- Abdomen packed with mops, soaked in hypertonic saline and area of cyst isolated. Cyst is punctured with a 14G needle fitted with a three way stopcock
- The fluid from the cyst is aspirated by a syringe, taking care so that it does not spill into the peritoneal cavity
- After the fluid has been aspirated the cyst cavity is then filled with a scolicidal agent like hypertonic saline and wait for 5 minutes
- The scolicidal solution is aspirated back
- An incision is made over the thinned out liver tissue up to the pericyst
- Once the pericyst is incised the laminated membrane is seen
- The laminated membrane is grasped with a sponge holding forceps and can be removed intact. In case of infected hydatid cyst laminated membrane may be required to be removed in piecemeal. All the daughter cysts are removed

- The thinned out liver parenchyma forming the pericyst is partially excised and hemostasis achieved with electrocautery or suture
- Look for any bile leakage in the hydatid cyst cavity. If minor bile leakage is found it may be under-run with suture. If major biliary communication is found a drainage procedure like Rou-en-Y cystojejunostomy will be required.

Q. How will you tackle the cavity of hydatid cyst following excision of the cyst?

Ans.

- *Small cavity may be obliterated* by deep stitches (Capitonnage)
- *Omentopexy:* Greater omentum may be mobilized and packed into the cavity of the cyst
- *External drainage:* The cavity is closed keeping a drain inside
- *Cystoenteric anastomosis (Roux-en-Y cystojejunostomy):* Particularly in the cyst with a major biliary communication
- *Marsupialization:* Usually not done nowadays. May be done in infected cyst in patients with poor general condition.

Q. What are the indications of segmental resection of liver?

Ans. If cyst is situated in peripheral part of the liver and not too large, excision of the cyst with a margin of liver is considered safe. There is no risk of spillage of contents of the cyst into peritoneal cavity.

    If there are multiple cysts in one lobe then a hepatic lobectomy may be considered.

Q. Which parasite causes hydatid disease?

- *Echinococcus granulosus*
- *Echinococcus multilocularis.*

Q. Who is the definitive host for the *Echinococcus?*

Q. Who is the intermediate host for the *Echinococcus?*

Q. How does the man get the infection?

Q. How does an adult *Echinococcus* look like?

Q. How is the life cycle of worm continued?

Q. Which other animals can act as intermediate host?

Q. How does a hydatid cyst develop in man?

Q. How does the different layer of the cyst develop?

Q. What are the functions of the endocyst?

Q. How does the daughter cyst develop?

Q. What is the characteristic of cyst formed by *Echinococcus multilocularis?*

Q. What is the characteristic of hydatid fluid?

For answers of this question, *See* Surgical Pathology Section, Page No. 889–893, Chapter 18.

Q. What are the usual presentations of patient with hydatid cyst of liver?

Ans.
- Asymptomatic in 75% cases
- An epigastric cystic lump is felt in relation to the liver
- Dull aching pain in right upper abdomen
- May present with some complications.

Q. What are the complications of hydatid cyst?

Ans. Hydatid cyst may lead to a number of complications:
- *Pressure effects:*
  - Pressure of cyst on bile duct—obstructive jaundice
  - Pressure of cyst on portal vein—portal hypertension.
- *Rupture:* It may rupture into
  - Peritoneal cavity: Symptoms and signs of generalized peritonitis/anaphylaxis
  - Into intestine or stomach—cyst content may be vomited out
  - Into biliary tree—biliary colic, fever and jaundice (cholangitis)
  - Into pleural cavity—empyema
  - Into lungs—cyst content and bile may be coughed out.
- *Infection and suppuration*—pain, rigor and fever.
- *Anaphylactic shock* due to rupture of the cyst.

Q. What are the sequelae of hydatid cyst?

Ans.
- Cyst may gradually enlarge
- The parasite may die, fluid is absorbed, the laminated membrane may calcify. A completely calcified cyst indicate a dead nonreactive cyst
- May lead to some complications.

Q. What are the features of intraperitoneal rupture of cyst?

Ans. Patient may present with acute abdominal pain and following signs:
- *Signs of shock*
  - Tachycardia
  - Hypotension
  - Air hunger.
- *Signs of diffuse peritonitis*
  - Tenderness all over abdomen
  - Rigidity all over abdomen
  - Absence of bowel sounds.
- *Skin manifestations*
  - Itching, urticaria.

Q. How will you treat intraperitoneal rupture of cyst?

Ans.
- Treatment of shock with:
  - IV fluid

- IV hydrocortisone, antihistaminic
- Oxygen inhalation.
- Exploratory laparotomy
  - Peritoneal lavage with scolicidal solution
  - Tackling of hydatid cyst.

Q. What are the characteristic of polycystic liver disease?

Ans.
- Honeycomb like liver with multiple cysts
- Lesion is diffuse throughout the liver sometimes only the right lobe is affected
  There may be cystic involvement of other organs. In 51% cases polycystic kidney disease may be associated
- May be rarely associated with biliary atresia, cholangitis, cleft palate, spina bifida cardiac defect and malrotation of gut.

Q. What may be the causes of acute pain in cystic lesion in the liver?

Ans.
- Torsion, if cyst is pedunculated
- Intracystic hemorrhage
- Intraperitoneal rupture
- Infection.

Q. In abdominal X-ray what is the implication of a calcified cyst?

Ans. A calcified cyst indicates a dead nonreactive cyst.

Q. What is camellotte sign?

Ans. Following intrabiliary rupture, gas may enter into the cyst leading to partial collapse of the cyst wall. This is called camellotte sign.

Q. How the immunological tests become positive in hydatid disease?

Ans. Although the cyst is isolated from the liver by an adventitial layer there is absorption of parasitic products throughout the pericyst, which acts as an antigenic stimulus.

This is reflected as a positive ELISA test in 90% cases and eosinophilia in 25% cases.

However, some cyst never leaks and so immunological tests will be negative in these cases.

Q. What is hydatid sand?

Ans. The brood capsules arise from germinal epithelium. The brood capsules undergo localized proliferation and invagination of their wall to form scolices. Some brood capsules separate from germinal membrane and settle at the bottom of the cyst cavity as fine granular sediment called hydatid sand.

Q. Why hydatid disease is not common in childhood?

Ans. The infection may be acquired in childhood, but the cyst grows very slowly in size. So symptom does not appear until adult life. An interval of 20–30 years has been known to exist between primary infection and manifestation of the symptoms.

Q. What are the different immunological tests for diagnosis of hydatid disease?

Ans.

+ *Casonis test*: Sensitivity 60–80%
    – Done by injecting sterilized crude hydatid fluid. Positive test is indicated by wheal and flare at the site of injection
    – Positive test may persist for several years after excision of the cyst
+ *Complement fixation test:* Positive in 70% of patients and may remain positive for 2 years after the elimination of infection.
+ *Indirect hemoagglutination test:* Positive in 90% cases. May remain positive for several years after eradication of the cyst
+ *Bentonite flocculation test* is positive in 71% cases
+ *Detection of circulating antigen* by countercurrent immunoelectrophoresis or ELISA appears to give the most reliable result
+ *A rapid test: Dot ELISA test* detects antibody to a purified parasite antigen in a small finger prick blood sample.

Q. What drug therapy is effective in hydatid cyst?

Ans.

+ *Mebendazole:* 60 mg/kg/day in 3 divided doses for 6–24 months.
+ *Albendazole:* 10–12 mg/kg daily for 28 days followed by a gap of 15 days and continued for 3 months. There has been regression of cyst in some cases.
    There is 30–40% chance of response to medical treatment for smaller cyst.

Q. What is echinococcosis?

Ans. Infestation of the principal host by adult worm is called echinococcosis.

Q. What is the rate of enlargement of hydatid cyst?

Ans. The cyst grows very slowly at a rate of 2–3 cm/year.

Q. What is exogenous daughter cyst?

Ans. The germinal epithelium usually causes inward pouching toward the lumen of the cyst to form the daughter cyst. Rarely, the germinal epithelium may cause protrusion outward toward the pericyst, which forms exogenous daughter cyst.

The exogenous daughter cyst may be found in 19–23% of patients undergoing cystoperi-cystectomy. These exogenous daughter cyst lies outside the ectocyst and may be left behind during operation, if pericyst is left intact and may be one reason for recurrence of the cyst following operation.

Q. What is the role of medical treatment in hydatid cyst?

Ans. The following are the important indications for medical treatment in hydatid disease:

+ Small hydatid cyst may resolve with drug treatment
+ Disseminated hydatid disease
+ Multiple recurrence of hydatid disease
+ Inaccessible cyst in liver
+ Intraperitoneal and intrathoracic rupture

- Patient unfit for surgery
- Preoperative preparation of the patient to prevent peritoneal dissemination and reduce the incidence of recurrent disease due to intraperitoneal spillage during surgery.

Q. What are the scolicidal agents?

Ans. These are substances which can kill the scolices and may be instilled into the cyst during operation or may be instilled into the cyst percutaneously.

The different scolicidal agents are:

- About 20% hypertonic saline
- Cetrimide solution
- Silver nitrate
- Formalin and
- About 95% alcohol.
  Hypertonic saline is commonly used.

Q. What is the role of percutaneous aspiration (PAIR) in treatment of hydatid cyst?

Ans. Percutaneous aspiration, injection of scolicidal agent and reaspiration (PAIR) has been proposed as an alternative treatment to surgery in selected cases of hydatid cyst.

Under ultrasound guidance percutaneous aspiration of the cyst is done. Installation of 20% hypertonic saline or 95% alcohol instillation into the cyst is done. The content is then reaspirated after 10 minutes. This has to be done on number of occasion. This combined with systemic therapy with albendazole has been successful in 70% of patients in some reports.

This may be effective in uncomplicated unilocular cyst, poor surgical candidate and patients with multiple previous operations.

This form of treatment is contraindicated in patients with multilocular cysts, cyst with secondary infection or cyst with suspected biliary communication.

Q. What is the recurrence rate after conservative surgery?

Ans. The chance of recurrence after conservative surgery is 16%.

Q. How will you take care to prevent recurrence?

Ans. Use of intraoperative USG to detect exogenous daughter cyst or other small cyst not detected by preoperative USG.

Q. What are the different options for surgical treatment of hydatid cyst?

Ans.

- Conservative surgery:
  - Cystectomy and evacuation
  - Capitonnage
  - Partial pericystectomy and omentoplasty
  - Pericystojejunostomy.
- Radical surgery:
  - Cystopericystectomy (Total/subtotal)
  - Wedge resection of liver
  - Major liver resection: Right or left lobectomy.

■ PSEUDOCYST OF PANCREAS

Q. What is your case? (Summary of a case of pseudopancreatic cyst)

Ans. A 35-year-old gentleman presented with the history of acute pain in abdomen 3 months back. Pain was sudden in onset, colicky in nature, started in the central part of the abdomen and then radiated to the whole of abdomen and back. Pain was increasing in intensity for 2 days and then subsided with treatment in 5 days' time. Patient has history of nausea and vomiting along with the pain. About 10 days following the onset of pain patient noticed a small swelling in the central part of the upper abdomen which was gradually increasing in size for last 2 months. For last 1 month the swelling has become static. Complains of dull aching pain over the swelling. Bowel and bladder habits are normal. No other systemic symptoms.

On examination general survey is essentially normal. On local examination of abdomen on inspection the shape of the abdomen is normal with slight fullness in the epigastric and the umbilical region. The umbilicus is pushed downwards and is slightly stretched. The skin of the abdomen is normal. A lump is palpable in the epigastric, umbilical and both hypochondriac region. The lump is intra-abdomianl, size is about 15 cm in diameter and is globular in shape. It is moving slightly up and down with respiration. Margins are rounded and well-defined. Surface is smooth. Consistency is tense cystic, nontneder. Liver and spleen are not palpable and no other mass is palpable. Systemic examination is normal.

In view of the possible past attack of acute pain and the subsequent appearance of the swelling and the other characteristics of the swelling this appears to be a case of pseudopancreatic cyst.

Q. What are the other possibilities?

Ans.
- Hydatid cyst of liver
- Simple cyst of liver
- Hydatid cyst of spleen
- Cystadenoma of pancreas
- Cystadenocarcinoma of pancreas
- Hydatid cyst of pancreas
- Mesenteric cyst

Q. How will you manage this patient?

Ans. I would like to confirm my diagnosis by doing some investigations.

I will suggest ultrasonography of upper abdomen. Ultrasonography may show the cystic lesion and its relation to the pancreas. Can exclude associated chronic pancreatitis and any intraductal calculi in the pancreas may be seen.

Q. What is the role of CECT scan in evaluation of pseudocyst?

Ans. CECT scan has increased sensitivity and specificity in diagnosis of pseudocyst. A mature pseudocyst appears as unilocular, round, fluid-filled sac lined by a contrast enhancing wall. It can show retroperitoneal extension of fluid collection and also show relationship between the adjacent bowel lumen and the cyst.

Q. What else would you like to do?

Ans. I would advise a MRCP in this patient. This is a noninvasive investigation and gives a very good delineation of bile duct and pancreatic duct. The pancreatic duct and cyst communication may be diagnosed.

Q. What is the role of ERCP for evaluation of pseudocyst of pancreas?

Ans. ERCP is indicated in symptomatic patient when some form of intervention is indicated.

Abnormalities of the pancreatic duct may be demonstrated well, e.g. dilatation of the pancreatic duct, or presence of any intraductal calculi.

Any communication of the pancreatic duct with the cyst may be seen.

In jaundiced patient ERCP may show any obstruction of the distal common bile duct.

Q. What are the problems of ERCP?

Ans. ERCP is an invasive investigation and may aggravate pancreatitis or it may introduce infection into the pseudocyst.

Q. How will you treat this patient?

Ans. This is a large cyst with a history of three months. So the cyst wall is likely to be mature. I will plan for surgical treatment in this case.

Q. What surgery may be undertaken?

Ans.

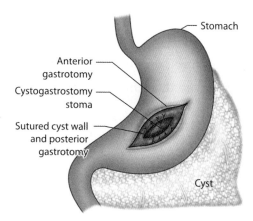

Fig. 3.45: Cystogastrostomy for pseudopancreatic cyst

* I will plan to do a cystogastrostomy
* Cysts situated in the epigastric region and adherent to the stomach are best drained by cystogastrostomy
* Cystogastrostomy involves an anterior gastrotomy. Aspiration confirms contiguity of the cyst wall to the posterior wall of the stomach. An eclipse of the adherent posterior wall of the stomach and the cyst wall is excised and sent for frozen section to exclude neoplasia. The stoma should be large and all collection and the debris within the pseudocyst is drained. Hemostasis along the cut edges is achieved by closely applied interrupted nonabsorbable sutures to appose the stomach wall and the wall of the pseudocyst. After completing the suture of the posterior gastric wall, the anterior gastrotomy is closed (Fig. 3.45).

Q. What is your diagnosis?

Ans. This is a case of obstructive jaundice due to choledocholithiasis.

Q. When will you consider a cystojejunostomy?

Ans. When the cyst is very large and extends beyond the epigastric region to the umbilical hypochondriac and lumbar region then a cystojejunostomy with a Roux-en-Y loop of jejunum is a preferred option.

Q. What operation is preferred for a cyst in the head of the pancreas?

Ans. The cyst in the head of pancreas usually gets adherent to the duodenum. This pseudocyst is best drained internally by a cystoduodenostomy. The technique of operation is same as cystogastrostomy. A duodenotomy is made in the anterior wall of duodenum. The common cyst wall between the duodenum and the cyst is exposed. An eclipse of the common wall is excised and the margin of the incised wall is over-run with sutures. Care should be taken to avoid injury to the intraduodenal part of the common bile duct and the gastroduodenal artery.

If a thick rim of pancreatic parenchyma intervenes between the cyst and the duodenal wall, this procedure is not suitable.

Q. What operation to be undertaken in a cyst in the body and tail of the pancreas?

Ans. Cysts in the body and tail of the pancreas are usually not adherent to the stomach so cysto-gastrostomy is not ideal in this situation. The cyst in the body and tail is best drained internally by cystojejunostomy to a Roux-en-Y loop of jejunum.

Q. What are the problems of cystogastrostomy for large pseudocyst?

Giant pseudocyst if treated with a cystogastrostomy there may be a tendency for the gastric and pancreatic secretions to pool in the dependent part of the cyst and result in an abscess. So giant cysts are best drained by a cystojejunostomy in the dependent part of the cyst.

Q. How will you treat pseudocyst associated with chronic pancreatitis?

Ans. Pseudocyst may be associated with chronic pancreatitis and the pancreatic duct may be dilated with intraductal calculi. In this situation a lateral pancreaticojejunostomy should be done concomitantly with a cystojejunostomy in the same Roux-en-Y loop.

Q. What is the role of endoscopic drainage of pseudocyst?

Ans. Chronic pseudocyst may be drained internally endoscopically. Cystogastrostomy or cystoduodenostomy may be done endoscopically. The cyst is localized endoscopically. The cyst is punctured endoscopically through the stomach or duodenal wall and by using a diathermy. A 1–2 cm opening is made in the cyst wall.

Q. What are the problems of endoscopic drainage?

Ans.
+ Unlike open drainage debridement is not possible endoscopically
+ Chance of bleeding from the cut margin is more with endoscopic drainage
+ Chance of leakage of cyst fluid into the peritoneal cavity.

Q. What is the role of percutaneous catheter drainage of pseudocyst?

Ans. Ultrasound or CT-guided percutaneous aspiration and placement of a catheter has been tried for pseudocyst of the pancreas. In uncomplicated pseudocyst without debris in the cyst the chance of success is high. But overall there is 70% chance of recurrence.

Q. What are the problems with percutaneous drainage?

Ans.
+ If only aspiration is done it needs repeated aspiration
+ Placement of catheter may lead to development of pancreatic fistula which might need surgical treatment
+ Chronic pseudocyst associated with pancreatic ductal obstruction and duct dilatation cannot be treated by percutaneous drainage alone.

Q. What are the indications of external drainage of pseudocyst?

Ans. The important indications for external drainage of pseudocyst are:
* Grossly infected cyst
* Cysts associated with hemorrhage
* Free rupture of the cyst requiring immediate laparotomy
* Cysts with a soft wall which will not hold sutures.

   After laparotomy the cyst wall is broken down, all debris removed and closed suction drain is placed in the cavity. If there is bleeding the cavity may be packed.

Q. What are the problems of external drainage?

Ans.
* 12–20% chance of development of pancreatic fistula. This usually closes within few months.
* Recurrence of pseudocyst: More common when the cyst communicates with a duct.
* Increased mortality and morbidity.

Q. What is the sequelae of pseudocyst?

Ans. More than 50% patients of acute pancreatitis develop some fluid collection in the lesser sac. Only when this fluid collection persists beyond 3 weeks a pseudocyst forms. About 50% of this acute pseudocyst resolves in 4–6 weeks.

Q. What is the timing for intervention of pseudocyst?

Ans. A waiting for a period of 6 weeks is recommended. Majority of the pseudocyst may resolve. If the cyst persists, the wall gets matured for safe internal drainage.

Q. When is early intervention indicated?

Ans.
* Increasing size
* Rupture of the cyst
* Infection
* Pressure effect—on duodenum causing gastric outlet obstruction or in the bile duct causing jaundice.

Q. Which pseudocyst are most likely to resolve spontaneously?

Ans.
* Cysts less than 5 cm in diameter
* Cysts with an indistinct interface between the cyst wall and the adjacent organ.

Q. Which pseudocyst are unlikely to resolve spontaneously?

Ans.
* Thick walled cyst on USG
* Associated with chronic pancreatitis
* Cysts that fail to show any decrease in size over 3–4 weeks rather show some increase is unlikely to resolve
* Traumatic pseudocysts are less likely to resolve.

Q. How do the pseudocysts resolves?

Ans. The cysts may resolve in different ways:
* Spontaneous transperitoneal resorption
* Decompression of the fluid into the pancreatic duct
* Erosion of cyst into an adjacent hollow viscus leading to a spontaneous cystoenteric fistula
* Free rupture of the cyst into the peritoneal cavity.

Q. What are the causes of pseudocyst formation?

Ans. Pseudocyst may form in a number of ways:
* As a complication of acute pancreatitis. There is acute fluid collection in lesser sac. The inflammatory cells and the granulation tissues form a membrane and encapsulate this fluid collection and the dead and devitalized tissue forming a pseudocyst
  - Another explanation of cyst formation is due to duct disruption with leakage of pancreatic juice into the surrounding tissues most often in the lesser sac. This also evokes an inflammatory response at the periphery and a membrane forms around this collection
  - The cyst takes about 4–6 weeks for maturation of its wall
* Following pancreatic trauma duct disruption leading to fluid collection in lesser sac. Trauma may be trivial and may even pass unnoticed
* Cysts may arise in the setting of chronic pancreatitis without an antecedent attack of acute exacerbation. There is obstruction and distension of the duct along with rupture of the duct and there is collection of pancreatic fluid within the substance of the gland or in the lesser sac and sometimes it is difficult to distinguish it from retention cyst.

Q. What are the natural courses of pseudocyst?

Ans. About 40–60% of acute pseudocyst undergoes spontaneous resolution in 6–8 weeks' time.

Q. What are the different types of pseudocyst?

Ans. D'Egidio and Schein (1991) have proposed a classification of pseudocysts based on the ductal anatomy, cyst duct communication and left branch of middle colic artery.

Type–I (Postacute pseudocyst):
* Develops following an attack of acute pancreatitis
* Pancreatic duct morphology is normal
* Cyst and duct communication found rarely
* No evidence underlying chronic pancreatitis.

Type–II (Postacute on chronic cyst):
* Develops following an attack of acute pancreatitis
* Pancreatic duct morphology is abnormal
* Cyst and duct communication found more frequently
* There is evidence of chronic pancreatitis.

Type III (Retention cyst):
* There is no history of acute pancreatitis
* There is duct stricture
* There is always a cyst duct communication
* There is evidence of chronic pancreatitis.

Q. What is the difference of true and pseudocyst of pancreas?

Ans.

* The pseudocyst of the pancreas is lined by a nonepithelialized wall of fibrous tissue
* The true cyst of the pancreas has an epithelial lining.

Q. How the patient with pseudocyst usually presents?

Ans.

* Suspected in patients of acute pancreatitis when symptoms fails to resolve in 7–10 days' time or there is deterioration of symptoms following initial recovery
* Persistent pain, nausea and vomiting are usual
* About 60% patients may have an epigastric mass
* Persistent hyperamylasemia following an attack of acute pancreatitis suggests development of pseudocyst
* May present with complications.

Q. What are the complications of pseudocyst?

Ans. In about 10% cases the pseudocyst may develop some complications:

* *Infection:* Fever and leukocytosis. Incidence 10–15%.
* *Obstruction:* The obstructive symptoms will depend on the site of pseudocyst. The most common site of obstruction is gastric outlet or the duodenum. Occasionally small or large bowel obstruction may occur. Large pseudocyst may cause obstructive jaundice due to CBD compression.
* *Hemorrhage:* Life-threatening complication with a mortality rate of 20%. The bleeding may be due to pseudoaneurysm formation or portal hypertension and rupture of a vessel across the stretched enlarging pseudocyst
* *Rupture:* The cyst may rupture into pleural or peritoneal cavity. Patient may present with S/S of acute peritonitis or may present in an indolent fashion with pancreatic ascites. The rupture may occur into stomach, duodenum or colon with significant hemorrhage. The internal rupture may sometime cause resolution of the cyst
* *Internal fistula:* Rupture into pleural cavity or peritoneal cavity may result in ductal communication with peritoneal or pleural cavity.

Q. Which pseudocysts need treatment?

Ans.

* Mature pseudocysts more than 6 cm in diameter
* Cysts showing increase in size
* Cysts with complications.

Q. What are other cystic lesions in pancreas?

Ans.

* *True cyst:* Having an epithelial lining.
* *Congenital cysts:*
  - Sequestration cyst
  - Enterogenous cyst
  - Dermoid cyst
  - Fibrocystic disease.

- *Neoplastic cysts:*
  - Serous cystadenoma
  - Mucinous cystadenoma
  - Cystadenocarcinoma
  - Cystic islet cell tumors.
- *Parasitic cysts:*
  - *Echinococcus* (Hydatid cyst)
  - Amebic
  - Cysticercosis.

Q. What are the characteristics of cystic neoplasms of the pancreas vis-a-vis the pseudocyst?

Ans. High suspicion of cystic neoplasm in following circumstances:
- No history of acute pancreatitis
- Internal septa or associated solid component seen in CT scan
- Calcification within the cyst or its wall
- Tumor marker CA 19-9 is elevated in cystic neoplasm
- Recurrence or persistence of the cyst after treatment—surgical or nonsurgical
- Cystic neoplasms should be treated by resectional surgery.

■ CARCINOMA OF COLON

Q. What is your case? (Summary of a case presenting with carcinoma descending colon)

Ans. A 52-year-old lady presented with occasional bleeding per rectum for last 1 year. Patient noticed passage of fresh blood per rectum for last 1 year. Initially patient used to pass blood at an interval of about 15–20 days and persist for 2–3 days each time. The bleeding occurs during defecation only. But for last 1 month patient is passing small amount of blood everytime she passes stool. Patient noticed a lump in left flank for last 8 months. The lump was about 4 cm in size at the onset and is gradually increasing in size for last 8 months. Patient complains of alteration of bowel habit for last 6 months. Patient used to pass stool twice a day, but for last 6 months patient noticed increasing constipation and she is passing stool once in 2–3 days and she has to take purgatives for bowel movement. Complains of dull aching pain in her left flank for last 3 months. She has some relief of pain with defecation. Complains of anorexia and weight loss for last 6 months. No urinary symptoms and no other systemic complaints.

On physical examination on general survey there is mild pallor and on abdominal examination the contour of the abdomen and umbilicus is normal. The abdomen is moving normally with respiration, no visible peristalsis and pulsatile movement is seen. The skin of abdomen is normal. There is a lump palpable in left lumbar region extending into the umbilical and left iliac fossa, the lump is intra-abdominal as is ascertained by leg rising test, the lump is globular in shape, 10 cm × 8 cm in size, surface is smooth, margins are rounded, consistency is firm, there is no mobility with respiration, the lump is slightly mobile from side to side and up and down. Liver, spleen and kidneys are not palpable. There is no other mass palpable. There is no free fluid in abdomen and normal bowel sounds are audible. Per rectal examination is normal except finger stall being smeared with blood. Per vaginal examination is normal (Undergraduate students can write P/R and P/V examination is not done). Systemic examination is normal.

Q. What is your diagnosis?

Ans. This is a case of carcinoma of descending colon.

Q. What are the points in favor of your diagnosis?

Ans.

* Elderly patient presented with:
  - Alteration of bowel habit, e.g. increasing constipation for last 9 months
  - History of bleeding P/R for last 9 months
  - History of passage of mucus with stool for last 9 months
  - Swelling in left side of abdomen for last 6 months, which is increasing in size
  - Pain in left side of abdomen for last 6 months.
* On examination:
  - Patient is anemic.
* On local examination of abdomen: There is a swelling in left lumbar region extending onto the umbilical and left iliac fossa. Intra-abdominal swelling free from skin and underlying structures mobile from side to side, nontender. P/R examination finger stall is smeared with blood.

Q. What are the other possibilities?

Ans.

* Left colonic tuberculosis
* Left colonic Crohn's disease
* Retroperitoneal tumor
* Lymphoma
* Differential diagnosis of a kidney lump.

Q. What investigation you will suggest in this patient?

Ans. I would like to confirm my diagnosis by:
Colonoscopy and biopsy from the lesion. Colonoscopy is a reliable investigation for evaluation of a patient with suspected carcinoma colon. The lesion can be seen and biopsy may be taken. The whole colon is examined and any metachronous cancer and associated polyp may be seen.

Q. How the extent of the disease may be assessed?

Ans. If the colonoscopy demonstrate the growth and biopsy report shows malignant lesion then some staging investigations are required.

The staging investigation of importance in evaluation of carcinoma colon includes:

* *Liver function test*: Elevated transaminase level, alkaline phosphatase and lactate dehydrogenase level may suggest liver metastasis.
* *CECT scan of abdomen:* CECT scan is a very good investigation to assess the extent of invasion by the primary tumor and to assess any intra-abdominal metastasis. In suspected locally advanced disease CECT scan is very essential.
* *Chest X-ray* to rule out pulmonary metastasis.

Q. Would you like to do a double contrast barium enema?

Ans. With advent of fiberoptic colonoscopy, the interior of the whole colon may be seen clearly. Along with improvement in imaging by CECT scan a barium enema study is no longer essential.

A double contrast barium enema may show an irregular filling defect due to growth or there may be a stenosing lesion. Associated polyps may also be seen in double contrast barium enema.

Q. What is carcinoembryonic antigen (CEA)?

Ans. It is a glycoprotein and is present in embryonic tissue and in colorectal cancers but is absent in normal colonic mucosa.

Q. What is the role of CEA estimation in colorectal cancer?

Ans. In patient with colonic cancer that has not penetrated the colonic wall the serum CEA level is not usually elevated.
* A preoperative CEA estimation is important as the baseline value
* The CEA level became normal after the surgical treatment provided there is no metastasis
* A rising CEA level in follow up period may suggest recurrence before the clinical disease becomes apparent.

Q. In which other conditions CEA level may be elevated?

Ans. Carcinoembryonic antigen may be elevated in other conditions like:
* Carcinoma stomach or pancreas
* Carcinoma breast or lung
* Benign conditions like—cirrhosis of liver, pancreatitis, renal failure, ulcerative colitis and in smokers.

Q. What other investigations you will do in this patient?

Ans. I would like to do some investigations to assess patient fitness for surgery:
* Blood for Hb% TLC, DLC and ESR
* Blood for sugar, urea and creatinine
* Stool for rectal examination and occult blood
* ECG.

Q. How will you treat this patient?

Ans. I will do exploratory laparotomy after proper preparation. If operable I will proceed with left hemicolectomy.

Q. How will you prepare this patient for surgery?

Ans.
* Patient is having anemia, so I will give preoperative blood or packed cell transfusion
* Gut preparation: This includes both mechanical cleansing and antibiotic preparation
  - Liquid diet 24 hours before surgery
  - Gut irrigation with polyethylene glycol. Polyethylene glycol is a balanced salt solution and a sachet of 100 g is administered by dissolving it in 2 L of water on previous evening. With intake of this solution patient passes almost clear motion. A dose of metoclopramide may be given beforehand to reduce the nausea.
* Antibiotic prophylaxis: Prophylactic antibiotic is given at the induction of anesthesia. A combination of broad spectrum antibiotic like injection cefuroxime and an aminoglycoside injection amikacin and injection metronidazole is administered at induction of anesthesia. The prophylactic antibiotic is given for 24 hours. If there is intraoperative contamination the antibiotic is to be continued for 3–5 days.

Q. What operation you will do for a growth in the descending colon?

Ans. The standard operation for a growth in the left colon is left hemicolectomy (Fig. 3.46). The structures to be removed are left one-third of the transverse colon, the whole of descending colon and proximal half of the sigmoid colon along with the part of the transverse mesocolon and sigmoid mesocolon and the regional lymph nodes.

Q. What should be the ideal proximal and distal line of resection in carcinoma of colon?

Ans. The proximal and the distal line of resection should be at least 5 cm from the tumor margin. However, margin as small as 2 cm may be adequate if adequate mesentery is resected with the gut. Wider margins are required for a poorly differentiated or anaplastic carcinoma.

Q. What are the indications for a total or subtotal colectomy in carcinoma of left colon?

Ans. If multiple colon cancer is present or if colonic carcinoma is associated with multiple neoplastic polyps then a subtotal or total colectomy with ileorectal anastomosis is to be considered.

Q. How will you assess operability?

Ans. On exploratory laparotomy the operability is assessed by:
- Examine the liver: Multiple secondaries in liver prohibit a curative resection, however if, growth is resectable it must be removed as resection provides best palliation.
- Disseminated peritoneal seedling, ascites and omental deposit suggest advanced disease and only palliative resection is advisable.
- Lymph node enlargement: Enlarged lymph node does not always mean that they are involved by metastasis as the enlargement may be inflammatory. Fixed metastatic lymph node indicates inoperability.
- Local fixation of the growth does not always imply inoperability: This fixation may be due to local inflammatory response.

Q. What is Turnbull's no touch technique for colonic resection?

Ans. While handling the tumor there is some chance of dissemination of the tumor cells by the bloodstream. Early division of blood vessel before the tumor is handled can reduce the chance of dissemination of tumor cells by the bloodstream during handling of the tumor.

Before the tumor is handled the blood vessel draining the site of growth is ligated. This is called Turnbull no touch technique of colonic resection.

Q. What is the extent of resection for carcinoma of cecum and ascending colon?

Ans. The standard resection is right hemicolectomy (Figs 3.46A to F).

Q. Which structures you will remove in right hemicolectomy?

Ans. Right hemicolectomy involves resection of terminal 10 cm of ileum, cecum, ascending colon, right colic flexure and right half of transverse colon. The ileocolic artery, right colic artery and the right branch of the middle colic artery are ligated and divided. Ileotransverse anastomosis is done.

Q. While doing right hemicolectomy what structures need to be identified to avoid injury?

Ans. Duodenum, ureter and gonadal vessels is to be identified to prevent injury.

Q. What is the extent of resection for growth in right colic flexure or right half of transverse colon?

Ans. The standard surgical treatment is extended right hemicolectomy. The trunk of the middle colic artery is tied and resection extended upto the proximal descending colon and an ileo descending anastomosis is done (Fig. 3.46B).

Q. What is the extent of resection for growth in midtransverse colon?

Ans. Extended right hemicolectomy resection being extended further down up to the mid descending colon (Fig. 3.46C).

Alternatively a segmental resection of the transverse colon with both right and left colic flexure may be done with anastomosis between the ascending and the descending colon.

Q. What is the extent of resection for growth in descending colon?

Ans. The standard resection is a left hemicolectomy. The trunk of left colic-artery and upper sigmoid arteries are ligated (Fig. 3.46E).

Q. What is the extent of resection for growth in sigmoid colon?

Ans. The standard resection is an extended left hemicolectomy or segmental resection of sigmoid colon (Fig. 3.46F).

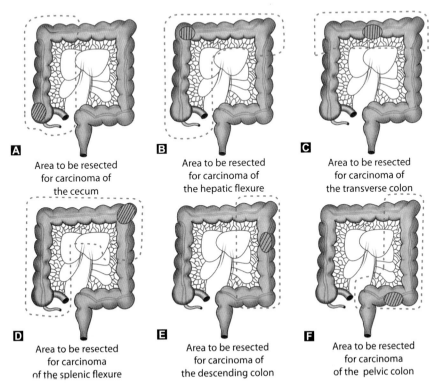

A Area to be resected for carcinoma of the cecum

B Area to be resected for carcinoma of the hepatic flexure

C Area to be resected for carcinoma of the transverse colon

D Area to be resected for carcinoma of the splenic flexure

E Area to be resected for carcinoma of the descending colon

F Area to be resected for carcinoma of the pelvic colon

Figs 3.46A to F: Resection of different portion of the colon when the growth is at the—(A) Cecum; (B) Hepatic flexure; (C) Transverse colon; (D) Splenic flexure; (E) Descending colon; (F) Pelvic colon

Q. How will you prevent intraluminal spread of tumor cells during operation?

Ans. During operation the intestine is encircled with ties both proximal and distal to the tumor to prevent intraluminal spread of the tumor cells during manipulation of the bowel.

Q. If growth in the descending colon is non-resectable what will you do?

Ans. I will do a transverse colostomy as a palliative measure.

Q. If a growth in the right colon is non-resectable what will you do?

Ans. I will do a palliative ileotransverse anastomosis.

Q. What may be the functional effect of right hemicolectomy?

Ans. The right colon absorbs approximately about one liter of fluid delivered from the ileum. After right hemicolectomy the stool is generally softer and an average volume of about 750 mL is passed in contrast to a normal volume of 250 mL. However, this is compensated with time as the ileum absorbs more water and bile salts.

Q. What may be the functional effect of left hemicolectomy or sigmoid colectomy?

Ans. This usually results in several small stools per day, but the volume is usually not increased.

Q. What may be the functional effect of total colectomy?

Ans. Patient usually has 4–10 bowel motions per day with an average volume of about one liter per day. However, with time ileum compensates and the number of bowel motions usually is lessened with lessening of stool volume.

Q. How will you treat hepatic metastasis from colonic carcinoma?

Ans.
* Single hepatic metastasis: May be resected during primary surgery
* Multiple hepatic metastases confined to one lobe/segment: During primary surgery a biopsy is taken and segmental resection or a lobectomy may be done later.
* Multiple painful hepatic metastases to both lobes need palliative treatment with cytotoxic chemotherapy, cryosurgery or laser therapy.

Q. What is the role of laparoscopic surgery in colonic carcinoma?

Ans. First laparoscopic colectomy for colonic carcinoma was done in 1991. Although there has been controversy regarding laparoscopic colectomy for carcinoma colon, there are reports in literature about laparoscopic colonic resection for carcinoma colon. However, this requires skill in advanced laparoscopy. The same principles of open operations apply for laparoscopic operation for carcinoma colon.

   If performed correctly the line of resection and lymph node harvest is said to be comparable to open surgery. Laparoscopic colon resection has been proven to be safe, efficacious, with decreased pain, early return of bowel function and shorter hospital stay.

Q. What adjuvant treatment you will plan for carcinoma colon?

Ans.

Stage I colonic cancer: Following adequate surgery, no adjuvant therapy is required.

Stage II colonic cancer: Following adequate surgery, the role of chemotherapy has been controversial. Current evidence, however, favors administration of adjuvant chemotherapy in stage II disease.

The chemotherapy regimen is:

+ 5 FU + leucovorin, Or
+ 5FU + leucovorin and oxaliplatin.

Stage III colonic cancer: There is clear benefit of chemotherapy in stage III disease.

The addition of oxaliplatin with 5FU and leucovorin has resulted in better disease free survival at 3 years.

Continuous infusion of 5FU is superior to bolus injection of 5 FU. An oral fluoropyrimidine capecitabine has been shown to be equivalent to IV 5 FU.

These chemotherapeutic drugs are given over a period of 6 months.

Q. How will you treat stage IV colonic cancer?

Ans. The treatment depends on the location and extent of the metastasis.

+ If the primary growth is resectable, resection provides best palliation
+ Isolated pulmonary or hepatic metastasis may be treated by resection
+ 5 FU-based chemotherapy in combination with leucovorin and oxaliplatin or irinotecan
+ Newer agents like monoclonal antibodies—Bevacizumab and cetuximab
  - Bevacizumab is a vascular endothelial growth factor inhibitor has shown improved survival when used in combination with 5 FU+ leucovorin and oxaliplatin or irinotecan
  - Cetuximab is a monoclonal antibody that binds to inhibit EGFR which are overexpressed in 60–80% patients of colonic carcinoma. Cetuximab is effective in tumors that do not have mutation of *KRAS* gene. So, genetic testing for *KRAS* gene is indicated before initiating treatment with these vascular endothelial growth factor inhibitors.

Q. What is the follow-up protocol for patient with carcinoma colon?

Ans. Patients who have been treated for carcinoma colon are at the risk of developing metachronous carcinoma, local recurrence or systemic metastasis. About 70% of recurrent disease becomes detectable in 2 years and about 90% is detectable in 4 years. Early detection of recurrent cancer can improve the prognosis in these patients and this justifies long-term follow-up of these patients.

During first 2 years, follow-up every 3 months and then every 6 months for next 3 years and then yearly.

Follow-up evaluation includes:

+ Clinical examination
+ Liver function test
+ CEA assay
+ Chest X-ray
+ Physical examination is of little value in detection of recurrent disease. Once the recurrent disease is palpable by clinical examination it is usually unresectable
+ Liver function test and CEA assay can indicate the presence of liver metastasis
+ A rising CEA level is an indication for colonoscopic examination or CT scan abdomen and chest X-ray

- Yearly CT scan abdomen for first 3 years
- Yearly colonoscopy to detect any metachronous lesion. After 3 years if colonoscopy is normal colonoscopy to be done every 5 years.

Q. What are polyps?

Ans. Polyps are any elevated tumor on the mucosal aspect.

Q. What are the different types of colonic polyps?

Ans. *See* Surgical Pathology Section, Page No. 876, 877, Chapter 18

Q. What are the macroscopic types of colonic carcinoma?

Ans. *See* Surgical Pathology Section, Page No. 879–882, Chapter 18

Q. What is the relative site distribution of colorectal carcinoma?

Ans. *See* Surgical Pathology Section, Page No. 879–882, Chapter 18

Q. What are the premalignant lesions in colon?

Ans. *See* Surgical Pathology Section, Page No. 879–882, Chapter 18

Q. How the carcinoma colon does spread?

Ans. *See* Surgical Pathology Section, Page No. 879–882, Chapter 18

Q. What is Dukes' staging for carcinoma of colon?

Ans. The Dukes staging system is a classification system for colorectal cancer. This system is now mainly of historical interest as it has largely been replaced by the TNM staging system. It is not recommended for clinical practice.

- Dukes A: Invasion into but not through the bowel wall (90%, 5 year survival)
- Dukes B: Invasion through the bowel wall but not involving lymph nodes (70%, 5 year survival)
- Dukes C: Involvement of lymph nodes (30%, 5 year survival)
- Dukes D: Widespread metastases.

Q. What is Astler and Coller modification for Dukes staging?

Ans. Astler and Coller (1954) adapted the original Dukes system as follows:

- Stage A: Tumor limited to mucosa
- Stage B1: Tumor extending into muscularis propria but not penetrating through it
- Stage B2: Tumor penetrating through muscularis propria
- Stage B3: Tumor involving adjacent organs
- Stage C1: Tumor B1 + Lymph nodes involved
- Stage C2: Tumor B2 + Lymph nodes involved
- Stage C3: Tumor B3 + Lymph nodes involved
- Stage D: Distant metastatic spread.

Q. What are the TNM classifications for colonic cancer?

Ans. The TNM classifications for colonic cancer are given in Table 3.12 and Anatomic staging is dissued in Table 3.13.

Table 3.12: TNM classifications for colonic cancer.

Primary tumor (T)

TX	Primary tumor cannot be assessed
T0	No evidence of primary tumor
Tis	Carcinoma in situ: Intraepithelial or invasion of lamina propria
T1	Tumor invades submucosa
T2	Tumor invades muscularis propria
T3	Tumor invades to the subserosa or through the muscularis propria into the pericolonic tissues in areas not covered by serosa
T4a	Tumor penetrates to the surface of the visceral peritoneum
T4b	Tumor directly invades or is adherent to other organs or structures

Regional lymph nodes (N)

NX	Regional lymph nodes cannot be assessed
N0	No regional lymph node metastasis
N1	Metastasis in 1–3 regional lymph nodes
N1a	Metastasis in 1 regional lymph node
N1b	Metastasis in 2–3 regional lymph nodes
N1c	Tumor deposit(s) in the subserosa, mesentery, or nonperitonealized pericolic or perirectal tissues without regional nodal metastasis
N2	Metastasis in 4 or more lymph nodes
N2a	Metastasis in 4–6 regional lymph nodes
N2b	Metastasis in 7 or more regional lymph nodes

Distant metastasis (M)

M0	No distant metastasis
M1	Distant metastasis
M1a	Metastasis confined to 1 organ or site (e.g. liver, lung, ovary, nonregional node)
M1b	Metastases in more than 1 organ/site or the peritoneum

Table 3.13: Anatomic staging

Stage	T	N	M	Dukes	MAC
0	Tis	N0	M0	--	--
I	T1	N0	M0	A	A
	T2	N0	M0	A	B1
IIA	T3	N0	M0	B	B2
IIB	T4a	N0	M0	B	B2
IIC	T4b	N0	M0	B	B3
IIIA	T1–T2	N1/N1c	M0	C	C1
	T1	N2a	M0	C	C1

Contd...

Contd...

Stage	T	N	M	Dukes	MAC
IIIB	T3–T4a	N1/N1c	M0	C	C2
	T2-T3	N2a	M0	C	C1/C2
	T1-T2	N2b	M0	C	C1
IIIC	T4a	N2a	M0	C	C2
	T3-T4a	N2b	M0	C	C2
	T4b	N1-N2	M0	C	C3
IVA	Any T	Any N	M1a	--	--
IVB	Any T	Any N	M1b	--	--

Q. What does L, V or R in staging denotes?

Ans. *See* Surgical Pathology: Carcinoma Colon, Page No. 882, Chapter 18.

Q. How does patient with right colonic carcinoma usually presents?

Ans.

- May present with vague symptoms like anemia, anorexia, and asthenia
- May present with a lump
- Cecal carcinoma may present with symptoms and signs of acute appendicitis
- May present with symptoms and signs of intestinal obstruction due to intussusception
- May present with symptoms and signs of advanced disease ascites, enlarged liver, metastasis to lungs, skin, brain and bone.

Q. How does patient with left colonic carcinoma usually presents?

Ans. Lesion in left colon is usually stenosing variety and usually presents with:

- Alteration of bowel habit increasing constipation is the usual mode of presentation in stenosing lesion of left colon. Patient needs increasing doses of purgative for bowel evacuation, which may sometime result in spurious diarrhea
- Pain may have dull aching pain or colic due to obstructive lesion
- May present with a lump
- May present with lower abdominal distension.

Q. If the growth is not resectable what will you do?

Ans.

- In right colonic growth a bypass ileotransverse anastomosis
- In left colonic growth a transverse colostomy
- In sigmoid or rectal growth a sigmoid colostomy proximal to the growth.

Q. What are the other methods of gut preparation?

Ans. The idea of gut preparation is to get an empty colon with reduced bacterial count. This reduces contamination during surgery and thereby incidence of wound infection following surgery is minimized. The different preparation includes:

- *Elemental or space diet*: For 5 days before surgery patient is given an elemental diet, which is predigested food and gets absorbed in small gut and renders the colon empty. But the bacterial count is not affected in this method so prophylactic antibiotic is necessary.
- *Liquid diet for 48 hours before surgery:* On day before surgery two sachets of Sodium picosulfate (Picolax) are then for good purgation. In addition enemas to clear the rectum provides adequate mechanical cleaning of the colon.
- *Whole gut irrigation:* Pass a Ryle's tube keeping the tip beyond the pylorus. Start administering normal saline through the Ryle's tube. Patient passes clear motion. Once the patient starts passing clear motion continue administering saline for one more hour.
- On an average 9–13 liters of normal saline is required for whole gut irrigation. This technique is not suitable in elderly and in patient with cardiac disease.

Urinary Cases

OUTLINE FOR WRITING URINARY CASES

▌HISTORY

1. **Particulars of the Patient**
2. **Chief Complaint(s)**
   - Pain in abdomen or loin for.............. months/years.
   - Swelling in abdomen or loin for.............. months/years.
   - Passage of blood in urine for............. months/years.
   - Increased frequency of micturition for.............. months/years.
   - Difficulty in passing urine for.............. months/years.
   - General symptoms like fever, anorexia, weight loss for.............. months/years.
3. **History of Present Illness**

Elaborate Each of these Chief Complaints

- *Pain*:
  - Duration
  - Onset: Sudden or gradual
  - Site: Abdomen or loin
  - Radiation: Loin to groin or scrotum
  - Character of pain: Dull aching, colicky or burning
  - Relation to micturition
  - Aggravating and relieving factors.
- *Swelling*:
  - Duration
  - Onset
  - Progress of the swelling: Slowly increasing or rapidly increasing
  - Any diminution of the size of the swelling with passage of urine
  - Any other swelling.
- *Passage of blood in urine*:
  - Red or dark in color

- Quantity: Slight or profuse
- Periodicity: Continuous since onset or intermittent/relation to micturition—before micturition, mixed with urine uniformly or bleeding after the urine is passed
- Any history of passage of clots
- Any pain during passage of blood in urine (clot colic).
- *Frequency of micturition*: Normal frequency is usually 5–6 times in 24 hours.
  - Any history of increased frequency of micturition: Diurnal, nocturnal or both
  - Any associated burning sensation during micturition.
- *Difficulty in passing urine*:
  - How is the stream: Any narrowing of stream
  - Any hesitancy: Patient has the desire to pass urine, he goes to the toilet, he takes more time and has to strain to initiate the act
  - Urgency: Once the patient has desire to pass urine, he has to rush to toilet otherwise he will spoil the underclothes.
- *History of incontinence*:
  - True incontinence: When urine dribbles in absence of a full bladder
  - False incontinence: Urine overflows from a distended bladder
  - Stress incontinence: Urine dribbles when the patient strains.
- Details of general symptoms:
  - Fever
  - Anorexia
  - Weight loss.
- *Other systemic symptoms*:
  - Gastrointestinal symptoms
  - Respiratory symptoms
  - Cardiovascular symptoms
  - Neurological symptoms.
4. **Past History**
5. **Personal History**
6. **Family History**
7. **Treatment History**
8. **History of Allergy.**

■ PHYSICAL EXAMINATION

1. **General Survey**
2. **Local Examination**

Examination of Abdomen and Loin

- *Inspection (Fig. 4.1)*:
  - Shape and contour of abdomen
    Umbilicus: Central/deviated
  - Movement of abdomen: Respiratory/peristaltic/pulsatile

- Skin over the abdomen: Scar/engorged vein/pigmentation
- Any swelling in abdomen: Position (in relation to abdominal regions)/size/shape/surface/margins/any movement with respiration/skin over the swelling
- Ask the patient to sit and look for any swelling in the loin and renal angle
- Inspection of external genitalia: Vulval region in female. Penis/testes/scrotum in male.

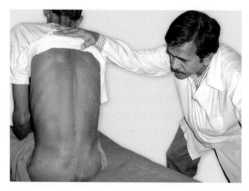

Fig. 4.1: Inspection of the renal angle area

- *Palpation:*
  - Temperature of the abdomen
  - Tenderness in the abdomen: Deep tender spots—gastric point/duodenal point/gallbladder point/McBurney's point/renal angle *(see* also Fig. 3.2)*;* (Figs 4.2A and B)

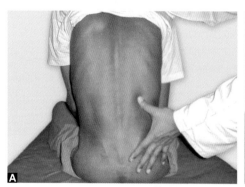 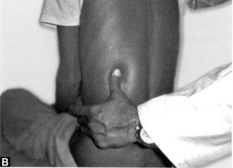

Figs 4.2A and B: Eliciting tenderness at renal angle

  - Palpable lump in abdomen. Details of the lump:
    - Temperature over the swelling—any rise of local temperature
    - Tenderness over the swelling
    - Position/extent/size/shape/surface—smooth, granular or nodular
    - Margin: Whether all the margins are palpable or not—margins well-defined/ill-defined/one margin passing under the costal margin or passing into the pelvis
    - Consistency: Soft, cystic, firm, hard or variegated (at places soft and at places firm or hard)
    - Any movement of the swelling with respiration/any mobility of the swelling: Side to side or up and down
    - Ascertain whether the swelling is intra-abdominal or parietal by doing rising test/if intra-abdominal ascertain whether the swelling is intraperitoneal or retroperitoneal by examination in knee elbow position

- Palpation of liver/spleen/kidneys
- Palpation of kidney (*see* also Figs 3.17 and 3.18; abdominal examination section).
- Palpation of urinary bladder: Normal urinary bladder is not palpable. Distended urinary bladder may be palpable in hypogastric region as a soft cystic swelling passing into the pelvis
- Palpation of the external genitalia:
  - Palpation of penis for any thickening or induration (Fig. 4.3)
  - Palpation of testes and the spermatic cord (Figs 4.4A and B).

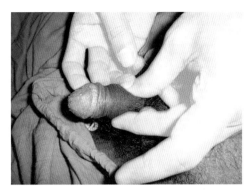

Fig. 4.3: Palpation of penis

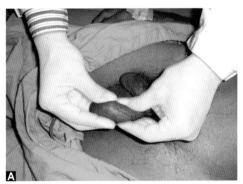
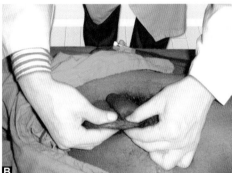

Figs 4.4A and B: Palpation of testes and spermatic cord

- ◆ *Percussion:*
  - General note of the abdomen
  - Upper border of liver dullness
  - Upper border of splenic dullness
  - Percussion over the lump or the kidney
  - Percuss at the renal angle: Normally renal angle area is resonant but in case of renal enlargement, this area usually becomes dull (Fig. 4.5).
- ◆ *Auscultation:*
  - Bowel sounds
  - Auscultate over the swelling for any bruit.
- ◆ *Per-rectal examination:*
  - Any rectal lesion
  - Palpation for prostate in male.

3. **Systemic Examination**

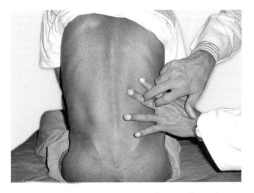

Fig. 4.5: Percussion over the renal angle

■ **SUMMARY OF THE CASE**

■ **PROVISIONAL DIAGNOSIS**

■ **DIFFERENTIAL DIAGNOSIS**

CLINICAL QUESTIONS

Q. How will you palpate kidney?

Ans. Patient should lie down in dorsal position. Kidney is best palpated bimanually. One hand is placed behind the loin in the area between the lower border of 12th rib and the iliac crest maintaining a forward pressure and the other hand is placed in the front of the abdomen below the costal margin. The patient is asked to take deep breathing and during expiration the hand in front is depressed, and the enlarged kidney may be palpated between the two hands. The extent of enlargement, size, shape, margins, surface and consistency of the swelling is assessed. Test whether the swelling is ballottable or not, once the swelling is palpable between the two hands, the anterior hand is placed on the front of the abdomen keeping the hand in such a way so that the swelling is not touching the anterior hand, the swelling is then pushed forward with the posterior hand, if the swelling touches the anterior hand then the swelling is said to be ballottable. A normal kidney is not palpable except in very emaciated patient (*see also* Figs 3.17 and 3.18, Page No. 99, Chapter 3).

Q. What do you mean by ballottability?

Ans. Once the swelling in the loin is palpable between the two hands then the anterior hand is placed on the front of the abdomen keeping the hand in such a way so that the swelling is not touching the anterior hand—the swelling is then pushed forward with the posterior hand. If the swelling touches the anterior hand then the swelling is said to be ballottable (Fig. 4.6).

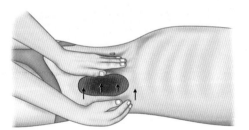

Fig. 4.6: Ballottability of the kidney

Q. What are the characteristics of a renal lump?

Ans. The enlarged kidney is palpated in the lumbar region and depending on the degree of enlargement may extend to hypochondriac, iliac fossa, epigastric and umbilical region. The characteristics of kidney lump are:

- The swelling is usually reniform in shape
- Lateral, medial, upper, and lower margins are usually palpable
- A notch may be present in the medial margin
- There may be slight mobility with respiration
- Swelling is bimanually palpable
- Swelling may be ballottable
- Hand can be insinuated between the costal margin and the lump

+ Renal angle is full
+ There is a band of colonic resonance in front of the swelling
+ The renal angle is dull on percussion.

Q. What is Murphy's kidney punch?

Ans. This is the method of eliciting of tenderness in the renal angle by pressing the thumb in the renal angle (*see* Figs 4.2A and B).

Q. What is renal colic?

Ans. This is acute colicky pain which starts in the loin and radiates to the groin or toward the inner side of thigh and testis (along the distribution of genitofemoral nerve). There is waxing and waning of the pain. There may be nausea, vomiting, rise of temperature and associated urinary symptoms like frequency, burning micturition, hematuria or pyuria.

Q. What is fixed renal pain?

Ans. This is a localized pain confined either in the loin near the renal angle or anteriorly below the costal margin, usually dull aching in nature and commonly due to stretching of renal capsule due to either tumor or hydronephrosis.

Q. What are the characteristics of bladder pain?

Ans. Pain arising out of the urinary bladder is usually felt in the hypogastrium. The pain is usually dull aching or burning in nature and the pain may be referred to the tip of penis.

Q. What are the characteristics of prostatic pain?

Ans. Prostatic pain is felt as a sensation of heaviness in the perineum. Throbbing pain in the perineum suggests prostatic abscess.

Q. What is hesitancy?

Ans. When patient has the urge for micturition and tries to pass urine, he has to wait longer to initiate the act of micturition.

Q. What is urgency?

Ans. When the patient has the urge for micturition then he has to rush to pass urine otherwise he will spoil the underclothes.

Q. What is stress incontinence?

Ans. In stress incontinence, there is involuntary passage of urine when the patient strains (either during coughing or sneezing or any other condition causing increased intra-abdominal pressure).

Q. What is urge incontinence?

Ans. When the patient has the urge to pass urine there is some involuntary passage of urine before the patient gets time to evacuate the bladder.

Q. What is overflow incontinence?

Ans. When the bladder is over distended due to chronic retention of urine then some amount of urine may be dribbled involuntarily. This is called overflow incontinence.

Q. What is true incontinence?

Ans. When there is involuntary passage of urine in spite of bladder being not full.

■ HYDRONEPHROSIS

Q. What is your case? (Summary of a case presenting with hydronephrosis).

Ans. This 35 years gentleman presented with pain in the right loin for last 1 year and swelling in the right loin for the same duration. Patient complains of gradual onset of pain in the right loin for last 1 year. The pain is dull aching in nature and persisted almost continuously for that period, sometimes patient has relief after passage of urine and with analgesics. Patient noticed a lump in the right loin for last 1 year, gradually increasing in size. There is no history of rapid increase in size of the swelling and there is no history of diminution of size with passage of urine. No history of hematuria. No history of difficulty in passing urine. Patient passes urine 5–6 times in 24 hours. No history of increased frequency of micturition. No history of fever. Patient has no other symptoms.

On physical examination, general survey is essentially normal except slight pallor. Blood pressure is 130/80 mm Hg. On local examination of abdomen, the inspection of the contour of abdomen and umbilicus are normal. There is slight fullness in the right lumbar region; also the right renal angle is full. On palpation, temperature of the abdomen is normal, there is no tenderness. The right kidney is palpable, reniform in shape, 9 cm × 6 cm in dimension, moving up and down with respiration. There is slight mobility of the swelling from side to side and from above downward, the medial lateral, upper and lower margin of the swelling is palpable and rounded, surface is smooth and consistency is tense cystic, the hand can be insinuated between the swelling and the right costal margin. On percussion, the swelling is dull and there is a band of resonance in the front of the swelling. Liver/spleen are not palpable, no other lump is palpable, no free fluid in abdomen. Systemic examination is normal.

Q. What is your diagnosis?

Ans. This is a case of right sided hydronephrosis.

Q. What is the differential diagnosis?

Ans.
* Simple cyst of kidney
* Polycystic disease of kidney. In bilateral disease, one side may contain large cysts and become palpable earlier than the other
* Tuberculous pyonephrosis
* Parapelvic cyst
* Hydatid cyst of kidney
* Retroperitoneal cyst
* Carcinoma of kidney.

Q. What investigations will you suggest in this patient?

Ans.
* I would like to do some investigations to confirm my diagnosis.
* Ultrasonography of abdomen.

Q. How ultrasonography (USG) will help in diagnosis?

Ans.
- To delineate the mass palpable
- To ascertain the organ from which it is arising
- If hydronephrosis is detected, degree of dilatation of pelvicalyceal system
- Assessment of thickness of renal cortical tissue
- whether the ureter is dilated or not
- Any calculus in the kidney or in the ureter
- The opposite kidney is also assessed.

Q. What other investigations would you suggest?

Ans. After ultrasound confirms this to be a kidney mass and shows features of hydronephrosis. I will advise for blood urea and creatinine estimation and an intravenous urography (IVU).

Q. How an intravenous urography (IVU) helps in diagnosis?

Ans. If the hydronephrotic kidney is functioning, then IVU may demonstrate:
- Dilatation of pelvis and calyceal system
- The normal cupping of the minor calyces is lost and the minor calyces become clubbed
- Dilated ureter may be seen and the site of obstruction may be localized
- In advanced hydronephrosis, the faint nephrogram around the dilated calyces may give a soap bubble appearance.
- Delayed film up to 24 hours may be taken to delineate the site of obstruction.

If the hydronephrotic kidney is nonfunctioning, then the pelvicalyceal system of the affected kidney will not be visible on IVU.

Q. How isotope renography is helpful in evaluation of patient with hydronephrosis?

Ans. 99mTc-labeled DTPA (diethylenetri-aminepentaacetic acid) is injected intravenously for radioactive renography. DTPA is filtered by the glomeruli and not absorbed hence is helpful for evaluation of patients with hydronephrosis and may delineate the site of obstruction. The passage of 99mTc-labeled DTPA is tracked using a gamma camera. If there is obstruction either at pelviureteric junction or at the ureter, the radioactive substance will be trapped proximal to the obstruction and will not be cleared even after administration of furosemide.

Using this radioisotopic scanning, the individual function of the kidneys may be assessed and the differential glomerular filtration rate may be calculated (Fig. 4.7).

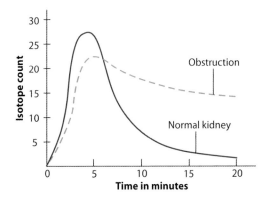

Fig. 4.7: Radioisotope renogram of patient with hydronephrosis

Q. When will you consider doing a retrograde pyelography?

Ans. If IVU shows the affected kidney is nonfunctioning and the site of obstruction cannot be localized, a retrograde pyelography may be helpful to delineate the site of obstruction.

Q. How retrograde pyelography is done?

Ans. Under local anesthesia cystoscopy is done. Ureteric orifices in the trigone of bladder are localized by viewing with the cystoscope. A fine ureteric catheter is introduced through the cystoscope into the ureteric orifice and upward into the ureter under fluoroscopic guidance. Urografin injected through the ureteric catheter will visualize the ureter and the dilated renal pelvis, and the site of obstruction in the ureter may be localized.

Q. What is the role of contrast-enhanced computed tomography (CECT) scan for evaluation of hydronephrosis?

Ans. Contrast-enhanced computed tomography scan after injection of IV contrast is helpful:
* To assess the functional status of the kidney
* May assess the renal cortical thickness
* May show the dilated pelvis and ureter
* The site of obstruction may also be localized.

Q. What other investigations will you do in this patient?

Ans.
* Blood urea and creatinine to assess any impairment of renal function
* Urine routine examination and culture sensitivity
* Apart from this routine investigations to assess patient's fitness for general anesthesia
* Complete hemogram/blood for sugar/chest X-ray/ECG.

Q. If the hydronephrosis is due to pelviureteric junction obstruction, what will you do?

Ans. If there is adequate renal function and there is reasonable thickness of functioning renal parenchyma, I will do Anderson-Hynes pyeloplasty (Fig. 4.8).

Anderson-Hynes pyeloplasty is a type of dismembered pyeloplasty. The kidney is exposed by a standard lumbar approach. The upper third of the ureter and the pelvis is dissected and mobilized. The redundant renal pelvis and the pelviureteric junction are excised. The cut end of the ureter is spatulated and the splayed ureter is anastomosed to the pelvis using 3-0 vicryl suture (polyglactin suture). The anastomosis is stented either by a double J stent or by a nephrostomy.

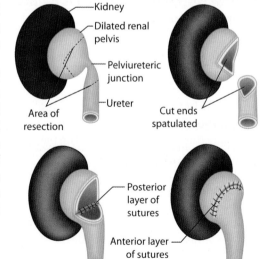

Fig. 4.8: Anderson-Hynes pyeloplasty

Q. What are the different types of pyeloplasty?

Ans. Pyeloplasty may be either:
* Dismembered pyeloplasty: Anderson-Hynes pyeloplasty
* Non-dismembered pyeloplasty: Includes Foley's Y-V pyeloplasty.

Q. What is the role of laparoscopy in hydronephrosis surgery?

Ans. Laparoscopic surgery is gaining popularity for treatment of hydronephrosis. Anderson-Hynes pyeloplasty may be done laparoscopically with equal success.

Q. What is endoscopic pyelolysis?

Ans. It is possible to dilate the pelviureteric junction by using a balloon passed either through a nephroscope or by passing the balloon up through ureteric orifice into the pelviureteric junction under fluoroscopic control. This minimal access surgery is gaining popularity, however, the long-term results are not yet certain.

Q. What is hydronephrosis?

Ans. Hydronephrosis is defined as aseptic dilatation of the pelvicalyceal system of kidney due to partial or complete obstruction to the outflow of urine.

Q. What are the important causes of unilateral hydronephrosis?

Ans.
- Obstruction in the lumen of the ureter due to a calculus or sloughed papilla.
- Obstruction due to some lesion in the wall of the ureter:
  - Transitional cell carcinoma, involving the ureter or bladder, invading the ureter
  - Inflammatory stricture in the ureter due to tuberculosis/following removal of ureteric calculus
  - Congenital stenosis of ureter or pelviureteric junction obstruction.
- Obstruction of the ureter due to some lesion adjacent to ureter.
  - Tumors of colon, rectum, cervix, prostate and cecum secondarily involving the ureter
  - Idiopathic retroperitoneal fibrosis.

Q. What are the important causes of bilateral hydronephrosis?

Ans. Bilateral hydronephrosis is due to distal obstruction either at the bladder neck or the urethra or bilateral ureteric obstruction due to the above causes. Important causes are:
- Meatal stenosis: Congenital or acquired
- Congenital posterior urethral valve
- Urethral stricture: Inflammatory or traumatic
- Prostatic enlargement: Benign hyperplasia or carcinoma
- Bladder neck obstruction due to congenital stenosis, Marion's disease or postoperative scarring.

Q. How patient with hydronephrosis does usually presents?

Ans. Patient may present in different ways:
- *Asymptomatic*: Diagnosed incidentally on ultrasonography
- *Lump in the loin*: The enlarged kidney may be palpable
- *Pain in the loin*: This may be dull aching pain or colicky pain
- *Dietl's crisis*: After an attack of renal colic a lump appears in the loin and after few hours the pain, and the swelling disappears with passage of large quantities of urine
- *In case of bilateral hydronephrosis* due to urethral obstruction, the predominant presenting features are due to bladder outflow obstruction—frequency, dysuria, hesitancy, urgency and chronic or acute on chronic retention of urine
- *In bilateral hydronephrosis* with gross deterioration of renal function symptoms and signs of chronic renal failure may be the presenting feature.

Q. What are the complications of hydronephrosis?

Ans.

- Infection of the hydronephrotic kidney—lead to pyonephrosis.
- Nonfunctioning kidney—long-standing hydronephrosis causes back pressure changes in the kidney leading to thinning of the cortex and ultimately nonfunctioning kidney.
- Chronic renal failure—in bilateral hydronephrosis with deterioration of renal function on both sides will ultimately lead to chronic renal failure.

■ CARCINOMA OF KIDNEY

Q. What is your case? (Summary of a case presenting with carcinoma of kidney.)

Ans. This 55-year-old gentleman presented with a swelling in the left loin for last 9 months. The swelling is gradually increasing in size. Patient complains pain in the left loin for last 6 months. The pain is dull aching in nature and is continuous for the above duration. There is no specific aggravating or relieving factors. Patient also complains of passage of blood in urine for last 6 months. Patient passes dark red urine, often associated with passage of clots. The passage of blood in urine is intermittent and is occurring at an interval of 10–15 days over the period and lasted for about 2–3 days each time. Patient complains of swelling in the left side of scrotum for last 2 months. The swelling in the scrotum gets aggravated during walking and diminishes on lying down position. Patient has no other complain.

On examination, general survey is essentially normal except patient is mildly anemic. On local examination of abdomen, shape and contour of abdomen and umbilicus are normal, no engorged vein or scar in abdomen. Abdomen is moving normally with respiration, no visible peristalsis is seen. The left kidney is enlarged and palpable extending from left lumbar region to epigastric, left hypochondriac and umbilical region. Medial, lateral, and lower margin is rounded and palpable but the upper margin is not palpable, surface is irregular, nontender, firm in consistency, moving slightly with respiration. The swelling on percussion is dull but there is a band of colonic resonance along the medial margin of the swelling but the renal angle is dull. The liver and spleen is not palpable and there is no other mass in the abdomen. On examination of the external genitalia, the testes and the penis are normal. There is moderate degree of varicocele on the left side. Per-rectal examination is normal. Systemic examination is normal.

Q. What is your diagnosis?

Ans. This is probably a case of carcinoma of left kidney.

Q. What are the points in favor of your diagnosis?

Ans. This elderly male patient presented with the triad of symptoms—lump in the loin, pain and hematuria for last 9 months. Patient also complains of a swelling in the left side of the scrotum.

On examination, patient is having pallor and the left kidney is enlarged and palpable. There is an associated varicocele on the left side.

So this is likely to be a case of left sided carcinoma of kidney with left sided varicocele.

Q. What are the other possibilities?

Ans. The other possibilities are:

- Hydronephrosis

* Tuberculosis of kidney
* Hydatid cyst of kidney
* Polycystic kidney
* Retroperitoneal tumor.

Q. How will you proceed to manage this patient?

Ans. I will do some investigations to confirm my diagnosis.
* Ultrasonography of abdomen and kidney region. Ultrasonography will show:
    – The organ of origin of the swelling
    – The nature of the swelling whether solid or cystic
    – The extent of involvement of the kidney whether the swelling arises either from the poles or involves the whole kidney
    – The size and shape of the opposite kidney may also be assessed
    – Any lymphadenopathy and liver enlargement may also be seen.
* Contrast-enhanced computed tomography scan of abdomen will show:
    – The exact extent of the involvement of the kidney
    – The function of the opposite kidney may also be assessed by the CECT scan
    – Invasion of the tumor along the renal vein or the inferior vena cava may also be seen by the CECT scan.

Q. Do you like to do an intravenous urography?

Ans. If a CECT scan is done then an IVU may not be required as the information obtained by IVU may be obtained from the contrast CT scan. The contrast CT scan in addition will be helpful for assessment of the renal mass.

Q. What other investigations will you do?

Ans.
* Chest X-ray to look for any metastasis (Cannonball like metastasis) may occur in carcinoma kidney
* Blood for complete hemogram [hemoglobin, total leukocyte count (TLC), differential leukocyte count (DLC), erythrocyte sedimentation rate (ESR), platelet]
* Blood for sugar, urea and creatinine and serum electrolyte level to assess renal function
* Liver function test
* Serum calcium level
* Urine for routine examination may reveal RBC in urine
* Exfoliative cytology of urine for malignant cells.

Q. Would you like to do a fine-needle aspiration cytology (FNAC)?

Ans. Carcinoma kidney is diagnosed on clinical ground and on radiological features. A FNAC is not indicated as it will breach the capsule and may cause seedling of tumor cells along the needle track.

Q. Would you like to do bone scan?

Ans. Bone scan is not indicated in all patients. Patient presenting with bone pain or advanced disease requires whole body bone scanning with 99mTc.

Q. Would you like to do a renal angiography?

Ans. With advent of good quality CECT scan, the renal angiography is not a routine investigation for evaluation of carcinoma of kidney. Renal angiography is indicated in patients with bilateral tumors and patient with solitary functioning kidney where nephron sparing surgery is contemplated.

However, if done, the renal angiography will show the extensive neovascularization and tumor blush. The venous phase will show the renal vein and the inferior vena cava and any extension of tumor thrombus may be seen.

Q. How will you treat this patient?

Ans. Contrast-enhanced computed tomography scan report is to be reviewed with particular attention to tumor extension beyond the renal capsule and into the renal vein or the inferior vena cava. If there is no extension to renal vein or inferior vena cava, I will plan to do radical nephrectomy.

Q. What structures will you remove in radical nephrectomy?

Ans. This involves en bloc removal of:
* Kidney with Gerota's fascia
* Removal of ureter
* Adrenal gland
* Renal vessels, and
* Local lymph nodes.

Q. How will you do radical nephrectomy?

Ans. I will proceed with a transperitoneal approach as it is possible to expose the renal vein and the inferior vena cava easily. The colon is mobilized medially. Before handling the tumor, the renal pedicle should be tackled first. The renal artery is dissected, ligated and divided. The renal vein is palpated and if there is no tumor extension into the renal vein, the vein is dissected, ligated, and divided. The kidney mass along with the perinephric fat is mobilized and dissected. There may be leash of new vessels around the tumor which needs ligation and division. The ureter is dissected as low as possible, ligated and divided.

Q. If there is extension of tumor into the renal vein or the inferior vena cava, how will you manage the case?

Ans. Tumor may extend into the renal vein or the inferior vena cava or sometimes up to the right atrium of the heart.
* If there is tumor extension into the renal vein only, the renal vein should be ligated proximal to the site of tumor extension.
* If there is tumor extension into the inferior vena cava then the inferior vena cava should be dissected and proximal control of vena cava should be achieved. The tumor extension from the inferior vena cava may be removed by a long venotomy.
* If there is extension of tumor into the right atrium, help of cardiac surgeon is necessary and the tumor extension from the vena cava and the right atrium may be removed under cardiopulmonary bypass.

Q. What is the role of therapeutic embolization?

Ans. Earlier therapeutic embolization was done more frequently as a preoperative measure to regress the tumor size as well as to reduce the vascularity to reduce bleeding during surgery.

However, this may also be considered as a palliative measure in locally advanced inoperable cases.

A selective renal arteriogram is done. Following this, particulate material like Gelfoam, muscle, metal coils may be injected through the angiogram cannula, which will block the vessels and cause infarction of the tumor mass.

Q. Where from the carcinoma of kidney arises?

Ans. Hypernephroma is an adenocarcinoma and arises from the renal tubular epithelial cells.

Q. What are the important etiological factors for development of carcinoma kidney?

Ans. The exact cause is uncertain. Some factors have been implicated to be associated with increased risk for development of carcinoma of kidney.
* *Smoking*: Associated with two-fold increased risk for development of carcinoma kidney.
* *Excessive coffee* consumption
* *Analgesic abuse*—phenacetin nephropathy
* *Occupational exposure* to cadmium, asbestos, and petroleum products
* *Exogenous estrogen*
* *HLA antigen BW 44 and DR8*
* *Von Hippel–Lindau disease*: a triad of bilateral renal cell tumors, retinal angiomata and cerebellar hemangiomata
* *Adult polycystic* kidney disease.

Q. How carcinoma of kidney does spread?

Ans. *See* Surgical Pathology Page No. 910, 911, Chapter 18

Q. What is the classical triad of presentation of carcinoma of kidney?

Ans.
* Painless hematuria
* Kidney mass
* Loin pain.

Q. What are the atypical presentations of carcinoma of kidney?

Ans.
* Constitutional symptoms like anemia, weakness, anorexia, and weight loss
* Hemoptysis due to pulmonary metastasis
* A pulsatile bone swelling due to bone metastasis or pathological fracture
* Pyrexia of unknown origin underlying carcinoma kidney may be one of the obscure cause
* Polycythemia may be a presentation in 4% of cases. This is due to increased production of erythropoietin by the tumor
* Nephrotic syndrome
* Hypertension due to increased renin production
* Hypercalcemia due to increased parathormone like substance secretion from the tumor cells
* May present with Cushing's syndrome
* Leukemoid reaction due to bone marrow stimulation
* Secondary amyloidosis in about 5% cases.

Q. What is tumor, node, and metastasis (TNM) classification of renal cell carcinoma (RCC)?

Ans.

Primary tumors (T)	
TX	Primary tumor cannot be assessed
T0	No evidence of primary tumor
T1	Tumor ≤7 cm in greatest dimension, limited to the kidney
T1a	Tumor ≤4 cm in greatest dimension, limited to the kidney
T1b	Tumor >4 cm but ≤7 cm in greatest dimension, limited to the kidney
T2	Tumor >7 cm in greatest dimension, limited to the kidney
T2a	Tumor >7 cm but ≤10 cm in greatest dimension, limited to the kidney
T2b	Tumor >10 cm, limited to the kidney
T3	Tumor extends into major veins or perinephric tissues but not into the ipsilateral adrenal gland and not beyond the Gerota fascia
T3a	Tumor grossly extends into the renal vein or its segmental (muscle-containing) branches, or tumor invades perirenal and/or renal sinus fat but not beyond the Gerota fascia
T3b	Tumor grossly extends into the vena cava below the diaphragm
T3c	Tumor grossly extends into the vena cava above the diaphragm or invades the wall of the vena cava
T4	Tumor invades beyond the Gerota fascia (including contiguous extension into the ipsilateral adrenal gland)
Regional lymph node (N)	
NX	Regional lymph nodes cannot be assessed
N0	No regional lymph node metastasis
N1	Metastasis in regional lymph node(s)
Distant metastasis (M)	
M0	No distant metastasis
M1	Distant metastasis

Anatomic stage	T	N	M
I	T1	N0	M0
II	T2	N0	M0
III	T1-2	N1	M0
	T3	N0-1	M0
IV	T4	N2	M0
	Any T	Any N	M1

Q. What is nephron sparing surgery for renal cell carcinoma?

Ans. Patient presenting with bilateral renal cancer or renal cancer in a solitary kidney, radical nephrectomy will render a patient anephric and will require lifelong dialysis or renal transplantation.

In these situations a nephron or parenchyma sparing surgery may be considered for RCC.

In this procedure the renal artery is temporarily occluded by a vascular clamp and the kidney is cooled down. A partial nephrectomy or a wedge resection is done. Frozen section of the resected specimen is done to ensure adequacy of resection. After restoration of circulation the cut margin and the renal capsule is sutured to achieve adequate hemostasis and proper healing.

Q. How will you treat metastatic disease?

Ans. In selected patients who have a solitary resectable metastasis, radical nephrectomy along with resection of the metastasis may be done. Some series reported 30–35% 5 years survival after resection.

Multiple metastasis, however, precludes any surgical intervention.

Q. What is the role of radiotherapy in carcinoma kidney?

Ans. Renal cell carcinomas are radioresistant. Good palliation may be achieved with radiotherapy in brain, bone or pulmonary metastasis.

Q. What is the role of chemotherapy in RCC?

Ans. Renal cell carcinomas are relatively chemoresistant and chemotherapy has not shown any benefit in RCC. Vinblastine used singly has shown a response rate of 10–15%.

Q. What is the role of hormone therapy?

Ans. Medroxyprogesterone acetate has been used in some cases. But the response rate is only 10–15%.

Q. What is the role of immunotherapy in RCC?

Ans. A number of agents has been used as immunotherapy:
* Interferon alpha, beta, and gamma
* Antilymphocyte serum
* Lymphocyte activated killer cells
* Interleukin II
* Interleukin II is currently used for metastatic RCC. This is a cytokine produced by activated T cells. This has marked immunomodulatory and antineoplastic properties.

Breast

■ HISTORY

1. **Particulars of the Patient**
2. **Chief Complaints**
   – Swelling in the right/left breast for last .... months/years.
   – Pain in the breast over the swelling for last .... months/years.
   – Ulceration over the breast for.............. months/years.
   – Nipple discharge for .... months/years.
   – Swelling in the axilla/neck for .... months/years.
3. **History of Present Illness**
   – *Detailed history about the swelling*:
     - Duration
     - Progress: Rate of growth
     - Any history of rapid growth
     - Any swelling in the opposite breast and axilla
   – *Pain*:
     - Duration
     - Site
     - Character
     - Relation with the swelling
     - Relation with menstrual cycle
   – *If ulcer is present—details about the ulcer*:
     - Duration
     - Progress
   – *Any nipple discharge*:
     - Duration
     - Type of discharge: Serous/blood/milky
     - From one duct opening or multiple openings
   – Any swelling in axilla and neck—details of the swelling
   – Chest pain/cough/hemoptysis

- Appetite/weight loss
- Any pain in abdomen, any history of jaundice
- Any history of low backache
- Any history of aches and pain in limbs
- Any history of headache/loss of consciousness/vomiting/weakness of any of the limbs.

4. **Past History**
5. **Family History**

    Detailed family history regarding similar illness or any history of gastrointestinal or ovarian malignancy in 2–3 generations. Any history of breast carcinoma or gastrointestinal or ovarian malignancy in sibling and cousins, in parents, aunts, and uncle and in grandparents.

6. **Personal History**
    - Details of menstrual history
    - Details of obstetrical history
        - Age at first pregnancy
        - Total number of pregnancy (P2+O)
        - Number of abortion
        - Mode of delivery
        - Last child birth
        - Any history of oral pill intake or hormone replacement therapy.

7. **Treatment History**
8. **History of Allergy**

■ PHYSICAL EXAMINATION

1. **General Survey**
2. **Local Examination**

Examination of Both Breasts

Inspection: Examination of diseased breast (right or left).

- Symmetry and position of breast in comparison to normal side
- Size and shape of breast in comparison to normal breast
- *Nipple*:
    - Position in comparison to the normal side
    - Drawn up or pushed down
    - Displaced inward or outward
    - Size and shape of nipple
    - Surface of the nipple: Any cracks or fissure
    - Any nipple retraction
    - Any discharge from nipple
    - Any ulcer over the nipple.
- *Areola*:
    - Size of areola
    - Any diminution of size due to retraction
    - Any cracks, fissure, ulcer or eczema
    - Any discharge.

- *Skin over the breast*:
  - Scar
  - Engorged vein
  - Pigmentation
  - Any redness or shininess
  - Any skin change dimpling, retraction, puckering, *peau d'orange*, nodule, ulceration (fungation), *cancer-en-cuirasse*
- *Any swelling in the breast*:
  - Position in relation to breast quadrant
  - Extent
  - Size and shape
  - Surface and margin
  - Skin over the swelling
- *Any ulcer over the breast or over a swelling in the breast*:
  - Position and extent
  - Size and shape
  - Margin
  - Floor
- *Any edema of the arm*:
  - *Inspection* of the breast with the arms raised over the head—to look for any nipple deviation or any skin changes.
  - *Inspection* with the patient sitting and leaning forward—to look for whether both the breast fall forward equally or there is fixity of the diseased breast.
  - *Inspection* with the patient sitting and pressing her waist with the hands—to look for any evident skin changes.
  - Other breast on inspection—normal.

Palpation: Normal breast palpated first—describe as normal.

Diseased breast (right or left):

- Temperature in all the quadrant of the breast
- Tenderness over the breast
- Any swelling, palpate, the details:
  - Position and extent in relation to the breast quadrant
  - Size and shape
  - Surface and margin
  - Consistency
  - Fixity to skin
  - Fixity to breast tissue
  - Fixity to underlying pectoral fascia and pectoralis major muscle
  - Fixity to chest wall
  - Fixity to serratus anterior muscle for lumps in outer quadrant of breast
  - If swelling is cystic—fluctuation and transillumination

If there is an ulcer over the breast—examination of ulcer:

- Site
- Size and shape

- Margin
- Floor
- Any discharge
- Surrounding area
- Tenderness
- Base of ulcer
- Mobility.

Examination of Regional Lymph Node

- *Level I*: Lymph node include anterior (pectoral), lateral and posterior group of axillary nodes. This group of lymph nodes lies lateral to the lateral border of pectoralis minor.
- *Level II*: Lymph node includes the central group of lymph nodes and lies behind the pectoralis minor.
- *Level III*: It is the apical group of lymph nodes and lies medial to the pectoralis minor.

Examination of supraclavicular lymph nodes:

Examination of opposite axillary lymph nodes: Level I to level III lymph nodes.

3. **Systemic Examination**
   Examine all the systems

▌SUMMARY OF THE CASE

▌PROVISIONAL DIAGNOSIS

▌DIFFERENTIAL DIAGNOSIS

▌INVESTIGATIONS SUGGESTED

Q. Write a complete diagnosis.

Ans.

- Carcinoma of breast right or left
- TNM definition of tumor, e.g. T1N1M0/ T4bN2M0
- Staging depending on T, N, M. Stage I/ II/III/IV, e.g. carcinoma of right breast in a postmenopausal woman—Stage 1 (T1N0M0).

Q. How inspection in different position does help?

Ans.

Inspection is done:

- With the arms by the side of the body (Fig. 5.1A).

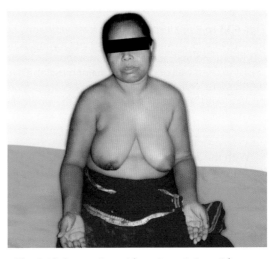

Fig. 5.1A: Inspection with patient sitting with arms by the side of body

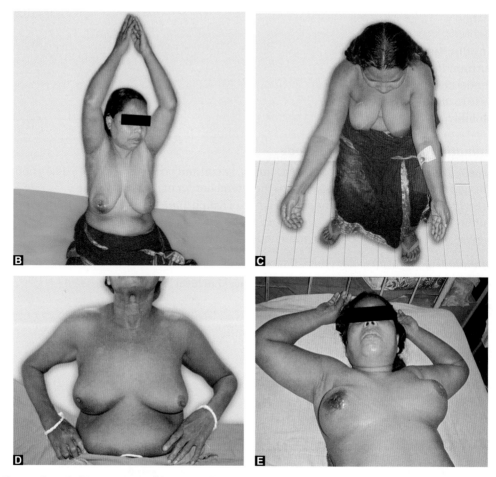

Figs 5.1B to E: (B) Inspection of breast with arms raised over the head. Note that the nipple retraction becomes more obvious in this posture; (C) Inspection with the patient leaning forward. Note that the left breast (normal side) is falling more forward than the diseased right breast (suggesting fixity of the breast to chest wall or pectoralis major muscle); (D) Inspection with patient sitting and the hands pressed on the waist. Note that skin dimpling becomes more obvious; (E) Inspection with patient in recumbent position with head end up by 45°. Note the whole breast including the inferior quadrant is seen better in this position

- With the arms raised over the head (Fig. 5.1B).
- Patient sitting and bending forward so that the breasts fall away (Fig. 5.1C).
- Patient sitting and hands pressed on the waist to contract the pectoralis major muscle (Fig. 5.1D).
- Patient recumbent with 45° head end elevation and both hands lying by the side of head (Fig. 5.1E).
- Any lump or skin dimples present will be more marked when the patient raises her arms above the head.
- Any nipple retraction or deviation of nipple will become more obvious as the patient raises her arms above her head.

- If the lump is fixed to the pectoral muscle or chest wall, this will become more obvious as the patient leans forward.
- The normal breast falls more forward than the diseased breast suggesting fixity of the breast or the lump to the pectoral muscle or the chest wall.
- As the patient presses the waist with her hands to contract the pectorals, the skin dimples may become more evident.
- Patient in recumbent position the inferior quadrant of the breast will be seen better particularly if the breast is pendulous.

Q. How will you ascertain displacement of nipple?

Ans.
- On inspection—deviation of nipple will be obvious if there is a gross deviation
- The upward and downward displacement of nipples may be ascertained by measuring the distance of the nipples from midclavicular point and comparing with the normal side
- The inward and outward displacement of nipple may be ascertained by measuring distance of the nipple from the midline (Fig. 5.2).

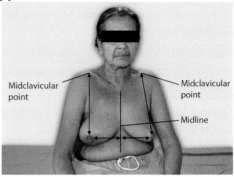

Fig. 5.2: Ascertaining displacement of nipple

Q. How do you divide the breast into different quadrants?

Ans. One vertical and one horizontal line are drawn through the nipple. The area surrounding the nipple and areola is included as (a) central quadrant.

The other quadrants are (Figs 5.3A and B):

b. Upper outer quadrant
c. Upper inner quadrant
d. Lower outer quadrant
e. Lower inner quadrant.

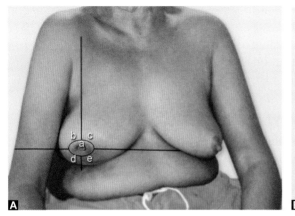
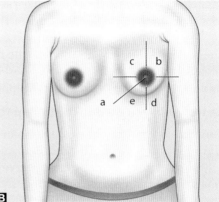

Figs 5.3A and B: Quadrants of breast—a, b, c, d, and e

Q. How will you palpate the breast?

Ans. Breast palpation is done systematically quadrant-wise with the palmar surface of fingers. The palpation may be done in sitting posture or patient in recumbent position. A neoplastic lump is easily felt with the palmar surface of the fingers. In fibroadenosis the breast feels granular and a lump may be palpable in between fingers but not with the palmar surface of fingers.

Q. How will you ascertain temperature over the breast?

Ans. Palpate with the dorsal aspect of the fingers in all quadrant of the breast and compare with the corresponding area of the normal breast (Fig. 5.4).

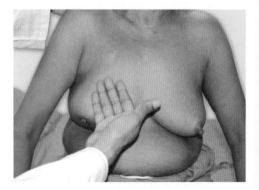

Fig. 5.4: Ascertaining temperature over the breast

Q. How will you demonstrate fixity of lump to breast tissue?

Ans. The breast tissue is fixed in between fingers of one hand and the lump is pushed to one side with the other hand. If the lump is fixed to breast tissue then the breast tissue moves along with the lump (Fig. 5.5).

Q. How will you demonstrate skin tethering?

Ans. As the malignant breast lump grows it may infiltrate the Cooper's ligament and make these strands inelastic and pulls the skin inward rendering puckering of the skin. At this stage the lump can be moved for limited distance independently of the skin.

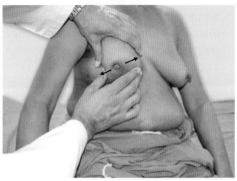

Fig. 5.5: Ascertaining the fixity of the lump to the breast tissue

The tethering can be demonstrated by moving the lump from side-to-side and observing if skin dimples appear at the extremes of movement (Fig. 5.6).

Tethering may also be demonstrated by asking the patient to lift her hands above the head or pressing the waist with both hands (*See* Figs 5.1B and 5.1D) when the skin dimple will appear.

Q. How will you demonstrate skin fixity?

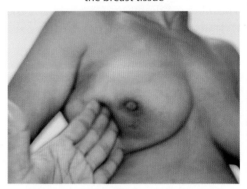

Fig. 5.6: Demonstration of skin tethering

Ans. Skin fixity implies direct infiltration of the skin by the underlying malignant tumor. When the lump is fixed to the skin, the lump and the skin cannot be moved independently.

The skin fixity is demonstrated by trying to lift the skin from the underlying lump in between fingers. If the skin is fixed to the underlying lump, the overlying skin cannot be lifted up from the underlying lump (Figs 5.7A and B).

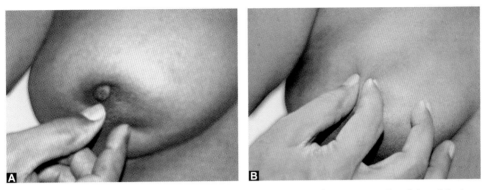

Figs 5.7A and B: (A) The skin cannot be lifted up from the underlying lump suggesting fixity of the lump to the overlying skin; (B) The skin can be easily lifted up from the underlying lump, suggesting no fixity of the lump to the overlying skin

Q. How will you demonstrate pectoral fixity of the lump?

Ans. Patient keeps her hands on the waist. The lump is moved along and across the direction of muscle fibers of pectoralis major keeping the pectoralis major muscle relaxed. If the lump is mobile, it indicates that the lump is not fixed to the chest wall. If the lump is immobile with the

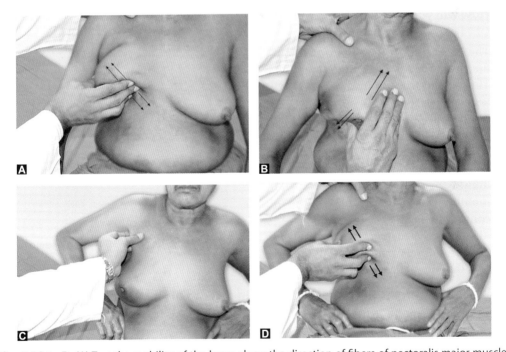

Figs 5.8A to D: (A) Test the mobility of the lump along the direction of fibers of pectoralis major muscle with muscle relaxed; (B) Test the mobility of the lump along the direction of fibers of pectoralis major muscle with muscle relaxed; (C) Ask the patient to press her waist with both hands and palpate the anterior axillary fold to confirm that the pectoralis major muscle is contracted; (D) Test the mobility again along the direction of the fibers of pectoralis major muscle

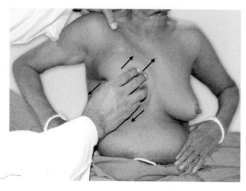

Fig. 5.8E: Test the mobility again across the direction of fibers of pectoralis major muscle

pectoralis major relaxed, then the lump is fixed to the chest wall. In that case testing mobility again with the muscle contracted is not required at all.

If the lump is mobile with the muscle relaxed, patient is then asked to press her hand against the waist, the pectoralis major muscle is made taut [confirmed by palpation of the anterior axillary fold (Fig. 5.8C)] and the lump is then moved again in the same direction and compare the range of mobility of the lump with muscle relaxed and contracted. The mobility will be restricted if the lump is fixed to the pectoralis major muscle (Figs 5.8A to E).

Q. How will you test fixity of the lump to serratus anterior?

Ans.

+ The lump situated in outer quadrant of the breast may be fixed to serratus anterior.
+ The mobility of the lump over the chest wall is tested in relaxed state
+ The patient is then asked to push the shoulders of the clinician with both hands in front and the mobility of lump is tested again on the contracted serratus anterior muscle. If the lump is fixed to serratus anterior then the mobility will be restricted with the muscle contracted (Fig. 5.9)
+ Alternatively, patient may be asked to push the wall in front and the mobility of the lump tested over the contracting serratus anterior muscle.

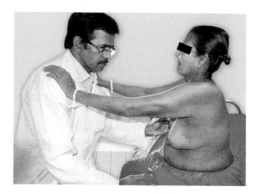

Fig. 5.9: Testing for fixity of the lump to serratus anterior muscle

Q. What is the implication of serratus anterior fixity of the lump?

Ans. Serratus anterior fixity of a lump denotes chest wall fixity, i.e. T4a. Pectoral muscle fixity does not alter T staging.

Q. How will you demonstrate peau d'orange?

Ans. Gross peau d'orange will be obvious on inspection. Peau d'orange may also be demonstrated by squeezing a segment of skin over the breast which will show the lymphedema in the skin with prominent hair follicles in between (Figs 5.10A and B).

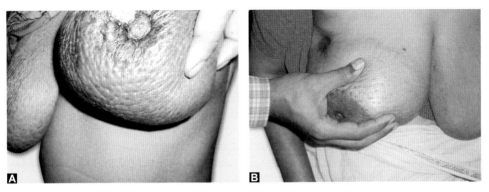

Figs 5.10A and B: (A) Gross peau d'orange; (B) Peau d'orange made obvious by palpation

Q. How will you palpate axillary lymph node?

Ans. Patient is in sitting posture facing the clinician, and proper exposure is done. The anterior, central, apical, and the lateral group of lymph nodes are palpated from the front and the posterior or subscapular group are palpated from the back of the patient. The right axilla is palpated with the left hand except the lateral and the posterior group which are palpated with the corresponding hand.

♦ *Palpation of the anterior group of axillary node and the Rotter's nodes*: The right hand of the clinician lift the right hand of the patient to expose the axilla. The index, middle and the ring finger of the left hand of the clinician is placed behind the anterior axillary fold and the thumb kept in front. The hand is then brought down to rest on the left forearm of the clinician. The right hand of the clinician is now steady the opposite shoulder. The anterior group of lymph nodes are now palpated between the thumb and the other fingers along the lateral border of pectoralis major muscle (Figs 5.11A and B).

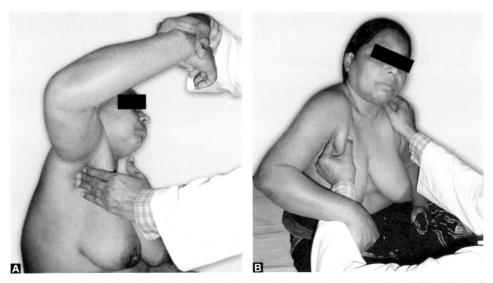

Figs 5.11A and B: (A) Lift the hand and place the fingers behind the anterior axillary fold; (B) Bring the hand down over the forearm of the clinician and palpate along the anterior axillary fold

To palpate the Rotter's node the fingers are pushed further inward and any enlarged node is palpated in-between the pectoralis major and minor muscle.

♦ *Palpation of central and apical group of lymph nodes*: Lift the right hand of the patient and place the left hand of the clinician in the center of the axilla. Bring the right hand down to rest on the left forearm of the clinician and the right hand of the clinician now steadies the opposite shoulder. The central group of lymph node is now palpated with the fingers against the lateral chest wall over the 2nd, 3rd, and 4th rib in the axilla (Figs 5.11C and D).

The *apical group of lymph nodes* is palpated by pushing the finger up in the apex of the axilla and keeping the right hand over the ipsilateral supraclavicular fossa (Fig. 5.11E).

♦ *Palpation of lateral group of axillary lymph nodes:* The lateral group of lymph nodes lies against the shaft of the humerus in the lateral wall of the axilla and is palpated on the right side with the right hand of the clinician against the shaft of humerus between two axillary folds. The left hand of the clinician steadies the right shoulder of the patient (Figs 5.11F and G).

♦ *The posterior or subscapular lymph node palpation:* The clinician stands on the back of the patient. For right side, the right hand is supported by the left hand of the clinician and the right hand of the clinician palpate the posterior group of lymph nodes along the posterior fold of the axilla along the subscapularis muscle (Figs 5.11H and I).

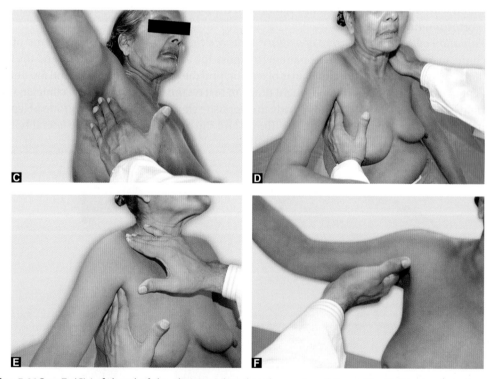

Figs 5.11C to F: (C) Left hand of the clinician placed in the center of the axilla; (D) The central group of lymph nodes are palpated against the 2nd, 3rd and 4th rib; (E) Palpation of the apical group of lymph nodes; (F) Lift the hand and place the right hand of the clinician in the lateral wall of the axilla in-between the anterior and posterior axillary folds

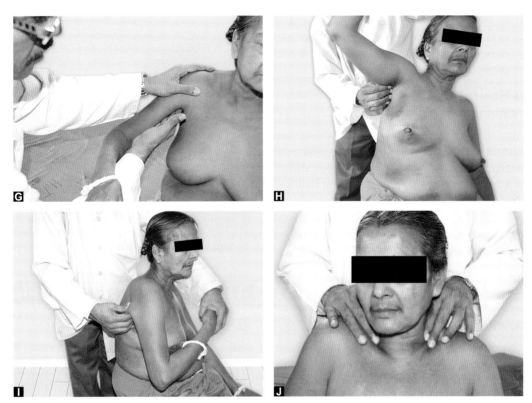

Figs 5.11G to J: (G) The clinician steadies the right shoulder with the left hand and right hand palpate the lateral group of axillary lymph nodes against the shaft of the humerus in-between two axillary folds; (H) For palpation of the posterior group of lymph nodes. Stand on the back of the patient. Lift the right hand with the left hand of the clinician and place the right hand of the clinician along the posterior axillary fold; (I) Bring the hand down and palpate along the posterior axillary fold; (J) Stand on the back of the patient and palpate at the supraclavicular fossa

- *Palpation of supraclavicular lymph nodes:* The clinician stands on the back of the patient. The supraclavicular lymph nodes are palpated in the supraclavicular fossa by asking the patient to shrug the shoulder up (Fig. 5.11J).

Q. What are the levels of lymph nodes in the axilla?

Ans. The axillary lymph nodes are divided into different levels depending on the location of the lymph nodes in relation to the pectoralis minor muscle.

- *Level I*: These lymph nodes lie lateral to the lateral border of pectoralis minor muscle. This includes anatomical anterior (pectoral), lateral and posterior group of lymph nodes.
- *Level II*: These lymph nodes lie behind the pectoralis minor muscle. This includes the anatomical central group of lymph nodes.

♦ *Level III*: These lymph nodes lie medial to the medial border of pectoralis minor muscle. This includes the anatomical apical group of lymph nodes.

Q. How to record the breast examination findings?

Ans. This can be done in a schematic diagram. The breast is divided into four quadrant, barring the nipple and areolar area which is marked as central quadrant. The axilla is marked as a triangular area. The palpable lump is shown in the particular breast quadrant and the palpable axillary lymph nodes are marked in the region of axilla (Fig. 5.12).

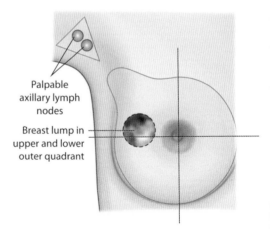

Palpable axillary lymph nodes

Breast lump in upper and lower outer quadrant

Fig. 5.12: Recording breast examination

EARLY CARCINOMA OF BREAST IN A PREMENOPAUSAL WOMAN

Q. What is your case? (Summary of a case of early carcinoma breast)

This 45-year-old premenopausal lady presented with a swelling in her right breast for last 8 months. The swelling was first noticed by the patient in her outer part of right breast and was about 1 cm in size at the onset. The swelling is gradually increasing in size. Patient complains of occasional dull aching pain over the swelling for last 1 month. She did not complain of any swelling in her axilla or opposite breast. No history of chest pain, cough, hemoptysis or breathlessness. Her appetite is normal. Bowel and bladder habits are normal. No other complaint. There is no family history of breast diseases.

On physical examination, general survey is essentially normal. On local examination of the breasts the left breast is normal. The position and symmetry of the right breast is normal. The nipple and areola is normal. On palpation a globular 3 cm × 3 cm lump is palpable in the upper outer quadrant of the right breast, the skin is free but the lump is fixed to the breast tissue. There is no chest wall and pectoral fixity of the lump. There is no fixity to muscle. The skin over the breast is normal. There is no palpable lymph node in the axilla and in the supraclavicular region. Systemic examination is normal.

Q. What is your diagnosis?

Ans. This is a case of early carcinoma of right breast. Stage IIA (T2N0M0).

Q. What are the other possibilities?

Ans.
♦ Fibroadenoma of breast
♦ Antibioma
♦ Chronic abscess
♦ Tuberculosis of breast
♦ Traumatic fat necrosis
♦ Fibroadenosis of breast with nodularity.

Q. How will you proceed to manage this patient?

Ans. I would like to do some investigations to confirm my diagnosis.
* Breast imaging with mammography.
* Core needle biopsy.

Q. How does mammography helps in diagnosis of carcinoma of breast?

Ans.
* In evaluation of patient with breast lump as part of triple assessment an imaging with mammography in patient older than 40 years is essential (Fig. 5.12A).
* Mammography may show a characteristic lesion suggestive of malignancy.
* Mammography can detect multicentric breast carcinoma which will preclude breast conserving therapy.
* May detect an impalpable lesion in the opposite breast.
* Digital mammography is superior to traditional screen film mammography in younger patient with dense breast.

Q. What are the characteristics of malignant lesion in mammography?

Ans.
* Architectural distortion of breast tissue
* Duct dilatation
* Dense stellate soft tissue mass with irregular margin and spiky projection
* *Microcalcification*: In elderly patients few microcalcification may be normal
* Stippled calcification is characteristic
* Increased thickness of skin due to lymphedema
* Nipple retraction may be seen.

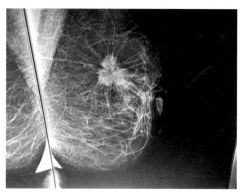

Fig. 5.12A: Mammography picture craniocaudal view showing distortion of architecture of the breast and a hyoerdense mass in upper quadrant of the breast. The mass is having a spiculated margin with areas of calcification. The nipple appears retracted. This is most likely to be a malignant mass in the breast

Q. Which views are essential for mammographic evaluation?

Ans. A craniocaudal and a mediolateral views are essential for mammographic evaluation.

Q. How reliable is mammography for evaluation of breast malignancy?

Ans.
* *Sensitivity (true-positive)*: 90%
* *False positive*: 10%
* *False negative*: 6–8%.

Q. What is BIRADS system of reporting of breast imaging?

Ans. The acronym BIRADS stand for Breast Imaging-Reporting and Data System and is proposed by American College of Radiology. This reporting system is applicable for ultrasonography (USG), mammography or magnetic resonance imaging (MRI). This system is useful for standardization of reporting of breast imaging. Other system is Nottingham classification.

Q. What is BIRADS category for breast imaging reporting?

Ans.

BIRAD category and definition:

- BIRADS 0: Incomplete assessment. Further imaging or information is required, e.g. magnification, special mammographic views, and ultrasound.
- BIRADS I: Negative. No masses, architectural distortion or suspicious calcifications present.
- BIRADS II: Benign findings. Benign masses with characteristic appearance. No mammographic evidence of malignancy.
- BIRADS III: Probably *benign*, short interval follow-up study suggested.
- BIRADS IV:
  - Suspicious mammographic abnormality of malignancy.
  - Biopsy should be considered for such a lesion
- These can be further classified as:
  - BIRADS IVa: Low level of suspicion for malignancy.
  - BIRADS IVb: Intermediate suspicion for malignancy.
  - BIRADS IVc: Moderate suspicion for malignancy.
- BIRADS V: There is a mammographic appearance which is highly suggestive of malignancy. Biopsy of the lesion should be done.
- BIRADS VI: Known biopsy proven malignancy.

Q. What is the risk of malignancy in different BIRADS lesion?

Ans.

- BIRADS III: Approximately 2%
- BIRADS IV: Approxinately 30%
- BIRADS V: 95%.

Q. What is the role of ultrasonography in evaluation of breast mass?

Ans.

In premenopausal women (<30 years) with dense breast tissue, mammography may not detect small lesion. In such situation USG is a better imaging modality to detect breast lesion.

- Ultrasonography (USG) can detect the mass as solid or cystic
- No radiation, cheap, easily available
- Useful in delineation of cystic lesion in breast
- USG-guided aspiration of cyst or USG-guided biopsy from solid lesion may be done
- May demonstrate solid lesion in breast but cannot detect lesion less than 1 cm in diameter.

Q. What are the characteristics of a benign lesion in USG?

Ans.

- Smooth contour of swelling
- Round or oval shape
- Week internal echoes and
- Well-defined anterior and posterior margins.

Q. What are the characteristics of malignant lesion in USG?

Ans.

- Elongated lesion—wider than tall

- Increased vascularity
- Jagged/irregular anterior and posterior wall
- Lesion is heterogeneous
- High internal echoes.

Q. How does Doppler flow study helps in diagnosis of breast lesion?

Ans.
- Malignant lesion has increased blood flow
- Malignant lesion shows signals of high frequency and amplitude with continuous flow through diastole. However, this is not very specific.

Q. What is the role of MRI in evaluation of breast mass?

Ans. Magnetic resonance imaging is also helpful for evaluation of breast mass. MRI is more useful in young patient with dense breast for detection of nonpalpable mass. The sensitivity of MRI for invasive cancer is 90% but for ductal carcinoma in situ (DCIS) the sensitivity is only 60%.

Q. Why do you prefer to do a core needle biopsy?

Ans.
- Core needle biopsy has become the standard of care for biopsy of breast lesion
- In core needle biopsy a number of wedge of tissue is taken
- A histological diagnosis of invasive or noninvasive carcinoma may be made
- The tumor grade and any lymphovascular invasion may be assessed
- The ER/PR and Her2-neu status may also be assessed in the core biopsy specimen.

Q. How is core biopsy done?

Ans.
- For a well-palpable lesion core biopsy can be done without image guidance. For small or nonpalpable lesion USG/mammographic or MRI-guided core biopsy may be done
- After antiseptic cleaning and draping, local anesthesia with injection of 2% lignocaine hydrochloride
- A small stab incision is made in the skin and a 11-G core needle biopsy needle is inserted into the lesion with vacuum assistance and tissue sample is obtained
- 6–8 biopsy sample is to be taken for histological examination.

Q. What is the role of FNAC in breast lesion?

Ans. Earlier fine needle aspiration cytology (FNAC) was the common method for diagnosis of breast mass. But FNAC could not differentiate between noninvasive and invasive breast carcinoma. Hormone receptor study is not possible in FNAC specimen. So, FNAC is now superseded by core needle biopsy.

Q. How FNAC is done?

Ans. Fine needle aspiration cytology is done by aspiration of the material from the tumor tissue by a fine needle of 22 G or 23 G attached to a syringe which is attached to a piston so that it can create a good vacuum for ease of aspiration of tissue from the tumor.

Q. What is the predictive value of FNAC?

Ans.
* Sensitivity (true positive): 80–98%
* False negative: 2–10%
* Specificity is almost 100% as false positive is very rare.

Q. What is the indication for incisional biopsy in breast lesion?

Ans. Core biopsy is helpful for diagnosis of carcinoma of breast in about 90% of cases. In about 10% cases when core biopsy is inconclusive, in such situation an incisional biopsy may be considered.

Q. What precaution should you take while taking incisional biopsy?

Ans.
* It is important to keep the incision for biopsy within the boundary of subsequent incision for mastectomy or wide local excision. Incision should be curvilinear (circumareolar) rather than radial
* Diathermy should not be used while taking biopsy specimen. Use of electrocautery may distort the histologic picture of the tumor and may invalidate tissue level of hormonal receptors.

Q. When will you consider excisional biopsy?

Ans. When lump is small (<4 cm) in size then whole lump with a 1 cm clear margin may be excised in a suspicious lesion.

Q. What is the value of frozen section biopsy in breast lesion?

Ans. In breast lesion it is difficult on frozen section biopsy to differentiate an invasive carcinoma from severe atypia or in situ disease. So frozen section biopsy is not very helpful in breast lesion.

Q. What other investigations you will do?

Ans. Routine preoperative investigations should include:
* Chest X-ray [posteroanterior view (PA)]
* 12-lead electrocardiography (ECG)
* Blood for hemoglobin, total leukocyte count (TLC), differential leukocyte count (DLC) and erythrocyte sedimentation rate (ESR)
* Blood for sugar, urea, and creatinine
* Blood for liver function tests (LFTs)
* Ultrasonography of abdomen.

Q. Why detail staging investigation is not required in patients with early carcinoma of breast?

Ans. In early carcinoma of breast with negative axilla, the chance of distant metastasis is remote. So whole body bone scanning, or computed tomography (CT) scan of abdomen and chest is not routinely required in these patients.

Q. What treatment do you plan for this patient?

Ans. I am planning to do breast conserving surgery in this patient as it is a case of early carcinoma of breast. I will do wide local excision of the lump with a clear 1 cm margin all around the lump. Through a separate incision in the axilla, axillary dissection removing level I and level II lymph nodes should be done. The subsequent treatment will depend on the histopathological examination of the excised specimen.

Q. How will you manage the defect after wide excision of breast lump?

Ans. Immediate reconstruction of the defect after lumpectomy is preferred over delayed reconstruction. This defect after lumpectomy may be reconstructed by local advancement flap or other oncoplastic surgical technique. This oncoplastic reconstruction is essential for a cosmetic outcome after wide excision. This reconstruction may be done by using a latissimus dorsi myocutaneous flap.

Q. What is a sentinel lymph node?

Ans.

- Sentinel lymph node is the lymph node which is in a direct drainage pathway from the primary tumor
- Sentinel lymph node is the first node encountered by the tumor cells and its histological status predicts distant lymph basin status with regard to metastasis (Fig. 5.13).

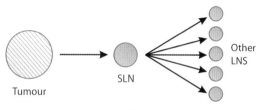

Fig. 5.13: Sentinel lymph node (SLN)

Q. What is the role of sentinel lymph node biopsy in early breast cancer?

Ans. In western centers and in specialized breast centers sentinel lymph node biopsy is the standard of care in patient with clinically negative axilla (No). If the sentinel lymph node is positive a formal axillary dissection should be undertaken. If the sentinel lymph node is negative, then further axillary surgery may be avoided.

Q. What are the advantages of sentinel lymph node biopsy?

Ans.

- Minimally invasive technique which can reduce morbidity and cost
- By identifying one or two lymph nodes most likely to be involved—more detailed histologic analysis is possible—micrometastases may be detected
- May obviate the need for axillary lymph node dissection (ALND) in breast cancer patient without compromising staging information, local control or long-time survival.

Q. When will you consider sentinel lymph node biopsy?

Ans. All patients with early carcinoma of breast T1 or T2. No stage on triple assessment.

Q. Why sentinel node biopsy is not suitable in clinically involved axilla?

Ans. If axillary lymph node is clinically palpable then sentinel lymph node biopsy may be fallacious. This may be due to a change in the lymphatic flow as a result of replacement of the sentinel node with metastatic deposit. The radioactive colloid or blue dye bypasses the sentinel node and move on to a nonsentinel lymph node.

Q. Why multifocal and multicentric diseases are not suitable for sentinel lymph node biopsy?

Ans. Multifocal tumors are likely to involve more than one lymphatic trunk from the mammary gland to the axillary node which may give rise to a false negative result.

Q. Which agents are used for localizing sentinel lymph node?

Ans. The agents in use are:
- ^{99m}Tc labeled as sulfur colloid. These particles are taken up by reticuloendothelial (RE) system and taken to sentinel lymph node which may be detected by hand held gamma probe. This radioactive particle finds the first draining lymph node irrespective of whether they are involved with carcinoma or not. They are lymph node seeking and not tumor seeking agents.
- Isosulfan vital blue dye injected into the peritumoral area and the success rate is 65% and sensitivity 75%. 3–5 mL of isosulfan blue is injected peritumorally and the area is massaged to facilitate passage of the dye through the lymphatics.

Q. How will you do sentinel lymph node biopsy?

Ans. The sentinel lymph node may be localized by blue staining of lymph node after blue dye injection or by hand held gamma probe after injection of radioactive colloid alone or in combination.

Q. When will you inject the radioactive substance?

Ans. The radioactive substance can be injected the day before operation or on the day of operation as per decided protocol.

Q. What are the sites of injection of radioactive substance?

Ans.
- Subdermal tissue overlying the tumor
- Intratumor injection
- Peritumor injection.

Q. How to determine the site of skin incision?

Ans. The location of radioactivity may be detected by the gamma probe and skin incision can be planned accordingly.

Q. How to identify the sentinel node?

Ans. After skin incision and dissection of subcutaneous tissue the sentinel node may be identified by the gamma probe and additional visual assistance from the blue staining of the lymph node when blue dye is injected.

Q. How will you confirm that sentinel node is excised?

Ans.
- After excision of sentinel node ex vivo radioactivity may be detected in the node
- After removing the sentinel node the probe is reapplied in the wound and a careful reassessment of the residual activity is done.

Q. What may be the cause of false negative results in sentinel lymph node biopsy?

Ans.
- Extensive infiltration by metastatic carcinoma in the sentinel lymph node can lead to directional flow change of lymph leading to a skip phenomenon whereby the sentinel node is bypassed and the radionuclide is taken up by a nonsentinel lymph node
- Fatty degeneration of sentinel lymph nodes happens in elderly patient, where fatty degeneration of axillary lymph node may cause poor uptake of the radioactive tracer which may make the probe localization difficult
- In upper quadrant breast lesion the radioactivity over the tumor tissue may interfere with localization of the sentinel lymph node. Breast retraction downward and medially may overcome the problem and enable the gamma probe detect the radioactivity in the axilla.

Q. In which other malignant lesions sentinel node biopsy is practiced?

Ans.
- Carcinoma of penis
- Malignant melanoma.

Q. What are the contraindications of sentinel lymph node biopsy?

Ans. In cases with clinically involved axilla and multifocal breast cancer, there is higher incidence of false-negative rate.

Q. How to enhance accuracy of sentinel lymph node biopsy?

Ans. Combination of preoperative lymphoscintigraphy, probe guided surgery in combination with blue dye technique is associated with higher detection rate and lower false-negative rate.

Q. What is the average number of sentinel lymph node?

Ans. This has been observed that there are 2–3 sentinel lymph nodes in each patient.

Q. What will you do if sentinel lymph node biopsy is positive?

Ans. If the sentinel lymph node is positive a formal axillary dissection is to be done removing level I, II, and III lymph nodes in the axilla.

Q. What is the strategy of management when the axillary lymph nodes are clinically palpable?

Ans. When the axillary lymph nodes are palpable clinically a formal axillary dissection may be done and further treatment will be planned depending on the histopathology report.

The centers who are practicing sentinel lymph node biopsy, when the axillary lymph nodes are clinically palpable, USG and FNAC of the axillary lymph node may be done. If the FNAC report is negative, the sentinel lymph node biopsy may be done. If the sentinel lymph node biopsy is negative, no further treatment of axillary lymph node is required.

Q. What is the optimal extent of axillary dissection?

Ans. In early carcinoma breast optimal axillary dissection will include dissection of level I and level II lymph nodes in the axilla.

However, if there is gross involvement of the axilla, the dissection may include level I to level III lymph nodes.

Q. What examinations are required of excised specimen?

Ans. The resected specimen is oriented and marked so that pathologist can identify the margins properly. If a particular margin is positive, re-excision may be done to allow breast conservation.

The specimen is to be sent for detailed pathological examination including:

* Histopathological type of the tumor
* Comment about resection lines both circumferential and deeper. Whether margin of excision is cancer-free
* *Grading of tumor*: Well-differentiated, moderately differentiated or poorly differentiated
* Any lymphovascular invasion
* Estrogen-receptor/progesterone-receptor (ER/PR) status
* Her2/neu status
* Axillary lymph nodal status
  - Number of lymph nodes dissected and number of lymph node showing metastatic deposit
  - Any capsular breach.

Q. What are the aims of treatment in early breast cancer?

Ans. The aims of treatment in early breast cancer are:
* Achieve cure
* Control of local disease in the breast and axilla
* Conservation of local form and function
* Delaying the development distant metastasis.

Q. Why do you want to do breast conserving surgery?

Ans. It has been studied and concluded in different trials that for early carcinoma of breast results of mastectomy and breast conserving surgery with adjuvant therapy are comparable with respect to both local recurrence and long-term survival. Recent studies have revealed that with lumpectomy and adjuvant radiation therapy the local recurrence rate is less than 5% at 10 years. As mastectomy lead to disfigurement and emotional upset in women, breast conserving surgery is gaining popularity.

Q. What are the criteria for planning breast conserving surgery?

Ans.
* Early breast cancer with lump up to 5 cm in diameter
* Excision with a clear margin and an acceptable cosmetic result after lumpectomy is achievable
* Clinically negative axillary node
* Breast of adequate size to allow uniform dosage of radiation
* Facility for radiation therapy is available
* Patient compliance for regular follow-up
* Patient's consent for breast conservation therapy.

Q. Which patients are most likely to be candidate for breast conservation surgery?

Ans.
* Mammographically detected lesion
* Small size of primary tumor (up to 5 cm)
* Low S-phase component in DNA flow cytometry.

Q. What are the indications of mastectomy in early carcinoma of breast?

Ans. Although breast conserving surgery is preferred, mastectomy is, however, still the most common operation performed for carcinoma of breast. The indications for mastectomy in early carcinoma breast are:
* Large tumor relative to the breast size
* Extensive calcification on mammography
* Following lumpectomy or segmentectomy resection lines are not free of tumor
* Multicentric disease
* Poorly differentiated tumor
* There is contraindication to postoperative radiation therapy (Collagen disease)
* Patient's choice. Following breast conserving surgery patient may worry about risk of local recurrence.

Q. What is quadrantectomy?

Ans. This is also a form of breast conserving surgery for early breast carcinoma. The entire segment of the breast containing the tumor is excised. The resultant defect should be reconstructed by oncoplastic technique.

Q. What is QUART?

Ans. QUART is quadrantectomy, axillary dissection (level I–III) and postoperative radiotherapy. This concept has been popularized by Umberto Veronesi from Milan.

Q. Why is axillary sampling essential?

Ans.
* Axillary lymph node status is one of the important prognostic markers in carcinoma of breast and an important factor for deciding about adjuvant therapy
* At least 10–15 nodes are sampled from the ipsilateral axilla by a separate incision
* A curvilinear incision between the lateral border of pectoralis major and latissimus dorsi 4–6 cm below the apex of the axilla is adequate for sampling.

Q. How will you plan adjuvant therapy after breast conserving surgery?

Ans. Patient undergoing breast conserving surgery will need adjuvant therapy.
* *Role of radiation therapy*: Adjuvant radiotherapy following breast conserving surgery has shown conclusive evidence of reduced incidence of local recurrence and improved overall outcome. Whole breast radiotherapy with 5000 cGy with boost to the tumor bed with 1000 cGy has been recommended as optimum radiation therapy following breast conserving surgery.

* *Role of systemic therapy*:
  - In spite of adequate locoregional treatment, women with breast cancer may die of metastatic disease 5–10 years after diagnosis. So systemic treatment with chemotherapy or hormone therapy is indicated both in early breast cancer to treat distance micrometastasis and in advanced breast cancer to treat the metastatic disease
  - As the lump is 3 cm, I will consider systemic chemotherapy in this patient
  - If the tumor is ER/PR positive, adjuvant hormone therapy is also indicated.

Q. What are the different regimens of chemotherapy for carcinoma breast?

Ans.

* A chemotherapy regime comprising *CMF (cyclophosphamide/methotrexate/5-fluorouracil)* as a monthly cycle for six cycle achieved a 30% reduction in the risk of relapse over 10–15 years.
  - Cyclophosphamide: 500 mg/m^2 of body surface area
  - Methotrexate: 10 mg/m^2
  - 5-fluorouracil: 500 mg/m^2.

These are administered every 21 days for a total of six cycles

* The alternative regime of chemotherapy *may be CAF (cyclophosphamide/Adriamycin/5-fluorouracil)*. Adriamycin instead of methotrexate.
  - Adriamycin at a dose of 50 mg/m^2
  - Cyclophosphamide and 5-fluorouracil at same dose for six cycles
* A chemotherapy based on AC (Adriamycin and cyclophosphamide) for four cycles has shown to be comparable to regime I and regime II.
  - Adriamycin 60 mg/m^2
  - Cyclophosphamide 600 mg/m^2
* TAC—docetaxel, doxorubicin, and cyclophosphamide
* TC—docetaxel and cyclophosphamide.

Q. What is the indication for using Trastuzumab?

Ans. When Her2-neu is positive, a trastuzumab-based chemotherapy is indicated for better response.
* AC followed by paclitaxel and trastuzumab
* TCH—docetaxel, carboplatin, and trastuzumab.

Q. What are the side effects of chemotherapy?

Ans.
* Nausea and vomiting
* Alopecia
* Myelosuppression
* Cardiac toxicity (Adriamycin)
* Premature menopause
* Second malignancy.

Q. What is the role of hormone therapy in early breast cancer patients?

Ans.
* Tamoxifen therapy is effective in both pre- and postmenopausal in most cases except ER negative tumor in premenopausal women

- Tamoxifen is a selective estrogen receptor modulator that has antagonistic and weak agonistic estrogen effect
- Tamoxifen reduces the risk of recurrence of breast cancer in ER/PR positive cases
- Tamoxifen has beneficial effect of reducing the incidence of contralateral breast cancer.
- At present tamoxifen therapy is given to both pre- and postmenopausal patients with positive of ER/PR status. Both in node negative and node positive cases.

Q. What is the optimum duration of tamoxifen therapy?

Ans. Tamoxifen is to be given in a dose of 20 mg/day for 5 years.

Q. How does tamoxifen act?

Ans. Activity of tamoxifen is closely related to ER/PR status of tumor. This blocks the uptake of estrogen by the target tissue after cytosol binding to the estrogen receptor.

Q. What are the side effects of tamoxifen therapy?

Ans.
- Nausea and vomiting
- Transient hypercalcemia
- Fluid and electrolyte retention
- Increased incidence of endometrial cancer
- Slight increase of thrombotic events.

Q. What other hormonal treatments are effective?

Ans.
- *Surgical oophorectomy*—has shown good response with decreased incidence of local recurrence and improved survival
- *Luteinizing hormone releasing hormone (LHRH) agonist, like goserelin*—induces reversible ovarian suppression, has beneficial effect in carcinoma of breast. This induces chemical castration in premenopausal women
- *Oral aromatase inhibitor, like anastrozole and letrozole*—induces blockade in estrogen synthesis by the adrenals is effective in postmenopausal women.

Q. What are newer drugs which has estrogen receptor modulatory effect?

Ans. Toremifene and raloxifene have effect identical to tamoxifen.

Q. What is Patey's modified radical mastectomy?

Ans.
- This entails en block resection of breast and axillary lymph node
- The line of resection of skin is 3–5 cm beyond the tumor margin to provide adequate clearance
- The pectoralis minor muscle is divided for adequate axillary dissection
- The limits of excision of breast are:
  - Laterally up to anterior margin of latissimus dorsi
  - Medially up to the midline
  - Superiorly up to subclavius muscle
  - Inferiorly up to caudal extension of breast 2–3 cm inferior to the inframammary fold.

Q. Describe the steps of modified radical mastectomy.

See Operative Surgery Section, Page. No. 1126–1128, Chapter 22.

Q. What structures are to be preserved during modified radical mastectomy?

Ans.

- ◆ Long thoracic nerve (supplies serratus anterior)
- ◆ Thoracodorsal nerve (supplies latissimus dorsi)
- ◆ Cephalic vein
- ◆ Axillary vein.

Q. When will you consider chemotherapy in node negative patients?

Ans. Chemotherapy may be indicated in node negative patients if other prognostic factors such as tumor grade/negative ER/PR/positive Her2-neu status infers a high-risk of recurrence.

Premenopausal women with moderately or poorly differentiated invasive tumors of larger than 1 cm, and negative hormone receptor status require adjuvant chemotherapy.

Patient more than 35 years of age, tumor size less than 1 cm, well-differentiated tumors and ER/PR positive tumors does not require adjuvant chemotherapy.

Q. What is the usual dose of radiotherapy?

Ans. Breast is irradiated to a dose of 4500–5000 cGy divided into 200 fractions per day and 5 days a week. Following breast conserving surgery, a local boost radiotherapy (at a dose of 1000 cGy) delivering high dose to the breast tissue is preferred.

Q. Is it mandatory to give radiotherapy after breast conserving surgery?

Ans. Different studies are on to compare results of lumpectomy alone and lumpectomy plus radiotherapy.

Long-term survival is comparable but there is more chance of local recurrence in non-radiated group. So, radiotherapy is advisable following breast conserving surgery.

Q. What is the indication of radiotherapy to axilla even after adequate axillary dissection?

Ans.

- ◆ After complete dissection of axilla from level I–III, axillary irradiation is not advisable as there is high incidence of lymphedema with combination therapy.
- ◆ If, however, pathological examination of axillary lymph node showed any extracapsular extension or tumor implantation seen in soft tissue of axilla then axillary irradiation should be combined with surgery.

Q. If after breast-conserving surgery resection line is not free of tumor what will you do?

Ans. The next step is re-excision of the scar with a clear 1 cm margin. If re-excision lines are not free of tumor, these patients are best treated by total mastectomy.

Q. Why radiation therapy is required after breast-conserving surgery?

Ans.

- ◆ In different trials it has been shown that results of total mastectomy, lumpectomy and radiotherapy or only lumpectomy are comparable in terms of long-term survival. But patients not receiving radiotherapy have higher incidence of local recurrence.

- So, lumpectomy and radiation therapy are an appropriate treatment for patients with early breast carcinoma with lump less than 5 cm in diameter with negative or positive axillary nodes.

Q. How will you plan adjuvant therapy in patient with invasive breast cancer?

Ans. Following adequate surgery patient has the risk of local recurrence and distant metastatic disease in follow-up. The requirement for adjuvant therapy is based on a number of factors:
- Size of the tumor
- Axillary lymph node status
- Age of the patient
- ER/PR/Her2-neu status of the tumor
- S-phase fraction/DNA ploidy/cerB and cathepsin D expression of the tumor.
  - Node negative patients (both pre- and postmenopausal women):
    - Tumor less than 1 cm with ER positive or negative tumor—no chemotherapy. Tamoxifen therapy to reduce the risk of opposite breast cancer
    - Tumor size more than 1 cm and ER positive—combination chemotherapy + tamoxifen therapy
    - Tumor size more than 1 cm and ER negative—combination chemotherapy.
  - Node positive patients:
    - Any tumor size and ER negative—multidrug combination chemotherapy in both pre- and postmenopausal women
    - Any tumor size and ER positive—multidrug combination chemotherapy + tamoxifen therapy in premenopausal women
    - Any tumor size and ER positive—tamoxifen ± multidrug combination chemotherapy in postmenopausal women.

LOCALLY ADVANCED CARCINOMA OF BREAST

Q. What is your case? (Summary of a case of locally advanced carcinoma of breast)

Ans. This 50-year-old postmenopausal lady presented with the swelling in her right breast for last 2 years. The swelling was about the size of about 3 cm when she first noticed the swelling 2 years back. The swelling was initially increasing in size gradually for last one and half years. But for last 6 months, the swelling is increasing rapidly in size and there was an ulcer over the swelling for last 3 months. Patient complained of serous discharge from the ulcer site. Patient complained of swelling in her right axilla for last 1 year which is also increasing in size. No complain of any swelling in the opposite breast or axilla. Her appetite is normal. Bowel and bladder habits are normal. No chest pain, cough, hemoptysis or breathlessness. No major ailment in the past. There is no history of breast diseases in her family (Fig. 5.14).

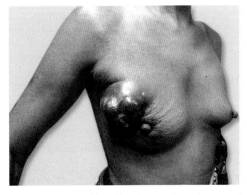

Fig. 5.14: Case of locally advanced carcinoma of right breast

On physical examination, general survey is essentially normal except presence of anemia. On local examination, the left breast is normal. The right breast is asymmetric drawn up; there is retraction of nipple and areola. There is a fungating mass in upper outer quadrant of the right breast about 10 cm in diameter. The tumor is fixed to skin and there is an ulcer over the swelling with serous discharge. The swelling is firm in feel and fixed to the underlying chest wall. On the right side multiple axillary lymph nodes are palpable which are firm in feel and fixed to each other. No supraclavicular lymph nodes are palpable. Systemic examination is normal.

Q. What is your diagnosis?

Ans. This is a case of locally advanced carcinoma of right breast. Stage III B (T4cN2M0).

Q. What do you mean by locally advanced carcinoma of breast?

Ans. Breast cancer with gross locoregional disease is said to be locally advanced disease. There is no evidence of distant metastasis.
* *Tumor characteristics*: T3 (tumor > 5 cm), T4a, T4b, T4c, and T4d tumor (tumor involving chest wall, skin involvement, ulceration, satellite nodules and inflammatory carcinoma).
* *Node characteristics*: N2 or N3 disease (bulky and fixed nodes). Clinically apparent internal mammary and supraclavicular lymph nodes.
  So this group includes:
  Stage IIB, IIIA, and IIIB tumors with:
  – T3 tumors with N1, N2, and N3 nodes
  – T4 tumors with any N nodes
  – Any T tumors with N2 or N3 nodes.

Q. Which locally advanced tumors are inoperable?

Ans. Locally advanced carcinoma may be operable or inoperable. Following characteristics makes a tumor inoperable:
* High tumor/breast ratio
* Extensive skin involvement including presence of satellite nodules
* Fixity of the tumor to the chest wall
* Fixity to the pectoral muscle does not indicate inoperability. However, wide excision of the muscle is required in such situation
* Fixed lymph nodes in the axilla preclude any sort of axillary surgery.

Q. How will you manage this patient with locally advanced breast cancer?

Ans. Confirmation of diagnosis by:
* Core biopsy from breast lump
* Mammography of both breasts.
  In locally advanced lesion there is high chance of distant metastasis. So I will advise some investigations for staging of the disease. The investigation for distant metastasis should include:
* Chest X-ray (PA view)
* Liver function test
* USG/CT scan of abdomen
* Whole body bone scanning.

Q. How will you manage patient with locally advanced breast cancer?

Ans. The aim of treatment in locally advanced carcinoma breast is palliation. The treatment planning depends whether the locally advanced lesion is operable or inoperable. The tumor in this patient is fixed to the chest wall, so is inoperable.

- After biopsy confirmation of the lesion, the primary treatment is systemic
- If the tumor is ER positive tamoxifen therapy is started
- Combination chemotherapy with CAF. With neoadjuvant chemotherapy, the tumor may regress and the lesion may become operable. Three to six cycles of neoadjuvant chemotherapy may be given depending on the response
- Once the lesion becomes operable and the axillary nodes become mobile modified radical mastectomy is done
- Postoperative radiotherapy to breast flap and lymph node fields
- Tamoxifen therapy is continued.

   If only three cycles of chemotherapy are given preoperatively, remaining cycles of chemotherapy is to be given in postoperative period.

Q. What regime of chemotherapy will you advise?

Ans. In locally advanced breast cancer a combination chemotherapy with:

- FAC (5-fluorouracil, adriamycin, and cyclophosphamide) or
- FEC (5-fluorouracil, epirubicin, and cyclophosphamide) has been claimed to be superior to CMF (cyclophosphamide, methotrexate, and 5-fluorouracil).

   Taxanes (paclitaxel and docetaxel), vinorelbine-based chemotherapy has also been used in locally advanced breast with good response.

Q. How will you treat a patient of carcinoma breast which is locally advanced but operable?

Ans.

- *Modified radical mastectomy*: Removal of the whole breast and the axillary lymph node (level I, II, and III)
- Histopathological examination of tumor tissue including ER/PR/Her2-neu status
- Postoperative adjuvant radiotherapy to breast flap and all lymph node fields
- Tamoxifen therapy if ER/PR status is positive
- Combination chemotherapy in premenopausal women and in postmenopausal women in selected cases.

Q. When will you consider chemotherapy?

Ans.

- In premenopausal women in view of locally advanced disease, the chance of distant spread is high, so adjuvant chemotherapy is recommended
- In postmenopausal women with ER negative status, adjuvant chemotherapy is advocated
- In postmenopausal patient with ER positive tumor, hormone therapy may be adequate.

Q. What is the role of axillary surgery in locally advanced breast cancer?

Ans.

- Fixed nodes in the axilla preclude any form of axillary surgery. If the axillary nodes become mobile after neoadjuvant chemotherapy, axillary dissection may be considered.

* Fixed nodes in the axilla may be treated with palliative radiotherapy.
* If the nodes are mobile during primary surgery, axillary dissection is to be done.

Q. What is the role of breast conservation in locally advanced breast cancer?

Ans. There are different trials claiming benefit of breast conserving surgery in locally advanced breast cancer. Patient is given neoadjuvant chemotherapy. If there is good response to chemotherapy and patient fills other criteria for breast-conserving surgery then breast-conserving surgery may be considered in locally advanced breast cancer.

Postoperative radiotherapy with a local boost at the tumor bed is to be given. Patient is to be given remaining cycles of chemotherapy.

Tamoxifen therapy in ER positive tumors.

Q. What is the result of treatment of locally advanced breast cancer?

Ans. With multimodal approach of treatment for locally advanced breast carcinoma:
* *Five years survival*: 45%
* *Ten years survival*: 28%.

Q. What is inflammatory carcinoma of breast?

Ans.
* This is an aggressive type of carcinoma breast where there is swelling of the whole breast with redness of the overlying skin and skin edema due to dermal lymphatic invasion
* Most patients with inflammatory breast cancer do not have a defined mass in the breast and usually the whole breast is enlarged
* This lesion is often confused with breast abscess. However, the differentiating features are absence of fever and presence of skin changes like peau d'orange
* The prognosis of this type of carcinoma is uniformly poor.

Q. What should be the plan for treatment of inflammatory carcinoma of breast?

Ans.
* Inflammatory carcinoma of the breast is a locally advanced disease and is clinically inoperable in view of wide area of skin involvement
* Combination chemotherapy using CAF showed dramatic response in patient with inflammatory carcinoma of breast in 60–75% patients. The breast lesion and skin changes as well as axillary lymph node may regress
* Following 2–6 cycles of chemotherapy if there is good response. Simple mastectomy with dissection of axillary node may be done followed by radiotherapy and remaining cycle of chemotherapy
* Postoperative tamoxifen therapy is to be started irrespective of ER/PR status.

When there is progression of disease with chemotherapy second-line chemotherapy with taxanes may be tried. Alternatively palliative radiotherapy may be helpful.

Q. What are the results of treatment in inflammatory carcinoma of breast?

Ans. With multimodal treatment, 5 years survival for inflammatory carcinoma may be 30%.

Q. What is toilet mastectomy?

Ans. In case of locally advanced breast cancer with fungation, palliative mastectomy is done to get rid of the foul smelling fungating mass. This is called toilet mastectomy.

MANAGEMENT OF CARCINOMA OF BREAST WITH DISTANT METASTASIS

Q. What is the incidence of metastatic breast cancer?

Ans. About 7% of newly diagnosed breast cancer patients have distant metastasis at the time of initial diagnosis. About 24–30% of patients with node negative disease and 50–60% of patients with node positive disease will develop distant metastasis at follow-up if they do not die of their disease.

Q. How will you manage a patient with carcinoma of breast with distant metastasis?

Ans. Detailed investigation to confirm the diagnosis and to assess the extent of distant spread:

- Core needle biopsy from breast lump and axillary lymph node. ER/PR/Her2-neu status of the tumor is also assessed
- Chest X-ray (PA view)
- Liver function test
- USG and CT scan of abdomen
- Whole body bone scanning
- Other investigations like CT scan brain/skeletal survey/CT scan of chest depending on the site of distant metastasis
- Base line investigations.

Q. What are the aims of treatment in advanced carcinoma of breast?

Ans.
- To provide palliation
- Symptomatic relief
- Relief of symptom due to growth in the breast which may be fungated.

Q. How will you treat this patient with fungating mass and distant metastasis?

Ans. Most patients with metastatic breast cancer will eventually die with the disease, however, palliative therapy may be provided with:
- Hormone therapy
- Chemotherapy
- Radiation therapy, and
- Limited surgery.

Q. What is the role of hormonal agents in metastatic breast cancer?

Ans. Hormone therapy is effective in women with ER-positive/PR-positive, ER-positive/PR-negative and ER-negative/PR-positive tumors. In 10% cases with ER-negative and PR-negative tumors may show objective response with hormone therapy.

Hormonal therapies for metastatic breast cancer include:

- *Premenopausal women*:
    - First-line therapy: Tamoxifen

– Second-line therapy: If there is response to tamoxifen ovarian ablation with surgery or radiation may be considered. Luteinizing hormone-releasing hormone analogues, like goserelin, brings about reversible chemical castration by suppressing gonadotropin release
– Third-line therapy: Progestins—megestrol acetate
- *In postmenopausal women*:
  – First-line therapy: Anti-estrogens (tamoxifen)
  – Second-line therapy: Aromatase inhibitors—anastrozole or letrozole
  – Third-line therapy: Progestin.

Aromatase is an enzyme which catalyzes synthesis of estrogen. Aromatase inhibitors block this enzyme and inhibit synthesis of estrogen. In postmenopausal women the source of estrogen is extraovarian so aromatase inhibitors like anastrozole or letrozole is effective in postmenopausal women.

Q. What is the role of chemotherapy in metastatic breast cancer?

Ans. Hormone refractory patients and patients with aggressive disease need treatment with combination chemotherapy.
   Regimes of chemotherapy: CMF, CAF or FC for 6–12 cycles.

Q. What newer chemotherapeutic agents are used in breast cancer?

Ans.
- Taxanes include paclitaxel and docetaxel. Used as a single agent in metastatic breast cancer
- Newer vinca alkaloids include vinorelbine
- Newer antifolate.

Q. What should be the initial treatment for metastatic carcinoma of breast?

Ans. A number of factors like:
  – Patient factors
  – Tumor biology
  – R/PR status
  – Disease free interval from initial treatment
  – Sites of distant metastasis
  – Determines the choice of initial treatment.

The initial treatment is systemic chemotherapy. In ER/PR +ve tumor hormone therapy is also considered.

Q. What is the role of high dose chemotherapy in carcinoma of breast?

Ans. There are trials with high dose chemotherapy with cyclophosphamide, cisplatin and carmustine and melphalan along with bone marrow support. A complete response was achieved in 55% with an overall response rate of 73%. The use of hematopoietic growth factor [granulocyte macrophage-colony stimulating factor (GM-CSF)] may allow multiple dose application of chemotherapy to allow enhanced cell kill with autologous marrow rescue. But the benefit of high dose chemotherapy has not been established in subsequent trials.

Q. What is the role of radiotherapy in metastatic breast cancer?

Ans.
- Radiotherapy to the breast and lymph node field in selected cases

- *Bone metastasis*: Local radiotherapy provides dramatic pain relief. The exact mechanism by which radiotherapy provides pain relief is not clear. Pain relief occurs due to tumor shrinkage that relieves periosteal tension and also direct inhibition of humoral factors such as prostaglandin
- Pathological fracture needs surgical stabilization
- *Brain metastasis*: Whole brain irradiation provides some palliation of symptoms. For solitary brain metastasis stereotactic radiotherapy or surgical excision
- *Spinal cord compression*: Early radiotherapy is very effective. For vertebral instability internal fixation is required
- *Liver metastasis*: Despite limitation it has been concluded that radiotherapy may provide effective palliation of symptoms in liver metastasis.

Q. What is the role of surgery in metastatic breast cancer?

Ans.

- *Primary lesion*: Simple or toilet mastectomy
- *Lung metastasis*: Resectable disease confined to one lobe or one lung resection has some role
- *Brain metastasis*: Solitary metastasis may have some benefit with surgery
- *Hepatic metastasis*: Indicated in those whose disease at other sites is controlled with systemic chemotherapy
- *Ovarian ablation:* Second-line of hormone therapy in premenopausal women. LHRH analog may bring about reversible chemical castration.

Q. What is thermography?

Ans.

- Malignant lesions are hypervascular. The transmission of heat may be detected on the surface of breast either by telethermography, contact thermography or computed thermography
- But this is very nonspecific, sensitivity is less than 50%.

Q. What is the role of MRI in breast lesion?

Ans.

- T1–T2-weighted image in coronal, sagittal, and axial cuts may be taken
- Malignant lesion may be seen as irregular mass with spiculated margin
- Secondary skin change, lymphedema, and nipple retraction may be seen
- Enlarged glandular tissue
- Suitable in detecting vertebral body metastasis.

Q. What is ductography?

Ans.

- It is a contrast study for evaluation of patient with nipple discharge
- The duct opening is gently dilated and a fine cannula is passed into the duct. About 0.1–0.2 mL of dilute contrast medium is injected into the duct and craniocaudal and mediolateral views are taken
- Intraductal papilloma may be seen as a filling defect within the duct
- Intraductal carcinoma may appear an irregular filling defect within the duct.

Q. How will you localize a nonpalpable breast lesion?

Ans.
- The lesion may be localized by mammography and a wire hook may be placed on the mass localized by mammography for identification of the site during taking biopsy
- The mass can be excised following the wire hook as the guide
- The X-ray of the specimen will confirm the mammographically detected mass
- The stereotactic placement of needle is another advancement in technique and can localize a nonpalpable mass in 90% of cases
- The specimen radiography will confirm that mammographically detected lesion has been removed and further directs the pathologist to the precise location of the abnormality in the tissue to ensure that appropriate sampling is obtained
- Stereotactic core needle biopsy is another alternative and can give good diagnostic yield and open biopsy is not required in majority.

Q. What precaution should you take when sending specimen for ER/PR study?

Ans.
- Electrocautery should not be used while cutting near the tumor as it may invalidate ER/PR activity
- Specimen should be rapidly frozen (–70°C) because decay in activity is noted within 20–30 minutes after extirpation of the neoplasm.

Q. What are the different ER status of breast carcinomas?

Ans.
- *ER positive*: Value of more than 10 femtomoles/ng (fmol/ng)
- *Borderline*: 5–9 fmol/ng
- *Negative*: 3–4 fmol/ng.

Q. What are the differences in pre- and postmenopausal women with regard to ER/PR expression?

Ans. Premenopausal women have lower incidence ER/PR positivity (about 30%) as compared to postmenopausal women who show about 60% ER/PR positivity.

Q. What are the prognostic factors in carcinoma of breast?

Ans.
- Tumor size is one very important prognostic marker
- Lymph node status is the second most important prognostic marker. Survival depends on node positivity and also on the number of lymph nodes involved
- *Estrogen and progesterone receptor status*:
  - ER positive PR positive: Good prognosis
  - ER negative PR negative: Bad prognosis
  - ER positive PR negative/ER negative/PR positive: Borderline
- *Histological grade of tumor (Table 5.1)*:
  - Well-differentiated tumor: Good prognosis
  - Poorly-differentiated tumor: Poor prognosis

- *Proliferating rate*:
  - DNA flow cytometry: Aneuploid—poor prognosis
  - S-phase fraction: Low S-phase—good prognosis
- *Oncogene product measurements*:
  - c-erbB (epidermal growth factor)
  - c-erbB2 (neu/Her2)
  - c-HRAS
- *Growth factors*:
  - Epidermal growth factor
  - Transforming growth factor-alpha
  - Transforming growth factor-beta
  - Placental growth factor
- *Chromosomal defect*:
  - Loss of allele length on chromosome 11: Poor prognosis.

Table 5.1: Histologic grade of tumor	
Histologic grade (G)	
GX	Grade cannot be assessed
G1	Low combined histologic grade (favorable)
G2	Intermediate combined histologic grade (moderately favorable)
G3	High combined histologic grade (unfavorable)

Q. What is Nottingham prognostic index?

Ans. Nottingham prognostic index (PI) is calculated as follows:
- Nottingham PI = (0.2 × tumor size in cm) + N (0 = 1, 1–3 = 2, >3 = 3) + G (1, 2, 3)
- Nottingham PI—<5.4. Good prognosis.
- Nottingham PI—>5.4. Bad prognosis. Overall survival less than 50% at 5 years.

Q. What is Bloom–Richardson grading system?

Ans. Bloom–Richardson grading system takes into account following factors:
- *Tubule formation*:
  - >75%—1
  - 10–75%—2
  - <10%—3
- *Nuclear pleomorphism*:
  - Regular uniform—1
  - Moderate pleomorphism—2
  - Marked pleomorphism—3.
- *Mitotic count*:
  - <10/10/hpf—1
  - 10–20/hpf—2
  - >20/hpf—3
- Well-differentiated (low grade): 3–5
- Moderately differentiated (intermediate grade): 6–7
- Poorly differentiated (high grade): 8–9.

Q. What is TNM staging for breast carcinoma?

Ans. TNM staging and classification for breast carcinoma have been described in Tables 5.2 and 5.3.

Table 5.2: TNM staging

Primary Tumor (T)

TX	Primary tumor cannot be assessed
T0	No evidence of primary tumor
Tis	Carcinoma in situ
Tis (DCIS)	Ductal carcinoma in situ
Tis (LCIS)	Lobular carcinoma in situ
Tis (Paget)	Paget disease (Fig. 5.15) of the nipple not associated with invasive carcinoma and/or carcinoma in situ (DCIS and/or LCIS) in the underlying breast parenchyma. Carcinomas in the breast parenchyma associated with Paget disease are categorized based on the size and characteristics of the parenchymal disease, although the presence of Paget disease should still be noted
T1	Tumor ≤ 20 mm in greatest dimension
T1mi	Tumor ≤ 1 mm in greatest dimension
T1a	Tumor > 1 mm but ≤ 5 mm in greatest dimension
T1b	Tumor > 5 mm but ≤ 10 mm in greatest dimension
T1c	Tumor > 10 mm but ≤ 20 mm in greatest dimension
T2	Tumor > 20 mm but ≤ 50 mm in greatest dimension
T3	Tumor > 50 mm in greatest dimension
T4	Tumor of any size with direct extension to the chest wall and/or to the skin (ulceration or skin nodules)
T4a	Extension to chest wall, not including only pectoralis muscle adherence/invasion
T4b	Ulceration and/or ipsilateral satellite nodules and/or edema (including peau d'orange) of the skin, which do not meet the criteria for inflammatory carcinoma
T4c	Both T4a and T4b
T4d	Inflammatory carcinoma

Regional Lymph Nodes (N)
Clinical

NX	Regional lymph nodes cannot be assessed (e.g. previously removed)
N0	No regional lymph node metastasis
N1	Metastasis to movable ipsilateral level I, II axillary lymph node(s)
N2	Metastases in ipsilateral level I, II axillary lymph nodes that are clinically fixed or matted or in clinically detected ipsilateral internal mammary nodes in the absence of clinically evident axillary lymph node metastasis
N2a	Metastases in ipsilateral level I, II axillary lymph nodes fixed to one another (matted) or to other structures
N2b	Metastases only in clinically detected ipsilateral internal mammary nodes and in the absence of clinically evident level I, II axillary lymph node metastases

Contd..

Contd..

N3	Metastases in ipsilateral infraclavicular (level III axillary) lymph node(s), with or without level I, II axillary node involvement, or in clinically detected ipsilateral internal mammary lymph node(s) and in the presence of clinically evident level I, II axillary lymph node metastasis; or metastasis in ipsilateral supraclavicular lymph node(s), with or without axillary or internal mammary lymph node involvement
N3a	Metastasis in ipsilateral infraclavicular lymph node(s)
N3b	Metastasis in ipsilateral internal mammary lymph node(s) and axillary lymph node(s)
N3c	Metastasis in ipsilateral supraclavicular lymph node(s)

Pathologic (pN)

pNX	Regional lymph nodes cannot be assessed (for example, previously removed, or not removed for pathologic study)
pN0	No regional lymph node metastasis identified histologically. Note: Isolated tumor cell clusters (ITCs) are defined as small clusters of cells ≤ 0.2 mm, or single tumor cells, or a cluster of < 200 cells in a single histologic cross-section; ITCs may be detected by routine histology or by immunohistochemical (IHC) methods; nodes containing only ITCs are excluded from the total positive node count for purposes of N classification but should be included in the total number of nodes evaluated
pN0(i−)	No regional lymph node metastases histologically, negative IHC
pN0(i+)	Malignant cells in regional lymph node(s) ≤0.2 mm [detected by hematoxylin-eosin (H-E) stain or IHC, including ITC]
pN0(mol−)	No regional lymph node metastases histologically, negative molecular findings [reverse transcriptase polymerase chain reaction (RT-PCR)]
pN0(mol+)	Positive molecular findings (RT-PCR) but no regional lymph node metastases detected by histology or IHC
pN1	Micrometastases; or metastases in 1–3 axillary lymph nodes and/or in internal mammary nodes, with metastases detected by sentinel lymph node biopsy but not clinically detected†
pN1mi	Micrometastases (> 0.2 mm and/or > 200 cells, but none >2.0 mm)
pN1a	Metastases in 1–3 axillary lymph nodes (at least 1 metastasis > 2.0 mm)
pN1b	Metastases in internal mammary nodes, with micrometastases or macrometastases detected by sentinel lymph node biopsy but not clinically detected†
pN1c	Metastases in 1–3 axillary lymph nodes and in internal mammary lymph nodes, with micrometastases or macrometastases detected by sentinel lymph node biopsy but not clinically detected†
pN2	Metastases in 4–9 axillary lymph nodes or in clinically detected‡ internal mammary lymph nodes in the absence of axillary lymph node metastases
pN2a	Metastases in 4–9 axillary lymph nodes (at least 1 tumor deposit > 2.0 mm)
pN2b	Metastases in clinically detected‡ internal mammary lymph nodes in the absence of axillary lymph node metastases

Contd..

Contd..

pN3	Metastases in ≥10 axillary lymph nodes; or in infraclavicular (level III axillary) lymph nodes; or in clinically detected‡ ipsilateral internal mammary lymph nodes in the presence of ≥ 1 positive level I, II axillary lymph nodes; or in > 3 axillary lymph nodes and in internal mammary lymph nodes, with micrometastases or macrometastases detected by sentinel lymph node biopsy but not clinically detected†; or in ipsilateral supraclavicular lymph nodes
pN3a	Metastases in ≥10 axillary lymph nodes (at least 1 tumor deposit > 2.0 mm); or metastases to the infraclavicular (level III axillary lymph) nodes
pN3b	Metastases in clinically detected‡ ipsilateral internal mammary lymph nodes in the presence of ≥ 1 positive axillary lymph nodes; or in > 3 axillary lymph nodes and in internal mammary lymph nodes, with micrometastases or macrometastases detected by sentinel lymph node biopsy but not clinically detected†
pN3c	Metastases in ipsilateral supraclavicular lymph nodes

Distant metastasis (M)

M0	No clinical or radiographic evidence of distant metastasis
cM0(i+)	No clinical or radiographic evidence of distant metastases, but deposits of molecularly or microscopically detected tumor cells in circulating blood, bone marrow, or other nonregional nodal tissue that are no larger than 0.2 mm in a patient without symptoms or signs of metastases
M1	Distant detectable metastases as determined by classic clinical and radiographic means and/or histologically proven > 0.2 mm

Table 5.3: Anatomic stage/prognostic groups

Stage	T	N	M
0	Tis	N0	M0
IA	T1	N0	M0
IB	T0	N1mi	M0
	T1	N1mi	M0
IIA	T0	N1	M0
	T1	N1	M0
	T2	N0	M0
IIB	T2	N1	M0
	T3	N0	M0
IIIA	T0	N2	M0
	T1	N2	M0
	T2	N2	M0
	T3	N1	M0
	T3	N2	M0
IIIB	T4	N0	M0
	T4	N1	M0
	T4	N2	M0
IIIC	Any T	N3	M0
IV	Any T	Any N	M1

Q. What are molecular subtypes of breast cancer?

Ans.

* *Luminal A*: ER/PR +ve, Her2 neu –ve, Ki 67 (proliferating index)—low.
* *Luminal B*: ER/PR +ve, Her2 neu +ve, Ki 67 (proliferating index)—high.
* ER/PR +ve, Her2 neu +ve
* Triple negative-ER/PR –ve, Her2 neu –ve
* Claudin-low-variant of triple –ve with low E-cadherin
* Molecular apocrine-ER –ve Luminal A, some apocrine marker +ve.

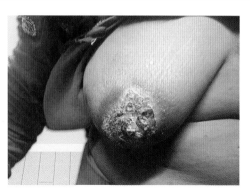

Fig. 5.15: Paget disease of nipple

Q. What is medical adrenalectomy?

Ans. After menopause adrenal gland is the major source of endogenous estrogen.

Aminoglutethimide (mitotane) blocks the enzymatic conversion of cholesterol to gamma 5 prednisolone and inhibits the conversion of androstenedione to estrogen in peripheral tissues.

After treatment with aminoglutethimide adrenal is suppressed with reduction of cortisone production which causes feedback increase of adrenocorticotropic hormone (ACTH). Increased ACTH may override aminoglutethimide block. Administration of cortisone prevents feedback rise of ACTH.

Adrenalectomy was done earlier in patient of carcinoma of breast in postmenopausal women who responded to estrogen therapy.

Q. What is the incidence of carcinoma of breast?

Ans.

* Accounts for 32% of all female cancer
* Accounts for 19% of all cancer related deaths in women.

Q. What do you mean by sporadic breast cancer?

Ans.

* A breast cancer patient with no family history of breast cancer in two generation
* Incidence is 68%.

Q. What do you mean by familial breast cancer?

Ans.

* A breast cancer patient with a positive family history of breast cancer or related malignancy in first or second-degree relatives
* No definite mode of inheritance
* Incidence is 23%.

Q. What is hereditary breast cancer?

Ans.

* A breast cancer patient with positive family history of breast cancer

- Related cancer like ovarian or colonic cancer in family
- Highly penetrating autosomal dominant mode of inheritance
- Increased incidence of bilateral cancer
- Increased incidence of multiple primary tumor
- Incidence is 8%.

Q. What is the role of genetic testing in breast cancer?

Ans.
- Inherited mutation in two breast, cancer gene *BRCA1* and *BRCA2* accounts for 4% of all breast cancer and 80% of familial and hereditary breast cancer
- *BRCA1* located in 17q chromosome linked to hereditary breast cancer and ovarian malignancy
- *BRCA2* located in 13q chromosome linked to most case of hereditary male breast cancer
- *BRCA1* and *BRCA2* are two important breast cancer susceptibility gene
- A part from *BRCA1*, *BRCA2* genome mutation, P53 suppressor gene, and a *BRCA3* gene has been implicated in breast cancer.
  However, a person with *BRCA1*, *BRCA2* gene negative cannot be assured 100%, as the person might be carrying some other as yet undiscovered genetic anomalies.

Q. Is estrogen all important for breast cancer development?

Ans.
- Estrogen has been incriminated for increased incidence of breast cancer
- Early menarche, late menopause and late first pregnancy all suggest increased estrogenic activity
- But there are some reverse observations also. In days before tamoxifen therapy, many subjective responses have been observed paradoxically in postmenopausal women with administration of estrogen
- If high estrogen would have been detrimental then pregnant patient should have a worse outcome which is not usual
- In premenopausal women treated with tamoxifen results in high level of circulating estrogen as it interferes with negative feedback mechanism
- So, the estrogen level alone does not decide about the course of disease.

Q. Is there any effect of timing of surgery with menstrual cycle?

Ans.
- It has been suggested that outcome of surgery is better if surgery is done during the luteal phase of menstruation rather than during the estrogenic phase.
- Estrogenic activity helps in angiogenesis and helps microscopic deposit to go on for an uncontrolled proliferation.

Q. Is dietary factor important for development of carcinoma of breast?

Ans. Diet high in fat and fried food has increased incidence of breast cancer. However, diet rich in omega-3 fatty acid has some protective effect.

Q. What is the relation between oral pill and breast cancer?

Ans. There is no increased risk of breast cancer in women taking oral pill in the age group between 25 years and 39 years. The slight increase in relative risk (RR 1.2) far outweighs the advantage of use of oral pills.

Q. What is the relationship of hormone replacement therapy (HRT) and breast cancer?

Ans. There is slight increase in relative risk of breast cancer in patient taking HRT particularly in patient with benign breast disease. But for potential effect of HRT with regard to osteoporosis and ischemic heart disease HRT therapy should not be denied when indicated.

Q. What is the relation of obesity and breast cancer?

Ans. Postmenopausal obese women have increased risk of breast cancer, 1.5–2 times higher than nonobese women.

Q. Does breastfeeding provide protection for breast cancer?

Ans. Earlier it was said that prolonged breastfeeding for more than 36 months reduces the incidence of breast cancer. Subsequent studies does not corroborate lower incidence of breast carcinoma in women who have breast fed their child for a long time.

Q. What is the relationship of menstruation and breast cancer?

Ans.
- Early menarche and late menopause has been found to be associated with increased incidence of breast cancer
- Artificial menopausal by surgery at an early age provides immunity against breast cancer.

Q. What is the relationship between parity and breast cancer?

Ans. Infertility and nulliparity is associated with higher incidence of breast cancer as compared to parous women. Full-term pregnancy before 18 years of age reduces the chance of developing breast cancer as compared to first pregnancy after 35 years of age.

Q. What is the risk of opposite breast cancer?

Ans. Women with breast cancer on one side has 3–4 times higher risk for development of opposite breast cancer particularly in patient with positive family history.

Q. What is the effect of ionizing radiation in breast cancer?

Ans.
- Atomic bomb survivor of Hiroshima and Nagasaki has increased incidence of breast cancer
- Repeated X-ray exposures for diagnostic chest X-ray increase the incidence of carcinoma of breast to some extent
- Radiotherapy for carcinoma in one breast poses increased risk of breast cancer in opposite breast.

Q. What are the different risk factors for developing breast cancer?

Ans.
- Old age
- High socioeconomic status
- Early menarche and delayed menopause
- Obese nulliparous patients
- Late first pregnancy
- First-degree relatives with history of breast cancer
- History of radiation to neck.

Q. What is the most important prognostic factor in breast cancer?

Ans. Apart from tumor size and histological grading, lymph nodes status is one of the most important prognostic markers of cancer breast.

*   *Node negative patient 5 years survival*: 75–80% and relapse rate—20–25%
*   *Node positive patient 5 years survival*: 45–50% and relapse rate—50–75%
*   *1–3 positive node 5 years survival*: 60%
*   *More than 4 node positive 5 years survival*: 30%.

Q. What is the implication of lymph node involvement at different levels?

Ans. Level III or apical lymph node involvement indicates worse prognosis.

Q. How many nodes should be removed for a sampling?

Ans. At least 10 lymph nodes have to be removed from level I and level II axillary nodes for proper sampling.

Q. What are the staging investigations for carcinoma of breast?

Ans.

*   History and clinical examination
*   Bilateral mammography
*   Hb% TLC, DLC, ESR
*   Liver function test
*   Chest X-ray
*   USG/CT scan of abdomen
*   Whole body bone scanning
*   CT scan of brain/CT scan of chest, if there is suggestive of brain or chest metastasis.

Q. When will you consider whole body bone scanning?

Ans.

*   Advanced local disease T3, T4 tumor
*   Lymph node metastasis
*   Clinical evidence of distant metastasis
*   Osseous symptom, bone pain
*   Palpable bony lesion.

Q. What are the causes of finding of hot spot in bone scanning?

Ans.

*   Metastatic deposit
*   Osteoarthritis
*   *Inflammatory lesion*: Osteomyelitis
*   Inflammatory lesion in soft tissue overlying the bone
*   Paget's disease of bone
*   Healing fracture.

Q. What are the causes of death following treatment of breast cancer patient?

Ans. Metastatic disease is the main cause of death for 5–10 years following mastectomy.

Q. How does peau d'orange develop?

Ans. With growth of tumor, the tumor cells involve and block the subdermal lymphatic and this causes cutaneous lymphatic edema. The skin areas tethered to sweat ducts cannot swell remains dimpled in between the areas of cutaneous lymphatic edema giving an appearance of orange skin.

Peau d'orange appearance may also develop over a chronic breast abscess.

Q. What are the causes of lymphedema of arm in breast carcinoma?

Ans.
* Formal dissection of axilla from level I to III may cause edema of the arm
* Treatment combining both surgery and radiotherapy for axillary lymph node leads to increased incidence of lymphedema
* Local recurrence of the disease causing metastatic infiltration of both lymphatic and venous flow.

Q. How will you treat lymphedema of arm?

Ans.
* Limb elevation
* Elastic arm stockinette
* Pneumatic compression device.

Q. How tumor does ulcerate?

Ans. As the tumor grows, the subdermal emboli of neoplastic cells fill the endolymphatic spaces and ultimately involve the corium of the skin. The tumor cell in the corium of skin continues to grow and result in skin ulceration.

As new areas of skin are invaded small satellite nodules appear near the ulcer crater.

Q. What are the common sites of distant metastasis from carcinoma of breast?

Ans.
* *Bones*: 50–65%
* *Lung*: 15–20%
* *Pleura*: 10–15%
* *Soft tissue*: 7–15%
* *Liver*: 5–15%
* Brain/adrenals.

Q. What are the patterns of recurrence in carcinoma of breast?

Ans.
* Local recurrence: 10–35%
* Distant metastasis: 60–75%
* Both local and distant: 10–30%.

Q. What is the role of axillary surgery in a case of carcinoma of breast?

Ans.
* Axillary lymph node status is one of the most important prognostic marker of carcinoma of breast (Flowchart 5.1)

Flowchart 5.1: An algorithm to manage axillary lymph node in carcinoma of breast

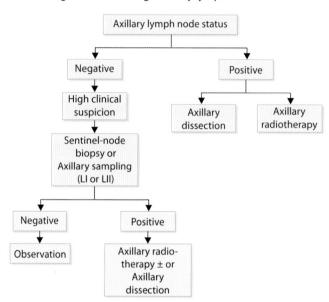

- In node negative axilla on clinical ground sentinel node biopsy is done.
  - If sentinel node is histologically negative, axillary dissection is not required. The axillary irradiation may or may not be given
  - If sentinel lymph node is positive either axillary dissection or radiotherapy is considered. The results of surgery and radiotherapy to the axilla are comparable
- In node negative axilla on clinical ground, axillary sampling may be done from level I and level II. At least 10 lymph nodes need to be removed for proper axillary sampling. If axillary nodes are histologically negative no treatment is required for axilla. If axillary nodes are positive axilla is treated either with formal axillary dissection or axillary radiotherapy
- In node negative axilla on clinical ground, formal axillary dissection from level I–III may be done
- In node positive axilla on clinical ground, either axillary dissection or radiotherapy is done.

Q. What is the justification for modified radical mastectomy in early carcinoma of breast?

Ans. The modern trend is toward breast conservation. But still there are indications for doing. Modified radical mastectomy in early carcinoma of breast:
- Patients desire for mastectomy as there is slight increased incidence of local recurrence with breast conserving surgery. Needs repeated follow-up and radiotherapy
- In patient with DCIS adjacent to the index lesion
- For lesion in central quadrant of breast
- Two or more primary lesion in breast as there is high chance of local recurrence
- Histology showed poorly differentiated tumor.

Q. Why breast carcinoma is considered as systemic disease?

Ans. Halstead concept regarding spread of carcinoma of breast is sequential spread from breast to the lymph node and then systemic spread.

Fischer concept is that there is preclinical spread of the disease to a distant site. So it is a systemic disease from the beginning.

Tumors less than 1 cm:
- Generally are not aggressive
- Usually well differentiated and low grade
- Rarely show axillary lymph node metastasis (4–15%)
- Curable in 90% with locoregional therapy and no systemic therapy is required
- Tumor more than 3 cm is often disseminated and difficult to control.

Q. What is the significance of multicentric cancer and local recurrence?

Ans.
- A striking feature of local recurrence is that it occurs in same region as primary tumor
- Different studies showed that multicentric foci are not always the site of local recurrence.

Q. What is transfection?

Ans. In breast cancer all metastases are not due to cellular dissemination.

Transfection is a phenomena whereby nuclear material from the primary malignant lesion infects the wandering cells of monocyte-macrophage system and are transported to distant site where local mesenchymal cells are transfected with genetic misinformation that activate the components of the genome to instruct these plastic cells also to express the phenotypic picture of dedifferentiated breast epithelial cell.

Q. When will you consider for breast reconstruction?

Ans.
- Patient undergoing mastectomy may be offered breast reconstruction. Breast reconstruction may be done immediately in same sitting as mastectomy or it may be delayed till radiation therapy or chemotherapy is completed (delayed reconstruction)
- Immediate breast reconstruction may be considered in patient undergoing mastectomy for DCIS, lobular carcinoma in situ (LCIS) or high-risk individual undergoing prophylactic mastectomy.

Q. How breast reconstruction is done?

Ans. Use of autologous tissue:
- By latissimus dorsi myocutaneous flap (LDMF)
- By transverse rectus abdominis myocutaneous (TRAM) flap
- Silicone gel implant under the pectoralis major muscle
- Nipple reconstruction may be done later or a prosthetic nipple may be fitted.

Q. What is the role of screening in breast cancer management?

Ans.
- There have been controversies regarding routine screening for breast cancers. A number of studies have shown that breast screening by mammography in women over 50 years reduce the cause specific mortality by 30%

- The advantage of screening program is early detection of the disease and improved survival in view of early treatment and reassurance if no disease is found
- The disadvantage is high cost involved, false reassurance if negative on screening as these patients may still develop carcinoma on later period. Not all patients DCIS or LCIS will develop invasive carcinoma. Women with stigmata of DCIS or LCIS carry stigmata of breast cancer for the rest of their life which may interfere with their social life
- In view of resource and cost involved routine screening is not advisable.

Q. Can you treat breast cancer patient without surgery?

Ans.

- This has been tried in early carcinoma of breast
- Three cycles of neoadjuvant chemotherapy is given. In 5% cases there may be complete response with disappearance of primary tumor and total sterilization of cancer cells. When combined with radiotherapy it may boost the nonsurgical treatment
- Longer treatment with chemotherapy and vigorous dose of radiotherapy may totally destroy a small carcinoma without the need for surgery
- Future development of brachytherapy and low toxicity chemotherapy in combination are all elements which might bring a new mode of minimal or no surgery for carcinoma of breast.

Q. How does carcinoma of breast behave in pregnancy?

Ans.

- Earlier, it was believed that carcinoma of breast has worse prognosis once it is associated with pregnancy
- More recent data indicate that carcinoma of breast in pregnancy is associated with a prognosis similar to the nonpregnant female
- But proportionally more patients are diagnosed in stage II or stage III during pregnancy than in nonpregnant women. The cause of this late diagnosis is uncertain, may be due to hormonal stimulation of pregnancy or diagnosis may be delayed because symptoms are masked by pregnancy.

Q. How will you diagnose carcinoma of breast during pregnancy?

Ans.

- History and physical examination
- Mammographic examination are less reliable because of extensive parenchymal change associated with gestation
- Core needle biopsy
- If inconclusive, an incisional biopsy.

Q. How will you plan treatment of carcinoma of breast in pregnant patients?

Ans.

- *Stage I or Stage II*: Modified radical mastectomy is the optimal treatment:
  - If node is positive adjuvant chemotherapy is delayed till second trimester of pregnancy as the chances of teratogenic effect due to chemotherapy is not usual in second or third trimester of pregnancy

* *Breast conservation surgery during pregnancy:*
  - In early carcinoma of breast, breast conserving surgery is only indicated when diagnosed in third trimester of pregnancy. Segmental mastectomy followed by radiation therapy 4–6 week later when pregnancy is over
  - In early pregnancy as radiotherapy could not be given, breast conserving surgery is not advisable.

Q. How will you treat advanced breast cancer during pregnancy?

Ans.
Operable advanced lesion:
* Simple mastectomy and level I axillary dissection
* Adjuvant chemotherapy in second and third trimester of pregnancy
* Radiotherapy to locoregional field at the end of pregnancy
* Hormonal therapy is not very effective during pregnancy as most tumors are ER/PR negative
* In first trimester both radiotherapy and chemotherapy are teratogenic.

Q. While in course of treatment of carcinoma breast, if patient becomes pregnant, what should be done?

Ans. During postoperative radiotherapy or chemotherapy for advanced primary disease, therapeutic abortion should be considered as both radiotherapy and chemotherapy are teratogenic in first trimester.

Q. Can women be advised pregnancy following treatment of breast cancer?

Ans. Previous history of breast cancer is not a contraindication for pregnancy. Proper counseling is required. Husband should bring up the child if the initial disease has a poor prognosis. It is advisable to wait for at least 2 years as it is within this period that most recurrence occurs.

Q. Why routine axillary lymph node dissection is not indicated in all cases of carcinoma of breast?

Ans.
* The results of different studies show that chance of lymph node positivity in axillary dissection depends on tumor size
* Tla—7%
* Tlb—19%
* Tlc—32%
* T2—51%
* In routine axillary lymph node dissection (ALND) up to 50% patients develop complication due to the operation such as postoperative pain, seroma formation, limitation of shoulder movements, lymphedema and increased hospital stay
* So routine ALND dissection has been questioned.

Thyroid

WRITING A LONG CASE OF THYROID DISEASE

▮ HISTORY

1. **Particulars of Patient**
2. **Chief Complaint(s)**
   In different thyroid diseases chief complaints may be:
   – Swelling in front and sides of the neck for...................
   – Pain over the swelling for...................
   – Hoarseness of voice for...................
   – Difficulty in swallowing for...................
   – Difficulty in breathing for...................
   – Bulging of eyes, trembling of limbs for...................

3. **History of Present Illness**
   – *Details about the swelling*:
     - Duration
     - Onset: Sudden or insidious
     - Site where first noticed: Front or on the side of the neck
     - Progress of the swelling:
       » Gradually increasing in size (benign swelling)
       » Rapidly increasing in size (malignant swelling)
       » Initially gradually increasing later rapidly increasing (benign turning malignant)
   – *Pain*:
     - Duration
     - Site
     - Character: Usually dull-aching
     - Any radiation
     - Relieving and aggravating factors
   – *Enquire about pressure symptoms with duration*:
     - Difficulty in swallowing: Solid or liquid
     - Difficulty in breathing
     - Alteration of voice, commonly hoarseness

- *Enquire about any symptom of hyperthyroidism or hypothyroidism*:
  - Appetite
  - Weight loss/weight gain
  - Bowel habits: Particularly enquire about diarrhea
  - Chest pain and its relation with exercise
  - Palpitation
- Any history of dropped beat (if patient can mention in history then only it is to be recorded)
- Breathlessness on exertion
- Any trembling of limbs
- Irritability on slight provocation
- Insomnia
- Weakness of limbs
- *Bulging of eyes*:
  - Duration and progress
  - History of redness of eye and watering
  - History of double vision
  - Loss of vision
- Increased sweating
- Heat intolerance
- Intolerance to heat or cold.

In a patient with thyrotoxicosis, some of these toxic symptoms may be present. If treated with antithyroid drugs, there may be some improvement. This should be included in history of present illness.

Enquire about symptoms suggestive of hypothyroidism: Weakness/lethargy/swelling of face, whole body or legs/intolerance to cold/menstrual problems/constipation.

4. **Past History**

   Any history of radiation exposure in the head, neck, and chest. Papillary carcinoma or mixed papillary and follicular carcinoma is common in post radiated patient. Most of these cancers are occult (<1.5 cm), more than 50% may have multifocal disease and about 20% has lymph node metastasis at diagnosis.

5. **Personal History/Menstrual History/Obstetrical History**

6. **Family History**

   Any history of thyroid disease in the family members or the neighborhood. Any history of thyroid cancer in family. Papillary carcinoma has been reported in family. Medullary carcinoma is familial in 20% cases usually as the component of multiple endocrine neoplasia (MEN 2).

   Additional features of MEN 2 may be pheochromocytoma in 50% cases and primary hyperparathyroidism in 15% cases.

7. **Treatment History**
   - *Enquire about any drug treatment*:
     - Eltroxin
     - Antithyroid drugs
     - Beta blockers.

8. **Any History of Allergy**

■ PHYSICAL EXAMINATION

1. **General Survey**
   - *Facies*: Thyrotoxic facies, myxedema facies
   - *Neck gland*: Thyroid gland is enlarged. Described under local examination
   - Pulse rate/minute rhythm regular, described in details in examination for toxic sign.
2. **Local Examination:** Examination of the Thyroid Region.

Inspection (Fig. 6.1)

Position and extent of the swelling: Swelling situated in the front and sides of the neck in the thyroid region extending laterally up to the sternomastoid, below up to the suprasternal notch and above up to the thyroid cartilage.

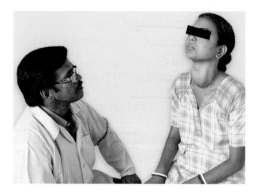

If both lobes of the thyroid gland are enlarged, describe the extent of each lobe upward, downward and laterally. Both lobes of the thyroid gland are enlarged and extend above up to the thyroid cartilage, below up to the sternoclavicular joint and laterally up to the posterior border of sternocleidomastoid.

Fig. 6.1: Inspection of thyroid region

- *Describe the extent of the isthmus in the midline*: Upper and lower extent. The isthmus of the thyroid gland is also enlarged and extends below up to the suprasternal notch and extends 3 cm above the suprasternal notch.
- *Shape*: If thyroid gland is enlarged as a whole, it may be described as a butterfly-shaped swelling. Otherwise describe the shape as it is seen.
- *Size*: If both lobes and isthmus are enlarged.

Describe vertical and horizontal dimension of each lobe and vertical and transverse dimension of the isthmus separately.
- *Surface*: Smooth/irregular/nodular.
- Margins
- *Skin over the swelling*: Scar/pigmentation/venous prominence.
- Any pulsation
- Movement of the swelling with deglutition
- In case of solitary thyroid swelling look for upward movement of the swelling on protrusion of the tongue to differentiate a thyroid nodule from thyroglossal cyst.
- If there is diffuse enlargement of the thyroid gland, movement of the swelling on protrusion of the tongue need not be tested as differential diagnosis with thyroglossal cyst is not required.
- Comment whether lower border can be seen as such or on swallowing.
- Any venous prominence over neck or chest wall.

Palpation

- Temperature over the swelling
- Tenderness

- Movement of the swelling with deglutition. Movement of the swelling on protrusion of the tongue, if it is a solitary swelling in the thyroid gland
- Position and extent of the swelling
- Shape
- Size
- Measurement of circumference of the neck at most prominent part of the swelling (measure with a tape in centimeters)
- Surface, margin
- *Consistency*: Hard, firm, soft cystic, and variegated
- Any pulsation
- Any thrill
- Any skin fixity
- *Mobility*: Mobility from side to side and up and down
- Relation of the swelling with sternocleidomastoid muscle
- *Note the positions of trachea and larynx*:
  - Any shifting to either side by the swelling
- *Test for tracheal compression*: Kocher's test—
  - The swelling is pressed slightly on either side of trachea. If trachea is already compressed, or if there is tracheomalacia, patient will have stridor
  - Kocher's test negative (no stridor)
  - Kocher's test positive (stridor on compression of both lobes)
- *Palpate the carotid pulsation*:
  - Carotid pulsation may be felt at normal site (at the anterior border of sternocleidomastoid at the level of the upper border of thyroid cartilage)
  - Carotid pulse is not palpable on the side of the swelling (Berry's sign positive)
  - Carotid pulse is palpable but is displaced laterally
- In a locally advanced thyroid carcinoma sympathetic trunk may be involved. Look for signs of sympathetic trunk palsy (Horner's syndrome):
  - Enophthalmos
  - Pseudoptosis (slight drooping of upper eyelid)
  - Anhidrosis (loss of sweating)
  - Miosis
  - Loss of ciliospinal reflex.

Percussion: Percussion over the manubrium sterni

Superior mediastinum is normally resonant. If there is retrosternal prolongation of goiter, the area may be dull.

Auscultation

- Any bruit audible or not
- In thyrotoxicosis, the bruit is audible near the upper pole of the thyroid lobes.

Examination of Cervical Lymph Nodes

- *Examination of all the cervical lymph node groups*: If lymph nodes are palpable then describe, which groups of lymph nodes are palpable.

- Number, site, surface, margin, consistency, and mobility.
- Write details about lymph node enlargement.

Examination for Toxic Signs

If toxic signs are present write in details:

- Pulse rate, rhythm, volume, any special character—collapsing or not
- Tremor in hands and tongue
- Thrill and bruit over the thyroid gland usually present at upper pole
- *Eye signs*:
  - *Exophthalmos*: Forward bulging of the eyeball.
  - *Dalrymple's sign*: Visibility of upper sclera due to spasm of upper eyelid. If present, the sign is positive.
  - *Von Graefe's sign*: If lid lag is present, the sign is positive.
  - *Joffroy's sign*: Loss of wrinkling of forehead on looking up—the sign is positive.
  - *Möbius sign*: If there is failure of convergence on accommodation at a near object from a distant object—the sign is said to be positive.
  - *Stellwag's sign*: Infrequent blinking—a stare look. If present, the sign is positive.

In advanced case:

- Chemosis
- Test for eye movement and comment about any palsy
- Look for diplopia. In thyrotoxicosis, diplopia may occur due to paralysis of inferior oblique and superior rectus muscle.

Examination for Retrosternal Prolongation

- Lower margin of swelling. Whether visible or not, as such or on deglutition.
- Any dilated vein over the neck and chest wall.
- *Pemberton's sign*: Ask the patient to raise both upper limbs above the head and keep it for 2-3 minutes. If retrosternal prolongation is there, patient will have congestion and puffiness in the face with respiratory distress. The Pemberton's sign is then positive.
- Percussion over the manubrium sterni—normally resonant. Dull note suggest retrosternal prolongation of goiter.

3. **Systemic Examination**

   Describe all systems.

■ SUMMARY OF THE CASE

■ PROVISIONAL DIAGNOSIS

- Primary thyrotoxicosis
- Nontoxic solitary nodular goiter
- Nontoxic multinodular goiter
- Carcinoma of thyroid.

■ INVESTIGATIONS SUGGESTED

♦ Investigation to confirm the diagnosis
♦ Investigations to stage the disease in case of carcinoma thyroid
♦ Baseline investigations.

■ DIFFERENTIAL DIAGNOSIS

Q. How will you palpate the thyroid gland? Say one method of palpation.

Ans. I will palpate the thyroid gland by Lahey's method.

Stand in front of the patient. To palpate the left lobe, push the right lobe to the left with the left hand so that the left lobe becomes prominent. The left lobe is then palpated with the right hand. The anterolateral surface and the posterior surface of the left lobe are then palpated (Fig. 6.2). Similarly, the right lobe is palpated by pushing the left lobe toward the right thereby making the right lobe prominent.

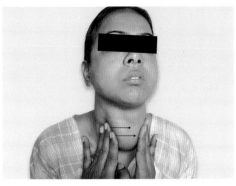

Fig. 6.2: Palpation of the thyroid gland—left lobe is palpated by the palmar aspect of the right fingers by pressing the right lobe with the other hand

Q. How will you palpate the posterior surface of the thyroid lobes?

Ans. This can be palpated either from the front or back. For palpating the posterior surface of the right lobe, the left lobe is pushed toward the right and the posterior surface is palpated by insinuating the fingers between the anterior border of sternocleidomastoid and the posterior surface of the thyroid lobe. Alternatively, the posterior surface may be palpated by fingers placed at the posterior border of the sternocleidomastoid (Fig. 6.3).

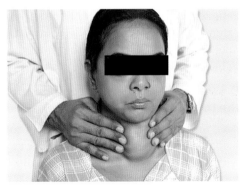

Fig. 6.3: Palpation of the posterior surface

Q. How will you palpate the isthmus of thyroid gland?

Ans.
♦ The isthmus is palpated in the midline against the trachea (Fig. 6.4).
♦ The normal thyroid gland is not palpable.

Q. What are other methods for palpation of the thyroid gland?

Ans. The gland may be palpated from the back with the neck flexed and turned to the side of palpation slightly. One lobe is pushed to the opposite side; the other lobe becomes prominent and palpated from the back (Fig. 6.5).

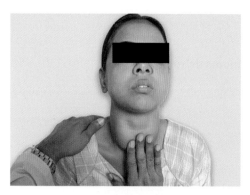

Fig. 6.4: Palpation of the isthmus of the thyroid gland

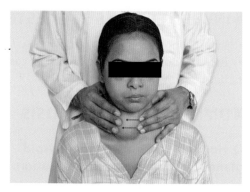

Fig. 6.5: Palpation of thyroid gland from the back. Keep the thumbs in the region of the occiput to steady the neck. The neck is slightly flexed and turned to the side of palpating finger

Q. What is Pizzillo's method for palpation for thyroid gland?

Ans. In obese patients with short neck, the thyroid gland may be palpated by Pizzillo's method. Patient keeps both his hands on the occiput and extends the neck. The slightly enlarged gland may be seen and palpated either from the front or back (Fig. 6.6).

Q. What is Crile's method for palpation of the thyroid gland?

Ans. Small swelling in thyroid gland may be palpated by Crile's method. Palpate the swelling with the pulp of the thumb. Place pulp of the thumb over the swelling and ask the patient to swallow as the swelling moves up and down. Palpate the surface of the swelling with the pulp of the thumb (Fig. 6.7).

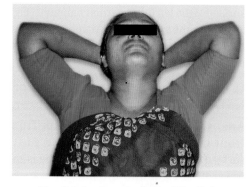

Fig. 6.6: In obese individual Pizzillo's method for palpation

Q. What other swelling apart from thyroid moves up and down with deglutition?

Ans.
* Subhyoid bursitis
* Prelaryngeal or pretracheal lymph node
* Any swelling arising from larynx or trachea
* Thyroglossal cyst.

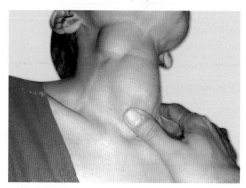

Fig. 6.7: Crile's method for palpation of thyroid gland

Q. Why the thyroid swelling moves up and down with deglutition?

Ans. The thyroid gland is enclosed by the pretracheal fascia. The pretracheal fascia is condensed posteromedially to form the ligament of Berry, which is attached to the cricoid cartilage. The pretracheal fascia is also attached to the trachea and larynx. During deglutition, the larynx and the cricoid cartilage moves up and down so the thyroid swelling moves up and down with deglutition due to its attachment to the larynx and the cricoid cartilage.

Q. Which thyroid swelling does not move up and down with deglutition?

Ans.
* Carcinoma thyroid with local infiltration
* Riedel's thyroiditis
* Huge goiter
* Retrosternal goiter with intrathoracic impaction.

Q. How do you ascertain any retrosternal prolongation of goiter?

Ans.
* *From history*: Patient may have respiratory distress and swelling of face and neck.
* On general survey, face may be puffy.
* *On local examination*:
  - There may be engorged vein over the neck or chest wall (Fig. 6.8).
  - The lower margin of thyroid gland is not visible and the lower margin could not be palpated.
  - On percussion over the manubrium sterni, the area is dull (Figs 6.9A and B).
  - Pemberton's sign is positive (Fig. 6.10).

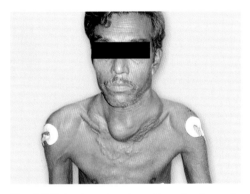

Fig. 6.8: Retrosternal prolongation of goiter: note the dilated veins over the chest wall, puffy face and overhanging enlarged thyroid gland over the suprasternal notch

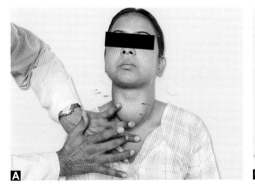
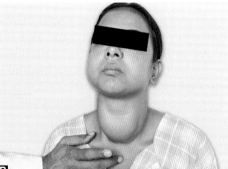

Figs 6.9A and B: Percussion over the manubrium sterni

Q. What is Pemberton sign?

Ans. Ask the patient to raise both arms over the head touching the ears and maintain this position of the arms above the head for 2–3 minutes. If there is retrosternal prolongation of goiter then there will be congestion of face, engorgement of vein in the neck and patient may have respiratory distress. Pemberton sign is said to be positive if there is retrosternal prolongation of goiter (Fig. 6.10).

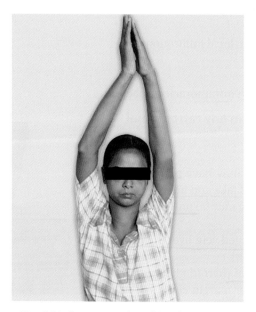

Fig. 6.10: Demonstration of Pemberton sign

Q. How will you demonstrate different eye signs?

Ans.

Demonstration of exophthalmos: Stand behind the patient. Look from behind with the neck of the patient slightly extended and look along superior orbital margin. Exophthalmos is present when the eyeball is seen beyond the superior orbital margin. This is called Naffziger method for demonstration of exophthalmos (Fig. 6.11).

Visibility of both upper and lower sclera, indicate presence of exophthalmos (Figs 6.12 and 6.13).

Von Graefe sign: Steady the patient's head with one hand and ask the patient to look at your finger held in front of the eye. Ask the patient to look up

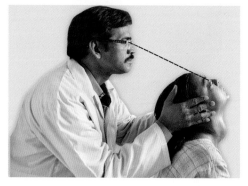

Fig. 6.11: Naffziger method for demonstration of exophthalmos

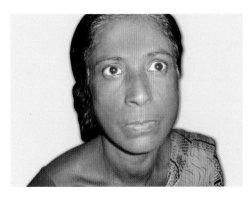

Fig. 6.12: Exophthalmos: Note the visibility of both upper and lower sclera.

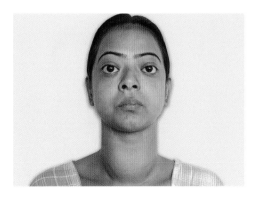

Fig. 6.13: Exophthalmos: Note the visibility of lower sclera

and down following your finger moving in front of the eye up and down quickly for 5–6 times. Normally, the movement of upper lid follows the movement of eyeball. In case of thyrotoxicosis, the lid may lag while the eyeball move downward and the upper sclera become visible. If the lid lag is present, the sign is said to be positive (Figs 6.14A and B).

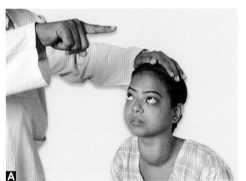

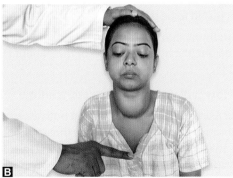

Figs 6.14A and B: (A) Steady the head and ask the patient to look up; (B) Ask the patient to look down—no lid lag present

Joffroy sign: Steady the patient's head with one hand. Ask the patient to look up at the ceiling. Normally there will be wrinkling of forehead while looking up. In case of thyrotoxicosis, there may be loss of wrinkling of forehead. If there is loss of wrinkling of forehead, the sign is said to be positive (Fig. 6.15).

Möbius sign: Patient is asked to look at a distant object (Fig. 6.16A) and then asked to look at the finger of the clinician brought suddenly in front of the eye from the side (Fig. 6.16B). Normally, there is medial convergence of both the eyeballs and constriction of the pupils due to accommodation

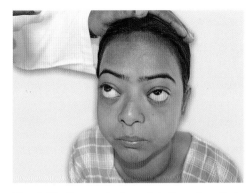

Fig. 6.15: Demonstration of Joffroy sign: Note the absence of wrinkling of forehead on looking up. Positive Joffroy sign.

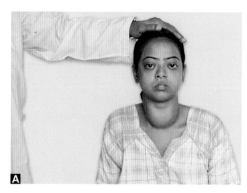
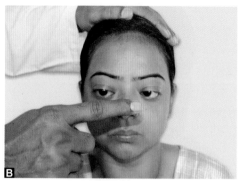

Figs 6.16A and B: (A) Patient is asked to look at a distant object; (B) Patient is asked to look at the finger brought close to the eye: note the failure of medial convergence in right eye. Demonstration of Möbius sign

reaction. In thyrotoxicosis, there is failure of medial convergence of the eyeball. If there is failure of medial convergence of the eyeball, the sign is said to be positive.

Stellwag sign or infrequent blinking may be made out just by observation of the patient (Fig. 6.17).

Q. How will you demonstrate tremor?

Ans. Ask the patient to stretch out both the upper limbs in front and spread out the fingers. Look at the fingers for presence of fine tremor (Fig. 6.18).

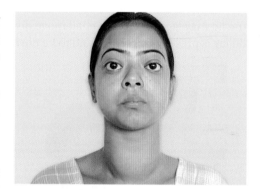

Fig. 6.17: Stellwag sign: Note the stare look

Patient is asked to put out the tongue resting on lower lip. Fine tremor may be observed in the tongue. In severe case whole body may tremble (Fig. 6.19).

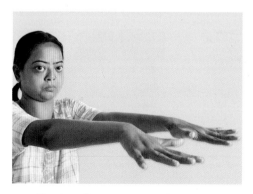

Fig. 6.18: Demonstration of tremor in outstretched hands

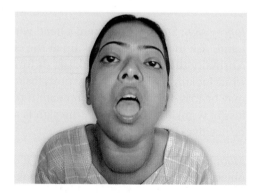

Fig. 6.19: demonstration of tremor in tongue: Keep the protruded tongue over the lower lip

Q. Where do you palpate the normal carotid artery?

Ans. At the level of upper border of thyroid cartilage along the anterior border of sternocleidomastoid (Fig. 6.20).

Q. What is Berry's sign?

Ans. When carotid pulse is impalpable due to infiltration of carotid sheath by a malignant thyroid swelling then it is called positive Berry's sign.

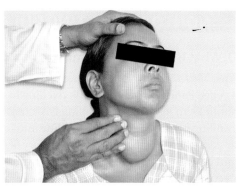

Fig. 6.20: Palpation of carotid pulse

Q. Where do you palpate for thrill over the thyroid gland?

Ans. Thrill over the thyroid gland is better palpated at the upper pole of the thyroid gland.

Q. Where do you auscultate for bruit over the thyroid gland?

Ans. The bruit is audible at the upper pole of the thyroid gland (Fig. 6.21).

Q. What may be the cause of sudden increase in size of the thyroid swelling?

Ans. The sudden increase in size of a preexisting thyroid swelling may be either due to hemorrhage or malignant change.

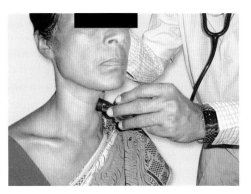

Fig. 6.21: Listening to bruit over the upper pole of the thyroid gland by placing the bell of the stethoscope

Q. What are the causes of respiratory distress in a patient with thyroid swelling?

Ans.

* Carcinoma thyroid causing bilateral recurrent nerve palsy or mechanical compression of trachea may cause respiratory distress
* Retrosternal goiter may cause tracheal compression and respiratory distress
* Long-standing multinodular goiter may cause tracheomalacia and respiratory distress. This may be more pronounced in postoperative period
* In patients with thyrotoxicosis congestive cardiac failure may cause respiratory distress.

Q. What are the different groups of lymph nodes in the neck?

Ans. *See* Page No. 18 Chapter 1.

Q. How will you palpate different levels of lymph nodes in the neck?

Ans. *See* Page No. 19 and 20, Chapter 1.

NONTOXIC MULTINODULAR GOITER OR COLLOID GOITER

Q. What is your case? (Summary of a case of nontoxic multinodular goiter)

Ans. This 45-year-old lady presented with a swelling in the front and side of the neck for last 4 years. Patient first noticed the swelling in the right side of the neck four years back, which was about 2 cm in size. The swelling is increasing in size very slowly over the last 4 years and the swelling has extended to the midline and to the left; there has been no history of rapid increase in size of the swelling. There is no history of pain over the swelling. Her appetite is normal. Bowel and bladder habits are normal. There are no symptoms pertaining to respiratory, cardiac and nervous system. There is no history of any major ailment in the past. There are no menstrual problems. No other in the family has similar swellings in the neck.

On physical examination, general survey is essentially normal. on local examination of the neck, there is a swelling in the front and sides of the neck in the thyroid region. The swelling is butterfly shaped and moves up and down with deglutition, suggesting this to be a thyroid swelling. The right half of the swelling measures 5 cm × 3 cm and the left half of the swelling measures 6 cm × 3 cm. The swelling in the midline measures 3 cm × 4 cm. On either side, the swelling extends above up to the upper border of the thyroid cartilage and below up to the clavicle.

In the midline, the swelling extends below up to the suprasternal notch and above about 4 cm above the suprasternal notch. The surface of the swelling is nodular. The margins are rounded and on the lateral sides the swelling passes under the sternocleidomastoid muscle. The swelling is firm in consistency and is nontender. The carotid pulse is palpable in the normal position on both sides. Cervical lymph nodes are not palpable. The circumference of the neck at the maximum extent of the swelling is ... cm. No toxic signs are found on examination. There is no clinical evidence of retrosternal prolongation (Fig. 6.22).

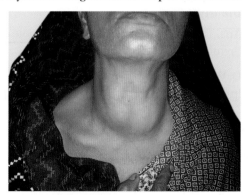

Fig. 6.22: Multinodular goiter.

Q. What is your diagnosis?

Ans. This is a case of nontoxic multinodular goiter involving both lobes and isthmus of the thyroid gland.

Q. What do you mean by goiter?

Ans. A generalized enlargement of thyroid gland is called a goiter.

Q. What do you mean by solitary or isolated swelling in thyroid?

Ans. When there is a palpable nodule in one lobe without any palpable abnormality in the rest of the gland then it is called a solitary or isolated swelling.

Q. What do you mean by a dominant swelling in the thyroid?

Ans. When there is a discrete swelling in the thyroid lobe with palpable abnormality in the rest of the gland then this swelling is said to be a dominant swelling.

Q. Why do you say that this is a thyroid swelling?

Ans. From history, patient complained of a swelling in front and side of the neck in the thyroid region which was gradually increasing in size. On examination, there is a butterfly-shaped swelling present in the thyroid region. The swelling moves up and down with deglutition. So, this is a thyroid swelling.

Q. What are the differential diagnoses for a nontoxic multinodular goiter?

Ans.
* Colloid nodule in right or left lobe or in both lobes
* Chronic thyroiditis
* Carcinoma of thyroid.

Q. What are the differential diagnoses of the solitary thyroid nodule?

Ans.
* Colloid nodule
* Benign tumor of thyroid gland—follicular adenoma
* Carcinoma of thyroid gland
* Thyroid cyst
* Hashimoto thyroiditis.

Q. How will you manage this case of multinodular goiter?

Ans. I would like to confirm my diagnosis by:
* Ultrasonography (USG) of thyroid gland.
* Fine needle aspiration cytology (FNAC) from different sites of the enlarged thyroid gland. Alternatively, USG-guided FNAC may be done.
* Thyroid-stimulating hormone (TSH).

Q. Does all patients with thyroid nodule need thyroid profile study?

Ans. Thyroid-stimulating hormone level estimation is required in all patients with thyroid nodule to detect hypo- or hyperthyroidism. If TSH is normal T3 or T4 level estimation is not necessary. But in suspected hypo- or hyperthyroidism thyroid profile (T3, T4, and TSH) is to be done.

Q. What are the normal levels of thyroid hormone?

Ans.
* *T3*: 1.5–3.5 nmol/L
* *T4*: 55–150 nmol/L
* *TSH*: 0.5–5 mIU/L
* *Free T3*: 3–9 pmol/L
* *Free T4*: 12–28 pmol/L.

Q. How does ultrasonography helps in evaluation of the patient?

Ans.
* Ultrasonography is an important investigation for evaluation of a thyroid swelling.
* It can detect nodules in the thyroid gland up to 2–3 mm in diameter.
* It can distinguish a solid and a cystic lesion.
* Some cysts are complex, i.e. there is both cystic and solid component. A complex cyst is highly suspicious of malignancy.

- It may guide FNAC from a deep small impalpable nodule.
- Useful also for follow-up of small nodule to assess any increase or decrease in size while being observed or treated with thyroid hormone.
- Useful to detect recurrence following thyroidectomy.
- It may demonstrate vascular invasion of thyroid mass to either internal jugular vein or the carotid.
- It can detect any enlarged cervical lymph node.

Q. What is TIRADS classification system for thyroid lesion on imaging?

Ans. A classification system has been proposed by Horvath et al. with a modification from Jin Kwak et al.

Similar to BIRADS (breast imaging-reporting and data system) category, sonographic TIRADS (thyroid image reporting and data system) classification is as follows:

- *TIRADS 1*: Normal thyroid gland
- *TIRADS 2*: Benign lesions
  - Avascular anechoic lesion with echogenic specks (colloid type I)
  - Vascular heteroechoic non-expansile, non-encapsulated nodules with peripheral halo (colloid type II)
  - Isoechoic or heteroechoic, non-encapsulated, expansile vascular nodules (colloid type III)
  - These conditions have 0% risk of malignancy benign lesions
- *TIRADS 3*: Probably benign lesion
  - Hyperechoic, isoechoic or hypoechoic nodules
  - Partially formed capsule and
    - Peripheral vascularity, usually in setting of Hashimoto's thyroiditis (Hashimoto's pseudonodule)
  - Modified TIRADS classification has simplified TIRADS 3 category as none of the suspicious malignant sonographic features described here.
  - These lesions are mostly benign with less than 5% risk of malignancy
- *TIRADS 4*: Suspicious lesions (subclassified as 4a, 4b, and later 4c with increasing risk of malignancy)
- *TIRADS 5*: Probably malignant lesions (>80% risk of malignancy).

TIRADS 4 and 5 categories are based on five suspicious sonographic features of malignancy:
1. Solid component:
   - High stiffness of nodule on elastography if available
2. Markedly hypoechoic nodule
3. Microlobulations or irregular margins
4. Microcalcifications
5. Taller-than-wider shape.
Subclassification:
- TIRADS 4a: One suspicious feature (5–10% risk of malignancy)
- TIRADS 4b: Two suspicious features
- TIRADS 4c: Three/four suspicious features (4b and 4c—10–80% risk of malignancy)
- TIRADS 5: All five suspicious features (>80% risk of malignancy)
- TIRADS 6: Biopsy proven malignancy.

Q. How FNAC helps in evaluation of a thyroid swelling?

Ans.

* FNAC is a good investigation for evaluation of thyroid nodule
* FNAC can differentiate between a benign and malignant nodule
* If papillary pattern is found, it is diagnostic of papillary carcinoma
* Follicular adenoma and follicular carcinoma cannot be differentiated on FNAC. The signs of malignancy in follicular carcinoma is vascular and capsular invasion
* It can diagnose a colloid nodule.

Q. What is the sensitivity and specificity of FNAC?

Ans.

* Sensitivity: 68–98%
* Specificity: 72–100%.

Q. What is Bethesda system of reporting for thyroid cytology on FNAC?

Ans.

* *Category I—nondiagnostic or unsatisfactory (ND/UNS)*
* *Category II—benign*: This category includes benign follicular nodule (adenomastoid nodule, colloid nodule), lymphocytic (Hashimotos) thyroiditis, and granulomatous (subacute) thyroiditis.
  The recommended management of this category is clinical follow-up.
* *Category III—atypia of undetermined significance or follicular lesion of undetermined significance (AUS/FLUS)*: Thyroid FNAs that do not fit into benign, suspicious or malignant categories are included here.
* *Category IV—FN or suspicious for a FN (FN/SFN)*: The aim of this category is to identify a nodule that might be a follicular carcinoma. Follicular carcinomas have cytomorphologic features that distinguish them from benign follicular nodules but do not permit distinction from a FA. They are reportable as FN or SFN.
* *Category V—suspicious for malignancy*: Many thyroid cancers, especially papillary thyroid carcinoma (PTC) can be diagnosed with certainty by FNA. May be suspicious of malignancy.
* *Category VI—malignant*: The general category malignant is used whenever the cytomorphologic features are conclusive for malignancy.
  The criteria for reporting medullary carcinoma are moderate to markedly cellular smears, with plasmacytoid, polygonal, round or spindle-shaped cells. Amyloid is often present and appears as dense amorphous material.
  The criteria for reporting anaplastic thyroid carcinoma are neoplastic cells arranged in groups or discretely. Individual cells being epithelioid, spindled, plasmacytoid or rhabdoid in shape. Nuclear pleomorphism, multinucleation and neutrophilic infiltration of tumor cell cytoplasm are other features. Mitotic activity will be numerous and abnormal.

Q. Is there any role of frozen section biopsy in thyroid nodule?

Ans. In cases where FNAC is inconclusive and there is clinical suspicion of malignancy, a lobectomy may be done and specimen subjected to frozen section biopsy. If malignancy is confirmed, proceed with total thyroidectomy. Frozen section biopsy may help in intraoperative decision for optimal surgical treatment.

Q. If FNAC is inconclusive what should be done?

Ans. If FNAC is inconclusive a core needle biopsy (trucut biopsy) may be considered. However, with trucut biopsy chance of complication like hemorrhage is more.

Q. What is the role of isotope scanning for a multinodular goiter?

Ans.

- Earlier it was one of the most common investigations for evaluation of thyroid nodule. However, nowadays a multinodular goiter rarely needs an isotope scanning for evaluation.
- The thyroid scan does neither always identify the presence of a nodule nor does it always distinguish between a benign from a malignant nodule.
- Radioiodine scanning cannot show nodule less than 1 cm in diameter.
- Warm nodules are not always delineated on thyroid scanning.
- However, isotope scanning is indicated for evaluation of a toxic nodular goiter or a toxic adenoma. In this situation, the whole radioactivity is taken up by the hyperfunctioning nodule and rest of the thyroid does not take up any radioactivity
- Ideal for follow-up evaluation of thyroid cancer patients.

Q. How will you do radioactive iodine uptake and radioactive thyroid scanning?

Ans.

- Material used ^{99m}Tc, ^{123}I or ^{131}I
- Thyroid gland takes up ^{99m}Tc exactly like radioactive iodine
- 5 μCi of radioactive iodine ^{123}I or ^{131}I is given orally. Radioactive iodine uptake by the thyroid gland is measured by a Geiger-Müller counter placed on the thyroid gland. The uptake over the thyroid gland is measured at 4-hour and 24-hour. The amount of radioactivity over the thyroid is expressed as percentage of the total dose given.
- Distribution of radioactivity over the thyroid gland is picked up by a gamma camera. This is represented as stipple lines showing the distribution of radioactivity over the thyroid gland. This is called thyroid scanning.

Q. How will you classify thyroid nodule by radioactive scanning?

Ans. The nodule may be:

- *Cold nodule*: Does not take up any radioactivity—80% is benign and 10–20% is malignant.
- *Warm nodule*: They take up same radioactivity as the rest of the gland.
- *Hot nodule*: The nodule takes up all radioactivities and rest of the gland is suppressed. Only 1% is malignant. Some may be toxic adenoma.
- *Nodule with discordant scans*: The nodule is hot or warm on ^{99m}Tc scan but cold on radioactive ^{123}I scanning. These nodules are most likely to be malignant.

Q. What other investigations would you like to do in this patient of nontoxic multinodular goiter?

Ans. Some routine investigations to assess patient's fitness for general anesthesia are required in this patient:

- *Complete hemogram*: Hb%, total leukocyte count (TLC), differential leukocyte count (DLC), and erythrocyte sedimentation rate (ESR).

- Chest X-ray [anteroposterior (PA) view]
- Electrocardiography
- X-ray neck (anteroposterior and lateral view)—look for tracheal deviation.
- Blood for sugar, urea and creatinine
- Urine and stool routine examination
- Ear, nose, and throat (ENT) check-up—indirect laryngoscopy to assess vocal cord movement.

Q. How does a simple or nontoxic multinodular goiter develop?

Ans. Simple multinodular goiter usually develops as a sequela of hyperplastic or parenchymatous goiter. When there is increased demand of thyroid hormone during puberty or pregnancy, there is diffuse hyperplasia of follicular cells and there are increased numbers of active follicles with uniform iodine uptake. This forms a hyperplastic goiter. As stimulation ceases, this phase can revert to normal. If there is fluctuation of stimulation, a mixed pattern develops. Some lobules remain active and some lobules become inactive.

Active lobules become more vascular and hyperplastic and afterward develop central necrosis and hemorrhage and becomes an inactive lobule with a surrounding rim of active follicles. The necrotic lobules coalesce and form nodules filled with iodine-free colloid. Continual repetition of this same process leads to a multinodular goiter. Most nodules are inactive and active follicles are present only in internodular tissue.

Q. What is a colloid goiter?

Ans. Colloid goiter is a late stage of diffuse hyperplastic goiter when TSH stimulation has subsided. Many active follicles become inactive and become full of colloid material.

Q. What are the characteristics of these nodules?

Ans.
- Nodules are multiple.
- Nodules may be colloid or cellular.
- Cystic degeneration and hemorrhage are common in this nodule.
- In endemic areas, this nodule may occur in early age group.

Q. If a single nodule is palpable, can it be still a multinodular goiter?

Ans. Yes, sometimes a single nodule is palpable and there may be other small nodules in other parts of the gland, which is not palpable but can be detected by USG.

Q. What are the complications of nodular goiter?

Ans.
- Tracheal obstruction—large swelling may compress trachea in a lateral direction, or a retrosternal goiter may cause compression anteroposteriorly. Hemorrhage in a nodule may cause acute tracheal obstruction.
- Secondary thyrotoxicosis—incidence 35%.
- Malignant change is uncommon but there is increased incidence of follicular carcinoma in endemic areas.

Q. What are the indications of surgical treatment in multinodular goiter?

Ans. The multinodular goiter is an irreversible stage but all patients do not require surgical treatment:

* Operation may be required for cosmetic reason.
* Retrosternal prolongation of goiter with compressive symptoms.
* Goiter with compressive symptoms—tracheal or esophageal compression.
* Multinodular goiter suspected to be neoplastic.

Q. What surgery do you consider in this patient?

Ans.

* Multinodular goiter involving both the lobes—subtotal thyroidectomy leaving behind normal amount of thyroid tissue in each lobe
* If one lobe is more affected than the other one, then lobectomy on one side and subtotal resection on the other side (Hartley Dunhill procedure).

Other Operations on Thyroid Gland

Hemithyroidectomy: Removal of one complete lobe with the isthmus of the thyroid gland is called hemithyroidectomy.

Near total thyroidectomy: Removal of almost whole of thyroid gland leaving behind a rim of thyroid tissue in each lobe to avoid injury to the recurrent laryngeal nerve and the parathyroid glands.

Total thyroidectomy: Complete removal of both the lobes and the isthmus of the thyroid gland.

Q. What is the optimum amount of thyroid tissue you will leave behind while doing subtotal thyroidectomy?

Ans. An amount of thyroid tissue filling the tracheoesophageal groove is left behind on each side while doing subtotal thyroidectomy. This also corresponds to about 4 g of thyroid tissue in each lobe or thumb size thyroid tissue left behind in the tracheoesophageal groove.

Q. Is there any role of total thyroidectomy in multinodular goiter?

Ans. Sometimes, the nodules involve both the lobes and there is hardly ever any normal tissue and leaving behind this nodular tissue may not function well. If the surgeon is experienced enough, a total thyroidectomy may be done.

Q. Do you want to give L-thyroxine following subtotal thyroidectomy in the postoperative period?

Ans.

* The role of L-thyroxine is uncertain.
* In endemic areas the chance of recurrence is more due to persistence of deficient factor. In this situation there is rationality for L-thyroxine in the postoperative period. However, the beneficial effect is not certain.
* In hypothyroid patient L-thyroxine is required in postoperative period.

SOLITARY THYROID NODULE

Q. What is your case? (Summary of a case presenting with solitary thyroid nodule)

Ans. This 30-year-old lady presented with a swelling in the front and right side of the neck for last 3 years. Patient noticed a swelling in the lower part of the right side of the neck 3 years back which was about 2 cm in size when first noticed. Since then, the swelling is gradually increasing in size to attain the present large size. There has been no history of rapid increase in size of the swelling. Patient has no difficulty in breathing, swallowing and there has been no change of voice during this period. Patient has no other systemic symptoms (Fig. 6.23).

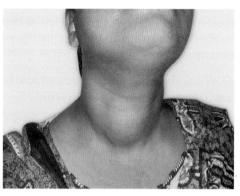

Fig. 6.23: Solitary thyroid nodule involving the right lobe

On examination, general survey is essentially normal. On local examination of the thyroid region, there is a swelling in the right side of the neck extending medially to about 1 cm to the left of midline laterally extends up to the anterior border of right sternomastoid, below extends up to the sternoclavicular joint region. The swelling moves up and down with deglutition, but does not move up with protrusion of tongue. The swelling is globular, margins are rounded, the overlying skin is normal, the swelling is firm in consistency, and is free from the skin and underlying structures. The carotid pulse is palpable. There are no toxic signs and there is no clinical evidence of retrosternal prolongation.

So this is a case of nontoxic solitary thyroid nodule involving the right lobe of the thyroid gland.

Q. What are the possible pathological diagnoses?

Ans.
- Colloid nodule
- Follicular adenoma
- Carcinoma thyroid
- Thyroid cyst.

Q. What is the most common cause of solitary or isolated nodule?

Ans. The most common cause of solitary thyroid nodule is a colloid nodule.

Q. How will you manage this patient?

Ans. I will do some investigations to confirm my diagnosis to find the pathological nature of the nodule:
- Ultrasonography of thyroid region
- USG-guided FNAC
- Thyroid-stimulating hormone (TSH) and free T4.

Q. Is it necessary to do thyroid profile study in all patients with solitary thyroid nodule?

Ans. Full thyroid profile study is not essential in all patients with thyroid nodule. Free T4 estimation may be a screening test for all patients with solitary thyroid nodule. Alternatively, TSH estimation may suggest hyper- or hypothyroidism.

T3, T4, and TSH study is required in patients with clinical features suggestive of hyper- or hypothyroidism.

Q. What should be the biochemical investigation in patients suspected to have medullary carcinoma of thyroid?

Ans. Serum calcium and calcitonin level study is to be done in suspected cases.

In patients suspected of having multiple endocrine neoplasia type 2 (MEN 2) syndrome, 24 hours urine examination for catecholamines for 3 days is to be done to exclude associated pheochromocytoma. The associated pheochromocytoma has to be excluded to avoid severe hypertensive crisis during surgery. If pheochromocytoma is present this should be treated first.

Q. Is it possible to differentiate follicular adenoma and follicular carcinoma in FNAC?

Ans. No, the FNAC picture of follicular adenoma and follicular carcinoma may be same. The diagnosis of follicular carcinoma is dependent on finding of capsular and vascular invasion by the neoplastic follicular cells. This cannot be commented from the FNAC.

Q. Why FNAC is the first-line investigation for evaluation of a solitary thyroid nodule?

Ans. A definitive tissue diagnosis permits the option of nonoperative management of patients with benign disease and also allows appropriate planning for surgical treatment in patients with thyroid cancers. The finding of thyroid lymphoma obviates requirement for unnecessary surgery.

Q. Would you like to do CT scan or MRI for evaluation of solitary thyroid nodule?

Ans. Computed tomography (CT) scan and MRI give excellent anatomical details of the neck structures but are not practiced routinely. This is indicated in selected patients to define the anatomical extent of a large cervical or retrosternal goiter.

Q. What is the role of radioisotope scanning for solitary thyroid nodule?

Ans. Earlier radioisotope scanning was the mainstay of investigation for a solitary thyroid nodule. Scintigraphy with ^{131}I or ^{99m}Tc provides only functional assessment and based on the uptake grouped as hot, warm or cold nodule. Isotope scanning does not provide a tissue diagnosis.

The possibility of malignancy occurring in a hot nodule is very rare. Malignancy may occur in a warm nodule (incidence 24%). The chance of malignancy in a cold nodule is less (incidence 14–22%).

Q. Which cold nodules are suspicious of malignancy?

Ans. A study of the dynamic phase in 99mTc scanning may provide some clue to the diagnosis of thyroid malignancy. On dynamic scanning the nodules may be classified as hyperperfused, normally perfused or hypoperfused. There is no risk of malignancy in hypoperfused nodules in dynamic scanning.

Q. What is the role of core biopsy or trucut needle biopsy in evaluation of thyroid nodule?

Ans.
* In cases where FNAC is inconclusive, a trucut needle biopsy may be done
* It is also indicated in anaplastic and locally advanced thyroid carcinoma
* Trucut biopsy produces a small cylinder of tissue which helps in histopathological examination
* Problems of trucut biopsy are pain, bleeding, tracheal injury, and recurrent laryngeal nerve palsy.
* Routine trucut biopsy of solitary thyroid nodule is not indicated.

Q. What may be the possibilities in a cold nodule?

Ans. The cold nodule in an isotope scan does not take up any isotope. The colloid nodule may be:
* Degenerating colloid nodule
* Follicular neoplasm
* Thyroid cyst
* Carcinoma thyroid
* Lymphocytic thyroiditis.

Q. When do you suspect malignancy in a solitary thyroid nodule?

Ans.
* Rapid increase in size of the nodule
* Obstructive symptoms—dysphagia, stridor
* Involvement of recurrent laryngeal nerve—hoarseness of voice
* Presence of enlarged significant lymph node in the neck
* History of irradiation at head, neck, and chest.

Q. What are the indications for surgical treatment of a solitary thyroid nodule?

Ans. All solitary thyroid nodules do not require surgical treatment. The indications for surgical treatment are:
* All proven malignant nodules
* Cytologically diagnosed follicular neoplasm
* Suspicious nodules on FNAC
* Cystic nodules which recur following aspiration
* Nodules producing obstructive symptoms
* Hyperfunctioning nodule resulting in hyperthyroidism
* Cosmetic reasons
* Patient's anxiety and wish for surgical treatment.

Q. What should be the extent of surgery for a solitary thyroid nodule?

Ans. This is to be guided by FNAC report:
* In most instances, a benign solitary thyroid nodule confined to one lobe is best treated with total thyroid lobectomy on the side with removal of the isthmus (hemithyroidectomy)
* Nodule in isthmus—isthmusectomy with a segment of each adjacent lobe
* FNAC diagnosed carcinoma—total thyroidectomy
* FNAC follicular adenoma—hemithyroidectomy—material is sent for frozen section biopsy. If malignancy is found proceed with total thyroidectomy.

Q. How reliable is frozen section biopsy in thyroid lesions?

Ans.

- Frozen section biopsy is advised for suspicious lesion if characteristic of malignant lesion is found, proceed with total thyroidectomy.
- However, in 10–15% cases of follicular carcinoma report may be inconclusive. In such situation do a hemithyroidectomy. If follicular carcinoma is found on histopathological examination completion of thyroidectomy is to be done.

Q. When will you consider nonsurgical treatment for solitary thyroid nodule?

Ans. When FNAC has excluded malignancy and there is no obstructive symptom patient may be treated conservatively.

The patients should be reviewed after 6 months and assessed clinically and repeat FNAC. If the report is equivocally benign then the patient may be reviewed annually.

Q. How will you treat a colloid nodule?

Ans. When colloid nodule is diagnosed in FNAC, patient can be offered nonoperative treatment with L-thyroxine. About 50% of patients respond to thyroxine treatment.

The indication of surgery in colloid nodule is cosmetic, nodules showing increase in size on follow-up and in patients with previous history of irradiation to the neck.

There has been conflicting views regarding the use of L-thyroxine in treatment of solitary thyroid nodule. Some reports suggest reduction in size of the significant numbers of solitary thyroid nodules. Others has reported that T4 therapy is not effective in reducing the size of the solitary thyroid nodule even when circulating TSH level is suppressed to below normal.

Q. What you should explain to the patient before you proceed with surgery for thyroid nodule?

Ans. Even in experienced hands there is chance of recurrent laryngeal nerve palsy. So patient should be counseled preoperatively with regard to the risk of recurrent laryngeal nerve palsy.

Q. What is the incidence of malignancy in solitary thyroid nodule?

Ans. The vast majority of solitary thyroid nodules are benign. About 15–20% solitary thyroid nodules may be malignant.

Q. What are the risk factors which may suggest a solitary thyroid nodule be due to malignancy?

Ans.

- There are two important risk factors which may arouse the suspicion of malignancy in a solitary thyroid nodule.
- The most important is past history of irradiation in the neck.
- Family history of thyroid cancer.
- About 6% of papillary carcinoma may be familial.
- Medullary carcinoma risk is the greatest if there is a history of medullary thyroid carcinoma in other family members as this is inherited by autosomal dominant gene.

Q. When will you suspect malignancy in a solitary thyroid nodule?

Ans. Apart from family history and history of irradiation to the neck, following will arouse the suspicion of malignancy:

- *Age*: Thyroid nodules in children and elderly may be malignant.

- Rapid enlargement of an old or a new thyroid nodule.
- *Symptom of local invasion*: Unilateral vocal cord paralysis.
- Compressive symptoms, such as dysphagia and dyspnea due to invasion to esophagus or trachea.
- A hard, fixed thyroid nodule also arouses the suspicion of malignancy.
- Presence of palpable cervical lymph node adjacent to the thyroid nodule raises the suspicion of malignancy.

Q. What is the incidence of thyroid cyst?

Ans.
- About 30% of solitary thyroid swelling is found to be cystic.
- About 50% cystic swelling is due to colloid degeneration.
- 10–15% of cystic swelling is malignant.
- Papillary carcinoma is often associated with cyst formation.

Q. What do you mean by a complex cyst?

Ans. A cyst with both solid and cystic component is called a complex cyst. This can be seen well in USG. Complex cysts are suspicious of malignancy.

Q. What should be the management strategy for thyroid cyst?

Ans.
- When a cyst is found on FNAC, it should be completely aspirated. This is curative in 75% cases of simple cyst. If the cyst refills, reaspiration may be done.
- If the cyst persists after three aspirations then unilateral thyroid lobectomy is recommended.
  If the cyst is complex containing both solid and cystic component and is larger than 4 cm then thyroid lobectomy is indicated as there is about 15% chance of these cysts being malignant.

PRIMARY THYROTOXICOSIS (GRAVES' DISEASE)

Q. What is your case? (Summary of a case of primary thyrotoxicosis)

Ans. This 35-year-old lady presented with a swelling in front and side of the neck for last 1 year which was gradually increasing size for 6 months since the onset of the swelling and remained static for last 6 months. Along with the onset of the swelling, patient complained of bulging of her both eyes for last 1 year. She also complains of trembling of limbs, generalized weakness, palpitation, and weight loss in spite of increased appetite. Again she complains of occasional diarrhea, heat intolerance, and increased sweating (mention the points present in your patient). Patient is taking antithyroid drugs for last 6 months. Her symptom has improved to some extent but is still persisting (Fig. 6.24).

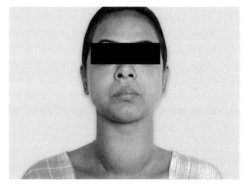

Fig. 6.24: Primary thyrotoxicosis.

On examination, general survey of patient revealed a typical thyrotoxic facies, pulse 110 beats per minute with high volume collapsing in character and warm moist hand.

On local examination, there is diffuse enlargement of the thyroid gland, which is moving up and down with deglutition. The margins are well defined, surface is smooth and nontender firm in consistency. Palpable thrill and audible bruit near the upper pole of the thyroid gland.

On examination for toxic signs, there is tachycardia with high volume collapsing pulse. Eye signs are present—visible exophthalmos, Von Graefe's sign is absent, Joffroy's sign, Möbius sign, Dalrymple sign, Stellwag's sign are all positive. There is tremor in outstretched hands and tongue. There is palpable thrill and on auscultation audible bruit near the upper pole of thyroid gland.

Q. What is your diagnosis?

Ans. This is a case of primary thyrotoxicosis.

Q. What is exophthalmos?

Ans. Exophthalmos is forward protrusion of the eyeball when a portion of the sclera is visible both above and below the cornea.

Q. What is the mechanism of development of exophthalmos in thyrotoxicosis?

Ans. Increase in retro-orbital fat, infiltration of retrobulbar tissue with fluid and round cells pushes the eyeball forward.

Q. Why there is diplopia in advanced exophthalmos?

Ans. In advanced exophthalmos there is edema and cellular infiltration of extrinsic muscles of the eyeball. The superior rectus and inferior oblique and sometimes lateral rectus are commonly involved resulting in diplopia more so when looking upward and outward.

Q. What are the causes of exophthalmos?

Ans.
* *Unilateral exophthalmos*:
  – Orbital tumor
  – Retrobulbar tumor
  – Unilateral cavernous sinus thrombosis
  – Some cases of thyrotoxicosis.
* *Bilateral exophthalmos*:
  – Thyrotoxicosis
  – Superior vena cava obstruction
  – Craniostenosis
  – Bilateral cavernous sinus thromboses
  – Cushing's syndrome.

Q. What are the different grades of exophthalmos in thyrotoxicosis?

Ans.
* *Grade 0*: No sign no symptom
* *Grade 1*: Only sign (lid retraction/lid lag) no symptom
* *Grade 2*: Soft tissue involvement
* *Grade 3*: Proptosis more than 22 mm (measured by exophthalmometer)

* *Grade 4*: External ophthalmoplegia (inferior oblique and superior rectus are commonly involved)
* *Grade 5*: Corneal ulceration
* *Grade 6*: Loss of vision.

Q. What do you mean by malignant exophthalmos?

Ans. A form of progressive exophthalmos with conjunctival edema, chemosis and ophthalmoplegia causing diplopia, corneal ulceration and visual loss. Mainly, the superior rectus and inferior oblique muscles are involved and the patient has diplopia on looking upward and outward.

Q. What may be the differential diagnosis of primary thyrotoxicosis?

Ans.
* *Anxiety neurosis*:
  - Appetite diminished
  - Hands are cold and moist
  - Tachycardia is present but sleeping pulse rate is normal
  - No goiter.
* Diabetes mellitus
* Pulmonary tuberculosis
* Malabsorption syndrome
* Pheochromocytoma.

Q. How will you proceed with the management of this patient with Graves' disease?

Ans.
* I would like to do a thyroid profile study T3, T4, and TSH.
* Ultrasonography of thyroid region to assess the thyroid swelling—any nodularity.

Q. What do you expect on thyroid profile study?

Ans. T3 and T4 elevated with very low level of TSH.

Q. Can total hormone level be normal in a patient with thyrotoxicosis?

Ans. Yes. It is the only free fraction of hormone which is important. If free fraction is more, it may cause thyrotoxicosis even if the total level of thyroid hormone is normal. So in selected cases of thyrotoxicosis free T3 and free T4 may need to be estimated.

Q. Is it necessary to do a radioactive iodine uptake test?

Ans. With advent of estimation of total and free T3 and T4, radioactive iodine uptake test is no longer required for diagnosis of thyrotoxicosis. If done, radioactive iodine uptake test shows increased uptake over the thyroid gland at 4 hours and 24 hours.

Q. Do you like to do a radionuclide thyroid scanning?

Ans. A radionuclide thyroid scanning is not very helpful in evaluation of a patient with primary thyrotoxicosis. It only shows a diffused increased uptake of the radioactivity over the thyroid gland. Radionuclide scanning is helpful for evaluation of toxic multinodular goiter or a solitary toxic nodule, which will show the sites of hyperfunctioning thyroid tissue which is required for planning surgical treatment.

Q. To which proteins T3 and T4 are bound?

Ans. These hormones are bound to thyroxine-binding globulin.

Q. In which conditions thyroxine-binding globulin may be altered?

Ans.
* In pregnancy and in patient taking oral pill thyroxine-binding globulin is raised. Total T3 and T4 increased but free T3 and T4 normal. So there are no features of toxicity.
* In some liver diseases thyroxine-binding globulin may be low. Total T3 and T4 may be low but free T3 and T4 are normal. So there are no features of hypofunction.

Q. Which thyroid antibodies are important clinically?

Ans. Serum titers of antibody against microsomes and thyroglobulin are useful in determining the cause of thyroid dysfunction and swelling.

Those antibodies are positive in autoimmune thyroiditis (chronic lymphocytic thyroiditis, Hashimoto's thyroiditis). However, some patients may be seronegative.

Q. What are the different modalities of treatment for thyrotoxicosis?

Ans.
* General measures
* Antithyroid drugs
* Surgical treatment
* Radioiodine therapy.

Q. How will you treat this patient of Graves' disease?

Ans. Patients admitted in surgical ward are usually admitted for surgical treatment. These patients either have failure with antithyroid drug treatment or a large unsighted goiter or are having poor response to drug treatment. This will be revealed in history of the patient.

I will prepare the patient for surgery. I will do some investigations to assess the patient's fitness for general anesthesia:
* Chest X-ray
* Electrocardiography
* Blood for complete hemogram
* Blood for sugar, urea and creatinine
* Urine for routine examination.

Q. What are the specific preparations for a thyrotoxic patient?

Ans. The antithyroid drug NeoMercazole 10 mg is given 6–8 hourly. It requires 6–8 weeks for symptomatic and biochemical improvement. The antithyroid drug that patient is taking is to be continued. Last dose of NeoMercazole should be given on the evening before the day of surgery.

Propranolol tablet is given in a dose of 20–40 mg twice or thrice daily to ameliorate the cardiovascular symptoms.

To reduce the vascularity of the thyroid gland and to minimize bleeding during surgery, patient is given Lugol's iodine 15 drops thrice daily for 10 days prior to surgery.

The thyroid status is determined by clinical assessment, by improvement of symptoms and signs, gain in weight, lowering of pulse rate and by serial estimation of thyroid hormones.

Q. What surgery will you plan for this patient?

Ans. I will do total thyroidectomy in this patient.

Q. What other surgery may be done in this patient?

Ans. The alternative may be subtotal or near-total thyroidectomy.

Q. What is the rationale for doing total thyroidectomy in thyrotoxicosis?

Ans. Total thyroidectomy has been practiced as a standard surgical procedure for Graves' disease particularly with eye signs. Total thyroidectomy provides total control of thyrotoxic features and eye signs regressed better following total thyroidectomy.

However, the problem is inherent complication of thyroidectomy particularly recurrent laryngeal nerve palsy and parathyroid insufficiency is more common following total thyroidectomy. Patient will need lifelong L-thyroxine replacement.

Q. Why do you want to do subtotal thyroidectomy?

Ans. Subtotal thyroidectomy preserving normal thyroid tissue in each lobe will provide effective control of thyrotoxicosis. In postoperative period no further drug treatment will be necessary.

Q. What is the advantage of surgery in thyrotoxicosis?

Ans.
- Surgery provides rapid cure by removing the goiter
- Recurrence is very rare if surgery is adequate
- In diffuse toxic goiter and toxic multinodular goiter or toxic adenoma surgery cures by removing the hyperactive tissues.

Q. What are the drawbacks of surgical treatment?

Ans.
- Recurrence rate following surgical treatment is 5–10%.
- Complication due to surgery like recurrent laryngeal nerve palsy, parathyroid insufficiency and bleeding even in experienced hands.
- Postoperative hypothyroidism may occur in 20–45% of patients after subtotal thyroidectomy and in all patients after total thyroidectomy.
- Long-term follow-up is required to detect late hypothyroidism or recurrence of hyperthyroidism.
- If total thyroidectomy is done, life-long supplement with L-thyroxine is required.

Q. What is rationale for drug treatment in thyrotoxicosis?

Ans.
- Antithyroid drugs are used to restore the patient to a euthyroid state and to maintain this for a prolonged period of time so that the patient may go into a phase of spontaneous remission.
- The production of thyroid stimulating antibody will diminish or cease.
- No surgery, no radioiodine so the side effects of surgery and radioiodine are avoided.

Q. Which antithyroid drugs are used?

Ans.

- *Antithyroid drug—NeoMercazole*—decreases hormone synthesis. It also has an immunosuppressive action on thyroid stimulating antibody production so thyroid-stimulating antibodies (TsAb) production will diminish or cease.
- NeoMercazole is given at a dose of 10 mg 6–8 hourly. There is a latent period of 7–14 days before any clinical improvement. The euthyroid state may be achieved in 6–8 weeks' time. Afterward a maintenance dose of NeoMercazole at a dose of 5 mg 8 hourly is to be continued for 12–18 months.
- When contemplating surgical treatment for Graves' disease, the patient should be initially treated with antithyroid drugs for 6–8 weeks to achieve a euthyroid or near euthyroid state before surgery to prevent development of thyroid crisis after surgery.

Q. What are other antithyroid drugs?

Ans.

- Methimazole—given in a dose of 5–20 mg daily.
- Propylthiouracil—given in a dose of 200 mg 8 hourly.

Q. What is the rationale for using beta blockers?

Ans. Beta adrenergic blocking drugs like propranolol or nadolol counteract the effects of thyroid hormones in the peripheral tissues.

Propranolol is given in a dose of 10 mg thrice daily and may be increased up to 240 mg daily. This may control symptoms like palpitation, tremor and sweating.

Q. What are the problems of treatment with antithyroid drugs?

Ans. Drug treatment is usually prolonged and it is not possible to predict which patient will go into the phase of remission.

After prolonged treatment for a period of 18–24 months there is 50% chance of relapse with stoppage of the drug.

Some goiter may enlarge and become very vascular during treatment with antithyroid drugs. This is probably due to the effect of TsAb and not the direct effect of the drug.

Rarely there may be reaction due to the drug itself, such as nausea, vomiting, skin rashes, agranulocytosis or aplastic anemia.

Q. If the patient develops reaction to the antithyroid drugs, how the patient may be prepared for surgery?

Ans. The patient may be prepared for surgery with use of beta blockers like propranolol or nadolol. These beta blockers do not reduce synthesis of thyroid hormones but counteracts the peripheral effects of thyroid hormones. These drugs need to be continued in the postoperative period.

Q. What is the role of radioiodine therapy in thyrotoxicosis?

Ans. Radioiodine in adequate dose can destroy the thyroid cells and control thyrotoxicosis. No surgery is required and prolonged drug therapy is not required.

Q. What are the drawbacks of radioiodine therapy?

Ans.
- Progressive increase in incidence of hypothyroidism about 75–80% patients develops hypothyroidism in 10 years.
- Prolonged follow-up is required.
- Radioiodine cannot be given in pregnancy or to young infants.

Q. Which group of patients may be treated with radioiodine?

Ans. Earlier it was not advised below the age of 45 years but the indication has been relaxed and younger patients are also now treated with radioiodine. Almost all patients above the age of 25 years are being treated with radioiodine.

Q. What is the dose of radioiodine for treatment of thyrotoxicosis?

Ans.
- 300–600 MBq is the usual dose
- A substantial improvement occurs between 8–12 weeks
- If there is no improvement in 12 weeks, the dose may be repeated.

Q. What are the different modalities for treatment of thyrotoxicosis?

Ans.
- *Surgery*:
  - In diffuse toxic goiter particularly with large goiter
  - Toxic multinodular goiter and toxic nodule
- *Radioiodine*:
  - Diffuse toxic goiter above age of 25 years
  - Toxic nodule above 25 years
- *Antithyroid drugs*:
  - Diffuse toxic goiter (small goiter)
  - For preoperative preparation of patients with toxic goiter
  - Toxic nodular goiter does not respond well to antithyroid drugs.

Q. How will you treat recurrent thyrotoxicosis following surgery?

Ans.
- Repeat surgery is very difficult
- Treated either with radioiodine or antithyroid drugs.

Q. How will you treat recurrent thyrotoxicosis following radioiodine therapy?

Ans. Repeat dose of radioiodine or surgery.

Q. What is the effect of antithyroid drugs on a toxic nodule?

Ans. Antithyroid drugs cannot cure a toxic nodule. The overactive thyroid tissue is autonomous and recurrence of thyrotoxicosis is certain when the drug is withdrawn.

Q. What are the complications of thyroidectomy?

Ans.

1. *General complications*:
   - Respiratory
   - Cardiac
   - Anesthetic.
2. *Local complications*:
   - Hemorrhage
   - Respiratory obstruction
   - Recurrent laryngeal nerve palsy unilateral or bilateral—hoarseness of voice or respiratory stridor
   - Thyroid insufficiency
   - Parathyroid insufficiency
   - Thyroid storm or crisis in patients with thyrotoxicosis
   - Wound infection
   - Stitch granuloma
   - Keloid scar.

Q. What are gastrointestinal symptoms in thyrotoxicosis?

Ans.

- Increased appetite
- Weight loss
- Diarrhea.

Q. What are cardiovascular manifestations in thyrotoxicosis?

Ans.

- Palpitation
- Exertional chest pain
- Exertional breathlessness
- Tachycardia with high volume and collapsing pulse
- *Arrhythmias*: Extrasystole, paroxysmal atrial tachycardia, paroxysmal atrial fibrillation, paroxysmal atrial fibrillation and persistent atrial fibrillation.

Q. What are neurological manifestations of thyrotoxicosis?

Ans.

- Insomnia, irritability, and easy excitability
- Hyperkinesia
- Increased sweating
- Trembling of upper and lower limbs and sometimes the whole body
- Proximal muscle weakness leading to difficulty in climbing stairs and standing from sitting posture
- Myasthenia like syndrome
- Exaggerated deep reflexes.

Q. Which features in thyrotoxicosis are not due to hormone?

Ans.
- Orbital proptosis
- Ophthalmoplegia
- Pretibial myxedema.

Q. What is thyrotoxic myopathy?

Ans.
- Weakness of proximal limb muscles
- Severe muscle weakness may resemble myasthenia like syndrome.

Q. What are ocular manifestations of thyrotoxicosis?

Ans.
- Exophthalmos—forward bulging of eyeballs. The proptosis is caused by infiltration of retrobulbar tissues with fluid and round cells.
- Other eye sign.

Q. What is the course of exophthalmos?

Ans.
- Exophthalmos tends to improve with time.
- Sleeping propped up and lateral tarsorrhaphy will help to protect the eye but will not prevent progression.
- Antithyroid drug therapy may aggravate exophthalmos.
- Improvement has been seen with high dose of steroid.
- Orbital decompression may be helpful if eye is in danger.

Q. What is pretibial myxedema?

Ans.
- Swelling of both lower limbs found in patients with thyrotoxicosis.
- In early stage, there are shiny red plaques of thickened skin with coarse hair.
- In severe case, the whole leg below the knee including the ankle and foot is swollen. It is due to deposition of mucin-like material in the subcutaneous tissue.

Q. What is thyroid acropachy?

Ans.
- Clubbing associated with thyrotoxicosis.
- Hypertrophic pulmonary osteoarthropathy may be found in thyrotoxicosis.

Q. What are the different types of hyperthyroidism?

Ans. There are two types of hyperthyroidism: (1) primary and (2) secondary. Hyperthyroidism, or overactive thyroid, is a disorder of the thyroid gland in which it produces high levels of thyroxine and/or triiodothyronine.

Q. What is primary hyperthyroidism?

Ans. Primary hyperthyroidism is due to the malfunctioning of the thyroid gland itself. The gland produces excess thyroid hormones and causes hypermetabolism.

The causes of primary hyperthyroidism include:
* Graves' disease
* Thyroiditis
* Multinodular goiter
* Single hyperfunctioning "hot" nodule.

Q. What is secondary hyperthyroidism?

Ans. Secondary hyperthyroidism is caused by dysfunctions outside the thyroid gland.

The main causes of secondary hyperthyroidism are:
* Thyroid-stimulating hormone secreting pituitary adenoma
* Other causes include:
  – Gestational thyrotoxicosis (hyperthyroidism during pregnancy) usually due increased hCG secretion by placenta
  – Human chorionic gonadotropin (hCG)-producing tumor.
  The symptoms of primary and secondary hyperthyroidism may be similar. Secondary hyperthyroidism is rare and less common than primary hyperthyroidism.

Q. What are the signs and symptoms of secondary hyperthyroidism?

Ans. The signs and symptoms of secondary hyperthyroidism may include:
* Rapid weight loss
* Diarrhea
* Irregular heartbeat, palpitations
* Fatigue
* Irritability, paranoia
* Heat sensitivity
* Tremors
* Sweating
* Thinning of skin.

Q. How is secondary hyperthyroidism diagnosed?

Ans. The diagnosis of secondary hyperthyroidism may require:
* Complete evaluation of medical history along with a thorough physical examination.
* Diagnostic tests for secondary hyperthyroidism include:
  – TSH blood test: High thyroid-stimulating hormone level may be observed
  – T3 and T4 test: High serum T3 and T4 may be observed
  – TRH test: Low levels of TRH (thyrotropin-releasing hormone) can be seen
  – Ultrasound scan of the thyroid gland
  – CT scan of head or MRI of brain to detect tumors in the pituitary gland.

Q. How is secondary hyperthyroidism treated?

Ans. Treatment of secondary hyperthyroidism includes:
* Antithyroid drugs and β-blockers can be used to control the symptoms of hyperthyroidism.
* Treatment of the cause responsible for secondary hyperthyroidism such as a removal of pituitary adenoma or hCG-secreting tumor.

Q. What is the prognosis of secondary hyperthyroidism?

Ans.

+ With appropriate treatment the prognosis of secondary hyperthyroidism is good.
+ The prognosis depends on the underlying cause of the condition.

CARCINOMA OF THYROID GLAND

Q. What is your case? (Summary of a case of carcinoma of thyroid gland)

Ans. This 45-year-old lady presented with a swelling in the front and sides of the neck for last 1 year which was initially increasing slowly in size but for last 4 months patient noticed that swelling is rapidly increasing in size. She complains of dull aching pain over the swelling for last 2 months. Patient also complains of slight hoarseness of voice for last 3 months. No difficulty in swallowing or breathing. There are no symptoms suggestive of hypo- or hyperthyroidism.

On examination, general survey is essentially normal. On local examination of the thyroid region, there is diffuse enlargement of the thyroid gland; right lobe is more enlarged than the left lobe. The enlarged right lobe measures 7 cm × 5 cm and the left lobe measures 4 cm × 2.5 cm and the isthmus region measures 2 cm × 2 cm. Surface is nodular, hard in consistency, moving up and down with deglutition, mobile, not fixed to the skin and underlying structures. There are no signs of toxicity and there are no signs of retrosternal prolongation. Multiple lymph nodes are palpable in the right deep cervical group at levels II and III. The lymph nodes are firm in consistency and are mobile. Systemic examination is normal (Fig. 6.25).

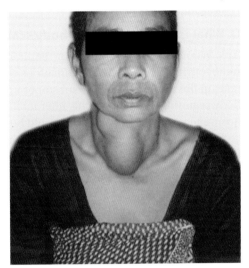

Fig. 6.25: Carcinoma thyroid with lymph node metastasis

Q. How will you proceed to manage this case?

Ans. I will like to do some investigations to confirm my diagnosis.

+ Ultrasonography of thyroid region to assess the extent of enlargement of the thyroid, any invasion of the gland to adjacent structure including extension into the internal jugular vein. The extent of lymph node enlargement.
+ USG-guided FNAC from the thyroid swelling and from the palpable lymph nodes.
+ *Thyroid profile:* T3, T4, and TSH.

Q. What are the other possibilities?

Ans.

+ Simple multinodular goiter
+ Granulomatous thyroiditis
+ Riedel's thyroiditis
+ Follicular adenoma.

Q. Would you like to do radioiodine scanning in this patient?

Ans. Radioiodine scanning is not required for preoperative evaluation of patient with carcinoma thyroid. If done failure to take up radioiodine is characteristic of all thyroid carcinomas. Rarely some differentiated carcinomas may take up ^{123}I.

Q. Which radiographic scanning is helpful for detection of medullary carcinoma of thyroid?

Ans.

* Indium-111 labeled octreotide scanning is useful in detection of medullary carcinoma of thyroid.
* Sensitivity being 70%.
* In postoperative patient with elevated calcitonin, Indium-111 labeled octreotide scintigraphy may indicate location of recurrent or metastatic foci of tumor not demonstrable by other imaging modalities.

Q. What is the role of whole body scanning in thyroid carcinoma?

Ans. Whole body scanning is not required preoperatively. Normal thyroid tissue uptake the radioactivity in preference to cancerous tissue so that normal thyroid tissue in the neck will take up the whole radioactive substance and the metastatic foci could not be detected. Whole body scanning is indicated only after total thyroidectomy. Patient should not be given thyroid hormone for 4 weeks (TSH level should be high).

Give 5 µCi of ^{123}I orally and measure radioactive uptake at 48–72 hours. Whole body scanning is obtained after 48–72 hours by using a gamma camera.

Q. What is the role of ^{99m}Tc sestamibi scan in thyroid carcinoma?

Ans. Hürthle cell tumor concentrates ^{99m}Tc sestamibi well and may be used for imaging of patient suspected of having a metastatic Hürthle cell tumor.

Q. Can thyroid antibody be raised in carcinoma thyroid?

Ans. Yes, thyroid antibody titers are often raised in carcinoma of thyroid.

Q. Is it possible to differentiate follicular adenoma and carcinoma by FNAC?

Ans. No, it is not possible to differentiate follicular adenoma and carcinoma by FNAC. The FNAC appearance of adenoma and carcinoma may be almost same. The follicular carcinoma may be diagnosed by demonstrating vascular and capsular invasion of the tumor in histopathological examination.

Q. What are the sites of primary carcinomas which may spread to thyroid?

Ans. Blood borne metastasis may occur in thyroid from primary carcinomas in colon, kidneys, and melanomas.

Q. What are the important causes for the development of thyroid carcinomas?

Ans.

* Irradiation in the neck is one of the important causes for development of papillary carcinoma of the thyroid.

- Follicular carcinomas may develop in areas of endemic goiter possibly due to continued TSH stimulation.
- Malignant lymphomas may develop in autoimmune thyroiditis or Hashimoto's thyroiditis.

Q. Does recurrent nerve invasion always cause hoarseness of voice?

Ans. Invasion of recurrent laryngeal nerve does not always cause vocal cord paralysis. Sometimes if one vocal cord is paralyzed the voice change may be subtle or even absent.

Q. Does bilateral recurrent laryngeal nerve palsy always require tracheostomy?

Ans. In bilateral recurrent laryngeal nerve palsy the cord may lie either in completely adducted position or in cadaveric position.

If the cords lie in completely adducted position, it will cause stridor and respiratory obstruction and will require urgent tracheostomy for relief of respiratory obstruction.

However, if the cord lies in a cadaveric position (midway between adduction and abduction) tracheostomy may be deferred.

Q. What is nonrecurrent laryngeal nerve?

Ans. The recurrent laryngeal nerve sometimes may not hook around innominate artery or the arch of aorta but may go directly to the larynx at higher level as a direct branch of the vagus. This is called a nonrecurrent inferior laryngeal nerve. This is often associated with absence of innominate artery.

Q. In which sex carcinoma thyroid is common?

Ans. Female:Male = 3:1.

Q. What is lateral aberrant thyroid?

Ans. In some cases of papillary carcinoma, the thyroid gland may be impalpable. Metastasis from occult papillary carcinoma may occur to cervical lymph node. The palpable lymph node due to metastasis from occult thyroid carcinoma is called a lateral aberrant thyroid.

Q. What are the different types of thyroid tumors?

Ans.
- Epithelial tumors
  - Benign
    - Follicular adenoma
    - Others including trabecular adenoma
  - Malignant
    - Follicular carcinoma: Minimally invasive, widely invasive and poorly differentiated
    - Papillary carcinoma: Microcarcinoma, follicular variant and sclerosing variant
    - Medullary carcinoma: Including mixed medullary and follicular
    - Others including anaplastic carcinomas
- Nonepithelial tumor
  - Benign: Hemangioma
  - Malignant: Angiosarcoma and others
- Malignant lymphoma
- Miscellaneous tumors.

Q. What is the etiology of thyroid cancer?

Ans.
- Radiation exposure to head, neck, and chest.
- Preexisting nodular goiter—usually predisposes to follicular carcinoma.
- Hashimoto thyroiditis may predispose to lymphoma.

Q. What are the histological features of papillary carcinoma?

Ans.
- Presence of papillae
- Ground glass clear nuclei in the cells
- Nuclear membrane irregularity
- Nuclear grooving of the cells
- Intranuclear or cytoplasmic inclusions.

Q. What is papillary microcarcinoma?

Ans.
- Initially regarded as occult carcinoma.
- Papillary carcinoma 1 cm or less in diameter is regarded as microcarcinoma.

Q. What is prognostic classification of thyroid tumors?

Ans.
- *Low-grade malignancy*:
  - Papillary carcinoma
  - Low-grade follicular carcinoma
  - Low-grade malignant lymphoma
- *Intermediate-grade malignancy*:
  - Tall cell and columnar variants of papillary carcinoma
  - Widely invasive follicular carcinoma
  - Medullary carcinoma
  - Mixed medullary and papillary carcinoma
  - Malignant lymphoma (large cell type)
- High-grade malignancy:
  - Undifferentiated carcinoma
  - Angiosarcoma
  - Other sarcomas.

Q. What are the relative incidences of different types of thyroid carcinomas?

Ans.
- Papillary carcinoma, 60–80%
- Follicular carcinoma, 5–25%
- Medullary carcinoma, 5–10%
- Undifferentiated (anaplastic) carcinomas, 4–10%.

Q. How will you treat this patient of papillary carcinoma with lymph node metastasis?

Ans. If confirmed by FNAC, I will do total thyroidectomy and modified radical neck dissection on the right side.

Q. If the tumor is confined to one lobe, what should be the operation?

Ans. If FNAC diagnosis is papillary carcinoma, the ideal surgical treatment is total thyroidectomy.

Q. What is the rationale of doing total thyroidectomy in differentiated thyroid cancer confined to one lobe?

Ans.
* This removes all intrathyroidal tumors including occult site of carcinomas in the other lobe and thereby decrease the possibility of recurrent cancer in the other lobe.
* Allows for whole body radioiodine scanning and ablation of metastatic disease with radioiodine.
* Renders serum thyroglobulin level more sensitive for detecting recurrent or metastatic disease.

Q. You have done lobectomy for a solitary thyroid nodule and the report has come as papillary carcinoma. How will you manage this patient?

Ans. This depends on histology report and some risk factors consideration.
* If the patient's age is less than 40 years, tumor is less than 1 cm, unifocal, intrathyroidal and well differentiated then lobectomy may be enough. Follow-up of the patient with full suppressive dose of L-thyroxine.
* If the patient is more than 40 years of age and the resected lobe shows multifocality, tumor is more than 1 cm in size, there is extrathyroidal extension of the tumor and the tumor is not well differentiated then completion thyroidectomy is to be done.

Q. Which factors are taken into consideration as prognostic marker for carcinoma thyroid?

Ans. The important risk factors are AGES:
* A = Age of the patient
* G = Grade of the tumor
* E = Extension of the tumor: Intrathyroidal or extrathyroidal
* S = Size of the tumor.

Q. What are the criteria of less risk-group (patient with good prognosis)?

Ans.
* A = Age less than 40 years in female and less than 50 years in male
* G = Grade of the tumor: Well differentiated
* E = Extent of the tumor: Intrathyroidal
* S = Size less than 1 cm for papillary carcinoma and less than 4 cm in follicular carcinoma.

Q. What are the criteria of high-risk group (patient with poor prognosis)?

Ans.
* A = Age more than 40 years in female and more than 50 years in male
* G = Grade: Poorly differentiated tumor
* E = Extent: Extrathyroidal
* S = Size more than 1 cm in papillary carcinoma and more than 4 cm in follicular carcinoma
* Presence of distant metastasis.

Q. What are the other risk factors assessment?

Ans.

* AMES:
  - A: Age less than 40 years better prognosis
  - M: Distant metastasis
  - E: Extent of primary tumor
  - S: Size of the primary tumor. Tumor less than 4 cm better prognosis
* MACIS:
  - M: Distant metastasis
  - A: Age of the patient
  - C: Completeness of resection
  - I: Local invasion/vascular invasion
  - S: Size of the tumour

Q. After hemithyroidectomy report has revealed it to be follicular carcinoma, what will you do?

Ans. If follicular carcinoma is of minimally invasive type then further surgery is rarely necessary and patient should be given full suppressive dose of L-thyroxine.

However, if follicular carcinoma is frankly invasive, completion thyroidectomy is to be done to facilitate subsequent management with whole body radioiodine scanning and follow-up with thyroglobulin study.

Q. What is the rationale of near-total thyroidectomy?

Ans. Thomas recommended near-total thyroidectomy for carcinoma thyroid. This procedure removes almost all parts of the thyroid except a rim of thyroid tissue along the tracheoesophageal groove to avoid injury to recurrent laryngeal nerve and to conserve the parathyroid glands.

Q. Which carcinoma of thyroid is grouped as differentiated thyroid carcinomas?

Ans. Papillary and follicular carcinomas are grouped as differentiated thyroid carcinomas.

Q. How will you treat lymph node in patients of differentiated thyroid carcinoma?

Ans.

* 40% of papillary carcinoma patient has lymph node metastasis at diagnosis.
* 10% of follicular carcinoma patient has lymph node metastasis at diagnosis.
* There is no role of prophylactic neck dissection in differentiated thyroid carcinomas.
* Once lymph nodes are involved, modified radical neck dissection is advisable with preservation of sternocleidomastoid muscle, internal jugular vein, and spinal accessory nerve.

Q. What is the role of L-thyroxine in follow-up of patients with differentiated thyroid cancer?

Ans. Differentiated thyroid carcinomas are TSH dependent. So in postoperative period supraphysiological dose of L-thyroxine is to be given to suppress endogenous TSH secretion. Dose up to 0.2–0.3 mg of L-thyroxine may be given to keep TSH level below 0.1 mIU/L or close to 0.01 mIU/L.

Q. When will you advise for whole body scanning following surgery?

Ans. Following total thyroidectomy, patient is not started on L-thyroxine supplement. Monitor TSH level. Usually in 4–6 weeks time, patient develops features of hypothyroidism and TSH level usually goes up to 100 mIu/L. Whole body scanning is to be done 4–6 weeks after total thyroidectomy. This will demonstrate any residual thyroid tissue in the thyroid region and may demonstrate any evidence of distant metastasis.

Q. When will you consider radioiodine scanning in follow-up?

Ans. If there is clinical evidence of recurrent or metastatic disease or thyroglobulin level shows an increase then radioiodine scanning is to be done to detect the site of metastatic disease.

Q. What precaution you should take while doing radioiodine scanning in follow-up period?

Ans. Patient on follow-up is usually kept on L-thyroxine replacement. Before doing radioiodine scanning L-thyroxine should be stopped for at least 4 weeks so that TSH level goes up. Patient may develop features of hypothyroidism during this period.

Triiodothyronine has a shorter half-life of about 7 days. Four to six weeks before radioiodine scanning patient may be switched on to triiodothyronine therapy instead of L-thyroxine and this can be discontinued for 7 days prior to radioiodine scanning.

Q. What is TNM staging for thyroid cancer? or, What is TNM staging for thyroid carcinoma?

Ans.
T: Primary tumor categories for thyroid cancer (other than anaplastic thyroid cancer)
- **TX:** Primary tumor cannot be assessed.
- **T0:** No evidence of primary tumor.
- **T1:** The tumor is 2 cm across or smaller and has not grown out of the thyroid.
  - **T1a:** The tumor is 1 cm across or smaller and has not grown outside the thyroid.
  - **T1b:** The tumor is larger than 1 cm but not larger than 2 cm across and has not grown outside of the thyroid.
- **T2:** The tumor is more than 2 cm but not larger than 4 cm across and has not grown out of the thyroid.
- **T3:** The tumor is larger than 4 cm across, or it has just begun to grow into nearby tissues outside the thyroid.
- **T4a:** The tumor is any size and has grown extensively beyond the thyroid gland into nearby tissues of the neck, such as the larynx, trachea, esophagus or the nerve to the larynx. Also called *moderately advanced disease.*
- **T4b:** The tumor is any size and has grown either back toward the spine or into nearby large blood vessels. This is also called *very advanced disease.*

T categories for anaplastic thyroid cancer:
- All anaplastic thyroid cancers are considered T4 tumors at the time of diagnosis.
- **T4a:** The tumor is still within the thyroid.
- **T4b:** The tumor has grown outside the thyroid.

N categories for thyroid cancer:

- **NX:** Regional lymph nodes cannot be assessed.
- **N0:** The cancer has not spread to nearby lymph nodes.
- **N1:** The cancer has spread to nearby lymph nodes.
  - **N1a:** The cancer has spread to lymph nodes around the thyroid in the neck (called *pretracheal, paratracheal,* and *prelaryngeal* lymph nodes).
  - **N1b:** The cancer has spread to other lymph nodes in the neck (called *cervical*) or to lymph nodes behind the throat (*retropharyngeal*) or in the upper chest (*superior mediastinal*).

M categories for thyroid cancer:

- **MX:** Distant metastasis cannot be assessed.
- **M0:** There is no distant metastasis.
- **M1:** The cancer has spread to other parts of the body, such as distant lymph nodes, internal organs, bones, etc.

Stage Grouping

Papillary or follicular (differentiated) thyroid cancer in patients younger than 45 years:

- Younger people have a low likelihood of dying from differentiated (papillary or follicular) thyroid cancer. The TNM stage groupings for these cancers take this fact into account. So, all people younger than 45 years with these cancers are *stage I* if they have no distant spread and *stage II* if they have distant spread.
- *Stage I (any T, any N, M0):* Tumor can be any size (any T) and may or may not have spread to nearby lymph nodes (any N). It has not spread to distant sites (M0).
- *Stage II (any T, any N, M1):* The tumor can be any size (any T) and may or may not have spread to nearby lymph nodes (any N). It has spread to distant sites (M1).
- *Papillary or follicular (differentiated) thyroid cancer in patients 45 years and older:*
- *Stage I (T1, N0, M0):* The tumor is 2 cm or less across and has not grown outside the thyroid (T1). It has not spread to nearby lymph nodes (N0) or distant sites (M0).
- *Stage II (T2, N0, M0):* The tumor is more than 2 cm but not larger than 4 cm across and has not grown outside the thyroid (T2). It has not spread to nearby lymph nodes (N0) or distant sites (M0).
- *Stage III:* One of the following applies:
  - *T3, N0, M0:* The tumor is larger than 4 cm across or has grown slightly outside the thyroid (T3), but it has not spread to nearby lymph nodes (N0) or distant sites (M0).
  - *T1 to T3, N1a, M0:* The tumor is any size and may have grown slightly outside the thyroid (T1 to T3). It has spread to lymph nodes around the thyroid in the neck (N1a) but not to other lymph nodes or to distant sites (M0).
- *Stage IVA:* One of the following applies:
  - *T4a, any N, M0:* The tumor is any size and has grown beyond the thyroid gland and into nearby tissues of the neck (T4a). It might or might not have spread to nearby lymph nodes (any N). It has not spread to distant sites (M0).
  - *T1 to T3, N1b, M0:* The tumor is any size and might have grown slightly outside the thyroid gland (T1 to T3). It has spread to certain lymph nodes in the neck (cervical nodes) or

to lymph nodes in the upper chest (superior mediastinal nodes) or behind the throat (retropharyngeal nodes) (N1b), but it has not spread to distant sites (M0).

- *Stage IVB (T4b, any N, M0)*: The tumor is any size and has grown either back toward the spine or into nearby large blood vessels (T4b). It might or might not have spread to nearby lymph nodes (any N), but it has not spread to distant sites (M0).
- *Stage IVC (any T, any N, M1)*: The tumor is any size and might or might not have grown outside the thyroid (any T). It might or might not have spread to nearby lymph nodes (any N). It has spread to distant sites (M1).

Medullary Thyroid Cancer

- Age is not a factor in the stage of medullary thyroid cancer (MTC).
- *Stage I (T1, N0, M0)*: The tumor is 2 cm or less across and has not grown outside the thyroid (T1). It has not spread to nearby lymph nodes (N0) or distant sites (M0).
- *Stage II*: One of the following applies:
  - T2, N0, M0: The tumor is more than 2 cm but is not larger than 4 cm across and has not grown outside the thyroid (T2). It has not spread to nearby lymph nodes (N0) or distant sites (M0).
  - T3, N0, M0: The tumor is larger than 4 cm or has grown slightly outside the thyroid (T3), but it has not spread to nearby lymph nodes (N0) or distant sites (M0).
- *Stage III (T1 to T3, N1a, M0)*: The tumor is any size and might have grown slightly outside the thyroid (T1 to T3). It has spread to lymph nodes around the thyroid in the neck (N1a) but not to other lymph nodes or to distant sites (M0).
- *Stage IVA*: One of the following applies:
  - T4a, any N, M0: The tumor is any size and has grown beyond the thyroid gland and into nearby tissues of the neck (T4a). It might or might not have spread to nearby lymph nodes (any N). It has not spread to distant sites (M0).
  - T1 to T3, N1b, M0: The tumor is any size and might have grown slightly outside the thyroid gland (T1 to T3). It has spread to certain lymph nodes in the neck (cervical nodes) or to lymph nodes in the upper chest (superior mediastinal nodes) or behind the throat (retropharyngeal nodes) (N1b), but it has not spread to distant sites (M0).
- *Stage IVB (T4b, any N, M0)*: The tumor is any size and has grown either back toward the spine or into nearby large blood vessels (T4b). It might or might not have spread to nearby lymph nodes (any N), but it has not spread to distant sites (M0).
- *Stage IVC (any T, any N, M1)*: The tumor is any size and might or might not have grown outside the thyroid (any T). It might or might not have spread to nearby lymph nodes (any N). It has spread to distant sites (M1).

Anaplastic (Undifferentiated) Thyroid Cancer

- All anaplastic thyroid cancers are considered stage IV, reflecting the poor prognosis of this type of cancer.
- *Stage IVA (T4a, any N, M0)*: The tumor is still within the thyroid (T4a). It might or might not have spread to nearby lymph nodes (any N), but it has not spread to distant sites (M0).

* *Stage IVB (T4b, any N, M0)*: The tumor has grown outside the thyroid (T4b). It might or might not have spread to nearby lymph nodes (any N), but it has not spread to distant sites (M0).
* *Stage IVC (any T, any N, M1)*: The tumor might or might not have grown outside of the thyroid (any T). It might or might not have spread to nearby lymph nodes (any N). It has spread to distant sites (M1).

Q. What should be follow-up protocol for differentiated thyroid carcinoma (DTC)?

Ans.

* After surgery whole body scanning with radioiodine is done after 4–6 weeks. If there is no residual thyroid tissue in the neck or no distant metastasis, keep the patient on full suppressive doses of L-thyroxine.
* Follow-up whole body radioiodine scanning after 6 month. Before whole body scanning, stop L-thyroxine for 1 month.
* Estimation of thyroglobulin.
* If both are normal, continue suppressive therapy with L-thyroxine.
* Continue follow-up with clinical evaluation and thyroglobulin study at 3 months interval for initial 2 years, then at 6 months interval for 3 years and then yearly.
* If thyroglobulin shows rising level then whole body radioiodine scanning is to be done. Before whole body scanning stop L-thyroxine for 1 month. If radioiodine scanning showed any metastasis, treat the metastasis with ablative dosages of radioiodine.

Q. How does papillary carcinoma spread?

Ans.

* *Local spread*: It may invade thyroid gland capsules and become extrathyroidal.
* *Lymphatic spread*: It spread to cervical lymph node.
* Blood spread is rare.

Q. How does follicular carcinoma spread?

Ans.

* Local spread
* Blood spread is common
* Lymphatic spread is rare.

Q. What are the advantages of using T3 in postoperative period over T4?

Ans. T3 may be used in a dose of 60–80 µg/day.

* Shorter acting and on stopping, the TSH and thyroid avidity for iodine recurs quickly so that radioiodine scan can be done after one week of stopping T3 therapy.
* Thus, patients are spared of thyroid insufficiency over weeks.

Q. What is the role of thyroglobulin assay in postoperative period?

Ans.

* Patient who has undergone total thyroidectomy has thyroglobulin level of less than 3 ng/mL. A high level of thyroglobulin suggests persistent, recurrent disease in the neck or metastatic disease.
* In follow-up of patient thyroglobulin should be estimated at 3 monthly intervals initially for 2 years and later on annually.

◆ Serial thyroglobulin assay may obviate the need for whole body radioiodine scanning, if thyroglobulin is normal. If thyroglobulin is raised, radioiodine scanning may be done to localize the metastatic disease.

■ DISCUSSION ON ANAPLASTIC THYROID CARCINOMA

Q. What are the important points for diagnosis of anaplastic carcinoma of thyroid?

Ans.
◆ Usually involves elderly female patients.
◆ Rapid increase in size of the swelling.
◆ Compressive symptoms like hoarseness of voice, difficulty in breathing and difficulty in swallowing may be present.
◆ On examination, there is hard, diffuse irregular enlargement of the thyroid gland, which is immobile being fixed to the underlying structures. The carotid pulses are not palpable. The cervical lymph nodes may be palpable.

Q. How will you treat patient with anaplastic carcinoma?

Ans. The diagnosis may be confirmed by a FNAC or trucut needle biopsy.
◆ A curative resection is not possible in majority of patients with anaplastic carcinoma as the tumor is aggressive in nature.
◆ Anisthmusectomy or isthmusectomy may be done to relieve tracheal compression and obtain tissue for histopathological examination.
◆ Tracheostomy is to be avoided.
◆ Palliative radiotherapy may be tried.
◆ Combination chemotherapy has been tried but not very effective.

Q. How will you manage residual thyroid tissue in the neck following near-total thyroidectomy for thyroid cancer?

Ans.
◆ Whole body radioiodine scanning and radioiodine uptake in the neck is done.
◆ Uptake in the neck 1% or less with a negative body scan—a dose of 29 mCi of ^{131}I is given to ablate the residual thyroid tissue (OPD treatment).
◆ Uptake in the neck more than 1% and/or if metastatic foci is found a larger therapeutic dose of 100–300 mCi of ^{131}I is given (requires isolation in hospital).
◆ If there is substantial amount of thyroid tissue in the neck reoperation and surgical ablation may be considered.

Q. What are Hürthle cell tumors?

Ans. This is a variant of follicular cell neoplasm. This arises from the oxyphilic cells of the thyroid gland. The functions of these cells are unknown but these cells have TSH receptors and secrete thyroglobulin.

Q. What is the behavior of Hürthle cell tumors?

Ans. Majority of the Hürthle cell tumors are benign. Only 20% of Hürthle cell tumors are malignant. Like follicular neoplasm, it is difficult to differentiate Hürthle cell adenoma and carcinoma in FNAC. In Hürthle cell carcinoma, there is evidence of capsular and vascular invasion.

Q. What are the characteristics of Hürthle cell carcinomas?

Ans. The Hurtle cell carcinomas are more often multifocal, bilateral, and there is higher incidence of lymph node metastasis (25%).

Q. Which radionuclide scan is helpful in the diagnosis of metastasis from Hürthle cell tumor?

Ans. 99mTc labeled sestamibi scan is required to detect metastatic foci from Hürthle cell tumor.

Q. How will you treat Hürthle cell tumors?

Ans.

* *Hürthle cell neoplasm confined to one lobe*: Hemithyroidectomy—if frozen section biopsy shows carcinoma, total thyroidectomy and central lymph node dissection.
* *Hürthle cell carcinoma diagnosed by trucut needle biopsy*: Total thyroidectomy with central lymph node dissection.
* If there are palpable lymph nodes, total thyroidectomy is to be combined with modified radical neck dissection.
* Patient should be given full suppressive dose of L-thyroxine postoperatively.

■ DISCUSSION ON MEDULLARY CARCINOMA OF THYROID

Q. Where from medullary thyroid carcinoma arises?

Ans. The medullary carcinoma of thyroid arises from parafollicular cell (or C cell) of thyroid gland. The C cells are derived from neural crest and from a part of APUD system (amine precursor uptake and decarboxylation). The highest concentration of cell is found near the upper pole of the thyroid gland.

Q. What is the background for suspecting a diagnosis of medullary carcinoma of thyroid?

Ans. It is difficult to give a clinical diagnosis of medullary carcinoma of thyroid. The diagnosis may be suspected in cases:

* Patients presents with symptoms and signs like carcinoma thyroid (increasing neck mass, features of compression—dyspnea, dysphagia, and hoarseness).
* In addition, there may be family history of thyroid carcinoma (in 30% cases).
* The lymph nodes are more commonly involved in medullary thyroid carcinoma.
* There may be history of hypertension due to associated pheochromocytoma or other features of multiple endocrine neoplasia.

Q. What is the genetic basis of MTC?

Ans. Apart from sporadic MTC, the other type of medullary carcinoma in MEN 2A and MEN 2B, and familial MTC has genetic basis. It has autosomal dominant inheritance. The RET proto-oncogene in chromosome number 10 is the genetic marker.

Q. What is the implication of C cell hyperplasia?

Ans. Medullary thyroid carcinoma is preceded by C cell hyperplasia and high-risk family members of MTC patients may exhibit C cell hyperplasia.

Q. What are the secretory products from C cells in MTC?

Ans. As a part of APUD system, C cells may secrete:
- Calcitonin
- Carcinoembryonic antigen (CEA)
- Histaminase
- Calcitonin gene-related peptide
- Serotonin
- Chromogranin
- Substance P
- Somatostatin
- Vasoactive intestinal peptide (VIP)
- Prostaglandin
- Adrenocorticotropic hormone (ACTH)
- Thyroid-stimulating hormone.

Q. What are the pathological features of MTC?

Ans.
- MTC is usually a circumscribed nonencapsulated white mass.
- In sporadic form it is mostly solitary.
- In familial form it is usually bilateral and multicentric.
- C-cell hyperplasia is present in familial MT.
- Microscopically MTC shows tumor cell in nests and sheets, nuclei are round or oval with chromatin. Binucleate cells and pseudoinclusion may be seen. The characteristic amyloid may be seen both in stroma and inside the cells
- Immunohistochemistry reveals calcitonin in amyloid.

Q. What are the different forms of MTC?

Ans. The different forms of MTC may be:
- *Sporadic*: 70%
  - Fifth decade
  - Presentation as a solitary thyroid nodule
  - 50% has lymphadenopathy
  - 30% has associated watery diarrhea
  - Rarely flushing and Cushing's syndrome
  - No positive family history.
- *MEN 2A*:
  - Third decade
  - Medullary thyroid cancer
  - 50% associated pheochromocytoma

- 30% parathyroid hyperplasia
- May be associated with amyloidosis or Hirschsprung's disease
* *MEN 2B*:
    - Second decade
    - MTC most virulent type
    - Pheochromocytoma (unilateral or bilateral)
    - Multiple intestinal mucosal and cutaneous neuromas
* *Familial medullary thyroid carcinoma (FMTC) without other endocrinopathies*:
    - Most indolent form of MTC
    - Runs in family
    - No other associated endocrine disease.

Q. FNAC from a solitary thyroid nodule revealed MTC. What should you do next?

Ans.

It is important to exclude other associated endocrine neoplasia.
* Take detailed family history to exclude any familial endocrinopathy.
* History of hypertension, headache to exclude pheochromocytoma.
* Tests for 24 hours urinary catecholamines, vanilylmandelic acid and metanephrine to exclude pheochromocytoma.
* Serum calcium and parathormone assay.

Q. How will you screen family members for MTC?

Ans.

* Test for RET proto-oncogene. If RET proto-oncogene is negative unlikely to inherit MTC
* Stimulated-calcitonin testing:
    - Estimate basal calcitonin
    - Pentagastrin injection given at a dose of 6 μg/kg subcutaneously. If there is rise of calcitonin, the test is positive
    - 50% sensitivity.

Q. Why it is important to exclude pheochromocytoma?

Ans. Associated pheochromocytoma should be excluded by relevant tests. Operation in a patient with undiagnosed pheochromocytoma may result in hypertensive crisis and death.

Q. If there is associated pheochromocytoma how will you proceed?

Ans. Treat pheochromocytoma first with adrenalectomy after proper preparation and then treat medullary carcinoma of the thyroid.

Q. How will you treat MTC?

Ans.

* Total thyroidectomy with central node dissection (level 6) even if there is no palpable nodes in the neck.
* If lymph node are palpable, total thyroidectomy with modified radical node dissection along with central node dissection.

Q. When will you consider prophylactic thyroidectomy in familial or MEN 2A or MEN 2B associated MTC?

Ans. If RET proto-oncogene is positive, total thyroidectomy may be considered as early as 5 years of age in family members of MEN 2A and FMTC. In MEN 2B, total thyroidectomy may be considered as early as first year of life.

Q. How will you manage parathyroid hyperplasia in MEN 2A setting?

Ans. There is associated parathyroid hyperplasia in MEN 2A. The options are:
- Total parathyroidectomy and autotransplantation of one parathyroid in nondominant forearm or sternocleidomastoid muscle.
- Subtotal parathyroidectomy with in situ preservation of half of one parathyroid gland.

Q. What happens to calcitonin level in MTC in postoperative period?

Ans. The hypercalcitoninemia persist in 50–80% cases of hereditary MTC and 50–55% cases of sporadic MTC in postoperative period.

Q. What should be the treatment for persistent hypercalcitoninemia?

Ans.
- The various treatment options for this include observation in asymptomatic or minimally symptomatic patients and reoperation in symptomatic case.
- Other nonsurgical options include radiotherapy, chemotherapy and interferon administration.
- Even after reoperation calcitonin rarely comes down to normal.

Q. What are the prognostic factors in MTC?

Ans.
- MEN 2A, FMTC has better prognosis than MEN 2B and sporadic form
- Tumor stage
- Plasma calcitonin level
- Plasma CEA level
- DNA ploidy.

Q. What are the blood supplies of parathyroid glands?

Ans.
- *Superior parathyroid gland*: Inferior or superior thyroid artery or an anastomotic loop between the two.
- *Interior parathyroid gland*: From inferior thyroid artery.

Q. Can all parathyroid gland be preserved during total thyroidectomy?

Ans.
- In cases without any invasion of parathyroid gland total thyroidectomy may be done preserving all parathyroid glands.
- The incidence of hypoparathyroidism after total thyroidectomy is less than 1%.

Q. If after total thyroidectomy blood supplies to the parathyroid glands are compromised, what will you do?

Ans. If blood supplies to the parathyroid glands are compromised, parathyroid glands appear dusky after 20–30 minutes. Parathyroid glands are removed, cut into fragments and implanted into sternocleidomastoid muscle or on nondominant forearm muscle.

Q. If there is extrathyroidal extension of thyroid cancer, how will you treat?

Ans. Differentiated thyroid cancers are usually slow growing. May invade the strap muscles or invade into the trachea, esophagus, larynx or major vessels in the neck.

- If invaded into the strap muscles, the strap muscles may be excised along with the thyroid gland.
- If invaded into trachea, esophagus or larynx, the trachea/esophagus/larynx may be resected along with the thyroid gland and reconstruction may be done.

Q. What is the role of L-thyroxine in follow-up of patient with differentiated thyroid carcinoma?

Ans.
- Following near-total and total thyroidectomy
- Thyroxine is required as a replacement therapy

In DTC, dose should prevent hypothyroidism and should keep TSH to low level less than 0.1 mIU/L.

- Data has shown that foci of DTC have regressed with thyroid hormone. Following hemithyroidectomy for differentiated thyroid cancer L-thyroxine is indicated in full suppressive dose and it has been found to be beneficial to prevent recurrence in the residual thyroid tissue and in presence of recurrence reduce the growth of the tumor.
- Clinical data establishes improved overall 10 years and 20 years survival rate in patients who are given thyroid hormone replacement therapy in postoperative period.

Varicose Veins

OUTLINE FOR WRITING A LONG CASE OF VARICOSE VEINS

■ HISTORY

- *Particulars of the patient*
- *Chief complaints:*
  - Swelling along the veins in (right/left) lower limb for .... months/years
  - Pain in right/left lower limb for ....
  - Pigmentation of skin in the leg for ....
  - Ulcer in right/left leg for ....
- *History of present illness*
  - *Swelling*
    - *Onset*—sudden or insidious
    - Duration
    - Where did it start and progress?
    - Relation of the swelling to standing, walking
    - Whether the swelling reduces or disappears on lying down
    - Any pain or color change along the course of the vein (suggesting thrombophlebitis).
  - Pain
    - Onset—acute or insidious
    - Site of pain
    - *Character of pain*—dull aching/cramping
    - Severity
    - *Time of occurrence*—on walking (intermittent claudication) or towards the end of the day
    - *Aggravating factors*—walking/standing
    - *Relieving factors*—lying down
    - Any night cramps.

    (Characteristics of pain in case of varicose vein—usually dull aching pain in the calves and lower legs, occurs towards the end of the day and is relieved by lying down for about 15–30 minutes).
  - Ulcer
    - *Mode of onset*—how it started
    - Duration

- Site
- Any associated pain
- Any discharge, bleeding.
- Any itching
- Any change in skin color
- Any pain in abdomen
- Any lump in lower abdomen
- *Bladder habit*—any obstructive symptoms
- *Bowel habit*—any history of increasing constipation
- Any other systemic symptoms.
- *Past history:*
  - Any major ailment in the past
  - Any history suggestive of deep venous thrombosis. Pain and swelling in the calf associated with fever
  - Any history of hospitalization or prolonged immobilization in bed.
- *Personal history:*
  - Any history of oral pill intake
  - Smoking
  - Does the occupation involve standing for long time?
- *Family history:*
  - Any family history of similar disease.
- *Treatment history:*
  - Any history of operation
  - Whether using elastic stockinette
  - Injection treatment.
- *History of allergy.*

PHYSICAL EXAMINATION

- *General survey*
- *Local examination:* Examination of both lower limbs.
  - *Inspection:* Describe the diseased limb first. Patient is initially examined in standing position and asked to lie down while eliciting some tests
  - Attitude of the limbs
  - Deformity
  - *Local gigantism*—compare two sides
  - Which venous system is affected:
    - Great saphenous system
    - Short saphenous system
    - Communicating veins and the tributaries
    - Both great and short saphenous system.
  - *Extent of involvement:* From dorsum of foot to the level above, e.g. varicosity of great saphenous system of vein extending from dorsum of foot to upper thigh. Some varicose communicating veins are also seen.

- Skin of the leg:
  - *Pigmentation*—dark red or black spots
  - Eczema in leg
  - *Ulcer in the leg (describe details of ulcer)*—site, shape, size, edge, floor, discharge, and area surrounding the ulcer
  - *Venous stars*—this consists of a number of minute veins radiating from a single feeding vein.
- Look for any cough impulse at saphenous opening (Morrissey's test).

Palpation

- Feel for any tenderness or thickening of veins along its course
- Feel for any cough impulse at saphenofemoral (SF) junction
- *Trendelenburg's test:* Positive or negative (+/+, +/-, and -/+).
  - Keeping the tourniquet tied if the superficial veins get distended then first component of Trendelenburg's test is said to be positive. This suggests perforator incompetence below the SF junction. Afterwards release tourniquet and look for further filling from above. If there is further filling from above, suggests SF incompetents.
  - On releasing the tourniquet immediately after standing—if the superficial veins get filled quickly from above, the second component of Trendelenburg's test is said to be positive. This suggests incompetence of SF junction.
- Two tourniquet test at the level of each known perforator—comment which perforators are incompetent
- *Schwartz test:* Positive or negative
- *Fegan's test:* Crescentic gap felt in the deep fascia. Comment at what level the gap is felt
- *Modified Perthes' test:* Positive or negative
- Palpation of the ulcer in the leg
- *Palpation of arterial pulses in the leg*—femoral/popliteal/posterior tibial/dorsalis pedis.

Auscultation

- *Along the dilated veins:* Presence of bruit suggest arteriovenous fistula.
- *Examination of other limb*—Normal.

■ VARICOSE VEINS

Q. What is your case? (Summary of a case of varicose vein)

Ans. This 45-year-old gentleman presented with insidious onset of swelling of veins along the inner aspect of the right leg for last 3 years. Patient noticed the swelling along the vein which started in the lower part of right leg around the ankle and later the swelling extended up to the upper part of the thigh. The swelling gets aggravated after prolonged standing and walking. The swelling along the vein reduces and sometimes disappears on lying down. Patient complains of dull aching pain in right calf region for last 2 years. The pain is experienced towards the evening. There is no history of intermittent claudication. Patient complains of dark pigmentation of skin around the ankle for last 1 year. There is no history of ulcer in the leg. His bladder and bowel habits are normal. He does not complain of any lump in abdomen and there are no other systemic complain. There is no history of major ailment in the past and there is no history suggestive of deep venous thrombosis. Patient's profession involves long hours of standing (waiter in a hotel) (Fig. 7.1).

On examination, general survey is essentially normal. On local examination of lower limbs, there is varicosity affecting the great saphenous system of the right lower limb along with some varicosity of communicating veins between the long and short saphenous system of veins. Some tributaries of great saphenous vein (GSV) in the thigh and leg are also found dilated. There is dark pigmentation in the right leg more marked around the ankle. Trendelenburg's test is positive suggesting incompetence at the SF junction and some perforator incompetence at the lower levels. Multiple tourniquet tests revealed perforator incompetence at adductor

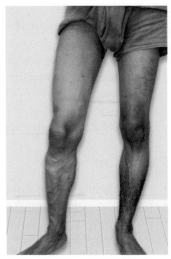

Fig. 7.1: Varicose vein affecting the right lower limb

canal, below knee perforator, and at 15 cm and 5 cm medial ankle perforator. Schwartz test is positive. Fegan's test is positive and a gap can be felt in the deep fascia at 15 cm and 5 cm above the medial malleolus. Modified Perthes' test is negative suggesting that deep veins are patent. Arterial pulses in the lower limbs are normal. There is no bruit on auscultation along the dilated veins in the leg. Systemic examination is normal.

Q. What is your diagnosis?

Ans. This is a case of varicose vein affecting great saphenous system of vein in right lower limb with perforator incompetence at SF junction, below knee perforator, and 5 cm ankle perforator without any clinical evidence of deep venous thrombosis.

As per clinical-etiologic-anatomic-pathophysiologic (CEAP) classification—$C_{S4a}E_pA_{SP}P_R$.

Q. How will you do inspection?

Ans. In inspection ascertain which system of veins is affected by varicosity. Look at the leg from front, back, and the side to ascertain which veins are affected by varicosity (Figs 7.2A to C).

Q. How will you do Trendelenburg's test?

Ans. There are two components of Trendelenburg's test:
1. Patient is asked to lie down and the superficial veins are emptied by elevating and milking the leg (Figs 7.3A to C). The tourniquet is tied below the saphenous opening and the patient is asked to stand (Fig. 7.3D). The tourniquet is kept tied for 2–3 minutes and the condition of the superficial veins are observed, then the tourniquet is released and look for filling from above.

If the veins start getting dilated with the tourniquet kept tied below the saphenous opening, this suggests there is some perforator incompetence below the SF junction. The Trendelenburg's test is said to be positive. Release the tourniquet. If there is further filling from above, this suggests there is incompetence of SF junction. The test may be described as positive and positive (+ +).

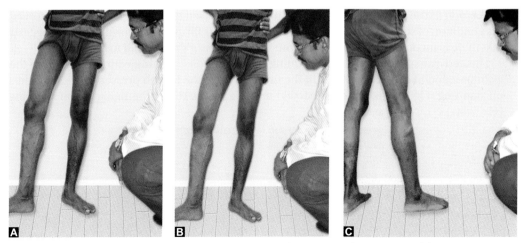

Figs 7.2A to C: (A) Look from the front; (B) Look from the sides to assess the varicosity of the communicating veins and the tributaries; (C) Look from the back to assess the varicosity affecting the short saphenous system

If on releasing the tourniquet there is no further filling from above, the test may be described as positive and negative (+ –).

If keeping the tourniquet tied, there is no filling of veins from below then the test is negative. If on releasing the tourniquet there is filling from above, the test may be described as negative and positive (– +).

2. Patient is asked to lie down on the bed. The veins are emptied by elevating the leg and by milking the vein (Figs 7.3A to C). A tourniquet is tied below the saphenous opening and the patient is asked to stand.

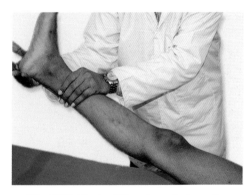

Fig. 7.3A: Start milking the vein from the region of ankle

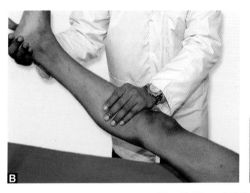

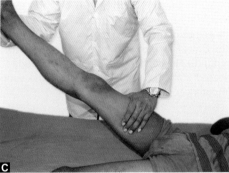

Figs 7.3B and C: Emptying the vein

As soon as the patient stands, the tourniquet is released quickly (Fig. 7.3E) and observed the condition of superficial veins. If the superficial veins fill quickly from above, this suggests that there is incompetence of SF junction. Trendelenburg's test is said to be positive.

This test can also be done by occluding the saphenous opening with the thumb of the examiner and like tourniquet test in the first test, keep the thumb pressed for 2–3 minutes on standing (Fig. 7.3F) and in the second test release the thumb immediately on standing (Fig. 7.3G).

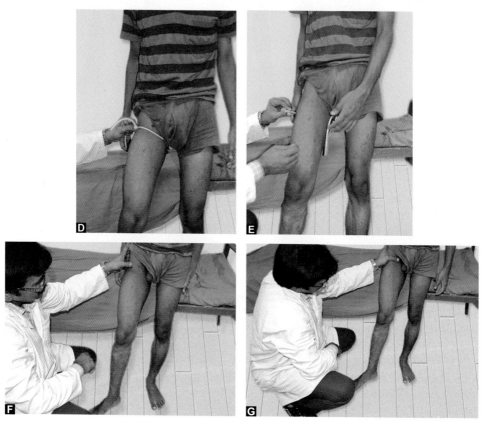

Figs 7.3D to G: (D) A tourniquet is tied and the patient is asked to stand, look for filling of vein from below; (E) On standing, the tourniquet is released immediately. if there is quick filling of vein from above, suggest incompetence of saphenofemoral junction; (F) Trendelenburg test: saphenous opening kept occluded by thumb. Note: Filling of vein from below suggests some perforator incompetence below the saphenous opening; (G) The saphenous opening is occluded by pressing with the thumb. On standing the thumb is released immediately. Quick filling of the varicosity from above suggests saphenofemoral junction incompetence

Q. How will you find the saphenofemoral junction?

Ans. The SF junction (termination of GSV into the femoral vein) lies at the saphenous opening which is situated 3.5 cm below and lateral to the pubic tubercle. Mark the pubic tubercle and measure 3.5 cm below the pubic tubercle and 3.5 cm lateral to it (Figs 7.4A and B).

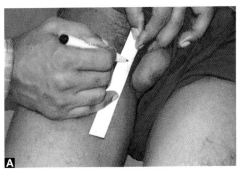 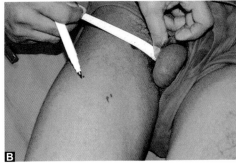

Figs 7.4A and B: Measure 3.5 cm below the pubic tubercle and mask the point; (B) Measure 3.5 cm laterally and the saphenous opening is marked

Q. How will you mark the pubic tubercle?

Ans. Pubic tubercle is found out by asking the patient to adduct the leg against resistance and follow the taut adductor longus tendon to reach the pubic tubercle (Fig. 7.5).

Q. How will you test for other perforator incompetence?

Ans. There are some constant perforators communicating the GSV to the deep vein. These perforators may be tested by two tourniquet test.

The veins are emptied and two tourniquets are tied one above and below and the perforator to be tested. When the patient is asked to stand, the segment of the vein between the two tourniquets will become varicose if the particular perforator is incompetent (Figs 7.6A to G).

Q. How will you do Schwartz test?

Ans. The patient is asked to stand. Keep one finger at the saphenous opening and tap the dilated vein lower down in the leg. The test is said to be positive when an impulse is palpable at the saphenous opening on tapping the vein at the lower level. Positive Schwartz test is found in gross varicosity of the veins (Figs 7.7A and B).

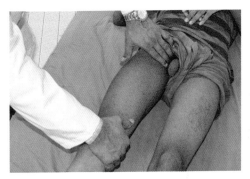

Fig. 7.5: Finding the pubic tubercle by following the taut adductor longus tendon

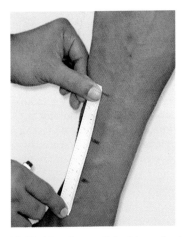

Fig. 7.6A: Marking the medial ankle perforators at 5 cm, 10 cm and 15 cm above the medial malleolus

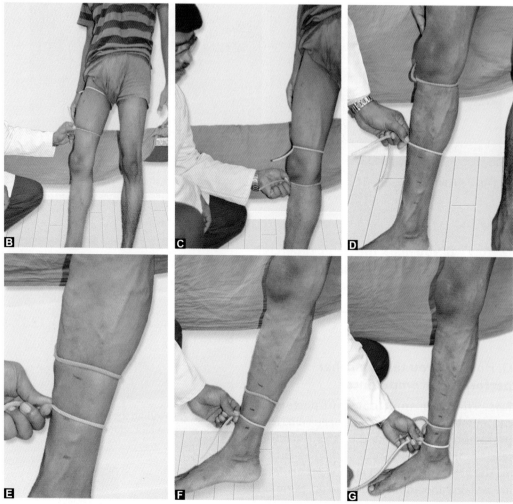

Figs 7.6B to G: (B) Testing the adductor canal perforator—no filling of vein in between the tourniquet—adductor canal perforator is competent; (C) Testing the above knee perforator—no filling of vein in between the tourniquet—above knee perforator competent; (D) Testing the below knee perforator. *Note*: The varicosity appearing keeping the tourniquet tied, suggesting incompetence of the below knee perforator; (E) Testing medial ankle perforator at 15 cm level. *Note*: No filling of vein in between the tourniquet—15 cm perforator is competent; (F) Testing medial ankle perforator at 10 cm level. No filling of vein in between the tourniquet—10 cm perforator is competent; (G) Testing medial ankle perforator at 5 cm level. Note: The filling of vein in between the tourniquet 5 cm perforator is incompetent

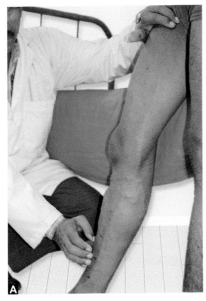 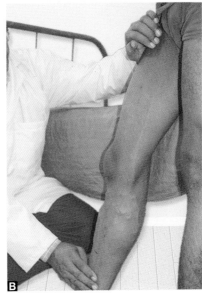

Figs 7.7A and B: Keep one hand at saphenous opening and tap the vein below; B) Keep one hand over the great saphenous vein above the ankle and tap over the great saphenous vein near the saphenous opening

Q. What is Fegan's test?

Ans. Fegan's test is a technique to localize the dilated perforating veins (The perforating veins connect the superficial veins to the deep veins and pierces the deep fascia of the leg to drain into the deep vein. When the perforating veins are incompetent and dilated this causes stretching of the deep fascia).

The course of the GSV is marked. The veins are emptied and the sites of known perforator area are palpated with a finger (Fig. 7.8). The sites where perforators are incompetent and dilated a crescentic gap may be felt in the deep fascia.

Q. How will you do modified Perthes' test?

Ans. A tourniquet is tied below the saphenous opening with the veins being full. Ask the patient to walk for about 3–5 minutes (Figs 7.9A to D).

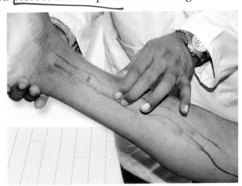

Fig. 7.8: Fegan's test

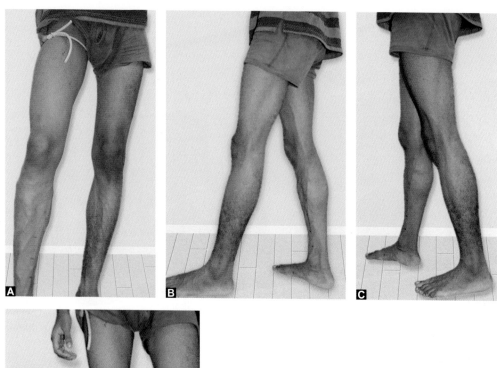

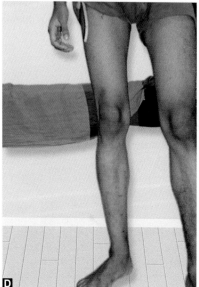

Figs 7.9A to D: (A) Tie tourniquet below the saphenous opening with the veins being full. The test is done in standing position; (B and C) Ask the patient to walk briskly for 2–3 minutes; (D) Observe the vein after walking. *Note:* The distended vein has collapsed after walking, suggesting that the deep veins are patent. Modified Perthes' test is negative

If the deep veins are patent, the dilated superficial veins will collapse. However, if the deep veins are occluded by thrombosis then the superficial veins will become more distended and patient will complain of bursting pain in the leg. This is said to be positive Perthes' test.

Q. What do you mean by positive Perthes' test?

Ans. In modified Perthes' test, a tourniquet is tied below the saphenous opening with the veins being full. Patient is asked to walk for few minutes. A positive Perthes' test means the superficial veins become further dilated and tortuous, and patient complains of severe bursting pain in the leg. This suggests an occluded deep venous system due to previous deep venous thrombosis.

Q. Do you like to demonstrate Homans' or Moses' sign to ascertain deep venous thrombosis in this patient?

Ans. No, because these signs are found only in acute deep venous thrombosis.

Q. What is CEAP classification of lower extremity venous disease?

Ans. The severity of venous disease is assessed by CEAP. The CEAP classification of varicose vein:
- *C: Clinical severity of the disease* expressed as C0–C6 and may be asymptomatic (A) or symptomatic (S)
  - *C0:* No apparent disease
  - *C1:* Telangiectasia or reticular veins
  - *C2:* Varicose veins
  - *C3:* Presence of edema
  - *C4:* Skin changes
  - *C4a:* Pigmentation/eczema
  - *C4b:* Lipodermatosclerosis/Atrophie blanche
  - *C5:* Healed ulcer
  - *C6:* Active venous ulcer
  - *Asymptomatic:* A
  - *Symptomatic:* S.
- *Etiologic classification: E:* Congenital, primary, or secondary
  - *Ec:* Congenital, present since birth
  - *Ep:* Primary—paucity of valves or weakness of veins
  - *Es:* Secondary—varicose vein secondary to deep vein thrombosis.
- *Anatomic classification: A:* May involve superficial, deep, or perforating veins alone or in combination
  - *As:* Involvement of superficial veins
  - *Ad:* Involvement of deep veins
  - *Ap:* Involvement of perforator veins.
  - The anatomical involvement may be alone or in combination.
- *Pathophysiologic classification: P:* Disease due to reflux of flow or obstruction alone or in combination
  - *PR:* Due to reflux
  - *PO:* Due to obstruction
  - *PRO:* Combination of reflux and obstruction.

Q. How will you manage this patient?

Ans. I will do some investigations to confirm my diagnosis.

Duplex imaging of the venous system of the lower limb.

* This is the combined study of veins with B-mode ultrasonography coupled with Doppler flow study with a Doppler probe.
* The anatomical delineation of the deep vein and the patency of the deep veins may be assessed. The normal deep veins are compressible. If the deep veins are occluded by thrombus, the vein is not compressible. The thrombus in the deep vein may be seen.
* The venous reflux may be demonstrated. The examination is done with the patient in standing position when the veins are full.
* The vein to be studied is imaged first. The Doppler ultrasound (US) probe is then applied over that vein and the calf muscle is squeezed to produce forward flow which is shown as blue in the color flow map. The calf is then released—the competent valves show no reverse flow but the incompetent valve allows reverse flow which is represented as red in the color flow map. The functional assessment and the site of reflux may be precisely localized. SF, saphenopopliteal reflux, and reflux at the sites of other perforators may be demonstrated.

Q. Would you like to do an ascending venography?

Ans. If the facility of duplex scanning is available it is possible to have good delineation of the vessel anatomy and ascending venography is not essential.

Q. What other investigations will you do in this case?

Ans. I will suggest some investigations to assess patient's fitness for anesthesia:

* Blood for complete hemogram Hb%, total leukocyte count (TLC), differential leukocyte count (DLC), and erythrocyte sedimentation rate (ESR)
* Blood for sugar, urea, and creatinine
* Chest X-ray
* Electrocardiography (ECG).

Q. How will you treat this patient?

Ans. This patient has varicosity of great saphenous system and there is perforator incompetence at SF junction, adductor canal, and 15 cm and 5 cm ankle perforator with a patent deep venous system.

* I will consider surgical treatment of the varicose vein in this patient
* I will do SF flush ligation, stripping of GSV up to the upper calf, and ligation of perforators at 15 cm and 5 cm above the ankle.

Q. What will happen if you ligate the great saphenous vein little away from the saphenofemoral junction?

Ans. The ideal procedure is flush SF ligation that is ligation of the GSV at its junction with the femoral vein. All the tributaries—superficial circumflex iliac veins, superficial epigastric veins, and the superficial external pudendal veins need to be ligated separately. If the saphenous vein is ligated little away from the junction keeping a stump of GSV then this segment of vein will continue to get dilated forming a saphena varix as the incompetent valve at SF junction remained and all the tributaries will also get dilated (Fig. 7.10).

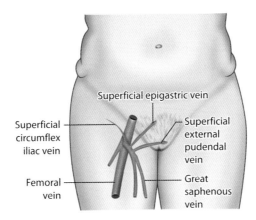

Fig. 7.10: Saphenofemoral junction

Q. Why the whole length of great saphenous vein is not stripped?

Ans. The saphenous nerve lies in close contact with the GSV in the leg. So, stripping of GSV in the leg may cause injury to the saphenous nerve. If individual incompetent perforators below the knee are ligated, this varicosity will disappear. So, stripping of GSV in the leg is not required.

Q. What is Trendelenburg's operation?

Ans. Trendelenburg's operation involves flush ligation of SF junction. An oblique incision is made over the groin below the inguinal ligament starting at the level of femoral artery and extending medially for 4 cm. The long saphenous vein, the superficial femoral vein, and common femoral vein are exposed by dissection. The tributaries of the saphenous vein superficial circumflex iliac, superficial epigastric, and the superficial external pudendal veins are dissected and ligated individually. The GSV is ligated and divided flush with the femoral vein (Fig. 7.11).

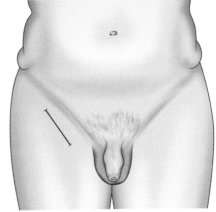

Fig. 7.11: Incision for Trendelenburg's operation

Q. How will you tackle the varicosity affecting the short saphenous system of vein?

Ans. The treatment involves flush ligation of the saphenopopliteal junction and stripping of the dilated segment of the short saphenous vein. The termination of the short saphenous vein is highly variable and ends at the popliteal vein at a variable point from 2 cm below the knee up to 15 cm above the knee joint line. The short saphenous vein is ligated flush with the popliteal vein. A metal stripper is inserted through the upper end of the divided short saphenous vein and retrieved at the lower end of the vein. A heavy suture is used to attach the vein to the upper end of the stripper and the vein is stripped by pulling the stripper from below, thereby inverting the vein.

Q. How will you tackle the small varicosities affecting the communicating veins?

Ans. The additional varicosities involving the small veins need to be stripped off. This can be achieved either by long skin incisions and then stripping the whole length of the vein. Alternatively, this can be achieved by hook phlebectomy. Skin incision of 1–2 mm is made over the varicose vein and an OESCH phlebectomy hook is inserted into the vein and the varicose vein is delivered into the wound and the vein may be grasped by a large artery forceps and the remaining vein may be teased and delivered through the tiny skin incision. Multiple such incisions may be made and veins stripped off by an OESCH phlebectomy hook.

Q. What are the different types of stripper used for stripping the varicose veins?

Ans.

+ *Babcock's or Meyer's stripper:* The conventional stripper is the Babcock's or Meyer's stripper which is a flexible wire, which is passed down the long saphenous vein up to the upper calf. The end of the stripper is retrieved at the upper calf by a small skin incision at the upper calf and by a venotomy at this level. An olive of about the size of 8 mm is attached to this retrieved end and the vein is stripped by pulling the stripper from above.
+ *Rigid metal pin stripper:* A rigid metal pin stripper is also used. This metal stripper is passed down the long saphenous vein and retrieved at the upper calf. A strong suture is passed through an eye at the end of the stripper and is then firmly ligated to the proximal end of the vein and by pulling the stripper from above the vein may be inverted and stripped off.
+ *OESCH phlebectomy hook:* An OESCH phlebectomy hook may be used to strip the small varicosities by a small skin incision of about 2 mm. The vein is delivered on the surface by the OESCH phlebectomy hook and grasped with the artery forceps and teased off.

Q. What will you do on the day of surgery before the patient is anesthetized?

Ans. The varicose main trunk of the vein along with the communicating vein should be marked with skin marker pen. The sites of perforator incompetence are also marked with skin marker pen for ease of identification during surgery.

Q. What is the postoperative management following varicose vein surgery?

Ans. Compression bandage is applied at the end of surgery to prevent bleeding and bruising. The compression bandage is kept for 2 days and then replaced with an elastic stockinette which is kept for about 7 days.

Q. What are the complications following varicose vein surgery?

Ans.

+ Bruising, bleeding, and hematoma
+ Pain
+ Injury to saphenous or sural nerve. Incidence is 4–8%
+ Venous thrombosis in residual varicose vein
+ Deep venous thrombosis.

Q. How will you manage small residual varicosities following surgery?

Ans. The residual minor varicosities following surgical treatment may be managed either by compression bandage or injection sclerotherapy.

Q. What is the role of conservative treatment for varicose veins?

Ans.
* *Secondary varicose veins:* Surgery is contraindicated in patient with varicose vein secondary to deep vein thrombosis as these are the sole channels for venous drainage from the lower limbs
* Patient unfit for surgery
* Patient refusing surgical treatment
* Patient waiting for surgery.

Graduated compression stockings are useful for varicose veins. The ankle compression pressure of 35–40 mm Hg is ideal.

Q. What are the recent advances in treatment of varicose veins?

Ans. There have been newer and less invasive treatment of varicose veins which include:
* Radiofrequency ablation (RFA) of varicose veins
* Endovenous laser ablation (EVLA) of varicose veins
* Foam sclerotherapy.

Q. What is the principle of radiofrequency ablation (RFA) in varicose vein?

Ans. This is a form of endothermal ablation of varicose veins. A radiofrequency catheter is introduced into the main trunk of the vein over a guidewire and the catheter is connected to a radiofrequency generator. The radiofrequency wave is delivered into the vein with a target temperature of 120°C, the vein walls are compressed by injecting tumescence anesthesia. The heat generated in the vein causes thermal injury to the vein wall. This thermal injury causes denaturation of the matrix protein and eventual fibrotic sealing of the lumen of the vein.

Q. How radiofrequency ablation treatment is done?

Ans. This is usually done under general anesthesia.

This is done under intraoperative mapping of varicose vein by using a duplex scan. The patient is placed in reverse Trendelenburg position for ease of cannulating the varicose vein.

The GSV is punctured at the upper calf percutaneously and a guidewire is passed upwards near the SF junction. The radiofrequency catheter (Berenstein catheter) is passed over the guidewire into the lumen of the vein. The placement of the catheter is done under duplex scanning. The tip of the catheter is placed 2 cm distal to the SF junction. The patient is then placed in Trendelenburg position to decompress the vein.

Tumescence anesthesia is injected along the length of great saphenous vein to be treated under US guidance. The recommended amount of tumescence fluid is 10 mL/cm vein to be treated.

After injection of tumescence anesthesia the catheter position is finally checked by US and tip is positioned 2 cm distal to the SF junction. External compression is applied so that the vein wall remains in contact with the catheter electrode. The radiofrequency generator is turned on and the first segment of the GSV close to the SF junction is treated twice. The process is repeated till the entire vein is treated and at each step 7 cm length of vein is treated.

The completion of ablation is confirmed by duplex scanning and US of the area to exclude thrombosis of SF junction and the deep vein.

Radiofrequency ablation treatment of perforator incompetence is now possible using new generation closure RFA stylet which are placed in the perforator vein under US guidance and treated with radiofrequency generator.

The side varicosities may be treated with hook phlebectomy or sclerotherapy.

Q. What is tumescence anesthesia?

Ans. Tumescence anesthesia is used during RFA and EVLA treatment. The tumescence solution is prepared by adding:
- 450 mL of Ringer's lactate solution
- + 50 mL of 1% lidocaine with epinephrine
- + 16 mL of sodium bicarbonate (8.4%).

About 10 mL of tumescence fluid is injected for each cm of vein to be treated. The tumescence fluid is injected under US guidance.

The tumescence anesthesia has number of effects:
- Compresses the vein so that the vein walls remain in contact with the catheter
- Prevent thermal injury to the skin
- Decrease nerve injury
- Provides local anesthesia.

Q. How will you treat short saphenous varicosity?

Ans. The technique of treatment is same but patient should be in prone position.

Q. What are the results of radiofrequency ablation (RFA) treatment of varicose vein?

Ans. Radiofrequency ablation treatment is a very effective recent modality of treatment for varicose vein. The immediate success rate is 98%. Using newer generation of Closure Fast catheter success rate at 6 months is said to be 99%.

Q. What are the complications of radiofrequency ablation (RFA) treatment?

Ans. The important complications of RFA treatment are:
- Deep vein thrombosis
- Pulmonary embolism
- Superficial thrombophlebitis
- Paresthesia due to nerve injury
- Skin burn
- Ecchymosis and seroma formation.

Q. What are the contraindications of radiofrequency ablation (RFA) treatment of varicose veins?

Ans.
- Arteriovenous malformation
- Acute deep vein thrombosis
- Patient on anticoagulant therapy
- Pregnant and nursing women
- Significant lower extremity of arterial insufficiency
- Large diameter of vein and after previous treatment.

Q. What is endovenous laser surgery?

Ans. Endovenous laser surgery (EVLS) is another recent modality of treatment of varicose vein. The mechanism of treatment is by thermal ablation. The steam bubbles generated at the tip of the laser fibers causes thermal injury to the vein endothelium and subsequently causes fibrotic sealing of the veins. The delivery of 60–100 J/cm of vein is effective for thermal ablation of the vein. The available laser generator has a wavelength of 800–1,470 nm. With newer endovenous laser catheter, it is also possible to treat the perforators.

Q. How endovenous laser surgery (EVLS) is done?

Ans. The treatment is limited to the above knee segment of the vein to avoid nerve injury.

The treatment is done under sedation or general anesthesia. The saphenous vein is mapped using US. The access site is chosen using US and the vein is punctured by a micropuncture needle. A guidewire is introduced through the needle and the microsheath is introduced over the guidewire. The microsheath is then replaced by the treatment sheath. The tip of the sheath is placed under US guidance at a point about 2 cm distal to the SF junction. The laser fiber is then advanced through the sheath so that the tip of the laser fiber project beyond the sheath.

The patient is placed in Trendelenburg position to empty the vein and like RFA tumescence anesthesia is injected between the vein and the skin under US guidance. The laser is activated to start the treatment. Manual pressure is also applied over the vein being treated. The laser tip is pulled back at a speed of 1–3 mm/sec with goal of delivering 60–100 J/cm of vein being treated. Circumferential compression bandage is applied on the treated limb from ankle to the groin.

Q. What are the results of treatment with endovenous laser surgery (EVLS)?

Ans. The occlusion of vein following EVLS varies between 77% and 100%. There is chance of recanalization and some series reported a recanalization rate of about 16% at 3 months. About 50% of these patients required surgical treatment and the remainder patient remained asymptomatic at 2 years follow-up.

Q. What is treatment result with radiofrequency ablation (RFA) versus endovenous laser surgery (EVLS)?

Ans. There are different randomized trials comparing the efficacy of RFA and EVLS. The data suggests better results with RFA in comparison to EVLS with respect to pain score, ecchymosis, and other complications.

Q. What are the indications of injection sclerotherapy?

Ans.
* Minor varicosities where the main trunks of great and short saphenous system are normal
* Residual varicosities following surgery.

Q. How does sclerotherapy cure varicose veins?

Ans. The sclerosant solution injected into the vein destroys the endothelial lining and results in fibrotic occlusion of the vein. To be effective the sclerosant solution has to be injected into the empty vein. The vein is then compressed so that the two walls remain in contact so that no thrombus is formed within the vein. The idea is to produce sclerosis and fibrotic occlusion of the vein so that no recanalization occurs.

Q. Which sclerosant solutions are used?

Ans. Sodium tetradecyl sulfate/polidocanol/phenol in olive or almond oil.

Q. How will you do sclerotherapy?

Ans. The varicose vein is marked. With the patient sitting or standing a 23-G or 25-G needle is introduced into the vein. The limb is elevated and the vein is emptied. A small volume of 0.5 mL of sodium tetradecyl sulfate is injected into the empty vein. Immediately after injection, the vein is compressed with the fingers and a firm bandage is applied keeping the vein completely compressed so that two walls remain in contact. A latex foam is applied over the injected vein and incorporated within the compression bandage.

The treatment is done in small segments of vein at a time and needs to be repeated at weekly intervals in the proximal segments of vein. The compression bandage has to be applied for 3–6 weeks following the injection of sclerosant so that vein is transformed into a fibrous cord by intimal damage of the apposed endothelium.

Q. What are the complications of sclerotherapy?

Ans.
+ Skin pigmentation
+ Ulceration of the skin if injected in extravenous space
+ Small region of superficial thrombophlebitis
+ Rarely deep venous thrombosis.

Q. What is microsclerotherapy?

Ans. The venous stars and reticular veins in the skin may be treated by microsclerotherapy. This technique involves injection of a small amount (0.1 ml) of very dilute solution of sclerosant (sodium tetradecyl sulfate or polidocanol) by a very fine needle of 30 G. The compression bandage applied after the injection is usually kept for 1–5 days. This is usually used as a cosmetic treatment.

Q. What is foam sclerotherapy?

Ans. Sclerotherapy was earlier used for treatment of minor varices involving the branches and telangiectatic veins. With development of foam sclerotherapy, the main trunk varicosities involving the GSV and small saphenous vein (SSV) are also being treated with foam sclerotherapy. The sclerosant agent like sodium tetradecyl sulfate or polidocanol when combined with air in a syringe forms a foam. When this foam sclerosant is injected into the vein, the foam displaces the blood and allows contact of the sclerosant with the endothelium of vein wall.

Q. How foam sclerotherapy is done?

Ans. The sclerosant is mixed with air in a syringe. The injection of foam sclerosant solution is done under US guidance. After the injection is made compression bandage is applied after waiting for about 1–10 minutes and the compression bandage is kept for 4 weeks.

The reported occlusion rate at 6 months of treatment is 88% for GSV and 82% for SSV. Some of these patients required a second treatment to obliterate the target vein.

Q. What are the complications of foam sclerotherapy?

Ans.

- Deep vein thrombosis
- Pulmonary embolism
- Superficial thrombophlebitis
- Headache
- Transient confusion
- Vasovagal reaction
- Visual disturbances
- Allergic reaction
- Skin pigmentation.

Q. What is subfascial endoscopic perforator surgery (SEPS) for treatment of varicose veins?

Ans. This is a minimally invasive surgery for varicose vein. .

The perforators are localized by preoperative duplex scanning and marked on the skin surface. Remote from the site of perforator through a small incision the videoendoscope is introduced into the subfascial plane. Through additional 5 mm ports using endodissector, the perforators are dissected, ligated, and divided under vision. This technique is used increasingly and has shown good early term results.

Q. What are the characteristics of varicose ulcer?

Ans. Venous ulcer is one of the important causes of leg ulcer. Venous ulcer is commonly situated just proximal to the medial or lateral malleolus but may extend to the ankle or the dorsum of the foot. Obvious varicose veins are demonstrable and there is associated lipodermatosclerosis and black pigmentation in the skin due to hemosiderosis. No associated arterial diseases as the peripheral pulses are normal.

Q. What are the other causes of leg ulcers?

Ans.

- Peripheral arterial diseases
- Diabetes mellitus
- Neuropathy
- Trauma
- Malignant ulcer—squamous cell carcinoma
- Infective ulcer
- Autoimmune diseases—systemic lupus erythematosus (SLE), systemic sclerosis.

Q. How does venous ulcer develop?

Ans. Due to incompetence of valves in the superficial or deep veins, there is reverse flow in superficial or deep veins. This is more marked during standing or walking and results in ambulatory venous hypertension. This venous hypertension is reflected on to the microcirculation. The capillaries in the skin enlarge in size and may become convoluted giving the appearance of glomerulus. Because of the increased pressure in the capillaries, there is extravasation of blood elements from the capillaries. A perivascular cuff is formed around the capillaries which consist of fibrin, collagen, and fibronectin. This fibrin cuff acts as a barrier to diffusion, preventing nutrient exchange between the capillaries, and the tissues resulting in tissue damage and ulceration.

The fibrin cuff hypothesis is not accepted by all. There is another explanation for development of venous ulcer by leukocyte trapping hypothesis. Venous hypertension causes leukocyte margination and sequestration in the capillaries. These marginated leukocytes become activated and release the proteolytic enzymes, oxygen free radicals which cause damage to the capillary endothelium and thrombosis in microcirculation and cause tissue damage resulting in skin ulceration.

Q. How will you manage venous ulcer?

Ans. In patients where the varicose ulcer is due to superficial varicosity, the ulcer heals well with surgical treatment of varicose veins. But varicose ulcer due to associated deep venous thrombosis, conservative treatment of ulcer is the only answer.

Q. What is the conservative treatment for varicose ulcer?

Ans. Local cleaning of the ulcer and dressing. Avoid using topical antibiotic which does not hasten healing and may leads to sensitization.

The most effective treatment for varicose ulcer is use of elastic stockinette to provide high level of compression at the site of ulcer. A pressure of 30–45 mm Hg applied at the ulcer site may hasten healing. Readymade elastic stockinette (Struva 35 or Norma 35) may be used. Below knee stockings are effective in healing of venous ulcer.

Q. How does compression bandaging helps in healing of ulcers?

Ans. A multilayered compression bandaging also helps in healing of venous ulcer. Optimum pressure should be applied at the site of ulcer as too high pressure may lead to leg injury or too low pressure may delay healing of ulcer. A four layer bandage technique, devised at Charing Cross Hospital, London, is very effective, which applies a pressure of about 45 mm Hg at the ulcer site.

Q. How will you prevent recurrence of venous ulcer?

Ans. Recurrence of varicose ulcer after conservative treatment is very high. Varicose ulcer associated with superficial varicosity needs surgical treatment of varicose vein to prevent recurrence. Varicose ulcer due to deep venous thrombosis needs supportive treatment with use of elastic stockinette and rest with foot end elevated.

Q. What drugs are effective in treatment of varicose ulcer?

Ans. No drug is as effective as compression bandaging. Antibiotics do not help in healing of ulcer. Antibiotics are indicated when there is associated cellulitis or there is infection in the ulcer. Some drugs have been used empirically like aspirin, pentoxifylline, diosmin, and calcium dobesilate. All these drugs have been said to have some effects in ulcer healing but their mechanism of action has not yet been substantiated.

Q. How will you treat varicose vein secondary to deep venous thrombosis?

Ans. In post-deep venous thrombosis of varicose vein, the superficial vein is the only channel for return of lower limbs blood to the heart. Stripping and ligation of varicose vein in this situation is contraindicated.

The conservative treatment for varicose vein is required in this situation—rest with foot end elevated/use of elastic stockinette.

Q. What is the role of direct venous surgery in deep venous obstruction?

Ans. Direct venous surgery is difficult due to absence of a suitable prosthetic graft and difficulty in reconstructing a venous valve.

In cases of iliac vein obstruction, a venous bypass graft between the femoral and the iliac vein proximal to the obstruction may be considered.

Alternatively, Palma's operation may be considered. This involves mobilizing the GSV of the opposite side, tunneling the distal end of the opposite saphenous vein along the suprapubic region, and inserting the saphenous vein into the femoral vein below the site of obstruction.

The segment of femoral vein blocked by previous thrombosis may be replaced by a segment of axillary vein. The risk of further deep venous thrombosis renders this operation unsuccessful in 50% of cases.

Q. How the damaged valves may be managed?

Ans. Although it is difficult to repair the damaged venous valve, the direct repair of the incompetent valves is being tried. If successful, this can lead to healing of venous ulcer.

Q. What are the complications of varicose veins?

Ans.
* Superficial thrombophlebitis
* Rarely may lead to deep venous thrombosis
* *Hemorrhage*—controlled by rest with elevation of leg and compression bandage
* Skin pigmentation, eczema
* Lipodermatosclerosis
* Varicose ulcer
* Periostitis.

Q. What are varicose veins?

Ans. When the vein becomes dilated, tortuous, and elongated then it is called varicose vein. The physiological definition of varicose vein is where there is reverse flow of blood in the superficial vein due to the incompetent valves.

Apart from varicosity of veins in the lower limb, there are other important sites where the veins may become varicose which are:
* *In esophagus*—esophageal varix
* *In rectum*—piles
* *In spermatic cord*—varicocele.

Q. What do you mean by primary varicose vein?

Ans.

- In this no obvious cause could be found to explain the varicosity
- Some changes in vein wall or valvular failure has been implicated
- A congenital predisposition with occupational influence leads to development of primary varicose vein.

Q. What is secondary varicose vein?

Ans. When varicose vein occurs due to some attributable cause:

- *Deep venous thrombosis*—leading to increased pressure in superficial vein–lead to valvular damage and formation of varicosity in the superficial veins.
- *Arteriovenous fistula*—arterializations of veins occur due to increased pressure in the veins leading to venous varicosity.
- *Obstruction to deep vein by a pelvic mass* may lead to superficial varicosity due to occlusion of the deep veins.
- *Pregnancy*—compression of the pelvic veins as well as hormonal effects of estrogen and progesterone which causes the smooth muscles in the vein wall to relax.
- *Inferior vena cava (IVC) thrombosis.*

Q. What is the normal physiology of venous drainage in lower limbs?

Ans. The pumping action of the heart allows the blood flow through the arteries. By the time blood reaches the capillaries, the pressure falls to about 20 mm Hg. But this is enough for the blood to return to the heart. In addition to this, there are muscle pumps in the lower limbs, muscles in the calf, and the thigh which help in propelling blood towards the heart. In addition, there is a foot pump which helps in propelling blood upwards due to pressure in the plantar veins during walking.

During exercise, the calf and thigh muscles contract compressing the veins and propel the blood towards the heart. The pressure in the calf compartment during walking and exercise may rise to as high as 200–300 mm Hg. During the relaxation of the muscles, the pressure in the calf muscles falls and the blood from the superficial veins flows into the deep veins through the perforating veins. The pressure in the superficial veins falls from resting pressure of 80–100 mm Hg to about 20 mm Hg during walking. In situations where this drop in pressure in the superficial veins is not possible during walking, due to reflux of blood, due to incompetence of the valves, or the perforating veins may rather lead to increased pressure resulting in dilatation and tortuosity of the superficial veins.

Q. How does the valvular failure occur?

Ans. There may be congenital paucity of valves. The valves may be damaged afterwards. A small gap appears between the valve cusps and the vein wall at the commissure. This gap extends and there is reflux of blood. The valves cusp degenerate and holes develop in the valve. Ultimately, the valve cusps may disappear leading to gross reflux resulting in varicose vein. The valves may be damaged as sequelae of deep venous thrombosis. After recanalization, the valvular function may be lost.

comission

Q. Why does pigmentation occur in patient with varicose vein?

Ans. Due to valvular incompetence or incompetence of the perforating veins, there is reflux of blood into the superficial system. Due to increased pressure of blood in the capillaries, there is leakage of blood from the capillaries. The red blood cells are broken down in the tissues. The hemosiderin derived as a breakdown product of the hemoglobin is deposited in the tissues to produce a brown pigmentation.

Q. How do you explain pain in patient with varicose veins?

Ans.
* Varicose veins are distended veins and stretching of vein wall may cause pain.
* There is leakage of fibrinogen from the blood at capillary, and the fibrin gets deposited around the capillaries forming a fibrin cuff, which acts as barrier for gaseous and nutritional exchange in the tissues, resulting in some degree of hypoxia which may explain pain to some extent.

Q. What are the usual presentations of patient with varicose veins?

Ans.
* *Incidental*—when varicose veins are found during a routine examination of the venous system. Patient is asymptomatic
* Tiredness and aching in the legs more towards the evening
* Swelling around the ankle more towards the evening
* Skin pigmentation
* Eczema
* Venous ulcer
* Cosmetic due to dilated veins in the legs.

Q. How will you do ascending venography?

Ans.
* This is done under fluoroscopic control. A tourniquet is tied above the ankle. A superficial vein on the dorsum of foot is cannulated keeping the cannula tip towards the distal foot.
* 20–30 mL of 60% urografin is injected into the superficial vein which is cannulated.
* Dye passes into deep vein.
* Deep veins can be seen clearly and deep venous thrombosis may be diagnosed.
* If there is any reflux due to incompetence of the perforator vein then that site can be seen and superficial vein will also be visualized.

Q. Why do you tie the tourniquet above the ankle?

Ans. By tying the tourniquet above the ankle, the dye is forced into deep vein from the superficial veins.

Q. What is dynamic venography?

Ans. After injecting dye patient is asked to stand on toes alternatively, thereby activating the soleus pump. The vein, its valve, and reflux may be seen better by this form of dynamic venography.

Q. What is descending venography?

Ans. Here a cannula is inserted into the femoral vein and with the patient standing. Dye is injected into the deep vein directly. The contrast material is heavier than blood and it may flow lower down in the leg if there are incompetent valves. The reflux in the superficial veins may also be demonstrated.

Q. What is varicogram?

Ans. The contrast material may be directly injected into a varicose vein and may be followed with fluoroscopy to identify its source.

Q. Do you require venography in all cases?

Ans.
* No, venography is not required in all cases
* Duplex scanning has replaced venography in most cases
* When duplex scanning facility is not available, ascending venography may be considered.

Q. What is saphena varix?

Ans. It is the dilated terminal end of the GSV where a thrill may be palpable. A cough impulse may be palpable over the saphena varix due to incompetence of valve at the SF junction.

Q. What are dermal flares or thread veins?

Ans. The varices of the smaller dermal vessels of size 0.5 mm in diameter appearing as purple or red spots are known as dermal flares or thread veins.

Q. What are reticular varices?

Ans. Smaller diameter subcutaneous vessels (1–3 mm in diameter) when become varicose give the appearance of reticular veins where fine dilated veins may be seen just deep to the skin.

Peripheral Vascular Disease

OUTLINE FOR WRITING A LONG CASE OF BUERGER'S DISEASE AND ATHEROSCLEROTIC PERIPHERAL VASCULAR DISEASE

■ HISTORY

- Particulars of patient
- Chief complaint(s)
  Usual chief complaints are:
  - Pain in right/left lower limb for......... (intermittent claudication/rest pain).
  - Ulceration at..... for...........
  - Black discoloration of toes/foot for..................
- *History of present illness:*
  - Pain
    - Site, character, and radiation of pain
    - Enquire whether patient has history of intermittent claudication or not.
      » *Site of pain*—foot/calf/thigh
      » Whether pain appears on walking, if so, after how long walking? Mention the distance he can walk before the pain starts (claudication distance) or after how long walking (time) he starts having pain?
      » What happen to pain if he continues walking? Does it compel him to take rest or the pain disappears on walking or the patient can continue walking in spite of pain?
    - *Progress of claudication*—is the claudication distance same from the onset or the claudication distance has reduced?
    - Enquire whether patient has rest pain or not
    If rest pain is present, site of rest pain in the toes/foot/calf/over the ulcer or gangrenous area.
  - How the patient does get relief? (Often patient has some relief by keeping the leg hanging below the bed or by application of warmth)
  - Write details about the ulceration or the gangrene
    - Duration and onset
    - Any history of trauma
    - Progress of ulceration or the gangrene
    - Any discharge
    - Any pain over the site, and adjacent area.

- Any history of superficial phlebitis. Ask whether patient has any pain, swelling, or discoloration along the course of superficial veins
- Any history of Raynaud's phenomenon.
  - Ask whether patient has pain, pallor on exposure to cold
  - And afterwards any bluish discoloration of toes or fingers and
  - Whether this is followed by dusky red congestion in the feet and hand
  - And any burning pain in the local site
  - Enquire whether gangrene at finger/toe tips has been preceded by such attack or not.
- Enquire about chest pain and its relation with exercise (suggesting anginal pain)
- Any history of blackout or loss of consciousness (suggesting any cerebrovascular disease)
- Any history of abdominal pain or other gastrointestinal symptoms
- Any tingling, numbness, or weakness of any of the limbs
- Any history of impotence (may suggest aortoiliac disease)
- Bladder and bowel habits.
- *Past history:*
  - Similar illness in any other limb in the past
  - Any history of hypertension or other cardiac disease
  - Any history of collagen disease.
- *Personal history:*
  - Detail history of smoking:
    - When did he start smoking?
    - How many cigarette/bidi per day?
    - Is he still continuing smoking or given up. If so, when? Any relief after that?
- *Family history:*
  - Enquire about peripheral vascular disease particularly atherosclerotic disease in the family.
- *Treatment history:*
  - Any drug treatment
  - Any surgical treatment already done.
- *History of allergy.*

PHYSICAL EXAMINATION

- *General survey:*
  - *Decubitus:* Patient may be comfortable with the affected legs hanging below the level of the bed
  - *Pulse:* Rate, rhythms, and character of pulse condition of arterial wall. Details of peripheral pulses are to be described under local examination.
- *Local examination:*
  Examination of both lower limbs
  Inspection: Keep both lower limbs side by side.
  - Attitude of limb
  - *Any deformity*—loss of toes or any other deformity
  - Any muscle wasting in thigh, calf, or foot
  - Condition of veins:
    - Whether normally filled veins are seen in both lower limbs

- Any discoloration along the veins
- Look for any guttering along the course of veins (In ischemic limb, the vein may remain collapsed and pale blue gutter may appear across the course of vein. This may appear with the patient in supine position or asking the patient to elevate his leg).
- Look for signs of peripheral ischemia:
  - Condition of skin:
    » Thin shiny skin
    » Loss of subcutaneous fat
    » Loss or diminished hair over toes, dorsum of foot.
  - *Changes in nail*—whether nails are brittle and there are transverse ridges on the nail
- Gangrene:
  - Site and extent of gangrene
  - Type (dry or moist)
  - Color of the gangrenous area
  - *Line of demarcation*—note the level and depth of demarcation—whether skin, muscle, or bone deep.
- Observe the limb above the gangrenous area—whether pale, congested, or edematous
- Look at the areas of pressure points—heel, malleoli, ball of the foot, and tip of the toes.

Palpation:

- *Skin temperature:* Start palpating from the foot and find at what level temperature becomes normal, comparing with the normal skin temperature of the patient.
- Gangrene:
  - Site
  - Sensation
  - Tenderness
  - Any local crepitus.
- Limb adjacent to gangrenous area:
  - Tenderness
  - Pitting edema.

Test for assessment of circulatory insufficiency.

- *Test for capillary refilling*—press the nail bed/or the pulp/and then release. Look for the rapidity of capillary refilling
- *Venous refilling (Harvey's sign)*—empty a segment of vein with two fingers and the distal fingers released—look for the timing of venous refilling.

Buerger's test (for assessment of vascular angle): In a normal person legs can be kept elevated at 90° angle without appearance of any pallor. Depending on the degree of ischemia pallor may appear on elevation of the limb to different angles. However, this test is not very helpful in dark-skinned individual as pallor is difficult to appreciate in dark skin individual.

- Raise legs gradually and keep at 30° angle to the bed for 2 minutes and look for pallor.
  - If no pallor, raise limb to 45°/60°/90° and look for pallor
  - Mention at what level pallor appears? This angle is called Buerger's angle of circulatory insufficiency.
- *Capillary filling time:* Normal or delayed.

♦ *Crossed leg test (Fuchsig's test):* This is an indirect test for assessment of presence of popliteal pulse.
  - *Method:* Patient sits on a chair with the legs crossed (*See* Figs 8.2A and B)—one knee resting on the other—divert attention—look for oscillatory movement of upper leg
  - If oscillatory movement is seen then popliteal pulse is present
  - If oscillatory movement is absent then popliteal pulse is absent.
♦ Movements of joints adjacent to gangrenous area:
  - Movement of interphalangeal joint
  - Midtarsal joint movement
  - Movement of ankle joint
  - Movement of knee joint
  - Movement of hip joint.
♦ Examination for nerve lesion in lower limbs:
  - Motor system of lower limbs:
    - Tone
    - Power of ankle dorsiflexor and plantar flexor
    - Power of knee flexor and extensor
    - Power of hip flexor/extensor/abductor/adductors
  - Sensory system in lower limbs:
    - Crude touch and fine touch
    - Pain sensation tested by pin prick
    - Temperature sensation.
  - Reflexes:
    - Ankle jerk/knee jerk
  - Plantar response
♦ Examination of regional lymph nodes:
  - Examination of inguinal lymph nodes
♦ Palpation of peripheral pulses:
  (++ normal; + palpable but feeble; – not palpable)

Pulse	Right	Left
1. Arteria dorsalis pedis		
2. Anterior tibial		
3. Posterior tibial		
4. Popliteal		
5. Femoral		
6. Radial		
7. Ulnar		
8. Brachial		
9. Axillary		
10. Subclavian		
11. Carotid		
12. Superficial temporal		

  - Condition of arterial wall
  - Palpate along the vessel for any tenderness
  - Auscultation along major arteries.

♦ *Systemic examination:*
  – Examination of abdomen
  – Examination of cardiovascular system
  – Examination of respiratory system
  – Examination of nervous system
  – Examination of spine and cranium.

■ SUMMARY OF THE CASE

■ PROVISIONAL DIAGNOSIS

■ DIFFERENTIAL DIAGNOSIS

■ INVESTIGATIONS SUGGESTED

■ BUERGER'S DISEASE

Q. What is your case? (Summary of a case of Buerger's disease)

Ans. This 28-year-old gentleman presented with history of pain in left lower limb in the region of calf during walking (intermittent claudication) for last 2 years. At the onset patient used to experience pain in the left calf region after walking for about 1 km but he continues to walk in spite of pain. Afterwards his symptoms have aggravated, and he started having pain after walking for about 200 meters; he has to take rest to get relief. For last 2 months, patient is having continuous dull aching pain in his left foot which disturbs his sleep. He has some relief of pain keeping his leg below the level of the bed. He had a history of trauma in his left second toe about 2 months back. Following this trauma he noticed gradual black discoloration of his left second toe associated with constant dull aching pain in the local site. The black discoloration progressed and involved the whole of the toe and 1 month later a part of the second toe automatically fell off (autoamputated). He has no history of pain in other limbs. No history of chest pain and breathlessness. Bladder and bowel habits are normal. No history of similar pain in the past in any of the other limbs. He is not a known hypertensive or diabetic. He is a smoker for last 10 years and used to smoke 20–25 bidis per day. For last 3 months, he has given up smoking. There is no family history of similar disease (Fig. 8.1).

On examination, general survey reveals mild pallor, pulse rate is 88 beats per minute, rhythm regular, and blood pressure is 130/80 mm Hg. On local examination of both lower limbs, the attitude of the lower limbs is normal. There is loss of second toe of the left foot. There are signs of

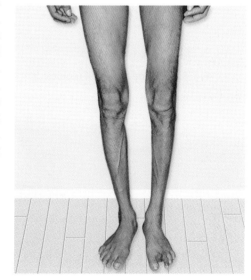

Fig. 8.1: Buerger's disease involving the left lower limb

ischemia in left lower limbs suggested by loss of hair on the dorsum of toes and the foot up to the level of ankle, the skin is thin and shiny, nails are brittle and there are transverse ridges in nails, temperature in the left foot is lower than the opposite side, and temperature is identical on both side from the mid-calf region. The distal part of the left second toe is absent. There is a dry gangrene involving the proximal part of the left second toe, it is tender to touch, and there is a clear line of demarcation between the gangrenous area and the normal skin. The area in the foot adjacent to the site of gangrene is edematous. On examination of peripheral pulses, there is absence of dorsalis pedis, posterior tibial pulses on the left lower limb but other peripheral pulses are normally palpable. The condition of the arterial wall is normal and there is no special character of the pulse. The adjacent joint movements in the left lower limb are normal and there is no neurological deficit in the lower limbs. Systemic examination is normal.

Q. What is your diagnosis?

Ans. This is a case of peripheral vascular disease affecting the left lower limb with ischemic gangrene of left second toe probably due to Buerger's disease.

Q. How will you assess for muscle wasting?

Ans. Inspect the thigh and calf region. Gross wasting may be ascertained on inspection (Figs 8.2A and B). The wasting may be confirmed by measuring the girth of the leg at thigh and calf during palpation (Figs 8.2C and D).

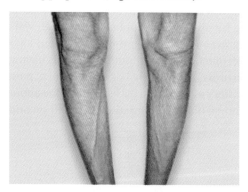

Fig. 8.2A: Inspect the calf region

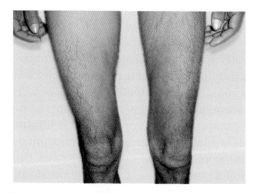

Fig. 8.2B: Inspect the thigh region for any wasting

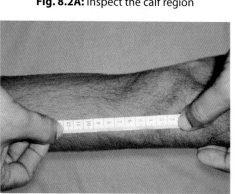

Fig. 8.2C: Assessment of muscle wasting at calf. Measure a distance from the tibial tuberosity towards the calf muscle

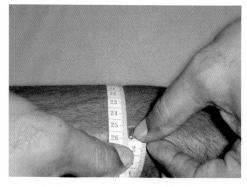

Fig. 8.2D: Measure the circumference of the limb at the calf, and compare the two sides

Q. How will you look for venous guttering?

Ans. In normal person, the veins are seen full on the dorsum of the foot and the leg. When the legs are raised above the level of heart, the vein collapses. However, if the circulation is normal the veins are not emptied completely.

In ischemic limbs, the veins may remain collapsed. In severe ischemic limbs on raising the limb to about 15–20°, pale blue gutter may appear along the course of veins. This is called guttering of veins (Fig. 8.3).

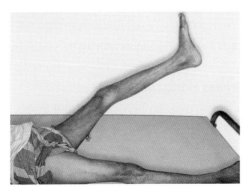

Fig. 8.3: Ask the patient to lift the leg above the level of bed and observe along the course of vein—Note the guttering appearing along the course of great saphenous vein

Q. How do you look for signs of peripheral ischemia?

Ans. Look at the foot for skin (thin and shiny), nail (note the brittle nails, the transverse ridges in the nail), and loss of hair on the dorsum of toes and foot (compare with the normal side), note the gangrenous area in second toe (Fig. 8.4).

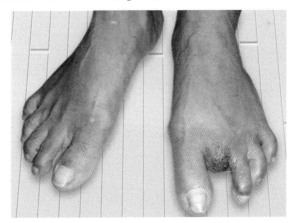

Fig. 8.4: Examination of foot for signs of peripheral ischemia

Q. How will you assess temperature of the limb?

Ans. Palpate with the dorsum of the fingers, start at the dorsum of the foot, and palpate upwards, compare the temperature in two limbs (Fig. 8.5).

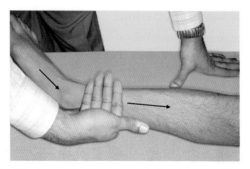

Fig. 8.5: Assess temperature with the dorsum of fingers

Q. How to assess tenderness along the veins?

Ans. Palpate along the course of great saphenous vein and assess for any tenderness or any cord-like feeling (suggesting thrombophlebitis) (Fig. 8.6).

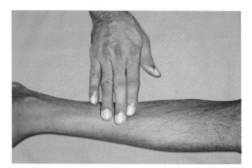

Fig. 8.6: Palpation along the course of great saphenous vein

Q. How would you palpate the gangrenous area?

Ans. The gangrenous area is palpated to ascertain any tenderness, any local crepitus, and sensation. The area adjacent to the gangrenous area is also palpated for any tenderness, pitting edema, and sensation (adjacent area may be hyperesthetic) (Figs 8.7A and B).

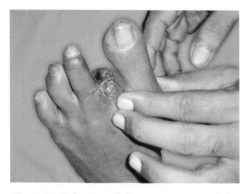

Fig. 8.7A: Palpation of the gangrenous and the adjacent area

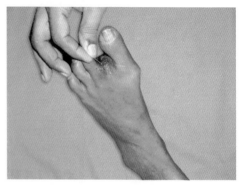

Fig. 8.7B: Assess the sensation of the gangrenous and adjacent area

Q. How will you test for capillary refilling?

Ans. Press the nail bed or tip of the pulp of the finger for 2–3 seconds and then release (Figs 8.8A and B).

In normal person, the blanching on pressure comes back to normal pink color immediately on release of pressure.

In ischemic limb—on release of pressure the return of normal pink color takes longer time—capillary refilling time is prolonged.

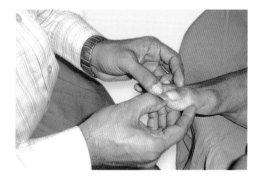

Fig. 8.8A: Press the nail bed—blanching appears

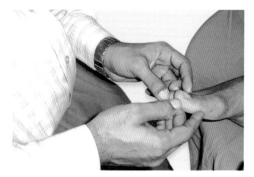

Fig. 8.8B: Release the nail and note the time required for return of normal pink color

Q. How will you assess venous filling time (Harvey's sign)?

Ans. Empty the segment of vein by milking with two index fingers. Release the distal finger, and note the time required for filling of the vein. In normal person, the veins get filled immediately on release of the distal finger. In ischemic limb this venous filling time may be prolonged (Figs 8.9A to C).

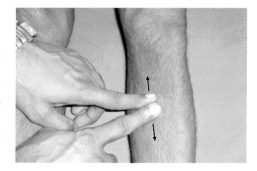

Fig. 8.9A: Place two index fingers side by side

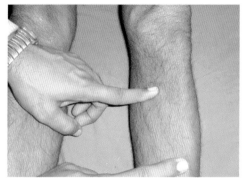

Fig. 8.9B: Empty the segment of vein by milking with the two index fingers

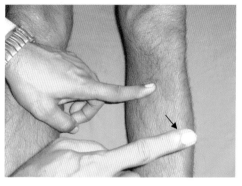

Fig. 8.9C: Release the distal finger and note the time required for venous refilling

Q. How will you assess Buerger's angle of circulatory insufficiency?

Ans. Keeping the patient supine in bed, raise the legs gradually and keep the leg at angle of 20° to the bed for 2 minutes, and observe for appearance of pallor or any discomfort (pain) (Fig. 8.10).

If no pallor appears at 20°, elevate the leg to 30°/45°/60° and 90°, and look for appearance of pallor or discomfort at a particular angle.

Mention the angle at which pallor appears or patient complains of discomfort (pain). This angle is called Buerger's angle of circulatory insufficiency.

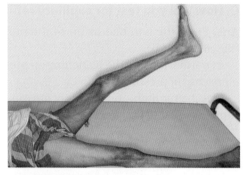

Fig. 8.10: Ask the patient to lift the leg at different angles and observe for appearance of pallor or discomfort (pain)

Q. How will you assess capillary filling time?

Ans. In normal person elevation of the leg to 90° or sitting with the leg dependent does not cause any appreciable color change and the limb remains pink throughout.

In ischemic limb on elevation, pallor may appear at a particular angle depending on the severity of ischemia. On sitting with the limb dependent, the limb becomes pink and with further time the limb becomes dusky red. The time required for the limb to become pink from pallor is called as capillary filling time.

The capillary filling time is prolonged in ischemic limb. A capillary filling time of more than 30 seconds suggest severe ischemia.

Ask the patient to elevate the limb above the bed level and see at what level pallor appears. Then ask the patient to sit with limb dependent (Fig. 8.11).

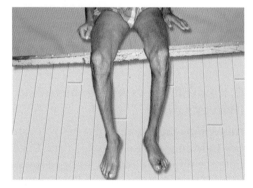

Fig. 8.11: Patient sitting with limbs dependent

Q. How will you do crossed leg test or Fuchsig's test?

Ans.

Method: Patient is asked to sit with legs crossed—one knee resting on the other, divert attention, and look for oscillatory movement of the leg (Figs 8.12A and B).

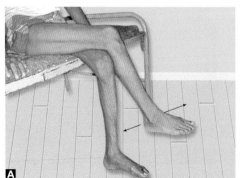
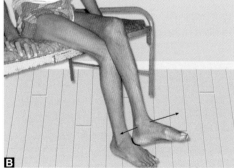

Figs 8.12A and B: Crossed leg test—Fuchsig's test

◆ If oscillatory movement is present—popliteal pulse is present
◆ If oscillatory movement is absent—popliteal pulse is absent.

Q. Where do you palpate the normal peripheral pulses?

Ans.

◆ *Arteria dorsalis pedis pulse:* This is palpated on the dorsum of the foot lateral to the tendon of extensor hallucis longus at the proximal intermetatarsal space (Fig. 8.13).

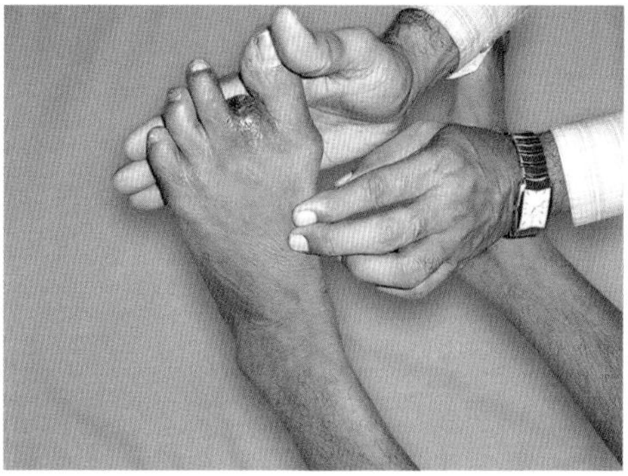

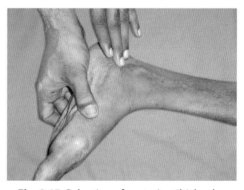

Fig. 8.13: Palpation of arteria dorsalis pedis

◆ *Anterior tibial artery pulse:* Anterior tibial pulse is palpated in front of the ankle midway between the two malleoli and just lateral to the extensor hallucis longus tendon (Fig. 8.14).
◆ *Posterior tibial pulse:* This is palpated in the medial aspect of the ankle midway between the tip of medial malleolus and the insertion of tendo-Achilles and slightly inverting the foot to relax the flexor retinaculum. Alternatively the posterior tibial pulse may be palpated at a point one-third of the way between the tip of medial malleolus and the point of the heel, slightly inverting the foot to relax the flexor retinaculum (Fig. 8.15).

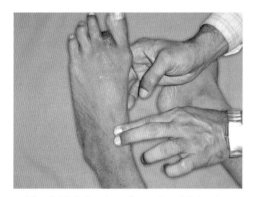

Fig. 8.14: Palpation of anterior tibial pulse

Fig. 8.15: Palpation of posterior tibial pulse

◆ *Popliteal pulse:* Patient supine, flex the knee to 135°, the popliteal artery is palpated against the tibia in between the medial and lateral condyles of tibia by placing the thumbs over the tibial tuberosity, and palpating fingers kept in the intercondylar area of the tibia (Fig. 8.16A). Alternatively patient lies prone-knee flexed, popliteal pulse may be palpated over the posterior surface of the lower end of femur (Fig. 8.16B).
◆ *Femoral pulse:* Palpated in the groin below the inguinal ligament at the level of the deep inguinal ring which is midway between the anterior superior iliac spine and the symphysis pubis (Figs 8.17A and B).
◆ *Radial pulse:* Palpated in the forearm just above the wrist joint in between the tendon of flexor carpi radialis and the lateral border of the lower end of the radius (Fig. 8.18).

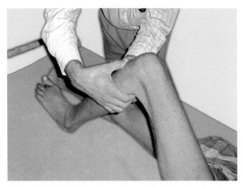

Fig. 8.16A: Palpation of popliteal pulse in the intercondylar area of tibia

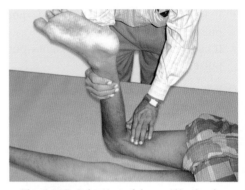

Fig. 8.16B: Palpation of the popliteal pulse against the lower end of the femur

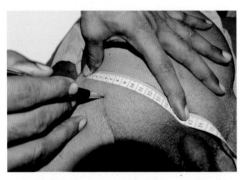

Fig. 8.17A: Find the midinguinal point by measuring the distance between the anterior superior iliac spine and the symphysis pubis

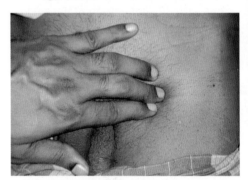

Fig. 8.17B: Palpate the femoral pulse at the midinguinal point below the inguinal ligament

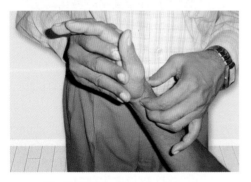

Fig. 8.18: Palpation of radial pulse

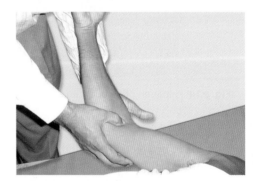

Fig. 8.19: Palpation of brachial pulse: Flex the elbow, support the forearm, and palpate at the elbow joint line medial to the tendon of biceps brachii

- *Brachial pulse:* Palpated in front of the elbow medial to the tendon of biceps brachialis (Fig. 8.19).
- *Axillary pulse:* Palpated in the lateral wall of the axilla against the shaft of humerus in between the two axillary folds (Fig. 8.20).

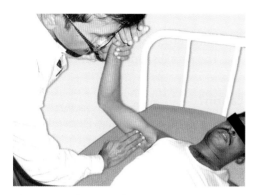

Fig. 8.20: Palpation of axillary pulse: Place the fingers in the lateral wall of the axilla in between the two axillary folds against the shaft of the humerus

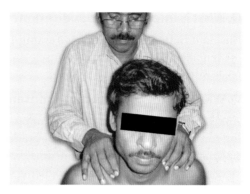

Fig. 8.21: Palpation of subclavian pulse: Keep the fingers at the supraclavicular fossa at midclavicular point (a point midway between the suprasternal notch and the angle of acromion) and ask the patient to shrug the shoulder up

* *Subclavian pulse:* Palpated in the supraclavicular fossa at the level of midclavicular point with the patient lifting the shoulder to relax the deep cervical fascia (Fig. 8.21).
* *Carotid pulse:* Palpated at the medial border of the sternocleidomastoid at the level of the upper border of thyroid cartilage (Fig. 8.22).
* *Superficial temporal pulse:* Palpated in front of the tragus over the zygomatic bone (Fig. 8.23).

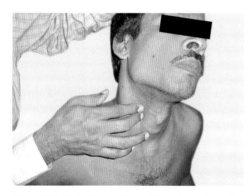

Fig. 8.22: Palpation of carotid pulse: place the fingers medial to the sternocleidomastoid muscle at the level of upper border of thyroid cartilage

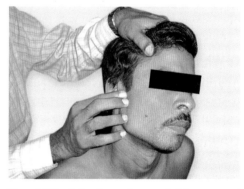

Fig. 8.23: Palpation of superficial temporal artery pulse: Place the fingers in front of the tragus over the zygomatic arch

Q. What is reactive hyperemia test?

Ans. Inflate the sphygmomanometer calf around the limb and inflate the cuff to about 250 mm Hg pressure and keep for about 5 minutes—a pallor will appear. Release the pressure in the cuff—pallor will change to a red flush. Record the time interval between the release of cuff and appearance of red flush in the skin. In presence of normal circulation, the red flush will appear within 1–2 seconds. In a severely ischemic limb, the appearance of red flush will take longer time.

Q. What is intermittent claudication?

Ans. Intermittent claudication is a cramp-like pain in the muscle during walking. This is due to inadequate blood supply in the muscle during exercise. The pain disappears when the patient takes rest and the muscle is relaxed.

Q. What are the grades of intermittent claudication?

Ans. Intermittent claudication is a cramp-like pain in the legs during walking. Depending on the severity of claudication it may be graded as:
- *Grade I:* After walking for some time patient has pain and pain disappears when the patient continues to walk. The pain producing substances are washed off by the adequate collateral supply.
- *Grade II:* Patient has pain after walking but he can continue to walk in spite of slight pain.
- *Grade III:* Patient has pain after walking for some time with continued walking, the pain aggravates, and patient has to take rest to get relief from pain.

Q. What is neurogenic claudication?

Ans. This is pain in the legs during walking due to some neurological causes and is usually due to nerve compression.

Q. How will you differentiate a neurogenic and vascular claudication?

Ans. In vascular claudication patient usually has pain after walking for some distance and patient gets relief by simply taking rest.

In neurogenic claudication patient usually has pain after walking for some distance often after taking few steps. Patient gets relief after taking rest and on assuming some posture so as to relieve compression of nerve. All peripheral pulses are palpable.

Q. What is rest pain?

Ans. Rest pain is defined as continuous pain in the limb present throughout day and night due to severe ischemia. The rest pain is due to ischemia of the nerves (crying of dying nerves) and patient may have some comfort by keeping the foot dependent below the level of bed.

Q. Why rest pain is worse at night?

Ans. Rest pain often awakens the patient from sleep. During sleep, there is diminution of heart rate and the blood pressure may also drop. This may result in further hypoperfusion and may aggravate the ischemic pain.

Q. How will you assess wasting of muscles in the limbs?

Ans. Muscle wasting can be assessed by inspection on comparing the two sides, if there is wasting on one side, if there is bilateral wasting it may be assessed by looking at the thinning of the limbs with bony prominence.

In unilateral wasting it can be further confirmed by measuring the circumference of the two limbs at same level from a bony point say 15 cm below the tibial tuberosity for assessing the calf muscle wasting.

Q. How will you grade muscle power?

Ans. While testing for muscle power, it can be graded as:
* *Grade 0:* No muscle contraction—complete paralysis
* *Grade 1:* Only flicker of contraction—No movement
* *Grade 2:* Can move only when the gravity is eliminated
* *Grade 3:* Can move against gravity but not against resistance
* *Grade 4:* Can move against some resistance
* *Grade 5:* Can move against normal resistance. Normal power.

Q. How will you proceed to manage this patient?

Ans. I will do a duplex scanning of arterial system of both lower limbs to corroborate my clinical diagnosis.

Q. How does duplex scanning helps in diagnosis of occlusive arterial diseases?

Ans.
* Duplex scanning is a combination of B-mode ultrasonography and Doppler study of the imaged vessels. B-mode ultrasonography provides the image of the vessels and the Doppler probe is applied over the imaged artery and the Doppler shift obtained is analyzed by a dedicated computer in the duplex scanner. This Doppler shift can give an assessment of the blood flow, turbulence, and the color coding may show visualization of blood flow on the image. Points of high velocity flow generally indicate stenosis.
* *Using the Doppler ultrasound probe, the following additional information may be obtained:* Listening to audible signal—Doppler ultrasound probe is placed over an artery if there is normal flow, normal signal may be audible. If the vessel is partially occluded, there may be audible turbulence. If there is complete blockage no signal will be audible. So listening to the audible signal, it is possible to assess the patency of the vessels.
* *Measurement of segmental blood pressure*—by applying cuff at the thigh, calf, or above the ankle and by listening with the Doppler probe, it is possible to measure blood pressure at the thigh, calf, and ankle.
  By measuring the ankle blood pressure and blood pressure at the arm (brachial blood pressure), it is possible to find the ratio of ankle and brachial blood pressure index (ABPI).
  ABPI = Ankle blood pressure/brachial blood pressure
* *Pulse wave tracing*—by placing the Doppler ultrasound probe over an artery, it is possible to record the pulse wave tracing. The waveform analysis may be helpful for assessment of occlusive arterial disease.

Q. What is the importance of measuring ankle brachial blood pressure index (ABPI)?

Ans.
* In a normal person, the ABPI is more than 1.
* Value of ABPI between 0.9 and 0.5 suggest mild occlusive disease usually presents with claudication.
* Value of ABPI between 0.5 and 0.3 suggest severe ischemia presents with rest pain.
* Value of ABPI less than 0.3 suggest critical ischemia and incipient necrosis.
* Measurement of ABPI after exercise is also important.

◆ Ankle brachial blood pressure index may be normal at rest with mild ischemia. After exercise in normal person ABPI will increase but in patient with occlusive arterial disease the ABPI will drop.

Q. Would you like to do an angiography in this patient?

Ans. With advent of duplex scanning, it is possible to get a good assessment of the peripheral blood vessels including the flow studies so angiography is usually not required. In Buerger's disease, the disease involves the medium and small-sized vessels and the direct arterial surgery is not feasible so angiography is not essential for evaluation of patients with Buerger's disease.

Q. What are the angiographic appearances in Buerger's disease?

Ans.
◆ There is affection of small and medium-sized vessels of the limbs. The proximal arteries are characteristically normal.
◆ Extensive collaterals give an inverted tree root or spider leg appearance of the vessels.
◆ The involved vessel may show a corkscrew appearance due to dilatation of vasa vasorum.
◆ Severe vasospasm may give a corrugated or ripple appearance of the artery.

Q. How can you assess the claudication distance?

Ans. Claudication distance may be assessed by a treadmill test and finding the point of time at which patient gets pain.

Q. What is Doppler shift?

Ans. In Doppler study, ultrasound signals are thrown over an artery as a transmitted beam and the reflected beam comes back. This difference in frequency between the transmitted and the reflected beam is called the Doppler shift. This Doppler shift is converted into an audible signal by a dedicated computer.

Q. What are the investigations required?

Ans. I will do following investigations to plan further treatment:
◆ Complete hemogram Hb%, total leukocyte count (TLC), differential leukocyte count (DLC), and erythrocyte sedimentation rate (ESR).
◆ Blood for fasting and postprandial sugar to exclude diabetes mellitus.
◆ Blood for lipid profile serum triglyceride, serum cholesterol including human low-density lipoprotein (HLDL), LDL, and very LDL (VLDL) to exclude any lipid abnormalities.
◆ Blood for urea and creatinine
◆ Chest X-ray
◆ Electrocardiography (ECG).

Q. How will you manage this patient?

Ans. I will take some general measures and some specific measures for treatment of the gangrene.
◆ *General measures:*
  – Patient is to be asked to stop smoking.
  – Blood sugar report is to be checked if he is diabetic; appropriate treatment of diabetes with diet and drugs.
  – If there is any lipid abnormalities, appropriate treatment with diet or drugs.
◆ *Drug treatment:*
  – Vasodilators drugs used earlier are not found to be beneficial.

- Pentoxifylline 400 mg twice daily has been tried. This has been claimed to improve microcirculation by reducing the blood viscosity.
- Cilostazol 100 mg twice daily has been claimed to be effective. This is a phosphodiesterase III inhibitor and improves circulation by inhibition of platelet aggregation.

* *Analgesics:* For rest pain analgesics like diclofenac or aceclofenac (100 mg twice daily) may be given. It is desirable to avoid narcotic analgesic because of addiction potential.
* Low-dose aspirin may be given for its antithrombotic activity. But if surgical treatment is contemplated aspirin should be withdrawn at least 72 hours before operation.
* *Specific measures:* The gangrenous area should be cleaned with antiseptic solutions like povidone-iodine and dry dressing is done with antibiotic powder.

Q. What surgical treatment will you consider in this patient?

Ans. As the disease involves the medium and small-sized vessels, direct arterial surgery is not very helpful. Lumbar sympathectomy may be helpful.

Q. How sympathetic fibers reach the lower limbs?

Ans. The preganglionic sympathetic fibers supplying the lower limbs arise from the lower four or five thoracic segments and the first lumbar segments. These preganglionic fibers reach the corresponding sympathetic ganglia via the white rami communicantes. These fibers descend in the sympathetic chain and synapse at the postganglionic cells in the lower lumbar and sacral ganglia. The postganglionic fibers emerge through the gray rami communicantes and join the plexus around the vessels. Removal of the 1st, 2nd, 3rd, and 4th lumbar ganglia causes sympathetic denervation of the whole lower limbs.

Q. How does lumbar sympathectomy help in these patients?

Ans. Lumbar sympathectomy results in cutaneous vasodilatation and may improve cutaneous circulation. Rest pain may be relieved. If an amputation is required, the level of amputation may be lowered following sympathectomy.

Q. Describe the steps of lumbar sympathectomy.

Ans. *See* Operative Surgery Section, Page No. 1128, Chapter 22.

Q. How will you manage the gangrenous toe?

Ans.
* Daily dressing.
* After sympathectomy a line of demarcation may appear between the gangrenous toe and the normal part and then a conservative amputation may be done. As the second toe is gangrenous, a ray amputation preserving the rest of the limb may be enough.

Q. If the patient's symptom is only claudication then how will you treat?

Ans. Lumbar sympathectomy is not very helpful for relief of claudication. So some general measures may help:
* *Reassurance:* Patient is to be reassured that walking is not doing harm. Encourage the patient to walk within his limit of claudication. With walking the collaterals will develop and the claudication will improve.
* Patient should stop smoking.
* *Drug treatment:* Drug treatment is not very helpful. Vasodilators used earlier like isoxsuprine causes generalized vasodilatation may steal the blood flow from the already ischemic limb

and may worsen the claudication so these are not used now. Pentoxifylline or cilostazol may be helpful in some cases.

◆ Treatment of underlying conditions like hypertension, diabetes, and any lipid abnormalities.

Q. Where do you find the lumbar sympathetic trunk?

Ans. The lumbar sympathetic trunk is found medial to the psoas muscle on the sides of the lumbar vertebral body. On the left side, it lies between the psoas muscle and the abdominal aorta and on the right side between the psoas muscle and the inferior vena cava. The inferior vena cava slightly overlaps the right sympathetic trunk.

Q. How will you differentiate between the sympathetic trunk and the lymphatic vessels?

Ans. Sometimes, it is difficult to differentiate between the sympathetic trunk and the lymphatic vessels. But, the sympathetic trunk may be identified by the presence of the distinct ganglia and the rami communicantes. Below the first lumbar segment there are only gray rami communicantes.

Q. What are the rami communicantes?

Ans. There are white and gray rami communicantes, which connects the sympathetic trunk with the spinal cord and the peripheral nerve. The white rami communicantes carries the preganglionic sympathetic fibers from the spinal cord to the sympathetic ganglia. The gray rami communicantes carry postganglionic fibers from the sympathetic ganglia to the peripheral nerve.

The white rami communicantes are present from T1 to L1 ganglia of the sympathetic trunk. The gray rami communicantes are present in all sympathetic ganglia—cervical, thoracic, and lumbar.

Q. Which sympathetic ganglia will you remove in lumbar sympathectomy?

Ans.
◆ If unilateral sympathectomy is done L1, L2, L3, and L4 ganglia need removal for sympathetic denervation of lower limb.
◆ If bilateral sympathectomy is done on one side L1 ganglion is to be preserved otherwise patient will develop impotence.

Q. What is chemical sympathectomy?

Ans. Lumbar sympathetic trunk may be blocked by injecting phenol into the lumbar sympathetic ganglion under fluoroscopic control. About 5 mL of phenol in water (1:16) is injected into the lumbar sympathetic trunk besides the bodies of the second and fourth lumbar vertebra taking care not to inject the chemical into the aorta or the inferior vena cava.

Q. How will you assess whether a proper sympathectomy has been done or not?

Ans. There is increase in skin temperature and the limbs become warm after sympathectomy and the rest pain disappears after a good lumbar sympathectomy.

Q. What is Buerger's disease?

Ans. Buerger's disease is a clinical condition characterized by:
◆ Occlusive disease of small and medium-sized vessels of the limbs.
◆ Thrombophlebitis of superficial or deep veins.

- Raynaud's phenomenon in male patient under the age of 30 years.
- Usually one, two, or all three manifestations are present.

Q. Which vessels are usually affected in Buerger's disease?

Ans.
- Medium and small-sized vessels like dorsalis pedis, posterior and anterior tibialis, radial, ulnar, and digital vessels are usually affected in Buerger's disease.
- Rarely mesenteric, cerebral, and coronary vessels may be affected.

Q. What are the pathological changes in the vessels?

Ans. Buerger's disease is a condition of panvasculitis, involving all the layers of the arteries and the veins, and leads to thrombotic occlusion of these vessels. The vessels are encased in a fibrous sheath and the nerves may also be encased.

There are inflammatory changes in all the layers of the vessels:

- *Tunica adventitia:* There is proliferation of vasa vasorum with lymphocytic infiltration and abundance of fibroblasts in this layer.
- *Tunica media:* There is lymphocytic infiltration.
- *Tunica intima:* There is intimal proliferation leading to intimal cushion formation and narrowing of lumen of the artery and there is lymphocytic infiltration.
    Adventitial fibrosis without medial fibrosis and swelling of endothelium of vasa vasorum are characteristics of Buerger's disease and helps to differentiate it from atherosclerosis.

Q. Which limbs are usually affected in Buerger's disease?

Ans. Buerger's disease may affect both lower and the upper limbs. But the lower limbs are affected more commonly than the upper limbs. Sometimes, all four limbs may be affected in one patient.

Q. What are the stages of chronic limb ischemia?

Ans. Fontaine's has described four stages of chronic limb ischemia in patients with atherosclerotic peripheral vascular disease:
1. *Stage I:* Asymptomatic disease
2. *Stage II:* Symptoms of intermittent claudication
3. *Stage III:* Symptoms of ischemic rest pain
    - *Stage IIIa:* Rest pain with ankle blood pressure more than 50 mm Hg
    - *Stage IIIb:* Rest pain with ankle blood pressure less than 50 mm Hg.
4. *Stage IV:* Either ischemic ulceration or gangrene.

Q. What is Buerger's exercise?

Ans. Patient with severe ischemia presenting with rest pain often gets some relief with Buerger's exercise. The patient alternately elevates the limb above the bed and depresses it below the level of the bed. The explanation for relief of pain is not clear.

Q. What is Raynaud's phenomenon?

Ans. These are sequences of changes in the limbs on exposure to cold.
- *Stage I—Stage of pallor or stage of local syncope:* When exposed to cold, the arterioles undergo spasm. This results in pallor of the fingers. This is also called stage of hypoxia.

◆ *Stage II—Stage of local cyanosis:* With accumulation of metabolite, there is dilatation of the capillaries and the capillaries become filled with deoxygenated blood; the digits therefore become blue.

◆ *Stage III—Stage of red engorgement:* As the attack passes off the precapillary sphincter relaxes but the postcapillary sphincter remains in spasm. The capillary bed now gets filled up with oxygenated blood and there is congestion of the local area with red blood, the digits become swollen and appear dusky red.

Afterwards the postcapillary sphincter relaxes and the blood returns from the local site and the attack passes off.

◆ *Stage IV—Stage of ischemic gangrene or resorption of terminal phalanx:* Repeated such attacks may lead to ischemic changes in the limbs and there may be resorption of the terminal phalanx.

Q. What is omentoplasty?

Ans. When sympathectomy has been already done and patient has relapse of symptoms omentoplasty may be done to improve the circulation to the limbs. A pedicled greater omentum is brought down up to the level of ankle by creating a subcutaneous tunnel. This has been claimed to improve the circulation.

Q. How does Ilizarov technique of bone lengthening may help in patients with Buerger's disease?

Ans. Ilizarov technique for bone lengthening has been tried for improving the blood supply to the ischemic limb in Buerger's disease. The beneficial effects of this technique are not only for relief of rest pain but also helps in improvement of claudication distance. Ilizarov technique of bone lengthening produces neo-osteogenesis and this also results in improvement of vascular supply of the limb. A longitudinal osteotomy is done, widening the upper part of the tibia, and the tissue regenerate in the gap created helps to improve the blood supply of the lower limb. This has beneficial effect in improving the rest pain as well as improvement of the claudication distance.

Q. What is the role of direct vascular surgery in Buerger's disease?

Ans. As the disease involves mainly the small and medium-sized vessels direct arterial surgery is not very helpful in Buerger's disease. Various types of surgery have been tried like:
◆ Arterial bypass graft (femorocrural)
◆ Arterialization of saphenous vein
◆ Profundoplasty
◆ Arterialization of popliteal vein.

Q. What is the role of gene therapy in Buerger's disease?

Ans. Isner et al. have tried gene therapy for improvement of vascular supply of the lower limbs. A vascular endothelial growth factor (VEGF) is secreted by endothelial cell mitogens that promote angiogenesis.

An intramuscular injection of phVEGF165 has been tried in critical limb ischemia. There was significant improvement in ABPI, ulcer healing, and limb salvage. This is still at an experimental stage and is not available for clinical use.

Q. What are the indications of amputation in Buerger's disease?

Ans. When there is ischemic gangrene of the limb, the gangrenous area needs to be treated by amputation. However, the amputation is to be considered after sympathectomy as the sympathectomy may improve the blood supply and may lower the level of amputation. In Buerger's disease, the level of amputation should be conservative.

■ ATHEROSCLEROTIC PERIPHERAL VASCULAR DISEASE

Elderly patient (>50 years) presenting with peripheral vascular disease involving the medium and large-sized vessels are usually due to atherosclerotic peripheral vascular disease. These are not to be diagnosed as Buerger's disease.

In addition to history of peripheral vascular disease, details history of any cardiac disease, any cerebrovascular disease, and mesenteric vascular disease (see Buerger's disease) is to be taken.

Examination is same as for Buerger's disease.

■ DIABETIC FOOT

When presents with a foot infection, ulceration or gangrene, Enquire about:
- *History*
    - Onset: History of trauma, any injury during cutting nail, injury due to soaking of foot in warm bath or application of heat pad, injury while walking or using an ill-fitting shoes.
    - Any swelling in the foot or leg, duration, progress of the swelling, any pain in the foot or leg, any purulent discharge.
    - Duration of the ulcer (Long standing non-healing ulcer is strongly suggestive of underlying arterial insufficiency)
    - History of intermittent healing and ulceration usually suggest underlying infection (Failure of healing after a podiatric procedure suggest underlying arterial insufficiency)
    - History of intermittent claudication, or rest pain (Diabetic neuropathy may obscure these symptoms even in presence of arterial insufficiency). Presence of rest pain often ascribed due to neuropathy may be due to underlying ischemia.
    - Any black discoloration of toes or foot—onset, progress.
    - Details history about the diabetes mellitus, age of onset, whether controlled or uncontrolled, treatment followed—oral hypoglycemic or insulin.
    - Any recent history of hyperglycemia, any history of increased insulin requirement.
    - Any symptoms of weakness, confusion and altered mental status (which may suggest diabetic ketoacidosis or non-ketotic hyperglycemic coma or may be a feature of systemic sepsis).
    - Any history of deformity in the toes, foot or leg, loss of sensation, loss of sweating (suggestive of neuropathy).
    - Any history of fever, chills and night swaets (May suggest systemic sepsis. In presence of ischemia and neuropathy the classic symptoms of infection like fever and pain may be absent).
    - Enquire about any problems in the opposite leg. History of revascularization in opposite leg may suggest arterial insufficiency in the diseased leg.
    - As diabetes may affect all organ system a detail enquiry should be made about any systemic symptoms.
    - Any history of cardiac disease, hypertension, ischemic heart disease (anginal pain or acute myocardial infarction).
    - Enquire about other systemic symptoms like chest pain, breathlessness (suggestive of ischemic heart disease).

- – Any history of deteriorating renal function, any history of dialysis. Deteriorating renal function may require alteration of antibiotic therapy and cautious use of contrast for angiography.
- – Enquire about previous foot problems. Any history of ulceration, how long it took to heal, any history of surgical intervention in the foot. Spontaneous healing of ulcer usually indicates adequate blood supply. Any history of revascularization procedure.
- – Any history of smoking or lipid abnormalities.
- ✦ *Physical examination*
  - – A detail general survey of the patient
  - – Look for signs of systemic sepsis—Fever, tachycardia and hypotension is suggestive of underlying deep infection.
  - – Assess for BMI (Body mass index)
  - – Assessment of functional status of the patient is important. Fully ambulatory patient should be considered for limb salvage. A bed ridden patient with other comorbidites may be better salvaged by amputation.

■ LOCAL EXAMINATION—EXAMINATION OF BOTH LOWER LIMBS

Inspection and Palpation

- ✦ Attitude and any deformity of the limb
- ✦ The entire foot, the nail beds and web spaces are examined.
- ✦ Look for any puncture wounds or ulcer in the dorsum or ventral aspect of foot or webspace.
- ✦ Any black discoloration of the toes or foot- extent.
- ✦ Any swelling in the foot

Examine the ulcer

- ✦ Site and extent
- ✦ Size and shape
- ✦ Edge and margin,.
- ✦ Floor and base (Necrotic, granular or fibrotic) of the ulcer.
- ✦ Color

Assessment for infection

- ✦ Look for edema (Presence of edema may suggest deep infection)
- ✦ Purulent discharge
- ✦ Crepitus
- ✦ Tenderness
- ✦ Erythema
- ✦ Sinus formation
- ✦ Look for cellulitis
- ✦ Any bone expose at the depth of the wound (May suggest osteomyelitis)
- ✦ Probing the ulcer –if bone is felt may suggest osteomyelitis.

Assess for neuropathy

- ✦ Protective sensation tested by Semmes-Weinstein 5.07 monofilament (Inability to feel the monofilament indicates sensory loss and is associated with increased risk of ulceration).

- Look for claw foot (found in advanced sensorimotor neuropathy due to atrophy of intrinsic muscles of the foot). Any osseous prominence, any pressure sore.
- Look for Charcot's joint deformity—bone and joint destruction at midfoot.
- Look for pressure points which may be the site of foot ulceration.

Assessment for arterial insufficiency

- Signs of peripheral ischemia- decreased temperature, loss of hair, opaque brittle nails, shiny skin, delayed capillary refilling, pallor on elevation, venous guttering.
- Presence of ulcer or gangrene at the tip of finger or dorsum of foot, absence of granulation tissue.
- Examination of all the peripheral pulses with special emphasis of lower limb pulses:
  - Femoral
  - Popliteal
  - Posterior tibial
  - Anterior tibial
  - Peroneal
  - Dorsalis pedis artery.

When pulse is not palpable ischemia is presumed to be present.

Palpation of peripheral pulses: *See* Page No. 348.

Systemic examination

Examination of all the system.

Summary of a Case Presenting with Diabetic Foot

This 65-year-gentleman presented with complains of pain and swelling in right lower limb for last 10 days. The pain and swelling started following a trivial trauma to right foot. The pain was acute in onset, progressively increasing in intensity, severe throbbing in nature, continuous, and gets relieved to some extent with analgesics. The swelling started in the sole of the right foot and is progressively increasing, initially involving the area around the trauma site and then involved the whole of the foot, and now extending up to midleg. Complains of fever for last 7 days , low grade intermittent fever. Patient is a known diabetic for last 5 years. He is on irregular treatment with oral hypoglycemics and blood sugar is not properly controlled. There is no history of intermittent claudication or Raynaud's phenomenon. No history of any cardiac disease. No other systemic symptoms. Patient is a known smoker for over 20 years.

On examination, on general survey patient is febrile, pulse is 100/min and mild pallor is present. On local examination, left limb is normal. Right limb is swollen. The swelling involves the both plantar and dorsal aspect of the foot and extends upto the midleg. The skin over the dorsum of the foot and lower leg is shiny skin and there are few blisters over lower part of leg. On palpation, local temperature is raised, tenderness is present. There is no visible gangrene in the area. Peripheral pulses of right lower limb were palpable till popliteal artery. PTA and DPA could not be assessed due to tenderness. Bilateral upper limb pulses are normal. Movement of the ankle, midtarsal, metatarsophalangeal and interphalangeal joints are painful. There is no neurological deficit in lower limbs. Systemic examination is normal.

Provisional diagnosis

This is a case of right sided diabetic foot infection with cellulitis extending upto the midleg associated with uncontrolled diabetes.

What are the problems in this patient?

The patient is having :
* Uncontrolled diabetes mellitus
* There is infection at the foot
* Spreading cellulitis upto the midleg.
* Some signs of systemic sepsis

Q. How will you ascertain infection in diabetic foot?

Ans. Infection in foot may range from mild infection to severe infection with necrosis of tissues in the foot, or there may be spreading of infection with systemic sepsis.

Diagnosis of DFI is based on a comprehensive history and physical examination.

In addition a laboratory evaluation, microbiology assessment, and diagnostic imaging are required.

Symptoms of infection include:
* Pain
* Swelling in the feet
* Blister formation or
* Ulcer in the foot
* Edema may suggest deep infection
* Presence of crepitus may suggest infection with gas forming organisms
* Purulent discharge.

Signs of infection:
* Fever
* Tachycardia
* Hypotension (may be due to systemic sepsis)
* *Two or more signs of inflammation:* Tenderness, erythema, tenderness, warmth, or induration.

Q. How will you manage this patient?

Ans. This patient of diabetes presented with infection in the left foot with spreading cellulitis extending to midleg with evidence of systemic sepsis. Patient will need intensive treatment.

The treatment will include:
* Hospitalization
* Relevant investigations
* Bed rest with foot elevation
* Antibiotic therapy
* Correction of systemic abnormality—control of diabetes
* Incision and debridement
* Regular dressings
* Skin coverage or reconstruction
* Revascularization if required.

Q. Which diabetic foot patient will need admission?

Ans.
* Patient with ulceration, gangrene with deep infection affecting tendon, muscles or bone, or systemic sepsis needs hospitalization.
* Patient with superficial infection may be treated as outpatient basis.

Q. What investigations may help in evaluation of diabetic foot infection?

Ans.
- Blood for fasting and postprandial sugar
- Hemoglobin A1c (HbA1c) to assess average blood sugar in previous 3 months
- Hemoglobin%, TLC, DLC, and ESR
- Lipid profile to assess any lipid abnormalities
- Blood urea and creatinine to assess renal function
- Pus C/S for both aerobic and anaerobic organism culture
- Duplex study of arterial system of both lower limbs
- X-ray of the local part to assess for osteomyelitis
- Magnetic resonance imaging (MRI) of local part for assessment of osteomyelitis
- Chest X-ray
- Electrocardiography
- Echocardiography.

Q. What are the usual organisms for infection?

Ans. Superficial infection and mild infection is usually caused by Gram-positive cocci—*Staphylococcus aureus* and Streptococci.

Deep and life-threatening infection is caused by mixed flora.

These include:
- *Gram-positive cocci:* Methicillin-resistant *Staphylococcus aureus* (MRSA) is increasingly important for infection, particularly in hospitalized patient and patients who has received antibiotics earlier.
- *Gram-negative bacilli: Escherichia coli, Klebsiella, Enterobacter aerogenes, Proteus mirabilis,* and *Pseudomonas aeruginosa.*
- Enterococci may be isolated.
- *Anaerobes: Bacteroides fragilis* and *Peptostreptococcus.*

Q. How to choose antibiotics?

Ans. Initial antibiotic choice is based empirically on the usual organisms responsible for infection. Once the culture sensitivity report is available antibiotics should be changed based on the C/S report.

For *Staphylococcus aureus* and Streptococci, a dual antibiotic—cephalosporin and beta-lactam antibiotic may be the initial choice.

For MRSA tetracycline or trimethoprim and sulfamethoxazole may be started.

A combination of fluoroquinolone and linezolid may also be an alternative choice.

For deep infection and chronic recurrent infections are typically polymicrobial.

The appropriate antibiotic option may be:
- Vancomycin + beta-lactam antibiotic with beta-lactamase inhibitor (piperacillin + tazobactam)
- Vancomycin + metronidazole + a quinolone.

Antibiotic should be continued till the wound is clean and cellulitis has resolved usually for 10–14 days.

If osteomyelitis is present antibiotic should be given for prolonged period (4–6 weeks).

Q. How will you diagnose osteomyelitis?

Ans.

* Clinically deep infection.
* Probing will reveal bone.
* Isolation of bacteria on bone biopsy confirms diagnosis of osteomyelitis.
* *Plain X-ray:* Bony changes may not be apparent in initial 2 weeks.
* Computed tomography (CT) scan provide good image showing cortical destruction, periosteal reaction, and soft tissue changes.
* Nuclear imaging may provide clue to diagnosis of osteomyelitis.
* Magnetic resonance imaging is a superior imaging modality for diagnosis of osteomyelitis. Early diagnosis possible with MRI.

Q. How will you treat diabetic foot infection?

Ans. Infection: Almost all diabetic foot are associated with infection. The antibiotics selected should achieve adequate level in both soft tissue and bone.

Wide debridement of all infected and necrotic tissue is of paramount importance for treatment.

Q. How will you manage diabetes?

Ans.

* Proper diabetic control is essential for management.
* Hyperglycemia is often associated with infection.
* Severe hyperglycemia may be associated with ketotic or nonketotic hyperosmolar states.
* Blood sugar should be gradually corrected.
* Most patients will need treatment with regular insulin.
* Dehydration is often present and needs correction with oral/intravenous (IV) fluids.
* A urinary catheter is a helpful guide to assess response to fluid therapy.
* Serum electrolytes, magnesium, and creatinine are to be measured to assess serum osmolality and to achieve correction of hyperosmolar states.
* Critically-ill patients will need cardiac monitoring and central venous pressure (CVP) or pulmonary capillary wedge pressure (PCWP) measurement for optimal fluid therapy.

Patient usually needs treatment with regular insulin. Insulin dose can be adjusted by regular blood sugar monitoring.

Q. What are the characteristics of mild infection?

Ans. Mild infections manifest as:

* Limited (<2 cm) cellulitis. Penetration confined to subcutaneous tissues.
* Wound with purulent discharge.
* At least two of the classic signs or symptoms of a host inflammatory response.
* No lymphangitis or regional lymphadenopathy.
* No systemic signs or symptoms of infection.
* Patient's white blood cell count and metabolic parameters are in or near the usual range.

Q. How will you treat mildly infected diabetic foot infection?

Ans. Mildly infected diabetic wounds can usually be treated:

* On an outpatient basis.

◆ With oral antibiotic therapy. Antibiotic therapy should usually be directed against *Staphylococcus aureus* and *Streptococcus* species., with the caveat that there are increasing rates of MRSA in these patients.
◆ Many patients will need some minor surgical procedure (e.g. debridement, incision, and drainage for a small abscess)
◆ Pressure offloading.
◆ Patient should be properly followed up in a few days to review the results of culture and sensitivity tests and to ensure there has been a clinical response to treatment.

Q. What are the characteristics of moderate and severe infection?

Ans. The characteristics of moderate infection are:
◆ Cellulitis extending more than 2 cm.
◆ Evidence of significant proximal spread.
◆ Penetration of infection into the deeper tissues, such as fascia, tendon, muscle, or bone.
◆ Lymphadenopathy or lymphangitis may be present.
◆ Patient is systemically well and metabolically stable.
◆ Mild elevation of the white blood cell count, and blood glucose levels may be higher than the patient's usual values.

Q. What are the characteristics of severe infection?

Ans.
◆ Infections similar to moderate infections.
◆ Evidence of a systemic sepsis.
◆ The patient may be febrile, hypotensive, and confused.
◆ Significant metabolic imbalance (e.g. azotemia and acidosis).
◆ Presence of severe peripheral arterial insufficiency of the affected leg increases the risk of adverse outcomes with severe infection.
◆ Moderate infections may be limb-threatening, severe infections may also be life-threatening.
◆ Severe infections are more often polymicrobial, including *Staphylococcus aureus* and Streptococci, as well as Gram-negative and/or obligately anaerobic organisms.

Q. What are the usual organisms for infection?

Ans.
◆ Superficial infection and mild infection is usually caused by Gram-positive cocci—*Staphylococcus aureus, Staphylococcus epidermidis*, and Streptococci. MRSA is increasingly important for infection, particularly in hospitalized patient and patients who has received antibiotics earlier.
◆ Deep ulcers, limb, and life-threatening infection is caused by mixed flora.
◆ *Gram-positive organisms: Staphylococcus aureus*, Streptococci including MRSA.
◆ *Gram-negative bacilli: Escherichia coli, Klebsiella, Enterobacter aerogenes, Proteus mirabilis*, and *Pseudomonas aeruginosa*.
◆ Enterococci may be isolated.
◆ *Anaerobes: Bacteroides fragilis* and *Peptostreptococcus*.
There is an increasing incidence of infection by resistant organisms.

Q. How will you treat diabetic foot infection?

Ans. Patient will need intensive medical treatment for stabilization and local wound care.

Q. How will you stabilize the patient of diabetic foot?

Ans.

- Patient with diabetic foot needs intensive medical management for stabilization.
- Hyperglycemia needs to be controlled with regular insulin.
- *Serum electrolytes*—Na, K, Ca and magnesium level measured and any electrolyte abnormality is quickly corrected.
- In ketotic patient dehydration is common need for correction with adequate IV fluid.
- Hydration status may be checked by urinary output, CVP, or PCWP measurement.
- Aspirin and beta blocker if not otherwise contraindicated.
- *Statin:* Improve dyslipidemia, stabilize coronary artery plaques, and improve patency of infrainguinal reconstruction.
- Antibiotics.

Q. How will you choose antibiotic therapy?

Ans. Initial antibiotic choice is based empirically on the usual organisms responsible for infection. Deep infection and chronic recurrent infections are typically polymicrobial.

Once the culture sensitivity report is available antibiotics should be changed based on the C/S report.

- For *Staphylococcus aureus* and Streptococci, a dual antibiotic—cephalosporin and beta-lactam antibiotic may be the initial choice.
- For MRSA tetracycline or trimethoprim and sulfamethoxazole may be started.
- A combination of fluoroquinolone and linezolid may also be an alternative choice.

The appropriate antibiotic option may be:

- Vancomycin + beta-lactam antibiotic with beta-lactamase inhibitor (piperacillin + tazobactam).
- Vancomycin + metronidazole + a quinolone.

Q. What is the optimal duration of antibiotic therapy?

Ans. Optimal duration of antibiotic therapy has yet to be defined based upon clinical studies. Antibiotic should be continued till the wound is clean and cellulitis has resolved usually for 2–4 weeks.

If osteomyelitis is present antibiotic should be given for prolonged course (4–6 weeks).

Q. How to plan antibiotic therapy?

Ans. Empiric therapy of DFIs should ideally be guided by:

- Severity of the infection.
- Likely microbiology of the wound.
- Acute, relatively mild infections in patients who have not recently received antibiotic therapy can often be solely directed at aerobic Gram-positive cocci.
- Infections that are chronic, moderate or severe, or that occur in patients who have failed previous antibiotic treatment should usually be more broad spectrum.
- Need to cover MRSA [or extended spectrum beta-lactamase (ESBL)] isolates depend on the likelihood of these pathogens in any given patient.
- Definitive therapy, to complete the appropriate course, should be based on both the clinical response to empiric therapy and the results of the culture and sensitivity report.

◆ In polymicrobial infections, some organisms may represent contaminants or colonizers, and may therefore not need to be specifically covered by the antibiotic regimen.

Q. What should be the duration of antibiotic therapy?

Ans. The duration of antibiotic therapy for soft tissue infections is governed by the resolution of signs and symptoms of infection. Thus, clinical judgment plays an important role. Generally, when the patient is metabolically stable and the cardinal signs of infection have resolved, systemic antibiotic therapy can be discontinued.

The optimal duration of therapy for mild and superficial infection is 2–4 weeks. For deep infections and osteomyelitis therapy it may be needed for at least 6 weeks or more. Antibiotics are designed to cure infections, not to heal wounds, which usually takes many weeks. No data support continuing to treat wounds with antibiotics after evidence of infection resolves, in an attempt to either hasten healing or to prevent recurrent infection.

Q. When will you consider incision and drainage in diabetic foot infection?

Ans. Incisions and drainage should be considered in presence of an abscess or deep space infection. Wide debridement of all infected and necrotic tissue is of paramount importance for treatment. Culture should be obtained from debrided deep tissue.

Abscess in medial, central, and lateral compartment in the sole of the foot should be drained by a longitudinal incision extending along the entire length of the abscess.

Drainage incision on the dorsum of the foot is usually not required.

Q. How will you manage deep infection and abscess?

Ans. Immediate incision and drainage is essential for abscess or deep space infection. Incision should be adequate to drain the abscess completely and all necrotic tissue should be debrided. The incision should allow for dependent drainage. Pus from deep tissue should be sent for C/S.

Q. How will you plan incision for diabetic foot infection?

Ans. The abscess at the foot may be either in medial, central, or lateral compartment. The incision should be vertical and along the neurovascular bundle. The abscess at the medial and central compartment is drained by an incision at the medial side of the foot and abscess at the lateral compartment is drained by a lateral incision. The incision should be deepened up to the plantar fascia. All necrotic tissue should be removed.

The web space infection should be drained through an incision at the plantar aspect.

Drainage incision on the dorsum of the foot is usually not required.

Q. When will you consider further debridement?

Ans. Further necrosis after initial debridement indicates undrained infection or continuing ischemia. This will need further debridement.

Foot infections can extend proximally into the leg through the tarsal tunnel, resulting in rapidly ascending limb and life-threatening infection. Early surgical treatment of DFI may reduce the need for major amputations.

Q. What is the incidence of osteomyelitis in diabetic foot infection?

Ans. Infection of bone usually occurs by contiguous spread from soft tissue. This process usually takes days or weeks, and is uncommon in acute infections. In most centers, approximately 20%

of patients who present with a DFI have involvement of the underlying bone. Some studies have suggested that in selected populations up to two-thirds of patients with a diabetic foot wound have osteomyelitis. The presence of osteomyelitis increases the likelihood of treatment failure and lower extremity amputation. Thus, accurately diagnosing and treating this complication is crucial.

Q. How will you do culture in osteomyelitis?

Ans.

- Several recent studies suggest that a carefully obtained culture of a sinus tract correlates well with concomitant bone cultures.
- Bone biopsy with culture or histopathology is still considered as the criterion standard for diagnosing diabetic foot osteomyelitis.
- In addition to confirming the presence of bone infection, only a bone biopsy can provide the causative pathogen and its antibiotic susceptibilities.
- Bone culture-based antibiotic therapy was the only variable significantly associated with remission of infection.

Q. Can osteomyelitis be treated nonsurgically?

Ans. Although osteomyelitis has traditionally been considered a surgical disease, several studies have demonstrated the possibility of antibiotic-only management. Highly bioavailable antibiotics that are effective in the presence of biofilm and can enter host cells have changed the way we think about treating chronic osteomyelitis and may make nonsurgical management feasible in some cases. A recent systematic review found that there is currently no evidence that surgical debridement of the infected bone is routinely necessary. The optimal duration of antibiotic therapy is 6 weeks. In some cases more prolonged therapy may required even up to 40 weeks. The drug is preferably administered parenterally. In some cases, oral antibiotics have also be found to be effective.

Q. What are the antibiotics used for osteomyelitis?

Ans. The most commonly used antibiotic agents were:
- Amoxicillin/clavulanate
- Combination of clindamycin with either ofloxacin or ciprofloxacin
- Doxycycline and trimethoprim/sulfamethoxazole were used for patients infected with MRSA.

Q. When will you consider amputation?

Ans.

- Unsalvageable foot
- Fulminant sepsis
- Hemodynamic instability
- Severe acid base and electrolyte abnormalities.

    In presence of severe sepsis and unsalvageable limb immediate guillotine amputation is to be done to remove the source of sepsis.

    Administration of systemic antibiotics, correction of dehydration and electrolyte abnormalities, and continuous monitoring are essential for management.

Q. How will you assess arterial ischemia in diabetic foot?

Ans.

- A detail history and clinical examination is the first step for evaluation of ischemic limb.

- Absence of peripheral pulses is one important sign of peripheral ischemia.
- Duplex study is noninvasive test for diagnosis of ischemic limb. Duplex study is useful for measurement of segmental blood pressure in limb, ABPI, arterial waveforms, and pulse volume recordings.
- Arteriography to exactly localize the site of arterial disease. Arteriography is done after the infection is controlled and systemic toxicity is resolved.
- Digital subtraction angiography is the gold standard for assessment of ischemia in the lower limb. This newer imaging modality provides better visualization of the vessels delineated by the contrast by subtracting the bone and soft tissue images.
- Magnetic resonance angiography (MRA) is an alternative to invasive contrast angiography. However, MRA provides good visualization up to tibial vessels but digital vasculature are not well delineated.

Q. How segmental blood pressure is measured?

Ans. Segmental blood pressure is the systolic blood pressure measured at thigh, calf, and ankle. The ankle blood pressure is slightly higher than the brachial blood pressure. The difference in segmental blood pressure should not be more than 20 mm Hg.

Q. What is ankle brachial blood pressure index (ABPI)?

Ans. Ankle brachial blood pressure index is calculated by:

$$ABPI = Ankle\ blood\ pressure/brachial\ blood\ pressure$$

- Ankle brachial blood pressure index more than 0.9 indicates normal perfusion.
- Ankle brachial blood pressure index—0.5–0.9 indicates moderate ischemia.
- Ankle brachial blood pressure index less than 0.40—indicates critical ischemia with rest pain and gangrene.

Q. Why ankle brachial blood pressure index (ABPI) is not an ideal method to assess ischemia in diabetic foot?

Ans. An ABPI value less than 0.90 or more than 1.30 is indicative of peripheral arterial disease (PAD).

Ankle brachial blood pressure index may be falsely elevated in diabetic patient secondary to medial arterial calcification.

Measurement of toe pressures is better in prediction of patients at risk for ulceration and potential for wound healing.

An absolute toe pressure of more than 70 mm Hg is normal.

The toe brachial index (TBI) may be substituted in those patients with elevated ABPIs secondary to lower extremity arterial calcification.

A normal TBI of more than 0.7 has been shown to be superior to ABPI for excluding the presence of PAD as calcification is not usually present in digital vessels.

Q. What is the importance of transcutaneous oxygen tension (TcPO$_2$) measurement?

Ans. Transcutaneous oxygen tension (TcPO$_2$) measurement can be performed, regardless of arterial calcification in major pedal arteries.

Although not highly prognostic of wound healing potential, TcPO$_2$s are predictive of wound healing failure at levels below 25 mm Hg.

Q. What is the importance of skin perfusion pressure (SPP) measurement?

Ans. Skin perfusion pressure (SPP) utilizes a laser Doppler measurement to indicate the presence or absence of perfusion in the lower extremities through cutaneous capillary circulation.

Skin perfusion pressure measurement requires a specialized equipment, it has proven more sensitive than other vascular tests for evaluation and diagnosis of PAD.

Q. What arterial waveform changes occur in ischemic limb?

Ans. Arterial waveforms are graphic representation of Doppler shift as blood flow through the arteries. Normal waveform is triphasic. During systole forward flow of blood results in a sharp upstroke. During early diastole, the vessels recoil from distension and there is a downward stroke going below the baseline. In late diastole as the ventricular filling occurs, there is transmission of the wave to the artery resulting in a small positive deflection. These three phases produces the classic triphasic waveform in normal vessels. Worsening stenosis results in failure of flow reversal and results in a monophasic waveform suggesting severe arterial disease.

Q. What are the important factors for development of diabetic foot ulceration?

Ans. About 10–26% of diabetic patients are at risk of developing foot ulcers. The major factors for developing diabetic foot ulcers (DFUs) are:
- Diabetic neuropathy with associated deformity.
- There is both sensory and motor neuropathy.
- Loss of sensation results in repeated trauma due to ill fitting shoes, foreign bodies, or thermal injury.
- Motor neuropathy results in Charcot's foot deformity. There is collapse and deformity of metacarpophalangeal and interphalangeal joints resulting in pressure over certain areas resulting in callosity and subsequent ulceration.
- Ischemia: There is combination of microvascular and macrovascular angiopathy and Infection.

Q. How will you take care of wound in the foot?

Ans. Repeated debridement of wound till healthy and bleeding tissue is seen is the mainstay of local treatment. Wound should be kept moist. A wet dressing with normal saline is ideal.

Q. What are the other modalities for wound care?

Ans. There are different adjunctive modalities for wound care which provides benefit in terms of wound healing. But these are not routinely recommended in all patients.
- Use of chemical debriding agents.
- Use of local growth factors.
- Hyperbaric oxygen therapy.
- Negative pressure system wound therapy—vacuum-assisted closure (VAC).

Q. What is the role of offloading?

Ans. Offloading by using special orthotic appliance is useful for relieving the pressure over the ulcerated area.

Q. What are the roles of topical application?

Ans. Following topical agents have been shown to improve the wound healing in diabetic foot ulceration:
- Platelet-derived growth factor (PDGF)
- Granulocyte-macrophage colony-stimulating factor

* Engineered skin allograft substitute
* Chemical enzymatic substances as medical debriding agent
* Hyperbaric oxygen therapy.
  These are usually expensive and routine use is not advisable. Normal saline dressing is ideal.

Q. How is vacuum-assisted closure (VAC) helps in wound healing?

Ans. Vacuum-assisted closure system for chronic and complex wound has shown advantages over wet dressings.

A sealed dressing is applied and a vacuum pump is attached underneath the sealed dressing to provide a constant or intermittent negative pressure. This negative pressure environment helps in wound healing in both chronic and acute wounds.

The VAC helps in following ways:

* Optimizes blood flow in the wound area
* Decreases tissue edema
* Removes exudates including the proinflammatory cytokines and the bacteria from the wound environment.
  Vacuum-assisted closure system is applied after the debridement and continued till the red granulation appears on the surface of the wound. Different studies have established the benefit of vacuum-assisted wound closure.

Q. Which factors impair healing in diabetic foot ulceration?

Ans. Following factors impair healing of ulcer:

* Poorly controlled diabetes.
* *Nutritional status:* Malnutrition adversely affects wound healing
* Unrecognized ischemia
* Ongoing infection
* Failure of proper wound care.

Q. How to treat heel ulcer?

Ans. Heel ulcer is a difficult problem to treat.
Dry eschar without any associated deep infection may be treated with offloading.

In patient having chronic ulceration with associated calcaneal osteomyelitis—partial calcanectomy with excision of the ulcer may be an option.

Q. How will you cover defect in heel?

Ans. Primary closure is difficult in most situations. The coverage may be achieved with a vascularized skin flap either local or a free flap.

Q. What is the role of offloading?

Ans. Offloading by using special orthotic appliance is useful for relieving the pressure over the ulcerated area.

Q. When will you consider revascularization of the ischemic limb?

Ans.

* Patient with critical limb ischemia
* Ischemic ulceration of the limb.

Q. What are the different revascularization techniques?

Ans. The different techniques of revascularization of the limbs include:
* *Endovascular techniques:* Angioplasty and stenting.
* *Bypass grafting:* By autologous venous grafting or prosthetic grafting.
* Combination of endovascular technique and bypass grafting.

Q. What measures to be taken for preventing foot ulceration?

Ans. Once the ulcer has healed some measures are to be taken to prevent recurrent ulceration:
* Patient counseling and education.
* Daily washing of foot and use of moisturizer.
* Daily inspection of the foot for any cuts or sores.
* Avoid walking barefoot.
* Well-fitting shoes.
* Avoid using any counterirritant for foot care.
* If there is associated neuropathy—chance of recurrent ulceration is more.
* Foot deformity may cause abnormal pressure points, which may be the site of future ulceration—needs custom made shoes and insoles for offloading.

Q. What is the pathogenesis of diabetic foot ulcer and infection?

Ans. Several factors predispose to DFU and infection namely:
* Neuropathy
* Vasculopathy and
* Immunopathy.

Q. How neuropathy affects diabetic foot ulcer and infection?

Ans. Peripheral neuropathy is considered as the most prominent risk factor for DFUs.

Diabetic patients with impaired protective sensation and altered pain response are vulnerable to trauma and extrinsic forces from ill-fitting shoes.

Motor neuropathy causes muscle weakness and intrinsic muscle imbalance leading to digital deformities such as hammered or clawed toes.

Autonomic dysfunction leads to changes in microvascular blood flow and arteriolar-venous shunting.

There is diminishing effectiveness of perfusion and elevation of skin temperatures.

There is loss of sweat and oil gland function. The skin becomes dry and keratinized with cracks and fissure which becomes the portal of entry for infection.

Q. How angiopathy affects foot ulcer and infection?

Ans. Diabetic angiopathy is the most frequent cause of morbidity and mortality in diabetic patients.

Macroangiopathy manifests as a diffuse multisegmental involvement typically involving the infrapopliteal vessels.

There is also associated compromised collateral circulation.

Associated atherosclerosis also leads to PAD of the lower extremities.

Peripheral arterial disease is an independent risk for DFI.

Microangiopathy results in thickening of capillary bed leading to tissue hypoxia and microcirculation ischemia.

Q. How immunopathy affects foot ulcer and infection?

Ans. Immunopathy in diabetic patient results in inherent susceptibility to infection as well as the potential to mount a normal inflammatory response.

Impaired host defenses secondary to hyperglycemia include defects in leukocyte function and morphologic changes to macrophages.

Leukocyte phagocytosis was significantly reduced in patients with poorly controlled diabetes. Improvement of microbiocidal rates was directly correlated with correction of hyperglycemia.

Decreased chemotaxis of growth factors and cytokines, coupled with excess of metalloproteinases, impede normal wound healing by creating a prolonged inflammatory state.

Fasting hyperglycemia and the presence of an open wound create a catabolic state.

Negative nitrogen balance ensues secondary to insulin deprivation, caused by gluconeogenesis from protein breakdown.

This metabolic dysfunction impairs the synthesis of proteins, fibroblasts, and collagen.

There is an impairment of the immune system with serum glucose levels more than 150 mL/dL.

Patients with diabetes tolerate infection poorly and infection adversely affects diabetic control. This repetitive cycle leads to uncontrolled hyperglycemia, further affecting the host's response to infection.

Q. What are the different classification systems of diabetic foot?

Ans. Wagner's grading system

Wagner classification system based on severity of diabetic foot lesion:

0   Preulcerative area without open lesion
1   Superficial ulcer (partial/full thickness)
2   Ulcer deep to tendon, capsule, and bone
3   Stage 2 with abscess, osteomyelitis, or joint sepsis
4   Localized gangrene
5   Global foot gangrene.

Table 8.1: University of Texas Health Science Center San Antonio classification system

	0	1	2	3
A	No open lesion	Superficial wound	Tendon/capsule	Bone/joint
B	With infection	With infection	With infection	With infection
C	Ischemic	Ischemic	Ischemic	Ischemic
D	Infection/ischemia	Infection/ischemia	Infection/ischemia	Infection/ischemia

The more recent and popular DFU classification is the University of Texas (UT) Health Science Center San Antonio classification system. This system incorporates four grades of wound depth with subgroups to denote the presence of infection, ischemia, or both.

Wounds with frank purulence and/or two or more local signs of inflammation such as warmth, erythema, lymphangitis, lymphadenopathy, edema, pain, and loss of function may be classified as "infected".

Lower extremity vascular insufficiency is diagnosed by a combination of one or more clinical signs or symptoms of claudication, rest pain, absent pulses, dependent rubor, atrophic integument, absence of pedal hair, or pallor on elevation coupled with one of more noninvasive values such as a $TcPO_2$ less than 40 mm Hg, ankle brachial index (ABI) less than 0.8, or absolute toe systolic pressure less than 45 mm Hg.

Diabetic foot infection classification schemes: Infectious Diseases Society of America (IDSA).

Mild infections are characterized by less than 2 cm of erythema while moderate infections have more than 2 cm of erythema. Severe infections are associated with systemic toxicity and/or metabolic instability (Table 8.2).

Table 8.2: Diabetic foot infection classification schemes: Infectious Diseases Society of America (IDSA)		
Clinical description	Infectious Diseases Society of America	International Working Group on the Diabetic Foot
Wound without purulence or any manifestations of inflammation	Uninfected	1
≥2 manifestations of inflammation (purulence or erythema, pain, tenderness, warmth, or induration); any cellulitis or erythema extends ≤2 cm around ulcer, and infection is limited to skin or superficial subcutaneous tissues; no local complications or systemic illness	Mild	2
Infection in a patient who is systemically well and metabolically stable but has ≥2 cm; lymphangitis; spread beneath fascia; deep tissue abscess; gangrene; muscle, tendon, joint, or bone involvement	Moderate	3
Infection in a patient with systemic toxicity or metabolic instability (e.g. fever, chills, tachycardia, hypotension, confusion, vomiting, leukocytosis, acidosis, hyperglycemia, or azotemia)	Severe	4

Q. How will you predict poor outcome in diabetic foot infection?

Ans.

- *Increased white blood cell:* In one study, the mean white blood cell (WBC) was 9,777 cells/mm³ for those patients who failed treatment compared to 7,933 cells/mm³ for those with a favorable response.
- *Severe UT wound grades 2 and 3:* Clinical failure was noted in 23% of the patients with UT wounds 2 BD and 3 BD compared with 11% with a wound stage of 0 or 1.
- C-reactive protein (CRP) and ESR values greater than 9.1 and 54.4 respectively were associated with treatment failure.
- Isolation of MRSA was found to be a significant factor associated with treatment failure.
- Absence of OM did not impact the outcome.
- In one study outcome of DFIs treated conservatively, fever, increased serum creatinine, prior hospitalization for DFI, and gangrenous lesions were independent factors associated with treatment failure.

Skin and Subcutaneous Tissue

Chapter

9

One student is expected to present three short cases for examination. About 5–10 minutes are allotted for a short case examination. The student is expected to take a short history and do a relevant clinical examination. The history will include details about the presenting complaint and relevant systemic complaints. A detail general survey is not required for short case examination. Depending on the particular case do relevant general survey.

A detail local examination is required following the standard steps of inspection and palpation. Percussion and auscultation in selected cases.

The history in short case usually includes:

- *Swelling with duration*—Onset, site, and progress of the swelling (size at the onset and how is the size at present). Any history of rapid increase in size. Any other swelling in other parts of the body.
- *Any secondary changes over the swelling*—Ulceration, satellite nodules—ask when these changes has occurred.
- Pain over the swelling. Duration, site, character of pain, and relation of pain with the swelling.
- In suspected hernia swelling enquire about any alteration of the size of the swelling with strenuous activities and what happens to the swelling on lying down.
- *In case of congenital swelling*—Enquire about any other congenital anomalies.
- *In suspected malignant swelling*—Enquire about symptoms suggestive of metastasis—appetite, weight loss, jaundice, abdominal distension, chest pain, cough, hemoptysis, bone pain, headache, vomiting, convulsion, loss of consciousness, and weakness of any of the limbs.
- *Ulcer*—Duration, onset, progress, and any discharge.

Other Relevant Symptoms are Discussed with Each Short Case

Physical Examination

General Survey

Detailed general survey is not required. Only relevant points depending on the case.

Local Examination

- *Inspection:*
  - Site and extent of the swelling
  - Shape and size
  - Surface and margin
  - Skin over the swelling
  - *Any secondary changes over the swelling*—Ulceration, satellite nodules
  - *Any cough impulse*—In suspected hernia swellings
  - *Ulcer*—Site and extent, shape and size, margin and edge, floor, any discharge, and condition of adjacent area
- *Palpation:* Corroboration of inspectory findings.
  - Site and extent
  - Shape and size
  - Surface and margin
  - Consistency
  - Fluctuation
  - Transillumination
  - *Pulsation*—If present—transmitted or expansile
  - Skin fixity
  - Fixity to underlying muscle or bone
  - Reducibility
  - Compressibility
  - *If an ulcer is present*—Corroboration of inspectory findings, base of the ulcer, and mobility.
- *Percussion:* In selected cases.
- *Auscultation:* In selected cases.
- Examination of regional lymph nodes.

SKIN AND SUBCUTANEOUS TISSUE

▌DERMOID CYST

Clinical Examination

- *History:*
  - *About the swelling*—Onset, duration, progress of the swelling, any history of rapid growth, and any pain over the swelling. Any other swelling in the body.
  - Any other complaint.
- On local examination
- *Inspection:*
  - Position and extent of swelling (dermoid cyst usually lies in the midline, and along the lines of embryonic fusion)
  - Size (usually variable) and shape (usually globular)
  - Surface and margin (smooth surface and well-defined margin)
  - Skin over the swelling (usually normal).

* *On palpation:*
  - Temperature
  - Tenderness
  - Position and extent
  - shape and size
  - surface
  - margin
  - Consistency (soft cystic in feel)
  - Fluctuation (fluctuation is usually positive)
  - Transillumination (usually not transilluminant)
  - *Test for mobility*—Fixity to skin (usually free from skin)
  - Fixity to underlying bone (usually not fixed to the underlying bone)
  - Any bony guttering (long-standing dermoid cyst may cause bony guttering at the margin of the swelling).

Q. What is your case? (Summary of a case with dermoid cyst in the lateral angle of left orbit)

Ans. This 20-year-old boy presented with a painless swelling in the lateral angle of left orbit for last 5 years, which is gradually increasing in size. No pain over the swelling. No other swelling in other parts of the body (Fig. 9.1).

On examination, there is a soft cystic swelling at lateral angle of the left orbit, globular in shape, and 3 cm × 3 cm in size. The swelling is fluctuant but transillumination is negative. The overlying skin is free. The cyst indents on pressure. There is a bony indentation at the margin of the orbit around the swelling.

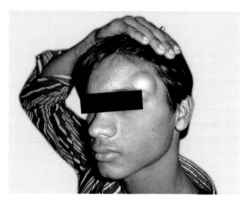

Fig. 9.1: Dermoid cyst in the lateral angle of left orbit

Courtesy: Prof Sukumar Maiti, Calcutta Medical College, Kolkata

Q. What is your diagnosis?

Ans. This is a case of dermoid cyst in the lateral angle of left orbit.

Other diagnosis may be:

* Dermoid cyst in the center of forehead
* Dermoid cyst in the lateral angle of right orbit
* Retroauricular dermoid cyst on the right/left side (Fig. 9.2)
* Dermoid cyst in the scalp (Fig. 9.3A)
* Preauricular dermoid cyst (Fig. 9.3B).

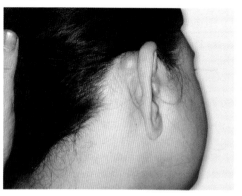

Fig. 9.2: Postauricular dermoid cyst

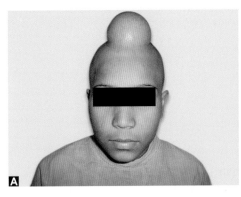 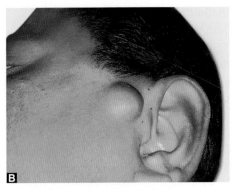

Figs 9.3A and B: (A) Dermoid cyst in scalp; (B) Preauricular dermoid cyst

Courtesy: Prof Abhimanyu Basu, Malda Medical College, West Bengal

Q. What are the other possibilities?

Ans.
- Sebaceous cyst
- Meningocele
- Lipoma
- Fibroma
- Neurofibroma.

Q. How will you demonstrate fluctuation in a small swelling?

Ans. The fluctuation in a small swelling may be demonstrated by placing index finger of one hand as watching finger and index finger of the other hand as displacing finger.

Alternatively, the index and the middle fingers of the left hand are placed apart over the swelling as watching fingers and the index finger of the right hand presses over the center of the swelling acting as the displacing finger (*see* Fig. 1.30, Page No. 30, Chapter 1).

This can also be demonstrated by Paget test. A soft cystic swelling is softer at the center than at the periphery.

Q. How will you demonstrate bony guttering?

Ans. The bony guttering may be demonstrated by placing the finger between the margin of the swelling and underlying bone. The bony indentation is usually found in the dermoid cyst developing over many years (*see* Fig. 1.30, Page No. 30, Chapter 1).

Q. Will you get a positive transillumination test in dermoid cyst?

Ans. The dermoid cyst usually contains a turbid fluid containing sebum and desquamated epithelial cells and is usually not transilluminant.

Rarely, the dermoid cyst may contain a clear fluid and in that case the dermoid cyst may show positive transillumination.

Q. How will you differentiate dermoid cyst and sebaceous cyst?

Ans. Dermoid cyst occurs at the lines of embryonic fusion, whereas sebaceous cyst may occur at any site.

Dermoid cyst lies in subcutaneous tissue and is free from the skin. The sebaceous cyst lies deep to the epidermis and the skin is usually fixed to the cyst and there is usually punctum over the skin.

Q. How will you differentiate dermoid cyst and meningocele?

Ans. The meningocele may be differentiated from dermoid cyst by:
* Presence of cough impulse
* Bony gap is palpable
* Swelling is transilluminant.

Q. What type of dermoid it is?

Ans. This is a sequestration dermoid.

Q. Why this is called a sequestration dermoid?

Ans. This is called a sequestration dermoid because it is formed by sequestration of some ectodermal cells into deeper layer during embryonic development. These sequestrated cells later proliferate and liquefy to form a sequestration dermoid.

Q. What are the pathological features of a sequestration dermoid?

Ans. The cyst is lined by stratified squamous epithelium, which may contain hair follicles, sweat glands, and sebaceous glands. The cyst contains a toothpaste-like material, which is a mixture of desquamated epithelial cells, sweat, and sebum.

Q. Why do you find bony indentation in sequestration dermoid?

Ans. During development of the cyst, the surrounding mesodermal tissue may be compressed causing indentation on the bone, which develops from mesoderm.

Q. What are the common sites of sequestration dermoid?

Ans. The common sites of sequestration dermoid are:
* *In the midline*—Forehead, root of nose, or in the neck
* *At the sites of fusion of skull bones*—Postauricular dermoid
* At the inner or outer angle of the orbit
* At the anterior triangle of the neck.

Q. Why dermoid cyst is called a true cyst?

Ans. This is called a true cyst because it is lined by squamous epithelium with hair follicles, sebaceous glands, and sweat glands. The wall of the cyst is lined by a layer of epidermis oriented with the basal layer superficially and more mature layers lying deep.

Q. What is false cyst?

Ans. The false cyst is a fluid-filled sac not lined by epithelium. This may be lined by granulation tissue or fibrous tissue. This includes pseudopancreatic cyst, cystic degeneration of a tumor.

Q. What is the content of a dermoid cyst?

Ans. The dermoid cyst contains a toothpaste-like material, which is formed by desquamated epithelial cells with or without hair.

Q. How will you treat this patient?

Ans.

◆ I will do an X-ray of skull both anteroposterior (AP) and lateral view to look for any bony gap in the skull, through which the cyst may extend intracranially.

◆ If there is no bony gap suggesting no intracranial extension, simple excision of the cyst is the treatment.

Q. What will you do if there is suspicion of intracranial extension?

Ans.

◆ Computed tomography (CT) scan of cranium is required to assess the extent of intracranial extension.

◆ Excision of the cyst—Both extracranial and intracranial part by raising an osteoplastic flap or by craniectomy.

Q. How will you excise the cyst?

Ans.

◆ Usually done under local anesthesia but may be done under general anesthesia if there is intracranial extension.

◆ An elliptical skin incision is made keeping an island of skin over the swelling. The two skin flaps are raised on either side up to the margin of the cyst. The cyst is then excised and hemostasis is secured. Skin is closed by interrupted nonabsorbable sutures (Figs 9.4A to D).

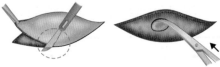

A–Elliptical skin incision   B-Skin flaps dissected

C-Cyst dissected all around   D-Any blood vessels ligated and divided

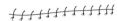

Figs 9.4A to D: Excision of dermoid cyst. Skin is closed by interrupted sutures

Q. What are other types of dermoid cyst?

Ans. Apart from sequestration dermoid, dermoid cyst may develop as:

◆ *Implantation dermoid:* Cyst develops due to implantation of epidermal cells into the deeper tissue usually due to a pinprick.

◆ *Tubulodermoid:* Cysts developing from a nonobliterated portion of a congenital ectodermal duct. The cyst is formed by accumulation of secretions of the lining ectodermal cells, e.g. thyroglossal cyst.

◆ *Teratomatous dermoid:* Cyst developing from totipotential cells and contains different structures arising from ectodermal, mesodermal, and endodermal elements. The cyst may contain hairs, bones, teeth, and other elements.

Q. Where do you find teratomatous dermoid?

Ans.

◆ *In ovary:* Dermoid cyst

◆ *Testis:* Teratoma

◆ *Mediastinum:* Mediastinal cyst

◆ *Retroperitoneum:* Retroperitoneal cyst

◆ Postanal dermoid.

Q. In dermoid cyst of scalp expansile impulse on cough is present. What is the implication?

Ans. When there is expansile impulse on cough it indicates that there is intracranial extension of the cyst.

Q. What are the complications of dermoid cyst?

Ans.
◆ Infection
◆ Hemorrhage
◆ Pressure effect on adjacent structure
◆ Calcification
◆ Rupture and surface ulceration.

■ IMPLANTATION DERMOID

Clinical Examination

◆ *History:*
  – About the swelling (*see* Page No. 382).
  – Any history of prick or cut injury which might drive epithelial cells into the depth.
  – Any history of pain (implantation dermoid may be painful).
◆ *Examination:* Same as swelling (*See* Page No. 382).
  – The implantation of dermoid may feel tense, firm, or hard.
  – As the swelling is very small fluctuation is not demonstrable.
  – The cyst is not transilluminant and is free from the skin and underlying tissues.

Q. What is your case? (Summary of a case of implantation dermoid)

Ans. This 50-year-old gentleman tailor by occupation presented with a swelling in the left palm for last 4 years. He had a history of needle prick in his palm 4.5 years back. He noticed a swelling in his palm 4 years back, which was about 1 cm in size at the onset. The swelling is increasing slowly in size to attain the present size of about 3 cm. There is no pain over the swelling. There is no other swelling in the body (Fig. 9.5).

On examination, there is a swelling in the middle of the left palm, globular in shape 3 cm in diameter, nontender, firm in feel, free from skin, and underlying structures.

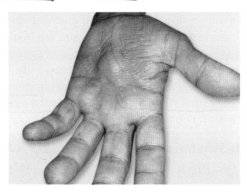

Fig. 9.5: This is a case of implantation dermoid on the palmar aspect of left hand

Courtesy: Prof Bitan Kumar Chattopadhyay, Institute of Postgraduate Medical Education and Research (IPGMER), Kolkata

Q. What is implantation dermoid?

Ans. This is an acquired cyst, which is formed by in-driving of surface epithelium usually due to a pinprick. It is common in tailors and gardeners.

Q. What is the pathology of implantation dermoid?

Ans. The cyst is lined by squamous epithelium. There are no hair follicles, sweat glands, or sebaceous glands. The cyst contains an amorphous material, which is formed by the desquamated epithelial cells.

Q. How will you treat this patient?

Ans. Excision of the cyst under local anesthetic block. The digital vessels and nerves are to be preserved.

Q. What are the complications in implantation dermoid?

Ans.
♦ Infection
♦ Rupture
♦ Pressure effect on digital nerves.

■ SUBMENTAL DERMOID

Q. What is your case? (Summary of a case of submental dermoid)

Ans. This 25-year-old gentleman presented with a swelling in submental region for last 6 years, which is gradually increasing in size. No pain over the swelling. No other swellings in other parts of the body (Fig. 9.6).

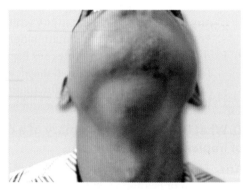

Fig. 9.6: This is a case of submental dermoid cyst. *Courtesy:* Dr Samik Kumar Bandyopadhyay, RG Kar Medical College, Kolkata

On examination: The swelling is situated in submental region in the midline and extending on either side. The swelling is globular in shape 7 cm in diameter, soft cystic, and fluctuation is positive but transillumination is negative. The overlying skin is free and there is no fixity to the underlying structures. The swelling does not move up with deglutition nor does the swelling move up on protrusion of tongue.

Q. What is your diagnosis?

Ans. This is a case of dermoid cyst in submental region.

Q. What else the swelling could be?

Ans.
♦ *Suprahyoid thyroglossal cyst:* Moves up and down with deglutition and moves up with protrusion of tongue.
♦ *Ectopic thyroid gland:* Moves up and down with deglutition but does not move up on protrusion of tongue.
♦ Submental lymph node enlargement may be due to chronic septic foci in oral cavity or Koch's lymphadenitis.
♦ Sebaccous cyst.

Q. How will you treat this patient?

Ans.
- I will do complete excision of the cyst under general anesthesia.
- A curved incision is made along the Langer's line over the cystic swelling. Skin flaps are raised. The deep fascia is incised along the line of skin incision and the cyst is removed by dissection all around the margin of the cyst.

Q. What are the complications of submental dermoid?

Ans.
- Infection
- If very big may cause difficulty in swallowing
- Prone to repeated trauma.

Q. What type of dermoid cyst it is?

Ans. This is a type of congenital sequestration dermoid and arises due to sequestration of surface ectodermal cells during fusion of 1st and 2nd branchial arches.

■ SEBACEOUS CYST

Clinical Examination

See Page No. 382.

Q. What is your case? (Summary of a case of sebaceous cyst)

Ans. This 30-year-old lady complains of a slowly growing swelling on the back of chest on the left side for last 3 years. The swelling was about 1 cm in size when she first noticed the swelling and since then is growing slowly in size. Patient complains of occasional discharge of greyish-white material from the swelling, which has offensive smell. There is no other swelling in other parts of the body (Fig. 9.7).

On examination: A globular soft cystic swelling 3 cm in diameter is found on the back of the chest on the left side. Surface is smooth, margins are well defined. There is a punctum on the surface of the swelling and the skin is fixed to the swelling. The swelling can be indented by pressure. Transillumination is negative (In big cyst, fluctuation may be positive).

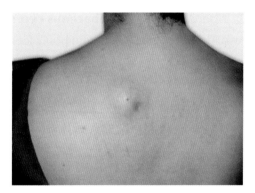

Fig. 9.7: Sebaceous cyst in back of chest on the left side (note the punctum)

Courtesy: Dr SN Chander, Institute of Postgraduate Medical Education and Research (IPGMER), Kolkata

Q. What is your diagnosis?

Ans. This is a case of sebaceous cyst in back of the chest on the left side.

Q. What else this can be?

Ans.
- Dermoid cyst
- Lipoma
- Fibroma
- Neurofibroma.

Q. What is sebaceous cyst?

Ans. This is a retention cyst in relation to sebaceous gland due to blockage of sebaceous duct and accumulation of secretion within the gland.

Q. Where sebaceous glands are located?

Ans. The sebaceous glands are situated in the dermis and their ducts open either into a hair follicle or directly on to the skin surface and it secretes sebum.

Q. Where sebaceous glands are absent?

Ans. Sebaceous glands are present throughout the body except in palms and soles.

Q. Why sebaceous cyst is also called an epidermoid cyst?

Ans. The sebaceous cyst is located in the dermis and is lined by superficial squamous epithelial cells of the epidermis, so it is called an epidermoid cyst.

Q. What is the content of a sebaceous cyst?

Ans. The sebaceous cyst contains a greyish-whitish cheesy material with an unpleasant smell. The material does not contain sebum and contains mainly epithelial debris.

Q. Where do you find sebaceous cyst commonly?

Ans. The sebaceous cyst is commonly found in scalp, face, neck, scrotum, chest, breast, and shoulder regions.

Q. What organism may be found in sebaceous cyst?

Ans. An organism called *Demodex folliculorum* may be found in the wall of the sebaceous cyst.

Q. How will you treat this patient?

Ans.
- Blood sugar estimation if patient is elderly
- I will do excision of the cyst, under local anesthesia.

Q. How will you excise the swelling?

Ans. Local anesthesia—By injection of 1% lignocaine hydrochloride. The local anesthetic is injected by ring block technique.

An elliptical incision is made over the swelling keeping a rim of skin around the punctum. The skin flaps are dissected off from the cyst wall. The cyst along with the rim of skin is dissected free from the underlying subcutaneous tissue and the cyst is removed intact along with its lining wall.

Q. What is the other technique of excision of sebaceous cyst?

Ans. It can be excised by incision and avulsion. Under local anesthesia an incision is made over the skin. The cyst content is squeezed out. The cyst wall is then held up with a hemostatic forceps and removed by avulsion.

Q. What are the complications of sebaceous cyst?

Ans.
* Infection
* Ulceration
* Cock's peculiar tumor
* Sebaceous horn formation
* Rarely malignant change may occur. Usually a basal cell carcinoma (BCC).

Q. What are the features of infected sebaceous cyst?

Ans.
* Patient complains of pain over the swelling and there is recent increase in size of the swelling.
* On examination, the overlying skin is red, inflamed. The cyst is tender and on squeezing, the cyst pus may be expressed through the punctum.

Q. How will you treat an infected sebaceous cyst?

Ans.
* Antibiotics
* After the infection is controlled—excision of the cyst
* If pus is already pointing, in addition to antibiotics, incision and drainage of pus, and avulsion of cyst wall may be done.

Q. What is Cock's peculiar tumor?

Ans. This is a complication found commonly in the sebaceous cyst of scalp. There is infection in the cyst and there is ulceration on the surface of the sebaceous cyst. There is escape of cyst content on the surface through the ulcer on the cyst wall. Chronic irritation may lead to formation of a granuloma on the surface of the sebaceous cyst. This may mimic like an epithelioma. This appearance of the cyst is called a Cock's peculiar tumor.

Q. What is sebaceous horn?

Ans. The sebaceous material may escape through the punctum and accumulate on the surface of the sebaceous cyst and gets dried in successive layers and form a horny projection on the surface of the sebaceous cyst. This appearance is called a sebaceous horn.

Q. How will you differentiate a scalp dermoid from a sebaceous cyst?

Ans.
* The sebaceous cyst is tethered to the skin but dermoid cyst is subcutaneous and skin is free in the dermoid cyst.
* Bony indentation is not found in the sebaceous cyst but usually found in the dermoid cyst.

Q. What are the characteristics of scrotal sebaceous cyst (Fig. 9.8)?

Ans.

* Usually multiple
* May feel solid
* No punctum is usually seen.

Q. How will you treat scrotal sebaceous cyst?

Ans.

* *Single cyst:* Excision
* *Multiple cysts confined to one segment of the scrotum:* Excision of that segment of scrotal skin along with the cyst
* *Multiple cysts involving whole of scrotum:* Total scrotectomy with all cysts. Testes may be implanted in a subcutaneous tunnel on the medial aspect of the thigh.

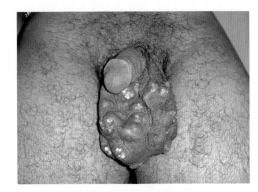

Fig. 9.8: Multiple sebaceous cysts in scrotum

Courtesy: Dr Sohabrata Mukherjee, Calcutta National Medical College, Kolkata

■ LIPOMA

Clinical Examination

See Page No. 382.

Q. What is your case? (Summary of a case of lipoma)

Ans. This 30-year-old gentleman presented with a gradually increasing swelling in the back of the neck for last 4 years. The swelling was about 2 cm in size at the onset and then gradually increased in size to attain the present size of about 5 cm, no history of rapid increase in size of the swelling. No pain over the swelling. No other swelling in other parts of the body (Fig. 9.9).

On local examination: A soft, globular swelling, 5 cm in diameter is found in the back of the nape of the neck. Surface is lobulated and the margins are rounded, well defined, and slips under the finger. Fluctuation and transillumination are negative. The skin is free and the swelling is freely mobile on the underlying structures. The swelling becomes more prominent on contraction of the underlying trapezius muscle.

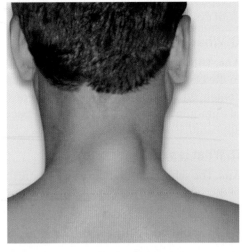

Fig. 9.9: Lipoma at the back of neck

Courtesy: Prof Prasanta Kumar Bhattacharya, Institute of Postgraduate Medical Education and Research (IPGMER), Kolkata

Q. What is your diagnosis?

Ans. This is a case of subcutaneous lipoma in the nape of the neck.

Q. How will you demonstrate that the surface of lipoma is lobulated?

Ans. In large lipomas, this can be ascertained on inspection.

Sometimes, the surface feels smooth. Firm pressure with one hand at the margin of the swelling will make these lobules more prominent and the lobulated surface may then be appreciated by palpating with the palmar surface of the fingers of the other hand.

Q. How will you demonstrate slip sign?

Ans. Lipomas are freely mobile swellings. When the edge of the swelling is pressed with the finger, the swelling along with the edge gets displaced by the palpating finger. This is called slip sign.

Q. Do lipomas show fluctuation?

Ans. Lipomas are soft in feel. Some lipomas are very soft and there may be an impression that there is positive fluctuation. On pressing on one side of the swelling, the swelling may yield on pressure. The swelling, however, does not become tense and prominent in a plane at right angles to the palpating fingers. So, this is often described as pseudofluctuation.

Q. Can lipomas show positive transillumination?

Ans. Sometimes in large lipomas, the light beam thrown from a torch light may pass right across the swelling and the swelling may show positive transillumination. However, all lipomas do not show positive transillumination.

Q. What else this swelling can be?

Ans.
- Neurofibroma
- Fibroma
- Sebaceous cyst
- Rhabdomyoma.

Q. How will you treat this patient?

Ans. I will do excision of the swelling.

The operation is done under local anesthesia unless the swelling is very big. A ring block with 1% lignocaine injection is used.

A skin incision is made along the Langer's line. The incision is deepened till the capsule is reached. The skin flaps are then raised on either side and lipoma along with the capsule is dissected off from the underlying subcutaneous tissue. Hemostasis is secured. Skin is closed with interrupted silk suture.

Q. What is lipoma?

Ans. Lipoma is a benign tumor arising from mature fat cells.

Q. Why this is called universal tumor?

Ans. This is the most common benign soft tissue tumor and can occur anywhere in the body. So, it is called universal tumor.

Q. What are the complications of lipoma?

Ans. The lipoma of long duration may undergo some secondary changes:

* May attain huge size and cause cosmetic deformity
* Saponification and calcification
* Rarely malignant change—Liposarcoma
* Myxomatous degeneration
* Infection
* Hemorrhage.

Q. Where do you find lipomas commonly?

Ans. The lipoma may be found anywhere in the body. It is commonly found in the subcutaneous tissues of trunk, neck, and limbs.

Q. Which lipomas commonly undergo malignant change?

Ans. Retroperitoneal lipomas; lipomas in the thigh and lipomas in the shoulder region more commonly undergo malignant change.

Q. When would you suspect a sarcomatous change in a lipoma?

Ans.

* History of rapid increase in size
* Swelling may become painful
* There may be symptoms due to distant metastasis
* The temperature over the swelling may be raised
* There may be dilated veins over the swelling
* There may be infiltration to deeper structure or to the skin—swelling may become fixed to the deeper structure or to the skin.

Q. How lipomas are classified according to their anatomical location?

Ans.

* *Subcutaneous:* Lipomas arising in subcutaneous tissue plane.
* *Subfascial:* Lipomas arising from fat cells lying deep to the deep fascia.
* *Intramuscular:* Lipomas arising from the fat cell lying in between the muscle fibers.
* *Subserous:* Lipoma arising from the fat cells lying in the subserous plane of the gut.
* *Submucus:* Lipoma arising from the fat cells lying in the submucus layer in respiratory and gastrointestinal tract.
* *Subsynovial:* Lipoma arising from fat cell lying deep to the synovial membranc lining the joint.
* *Parosteal:* Lipoma arising from fat cells lying deep to the periosteal lining the bone.
* *Intra-articular:* Lipomas arising from fat cells lying within the joint.
* *Extradural:* Lipomas arising from the fat cells lying in the extradural space in the spinal canal. Intracranial extradural lipoma does not occur as there is no fat cell in the cranial cavity.
* *Intraglandular:* Lipomas arising from the fat cells lying within the gland—breast and salivary glands.

Q. What is fibrolipoma?

Ans. Lipomas containing both fatty and fibrous tissue components are called fibrolipomas.

Q. What is nevolipoma?

Ans. Lipoma containing both fatty and hemangiomatous tissues. There may be telangiectasia of the overlying skin and the swelling may be partially compressible.

Q. What is neurolipoma?

Ans. Lipoma containing both fatty and neural components. This condition may be multiple and painful, called neurolipomatosis.

Q. What is Dercum's disease or adiposis dolorosa?

Ans. This is painful, tender, diffuse, or nodular deposits of fat in trunk or limb. Commonly found in women particularly affecting trunk, buttocks, and thigh. There are no capsules around these fatty deposits so they are also called false lipoma.

■ KELOID

Clinical Examination

History

♦ *Scar*—How scar occurred (following operation or a trauma)?
♦ Duration of enlargement of the scar (a keloid continues to grow beyond 6 months).
♦ Any extension of the scar to the normal tissue (a keloid scar grows into the normal tissue).
♦ Any systemic disease (tuberculosis, diabetes, and hypertension). Any family history of such disease.

Examination—Inspection/Palpation

♦ Site, extent of enlargement of the scar
♦ Does it extend into the normal tissue? Any other scar in the body showing similar change.

Q. What is your case? (Summary of a case of keloid)

Ans. This 20-year-old female patient complains of a gradually increasing scar in the front of her chest wall for last 8 years following excision of a swelling in this site about 8-year back. She complains of itching over the local site (Fig. 9.10).

The scar is raised from the surface, extends to the normal tissues. It is pink in color and the local temperature is slightly raised.

Q. Why it is not a hypertrophic scar?

Ans. Hypertrophic scar does not extend into normal tissue, has no claw-like extension, no itching, no sign of increased vascularity, and gradually regresses after 6 months. Usually does not get worse after 1 year.

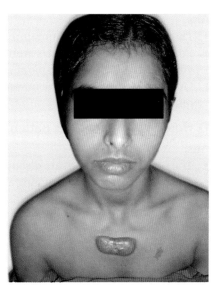

Fig. 9.10: Keloid in chest wall in front of manubrium sterni

Courtesy: Dr Samik Kumar Bandyopadhyay, RG Kar Medical College, Kolkata

Q. What is keloid?

Ans. Keloid is defined as a condition of proliferation of fibroblast, collagen fibrils, and immature blood vessel usually on a preexisting scar.

Q. What is spontaneous keloid?

Ans. When there is no history of injury or operation and as such there is no scar, the fibroblastic proliferation starts spontaneously and leads to formation of a keloid. This is common in Negro population.

Q. What is nonprogressive keloid?

Ans. Majority of the keloid shows continuous growth with extension into the normal tissues in a claw-like fashion. Some keloids, however, may stop growing after initial growth. Keloids showing no sign of progressive growth are called nonprogressive keloid.

Q. Which factors are responsible for development of keloid?

Ans. The definite cause for development of keloid is not known. A number of factors have been incriminated as etiological factors:
- *Race:* It is more common in Negro population
- *Sex:* Females are more affected than male
- *Familial:* Familial predisposition in some cases
- *Site of scar:* Incision across Langer's line increases chance of keloid formation
- *Tuberculosis:* Increased incidence of keloid formation in patients suffering from tuberculosis.

Q. What are the pathological characteristics of keloid?

Ans.
- There is proliferation of immature fibroblasts in abundance
- Proliferation of blood vessels around the base of sebaceous and sweat glands
- Fibroblasts are disposed in parallel sheets and embedded in a stroma of collagen
- Due to presence of plenty of immature blood vessels, the keloid is vascularized and there is pink discoloration.

Q. How will you treat this patient?

Ans.
- The results of treatment are disappointing
- The patient complains of itching at the local site
- Local steroid cream application (betamethasone or dexamethasone cream) may help to reduce the itching
- If local application of steroid fails or the patient complains of severe itching, intrakeloid injection of steroid, e.g. injection of triamcinolone into the keloid may help. Injection is done at weekly interval for 4–6 weeks.

Q. What other injection may help?

Ans.
- Intrakeloid injection of hyaluronidase
- Intrakeloid injection of vitamin A
- Intrakeloid injection of methotrexate.

Q. What is the role of surgical treatment?

Ans. Surgery has a very limited role in the management of keloid as there is high chance of recurrence following surgery.

The surgery commonly practiced is intrakeloid excision and approximation of the margin by suturing or split skin grafting.

Q. What is the role of deep X-ray therapy in treatment of keloid?

Ans. Earlier deep X-ray therapy has been used for treatment of large keloid lesion and has shown some benefit. Radiation suppresses the proliferation of fibroblasts and blood vessels, and helps in regression of keloid. But in view of side effects of radiation therapy its use for benign condition has been abandoned.

Q. What is the role of compression bandaging in treatment of keloid?

Ans. Pressure garments maintaining pressure over the keloid scar may help in some cases.

Q. What are the complications of keloid?

Ans.
+ Infection and suppuration
+ Ulceration due to itching or trauma. Rarely Marjolin's ulcer may develop
+ Recurrence after excision.

Q. What are the characteristics of hypertrophic scar?

Ans. Hypertrophic scars are more cellular and vascular than the mature scars. There is increased collagen production and breakdown. Hypertrophic scars appear as:
+ Scar raised above the surface
+ Does not extend to normal tissues
+ Does not worsen after 6 months.

■ POSTBURN CONTRACTURE

Clinical Examination

History
+ *Presenting complaints:*
    – Restriction of neck movement
    – Difficulty in closing mouth
    – Difficulty in drinking liquids/difficulty in chewing food
    – Any problem in the limbs (in case of contracture involving the limbs)
    – *History of burn injury*—Details of the mechanism of burn injury, treatment done for the burn injury.

Examination—Inspection/Palpation
+ Look for the burn scar
+ Look for the deformity
+ Assess neck movement
+ In case of contracture involving the limbs—assess movement of the local joints.

Q. What is your case? (Summary of a case of postburn contracture involving the face and neck)

Ans. This 20-year-old lady sustained flame burn injury 14 months back, involving the face, neck and chest, and both upper limbs. She was admitted in a hospital and was treated with intravenous fluid, antibiotics, and regular dressings. The wound took a long time of about 3 months for complete healing. Afterwards patient noticed that the scar tissues are getting gradually thickened and there is bending of neck. Patient cannot move the neck freely. Patient also could not lift her left upper limb freely. She has difficulty in eating and drinking for last 6 months. Patient also complains of drooling of saliva from the angle of mouth and has difficulty in speech. Patient also complains of itching over the scar (Fig. 9.11).

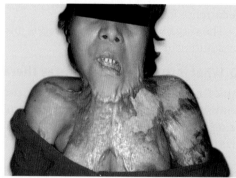

Fig. 9.11: This is a case of postburn contracture involving the face, neck, and axilla.

Courtesy: Prof Arindam Sarkar, Institute of Postgraduate Medical Education and Research (IPGMER), Kolkata

On examination: Patient is poorly nourished, there is gross thickening of scar tissue in the face, neck, and chest. The neck is slightly flexed and the patient is unable to extend and rotate the neck. The lower lip is everted. There is gross contracture of the scar tissue. The patient cannot appose both the lips and there is constant drooling of saliva from the mouth. There is a thickened scar in the region of the left axilla and there is restriction of left shoulder movement. The systemic examination is normal.

Q. What is your diagnosis?

Ans. This is a case of postburn contracture involving the face, neck, chest, and left axilla.

Q. How the postburn contracture develops?

Ans. In deep burns, there is destruction of all epithelial elements. In deep burns involving the full thickness of skin, healing occurs by fibrosis and not by epithelialization. For proper healing of deep burn areas, resurfacing is required either with split thickness skin graft or coverage with skin flaps. If proper resurfacing is not done these areas of deep burns heals by formation of granulation tissue and fibrosis, resulting in gross scarring. All scar contract as they mature and this phenomenon leads to formation of postburn contracture.

If superficial burn is infected, it may cause sloughing of deeper tissues, which then heals by fibrosis resulting in contracture, in spite of burn being superficial.

Q. How could you prevent this contracture?

Ans. The postburn contracture may be prevented by proper treatment of primary burn injury.

In case of deep burns, especially involving the joints of extremities, neck, hands, and face should be properly splinted during healing.

Once there is formation of granulation tissue, the wound should be covered with split thickness skin graft and should not be allowed to heal by fibrosis.

After skin grafting these areas should be properly splinted and intensive physiotherapy should be done to prevent secondary graft contracture.

The superficial burn wound should be treated properly and infection should be prevented by administering prophylactic antibiotics. The joint area should be splinted to prevent development of contracture during healing.

Q. What are the problems in patients with burn contracture?

Ans.
- Gross cosmetic deformity
- Limitation of anatomical movement of joints
- In contracture involving the neck there is gross restriction of neck movements resulting in restriction of normal activities. The range of vision is also restricted.
- The lip is everted and proper closure of oral orifice is hampered resulting in constant drooling of saliva.
- There may be difficulty in sucking and chewing food.
- In burn contracture involving the shoulder and axillary region will restrict the movement of upper limbs.
- Burn contracture involving hands and feet will cause impairment of functions of fingers and toes.

■ QUESTIONS ABOUT BURNS

Q. How will you assess the amount of burn area?

Ans. *See* Surgical Problems Section, Page No. 720–722, Chapter 16.

Q. What are the different grades depending on the depth of burn injury?

Ans. *See* Surgical Problems Section, Page No. 720–722, Chapter 16.

Q. What are the causes of burn shock?

Ans. *See* Surgical Problems Section, Page No. 720–722, Chapter 16.

Q. How will you manage burns shock?

Ans. *See* Surgical Problems Section, Page No. 720–722, Chapter 16.

Q. How will you treat this patient?

Ans. I would suggest some baseline investigations to assess fitness of the patient for anesthesia and surgery:
- *Complete hemogram*—Hemoglobin (Hb)%, total leukocyte count (TLC), differential leukocyte count (DLC), and erythrocyte sedimentation rate (ESR)
- Blood for sugar, urea, and creatinine
- *Blood for serum proteins*—Albumin and globulin
- X-ray of neck AP and lateral view to assess any bony deformity
- Chest X-ray posteroanterior (PA) view.

Q. What should be the optimum timing for release of postburn contracture?

Ans. Postburn contracture release should be planned after the scar tissue has matured. The scar maturation takes about 6 months to 1 year. Mature scar has a whitish hue, is soft, and supple in texture.

Q. What are the problems of anesthesia in these patients?

Ans. Because of contracture in the neck, there is great difficulty in endotracheal intubation.
* If there is facility for fiberoptic bronchoscopy, endotracheal intubation should be done in these patients with assistance of fiberoptic bronchoscopy.
* Blind nasotracheal intubation is sometimes successful.
* Alternatively, the neck contracture may be released partially under local anesthesia and then oral endotracheal intubation may be done in the usual way.

Q. How will you release these contractures?

Ans.
* *For neck:* Incise through the fibrotic scar tissue at the point of maximum tension up to the healthy soft tissue extending from the posterior border of sternocleidomastoid to the posterior border of other sternocleidomastoid. The release incision should be deepened up to the strap muscles. The raw surface should be covered with split-thickness skin grafting.
* *For contracture at the axilla or limbs:* The contracture may be released by single or multiple Z-plasty.
* *For contracture along the joints:* The scar tissue is released. The joints are manipulated under anesthesia. The resurfacing is done with split-thickness skin grafting or by using skin flaps. The joints need to be splinted during the phase of healing.
* *Coverage of difficult areas:* If after release of the contracture the bed is relatively avascular or there is bare bone, cartilage, or tendon, then the raw area should be covered with skin flap either a local or distant pedicle skin flap.

Q. How will you take care in the postoperative period?

Ans.
* Postoperative splinting is essential for proper healing:
    - *Neck:* Moulded cervical collar for 6 months.
    - *Axilla:* Abduction splint for 3–6 months.
    - *Elbow and knee:* Static extension splint (functional brace) for 3–6 months.
    - *Hand:* Keep hand in position of function for 2–3 months with active physiotherapy.
    - *Wrist:* Splint in 10–15° of extension.
    - *Thumb:* Splint in palmar abduction.
    - *Fingers:* Splint with metacarpophalangeal joints in 80–90° flexion and interphalangeal joints in extension.
* *Postoperative physiotherapy:* Supervised physiotherapy particularly for limb contracture.

■ MALIGNANT MELANOMA

Clinical Examination

History

* *Swelling*—Onset and progress of the pigmented lesion.
* Any history of presence of a preexisting pigmented lesion.
* If so, enquire about the secondary changes—itching, increase in size, change of shape, surface, and thickness. Any change in color.
* Any surface ulceration.
* Any bleeding.

- Enquire about any local spread.
- Any discoloration around the primary lesion (brown halo).
- Any satellite nodule around the primary lesion or along the lymphatic channels from the primary lesion (in-transit nodules).
- Any swelling at the regional lymph nodes site.
- Any systemic complaints:
  - Chest pain, cough, and hemoptysis.
  - Abdominal distension, jaundice.
  - Headache, vomiting, convulsion, loss of consciousness, and any focal neurological symptoms.

Examination

- *Examination of the swelling in the usual way*—Inspection/Palpation (*See* Page No. 381)
  - Look for color, any brown halo around the primary tumor.
  - Any satellite or in-transit nodules
  - Examine the skin and subcutaneous tissue between the primary tumor and the regional lymph nodes.
- Examine the regional lymph nodes.
- *Examination of abdomen*—Hepatomegaly, ascites.
- *Examination of chest*—Pleural effusion or lung collapse.
- *Examination of nervous system*—Higher functions, cranial nerves, and examination of limbs.

Q. What is your case? (Summary of a case of malignant melanoma)

Ans. This 50-year-old gentleman complains of a pigmented lesion on the heel of right foot for last 1 year. The pigmented lesion was about 1 cm in diameter at the onset and the swelling was growing slowly. For the last 2 months the swelling is growing rapidly and the pigmented area has spread to involve the whole of heel and part of the sole. The swelling has darkened in color. There is ulceration over the swelling for last 1 month and the ulcer is also increasing in size to involve the adjacent area. Patient also complains of dull aching pain over the swelling and complains of itching at the local site (Fig. 9.12).

On examination, there is a darkly pigmented nodular solid lesion 7 cm × 6 cm in size, firm in consistency. The floor of the ulcer is covered by necrotic tissue and the base is indurated but not fixed to the underlying calcaneus. The surrounding pigmentation involves about 4 cm all around the nodular lesion. The joint mobility is normal. There is no lymph node enlargement in popliteal fossa and inguinal region.

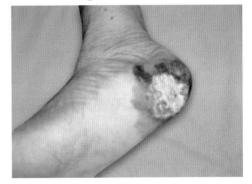

Fig. 9.12: The case of malignant melanoma involving the right heel

Courtesy: Prof Amitabha Sarkar, Institute of Postgraduate Medical Education and Research (IPGMER), Kolkata

Q. What is your diagnosis?

Ans. This is a case of malignant melanoma on the heel of the right foot without any lymph node metastasis.

Q. What are the other possibilities of such a pigmented lesion?

Ans.

- Angioma
- Pyogenic granuloma
- Pigmented BCC
- Pigmented squamous papilloma
- Glomus tumor
- Kaposi's sarcoma
- Pigmented senile keratosis.

Q. How will you manage this patient?

Ans. Clinically this appears to be malignant melanoma, so I will consider surgical treatment in this patient.

I will advise:

- Baseline investigations [complete hemogram, blood for sugar, urea and creatinine, chest X-ray, and electrocardiogram (ECG)]
- As the lesion is large I will advise an incisional biopsy from the margin of the lesion.

Q. What treatment will you plan for this patient?

Ans. Once the biopsy report confirms malignant melanoma I will plan to do a wide local excision with a 2 cm clear margin all around. The resultant defect needs coverage. The coverage may be achieved by a skin flap. As the heel is a weight-bearing area a split-thickness skin grafting may not be suitable.

The lymph nodes are not involved clinically but the lesion is large. I will consider for a sentinel lymph node biopsy. If lymph node is positive on sentinel lymph node biopsy I will advise ilioinguinal lymph node dissection.

Q. In which cases you will consider an incisional biopsy?

Ans.

- Incisional or punch biopsy is indicated in large pigmented lesions.
- Lesion in areas of cosmetic importance where primary closure will be difficult.
- Biopsy of suspected malignant melanoma is also indicated in lesions, which show recent change in growth, pigmentation, pruritus, or bleeding lesion.

Q. Why it is not necessary to do excision of deep fascia when excising a malignant melanoma?

Ans. The malignant melanoma does not usually invade the deep fascia and so excision of the deep fascia is not required in most cases.

Q. Why the resultant defect is better covered with a split skin graft?

Ans. It is better to cover the defect with a split skin graft particularly in nonweight-bearing areas. If a full thickness or pedicle graft is used, the diagnosis of local recurrence may be delayed.

Q. What is the management strategy for uninvolved lymph nodes?

Ans. If the lymph nodes are not clinically involved, patient can be kept under close follow-up. If in follow-up, the lymph nodes are found to be involved; a therapeutic block dissection will be required.

Alternatively, a sentinel lymph node biopsy may be considered. If sentinel lymph node biopsy is positive, a therapeutic lymph node dissection is to be done.

Q. What do you mean by elective lymph node dissection?

Ans. Elective lymph node dissection (ELND) involves dissection of primary draining lymph nodes when it is clinically negative.

Q. What are the rationalities of elective lymph node dissection?

Ans. Although, the role of ELND is controversial, the proponents of ELND agrees that ELND removes all the lymph nodes, which are not yet involved by metastatic deposits, thereby reducing the chance of recurrence of the disease at the lymph node site.

The cutaneous melanomas spread initially to the lymph nodes and then spread systemically. The interruption of the lymph node basin by prophylactic dissection will interrupt the progression in a proportion of patients in early stage and in some cases, improve survival.

Q. What are the problems of elective lymph node dissection?

Ans. In about 80% cases of ELND, the lymph nodes are found to be histologically negative. So in vast majority of cases, the surgery is unnecessary. This adds to increased cost of surgery, prolonged hospital stay.

Postoperative wound infection, wound dehiscence, and symptomatic lymphedema may occur following ELND.

Moreover, removal of the regional lymph nodes may hamper the immunological response to the tumor antigen.

Q. What are the indications for ELND?

Ans. There is a consensus that melanomas less than 1 mm in thickness does not benefit from ELND. ELND is also not beneficial in patients with melanoma more than 4 mm thickness, as the chances of systemic metastasis in these patients are very high and ELND does not improve survival. ELND has been considered in following situations:
- Intermediate thickness melanomas 1–2 mm thick has been claimed to benefit from ELND
- Difficulty in regular follow-up.
  However, there is no survival advantage following ELND.

Q. What is monoblock dissection?

Ans. When the primary lesion and the metastatic lymph nodes are lying in close proximity then a radical surgery of the primary lesion and incontinuity lymph node dissection is to be done along with the intervening lymphatic channels. This is called monoblock dissection.

If the lesion is in groin with involvement of inguinal lymph nodes, a monoblock dissection involves wide excision of the primary lesion along with ilioinguinal block dissection and intervening lymphatic channel.

Q. What is a sentinel lymph node?

Ans. Sentinel lymph node is one which receives the lymphatics from the area of the primary lesion in the skin. The sentinel lymph node is the first node in the lymphatic chain, which will receive the tumor cells from the primary site.

Q. What is the importance of sentinel lymph node?

Ans. If the sentinel lymph node is free of tumor it is likely that the rest of the lymph node basin is also free of tumor. Biopsy of this sentinel lymph node helps in assessing lymph node basin status thereby sparing lymphadenectomy for lymph node-negative patients.

Q. What are the advantages of sentinel lymph node biopsy?

Ans. If the sentinel lymph node is free of tumor it is unlikely to have metastasis in other lymph node in the lymph node basin at the site. So if sentinel lymph node biopsy reveal no tumor deposit a formal lymph node dissection may be avoided and block dissection is to be considered in patients only when there is a positive sentinel lymph node.

Q. In which other cancers sentinel lymph node biopsy is practiced?

Ans. Sentinel lymph node biopsy is also practiced in:
* Carcinoma penis
* Carcinoma breast.

Q. If the inguinal lymph nodes are palpable how will you proceed to manage this patient?

Ans. If the palpable inguinal lymph nodes are clinically significant and are most likely to be metastatic so fine-needle aspiration cytology (FNAC) is not required for diagnosis of metastatic deposits.
For metastatic lymph node: I will consider inguinopelvic block dissection.

Q. Why do you want to do inguinopelvic block dissection?

Ans. As the inguinal lymph node is involved, there is high chance of spread of the disease to pelvic lymph node and so for proper clearance an inguinopelvic block dissection is to be done. Different studies have revealed better survival in patients who have undergone inguinopelvic dissection than the patients who have undergone an inguinal block dissection only.

■ MALIGNANT MELANOMA WITH LYMPH NODE METASTASIS

Q. What is your case?

Ans. This is a case of malignant melanoma on the scalp in right frontoparietal region (Fig. 9.13) with metastasis in the right cervical lymph nodes at level II and III. The primary lesion is 7 cm in diameter.

Q. How will you manage this patient?

Ans. For primary lesion: In addition to baseline workup, I will do an incisional biopsy from the margin of lesion. If the histology report is malignant melanoma, I will consider wide local excision of the primary lesion with a 2 cm clear margin.

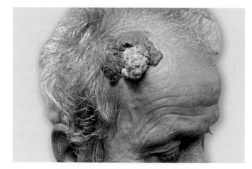

Fig. 9.13: Malignant melanoma in scalp in right frontoparietal region with lymph node metastasis in the right-sided cervical lymph nodes at level II and III

Courtesy: Dr AN Acharya, Institute of Postgraduate Medical Education and Research (IPGMER), Kolkata

For lymph nodes: If the palpable lymph nodes are clinically significant, I will consider doing a modified radical neck dissection removing levels I, II, III, IV, and V lymph nodes.

Q. What is malignant melanoma?

Ans. This is a malignant tumor of skin arising from melanoblasts or melanocytes.

Q. What are melanocytes?

Ans. Melanocytes are derived from the neural crest, which migrates during embryonic life and are located mainly in the skin at the dermoepidermal junction.

Q. What are the different sites where malignant melanoma may arise?

Ans. It may arise from melanoblast in any site of skin or may arise from pigmented regions of the eye. The sites distribution are:
- *Head and neck*—25%
- *Trunk*—25%
- *Lower extremity*—25%
- *Upper extremity*—11%
- *Other sites*—14%.

Q. What is amelanotic melanoma?

Ans. The malignant melanoma arising from melanoblasts may not always contain melanin pigment. These lesions are called amelanotic melanoma.

Q. In which age, malignant melanoma is more common?

Ans. Malignant melanoma is common after puberty, usually in the age group between 20 years and 40 years.

Q. What are the important etiological factors for development of melanoma?

Ans. A number of factors have been incriminated for development of malignant melanoma:
- *Genetic:* About 5–10% of melanoma patients has a family history of disease independent of other factors.
- *Exposure to sunlight:* Exposure to ultraviolet radiation of wavelength 290 nm (B wave), 375 nm (A wave), and 600 nm (visible light) has all been incriminated for increased risk of malignant melanoma. People who get sunburned easily are at an increased risk for melanoma.
- *Preexisting benign nevi:* About 90% of malignant melanoma arises from preexisting pigmented nevus. The malignant melanoma may arise from junctional nevus, compound nevus, congenital melanocytic nevi, or dysplastic nevi. The number of nevi rather than their size have been related to higher risk of malignant melanoma.
- *Immunosuppressive states:* Renal transplant recipient, patient with lymphoma, and patient taking immunosuppressive drugs are at increased risk for development of malignant melanoma.
- *Xeroderma pigmentosum and nonmelanoma skin cancer.*

Q. Why the incidence of malignant melanoma is increasing?

Ans. Over last few decades, the incidence of malignant melanoma is gradually increasing. Environmental pollution and progressive depletion of ozone layer allows more ultraviolet rays from the sun to reach the earth's surface and exposure to these ultraviolet radiation has been attributed to increasing incidence of malignant melanoma.

Q. What are the different types of melanoma?

Ans. There are four subtypes of malignant melanoma:
1. Superficial spreading melanoma
2. Nodular melanoma
3. Acral lentiginous melanoma
4. Lentigo maligna melanoma.

Q. How does the melanoma grow?

Ans. There are two phases of growth:
1. *A radial or horizontal phase of growth:* The melanoma grows in the epidermis. During this phase of growth, the melanoma does not invade the blood vessels or the lymphatic vessels.
2. *A vertical phase of growth:* During this phase of growth, the melanoma invades the dermis and the deeper tissues. During this phase of growth, the melanoma invades the blood vessel or the lymphatic channels and may lead to metastasis.

Q. What are the characteristic features of superficial spreading melanoma?

Ans.
- Most common variety (70% of all variety)
- May occur in any part of the body but commonly found in the trunk or the extremities
- Lesion is usually flat, with irregular margin, variegated color—may be brown, blue, or black
- Lesion is usually greater than 6–8 mm and nodule may develop later
- Less aggressive and prognosis is better.

Q. What are the characteristics of nodular melanoma?

Ans.
- Younger age group affected
- Incidence 15–30%
- May occur in any part of the body, legs and trunk are commonly affected
- Mucosal melanoma occurring at anal canal and genitalia are usually of nodular type
- *Uniform color*—Blue, gray, or black
- Clinically present as a raised nodule or papule and surface ulceration and bleeding may occur
- Lymph node involvement is common
- Usually aggressive and prognosis is poor.

Q. What are the characteristics of lentigo maligna melanoma?

Ans.
- Also known as Hutchinson's melanotic freckle
- Usually accounts for about 7–15% cases
- *Common in parts of body exposed to sun*—head, neck, and arms are the common sites
- The precursor lesion (lentigo maligna) usually begins as an irregularly pigmented tan to brown macule or patch, which grows slowly and may attain large size (3–6 cm in diameter) over 10–15 years
- Malignant change is marked by thickening and development of discrete tumor nodule within the precursor lesion.

Q. What are the features of acral lentiginous melanoma?

Ans.
+ Least common variety (2–8%)
+ Usually occurs in sole and palm, and may occur under the nail (subungual melanoma)
+ The lesion is usually large (>3 cm) and shows irregular pigmentation
+ Prognosis is poor and grows like a nodular melanoma.

Q. What changes in a benign mole suggest a malignant change?

Ans.
+ Sudden increase in size
+ *Change in outline:* The margin becomes irregular and the lesion becomes asymmetric
+ *Changes in color:* Increasing pigmentation, depigmentation, or irregular pigmentation
+ *Changes in thickness:* The lesion become thicker and nodular
+ *Changes in surface:* Scaling, crusting, erosion, ulceration, and bleeding
+ *Change in adjacent area:* Pigmented halo, satellite nodules, and spread of pigmentation from the lesion to the normal skin
+ The lesion becomes itchy and may bleed
+ Regional lymph node may be enlarged.

Q. What is the natural course of a malignant melanoma?

Ans. The behavior of malignant melanoma is unpredictable and varies in different individual. It grows both radially (along the epidermis) and vertically (dermal invasion). The tumor may progress rapidly with regional and distant spread causing death. In other extreme situation, some tumor may show spontaneous regression. Superficial spreading melanoma and lentigo maligna melanoma may show spontaneous regression, which may be partial or complete.

Q. What are the different levels of invasion of malignant melanoma?

Ans. Clark (1975) described both growth of melanoma and dermal invasion of melanoma depending on microinvasion. Clark has classified five different levels of invasion (Fig. 9.14):

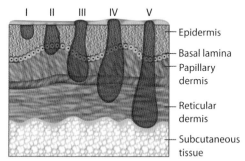

Fig. 9.14: Levels of invasion of malignant melanoma

1. *Level 1:* Tumor confined to the epidermis above the basement membrane (melanoma in situ).
2. *Level 2:* Tumor cell invasion to the papillary dermis.
3. *Level 3:* Tumor cells extending up to the interface between papillary dermis and reticular dermis.
4. *Level 4:* Tumor cells extending to the reticular dermis.
5. *Level 5:* Tumor cells extending to the subcutaneous tissue.

Q. What is the importance of different levels of invasion?

Ans. The deeper the levels of invasion more are the chance of having regional and distant metastasis. The survival rate worsens with increasing levels of invasion of melanoma cells.

Q. What is the importance of tumor thickness in malignant melanoma?

Ans. Tumor thickness is one of the prognostic markers of malignant melanoma. Breslow described different thickness of the tumor, which is measured by an optical micrometer. Depending on the tumor thickness, Breslow has described following groups:
- Tumor thickness—less than 0.75 mm
- Tumor thickness—0.76–1.5 mm
- Tumor thickness—1.6–3.0 mm
- Tumor thickness—more than 3.0 mm.

However, the current breakpoints of classification depending on the tumor thickness are:
- Tumor thickness of 0.75 mm
- Tumor thickness of 1.5 mm
- Tumor thickness of more than 4.0 mm.

Q. What is the importance of tumor thickness?

Ans. The tumor thickness predicts the risk of metastasis more precisely than the Clark's level of invasion. It is also a better predictor of survival. Tumor thickness of more than 4.0 mm suggests worst prognosis.

Q. What is the tumor, node, and metastasis (TNM) staging for malignant melanoma?

Ans. The tumor, node, and metastasis (TNM) staging for malignant melanoma is described in Tables 9.1 to 9.3.

Table 9.1: Tumor, node, and metastasis (TNM) staging for malignant melanoma	
Primary tumor (T)	
TX	Primary tumor cannot be assessed
T0	No evidence of primary tumor
Tis	Melanoma in situ
T1	Melanoma ≤ 1.0 mm in thickness • *T1a:* Without ulceration and mitoses < 1/mm² • *T1b:* With ulceration or mitoses ≥ 1/mm².
T2	Melanomas 1.01–2.0 mm in thickness • *T2a:* Without ulceration • *T2b:* With ulceration.
T3	Melanomas 2.01–4.0 mm in thickness • *T3a:* Without ulceration • *T3b:* With ulceration.
T4	Melanomas > 4.0 mm in thickness • *T4a:* Without ulceration • *T4b:* With ulceration.
Regional lymph nodes (N)	
NX	Patients in whom the regional nodes cannot be assessed (i.e. previously removed for another reason)
N0	No regional metastases detected

N1–3	Regional metastases based upon number of metastatic nodes and presence or absence of intralymphatic metastases (in-transit or satellite metastases)
N1	One lymph node • *N1a:* Micrometastases • *N1b:* Macrometastases.
N2	Two or three lymph nodes • *N2a:* Micrometastases • *N2b:* Macrometastases • *N2c:* In-transit met(s)/satellite(s) without metastatic lymph nodes.
N3	≥ Four metastatic lymph nodes, or matted lymph nodes, or in-transit met(s)/satellite(s) with metastatic lymph node(s)

Distant metastasis (M)	
M0	No detectable evidence of distant metastases
M1a	Metastases to skin, subcutaneous, or distant lymph nodes, normal serum lactate dehydrogenase (LDH) level
M1b	Lung metastases, normal LDH level
M1c	Metastases to all other visceral sites or distant metastases to any site combined with an elevated serum LDH level

Table 9.2: Clinical staging

Stage	T	N	M
0	Tis	N0	M0
IA	T1a	N0	M0
IB	T1b	N0	M0
	T2a	N0	M0
IIA	T2b	N0	M0
	T3a	N0	M0
IIB	T3b	N0	M0
	T4a	N0	M0
IIC	T4b	N0	M0
III	Any T	N1, N2, or N3	M0
IV	Any T	Any N	M1

Table 9.3: Pathologic staging

Stage	T	N	M
0	Tis	N0	M0
IA	T1a	N0	M0
IB	T1b	N0	M0
	T2a	N0	M0
IIA	T2b	N0	M0
	T3a	N0	M0
IIB	T3b	N0	M0
	T4a	N0	M0
IIC	T4b	N0	M0
IIIA	T(1–4)a	N1a	M0
	T(1–4)a	N2a	M0
IIIB	T(1–4)b	N1a	M0
	T(1–4)b	N2a	M0
	T(1–4)a	N1b	M0
	T(1–4)a	N2b	M0
	T(1–4)a	N2c	M0
IIIC	T(1–4)b	N1b	M0
	T(1–4)b	N2b	M0
	T(1–4)b	N2c	M0
	Any T	N3	M0
IV	Any T	Any N	M1

Mitotic rate assessment: For mitotic rate assessment, the pathologist counts the number of cells in a certain amount of melanoma tissue that are in the process of dividing. A higher mitotic rate means that the cancer is more likely to grow and spread. The mitotic rate is used to stage thin melanoma (Table 9.4).

Table 9.4: Mitotic rate assessment for pathologic staging

Pathologic stage	Tumor	Node	Metastasis
0	Tis	N0	M0
IA	T1a	N0	M0
IB	T1b	N0	M0
	T2a	N0	M0
IIA	T2b	N0	M0
	T3a	N0	M0
IIB	T3b	N0	M0
	T4a	N0	M0
IIC	T4b	N0	M0
IIIA	T1a–T4a	N1a/N2a	M0
IIIB	T1b–T4b	N1a/N2a	M0
	T1a–Ta	N1b.N2b	M0
IIIC	T1b–T4b	N1b.N2b	M0
	Any T	N3	M0
IV	Any T	Any N	M1

Q. What is the prognosis of different stage of the disease?

Ans. The 5-year survivals of different stages are:
* *Stage I*—more than 90%
* *Stage II*—70%
* *Stage III*—35%
* *Stage IV*—less than 2%.

Q. How does malignant melanoma spread?

Ans. This may spread in following ways:
* *Local spread:* Spread radially and vertically to adjacent area and to depth of skin; it does not usually invade the deep fascia.
* *Lymphatic spread:* Main spread is by lymphatics; spread by both lymphatic embolization and lymphatic permeation.
  – Local satellite nodule and in-transit nodules are due to lymphatic spread.
* *Blood-borne metastasis:* To lungs, liver, brain, and skin. Rarely may spread to sites like breast, intestine.

Q. What is the relation between the tumor thickness and nodal metastasis?

Ans. The most common site of metastasis is the regional lymph nodes. The risk of nodal metastasis is related to the depth of primary lesion:
* *Lesion less than 1 mm thickness*—2–10% chance of nodal metastasis.
* *Lesion between 1 mm and 4 mm thickness*—20–25% chance of nodal metastasis.
* *Lesion more than 4 mm thickness*—50–60% chance of nodal metastasis.

Q. What is the importance of number of lymph node involvement?

Ans. The prognosis of the patient depends on the number of lymph nodes showing metastatic deposit (Table 9.5).

Q. What is melanuria?

Ans. Presence of melanin pigment in urine is called melanuria. This is present in cases with extensive hepatic metastasis from a malignant melanoma.

Table 9.5: Number of lymph nodes showing metastatic deposit.

Number of lymph nodes positive	5-year survival
1	50%
2–4	20–40%
>5	<20%

Q. How to confirm diagnosis of malignant melanoma?

Ans.
- In most cases diagnosis is made on clinical grounds.
- Incisional biopsy is required only in doubtful case and in cases where benign mole has shown some changes and lesion in sites where wide local excision will cause cosmetic deformity.

Q. What should be treatment strategy for the primary lesion in malignant melanoma?

Ans. Surgical excision of the primary lesion with adequate margin is the mainstay of treatment.

Q. What should be the margin of excision in malignant melanoma?

Ans. Earlier a wide excision with a margin of about 5 cm was the standard treatment. This results in a wide gap requiring skin grafting. However, subsequent study showed that the tumor thickness is one of the determinant factors for margin of excision of the tumor.

The recommended margin of excision depending on tumor thickness:
- *Tis*—margin of 5 mm is adequate
- *Less than 1 mm thickness*—1 cm margin
- *About 1-2 mm thickness*—1-2 cm margin
- *More than 2 mm thickness*— + more than 2 cm margin of excision are required.

It is not necessary to excise the deep fascia as the malignant melanoma rarely invades the deep fascia.

Q. What is the role of adjuvant therapy in malignant melanoma?

Ans. There have been reports of better survival with use of interferon alpha-2 as adjuvant treatment in melanomas with nodal metastasis or thick melanomas. However, subsequent studies do not show consistent benefit for interferon adjuvant therapy.

Current recommendation for adjuvant treatment with interferon is in melanoma stage IIC and stage III.

Q. There is a lesion on the dorsum of the foot with in-transit nodule. How will you treat?

Ans.
- Wide excision of the primary lesion along with in-transit nodule.
- Isolated limb perfusion is effective in some cases (45% CR and 40% PR).
- Superficial electron beam radiotherapy may help.

Q. How will you treat metastatic malignant melanoma?

Ans. Malignant melanoma is usually radioresistant and relatively chemoresistant. The role of immunotherapy is also not well established.

Although, relatively chemoresistant, systemic chemotherapy is the mainstay of treatment.

- Drugs used include combination chemotherapy with cisplatin, vinblastine, and dacarbazine (CVD) combined with interferon alfa or interleukin-2.
- High-dose interleukin-2 therapy has been used with 40% success rate.

Q. What is the role of immunotherapy in malignant melanoma?

Ans.

- Immunotherapy has been tried in the treatment of malignant melanoma.
- Intralesional Bacillus Calmette-Guérin (BCG) vaccination has been used with some success in some cases.
- Other agents used include intralesional purified tuberculin, *Corynebacterium parvum.* levamisole is also used as a nonspecific immunostimulant.

Q. What is regional limb perfusion?

Ans. The tumor confined to the limb with in-transit nodule and recurrent tumor in the limb may be treated by this method.

The artery and the vein supplying the limb is cannulated and connected to extracorporeal circulation machine. The venous blood is oxygenated by passing through a membrane oxygenator and mixed with chemotherapy, thus high-dose chemotherapy may be delivered to the limb. The oxygenated blood is returned into the lower limb.

Q. What are the prognostic factors in malignant melanoma?

Ans.

- *Level of invasion and tumor thickness:* Clark has shown that the survival rates worsened with increasing level of invasion of the tumor. Breslow's tumor thickness is an important prognostic marker. Prognosis worsens with increasing thickness of the tumor.
- *Ulceration of the tumor* is an important prognostic factor and the prognosis is worse when the tumor is ulcerated.
- *Lymphocytic infiltration* suggests a favorable prognosis.
- *Number of mitotic figures* is also an important prognostic marker and prognosis worsens with increased mitotic figures.
- *Presence of metastasis.* Once tumor shows metastasis the prognosis is worsened. The lymph node is the first site of metastasis. The number of lymph nodes positive is an important prognostic marker and prognosis worsens with more number of lymph node involvements.

Q. How will you follow-up patient with malignant melanoma?

Ans. Melanoma patient has an unpredictable clinical course and needs regular follow-up for early detection of local recurrence and metastasis.

- *During first 2 years*—follow-up at an interval of 3–4 months
  - *3rd year to 5th year*—follow up at an interval of 6 months
  - Thereafter, follow-up at yearly interval.

Follow-up evaluation will include:

- Detail physical examination—of local site, regional lymph nodes—in-transit area for any nodules.

- Detail systemic examination:
  - Chest X-ray
  - Serum lactate dehydrogenase (LDH) level
  - Ultrasonography (USG)/computed tomography (CT) scan/positron emission tomography (PET)-CT scan in selected cases.

Q. Where do you find melanin producing cells in the body?

Ans.

- In skin
- Choroid of the eye
- Rarely in meninges, medulla, tela choroidea, and mucocutaneous junction of vagina and in nail bed.

Q. What are the sites of origin of the melanin producing cells?

Ans. The melanin producing cells melanoblasts arises from either:

- Surface epithelial cells
- Neuroectoderm of nervous system.

Q. How melanin is synthesized?

Ans. Synthesis occurs in melanocyte from tyrosine present in the cell.

$$\text{Tyrosine} \xrightarrow{\text{Tyrosinase}} \text{Dopa} \xrightarrow{\text{Dopa oxidase}} \text{Melanin}$$

Q. Which hormones control melanin production?

Ans.

- Melanocyte-stimulating hormone (MSH) secreted from anterior pituitary
- Adrenocorticotropic hormone (ACTH)
- *Sex hormones*—estrogen and androgen.

■ BENIGN PIGMENTED NEVUS

Clinical Examination

See Page No. 382.

Q. What is your case? (Summary of a case of benign nevus)

Ans. This 45-year-old lady presented with a pigmented patch on her neck and face since her childhood. The pigmented area was gradually increasing in size for last 30 years. But for last 3 years this remained static. She has no other complaints (Fig. 9.15).

On examination: There is a flat, circumscribed bluish patch in the skin of front, sides, and back of the neck. The lesion has extended on to the

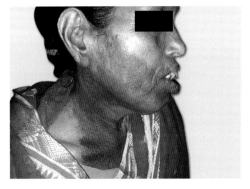

Fig. 9.15: Benign pigmented nevus

Courtesy: Dr Alok Kumar Biswas, Institute of Postgraduate Medical Education and Research (IPGMER), Kolkata

right side of the face and involved the lips and also extended into the right infraclavicular area. The lesion is not raised from the surface. Surface is smooth. The regional lymph nodes are not enlarged or palpable.

Q. What is your diagnosis?

Ans. This is a case of benign pigmented nevus involving the neck, face, and upper chest.

Q. How will you treat this lesion?

Ans. This is a benign lesion, remained static for last 3 years but the patient is concerned about the cosmetic problem, I will consider complete excision of the pigmented patch and skin drafting.

Q. What are the indications of surgery in benign nevus?

Ans.
* Cosmetic reason
* If the area is subjected to repeated trauma
* Suspicion of malignant change.

Q. Does trauma have any relation to malignant change?

Ans. Repeated trauma has not been proved to be a factor for malignant change in a benign nevus.

Q. What are the different types of simple melanocytic tumors or benign melanomas?

Ans. The melanocytes are situated in the basal layer of the epidermis. Increased number of melanocytes in the layers of the skin forms the benign pigmented nevi (moles).

The different types of benign mole include:
* *Hutchinson's melanotic freckle*—Melanocytes are present only in the basal layer of the epidermis in normal numbers and normal location but secretes excessive melanin. This is a benign nevus where proliferated melanocytes lie only in the basal layer of the epidermis.
* *Lentigo*—There are increased numbers of melanocytes, which are present in the basal layer of the epidermis. Each cell produces normal amount of melanin.
* *Moles or pigmented nevi*—There are increased numbers of melanocytes in abnormal clusters in both epidermis and dermis, and produces excess quantities of melanin. These are further subclassified as:
  - *Intradermal nevi:* Cluster of melanocytes are present only in the dermis. Most moles in face, arm, and trunks are of this variety. They may be flat or raised, smooth or warty, hairy, or nonhairy. They rarely turn malignant.
  - *Junctional nevi:* Aggregation of the melanocytes in the epidermis which projects into the dermis. The proliferated melanocytes lie confined to the dermis only. There is an increased risk of malignant change.
  - *Compound nevi:* Show features of both junctional and intradermal nevi. There are clusters of proliferated melanocytes in both epidermis and dermis.

Q. Which type of nevus is more likely to undergo malignant change?

Ans. Junctional nevus and compound nevus are more likely to undergo malignant change.

Q. What are the characteristics of a junctional nevus?

Ans.
- *Pigmented*—Light brown to black-colored lesion
- May occur anywhere on the body but is commonly found in soles, palms, digits, or genitalia. The lesion is smooth, flat, or slightly raised from the surface, usually hairless
- May undergo malignant changes.

Q. What are the characteristics of dermal nevus?

Ans.
- *Appear as pigmented lesion*—light brown in color, may be hairy
- The lesion is usually soft and smooth but may be warty and raised from the surface
- Commonly found on the face or other parts of the body but is not found in soles or palms.

Q. What are the characteristics of compound nevus?

Ans.
- Common in older children or adults
- Appear as round or elliptical elevated lesion, light brown in color
- It may grow and form a papillary lesion.

Q. What are the characteristics of lentigo maligna or Hutchinson's melanotic freckle?

Ans.
- Common in elderly
- Appear as dark pigmented, smooth lesion not raised from the surface
- Commonly occurs on the face and neck
- Usually shows continual centrifugal growth
- Prone to undergo malignant change.

Q. What is a blue nevus?

Ans.
- This is a type of dermal nevus
- Either flat or slightly raised bluish pigmented lesion
- Surface is smooth and shiny
- Commonly seen on face, dorsum of hands, feet, and buttocks (also known as Mongolian spots)
- May undergo spontaneous regression
- May rarely undergo malignant change.

Q. Which features suggest malignant change in a benign mole?

Ans.
- Increase in size of the lesion
- Involvement of the adjacent area
- Edges of the lesion becoming irregular
- Lesion becoming thicker and nodular
- Increasing pigmentation, depigmentation, or irregular pigmentation
- Scaling, ulceration, crusting, oozing, and bleeding of the surface
- Regional lymph node enlargement
- Microscopically, there may be hyperchromasia, pleomorphism, anaplasia, and mitotic figures.

Q. What are the principles of excision of benign pigmented lesion?

Ans.

- *Nevi appearing at birth or before puberty*—Complete excision close to the margin of the lesion
- *Suspicious nevi*—Complete excision with a 0.5 cm margin of healthy skin.

■ SQUAMOUS CELL CARCINOMA

Clinical Examination

See Page No. 382.

Summary of a Case of Squamous Cell Carcinoma

History: This 45-year-old gentleman presented with a swelling on the dorsum of left foot for last 2 years. The swelling was gradually increasing in size for last 1.5 years. But for last 6 months, the swelling is rapidly increasing in size with central ulceration and serosanguineous discharge (Fig. 9.16).

Local examination: There is a swelling on the dorsum of left foot; the swelling is about 6 × 5 cm. The swelling is irregular in shape with a rolled out everted margin. There is a central ulceration

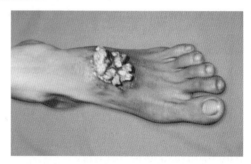

Fig. 9.16: Squamous cell carcinoma in left foot

and serosanguineous discharge from the surface of the swelling. The base is indurated. The swelling is not fixed to the underlying bone. The popliteal and the inguinal lymph nodes are not palpable.

Q. What is your diagnosis?

Ans. This is a case of squamous cell carcinoma on left foot without any evidence of lymph node metastasis in a 45-year-old male patient.

Q. How will you manage this patient?

Ans. I would like to confirm my diagnosis by taking biopsy.

Q. From which part of the lesion will you take the biopsy?

Ans. I will take an incisional biopsy from the junction of tumor and the normal skin, i.e. from the margin of the tumor.

Q. How will you treat this patient?

Ans.

- This is a lesion in the peripheral part of the limb, so I will consider surgical treatment in this patient.
- I will do a wide excision of the tumor with a 1 cm clear margin all around up to the deep fascia.
- The resulting defect will be covered by a split-thickness skin graft.

Q. How will you treat the lymph nodes in this patient?

Ans. As the lymph nodes are not involved, I will not do an ELND. I will follow-up the patient and subsequently if lymph nodes are involved, I will consider an appropriate lymph node dissection.

Once the inguinal lymph nodes are involved, I will do an inguinopelvic lymph node dissection.

Q. What is the indication for amputation in such distal lesion in leg or foot?

Ans. In locally advanced tumor when the tumor has invaded the deeper structure including the bone then for curative resection an amputation is advisable.

Q. How will you follow-up this patient?

Ans. I will review the histological report; if margins are free of tumor and tumor is well differentiated, I will follow-up the patient at regular intervals.

If the tumor is poorly differentiated, I would consider postoperative radiotherapy to the local part.

I will do regular follow-up at an interval of 3 months for the first 3 years and then every 6 months for next 2 years and then yearly. Examination of the local site for any local recurrence and also examines the regional lymph node for any evidence of metastatic enlargement.

If the lymph node becomes enlarged due to metastasis, I will consider inguinopelvic block dissection.

Q. If the histology report shows that the resection lines are not free of tumor what will you do?

Ans. In this situation, resurgery with a wider excision of 2 cm margin is to be done. Alternatively, postoperative radiotherapy may be given.

Q. Do you like to do elective lymph node dissection?

Ans. The squamous cell carcinomas are very slow growing tumor. Prophylactic lymph node dissection does not provide any survival advantage and in addition there is increased morbidity associated with ELND. So, an ELND is not advisable.

Q. What may be the cause of lymph node enlargement in patient of squamous cell carcinoma?

Ans. The lymph node enlargement may be due to:
* *Infection*—Respond to broad-spectrum antibiotic therapy
* *Metastatic*—Does not respond to antibiotic therapy and needs appropriate lymph node dissection.

Q. How does squamous cell carcinoma spread?

Ans.
* Local spread by continuity and contiguity
* Lymphatic spread both by lymphatic permeation and embolization
* Blood spread is extremely rare.

Q. Where from the squamous cell carcinoma arises?

Ans.
* In skin, the squamous cell carcinoma arises from the malpighian or spindle cell layer of the epidermis.

- In mucous membrane, squamous cell carcinoma may arise from the stratified squamous epithelium lining.
- The squamous cell carcinoma may also arise from metaplastic columnar epithelium.

Q. What are the other sites from where squamous cell carcinoma may arise?

Ans.
- From any part of the skin
- Mucus surface lined by stratified squamous epithelium, buccal cavity, pharynx, esophagus, larynx, upper nasal passage and tongue, anal canal, and vagina
- *Squamous metaplasia of columnar epithelium*—Gallbladder, bronchus
- *Squamous metaplasia of transitional epithelium*—Renal pelvis and urinary bladder.

Q. What are the histological characteristics of squamous cell carcinoma?

Ans.
- This arises from spindle cell layer of the epidermis.
- The cells invade the underlying connective tissue as solid irregular strands or column.
- The individual cells vary from large, well-differentiated cell with vesicular nucleus with prominent nucleoli and abundant cytoplasm.
- The cells may be anaplastic with a large nucleus and scanty cytoplasm.
- There are epithelial pearls or cell nests consisting of central keratin surrounded by eosinophilic prickle cells, which has hyperchromatic nuclei with mitotic figure and separated from one another by connective tissues.
- The epithelial pearls penetrate into the dermis.

Q. What are the histological characteristics of well-differentiated squamous cell carcinoma?

Ans.
- The cells are well-differentiated squamous epithelial cells
- Cell nests are well formed.

Q. What are histological characteristics of poorly differentiated squamous cell carcinoma?

Ans.
- The cells are grossly undifferentiated pleomorphic cells
- The epithelial pearls or cell nests are scanty or absent.

Q. Where else such epithelial pearls or cell nests may be found?

Ans. In pleomorphic salivary adenoma and teratoma testis.

Q. How will you stage squamous cell carcinoma?

Ans. The TNM classification of squamous cell carcinoma of skin:
- *T:* Primary tumor
  - *TX:* Primary tumor cannot be assessed
  - *T0:* No evidence of primary tumor
  - *Tis:* Carcinoma in situ
  - *T1:* Tumor less than or equal to 2 cm in greatest dimension with at most one of the high-risk features

- *T2:* Tumor more than 2 cm in greatest dimension with or without one additional high-risk feature, or any size with more than 2 cm high-risk features
- *T3:* Tumor with invasion of any of the facial bones (maxilla, mandible, orbit, or temporal bone)
- *T4:* Tumor with invasion of skeleton (axial or appendicular) or perineural invasion of skull base.

High-risk features include:

- Depth (>2 mm thickness; Clark level IV)
- Perineural invasion
- Location (primary site ear, primary site nonglabrous lip)
- Differentiation (poorly differentiated or undifferentiated).
- *N:* Nodal status
  - *NX:* Regional lymph nodes cannot be assessed
  - *N0:* No regional lymph node metastasis
  - *N1:* Metastasis in single ipsilateral lymph node, less than 3 cm in greatest dimension
  - *N2:* Metastasis in single ipsilateral lymph node, more than 3 cm but less than 6 cm in greatest dimension or in multiple ipsilateral lymph nodes, none more than 6 cm in greatest dimension or in bilateral or contralateral lymph nodes, none more than 6 cm in greatest dimension
  - *N2a:* Metastasis in single ipsilateral lymph node, more than 3 cm but not more than 6 cm in greatest dimension
  - *N2b:* Metastasis in multiple ipsilateral lymph nodes, none more than 6 cm in greatest dimension
  - *N2c:* Metastasis in bilateral or contralateral lymph nodes, none more than 6 cm in greatest dimension
  - *N3:* Any metastasis in lymph node, more than 6 cm in greatest dimension.
- *M:* Distant metastasis
  - *Mx:* Distant metastasis cannot be assessed
  - *M0:* No distant metastasis
  - *M1:* Distant metastasis present.

Stage grouping for cutaneous squamous cell carcinoma:

- *Stage 0:* Tis N0 M0
- *Stage I:* T1 N0 M0
- *Stage II:* T2 N0 M0
- *Stage III:* T3 N0 or T1 N1 M0 or T2 N1 M0
- *Stage IV:* T1, 2, or 3 N2 M0
  - Any T N3 M0
  - T4 Any N M0
  - Any T Any N M1.

Q. What are the premalignant lesions in the skin?

Ans.

- *Bowen's disease:* It is actually a squamous cell carcinoma in situ, which may later progress to invasive carcinoma
- *Radiodermatitis*

- *Solar keratosis*
- *Leukoplakia*
- *Xeroderma pigmentosum*
- *Chronic ulcer in the skin*—Venous ulcer, chronic ulcer secondary to long-standing osteomyelitis
- *Old scar secondary* to burns
- *Chronic skin irritations due to chemicals*—Tars, oils, soot, and aniline dyes
- *Chronic skin irritations due to local heat* application (Kangri cancer).

Q. What is the relation of sunlight exposure and squamous cell carcinoma?

Ans. Exposure to sunlight is one of the important factors for development of squamous cell carcinoma. An exposure for a long period of about 10–20 years is required for sun-related damage to become evident. So, squamous cell carcinoma secondary to solar keratosis is common in men more than 60 years.

Q. What are the sequences of change following exposure to sunlight?

Ans. On prolonged exposure to sunlight, grossly there are well-circumscribed erythematous maculopapular lesions. The color may be reddish to light brown and the lesion may be dry and scaly. Microscopically there is hyperkeratosis, parakeratosis and dyskeratosis, and acanthosis. There may be an associated inflammatory infiltrate consisting of lymphocytes.

Q. What are the options for treatment of solar keratosis?

Ans.
- Curettage and electrodesiccation
- Cryosurgery with liquid nitrogen
- Chemical peel and dermabrasion
- Local application of 1–5%, 5-fluorouracil cream has been found to be very effective.

Q. What is Bowen's disease?

Ans.
- Bowen's disease is an intraepithelial squamous cell carcinoma and may involve the skin and mucous membrane.
- The lesion is usually solitary.
- Well-defined erythematous, dull scaly plaque.
- There may be superficial crusting or oozing from the surface.
- Microscopic examination reveals:
  - Hyperkeratosis, parakeratosis, dyskeratosis, and acanthosis.
  - Cells are keratinized with bizarre hyperchromatic nuclei and there are increased mitotic figures.
  - There is no dermal invasion.
  - There may be infiltration of the papillary dermis with multinucleated giant cells.

Q. How will you treat Bowen's disease?

Ans.
- Curettage and electrodesiccation.
- Surgical excision with a healthy margin.

Q. What are the characteristics of a leukoplakic patch?

Ans. Leukoplakia (white patch) may be found in skin or mucous membrane. The lesion is usually elevated, sharply defined areas of keratinization, lighter than the color of the adjacent area, and is of variable thickness.

Microscopically, the leukoplakic patch shows hyperkeratosis, parakeratosis, dyskeratosis and acanthosis, and an inflammatory infiltrate in the papillary dermis.

The squamous cell carcinoma developing from malignant transformation of a leukoplakic patch behaves more aggressively.

Q. What is pseudoepitheliomatous hyperplasia?

Ans. Pseudoepitheliomatous hyperplasia is seen in long-standing chronic ulcers and appears as epidermal thickening and may appear like a squamous cell carcinoma grossly.

Microscopically, it shows downward proliferation of epithelial cell with some cellular atypia and an inflammatory infiltrate. But the cells do not show typical characters of squamous cell carcinoma.

Q. What are the different types of squamous cell carcinoma?

Ans. There are two main types of squamous cell carcinoma:
1. *Exophytic type:* The verrucous and the exophytic type grow very slowly. It is locally invasive but chance of metastasis much less.
2. *Ulcerative type:* This starts as a nodular lesion and grows rapidly, ulcerates early. Invades the local tissues early and chance of metastasis is also high.

Q. What should be the margin of excision in squamous cell carcinoma?

Ans.
+ For well defined and smaller lesion an excision with a healthy margin of 0.5 cm is adequate.
+ For larger lesion, aggressive lesion, or recurrent lesion an excision with a healthy margin of 1 cm is adequate.

Q. What are the risk factors for recurrence of squamous cell carcinoma?

Ans.
+ Degree of cellular differentiation is one important factor determining the local recurrence.
+ Perineural invasion of the tumor is associated with increased incidence of local recurrence of squamous cell carcinoma.

Q. What is Mohs micrographic surgery?

Ans.
+ Mohs micrographic surgery involves serial tangential excision of the lesion and examination of the specimen by fresh frozen technique till a healthy margin is reached.
+ This technique is useful for large primary lesion with poorly delineated border or perineural invasion, for treatment of sclerosing BCC, and in dealing with a recurrent lesion.

Q. What is the role of radiotherapy in the treatment of primary lesion in squamous cell carcinoma?

Ans. For primary lesion, after biopsy confirmation, some lesion may be treated only with radiotherapy:
+ Squamous cell carcinoma in head and neck may be treated only with radiotherapy

- Smaller lesion may be solely treated with radiotherapy
- Anaplastic carcinoma may be treated with radiotherapy
- Postoperative radiotherapy to local site if the resected margins are not free of tumor and tumor histology revealed it to be anaplastic.

Q. What is the management of lymph node metastasis?

Ans.

- In negative nodes treatment is regular follow-up.
- When the lymph nodes are positive for metastasis block dissection of the lymph is the preferred treatment and radiotherapy is usually not indicated.
- In cases where lymph nodes are fixed and inoperable, local radiotherapy may cause some regression and lymph nodes may become mobile; palliative lymph node dissection may be attempted.

■ BASAL CELL CARCINOMA

Clinical Examination (*See* Page No. 382)

History:

- Swelling or ulcer onset, progress, any discharge, and any itching.
- Any history of prolonged exposure to sunlight.

Examination of the ulcer—Inspection/Palpation:

- Site, size, shape, margin, floor and the base of the ulcer, and color.
- Depth of the ulcer.
- Most BCC are superficial and are confined to the skin but long-standing BCC may invade the underlying bones, fascia, and muscles.
- Examination of regional lymph nodes.
  Lymph nodes are not usually involved in BCC.

Q. What is your case? (Summary of a case of basal cell carcinoma)

Ans. This 60-year-old gentleman presented with a gradually progressive ulcerative lesion in the left side of face below the left orbit for last 2 years. Patient noticed an ulcer on the left side of the face above the left ala nasi, which was 5 mm in size at the onset of 2 years back, which was increasing very slowly in size. But for last 6 months, the ulcer is increasing rapidly. Apart from this ulcerative lesion, patient has no other complain (Fig. 9.17).

On examination: There is an irregular ulcer at the left side of face below the left orbit. The ulcer margin is raised and rounded and there are

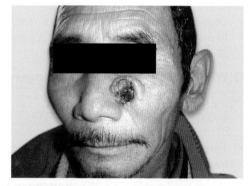

Fig. 9.17: Basal cell carcinoma in the left side of the face

Courtesy: Dr Basudev Sil, Institute of Postgraduate Medical Education and Research (IPGMER), Kolkata

beaded appearances of the ulcer margin. The floor of the ulcer is covered by a scab. On removing the scab from the floor of the ulcer there is slight bleeding. The base of the ulcer is indurated. The regional lymph nodes in the neck are not palpable.

Q. What is your diagnosis?

Ans. This is a case of basal cell carcinoma involving the left side of the face without any lymph node metastasis.

Q. How will you manage this patient?

Ans. I would like to confirm my diagnosis by doing a biopsy from the ulcer margin.

Q. How will you treat this patient if it is basal cell carcinoma?

Ans. I will do complete excision of the lesion with a healthy margin of 5 mm all around. The depth of excision will depend on the depth of invasion of tumor.

The resulting defect will be covered by split skin graft.

Q. Is it possible to treat this lesion with radiotherapy?

Ans. Basal cell carcinoma is very radiosensitive but as the lesion is close to the eye it is better to avoid radiotherapy due to risk of radiation damage to the eye.

Q. What is the role of local application of 5-fluorouracil?

Ans. For small and superficial lesion success has been achieved with local application of 5-fluorouracil cream.

Q. What is the role of cryosurgery in basal cell carcinoma?

Ans.
- Small nodular or ulcerative lesion located over the bone or cartilage or over the eyelid or nose may be ablated by cryotherapy.
- Liquid nitrogen is applied with a cotton tipped applicator and the tumor is frozen with a 5 mm area of normal tissues for a duration of about 30 seconds.
- There is immediate edema, exudation, subsequent necrosis, eschar formation, and later healing.
- Biopsy proof of the lesion is essential before this form of treatment.

Q. What is the role of curettage?

Ans. Small superficial lesion less than 1 cm in diameter may be managed by curettage and diathermy ablation to achieve a cure.

Not suitable for lesion situated over a bone or cartilage.

Q. How the defects following surgical excision may be covered?

Ans.
- *Split thickness skin grafting* is most commonly done. This is not suitable over a bone or cartilage
- *Skin flaps*—a cutaneous or musculocutaneous flaps provides better closure for large defects of the head and neck. It is useful particularly over a bone or cartilage
- *Distant skin or musculocutaneous flaps,* using a microvascular technique, are suitable for large defects.

Q. What is the role of radiotherapy?

Ans.
* Basal cell carcinoma is highly radiosensitive
* Most of the lesion may be treated solely by radiotherapy. This does not produce any disfigurement.

Q. What are the limitations of radiotherapy?

Ans.
* Lesions which have involved the underlying bone are not suitable for radiation treatment.
* Radiation treatment should better be avoided in lesion close to the eye to prevent radiation damage to the eye.

Q. Why basal cell carcinoma is also known as a rodent ulcer?

Ans.
* The basal cell carcinoma starts as a nodule. As the lesion grows there is central ulceration and this ulcer grows by invading the deeper tissues and resembles the deep burrows made by the rat (a rodent), so it is called a rodent ulcer.

Q. What is "field fire" type of basal cell carcinoma?

Ans. An unusual type of BCC, where there is healing at center with spread of ulcer centrifugally or the ulcer may heal at one margin and extend further in the other margin with a spreading edge. This resembles a field fire and is so named as field fire type of BCC.

Q. What are the common sites of basal cell carcinoma?

Ans. It is common in the face and is found most frequently in the face above an imaginary line joining the angle of the mouth and the ear lobule. Approximately 93% BCC occurs in the head and neck region. The common sites are:
* In the inner or outer angle of the orbit
* Nose, forehead, and on the cheek.

Q. What are the other sites where basal cell carcinoma may occur?

Ans.
* Other sites of the face, neck, and scalp
* Rarely trunk and the extremities.

Q. What are the gross types of basal cell carcinoma?

Ans. Grossly BCC may be of following types:
* *Nodular:* Well defined, elevated lesion. Begin as a small papule, grow slowly, and tend to ulcerate. As the lesion grows there is appearance of nodules along the margins. Distinct blood vessels may be seen across the surface of the tumor.
* *Cystic type:* Dark cystic swelling with or without tiny venules crossing over the surface.
* *Morphoeic type:* Appear as firm, raised, and red plaques.
* *Pigmented lesion:* Lesion like nodular ulcerative type associated with a deep brownish-black pigmentation.
* *Superficial type:* Lesions are usually multiple in the trunks and appear as lightly pigmented, erythematous, scaly, and patch like.

◆ *Sclerosing basal cell carcinoma:* Lesions are usually yellow-white epitheliomas associated with peripheral growth and central sclerosis and scarring.

Q. What are the histological features of basal cell carcinoma?

Ans.

◆ Basal cell carcinoma arises from the pleuripotential cells of the basal layer of the epithelium or from the root sheath of the hair follicle
◆ Composed of closely packed islands of polyhedral cells containing a large basophilic nucleus
◆ Consists of irregular masses of basaloid cells in the dermis with characteristic palisade arrangement of tumor cells in the periphery in an organized connective tissue stroma
◆ Prickle cells and epithelial pearls are absent.
  There is chronic inflammatory infiltrate and fibrosis in the connective tissue stroma.

Q. What are the different techniques of biopsy from the skin lesion?

Ans.

◆ *Curettage and biopsy:* The surface of the tumor is scraped with a curette and the curetted specimen is examined
◆ *Punch biopsy:* Usually 3 or 4 mm diameter provides a specimen for histologic examination
◆ *Deep wedge biopsy:* Gives valuable information regarding depth of infiltration of the tumor
◆ *Incisional biopsy:* From the margin of the swelling
◆ *Excisional biopsy:* Indicated when the lesion is small, involves complete excision of the tumor with a healthy margin of 3–5 mm all around.

Q. How does basal cell carcinoma spreads?

Ans.

◆ *Direct spread:* The BCC spreads mainly by direct spread. It grows centrifugally and also grows deeper to involve the subjacent connective tissue and the underlying bone.
◆ *Lymphatic spread:* May spread to regional lymph nodes rarely.
◆ *Blood spread:* Extremely rare, but has been reported in some cases.

Q. What are the sites of basal cell carcinoma, which are more prone for recurrence?

Ans. Basal cell carcinoma at the center of the face, postauricular region, pinna, and forehead are more prone to have recurrence.

Q. What is turban tumor?

Ans.

◆ May be a variety of BCC. Others regard it as endothelioma
◆ Stroma is arranged in a peculiar transparent cylinders
◆ Forms an extensive turban like swelling over the scalp
◆ Ulceration may occur.

■ MARJOLIN'S ULCER

Clinical Examination (*See* Page No. 382)

History:

* How did the scar occur?
* *History of ulcer*—onset, progress.
* Any discharge.
* Any pain over the ulcer (usually painless).

Examination—Inspection/Palpation:

* *Scar*—Site and extent.
* Details examination of ulcer.
* Site and extent, size and shape, margin, edge, and floor of the ulcer.
* Palpate the base of the ulcer.
* Any discharge from the ulcer.
* Whether the ulcer extends to the normal tissue or not.
* Examination of regional lymph nodes (usually regional lymph nodes are not involved in Marjolin's ulcer unless there is extension of ulcer to the normal tissue when the regional lymph nodes may be involved).

Q. What is your case? (Summary of a case of Marjolin's ulcer)

Ans. This 25-year-old lady complains of a gradual onset of ulceration over a preexisting burn scar in her left thigh for last 2 years. The ulcer is gradually increasing in size and there is serous discharge from the ulcer. Patient had burn injury in her left lower limb 5 years back, which healed with scarring. She does not complain of any swelling in the groin (Fig. 9.18).

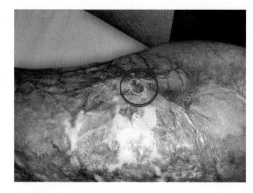

Fig. 9.18: Marjolin's ulcer involving the burn scar in left thigh

Courtesy: Dr Partha Bhar, Institute of Postgraduate Medical Education and Research (IPGMER), Kolkata

On examination: There is a large area of scar in the left thigh. There is an ulcer over the scar, irregular in shape, and size is 3 × 2.5 cm. The margin of the ulcer is rolled out. The floor of the ulcer is covered by necrotic tissue. The base of the ulcer is indurated but free from the underlying structures. The ulcer has not extended to the normal skin. There are no palpable lymph nodes in the inguinal region.

Q. What is your diagnosis?

Ans. This is a case of Marjolin's ulcer in the left thigh developing on a postburn scar without any evidence of lymph node metastasis.

Q. What is Marjolin's ulcer?

Ans. Marjolin's ulcer is a low-grade squamous cell carcinoma, which develops on a chronic benign ulcer or a long-standing scar tissue.

Q. What are the possible causes of development of Marjolin's ulcer?

Ans. Marjolin's ulcer may develop in:
- Postburn scar
- Long-standing venous ulcer
- Chronically discharging osteomyelitic sinus
- Postradiation ulcer
- Chronic ulcer due to trauma.

Q. What are the peculiarities of Marjolin's ulcer?

Ans.
- Slowly growing as the scar tissue is relatively avascular
- Painless as there are no nerves in the scar tissue
- Secondary deposits are usually not found in the regional lymph node as there are no lymphatic vessels in the scar tissue
- If the ulcer invades the normal tissue, then only lymph node may be involved by lymphatic spread.

Q. How will you treat this patient?

Ans.
- I will confirm my diagnosis by taking an incisional biopsy from the margin of the ulcer.
- If diagnosis is confirmed, I will do wide excision of the ulcer with at least 1 cm margin all around and the resulting defect will be bridged by split-thickness skin grafting.

Q. What is the role of radiotherapy in Marjolin's ulcer?

Ans. As the scar tissue is relatively avascular the Marjolin's ulcer developing on a scar is usually not sensitive to radiotherapy.

Q. What are the carcinogens responsible for the development of cutaneous malignancies?

Ans.
- *Exposure to sunlight:* Ultraviolet (UV) rays of different wavelengths are filtered by the ozone layer. Due to the breach in the ozone layer, more UV rays may reach the earth's surface. The detrimental effect of UV rays depends on the melanocytes content of the skin. In white-skinned individuals where the melanocytes content is low have higher incidence of cutaneous malignancy.
- *Ionizing radiation:* Ionizing radiation includes X-rays, gamma rays, and particulate radiation (electrons, protons, and neutrons). Cutaneous malignancy may develop after a long latent period of radiation exposure.
- *Chemical carcinogens:* Arsenic, psoralens, nitrogen mustard, and the atmospheric pollutant are important carcinogens, which may lead to cutaneous malignancies.

Q. Which inherited conditions may be associated with cutaneous malignancy?

Ans.

* *Xeroderma pigmentosum*—Autosomal recessive disorder associated with defective deoxyribonucleic acid (DNA) repair mechanism and has increased susceptibility to squamous cell carcinoma.
* *Albinism causes hypopigmentation* of skin, hair, and eyes and increases the risk of both squamous cell carcinoma and BCC.
* *Basal cell nevus syndrome (Gorlin syndrome):*
  – An autosomal dominant disorder.
  – Three characteristic findings include:
    1. Multiple basal cell nevi in the skin.
    2. Which undergoes malignant change by puberty.
    3. Jaw cysts.

Other inherited conditions include:

* Epidermodysplasia verruciformis
* Porokeratosis
* Muir-Torre syndrome.

■ SOFT TISSUE SARCOMA

Clinical Examination (*See* Page No. 382)

History:

* Age (may occur at any age, but common in elderly).
* Duration and progress [swelling may be present for long duration or history may be short Swelling may grow rapidly from the onset, swelling may grow slowly initially and later progresses rapidly, some soft tissue sarcoma (STS) may continue to grow slowly for long duration].
* Pain (local pain may be due to stretching or pain may be due to infiltration of local tissues and nerves).
* Any muscle weakness (muscle weakness may be due to muscle infiltration or due to nerve infiltration).
* Any swelling of the limbs distal to the swelling (may be due to invasion of the vessels).
* Any swelling of the lymph nodes at the draining site (some STS may spread to the regional lymph nodes).
* Any symptoms due to metastasis.
* Chest pain, cough, hemoptysis, and breathlessness due to chest metastasis.
* Bone pain due to bone metastasis.
* Headache, vomiting, and visual disturbances due to brain metastasis.
* Anorexia, weight loss, and general debility due to multiple metastasis.
* Abdominal distension, jaundice due to liver metastasis.

Examination—Inspection/Palpation:

* Position
* Extent
* Size
* Shape

- Surface
- Margin
- Skin
- Any palpation:
  - Swelling site and extent (STS may occur at any site of the body, but is more common in the extremities)
  - Temperature (STS are usually vascular and appears warmer than the surrounding tissues)
  - Tenderness (usually nontender except in rapidly growing tumors)
- Size (variable may attain large size)
- Shape (variable may be spherical or irregular in shape)
- Surface (usually smooth in slowly growing tumors, but may appear irregular with rapid growth)
- Margins (in slow growing tumors the margins are usually well defined, but in rapidly growing tumors and invasive tumors the margins are usually ill defined)
- Consistency (usually firm or hard, some STS may feel variegated)
- Skin over the swelling (there may be engorged veins over the swelling and in rapidly growing tumors the swelling may appear stretched and shiny)
- Pulsation (some STS may be highly vascular and may show pulsation, thrill may be palpable and a bruit may be audible over the swelling)
- *Mobility*—Test for fixity to the skin and underlying bone and muscles (swelling may be mobile, or in rapidly growing and invasive tumors the swelling may become fixed to the underlying muscles and bones, in rapidly growing and invasive tumors the skin may become fixed to the swelling)
- Examine the pulse distal to the swelling (in invasive tumors the distal arterial pulse may be absent)
- Examine the nerve distal to the swelling (invasion of the nerve may cause corresponding nerve deficit)
- Examine the regional lymph nodes (some STS may spread to the regional lymph nodes). Relevant systemic examination to exclude any distant metastasis.

Q. What is your case? (Summary of a case of soft tissue sarcoma in the left thigh) (Fig. 9.19)

Ans. This 40-year-old gentleman presented with a swelling in his left thigh for last 6 months. The swelling was insidious in onset and about 2 cm in diameter initially. Afterwards the swelling is rapidly increasing in size to attain the present size. Patient complains of dull aching pain over the swelling for last 3 months. No complaint of any swelling in the groin. No pain in abdomen, no history of groin swelling. No history of jaundice, abdominal distension. No history of chest pain, cough, and hemoptysis. No neurological symptoms.

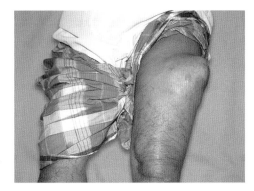

Fig. 9.19: Soft tissue sarcoma involving the left thigh

Courtesy: Dr Soumen Das, Institute of Postgraduate Medical Education and Research (IPGMER), Kolkata

On physical examination, general surgery is essentially normal. On local examination of lower limb, there is a swelling in left thigh located in anterolateral aspect of mid-thigh. Irregular in shape, 10 cm × 8 cm in size. Temperature over the swelling is raised, no tenderness. There is no fixity of the swelling to the overlying skin and underlying muscle and bone. No inguinal lymph nodes are palpable. Systemic examination is normal.

Q. What is your diagnosis?

Ans. This is a case of STS involving the left thigh.

Q. What is the clinical stage of the disease?

Ans. $T_{2b}N_0M_0$.

Q. What are the different soft tissue sarcomas?

Ans.
* In adults, the most common STS is malignant fibrous histiocytoma.
* Other STSs involving the limbs include:
    – Rhabdomyosarcoma
    – Liposarcoma
    – Synovial sarcoma
    – Fibrosarcoma
    – Neurofibrosarcoma
    – Hemangiosarcoma
    – Lymphangiosarcoma.

Q. How will you demonstrate fixity of lump to the underlying structures?

Ans. Try to move the lump with the muscle relaxed. If the lump cannot be moved at all then the lump is fixed to the underlying bone.

    If the lump is mobile with the muscle relaxed, ask the patient to contract the muscle against resistance and test the mobility of the lump with the muscle contracted. If the mobility gets restricted with the muscle contracted then the lump is fixed to the underlying muscle.

Q. How will you demonstrate skin fixity of the lump?

Ans. Try to pinch the skin up from the swelling. If the skin can be lifted from the swelling then the lump is not fixed to the skin.

Q. How will you manage this patient?

Ans. I would like to:
* Confirm my diagnosis
* Assess the local extent
* Assess for any evidence of distant spread of the disease.

For confirmation of diagnosis:
* *Magnetic resonance imaging (MRI) of thigh:*
    – MRI should be done before any invasive investigations like core biopsy or FNAC.
    – MRI is the most useful imaging modality for STS of the extremities.
    – MRI accurately delineates the muscle groups in the thigh.

- The tumor may be well seen and relation of the tumor with the adjacent structures may be better delineated using coronal and sagittal and transverse views.
- Soft tissue sarcoma appears as a heterogeneous mass.
- Hemorrhage, necrosis, and cystic changes may also be well seen.
- The relation of tumor with the adjacent neurovascular bundles may be well seen.
- Magnetic resonance imaging can demonstrate tumor regression with chemotherapy.
- *Core needle biopsy:* Core needle biopsy is the preferred technique for diagnosing STS. The histological types and grading can be done in core biopsy sample. The cytogenetic analysis and immunohistochemistry may also be done with the core biopsy specimen.

   Core biopsy under USG or CT guidance is better as it avoids taking biopsy from necrotic or cystic areas. Guided biopsy is also better in deep-seated lesion.

For assessment for distant metastasis:

- Chest X-ray.
- CT scan of chest in suspected cases.
- CT scan of abdomen.
- CT scan of brain if there are central nervous system (CNS) symptoms.

Q. What is the role of contrast-enhanced CT (CECT) scan in evaluation of local tumor?

Ans. Contrast-enhanced CT may be useful in evaluation of STS where MRI could not be done. CT is the preferred imaging technique for evaluation of retroperitoneal sarcoma. CT can delineate the mass and relation with the adjacent structures and vessels may be well seen. CT-guided FNAC/core biopsy may be done for deeper tumors.

Q. What is the role of contrast-enhanced CT (CECT) scan of chest?

Ans. In suspected case of chest metastasis and in patient with T2 tumors and patient having intermediate or high-grade tumors (G2 or G3) a CECT of chest is part of metastatic workup. CECT scan is more sensitive than chest X-ray to demonstrate parenchymal lesion and subpleural nodules.

Q. What is the role of positron emission tomography (PET)-computed tomography (CT) in the evaluation of soft tissue tumor (STS)?

Ans. Positron emission tomography is a functional imaging that measures the tumor uptake of glucose analog fluorodeoxyglucose (FDG) and allows imaging of the whole body. FDG/PET-CT is currently not recommended as the primary investigation for staging.

Q. When will you do incisional biopsy?

Ans. If trucut biopsy is inconclusive and the lesion is more than 5 cm an incisional biopsy may be done. Incisional biopsy, however, has some disadvantages. Complications like hematoma, infection, and tumor fungation may delay the primary treatment. Inappropriately placed incision for open biopsy may require a wider excision for covering the biopsy site.

Q. What precaution you will take while taking incisional biopsy?

Ans. While doing incisional biopsy the incision should be made vertically over the swelling in case of limbs so that the biopsy incision scar may be excised during the definitive surgery. Skin flaps should not be raised. Meticulous hemostasis is to be achieved while taking biopsy to prevent dissemination of the tumor cells into adjacent tissue planes by the hematoma.

Q. What is the role of fine-needle aspiration cytology (FNAC) in diagnosis of soft tissue sarcoma?

Ans. Fine-needle aspiration cytology is a useful modality for diagnosing soft tissue tumors. But exact histologic type and grading could not be done in a FNAC sample. However, FNAC may be useful for diagnosing metastasis and local recurrence.

Q. What is the role of excision biopsy in soft tissue sarcoma (STS)?

Ans. Excisional biopsy may be done for superficial lesion in the extremities which are less than 3 cm in diameter. However, the excisional biopsy provides no benefit over other biopsy technique. If diagnosed as STS re-resection with a wider margin will be required.

Q. What information is required from the pathological examination of tumor?

Ans. The pathologic reporting of sarcoma should include:
- Primary diagnosis
- Anatomic site
- Depth
- Size
- Histologic grade
- Presence or absence of necrosis
- Status of excision margin
- Lymph node status
- Mitotic rate
- Presence or absence of vascular invasion.

Q. What other investigations will you suggest?

Ans. Baseline investigations to assess patient's fitness for anesthesia and surgery—Hemogram, blood sugar, urea, and creatinine, liver function test.

Q. How will you treat this patient?

Ans. The tumor is localized to soft tissue and has not involved the bones. I will review the metastatic workup. If there is no evidence of distant metastasis I will consider wide local excision of the tumor along with the adjacent muscles. The goal of local therapy is to resect the tumor with a 2 cm normal surrounding tissue. The biopsy site should be resected en bloc with the tumor.

With growth of the tumor a zone of compressed reactive tissue forms a pseudocapsule surrounding the tumor. The excision should be outside the pseudocapsule.

Surgical clips are applied in the periphery of the tumor bed to guide postoperative radiotherapy.

Q. What is the role of adjuvant therapy in this patient?

Ans. As the tumor is more than 5 cm, I will consider postoperative radiotherapy to the tumor bed to achieve better local control and to reduce the chance of local recurrence.

Q. What should be the resection margin in soft tissue sarcoma (STS)?

Ans. The goal of wide excision is tumor excision with 1–2 cm of surrounding normal soft tissue. If the tumor is close to uninvolved neurovascular bundle narrower margin with preservation of neurovascular bundle may be adequate. Adventitia of vessel and perineurium of nerve should be removed.

Q. What is the surgical strategy for large tumors abutting the neurovascular bundles?

Ans. If the tumor is adjacent to the neurovascular bundle or displacing it—wide excision with adventitia or perineurium should be done.

If there is gross vascular invasion—compartment excision with vascular reconstruction may be done.

The incidence of postoperative complications is higher in patients requiring vascular resection. However, the incidence of local recurrence and overall survival is comparable to patients not requiring vascular resection.

Resection of nerves (sciatic, femoral, tibial, and peroneal) with appropriate reconstruction may provide acceptable functional outcome.

Q. What is the management strategy for bone involvement?

Ans. Bone involvement in extremity sarcoma may be delineated by cross-sectional MRI. STS abutting on the bone without cortical destruction and wide excision with periosteum provide adequate margin.

If there is cortical bone destruction, bone resection is required to obtain adequate margin. The resected bone has to be reconstructed. Patients undergoing bone resection has higher incidence of postoperative complications and less favorable functional outcome.

Q. What is the role of amputation in extremity sarcoma?

Ans. Earlier amputation was done in majority of patient presenting with extremity sarcoma. There have been several reports of limb sparing surgery with radiotherapy for extremity sarcoma with favorable outcome.

The consensus at present is limb sparing surgery for extremity sarcomas. In patients whose tumor cannot be grossly resected with a limb sparing procedure with preservation of function, only in those situations amputation is justified (5%).

National Cancer Institute study comparing amputation versus limb sparing surgery + adjuvant radiotherapy between 1975 and 1981, demonstrated no significant difference between the two groups in terms of overall survival. However, there is slight risk of local recurrence in limb sparing group (8% vs 0%).

Q. What is the role of regional lymphadenectomy?

Ans. There is no role of prophylactic lymph node dissection. Clinically and radiologically suspected lymph node needs confirmation by USG-guided FNAC. If the lymph nodes are metastatic therapeutic lymph node dissection should be carried out. The prognosis, however, is worse if the lymph nodes are involved.

Q. What is the role of sentinel lymph node biopsy in soft tissue sarcoma (STS)?

Ans. The role of sentinel lymph node biopsy is controversial. There have been no studies to ascertain the sensitivity and specificity of sentinel lymph node biopsy in STS.

Q. What is the role of radiotherapy in the management of soft tissue sarcoma?

Ans. The role of routine postoperative radiotherapy in all patients of STS is controversial.

As per National Comprehensive Cancer Network (NCCN) guidelines radiotherapy is not required in:

- Small STSs (<5 cm).
- Low-grade tumors.
- Resected with a widely negative margin.
- However, for such tumors radiotherapy is strongly recommended when margins of resection are close to the tumor or margins are positive or uncertain.

Adjuvant radiotherapy is indicated in:

- Soft tissue sarcoma more than 5 cm in size.
- High-grade lesion.
- This is beneficial in terms of local recurrence and overall survival.
- However, radiotherapy does not compensate for a suboptimal resection.

Q. What is the role of preoperative radiotherapy in soft tissue sarcoma (STS)?

Ans. In patients with large marginally resectable lesion and unresectable, a course of preoperative radiotherapy may allow the likelihood of a margin negative resection and greater likelihood of function preservation.

A dose of 50 Gy over a period of 5 weeks (1.8–2 Gy per day for 5 days a week).

A margin of 5–7cm is adequate. Surgery is planned 4–8 weeks after completion of radiotherapy to allow radiation reaction to subside.

Q. What are the different techniques of radiotherapy in soft tissue sarcoma (STS)?

Ans.

- External beam radiotherapy
- Brachytherapy
- Intensity modulated radiotherapy (IMRT).

Q. What is the role of brachytherapy in soft tissue sarcoma?

Ans. Brachytherapy has been shown to be as effective as external beam radiation in STS. A number of catheters are placed in the tumor bed with a 2 cm margins all around. After 5th postoperative day, the catheters are loaded with radioactive wires (Iridium-192) delivering 42–45 Gy to the tumor bed over 4–6 days. The duration of treatment with brachytherapy is smaller and there is less radiation scatter to the normal anatomic regions.

Q. What is the role of chemotherapy in soft tissue sarcoma?

Ans. The role of chemotherapy in STS is controversial. Combination chemotherapy with doxorubicin, dacarbazine, and ifosfamide has been used. Chemotherapy is indicated in high-risk group.

High-risk patient includes:

- Metastasis at diagnosis.
- Nonextremity sarcomas.
- Intermediate or high-grade histology.
- Large (T2) tumors.

Doxorubicin-based chemotherapy reduces the incidence of local recurrence. However, the absolute benefit of overall survival is not changed.

In general chemotherapy is often useful in young, healthy patients with high-risk tumors who are likely to tolerate the therapy well. Patients with cardiac disease and other comorbidities are not suitable candidates for adriamycin-based chemotherapy.

Q. What is the role of neoadjuvant chemotherapy?

Ans. Preoperative chemotherapy has been used in locally advanced sarcomas either alone or in combination with radiation therapy. The rates of disease response with combination of chemotherapy and radiotherapy have been found to be promising. As there is lack of randomized data, the role of chemotherapy is still investigational. The neoadjuvant therapy may allow limb preservation with superior long-term functional outcome in cases with locally advanced disease and in patients with high-grade sarcomas and sarcomas in relation to critical structures.

Q. What are the different regimens of preoperative chemotherapy?

Ans. MD Anderson Cancer Center uses a combination chemotherapy with doxorubicin, dacarbazine, cyclophosphamide, and ifosfamide for three cycles.

A continuous infusion of adriamycin with concurrent radiotherapy has also been used at MD Anderson Cancer Center. Macroscopic tumor resection was possible in all patients.

De Laney used a combination chemotherapy with mesna, adriamycin, ifosfamide, and dacarbazine alternating with radiotherapy. With this regime 5-years local control, freedom from distant metastasis, disease-free survival, and overall survival were improved (58% vs 87%) in comparison with controls.

Q. What are the patterns of recurrence in soft tissue sarcoma (STS)?

Ans. The recurrence may be:
- Local recurrence
- Isolated distant metastasis
- Widely disseminated disease.

Q. How will you treat local recurrence?

Ans. Patient with a local recurrence should be evaluated with clinical examination and imaging. The local recurrence without distant metastasis should be treated like a new primary.

Q. How will you manage metastatic disease?

Ans. Isolated metastasis may be treated with metastasectomy with or without pre or postoperative chemotherapy or radiotherapy.

In patients with disseminated disease palliative therapy includes:
- Surgery
- Chemotherapy
- Radiotherapy
- Embolization and ablative therapy
- If patient is asymptomatic observation may also be an option of palliative treatment.

Q. What is the follow-up protocol for soft tissue sarcoma (STS)?

Ans. National Comprehensive Cancer Network guidelines include follow-up with history and physical examination:
- Every 3–6 months for 2–3 years
- Every 6 months for next 2 years
- Then annually.

Chest imaging (X-ray or CT scan):

◆ For stage I tumors every 6–12 months
◆ For stage II and III tumors every 3–6 months for 5 years and then annually.
◆ Periodic imaging of the local site (CT or MRI) is to be done in high-risk patients especially if the location or depth of lesion makes physical examination unreliable for detection of local recurrence.

If the patient remains disease free for 10 years, the chance of recurrence becomes much smaller and subsequent follow-up should be individualized.

Q. What is the tumor, node and metastasis (TNM) staging for soft tissue sarcomas?

Ans. The American Joint Committee on Cancer (AJCC) staging for STS includes:

Primary tumor:

◆ *Tx*—Primary tumor cannot be assessed.
◆ *T0*—No evidence of primary tumor.
◆ *T1*—Tumor less than or equal to 5 cm in greatest dimension.
  – *T1a*—Superficial tumor
  – *T1b*—Deep tumor.
◆ *T2*—Tumor more than 5 cm in greatest dimension.
  – *T2a*—Superficial tumor
  – *T2b*—Deep tumor.

Regional lymph nodes:

◆ *Nx*—Regional lymph nodes cannot be assessed
◆ *N0*—No regional lymph nodes
◆ *N1*—Regional lymph nodes metastasis.

Distant metastasis:

◆ *Mx*—Distant metastasis cannot be assessed
◆ *M0*—No distant metastasis
◆ *M1*—Distant metastasis.

Q. What are the stagings of soft tissue sarcoma?

Ans. Stage grouping of STS takes into account the tumor grade, tumor size, regional lymph node metastasis, and distant metastasis.

◆ *Stage IA*	G 1–2	T1a–1b	N0	M0
◆ *Stage IB*	G1–2	T2a	N0	M0
◆ *Stage IIA*	G1–2	T2b	N0	M0
◆ *Stage IIB*	G3	T1a–1b	N0	M0
◆ *Stage IIC*	G3	T2a	N0	M0
◆ *Stage IIIA*	G3	T2b	N0	M0
◆ *Stage IIIB*	Any G	Any T	N1	M0
◆ *Stage IV*	Any G	Any T	Any N	M1.

Q. What are the different gradings for soft tissue sarcomas?

Ans. Depending on the mitotic figures (fewer than 10 or more mitosis per high-power field), cellularity (hypocellular versus hypercellular), necrosis (absent or present) and stromal content (abundant stroma versus less stroma), and differentiation (well differentiated versus poorly differentiated), the tumor may be graded as:

- *Gx*—Grade cannot be assessed.
- *G1*—Well differentiated (low grade)
- *G2*—Moderately differentiated (intermediate grade)
- *G3*—Poorly differentiated (high grade).

High-grade tumors are associated with poor prognosis and there is increased chance of metastasis.

Low-grade tumors have better prognosis and there is less chance of distant metastasis.

Q. How will you manage recurrent soft tissue sarcoma?

Ans. Recurrent soft tissue sarcoma usually presents as a nodular mass or multiple nodules in the operative scar. In recurrent retroperitoneal sarcomas, it present as recurrent abdominal mass with vague symptoms.

- Evaluation for extent of the local disease and any evidence of distant metastasis.
- Re-resection is the treatment of choice.
- In extremity recurrent sarcomas the likelihood of amputation is increased.
- In recurrent retroperitoneal sarcomas the adjacent organs may need resection.
- Adjuvant radiotherapy may be considered.

Q. What are the predisposing factors for development of soft tissue sarcomas?

Ans.

- *Genetic factors:*
  - Neurofibromatosis (von Recklinghausen's disease) associated with neurofibroma and neurofibrosarcoma.
  - Li–Fraumeni syndrome associated with p53 tumor suppressor gene for germline mutation. Increased incidence of STS.
  - Retinoblastoma 1 tumor suppressor gene for germline mutation associated with sarcoma of the eye in infancy and childhood.
- *Radiation exposure* is associated with increased incidence of STS and usually occurs 10–20 years after treatment.
- *Lymphedema due to filariasis*, postradiation, or postsurgical is associated with increased incidence of STS and manifests about 10–20 years after the onset of lymphedema.
- *Trauma*—Repeated trauma due to pregnancy is associated with increased incidence of desmoid tumor of abdominal wall.
- *Certain chemical carcinogens* like arsenic, polyvinyl chloride, and tetrachlorodibenzodioxin exposure are associated with increased incidence of STS.

Q. What are the usual distributions of soft tissue sarcomas?

Ans. Soft tissue sarcoma arises from the embryonic mesodermal cells. The relative site distributions are:

- *Extremities:* 50–60%
- *Trunk:* 19%
- *Retroperitoneum:* 15%
- *Head and neck:* 9%.

Q. What are the common pathological types of soft tissue sarcoma (STS)?

Ans. The pathological subtypes of STS include:
- *Malignant fibrous histiocytoma:* 28%
- *Liposarcoma:* 15%
- *Leiomyosarcoma:* 12%
- *Synovial sarcoma:* 10%
- *Malignant peripheral nerve sheath tumor:* 6%.

Q. What are the prognostic factors in soft tissue sarcoma (STS)?

Ans.
- *Histologic grade:* Most important prognostic factor in STS. Features defining grades are:
  - Cellularity
  - Differentiation (good, moderate, or poor/anaplastic)
  - Pleomorphism
  - Necrosis (absent, <50%, and >50%)
  - Number of mitoses per high-power field (<10, 10–19, and >20).

  The different grades are:
  - *Grade 1:* Well differentiated. Risk of metastasis—5–10%. 5-year survival—90%
  - *Grade 2:* Moderately differentiated. Risk of metastasis—25–30%. 5-year survival—70%
  - *Grade 3:* Poorly differentiated. Risk of metastasis—50–60%. 5-year survival—40%.
- Tumor size and location:
  - T1 tumors less than 5 cm
  - T2 tumors more than 5 cm
  - Superficial tumors (superficial to deep fascia) marked by "a" in T category
  - Deep tumors (deep to deep fascia) marked by "b" in T category
  - Large tumors and deep tumors have worse prognosis.
- *Nodal metastasis:*
  - Lymph node metastasis is rare in STS. Positive lymph node metastasis now grouped as stage III instead of stage IV. The prognosis in isolated lymph node metastasis is better than in patients with distant metastasis.
- *Distant metastasis:*
  - Distant metastasis may occur in lungs (most common site), bone, brain, and liver. Presence of distant is associated with poorer outcome.
- *Patient factors:*
  - Older age and male sex are a bad prognostic marker.
  - Recurrent tumors have bad prognosis with poor survival.
  - Positive microscopic margin—is associated with poor survival.
  - Over expression of Ki67, E-cadherin, and catenins high CD100 expression are all associated with poor prognosis.

Blood Vessels and Nerves

Chapter 10

▮ HEMANGIOMA

Clinical Examination

History: History of swelling (*See* Page No. 382, Chapter 9)
- Duration and onset
- Progress of the lesion
- Any history of trauma
- Any color change
- Any history of bleeding
- Any other lesion in the body.

Examination—Inspection/Palpation
- Examination of swelling—Site, size, shape, surface, margins, skin over the swelling and consistency
- Any pulsation
- Test for compressibility.

Q. What is your case? (Summary of a case of hemangioma)

Ans. This 20-year-old girl presented with a swelling on the right side of the neck for last 5 years. The swelling was about 2 cm in size at the onset and the swelling is gradually increasing in size to attain the present size of about 6 cm. Patient says that the swelling diminishes on pressure over the swelling. There is gradual dark discoloration of skin over the swelling during this period. There is no pain over the swelling and there is no other swelling in other parts of the body (Fig. 10.1).

On examination: There is a subcutaneous swelling in the right side of the neck, which is oval in shape 6 cm × 4 cm in size, soft in feel, surface is

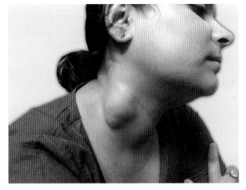

Fig. 10.1: Hemangioma in right side of the neck
Courtesy: Dr Prakash Bhagat, IPGME and R, Kolkata

smooth, margins are well-defined and the swelling is compressible (i.e. the swelling disappears on compressions and reappears on release of compression). There is dark discoloration of the overlying skin. The swelling is not fixed to the skin and underlying structures.

Q. What is your diagnosis?

Ans. This is a case of hemangioma in right side of the neck.

Q. How will you demonstrate sign of compressibility?

Ans. The swelling is pressed with the fingers. In compressible swelling, the swelling will diminish in size or may disappear and the swelling reappears on release of pressure (*See* Figs 1.36A to D and 1.37A to C, Page No. 34, Chapter 1).

Q. What is a hemangioma?

Ans. Hemangioma is a type of hamartoma arising from blood vessels. It is actually not a tumor.

Q. How will you treat this patient?

Ans. In view of the clinical sign of compressibility, the swelling is likely to be a hemangioma. I would like to do a color Doppler study to confirm my diagnosis. The color Doppler study will show the vascular lesion.

　　As the swelling is large, I will first give sclerosant injection and then plan for excision of the mass.

Q. How sclerotherapy is done?

Ans. I will inject 1% polidocanol into the swelling once a week for 4–6 weeks.

Q. What other sclerosants are used?

Ans. Hypertonic saline, sodium tetradecyl sulfate and boiling water may also be used as sclerosant.

Q. How does sclerotherapy help?

Ans.

Small swelling: May disappear with sclerotherapy.

Large swelling: Size of the lesion may diminish due to fibrosis and destructions of vascular spaces. Resection becomes easier and bleeding during surgery is reduced.

Q. What surgery will you do?

Ans.

- Excision of the swelling
- Alternatively feeding vessels are ligated and the hemangiomatous mass is then excised
- Bleeding may be controlled with diathermy or ligation.

Q. How else the hemangioma may be treated?

Ans.

- Laser beam therapy may be effective in small hemangiomas
- Embolization of the feeding vessels may cause some regression of the mass rendering surgical excision easier.

Q. What are the different types of hemangioma?

Ans. Depending on the nature of blood vessels involved, there are three types of hemangioma:
1. Capillary hemangioma
2. Cavernous hemangioma
3. Arterial or *plexiform hemangioma.*

Q. What type of hemangioma is this?

Ans.
* This is likely to be a cavernous hemangioma.
* Swelling is present for a long time and is gradually increasing in size.
* The swelling is raised from the surface of skin and there is bluish discoloration of the overlying skin.
* Feels soft and spongy
* No pulsation over the swelling
* The swelling is compressible.

Q. What are the common sites where cavernous hemangioma may be found?

Ans.
* It may be found in the subcutaneous tissues of the face, ear and lips.
* In the mucous membrane of tongue, mouth and lips
* In the internal organs, such as liver, kidneys, intestine and brain.

Q. What is capillary hemangioma?

Ans.
* It is a hamartoma arising from the capillaries.
* These are usually flat, not raised from the surface and non-pulsatile.

Q. What are the different types of capillary hemangiomas?

There are different types of capillary hemangiomas:
* Salmon patch
* Port wine stain
* Strawberry angioma
* Spider nevus.

Q. What is salmon patch?

Ans. This is a pigmented spot present at birth usually seen in the midline in the forehead or in the occipital region and usually disappears by 1 year.

Q. What is port wine stain (or nevus flammeus)?

Ans.
* Present since birth.
* Usually a deep red or purple discoloration situated in face, lip, cheek or neck.
* The color diminishes on pressure but reappears on release of pressure.
* The lesion does not show any change during the rest of life.

Q. What are the characteristics of strawberry angioma?

- A red pigmented lesion is usually noticed 1–3 weeks after birth and gradually increases in size for about a year forming a strawberry like swelling.
- Swelling is raised from the surface, surface is irregular and there may be small areas of ulceration, which is covered with scab.
- The swelling is soft, non-pulsatile and compressible
- Strawberry angioma can occur in any part of the body but is commonly seen in head, face and neck.
- After 1 year, the swelling starts regressing and may involute by the age of 7–8 years
- The lesion is composed of immature vascular tissue.

Q. How will you treat port wine stain?

Ans.
- May be left as such
- Suitable cosmetics to mask the color
- Laser therapy
- Excision with skin grafting may be considered in selected case.

Q. How will you treat strawberry angioma?

- Wait and watch till 7–8 years of age for spontaneous involution to occur
- Sclerosant injection may be tried
- Cryosurgery by application of carbon dioxide snow
- Laser therapy using carbon dioxide or Nd:YAG laser
- Excision and skin grafting in selected cases.

Q. What is Sturge-Weber syndrome?

Ans. Association of capillary hemangioma with:
- Hemangioma in cerebral hemisphere
- Mental retardation
- Jacksonian epilepsy
- Eye complication like glaucoma and buphthalmos.

Q. What is Osler-Rendu-Weber syndrome?

- Also called hereditary hemorrhagic telangiectasia
- Multiple small aneurysmal telangiectasias are seen in skin and mucous membrane of oral cavity, gastrointestinal tract, urinary tract, liver, spleen and in brain
- Present at birth and transmitted by autosomal dominant trait
- May present with hemorrhage due to rupture of the aneurysmal vessels.

■ PLEXIFORM HEMANGIOMA (CIRSOID ANEURYSM)

Q. What is your case? (Summary of a case of cirsoid aneurysm)

This 40-year-old gentleman complains of a swelling in forehead since childhood, which was gradually increasing in size. The swelling gets aggravated when the patient lies down, lowers his head and reduces to some extent on standing. There is no other swelling in other parts of the body (Fig. 10.2).

On examination: There is a diffuse swelling over the scalp. The swelling feels like a bag of pulsating earthworms, swelling is compressible, a systolic thrill is palpable and, on auscultation over the swelling, a bruit is audible. Bony indentation is palpable at the margin of the swelling.

Q. What is your diagnosis?

Ans. This is a case of cirsoid aneurysm in the scalp in forehead.

Q. What is cirsoid aneurysm?

Ans. This is a condition of congenital arteriovenous fistula. There is arterialization of veins. The vein becomes dilated, tortuous, thickened and pulsatile.

Q. How will you treat this patient?

Ans.

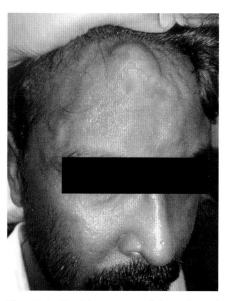

Fig. 10.2: Cirsoid aneurysm of the scalp and forehead

Courtesy: Dr Dev Kumar, IPGME and R, Kolkata

* Ligation of feeding vessel and excision of the mass
* Therapeutic embolization of feeding artery may help and may render the excision easier.

Q. What are the complications of hemangioma?

Ans.

* Hemorrhage
* Thrombosis
* Calcification
* Ulceration of overlying skin
* Pressure effects
* Rarely malignant change
* Infection.

Q. What are hamartomas?

Ans. A hamartoma is a developmental malformation leading to a tumor like overgrowth of tissue or tissues, which is the normal constituent of that particular organ.

Q. What are the characteristics of hamartomas?

Ans.

* Most hamartomas are present at birth or appears in early childhood.
* The hamartomas grow along with the growth of the normal tissues and the growth ceases after adolescence when the physiological growth ceases.
* Hamartomas are benign lesion but may rarely undergo malignant change
* Some hamartomas may regress spontaneously

- Some hamartomas may be multiple, e.g. neurofibromas
- There is no definite capsule around a hamartoma, it grows into the surrounding tissues.

Q. What are different hamartomatous lesions?

Ans.

- *Vascular hamartomas*: Hemangiomas, pigmented moles, glomus tumor.
- *Lymphatic tissues*: Lymphangiomas.
- *Neural tissues*: Neurofibromas.
- *Skeletal tissues*: Exostosis.

■ GLOMUS TUMOR

Q. What is your case? (summary of a case of glomus tumor)

History: This 30-year-old gentleman presented with a small bluish circumscribed swelling at the tip of the right index finger under the nail bed for last 1 year, which is growing very slowly. Patient complains of pain over the site of the tumor and pain gets aggravated by pressure over the local site or by exposure of the part to sudden changes in temperature (Fig. 10.3).

On examination: There is a very small, about 5 mm in diameter, bluish pigmented lesion situated at the tip of the right index finger deep to the nail. The site is extremely tender on touch and pressure.

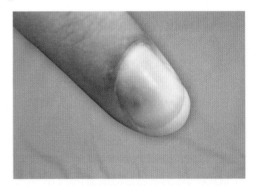

Fig. 10.3: Glomus tumor

Q. What is your diagnosis?

Ans. This is a case of glomus tumor (glomangioma) under the nail of right index finger.

Q. What is glomus body?

Ans. The glomus body is a specialized structure, which is composed of a tortuous arteriole and communicates directly with a venule, and is surrounded by a network of nerves.

Histologically, the tumor consists of a mixture of blood spaces, nerve tissues and muscle fibers derived from the wall of the arteriole. So this is also known as angiomyoneuroma. There are also large cuboidal cells with a dark central nucleus called glomus cells.

Q. Where do you find cutaneous glomus body commonly?

Ans. The glomus body is commonly found in nail bed at tips of fingers and toes, and at the palmar surface of the phalanges.

Q. What is the function of glomus body?

Ans. The glomus body helps in regulation of body temperature.

Q. What are the other possibilities?

* Subungual melanoma
* Pyogenic granuloma
* Squamous papilloma.

Q. How will you treat this patient?

* Excision of the tumor
* A wedge of nail is excised and the underlying lesion is excised all around under digital nerve block.

■ RAYNAUD'S DISEASE/RAYNAUD'S SYNDROME

Clinical Examination

History

* Onset and duration of the attack.
* What occurs on exposure to cold.
    – Sequence of changes—
        - Paleness of fingers or toes
        - Blueness and
        - Later red engorgement.
* Any associated pain during the red engorgement stage.
* Any history of ulceration at the tip of fingers or toes.
* History of resorption of terminal phalanges causing shortening of the terminal phalanges.
* Any history of cervical spondylosis—
    – Pain in the neck—duration, character of pain, radiation of pain in the upper limb.
    – Any difficulty in neck movements.
* Any history suggestive of scleroderma—
    – Any skin changes in the limbs or face
    – Any history of dysphagia.
* Any swelling in the supraclavicular fossa—may suggest cervical rib.
* Any history of rest pain or gangrene at the tips of fingers or toes.
* Any history of diabetes, hypertension or hypothyroidism.

Examination—Inspection/Palpation

* Attitude of the limb
* Any wasting or resorption of the fingers (pulp of the fingers may become wasted and the terminal phalanges may become conical)
* Temperature of the hand (may feel colder)
* Look for any scar or ulcer at the tips of fingers
* Look for stigma of scleroderma-skin changes and narrowing of oral orifice
* Examine the supraclavicular fossa for any bony swelling (suggestive of cervical rib)
* Examine neck for any evidence of cervical spondylosis. Any restriction of neck movements

- Any neurological deficit in the upper limbs
- Examine all the peripheral pulses (in Raynaud's disease all pulses are normal)
- Adson's test—to assess any thoracic outlet syndrome.

Q. What is your case? (Summary of a case of Raynaud's disease)

Ans. This 35-year-old lady presented with recurrent attacks of some color changes in her fingers of both upper limbs on exposure to cold for last 2 years. She says that her fingers become pale on exposure to cold. Later, they become blue and then become red again with burning pain. These attacks are occurring for last 2 years more during winter season. Patient noticed that the terminal phalanx of all the fingers getting shorter over these periods of time. She has no complain in her lower limbs. She has no symptom suggestive of collagen disease (Fig. 10.4).

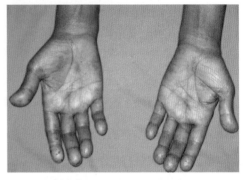

Fig. 10.4: Raynaud's disease involving the fingers of both hands. Note resorption of terminal phalanx of the fingers

Courtesy: Prof Alokendu Ghosh, IPGME & R, Kolkata.

On examination: General survey is normal. On local examination of the upper limbs, there is resorption of terminal phalanges of all the fingers in both hands and the tips of the fingers appear conical. There is slight tenderness in the tips of fingers. All the peripheral pulses are normal.

Q. What is your diagnosis?

Ans.
- This is a case of Raynaud's disease affecting both upper limbs with ischemic resorption of terminal phalanges of all the fingers.
  In patients with similar presentation—when there is a cause found the diagnosis should be Raynaud's syndrome.
  This is a case of Raynaud's syndrome secondary to scleroderma with ischemic resorption of terminal phalanges of all the fingers in both upper limbs.

Q. What is Raynaud's phenomenon?

Ans. Raynaud's phenomenon is a sequence of color changes in the fingers due to spasm of digital vessels. These color changes occur in number of stages:
- Stage I: Stage of local syncope or stage of pallor
- Stage II: Stage of local cyanosis
- Stage III: Stage of red congestion
- Stage IV: Stage of ischemic gangrene.

Q. What are the explanations for different color changes in Raynaud's phenomenon?

Ans.
- *Stage I (Stage of local syncope or pallor):*
  - On exposure to cold, there is spasm of the digital blood vessel.
  - As the vessel goes into spasm, there is reduced blood supply to the digits leading to pallor.

- *Stage II (Stage of local cyanosis):*
  - Due to reduced blood supply the local area suffers from anoxia and there is accumulation of tissue metabolite.
  - The accumulated tissue metabolite causes dilatation of capillaries, which becomes filled with slowly flowing deoxygenated blood resulting in local cyanosis.
  - During this phase both precapillary and postcapillary sphincter remains in spasm.
- *Stage III (Stage of red engorgement):*
  - As the attack passes off, the precapillary sphincter relaxes but the postcapillary sphincter still remains in spasm.
  - Oxygenated blood enters into the dilated capillary bed. As the postcapillary sphincter remains in spasm, there is red engorgement of the area due to over distension of the capillary bed with oxygenated blood.
  - There is burning pain in the local area due to partly increased tension in the capillaries and partly due to accumulation of tissue metabolites.
- *Stage IV (Stage of ischemic gangrene):*
  - As attacks are repeated there is resorption of the terminal pulp space and the tips of digits appear conical.
  - Persistent spasm of the digital vessel may result in ischemic gangrene.

Q. What is Raynaud's disease?

Ans. When Raynaud's phenomenon occurs in a patient, where no cause is discernible, it is called Raynaud's disease.

Q. What are the causes of Raynaud's phenomenon?

Ans. Raynaud's phenomenon may occur secondary to following conditions:
- *Autoimmune diseases.*
  - Scleroderma
  - Systemic lupus erythematosus
  - Polyarteritis nodosa
  - Rheumatoid arthritis
  - Dermatomyositis.
- *Occlusive arterial disease:*
  - Buerger's disease
  - Atherosclerotic vascular disease.
- *Drugs*
  - Ergot preparations
  - Propranolol
  - Methysergide
  - Cytotoxic drugs.
- *Blood disorders:*
  - Cold agglutinins
  - Cryoglobulinemia.
- *Miscellaneous:*
  - Working with vibrating tools
  - Atrophic changes in the limb due to poliomyelitis
  - Thoracic outlet syndrome.

Q. How will you manage this patient?

Ans. I would like to do some investigations:
- X-ray of cervical spine (anteroposterior and lateral view) to exclude cervical rib and associated cervical spondylosis.
- Doppler ultrasonography of upper limb arterial system to exclude disease of major blood vessels.
- Blood for lupus erythematosus cell (LE cell), antinuclear factor, rheumatoid factor to exclude collagen vascular disease.

Q. How will you treat this patient?

Ans. I will initially try conservative treatment:
- Avoid exposure to cold. To use gloves and socks during winter for protection of hands and feet from cold.
- *Drug treatment*: A number of drugs have been tried. Calcium channel blocker like nifedipine may have some beneficial effect.
- Cilostazole (a phosphodiesterase inhibitor) administered 100 mg twice may be helpful in some cases.
- Early treatment of nail bed infection.

Q. What is the role of vasodilator drugs?

Ans. The vasodilator drugs like isoxsuprine are not beneficial as it causes generalized vasodilation and may steal the blood flow from the ischemic limb.

Q. What is the role of cervicodorsal sympathectomy in Raynaud's disease?

Ans. Earlier cervicodorsal sympathectomy was routinely done in Raynaud's disease. But recently, it has been observed that it is not very effective and cervicodorsal sympathectomy is being considered in selected cases.

Q. What may be the possible benefits of sympathectomy?

Ans.
- Raynaud's disease is a vasospastic disease involving the digital vessels.
- Sympathectomy causes loss of vasomotor supply of cutaneous vessels and thereby causes vasodilatation of cutaneous vessel and the skin blood supply increases to some extent.
- But in majority, the symptoms may return within 5 years of sympathectomy.

Q. When will you consider cervicodorsal sympathectomy?

Ans. If the conservative measures fail and the patient has recurrent attacks of vasospasm then cervicodorsal sympathectomy may be helpful.

Q. What do you remove in cervicodorsal sympathectomy?

Ans. For complete denervation of the upper limb, the lower half of the stellate ganglion and the second and third thoracic sympathetic ganglia are to be divided along with both the gray and white rami communicantes. The nerve of Kuntz is a gray ramus running upward from the second thoracic ganglion to the first thoracic nerve, is also to be divided.

Q. What are the different approaches for cervicodorsal sympathectomy?

Ans.

* Supraclavicular approach by a transverse supraclavicular neck incision
* Transthoracic approach through lateral thoracotomy
* Axillary approach through an axillary incision at the third intercostal space
* Video-guided endoscopic surgery for cervicodorsal sympathectomy.

Q. Where do you find the stellate ganglion?

Ans. Stellate ganglion is formed by the joining of eighth cervical ganglion with the first thoracic ganglion and it lies against the neck of the first rib.

The clavicular part of the sternocleidomastoid muscle is divided. The inferior belly of the omohyoid and the scalenus anterior muscle is divided, and preserving the phrenic nerve. The subclavian artery is depressed and the suprapleural membrane is divided and the apex of the pleura is depressed downward. The stellate ganglion is identified against the neck of the first rib.

Q. How will you treat Raynaud's syndrome secondary to some causes?

Ans.

* Treatment of the underlying condition
* Above conservative measures are helpful. Steroid, immunosuppressant drugs for collagen diseases
* Cervicodorsal sympathectomy is usually not helpful.

Q. What is acrocyanosis?

Ans. Acrocyanosis is a condition of painless persistent blueness of fingers and toes. This cyanosis is exacerbated by exposure to cold. There may be associated paresthesia.

This condition is due to arteriolar spasm with associated capillary dilatation resulting in pooling of deoxygenated blood in the capillary bed.

Q. How will you treat acrocyanosis?

Ans. Avoidance of cold exposure may be helpful in some cases.

In severe case, cervicodorsal sympathectomy for upper limb disease and lumbar sympathectomy for lower limb disease may be helpful.

■ ARTERIOVENOUS FISTULA

Clinical Examination

See Page No. 382, Chapter 9.

History

* Onset, progress of the swelling along the veins. Whether from birth or not.
* Any history of trauma
* Any overgrowth of limb
* Any ulceration in the area distal to the site of fistula
* Any systemic symptoms like palpitation and breathlessness.

Examination: Inspection/Palpation

* Examine the pulse.
* Look for collapsing character of the pulse.
* Measure blood pressure—there may be wide pulse pressure.
* Details about the dilated veins—site and extent of involvement of the veins.
* Temperature of the limb (may feel warmer).
* Any evidence of local gigantism (usually found in congenital arteriovenous fistula).
* Look for Nicoladoni's or Branham's sign.

Q. What is your case? (Summary of a case of traumatic arteriovenous fistula)

Ans. This 30-year-old gentleman presented with swelling of veins in his left upper limb for the last 3 years. Patient had a history of trauma in his left upper limb 3 years back due to fall from a height. Fifteen days following the trauma patient noticed swelling of veins in his forearm which is gradually increasing in size and numbers and also extends upward in the arm and dorsum of hand. Patient complains of palpitation on exertion for last 6 months (Fig. 10.5).

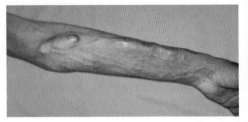

Fig. 10.5: Traumatic arteriovenous fistula involving the left forearm

Courtesy: Dr Nemai Nath, NRS Medical College, Kolkata.

Examination: On general survey, pulse is 90 beats/min, high volume collapsing in character. Blood pressure is 130/40 mm Hg. On local examination, there are dilated tortuous veins on the left forearm, dorsum of hand of the patient. The right upper limb feels warmer than the left. A thrill is palpable at the lower end of the forearm over the site of the arteriovenous fistula and, on auscultation, there is a continuous machinery murmur which is audible. Branham's sign is positive.

Q. What is your diagnosis?

Ans. This is a case of traumatic arteriovenous fistula in left upper limb.

Q. What is Branham's or Nicoladoni's sign?

Ans. Pressure on the artery proximal to the fistula causes:
* The venous swelling to diminish
* Thrill and bruit disappears
* Pulse rate falls
* Pulse pressure returns to normal.

  This is called Branham's sign or Nicoladoni's sign.

  In patient, pressure over the brachial artery, at the elbow region causes diminution of venous swelling over the forearm and dorsum of the hand. Thrill and bruit also disappeared and the pulse rate falls.

Q. What are the structural effects of arteriovenous fistula?

Ans. The veins become dilated tortuous and thick walled. This is called arterialization of veins. The venous dilatation gradually involves other superficial veins and the lesion becomes more diffuse.

In congenital arteriovenous fistula, the venous dilatation is more diffuse, may involve the veins in the bone and may result in local gigantism.

Q. What are the physiological effects of the arteriovenous fistula?

* There is an uncontrolled leak from the high pressure arterial system into the veins and the consequent increased venous pressure causes increased venous return to the heart. This results in increase in pulse rate and increased cardiac output. The pulse pressure is high due to large persistent shunt. Left ventricular hypertrophy and later cardiac failure may occur.
* A congenital arteriovenous fistula may cause overgrowth of a limb.
* An indolent ulcer may develop in large arteriovenous fistula of limb due to relative ischemia below the short circuit.
* Q. How will you manage this patient?
* **Ans.** I will do some investigation to confirm my diagnosis and plan the treatment:
* An arteriography is required to confirm the diagnosis. There is quick venous filling during arteriography. Sometime, it is difficult to pinpoint the site of the fistula.
* Chest X-ray to look for any cardiac enlargement.
* ECG
* Other baseline investigations.

Q. How will you treat this patient?

Ans. This is traumatic AV fistula and the site of the fistula is to be localized by clinical examination and by arteriography. I will treat this patient by quadruple ligation with a bypass graft for the artery segment. The site of the fistula is dissected and the artery and the veins below and above the site of fistula are also delineated. The artery and the vein are ligated above and below the site of fistula. The ligated arterial segment is bypassed using either a Dacron graft or a segment of a vein (Fig. 10.6).

Q. What are the characteristics of congenital arteriovenous fistula?

Ans. Congenital arteriovenous fistula is more extensive. The dilated veins may affect the bones

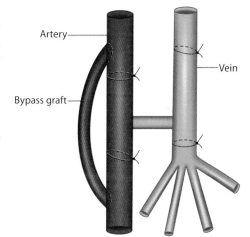

Fig. 10.6: Quadruple ligation

and may result in increased bone growth. Presence of port wine stain or superficial angiomata may be present in congenital AV fistula. Local gigantism is more common in congenital arteriovenous fistula.

Q. What are the problems of treatment of congenital arteriovenous fistula?

Ans. There are sites of multiple communications and the malformation is very extensive. So direct surgery is very difficult.

Selective embolization may help in some cases.

Q. What is Klippel-Trenaunay syndrome?

Ans. This is characterized by:

* Varicose veins on the lateral aspect of the leg.
* Local gigantism—Overgrowth of the limb.
* Presence of cutaneous angiomata.

Q. What is Cimino's fistula?

Ans. This is an iatrogenic arteriovenous fistula created by surgery. This is usually done at the wrist between the radial artery and a tributary of the cephalic vein. This results in dilatation and tortuosity of the veins around the wrist, which are utilized for easy access for hemodialysis. This can also be done at the ankle between the posterior tibial artery and an adjacent vein.

This can be easily reversed. The fistulous sac is excised and the rent in the artery and vein sutured.

Q. What are the indications of amputation in a case of arteriovenous fistula?

Ans.

* Cases with severe pain and ischemic gangrene
* Cases with intractable cardiac failure due to hyperdynamic circulation
* Giant limb incapacitating the patient
* Failure of surgical treatment by ligation or embolization.

■ NEUROFIBROMA

Clinical Examination

See Page No. 382, Chapter 9.

History

* History about the swelling
* Any pain, tingling or numbness in the area distal to the swelling
* Enquire about presence of swelling in other parts of the body (neurofibromas may be multiple and may be present throughout the body in Von Recklinghausen's disease).
* Any history of rapid growth of the swelling.
* Any headache, vomiting to exclude presence of any intracranial neurofibroma or meningioma.
* Any pain or weakness of the limbs to exclude any spinal neurofibroma.

Examination—Inspection/Palpation

* *Examination of swelling*: Site, extent, shape, size, surface, margin, skin over the swelling
* Mobility (neurofibromas are more mobile across the axis of the nerve than along the axis of the nerve).
* In generalized neurofibromatosis measure blood pressure to exclude pheochromocytoma.
* Test for hearing to exclude acoustic neuroma.
* Examine limbs for any neurological deficit to exclude a dumb bell neurofibroma.

Q. What is your case? (Summary of a case of neurofibroma)

Ans.

History: This 45-year-old gentleman complains of a swelling in right forearm for last 2 years. The swelling was about 1 cm in size at the onset and for last 2 years the swelling is increasing very slowly in size. He complains of dull aching pain over the swelling and tingling sensation along the outer aspect of the left forearm. There is no other swelling in the body. He has no systemic complaints (Fig. 10.7).

On examination: There is a firm globular swelling in the extensor aspect of left forearm, 3 cm x 3 cm in size, smooth surface and well-defined

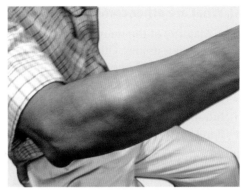

Fig. 10.7: Neurofibroma on the extensor surface of right forearm

Courtesy: Dr Subhashis Karmakar, RG Kar Medical College, Kolkata

margin. The overlying skin is free, the swelling is mobile but it is better moved transversely than vertically. Swelling is slightly tender. There may be sensory or motor deficit along the distribution of the particular nerve involved. There are no other swellings in other parts of the body.

Q. What is your diagnosis?

Ans. This is a case of neurofibroma in left forearm.

Q. What else this swelling can be?

- Lipoma
- Fibroma
- Enlarged lymph node
- Hemangioma
- Cystic lesion like sebaceous cyst, dermoid cyst or subcutaneous bursa.

Q. How will you treat this patient?

Ans. The swelling is painful so I will consider excision of the tumor with care not to damage the nerve.

Q. How will you excise the swelling?

Ans. I will excise the swelling under local anesthesia. After antiseptic cleaning and draping I will inject 1% lignocaine circumferentially around the tumor to achieve a ring block.

A transverse incision is made over the swelling and the incision deepened up to the subcutaneous tissue. The skin flaps are raised and the tumor is dissected off from the subcutaneous tissue and excised. Hemostasis is achieved and the skin closed with interrupted silk sutures.

Q. What is neurofibroma?

Ans. Neurofibromas are regarded as hamartomas rather than true neoplasms. Neurofibromas arise from endoneurium which is the innermost connective tissue covering of the nerve fibers.

Q. What are other common sites of neurofibroma?

Ans. Majority of the neurofibromas arise from the peripheral nerves and are present in the subcutaneous tissues. Other important sites where neurofibroma may be found are:
* From the cranial nerves—most commonly eighth nerve—acoustic neuroma, may also arise from fifth or ninth cranial nerve
* From dorsal nerve root ganglion
* Intramuscular
* Rarely in the bone.

Q. Can neurofibroma cause neurodeficit?

Ans. As the neurofibroma arises from the connective tissue of the nerve sheath, it may cause compression of the nerve fibers and interfere with function of that particular nerve leading either to motor or sensory deficit.

Q. What are the complications of neurofibroma?

Ans.
* Cystic degeneration
* Infection
* Sarcomatous changes.

Q. What are the different types of neurofibroma?

* Localized neurofibroma or solitary neurofibroma
* Generalized neurofibromatosis or Von Recklinghausen's disease
* Plexiform neurofibromatosis (pachydermatocele)
* Elephantiasis neurofibromatosa
* Cutaneous neurofibromatosis (molluscum fibrosum).

Q. What are the indications for excision of a solitary neurofibroma?

Ans. All solitary neurofibromas do not need excision. The indications for excision are:
* Painful neurofibromas
* Neurofibromas causing pressure symptoms
* Neurofibromas showing signs of malignant change
* Cosmetic deformity.

■ PLEXIFORM NEUROFIBROMATOSIS (PACHYDERMATOCELE)

Q. What is your case? (Summary of a case of plexiform neurofibromatosis)

This 20-year-old boy has presented with swelling in left side of the face for last 5 years. The swelling started in the left side of the cheek 5 years back which was about 3 cm in size at the onset and since then this swelling was gradually increasing in size and involved the whole of left side of the face, both lips and the left periorbital area. There is no headache, vomiting, any pain or weakness of any of the limbs. There is no history of hypertension (Fig. 10.8).

On examination: There is diffuse swelling involving the whole of the left side of the face. The skin appears thickened, and because of the extensive swelling the skin is showing a number of folds and appears pendulous. On palpation, temperature over the swelling is normal and the swelling is non-tender. The surface of the swelling is smooth. The skin is thickened. The overlying skin is hyperpigmented. The margins are ill-defined.

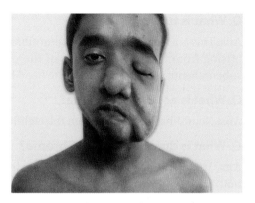

Fig. 10.8: Plexiform neurofibromatosis involving the left side of the face

Courtesy: Dr Arijit Mukherji, Calcutta Medical College, Kolkata

Q. What is your diagnosis?

Ans. This is a case of plexiform neurofibromatosis (pachydermatocele) involving the left side of the face.

Q. What are the common sites of plexiform neurofibromatosis?

Ans.
* This is commonly seen in the face in connection with branches of trigeminal nerve.
* It may also occur in the arm or thigh along the distribution of cutaneous nerves.

Q. What else could it be?

Ans.
* Hemangioma
* Lymphangioma
* Squamous papilloma.

Q. How will you treat this patient?

* This is cosmetically disfiguring and needs to be treated.
* As the lesion is extensive surgical treatment, involves staged excision and skin grafting.

Q. What is elephantiasis neurofibromatosa?

Ans. It is a form of plexiform neurofibromatosis affecting the cutaneous nerves of the limbs. The skin and subcutaneous tissue is thickened, coarse and dry resembling elephant's skin.

Q. What are the causes of elephantiasis of leg?

Ans.
* Filariasis
* Plexiform neurofibromatosis
* Elephantiasis graecorum or nodular leprosy
* Lymphatic obstruction due to malignancy, radiotherapy or lymph node dissection
* Arteriovenous fistula.

Q. What is turban tumor?

Ans. This is a form of cutaneous neurofibromatosis affecting the scalp. Multiple neurofibromas arising from terminal branches of the cutaneous nerves of the scalp may form multiple subcutaneous nodules covering the head like a turban so it is called turban tumor.

Q. What is acoustic neuroma?

Ans. Neurofibroma arising from the eighth cranial nerve is called acoustic neuroma.

Q. What is dumbbell neurofibroma?

Ans. The dumbbell neurofibroma arises from the dorsal nerve root. This neurofibroma grows both toward the spinal canal, and may cause cord compression and grows outward outside the vertebral foramen giving an appearance of dumbbell.

Q. What is neuroma?

Ans. A benign tumor arising from a nerve is called neuroma.

Q. What are false neuromas?

Ans. The nerve tumor, which arises from the connective tissue sheath of the nerve fibers, is called false neuromas. Neurilemmomas and neurofibromas are false neuromas.

Q. What are Schwannomas?

Ans. Schwannomas or neurilemmomas arise from the Schwann cell present in the nerve sheath. It is a benign, well-encapsulated tumor. This may involve cranial nerves or peripheral nerves in the mediastinum or the retroperitoneum.

Q. What are true neuromas?

Ans. True neuromas arise from the neural tissues derived from the neural crest, which forms the sympathetic nervous system.

Q. What are chromaffinomas or pheochromocytomas?

Ans. These are tumors arising from the chromaffin tissues in the adrenal medulla.

Q. What are neuroblastomas?

Ans. These are tumors of adrenal medulla arising from the primitive neuroblasts, which are derived from the neural crest.

Q. What are ganglioneuromas?

Ans. These are tumors arising from the mature sympathetic ganglion cells present in the sympathetic chain.

■ GENERALIZED NEUROFIBROMATOSIS (VON RECKLINGHAUSEN'S DISEASE)

Q. What is your case? (Summary of a case of generalized neurofibromatosis)

Ans. This 55-year-old gentleman complains of multiple swellings in different parts of the body since childhood, which was slowly increasing in size since then. Apart from the presence of the swelling, patient has no other complain. Patient's daughter has similar swellings in the body (Fig. 10.9).

On examination: multiple nodules of varying sizes are found throughout the body. The nodules are firm in consistency, mobile, and there are dark pigmented patches in the skin of the abdomen and in the buttocks (café au lait spots).

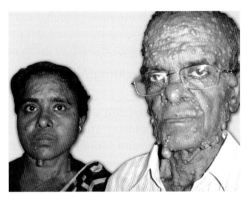

Fig. 10.9: Cases of Von Recklinghausen's disease. These cutaneous lesions are present throughout the body. Father and daughter have identical disease

Courtesy: Dr Anadi Nath Acharya, R G Kar Medical College, Kolkata

Q. What other lesion may be associated with Von Recklinghausen's disease?

Ans.
- Von Recklinghausen's disease may be associated with pheochromocytoma
- Neuromas affecting the cranial and spinal nerve
- Skeletal deformities like scoliosis or kyphosis
- Lisch nodules
- Retina—blindness
- Pseudoarthroses
- Local gigantism.

Q. What is the mode of inheritance?

Ans. This disease is transmitted as an autosomal dominant trait.

Q. What is the incidence of malignant change in a neurofibroma?

Ans. About 5% cases may show malignant change.

Q. Which features suggest sarcomatous change in a neurofibroma?

Ans.
- Swelling becoming painful
- Sudden and rapid increase in size of the swelling
- Swelling becomes more vascular
- Swelling becoming fixed to adjacent structures
- There may be signs of motor or sensory deficit along the distribution of the nerve.

Q. How will you treat this patient?

Ans.
- As such no surgery is required for multiple neurofibromas present throughout the body.
- I will reassure the patient keep him under regular follow-up.

Q. What are the indications of surgery for generalized neurofibromatosis?

Ans. As neurofibromas are present throughout the body excision of all such tumors are not indicated. Surgery for excision of the tumor is indicated when:
- The swelling becomes painful.

- The swelling shows signs of malignant change.
- The swelling is causing pressure symptoms.
- The swelling is large enough to cause mechanical problems.

Q. What is Von Recklinghausen's disease of bones?

Ans.

- Von Recklinghausen's disease of bone (osteitis fibrosa cystica) results from primary hyperparathyroidism. The disease is characterized by:
  - Gross resorption of bone due to demineralization
  - Pathological fracture of bones
  - Recurrent renal calculi
  - Peptic ulceration
  - This may be associated with other endocrine abnormalities as part of multiple endocrine neoplasia.

■ MENINGOCELE/MENINGOMYELOCELE

Clinical Examination

See Page No. 382, Chapter 9.

History—History of swelling

- Onset of swelling (present since birth)
- Progress of the swelling
- Relation of swelling with crying and coughing (swelling gets aggravated on straining—crying, coughing).
- Any weakness of the lower limbs (in meningocele usually no neurodeficit is found, in meningomyelocele—lower limb weakness, bladder and bowel incontinence is common).
- History of any maternal disease during pregnancy.
- Any drug intake by mother during pregnancy (steroid, phenytoin or carbamazepine).
- Type of delivery—full term, preterm. Normal delivery or cesarean section.

Examination—Inspection/Palpation

- Details of swelling
- Site and extent
- Size and shape
- surface and margin
- Skin over the swelling
- Consistency (usually soft cystic swelling)
- Fluctuation (positive)
- Transillumination (meningocele are brilliantly transilluminant, whereas meningomyelocele through transilluminant show fine strands of fibers within).
- Examine the head—Measure head circumference. Palpate fontanel to exclude hydrocephalus.

* Examination of lower limbs—tone, movement of the limbs—spontaneous and on pinching.
* Assess the anal sphincter tone.
* Look for any other congenital anomalies—cleft lip, cleft palate, anorectal malformations or vertebral anomalies.

Q. What is your case? (Summary of a case of meningocele)

Ans. This 3-month-old male infant presented with a swelling in lumbosacral region since birth. The swelling further increases during crying. The child moves all the four limbs normally.

On examination: There is a swelling in midline over the lumbosacral region, which is soft, cystic in consistency, fluctuation is positive, brilliantly transilluminant, swelling is compressible. the overlying skin is adherent to the swelling. The underlying bony defect is felt at the margin of the swelling. There is no neurological deficit.

Q. What is your diagnosis?

Ans. This is a case of lumbosacral meningocele.

Q. Why do you say it is lumbosacral meningocele?

Ans. The swelling is situated in the lumbosacral vertebral level.

The swelling is situated below the transcristal line (level L4) and extends up to the body of sacrum. So, this is a lumbosacral meningocele.

Q. Why do you want to exclude hydrocephalus in this patient?

Ans. Hydrocephalus may be associated with 80–85% cases of meningocele. If hydrocephalus is present, it needs treatment before excision of meningocele.

Q. Is it common to have neurodeficit in patients with meningocele?

Ans. No. Neurodeficit is more common in patients with meningomyelocele.

Q. What investigations would you like to do in this patient?

Ans. I will do a computed tomography (CT) scan of brain to exclude associated hydrocephalus. If necessary, magnetic resonance imaging (MRI) of the lumbosacral region and the craniovertebral junction area can be done. Magnetic resonance imaging of local area is necessary for:
* Clear delineation of the swelling
* Relation of the swelling to the neural structures
* Position of the lower end of the conus medullaris and presence of any cord tethering.

Magnetic resonance imaging of the craniovertebral junction is necessary for exclusion of associated Arnold-Chiari malformation.

Q. How will you treat this patient?

* Base line integration
* I will proceed for operative repair of the meningocele.

Q. When will you operate?

Ans. The operation has to be done as early as possible to avoid complications. An informed consent should be taken before operation. If there is associated neurodeficit, the neurodeficit may not recover following operation.

Q. What are the risks of anesthesia in this age group of patients?

Ans. Hypothermia and hypoglycemia are two important risk factors in this age group of patients.

Q. What operation will you do?

Ans.
+ Excision of meningocele and repair of the defect
+ The operation is done under general anesthesia
+ The skin flaps are raised. The meningocele sac is dissected and excised. The dural covering is repaired. The erector spinae muscle is apposed over the bony gap. The skin margins are then apposed if necessary by a lateral release incision.

Q. What are the postoperative complications?

Ans.
+ Wound infection
+ Wound dehiscence
+ Cerebrospinal fluid (CSF) leakage
+ Meningitis.

Q. What will you do if there is associated hydrocephalus?

Ans. Excision of meningocele will aggravate the hydrocephalus. So a ventriculoperitoneal shunt is to be done before undertaking the repair of meningocele. Ventriculoperitoneal shunt and excision of the meningocele can be done in the same sitting.

Q. How will you treat associated Arnold-Chiari malformation?

Ans. Arnold-Chiari malformation is to be treated before excision of meningocele.

Treatment of Arnold-Chiari malformation is by decompression of foramen magnum along with durotomy and duroplasty.

Q. What is meningocele?

Ans. This is a condition of protrusion of meninges through a bony gap in the vertebral canal or the cranium producing a cystic swelling containing cerebrospinal fluid.

Q. What are the coverings of meningocele?

Ans. The meningocele is covered by pia mater and the arachnoid mater. The dura mater extends up to the margin of the defect. The overlying skin is intact but there may be surface ulceration.

Q. What are the common sites of meningocele?

Ans. The common sites of meningocele are:
+ Lumbosacral region
+ Root of nose
+ Occipital region.

Q. What are the complications of meningocele?

Ans.
+ Ulceration
+ Infection

◆ Rupture
◆ May be associated with hydrocephalus and Arnold-Chiari malformation.

Q. How does meningocele develop?

Ans. This is a variety of neural tube defect. Meningocele develops due to failure of closure of the neural tube. This is most commonly found in the proximal region (occipital meningocele) or may occur in distal part (lumbosacral meningocele).

◼ MENINGOMYELOCELE

Q. What is your case? (Summary of a case of meningomyelocele)

Ans. This 2-month-old male infant presented with a swelling in lumbosacral region since birth which is gradually increasing in size. The swelling gets aggravated when the child strains during coughing or crying. There is an ulcer over the swelling for last 1 month and there is some serous discharge from the ulcer. The child could not move both lower limbs properly and the child is incontinent of stool and urine (Fig. 10.10).

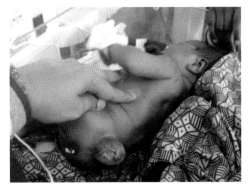

On examination: There is soft cystic swelling in the midline over the lumbosacral region, fluctuation is positive, transillumination is positive and during transillumination fine bands are seen within the swelling, the swelling is partially compressible.

Fig. 10.10: Lumbosacral meningomyelocele
Courtesy: Dr Kalyani Saha basu, NRS Medical College, Kolkata

Both the lower limbs are flaccid and sensation of lower limbs appears to be less than the upper limbs and there is bilateral club foot. A bony gap can be felt at the margin of the swelling.

Q. What is your diagnosis?

Ans. This is a case of lumbosacral meningomyelocele with neurodeficit in both lower limbs.

Q. What is meningomyelocele?

Ans. This is a congenital condition where there is protrusion of spinal membranes along with spinal cord or nerves of cauda equina through a gap in the neural arch.

Q. What investigations you will suggest in this patient?

◆ Computed tomography scan of brain. To exclude associated hydrocephalus.
◆ Magnetic resonance imaging (MRI) of cranioVertebral junction and the lumbosacral region.

Q. How will you treat this patient of meningomyelocele?

Ans.
◆ I will prepare the patient for early operation.
◆ The operation may be performed under general/local anesthesia.
◆ The sac is opened and the redundant membrane is excised.

- The nerves are separated from the membrane and replaced within the spinal canal.
- The cut margins of the membrane are sutured over the cord.
- The erector spinae muscles with the overlying fascia are closed over the defect. To reduce tension on the suture line, lateral release incision may be made.
- The skin is sutured. If there tension during skin closure, the skin defect may be closed by a rotation flap.

Q. If CT scan shows hydrocephalus what will you do?

Ans. If there is hydrocephalus in CT scan then a ventriculoperitoneal shunt is required before excision and closure of meningomyelocele otherwise the hydrocephalus will aggravate.

Q. How will you follow-up these patients?

Ans. Regular follow-up to assess development of milestones.

Q. What is syringomyelocele?

Ans. This is a congenital condition where there is protrusion of spinal cord along with dilatation of central canal of spinal cord. There is associated neurological deficit.

Q. What is myelocele?

Ans. This is a congenital condition where there is failure of development of the dorsal wall of the neural tube resulting in exposure of spinal cord and the central canal of the spinal cord is exposed on the dorsal body surface. This is associated with gross neurological deficit.

NERVE INJURIES

Clinical Examination

History

- Details of the history of injury
- Blunt or penetrating trauma (stab or gunshot wound or glass cut wound)
- Any history of fracture—site of fracture and details of treatment
- Enquire about weakness of the limbs
- Any history of loss of sensation
- Any history of pain along the distribution of the nerve involved (suggest causalgia).

Examination of the limb involved—Inspection/palpation

- Any obvious deformity—malunited fracture
- Any scar of previous injury
- Any obvious muscle wasting
- Any skin changes
- Test for individual nerves—
  - Motor—tone and muscle power
  - Sensory—Test for sensation—crude touch, fine touch, pain sensation and joint and vibration sense.
  - Test for reflexes.

∎ RADIAL NERVE INJURY

Q. What is your case? (Summary of a case of radial nerve injury)

Ans. This 35-year-old gentleman sustained an injury in his right arm with fracture of the shaft of the right humerus following a road traffic accident 1 month back. He was treated with plastering for his fracture shaft. Following the accident and immobilization with plastering patient noticed that he has wrist drop on right side and is unable to extend his wrist. He also has difficulty in extending his joints of fingers (Fig. 10.11).

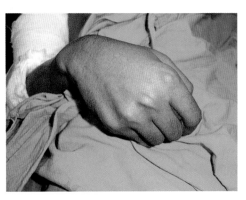

Fig. 10.11: Wristdrop in patient with right-sided radial nerve injury

Courtesy: Prof SS Chatterjee, IPGME and R, Kolkata

On Examination

On inspection:
* There is wrist drop with flexion of wrist and metacarpophalangeal joints of the hand.
* There is wasting of muscles on the extensor surface of the forearm.
* No apparent skin changes.
* There is plaster in his right upper arm.

On palpation:
* Patient cannot extend the wrist.
* Patient cannot extend the thumb.
* No extension is possible at the metacarpophalangeal joints of the fingers.
* There is paralysis of brachioradialis muscle on the right side
* Patient cannot supinate the forearm.
* The triceps power is normal and patient can flex and extend the elbow normally.
* There is loss of sensation over the anatomical snuff box and on the dorsal aspect of first web space.
* The passive movements of the wrist joint and the metacarpophalangeal joints are normal.

Q. How do you grade the muscle power?

Ans. The muscle power can be assessed by clinical examination:
* Grade 0: Complete paralysis, no contraction of muscle
* Grade 1: Only flicker of contraction
* Grade 2: Contraction of the muscle and joint movement possible only when gravity is eliminated
* Grade 3: Contraction of the muscle and movement of joint against gravity possible
* Grade 4: Contraction of the muscle and movement of joint against gravity and some resistance
* Grade 5: Strong movement but not normal
* Grade 6: Contraction of the muscle and movement of joint against powerful resistance— normal power.

Q. What is Medical Research Council (MRC) classification for sensory nerve dysfunction?

Ans.

◆ S0: No sensation
◆ S1: Deep pain sensation
◆ S2: Skin pain, touch and temperature sensation
◆ S3: S2 with accurate localization but deficient stereognosis
◆ S3+: Object and texture recognition but not normal. Two point discrimination good but not normal.
◆ S4: Normal sensation.

Q. What is your diagnosis?

Ans. This is a case of right-sided radial-nerve injury at the arm due to fracture of the shaft of humerus.

Q. How do you test for triceps muscle?

Ans. Patient is asked to extend his elbow. If the patient can extend his elbow then ask him to extend his elbow against resistance. If patient can do this then triceps power is normal (Figs 10.12A to C).

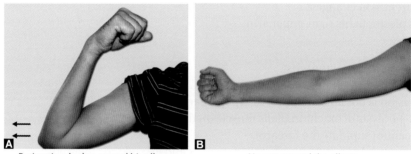

Patient is asked to extend his elbow   He can extend the elbow

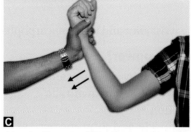

Patient is asked to extend his elbow against resistance

Figs 10.12A to C: Test for triceps muscle

Q. Why triceps are not paralyzed in lesion of the radial nerve at the mid-shaft of humerus?

Ans. The branches of radial nerve supplying triceps arise high up near the axilla so the triceps are spared.

Q. How will you test for wrist extensors?

Ans. The forearm is steadied in prone position and the patient is asked to extend the wrist. If patient can extend the wrist then movement against gravity is possible (Figs 10.13A and B).

 If patient is unable to extend the wrist against gravity then the forearm is made mid-prone and patient is asked to extend his wrist with the gravity eliminated, and look, whether he can extend the wrist with the gravity eliminated or there is any flicker of contraction in the wrist extensors. If there is no flicker of contraction in the wrist extensors, then the wrist extensors are graded as grade 0 (Figs 10.13 C and D).

 If the patient can extend the wrist against gravity then apply resistance and ask him to extend the wrist and assess the muscle power of wrist extensor (Fig. 10.13E).

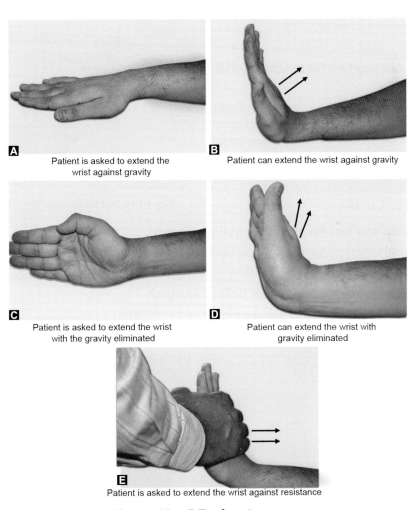

A   Patient is asked to extend the wrist against gravity

B   Patient can extend the wrist against gravity

C   Patient is asked to extend the wrist with the gravity eliminated

D   Patient can extend the wrist with gravity eliminated

E   Patient is asked to extend the wrist against resistance

Figs 10.13A to E: Test for wrist extensor

Q. How will you test for extension at the metacarpophalangeal joints?

Ans. With forearm in the prone position ask the patient to extend the metacarpophalangeal joints, and look, if he can move the joints.

If he can move the joints against gravity then apply resistance and ask him to extend the metacarpophalangeal joints against resistance and assess the muscle power (Fig. 10.14).

If he cannot extend against gravity, make the forearm mid-prone and ask him to extend the metacarpophalangeal joints with the gravity eliminated, and look, whether he can extend the joint with the gravity eliminated or there is any flicker of contraction in the extensor digitorum muscle and the muscle power is graded accordingly.

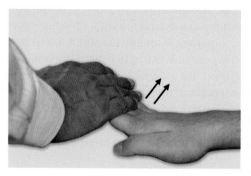

Fig. 10.14: Test for extension at the metacarpophalangeal joints (Extensor digitorum longus muscle)

Q. How would you test for brachioradialis muscle?

Ans. The brachioradialis muscle helps in flexion of the elbow when the elbow is in mid-prone position. Ask the patient to flex the elbow against resistance in mid-prone position, the contracted brachioradialis becomes prominent and if it is paralyzed, the contracted brachioradialis will not be palpable (Fig. 10.15).

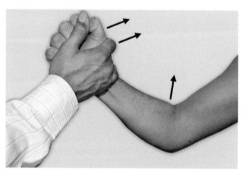

Fig. 10.15: Test for brachioradialis muscle

Q. How would you test for abductor pollicis longus?

Patient is asked to abduct the thumb. If he can abduct the thumb, ask the patient to maintain his thumb in abduction against the examiner's resistance (Fig. 10.16).

Q. How would you test for extensor pollicis longus?

Ans. Patient is asked to extend the thumb while the examiner attempts to flex it at the interphalangeal joint (Fig. 10.17).

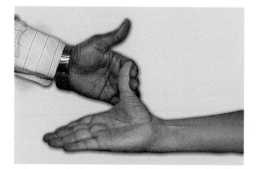

Fig. 10.16: Test for abductor pollicis longus

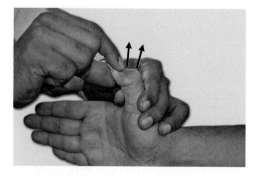

Fig. 10.17: Test for extensor pollicis longus

Q. How would you test for extensor pollicis brevis?

Ans. Patient is asked to extend the thumb while the examiner tries to flex the thumb at the metacarpophalangeal joint (Fig. 10.18).

Q. In radial nerve palsy, patient can extend the interphalangeal joints. How it is possible?

Ans. The interphalangeal joints are extended by the lumbrical muscles, which are supplied by the ulnar nerve. So, in radial nerve palsy, patient will be able to extend the interphalangeal joints.

Q. Where will you test for sensory supply of radial nerve?

Ans. In hand, the radial nerve supplies the area of anatomical snuff box on the dorsum. Radial nerve palsy will cause loss of sensation in this area (Fig. 10.19).

Q. How will you test for sensation?

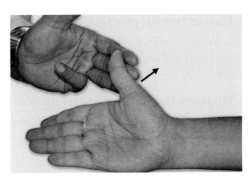

Fig. 10.18: Test for extensor pollicis brevis

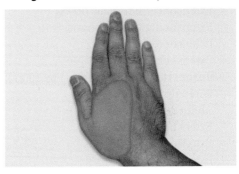

Fig. 10.19: Area of sensory loss in radial nerve injury

Ans. The different modalities of sensation which needs to be tested are—light or fine touch, deep or crude touch, pain sensation, temperature, vibration sense and position sense.

Q. How to test for light or fine touch?

Ans. Take a wisp of cotton wool. Ask the patient to close eyes. Touch the area of the limb with the cotton wool in a random manner and ask whether he can appreciate the sensation of cotton wool with his eyes closed. The area of sensory loss can thus be mapped out.

Q. How to test for deep or crude touch?

Ans. Press the area of the skin with a blunt object (blunt side of a pin) and ask whether patient can appreciate the object with his eyes closed.

Q. How to test for pain sensation?

Ans. This is assessed by pin prick. Ask the patient to close his eyes and press the area to be tested with the sharp end of the pin and assess whether he can appreciate the sharp prick of the pin.

Q. How will you test for temperature sensation?

Ans. Fill two test tubes—one with cold water and one with warm water. Touch the area of the skin to be tested alternately with the cold and the warm water filled test tube and assess whether patient can appreciate the difference in temperature of the two test tubes.

Q. How to test for vibration sense?

Ans. A vibrating tuning fork is placed over a bony prominence medial malleolus, subcutaneous surface of tibia and ask whether patient can appreciate the vibration of the tuning fork.

Q. How to test for position sense?

Ans. Ask the patient to close his eyes. Move the joint to be tested to extension (up) or flexion (down) and ask whether he can correctly say the position of the joint while in extension or flexion.

Q. What are the muscles in the back of the forearm?

Ans. The back of the forearm is the extensor compartment and the muscles include:

- Superficial muscles of the forearm (Fig. 10.20):
  - Anconeus
  - Brachioradialis
  - Extensor carpi radialis longus
  - Extensor carpi radialis brevis
  - Extensor digitorum longus
  - Extensor digiti minimi
  - Extensor carpi ulnaris.
- Deep muscles of the forearm (Fig. 10.21):
  - Supinator
  - Abductor pollicis longus
  - Extensor pollicis brevis
  - Extensor pollicis longus
  - Extensor indicis.

  All these muscles are supplied by the radial nerve.

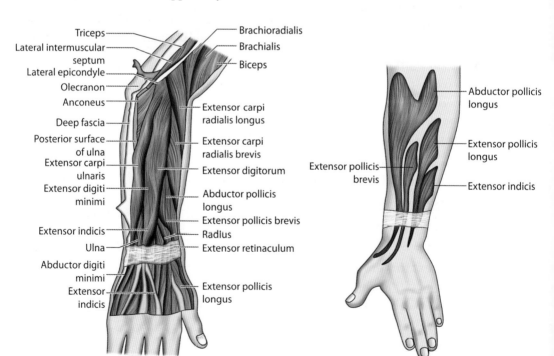

Fig. 10.20: Superficial extensor muscles of the forearm   **Fig. 10.21:** Deep extensor muscles of the forearm

Q. What is the distribution of the radial nerve?

* The radial nerve arises from the posterior cord of the brachial plexus (root value C5, C6, C7, C8 and T1)
* *In the arm:* Muscular branches to triceps, anconeus, lateral half of brachialis, brachioradialis and extensor carpi radialis longus
* Cutaneous branches to back of the arm and forearm
* *In the forearm:* Divides into posterior interosseous branch and superficial branch
  - Posterior interosseous nerve supplies all the extensor muscles in the back of the forearm.
  - Superficial branch supplies the skin over the lateral half of the dorsum of the forearm, over the anatomical snuff box and the first web pace.

Q. Which nerve roots form the brachial plexus?

Ans. The anterior primary rami of the cervical nerve roots C5, C6, C7, C8 and thoracic nerve root T1 contributes to the formation of brachial plexus (Fig. 10.22).

Q. What do you mean by a prefixed and a postfixed brachial plexus?

Ans. When the cervical nerve root C4 contributes to the formation of brachial plexus then it is known as a prefixed brachial plexus.

When the thoracic nerve root T2 contributes to the formation of brachial plexus then it is known as a postfixed brachial plexus.

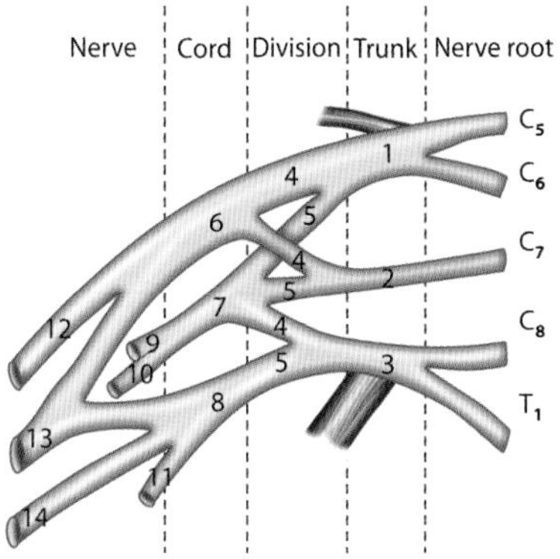

Fig. 10.22: Brachial plexus. 1. Upper trunk; 2. Middle trunk; 3. Lower trunk; 4. Anterior division; 5. Posterior division; 6. Lateral cord; 7. Posterior cord; 8. Medial cord; 9. Axillary nerve; 10. Radial nerve; 11. Medial cutaneous nerve; 12. Musculocutaneous nerve; 13. Median nerve; 14. Ulnar nerve

Q. How the trunks of brachial plexus are formed?

Ans. The nerve roots form three trunks of the brachial plexus—upper trunk, middle trunk and the lower trunk.
1. Upper trunk—formed by the C5 and C6 nerve roots
2. Middle trunk—formed by the C7 nerve root
3. Lower trunk—formed by the C8 and T1 nerve roots.

Q. How the cords of brachial plexus are formed?

Ans. Each trunk gives rise to an anterior and posterior division, and these divisions join to form the cords of brachial plexus.
* Lateral cord—formed by joining of the anterior division of upper and middle trunk
* Medial cord—formed by the anterior division of lower trunk
* Posterior cord—formed by joining of the posterior division of upper, middle and lower trunks.

Q. Which nerves arise from the medial cord?

Ans.
The medial cord gives rise to:
* Medial cutaneous nerve of the arm
* Ulnar nerve
* Medial cutaneous nerve of the forearm
* The medial root of the median nerve
* Medial pectoral nerve.

Q. Which nerves arise from the lateral cord?

Ans.

The lateral cord gives rise to:
* Musculocutaneous nerve
* Lateral root of the median nerve
* Lateral pectoral nerve.

Q. Which nerves arise from the posterior cord?

Ans.

The posterior cord gives rise to:
* Subscapular nerve
* Thoracodorsal nerve
* Radial nerve
* Axillary nerve.

Q. Which nerves arise from the roots of the brachial plexus?

* Dorsal scapular nerve arises from the C5 nerve root supplies the rhomboids muscle
* Long thoracic nerve arises from the C5, C6 and C7 nerve roots supplies the serratus anterior muscle.

Q. What are the root values of following important nerves?

Ans.
* Ulnar nerve—C8 and T1
* Median nerve—C5, C6, C7, C8 and T1
* Radial nerve—C5, C6, C7, C8 and T1
* Axillary nerve—C5 and C6.

Q. What is Saturday night palsy?

Ans. This is radial nerve palsy due to falling into deep sleep with the arm over the sharp back of a chair. This is due to prolonged compression of the nerve.

Q. How will you manage the patient presented?

Ans. This patient has complete paralysis of the muscles supplied by the radial nerve and there are no clinical signs of recovery. I would suggest:
* *Nerve conduction velocity (NCV)*: Recording of the sensory or motor nerve action potential and calculation of the conduction velocity for a given anatomical region to assess the degree of nerve injury and any evidence of recovery.
* *Electromyography (EMG)*: Recording of muscle action potential in response to voluntary activity. Denervation can be diagnosed and may also be differentiated from reinnervation.

Q. How will you repair the injured nerve?

Ans. I will consider exploration and repair of the injured nerve. The idea is to achieve a good coaptation of the nerve ends without tension. During operation, the nerve ends are exposed. There is some amount of fibrosis at the injured ends. The fibrous tissue is excised and the healthy margins of the proximal and distal ends of the nerves are exposed. If the freshened nerve ends can be opposed without tension then direct nerve suture is considered. The suturing should be done under microscope using 8-0 polypropylene sutures. Sutures are usually placed in the epineurium providing an epineurial repair of the severed nerve ends.

Q. If the nerve ends could not be opposed easily, what option remains?

Ans. It is not desirable to do nerve repair under tension. In such situation, nerve grafting should be done. An expendable nerve, like the sural nerve or medial cutaneous nerve of the forearm, may be used for nerve grafting. The nerve graft is usually cut up so that a number of strands can be used to build up a similar thickness to that of the nerve trunk, which is to be repaired.

Q. How will you take care in the postoperative period?

- Following nerve repair, the limb is to be splinted in a plaster cast for 3–4 weeks.
- Passive joint movements should be carried out to prevent joint stiffness.
- Afterwards gradual mobilization is allowed with active physiotherapy.

Q. How will you assess recovery following repair?

Patient should be evaluated clinically in respect of sensory or motor recovery.

Tinel's sign is a useful guide for recovery. On percussing over the nerve, patient has tingling sensation along the nerve. This usually proceeds from proximal to the distal end of the nerve usually at a rate of 1–2 mm/day.

Q. What is the structure of a peripheral nerve?

Ans. Nerve impulses are carried by axon. The neuron consists of a cell body, dendrites and axon.

The axons are surrounded by Schwann cells. A number of axons wrapped by a single Schwann cell along with endoneurial collagen fibers form the endoneurium.

A large number of nerve fibers grouped together in fascicles and surrounded by a connective tissue sheath form the perineurium.

A large number of nerve fascicles bound together by a connective tissue sheath is called epineurium.

Q. What are the different types of nerve injury?

Ans. Seddon classified nerve injuries into three types—neuropraxia, axonotmesis and neurotmesis.

Q. What is neuropraxia?

Ans. This is a transient nerve conduction block following a trauma. There is localized demyelination of the injured segment of the nerve. Wallerian degeneration does not occur in the distal segment. There is no discontinuity of the axons or the nerve itself.

Complete recovery occurs once the cause is removed usually in few days to several weeks.

Q. What is axonotmesis?

Ans. Axonotmesis denotes anatomical disruption of the axons and myelin sheaths. The supporting connective tissue sheaths endoneurium, perineurium and epineurium remains intact. Wallerian degeneration occurs in the distal segment of the injured nerve.

Recovery occurs by axon regeneration along the same endoneurial tube and results in good sensory and motor functional recovery.

Q. What is neurotmesis?

Ans. This is a more serious injury and there is complete severance of the nerve resulting in disruption of the axons and the connective tissue sheath. Wallerian degeneration occurs distal to the site of injury. Spontaneous recovery is impossible and appropriate surgical repair is required for recovery but complete recovery is unusual.

Q. What is Sunderland's classification for nerve injury?

Ans. Sunderland classified nerve injuries into five grades:
1. *First degree*: No anatomical disruption
2. *Second degree*: Axonotmesis—endoneurium, perineurium and epineurium intact
3. *Third degree*: Axonotmesis—perineurium and epineurium intact
4. *Fourth degree*: Neurotmesis—epineurium intact
5. *Fifth degree*: Complete disruption—no continuity at all.

Q. What changes occur in a peripheral nerve following an injury?

Ans. In neuropraxia, there is no appreciable change in the injured segment except localized demyelination of the injured segment.

In axonotmesis, there is Wallerian degeneration of the distal nerve segment. There is lysis of the axoplasm and fragmentation of the myelin sheath. The endoneurial tube with the Schwann cell sheath is left behind. The axons in the proximal segment of the nerve starts regenerating and find its way into the endoneurial tube of the distal nerve segment and subsequently make connections with the target organs.

In neurotmesis, Wallerian degeneration occurs in the distal segment of the injured nerve. However, in fifth degree injury, where the epineurial tube is disrupted and the regenerating axons do not find its way into the distal segment and spontaneous recovery is unlikely.

The regenerating axons grow at the rate of 1–2 mm/day.

Q. How will you manage nerve injury in a patient with open wound?

Ans. Early nerve repair provide the best chance of recovery. Once the patient is resuscitated well and general condition is satisfactory, surgical exploration of the nerve is advisable. If surgeon is experienced, an appropriate nerve repair is done. If the wound is very contaminated then primary nerve repair may not be appropriate.

If primary nerve repair is not done, the nerve ends are tied with a nonabsorbable suture and kept opposed to each other or the nerve end may be sutured to the local soft tissues to prevent retraction of the ends and easy identification during re-exploration.

Q. How will you manage nerve injuries due to blunt trauma?

Ans. Neuropraxia and axonotmesis usually recovers spontaneously. So a period of observation is required in such cases. Careful follow-up is essential. If there is no evidence of recovery after 2–3 months nerve conduction velocity and electromyography study is done. If there is no evidence of recovery then a surgical exploration is indicated. If there is evidence of recovery in 2–3 months then nonoperative management can continue. If the wound is explored for a skeletal or vascular injury then the nerve should also be explored.

Q. Which factors determine recovery following nerve repair?

Ans.

- *Age:* Children recover better than the adults.
- *Type of injury:* A clean cut injury has the best prognosis in terms of recovery of function. High velocity missile injuries or severe traction injuries has worst prognosis.
- *The level of injury:* The prognosis is worse in proximal lesion than in distal lesion.
- *The type of nerve:* Recovery is better in pure motor or sensory nerves than in a mixed nerve.
- *Associated injuries:* Associated vascular and skeletal injuries are associated with a worse prognosis than isolated nerve injuries.
- *Timing of repair:* Early repair of nerve within few days of injury is associated with good recovery than repaired after 2–3 months.

Q. What is causalgia?

Ans. This is a type of neuralgic pain associated with a major nerve injury which often may be partial. The pain is intense and burning in character. The pain, however, improves with recovery of nerve function.

Sympathectomy may be helpful in intractable cases of causalgia.

Q. What is Tinel's sign?

Ans. Percussion over the site of a nerve injury or nerve repair elicits a tingling or electric shock like sensation along the distribution of that nerve. An advancing Tinel's sign after nerve repair implies successful nerve regeneration toward the target organ. Although, sensory in nature, Tinel's sign is also found in regenerating motor nerves due to presence of proprioceptive afferent fibers within all motor nerves.

▮ ULNAR NERVE INJURY

Q. What is your case? (Summary of a case of ulnar nerve palsy)

Ans. This 30-year-old male patient sustained an injury in his right elbow region 6 months back following a fall for which his right forearm and the elbow joint was immobilized for 8 weeks. Following removal of plaster, patient noticed that he is unable to move his little finger and ring finger properly, and there is bending of these two fingers (Fig. 10.23).

On examination: There is wasting of muscles in the hypothenar eminence and interossei along with claw hand deformity involving the little finger and ring finger. There is paralysis of interossei muscles and adductor pollicis muscle. There is loss of sensation in the palmar aspect of the little finger and medial half of the ring finger.

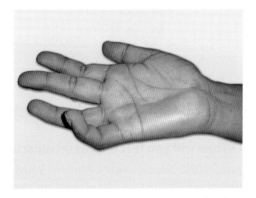

Fig. 10.23: Ulnar nerve injury—Note the claw hand involving the little and ring fingers
Courtesy: Prof SS Chatterjee, IPGME and R, Kolkata

Q. What is your diagnosis?

Ans. This is a case of ulnar nerve injury at the elbow region due to supracondylar fracture.

Q. Which muscles are supplied by the ulnar nerve?

Ans.

In the forearm:

* Flexor carpi ulnaris and the medial half of flexor digitorum profundus

In the hand:

* *Hypothenar muscles*: Flexor digiti minimi, abductor digiti minimi and opponens digiti minimi.
* *Interossei muscles*: Supplies all palmar and dorsal interossei
* *Thenar muscle*: Both head of adductor pollicis and deep head of flexor pollicis brevis.

Q. What are the sensory supplies of the ulnar nerve?

Ans. Sensory supplies the hypothenar area, medial aspect of the palm and palmar surface of the little finger and medial half of the ring finger. It also supplies articular branches to the elbow and wrist (Figs 10.24A and B).

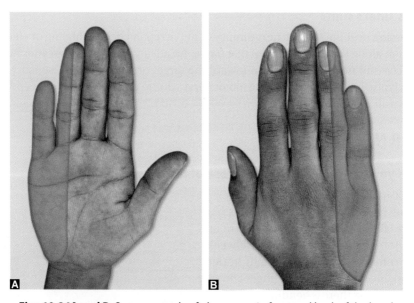

Figs 10.24A and B: Sensory supply of ulnar nerve in front and back of the hand

Q. How will you test interossei muscles?

Ans. Palmar interossei are adductors and dorsal interossei are abductors, along with lumbricals they also help in extension of proximal and distal interphalangeal joints.

* *Test for dorsal interossei:* Ask the patient to spread out his fingers. In paralysis of the dorsal interossei, patient cannot spread out his fingers (Figs 10.25Aand B). Ask the patient to spread out the fingers (abduct) against resistance (Fig. 10.25C).

♦ *Test for palmar interossei:* Card test—place a card in between the fingers and ask the patient to grip while trying to remove this card. In paralysis of the palmar interossei, patient will not be able to grip the card firmly (Figs 10.26A and B). Patient can hold the card firmly if palmar interossei are normal.

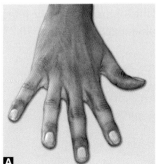

A Patient is ask to spread out the fingers

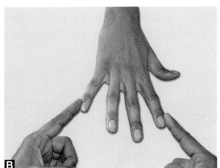

B Patient is asked to spread out the fingers against resistance

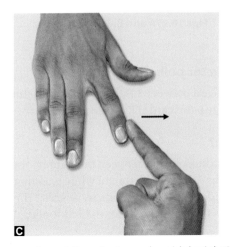

C Test for first dorsal interosseous muscle—ask the patient spread out (abduct) the index finger against resistance

Figs 10.25A to C: Test for dorsal interossei

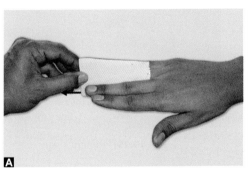

A

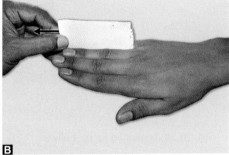

B

Figs 10.26A and B: Test for palmar interossei

Q. How will you test for the lumbricals?

Ans. Ask the patient to extend the interphalangeal joint keeping the metacarpophalangeal joint in flexed position (Fig. 10.27A).

Steady the patient's proximal phalanx and ask him to extend the proximal and distal interphalangeal joints against resistance. In paralysis of the lumbricals and the interossei, patient will be unable to extend the proximal and distal interphalangeal joints (Fig. 10.27B).

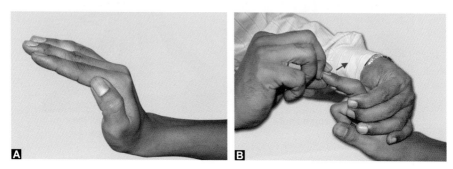

Figs 10.27A and B: Test for lumbricals

Q. How will you test adductor pollicis?

Ans. Ask the patient to grip a card between his thumb and the palm. In paralysis of the adductor pollicis, patient is unable to grip the card (Fig. 10.28).

Q. What is Froment's sign?

Ans. Ask the patient to grasp a book firmly between the thumbs and other fingers of both hands. In normal person, the thumbs will remain straight while grasping the book. In paralysis of the first palmar interosseous and the adductor pollicis, to grasp the book the terminal phalanx of the affected thumb will be flexed by the flexor pollicis longus. This is called Froment's sign (Fig. 10.29).

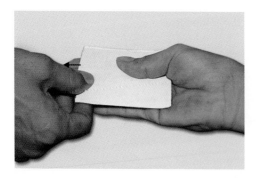

Fig. 10.28: Test for adductor pollicis

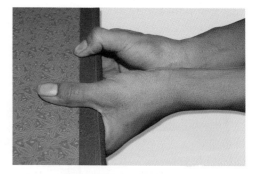

Fig. 10.29: Froment's sign

Q. How will you test for flexor carpi ulnaris?

Ans. Patient is asked to flex the wrist against resistance. In paralysis of flexor carpi ulnaris, the wrist will deviate toward the radial side.

Q. What are the common sites of ulnar nerve injury?

Ans.
+ Ulnar nerve is commonly injured at the elbow where it passes behind the medial epicondyle.
+ The nerve may also be injured at the wrist where it lies superficial to the flexor retinaculum.

Q. What are the characteristics of ulnar claw hand?

Ans. Hyperextension at the metacarpophalangeal joints, and flexion of the interphalangeal joints of the little and ring fingers. The intermetacarpal spaces are hollowed out due to wasting of interosseous muscles. Claw hand deformity is more obvious in wrist lesion as the profundus muscle is spared and there is marked flexion of the interphalangeal joints.

Q. Which lesions may cause claw hand?

Ans. Clawing of the hand may be caused by lesion of the ulnar nerve, Klumpke's paralysis, a combined lesion of ulnar and median nerves.

■ MEDIAN NERVE INJURY

Q. What are the motor supplies of median nerve?

Ans.
+ *In the forearm:* Pronator teres, flexor carpi radialis, palmaris longus, flexor digitorum superficialis, flexor pollicis longus, lateral half of flexor digitorum profundus and pronator quadratus.
+ *In the hand:* Abductor pollicis brevis, flexor pollicis brevis, opponens pollicis and the first and second lumbricals.

Q. What are the sensory supplies of median nerve?

Ans. It supplies the lateral half of palm and palmar, and dorsal aspect of the lateral three and half fingers (Fig. 10.30).

Q. What are the muscles in the flexor compartment of forearm?

Ans.
+ *Superficial muscles:* Pronator teres, flexor carpi radialis, palmaris longus, flexor carpi ulnaris.
+ *Intermediate muscles:* Flexor digitorum superficialis.
+ *Deep muscles:* Flexor digitorum profundus, flexor pollicis longus and pronator quadratus (Fig. 10.31).

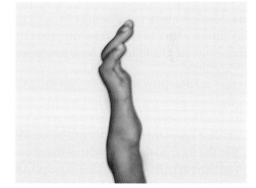

Fig. 10.30: Combined median and ulnar nerve injury
Courtesy: Prof SS Chatterjee, IPGME and R, Kolkata

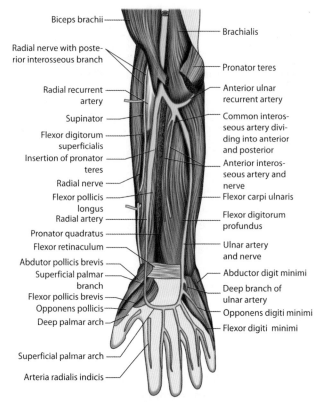

Fig. 10.31: Muscles in the flexor compartment of the forearm

Q. How will you test for median nerve palsy?

Ans. Median nerve palsy results in both motor and sensory loss in the areas supplied by the median nerve. The following tests are important for diagnosis:

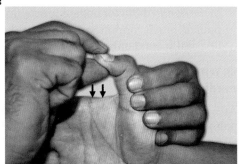

Fig. 10.32: Test for flexor pollicis longus

* *Test for flexor pollicis longus*: Steady the proximal phalanx of the thumb and ask him to flex the interphalangeal joint of the thumb against resistance. Patient will be unable to flex the interphalangeal joint of the thumb in median nerve lesion, resulting in palsy of flexor pollicis longus (Fig. 10.32).
* *Test for abductor pollicis brevis*: Patient is asked to keep the hand on a table with palm facing up. He is asked to move his thumb forward at right angle to the plane of the palm. He is asked to touch a pen held in front. Failure to do so indicates paralysis of abductor pollicis brevis (Fig. 10.33A). Alternatively patient is asked to abduct the thumb against resistance (Fig. 10.33B).
* *Test for opponens pollicis*: Patient is asked to touch the tip of other finger by the thumb. Paralysis of opponens pollicis results in failure of this opponent movement (Fig. 10.34A). Alternatively patient is asked to touch the tip of other fingers against resistance (Fig. 10.34B).

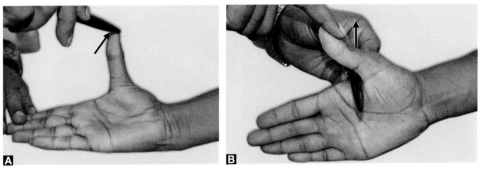

Figs 10.33A and B: Test for abductor pollicis brevis

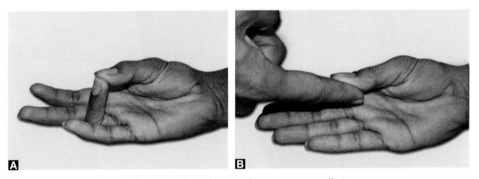

Figs 10.34A and B: Test for opponens pollicis

- *Test for flexor digitorum profundus (lateral half):* Steady the metacarpophalangeal joint and the proximal interphalangeal joint of the index finger and ask the patient to flex the distal interphalangeal joint. Failure of flexion of the distal interphalangeal indicates paralysis of flexor digitorum profundus (Fig. 10.35A). Alternatively, steady the metacarpophalangeal joint and the proximal interphalangeal joint of the index finger and ask the patient to flex the distal interphalangeal joint against resistance. Failure of flexion of distal interphalangeal joint is due to paralysis of the lateral half of flexor digitorum profundus (Fig. 10.35B)
- This is also tested by Ochsner's clasping test.
- *Ochsner's clasping test:* Patient is asked to clasp both the hands, all the fingers are flexed. Due to paralysis of the flexor digitorum profundus (lateral half) the index finger of the paralyzed side fails to flex and remains pointing (Fig. 10.36).
- *Test for flexor digitorum superficialis:* Patient is asked to flex the finger at the proximal interphalangeal joint against resistance with the examiners finger placed on the middle phalanx (Fig. 10.37).
- *Test for wrist flexors:* All the flexors of the wrist are supplied by the median nerve except flexor carpi ulnaris, which is supplied by the ulnar nerve. In median nerve palsy, there will be weakness of the wrist flexors. Patient is asked to flex the wrist against resistance or as such, and the wrist flexor power may be graded (Figs 10.38A and B).
- *Test for pronator teres:* In median nerve palsy, the forearm is kept supine by the unopposed action of supinator. The patient is asked to pronate the forearm. Failure of pronation implies paralysis of pronator teres (Figs 10.39A to C).

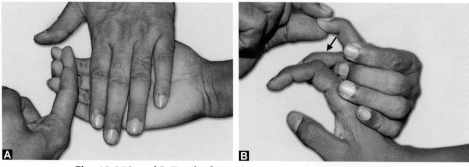

Figs 10.35A and B: Test for flexor digitorum profundus (lateral half)

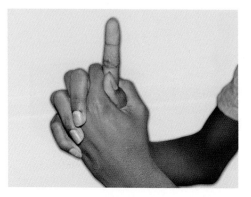

Fig. 10.36: Ochsner's clasping test

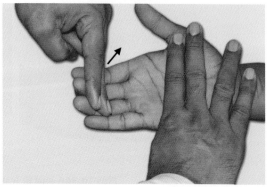

Fig. 10.37: Test for flexor digitorum superficialis

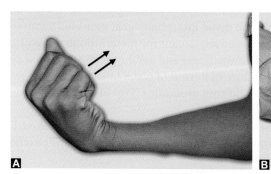

Figs 10.38A and B: Test for wrist flexors

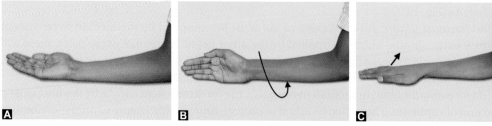

Figs 10.39A to C: Test for pronator teres

Q. What is the area of sensory supply of median nerve?

Ans. The median nerve supplies both the palmar and dorsal aspect of radial three and half fingers (Figs 10.40A and B).

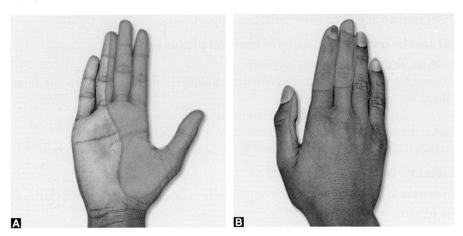

Figs 10.40A and B: Sensory supply of median nerve

Q. What are hypothenar muscles?

Ans. Four hypothenar muscles are:
1. Palmaris brevis
2. Abductor digiti minimi
3. Flexor digiti minimi
4. Opponens digiti minimi.
    All hypothenar muscles are supplied by the ulnar nerve.

Q. What are thenar muscles?

Ans.
* Abductor pollicis brevis
* Flexor pollicis brevis
* Opponens pollicis
* Adductor pollicis.
    All the thenar muscles are supplied by the median nerve except the adductor pollicis, which is supplied by the ulnar nerve.

Q. What are the causes of combined median and ulnar nerve palsy?

Ans. Supracondylar fracture, penetrating or missile injury in the elbow region may cause combined ulnar and median nerve palsy.

Q. What are the effects of combined ulnar and median nerve palsy?

Ans.
* *Classical claw hand deformity:* In this deformity, there is hyperextension of metacarpophalangeal joints due to unopposed action of the extensor digitorum, which

extends the proximal phalanx. The interphalangeal joints are flexed due paralysis of the lumbricals and the interossei.

* There is wasting of the flexors muscles of the forearm and both hypothenar, thenar and interossei muscles.
* Tests for median and ulnar nerve palsy (see above).

Q. What are the important causes of brachial plexus lesion?

Ans. Brachial plexus lesion may be caused by:

* Traction injury due to violent displacement of shoulder girdle and cervical spine. Road traffic accidents and obstetric injuries.
* Penetrating injuries in the neck by stab or missile wounds.
* Operative injury during lymph node dissection in the neck.
* Local infiltration by malignant tumors, e.g. carcinoma lung—Pancoast's tumor.

Q. What is Erb-Duchenne paralysis?

Ans. This is due to traction injury of the upper trunk of brachial plexus, which carries fibers of C5 and C6 roots.

This results in paralysis of deltoid, biceps, brachialis and brachioradialis and partly supinator and supraspinatus and infraspinatus.

Deformity:

* The arms hang by the side.
* There is failure of abduction and lateral rotation of the shoulder and the shoulder remains adducted and medially rotated.
* There is failure of flexion of the elbow joint and failure of supination of the forearm.
* The forearm remains extended and pronated.
* This typical appearance is called "policeman's tip hand".
* There is loss of sensation over a small area over the deltoid.

Q. What is Klumpke's paralysis?

Ans. This is also a traction injury due to hyperabduction of the arm. This may happen when a person catches something while falling from a height or due to birth injury. The lower trunks of the brachial plexus, carrying fibers from C8 and T1, are paralyzed.

This results in paralysis of the intrinsic muscles of the hand (supplied by T1 root), and paralysis of the ulnar flexors of the wrist and fingers.

Deformity:

* This results in claw hand with hyperextension of the metacarpophalangeal joints (due to unopposed action of the long extensor muscles, and flexion of the interphalangeal joints (due to unopposed action of the long flexors).
* There is also loss of sensation along the ulnar border of forearm and hand.

Q. What is the effect of complete brachial plexus injury?

Ans. There is complete paralysis of the whole upper limb. The upper limb is flaccid and hangs by the side and loss of all the movements and wasting of all the muscle groups and complete loss of sensation in the whole of upper limb.

Q. What is Horner's syndrome?

Ans. This is due to paralysis of cervical sympathetic, the fibers of which are derived from the T1 segment.

This results in:

◆ Enophthalmos
◆ Miosis
◆ Pseudoptosis
◆ Anhidrosis on the affected side of the face
◆ Loss of ciliospinal reflex.

Q. How will you manage traction injury of brachial plexus?

Ans. In severe traction injury, early surgery is indicated. Nerve grafting may be required in some cases.

Q. What is the effect of common peroneal nerve injury at the knee region?

◆ Patient will develop foot drop.
◆ There is paralysis of the dorsiflexor of the ankle. Patient is unable to dorsiflex the ankle.
◆ There is paralysis of the evertors of the foot. There is failure of eversion of the foot.
◆ There is sensory loss on the dorsum of the foot and toes.

Q. What is the effect of sciatic nerve palsy?

Ans. Motor deficit:

◆ Flexors of the knee are paralyzed. Some amount of flexion will be possible by the gracilis and sartorius.

Complete paralysis below the knee:

◆ Paralysis of both plantar flexor and dorsiflexors of the ankle. Foot drop due to gravity
◆ Paralysis of both the evertors and inverters of foot
◆ Paralysis of all flexors and extensors of the toes
◆ Paralysis of all intrinsic muscles of foot.

Sensory deficits:

◆ Complete loss of sensation below the knee, except the area on the medial aspect of the foot supplied by the saphenous nerve.

Neck Swellings

■ CYSTIC HYGROMA

Clinical Examination

See Page No. 382, Chapter 9.

History

* History about the swelling
* Onset (present since birth or appeared later)
* Progress of the swelling
* *Any associated complains*: Difficulty in neck movement, difficulty in swallowing, or difficulty in breathing
* Pain
* Any other swelling in the body.

Examination—Inspection/Palpation

* Site (commonly found in posterior triangle of neck) and extent
* Size and shape
* Surface (usually lobulated)
* Margins (usually well-defined rounded margins)/skin over the swelling
* Temperature over the swelling (usually normal)
* Tenderness (usually nontender)
* Consistency (soft in feel)
* Fluctuation (positive)
* Transillumination (brilliantly transilluminant)
* Test the relation of the swelling with adjacent muscle
* In neck test the relation with the sternocleidomastoid muscle. Ask the patient to look to opposite side and assess the relation of the swelling with the contracted muscle
* Test the relation of the swelling with the trapezius. Ask the patient to shrug the shoulder up against resistance and assess the relation of the swelling with the contracted muscle. If the swelling becomes less prominent after contracting the muscle—the swelling lies deep to the muscle
* *Examination of the regional lymph nodes*—usually the lymph nodes are not enlarged.

Q. What is your case? (Summary of a case of cystic hygroma)

Ans. This 10-month-old female child presented with a swelling on the right side of the neck since birth. The swelling is gradually increasing in size. There is no other complain.

On examination: There is a soft cystic swelling on the right side of the neck occupying the whole of the right side of the neck. Extending beyond the midline to the left side of the neck. The swelling is soft cystic in feel, nontender. The swelling is partially compressible. Fluctuation is positive and the swelling is brilliantly transilluminant. The swelling is passing deep to the sternocleidomastoid muscle. The swelling is free from the skin and the underlying structures (Fig. 11.1).

Q. What is your diagnosis?

Ans. This is a case of cystic hygroma on the right side of the neck.

Q. What are the other possibilities?

Ans.

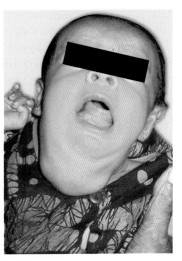

Fig. 11.1: Cystic hygroma in the right side of the neck

Courtesy: Dr Kalyani Saha Basu, NRS Medical College, Kolkata

* Branchial cyst
* Cold abscess in the neck
* Solitary lymphatic cyst.

Q. What are the other sites where cystic hygroma may be found?

Ans.

* Cheek
* Tongue
* Axilla
* Groin
* Mediastinum.

Q. What are the fates of cystic hygroma?

Ans. The cyst may:

* Expand rapidly and may cause respiratory obstruction
* Become infected and painful
* Undergo spontaneous resolution.

Q. How will you treat this patient?

Ans.

* I would like to do a chest X-ray to exclude any mediastinal cystic hygroma
* Blood for hemoglobin (Hb)%, total leukocyte count (TLC), and differential leukocyte count (DLC)
* Routine urine examination
* I would plan for complete excision of the cyst

◆ The main cyst usually has finger-like projection. All the finger projections are dissected carefully and removed.

Q. Do you like to give sclerosant injection?

Ans. Earlier sclerosants were used with the idea of reducing the size of the cyst. Hot water or hypertonic saline were used.

But sclerosants may destroy the normal tissue plane making the curative surgery difficult. So, sclerosants are not used routinely now.

Injection of sclerosant agents like bleomycin or OK-432 (a derivative of *Streptococcus pyogenes*) have been reported to cause regression of cystic hygromas.

Q. What are the indications for aspiration of the cyst?

Ans. Aspiration of the cyst does not provide cure. If the cyst increases in size rapidly so as to cause respiratory obstruction it may be aspirated to relieve the respiratory obstruction.

Q. As there is chance of spontaneous resolution do you like to wait?

Ans. If patient has no symptom due to compression, patient may be observed for about 2 years to see any spontaneous regression.

Q. What is a cystic hygroma?

Ans. Cystic hygroma is a congenital malformation of lymphatic channel that arise from the congenital lymphatic sacs, and clinically, appear as a soft fluctuant brilliantly transilluminant swelling commonly in the neck.

Q. What are the clinical characteristics of cystic hygroma?

Ans.
◆ May manifest in the neonate or early infancy
◆ Commonly found in the posterior triangle of the neck
◆ Swelling is soft, fluctuant, and brilliantly transilluminant
◆ May be slightly compressible and may increase in size slightly during straining.

Q. What are the pathological characteristics of the cyst?

Ans.
◆ Cystic hygroma consists of multiple cysts—larger ones situated towards the periphery and smaller ones towards the center
◆ These multiple cysts intercommunicate with each other
◆ The cysts contain clear or straw-colored fluid containing cholesterol crystals
◆ The cysts are lined by a single layer of columnar epithelium and covered externally by a rim of lymphoid tissue.

Q. How do lymphatic channels develop?

Ans. At 6th week of intrauterine life, three pairs of lymphatic sacs appear in the developing embryo, which develops into adult lymphatic channels:
◆ One pair of lymphatic sacs in the neck develops from the mesoblast situated at the junction of jugular and subclavian veins. These are called jugular lymphatic sacs
◆ One pair of lymphatic channel in the retroperitoneum develops into the thoracic duct
◆ One pair in the inguinal region—posterior lymphatic sacs.

Q. How does cystic hygroma develop?

Ans. During development there may be sequestration of a portion of jugular lymph sacs and some lymphatic channels from the main lymphatic system. The lining of epithelium secretes fluid. The sequestrated lymphatic channels filled with this secretion forms the cystic hygroma.

Q. What are the complications of cystic hygroma?

Ans.
* *Mechanical*: Because of huge size it may compress the trachea and cause respiratory obstruction or may cause dysphagia
* Cystic hygroma in the mediastinum may cause superior mediastinal syndrome
* Large cystic hygroma at birth may cause obstructed labor
* Infection.

Q. What may be good effect of infection?

Ans. Spontaneous recovery may occur following infection. Inflammation may lead to fibrosis and spontaneous regression of the swelling.

Q. Which other cyst fluid contains cholesterol?

Ans.
* Branchial cyst
* Dental cyst
* Hydrocele fluid
* Thyroglossal cyst
* Dentigerous cyst
* Cystic hygroma.

■ RANULA

Clinical Examination

See Page No. 382, Chapter 9.

History
* Details about the swelling
* Any fluctuation in size (some ranula may show spontaneous regression and reappears subsequently)
* Any pain (some ranula may be painful)
* Any associated swelling in the neck (in plunging ranula the swelling may project into the neck).

Examination—Inspection/Palpation
* Site and extent (usually lies in the floor of the mouth on one side of the midline)
* Color (usually semitransparent and bluish in appearance)
* Shape and size
* Surface (usually smooth) and margin

♦ Fluctuation (positive)
♦ In plunging ranula cross fluctuation will be positive
♦ Transillumination (usually transilluminant)
♦ Compressibility (usually noncompressible swelling).

Q. What is your case? (Summary of a case of ranula)

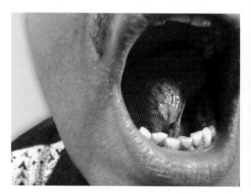

Ans. This 30-year-old gentleman presented with a swelling in the floor of the mouth on the right side for last 3 years. The swelling was about 2 cm in size at the onset and is slowly increasing in size to attain the present size. There is history of occasional diminution of the size of the swelling. No pain over the swelling, no swelling in the neck (Fig. 11.2).

On examination: There is a soft cystic swelling 4 cm × 3 cm on the right side of floor of the mouth between the under surface of the tongue and the inner surface of the mandible. The overlying mucous membrane is free and the swelling appears pale blue in color. Surface is smooth, nontender, fluctuation is present, and the swelling is transilluminant. Few dilated vessels are seen on the surface of the swelling.

Fig. 11.2: Ranula at the floor of the mouth on the right side

Courtesy: Dr Shyamal Kumar Halder, IPGMER, Kolkata

For plunging ranula: In addition to a swelling in the floor of the mouth another swelling is palpable on the same side of the neck in submandibular region. The swelling is also soft cystic in feel with positive fluctuation. Cross fluctuation is positive between the neck swelling and swelling in the floor of month (Figs 11.3A and B).

Q. What is your diagnosis?

Ans. This is a case of ranula on the floor of the mouth.

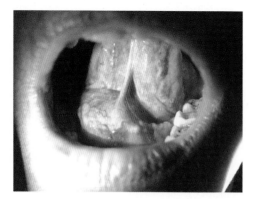

Fig. 11.3A: Plunging ranula in floor of the mouth
Courtesy: Dr Susnata De, IPGMER, Kolkata

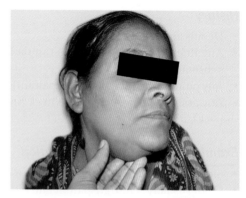

Fig. 11.3B: Plunging ranula—swelling in floor of the mouth and the right side of the neck
Courtesy: Dr Susnata De, IPGMER, Kolkata

If the ranula extend from the floor of the mouth to the neck then diagnosis should be plunging ranula.

Q. What is ranula?

Ans. Ranula is a mucous retention cyst arising from mucous glands in the floor of the mouth, arising from glands of Nuhn and Blandin. Ranula is also said to be extravasation cyst arising from a damaged sublingual gland situated in the floor of the mouth.

Q. Why it is called ranula?

Ans. The swelling resembles the belly of a frog (*Rana*), so it is called ranula.

Q. What is plunging ranula?

Ans. When the ranula extends to the neck into the submandibular region passing along the posterior border of mylohyoid then it is called plunging ranula. The cross fluctuation between the intraoral and the cervical swelling will be positive.

Q. What else this can be?

Ans.

+ *Sublingual dermoid:* Transillumination is negative.
+ *Hemangioma in the floor of the mouth:* Compressible, nontransilluminant swelling.
+ *Sublingual lymphangioma:* Like hemangioma it is compressible.

Q. How will you treat this patient?

Ans.

+ I will do baseline investigation and plan surgical treatment in this patient.
+ I will do complete excision of the swelling through intraoral route.

Q. If you cannot excise the swelling completely what will you do?

Ans. The swelling sometimes cannot be excised completely, as during dissection the cyst may be ruptured with extravasation of the cyst contents and then it is difficult to excise the remaining cyst wall. In such cases the alternative procedure is marsupialization. The cut edge of the cyst is sutured with the mucous membrane of the floor of the mouth. The bottom of the ranula becomes part of the floor of the mouth.

Q. How will you approach a plunging ranula?

Ans. The plunging ranula is excised through a cervical incision. The operation is done under general anesthesia. A transverse skin crease incision over the swelling is made and the skin flaps are raised. The deep fascia is incised. The cyst is dissected all around and the intraoral part of the swelling may also be dissected lateral to the mylohyoid muscle.

Q. What are the complications of ranula?

Ans.

+ Repeated rupture and reaccumulation of the cyst
+ Infection
+ A big ranula may cause functional difficulty during swallowing and speech.

■ THYROGLOSSAL CYST

Clinical Examination

See Page No. 381, Chapter 9.

History

* Detail history of swelling
* Any recent increase in size may indicate infection.

Examination—Inspection/Palpation

* Site (common site is usually in the midline between the level of thyroid isthmus and hyoid bone or just above the hyoid bone at the floor of the mouth, sometimes cyst may lie on one side of the midline) and extent
* Movement of swelling on swallowing
* Movement of swelling on protrusion of tongue
* Size and shape (usually globular)
* Surface (usually smooth) and margin
* Temperature and tenderness (usually nontender, presence of tenderness suggests infection in the cyst)
* Consistency (usually cystic, may feel tense cystic or sometimes may feel firm)
* Fluctuation (usually positive in very small swelling fluctuation cannot be demonstrated)
* Transillumination (majority are nontransilluminant, some cyst may contain clear fluid and may show positive transillumination)
* *Mobility*: Easily mobile from side to side, restricted mobility up and down
* Examination of cervical lymph nodes (usually cervical lymph nodes are not palpable)
* Examine the base of tongue for presence of any ectopic thyroid tissue.

Q. What is your case? (Summary of a case of thyroglossal cyst)

Ans. This 15-year-old boy presented with a swelling in the midline in front of the upper part of the neck for last 3 years, which is gradually increasing in size. There is no pain over the swelling and there is no history of any discharge from the swelling (Fig. 11.4).

On examination: There is a soft cystic swelling, in the midline of the neck in front of the thyroid cartilage, round in shape, 3 cm in diameter, surface is smooth, margins are rounded, and free from the skin and the underlying structures. Fluctuation is positive but transillumination is negative. The swelling moves up and down with deglutition and also moves up with protrusion of the tongue.

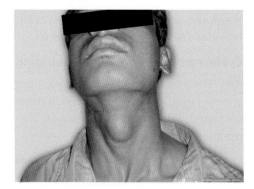

Fig. 11.4: Thyroglossal cyst (prelaryngeal type)
Courtesy: Prof Biswanath Mukhopadhyay, NRS Medical College, Kolkata

Q. What is your diagnosis?

Ans. This is a case of thyroglossal cyst situated in the prelaryngeal region.

Q. What are the other possibilities?

Ans.

- Cervical dermoid cyst
- Subhyoid bursal cyst
- Ectopic thyroid gland
- Solitary thyroid nodule from the isthmus of thyroid gland
- Enlarged prelaryngeal and pretracheal lymph node.

All the earlier swelling moves up with deglutition but does not move up with protrusion of tongue.

Q. How will you demonstrate that the swelling moves up with deglutition and protrusion of tongue?

Ans. Ask the patient to swallow and inspect the swelling moving up with deglutition.

Ask the patient to open the mouth slightly and keep the lower jaw still. Ask him to protrude the tongue outside the mouth and inspect the swelling moving up with protrusion of tongue. Hold the cyst between the thumb and index finger and ask the patient to protrude the tongue out of the already open mouth. The thyroglossal cyst will move up with protrusion of tongue (Fig. 11.5).

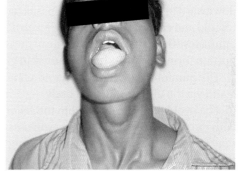

Fig. 11.5: Thyroglossal cyst—Note: Upward movement of the swelling with protrusion of tongue

Q. What other swelling moves up on protrusion of tongue?

Ans. Any other swelling attached to the hyoid bone will move up on protrusion of tongue, e.g. subhyoid bursitis and sublingual dermoid.

Q. What are the different sites where thyroglossal cyst may be situated?

Ans.

- At the base of tongue near the foramen of cecum
- In the floor of mouth
- Submental region
- Subhyoid region
- Prelaryngeal in front of thyroid cartilage
- At the level of cricoid cartilage (Fig. 11.6).

Q. What is the relation of thyroglossal duct with the hyoid bone?

Ans. The thyroglossal duct descends usually in front of the hyoid bone (Fig. 11.7A). The duct,

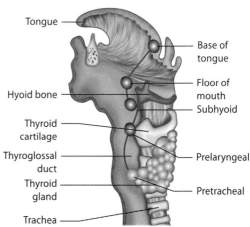

Fig. 11.6: Course of thyroglossal duct and locations of thyroglossal cyst

however, may form a retrohyoid loop and then descends downwards (Fig. 11.7C). Rarely the duct may pass through the hyoid bone (Fig. 11.7B).

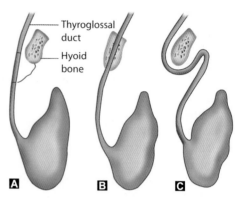

Thyroglossal duct

Hyoid bone

Figs 11.7A to C: Relation of thyroglossal duct with hyoid bone

Q. What is thyroglossal cyst?

Ans. Thyroglossal cyst is a cystic swelling which develops from the thyroglossal duct. It is a type of tubulodermoid.

Q. How does thyroid gland develops?

Ans. A diverticulum known as median thyroid diverticulum develops from the ventral portion of the endoderm between the first and second branchial arch. This median thyroid diverticulum forms the thyroglossal tract which descends downward in between the genioglossus muscle and then descends further down in front of the thyroid and cricoid cartilage to the level of 2nd, 3rd, and 4th tracheal rings. At this level the duct bifurcates. The lateral diverticula form the two lateral lobes of the thyroid gland. The intervening portion forms the isthmus of the thyroid gland.

The parafollicular cells of thyroid gland arise from the neural crest and reach the thyroid gland via the ultimobranchial body.

The hyoid bone develops from the second and third branchial arches come in close relation with the thyroglossal duct. The thyroglossal duct may descend either in front of the hyoid bone, may form a retrohyoid loop while descending in front of the hyoid bone or rarely it may pass through the body of the hyoid bone.

Q. What is the fate of thyroglossal duct?

Ans.
- Lower part forms the isthmus and two lateral lobes of thyroid gland
- Part from foramen cecum to the thyroid isthmus disappears
- Part from hyoid bone to the isthmus of thyroid gland may persist as a fibrous cord to form levator glandulae thyroideae
- Along the course of the duct ectopic thyroid tissue may develop in different sites—lingual thyroid, ectopic thyroid tissue in submental and subhyoid or prelaryngeal region
- A portion of the thyroglossal duct may remain unobliterated and accumulation of secretion may occur leading to formation of thyroglossal cyst.

Q. What is the pathology of thyroglossal cyst?

Ans. The thyroglossal cyst is lined by columnar or cuboidal epithelium. The cyst epithelium is surrounded by a rim of lymphoid tissue.

The cyst contains thick jelly-like fluid which may contain cholesterol crystals.

Q. How will you manage this patient?

Ans. I will advise for an ultrasonography (USG) of the thyroid region and the swelling. USG may show the normal thyroid lobes and the isthmus. The nature of the swelling may also be assessed.

Q. What is the role of radionuclide scanning?

Ans. Iodine-131 (^{131}I) scan may demonstrate presence of any ectopic thyroid tissue in the swelling. In case of ectopic thyroid tissue this may be the only functioning thyroid tissue and no thyroid tissue will be seen in the thyroid region.

So a ^{131}I radionuclide scanning is helpful for the evaluation of a patient with thyroglossal cyst.

Q. What operation will you do?

Ans. I will do Sistrunk operation. This operation involves complete excision of the cyst along with the thyroglossal tract. The body of the hyoid bone is excised. The excision of the body of the hyoid bone helps in excision of any retrohyoid part of the thyroglossal tract and also complete excision of the thyroglossal tract up to the foramen cecum.

The operation is done under general anesthesia. The head is extended by placing a sandbag in between the shoulder blades and head rest on a head ring. Head end of the bed raised by 15° to reduce venous congestion. An elliptical incision is made around the cyst and the skin flaps are raised. The cyst is dissected all around. The thyroglossal duct attached to the upper part of the cyst is dissected upwards.

Q. How can you visualize the thyroglossal tract during operation?

Ans. If methylene blue is injected into the thyroglossal cyst or fistula the thyroglossal tract may be seen during operation being stained with methylene blue.

Q. What are the complications of thyroglossal cyst?

Ans.
* Recurrent infection
* Fistula formation
* Rarely papillary carcinoma may develop in thyroglossal cyst.

■ THYROGLOSSAL FISTULA

Clinical Examination

History
* *Onset*: Fistula present since birth or developed as a sequelae of thyroglossal cyst
* Any history of preexisting swelling, infection and rupture, incision, and drainage of thyroglossal cyst may result in a fistula
* Incomplete excision of thyroglossal duct may result in a fistula
* Site of the opening
* Any history of discharge from the fistula opening (usually mucoid discharge).

Examination—Inspection/Palpation
* Site of the fistulous opening
* Any hood of skin (in thyroglossal fistula there is usually a hood of the skin around the upper margin of the fistulous opening)

♦ Ask the patient to swallow and appreciate the fistulous opening moving up with deglutition

♦ Ask the patient to protrude the tongue and assess the movement of the fistulous opening upwards.

Q. What is your case? (Summary of a case of thyroglossal fistula)

Ans. This 20-year-old boy presented with a discharging sinus in the midline of the front of the neck for last 3 years. The discharge is mucus. Patient had a swelling in the same region for last 5 years. The swelling became painful 3 years back and patient underwent drainage of abscess 3 years back. Following the operation patient noticed having this discharging sinus (Fig. 11.8).

On examination: There is a sinus opening at the level of lower border of cricoid cartilage situated in the midline and there is a hood of skin around the upper border of the fistula opening. The fistulous opening moves up on deglutition and on protrusion of tongue and hooding of skin become more prominent.

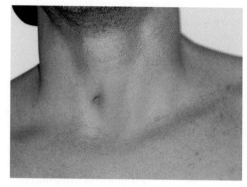

Fig. 11.8: Thyroglossal fistula

Courtesy: Dr sukumar Maiti, Calcutta Medical College, Kolkata

Q. What is your diagnosis?

Ans. This is a case of thyroglossal fistula with external opening at the level of upper border of thyroid cartilage.

Q. How does thyroglossal fistula develops?

Ans.

♦ Rarely it may be congenital, when the thyroglossal tract communicates directly with the skin at birth.

♦ More commonly, however, the thyroglossal fistula develops as a result of:
  – Infection and bursting of a thyroglossal cyst
  – Incision over thyroglossal cyst mistaking it as a simple abscess
  – Incomplete removal of thyroglossal tract during excision of thyroglossal cyst.

Q. How will you treat this patient?

Ans. I will do baseline investigations to assess patient fitness for general anesthesia.

I will do Sistrunk operation which involves complete excision of thyroglossal fistula tract from external opening up to foramen cecum with excision of the body of hyoid bone.

Q. What is the lining epithelium of thyroglossal fistula?

Ans. The fistula tract is lined by columnar epithelium and discharge is mucoid in nature.

■ BRANCHIAL CYST

Clinical Examination

See Page No. 302, Chapter 9.

History

* Detail history of swelling
* Age of onset (although present since birth, these cyst distend later and presents around the age of 20–25 years)
* Progress of the swelling (usually very slow growing)
* Pain (usually painless, presence of pain suggests infection).

Examination—Inspection/Palpation

* Site and extent (branchial cyst usually lies in the upper third of the neck behind the anterior edge of the sternocleidomastoid muscle)
* Tenderness (usually nontender—presence of tenderness suggests infection)
* Size and shape
* Surface and margin (usually smooth surface with well-defined margins all around)
* Consistency (usually soft cystic in feel, may feel tense cystic, or firm)
* Fluctuation (usually positive)
* Transillumination (usually contains a thick turbid fluid and does not show transillumination. Some cyst may contain clear fluid and may show positive transillumination)
* Mobility (branchial cyst is usually tethered to the local structures and show slight mobility side to side and above downwards)
* Test relation with the sternocleidomastoid muscle (the cyst becomes less prominent on contraction and the sternocleidomastoid muscle suggesting that the cyst lies deep to the sternocleidomastoid muscle)
* Examination of cervical lymph nodes (usually the lymph nodes are not enlarged—infection of the cyst may cause lymph node enlargement).

Q. What is your case? (Summary of a case of branchial cyst)

Ans. This 50-year-old lady presented with a swelling in the upper part of the lateral side of the neck on the left side for last 2 years, which is gradually increasing in size. No pain over the swelling. No other swellings in other parts of the body (Fig. 11.9).

On examination: There is a soft cystic swelling in the upper part of the left side of the neck medial to sternocleidomastoid muscle in its upper third. The swelling has smooth surface, rounded margin, free from skin, and underlying structures. Fluctuation is positive but transillumination is negative. No lymph nodes are palpable in the neck.

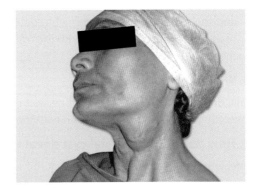

Fig. 11.9: Branchial cyst in the left side of the neck
Courtesy: Dr Subhasis Saha, IPGMER, Kolkata

Q. What is your diagnosis?

Ans. This is a case of branchial cyst in the left side of the neck.

Q. What are the other possibilities?

Ans.

- Chronic cervical lymphadenitis.
- *Cold abscess in the neck*: Adjacent matted cervical lymph nodes may be palpable. General features of tuberculosis will be present.
- *Cervical dermoid*: Lateral variety.
- *Plunging ranula*: Associated with a ranula in the floor of the mouth and transillumination will be always positive.
- *Cystic hygroma*: Usually present since birth and the swelling is brilliantly transilluminant.
- Carotid body tumor.
- *Submandibular salivary gland swelling*: Adenoma, carcinoma, or submandibular salivary calculi.

Q. How will you treat this patient?

Ans.

- I will prepare the patient for surgery. Routine investigations to assess patient's fitness for general anesthesia
- Complete excision of the cyst under general anesthesia is the ideal operation.

Q. What are the important steps of operation?

Ans.

- General anesthesia.
- Transverse skin incision over the swelling. The platysma is incised in the same line. The skin flaps are raised. The investing layer of the deep cervical fascia over the cyst along the anterior border of the sternocleidomastoid muscle is incised and the anterior wall of the cyst is exposed. The cyst is dissected all around. The dissection has to be continued upward to excise a track which passes from the swelling through the fork of the common carotid artery up to the lateral pharyngeal wall. It passes superficial to stylopharyngeus muscle and the glossopharyngeal nerve but deep to the hypoglossal nerve and the posterior belly of digastric muscle. The cyst with the tract is excised completely. If some part is left behind there is chance of recurrence.

Q. What is branchial cyst?

Ans. Branchial cyst is a cystic swelling arising from the persistent cervical sinus which is formed due to fusion of 2nd branchial arch with the 6th branchial arch.

Q. How does the branchial cyst develop?

Ans. During development of the neck the second branchial arch grows at a greater pace than the third and the fourth branchial arches. A diverticulum develops from the 2nd branchial arch which fuses with the 6th branchial arch. The intervening area forms the cervical sinus which lies superficial to the 3rd and 4th branchial arches but deep to the second branchial arch. Normally the cervical sinus disappears. If the cervical sinus persists there is accumulation of fluid from the epithelial lining and forms a cyst. This is called the branchial cyst (Figs 11.10A and B).

Q. What are the pathological characteristics of branchial cyst?

Ans. The branchial cyst is lined by stratified squamous epithelium. Sometimes it may be lined by columnar epithelium. The wall of the cyst contains large amount of lymphoid tissue and hence the cyst is prone to infection commonly.

The content of the cyst is viscid, cheesy material, and contains cholesterol crystals.

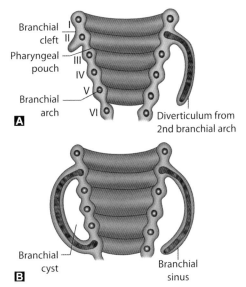

Figs 11.10A and B: Development of branchial cyst and fistula

Q. What is the usual age of presentation of branchial cyst?

Ans. Branchial cyst is a congenital cyst which develops due to the persistence of the cervical sinus. But usually presents at puberty between 20 years and 25 years of age.

Q. What is the relation of sternocleidomastoid muscle to the branchial cyst?

Ans. Branchial cyst lies at the level of the upper third of the sternocleidomastoid muscle. The sternocleidomastoid muscle develops from the myotome of the second branchial arch. So the cyst lies deep to the sternocleidomastoid muscle.

Q. Which cyst fluid may contain cholesterol crystals?

Ans.
- Branchial cyst
- Cystic hygroma
- Thyroglossal cyst
- Dental cyst
- Dentigerous cyst
- Hydrocele.

Q. What are branchial arches?

Ans. During development around the primitive pharynx six pairs of mesodermal condensation appear in the form of branchial arches. The branchial arches consist of mesodermal core and lined outside by the ectoderm and on the inside by the endoderm.

Q. What are branchial cleft and pharyngeal pouches?

Ans. There are depressions between the two adjacent branchial arches. These depressions are lined internally by the endoderm and are called pharyngeal pouches. These depressions are lined externally by the ectoderm and are called branchial clefts. The 5th arch disappears so there are four branchial clefts and four pharyngeal pouches.

Q. What are the constituents of the branchial arches?

Ans. The branchial arch consists of a central cartilage, a muscle mass, a nerve, and an artery.

Q. What are the derivatives of first arch or mandibular arch?

Ans.

- *Skeletal elements*: Malleus, incus, lingula of mandible and mental ossicles, anterior ligament of malleus, sphenomandibular ligament, body and ramus of mandible.
- *Muscular elements:*
  - Muscles of mastication—masseter, temporalis, medial, and lateral pterygoids.
  - Tensor palati, tensor tympani, mylohyoid, and anterior belly of digastric.
- *Neural element:* Mandibular branch of trigeminal nerve which supplies all the earlier muscles.
- *Vascular element:* Maxillary artery.

Q. What are the derivatives of second or hyoid arch?

Ans.

- *Skeletal elements:* Stapes, styloid process, stylohyoid ligament, lesser cornua of the hyoid, and the upper part of the body of hyoid.
- *Muscular elements:* Muscles of facial expression, occipitofrontalis, buccinator, platysma, stylohyoid, and stapedius.
- *Neural elements:* Facial nerve. Supplies all the earlier muscles.
- *Vascular element:* Stapedial artery.

Q. What are the derivatives of the third branchial arch?

Ans.

- *Skeletal elements:* Greater cornua and lower part of the body of the hyoid.
- *Muscular element:* Stylopharyngeus.
- *Neural element:* Glossopharyngeal nerve.
- *Vascular element:* Common carotid and the internal carotid artery.

Q. What are the derivatives of the fourth branchial arch?

Ans.

- *Skeletal elements:* Thyroid cartilage.
- *Muscular elements:* Inferior constrictor of pharynx and cricothyroid.
- *Neural elements:* Superior laryngeal nerve. Supplies the earlier muscles.
- *Vascular element:* On the right side it forms the first part of the subclavian artery and on the left side it forms the main part of the arch of the aorta.

Q. What are the derivatives of the sixth branchial arch?

Ans.

- *Skeletal elements:* Cricoid cartilage, arytenoid cartilage, and the rings of trachea.
- *Muscular elements:*
  - All the intrinsic muscles of larynx except cricothyroid.
  - All the muscles of pharynx except stylopharyngeus.
  - All the muscles of palate except the tensor palati.
- *Neural elements:* Recurrent laryngeal nerve, a branch of vagus carrying fibers from cranial accessory nerve.
- *Vascular elements:* The ventral part forms the main part of the pulmonary artery. The dorsal part on the left side persists as ductus arteriosus which closes after birth and remains as ligamentum arteriosum. The dorsal part on the right side disappears.

■ BRANCHIAL SINUS (FISTULA)

Clinical Examination

See Page No. 36, 37, Chapter 1.

History

◆ Onset (usually present since birth, may occur afterwards following infection and rupture of a branchial cyst or incomplete excision of a branchial cyst).
◆ *Site*: In congenital variety usually lies at the lower third of the anterior border of the sternocleidomastoid muscle. In acquired variety resulting as a complication of branchial cyst the opening lies along the anterior border of the sternocleidomastoid muscle at the upper third.
◆ Discharge (usually discharge is clear mucus, if infected may discharge pus).

Examination—Inspection/Palpation

◆ Site of sinus opening
◆ Any discharge
◆ Any hood of skin around the opening of sinus
◆ Any movement with deglutition or protrusion of tongue (no movement occurs with swallowing or protrusion of tongue)
◆ Examination of cervical lymph nodes.

Q. What is your case? (Summary of a case of branchial sinus)

Ans. This 8-month-old male child presented with a discharging sinus in the lower part of the neck on the right side since birth which discharges mucoid material occasionally. Sometimes the opening gets blocked and discharge stops but after varying interval of time there is recurrence of mucoid discharge from the same site (Fig. 11.11).

On examination: There is a tiny opening at the anterior border of the lower third of the right sternocleidomastoid muscle. There is no skin hood over the opening. The opening does not move up on protrusion of tongue. There is no swelling deep to the opening. Cervical lymph nodes are not palpable.

Q. What is your diagnosis?

Ans. This is a case of right-sided branchial sinus.

Q. What is branchial sinus?

Ans. Branchial sinus develops due to failure of fusion of the second branchial arch with the fifth arch and the disappearance of the second branchial cleft membrane.

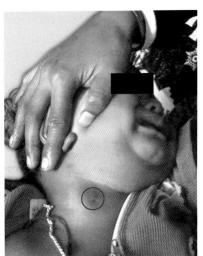

Fig. 11.11: Branchial sinus (external opening seen at the anterior border of the lower third of the sternocleidomastoid muscle on the right side)

Courtesy: Dr Kalyani Saha Basu, NRS Medical College, Kolkata

When an internal opening is found in the lateral pharyngeal wall then it is called a branchial fistula.

In most cases an internal opening is not found so this condition is better called as a branchial sinus rather than a fistula.

Q. How else branchial sinus may develop?

Ans. The branchial sinus may also develop due to rupture of an infected branchial cyst, due to inadvertent incision over an infected branchial cyst, or incomplete removal of a branchial cyst. This is also called *acquired branchial sinus.*

Q. Where does the external opening of a branchial sinus found?

Ans. In congenital variety the external opening is typically situated in the lower third of the neck at the anterior border of sternocleidomastoid.

In acquired variety the external opening is usually situated at the upper or middle third of the neck at the anterior border of sternocleidomastoid.

Q. Where is the internal opening of the branchial fistula found?

Ans. The internal opening of the branchial fistula is found in the lateral wall of the pharynx behind the tonsil and anterior to the posterior pillar of the fauces.

Q. What is the course of branchial fistula tract?

Ans.

* The external orifice of the fistula is usually located in the lower third of the neck near the anterior border of the sternocleidomastoid.
* The tract pierces the deep fascia at the level of upper border of thyroid cartilage. It passes through the fork of the common carotid bifurcation lying superficial to the internal carotid artery but deep to the external carotid artery.
* Further upwards the tract ascends towards the lateral pharyngeal wall and pierces the superior constrictor of pharynx and lies superficial to the stylopharyngeus muscle and glossopharyngeal nerve but lying deep to the hypoglossal nerve and the stylomandibular ligament.
* The internal orifice of the tract is located on the anterior aspect of the posterior pillar of the fauces just behind the tonsil. But more commonly the track ends blindly on lateral pharyngeal wall—when it is called a branchial sinus rather than a fistula (Fig. 11.12).

Q. What is the pathological feature of a branchial sinus?

Ans. The branchial sinus tract is lined by stratified squamous epithelium or pseudostratified ciliated columnar epithelium. There is a rim of lymphoid tissue around the fistulous tract.

The discharge is mucoid or mucopurulent.

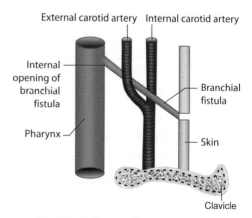

Fig. 11.12: Course of branchial fistula

Q. How will you treat this patient?

Ans. As the sinus is causing recurrent discharge, I will consider surgical treatment and complete excision of the fistula from the external opening up to the lateral pharyngeal wall.

Q. Do you like to do any investigation?

Ans.

+ A sinogram may be helpful to delineate the fistulous tract.
+ A radiopaque dye (meglumine iothalamate-280) 1–2 mL is injected through the external orifice and X-ray exposure is taken. This will delineate the tract.

Q. What are the steps of excision of a branchial sinus?

Ans.

+ General anesthesia with endotracheal intubation.
+ An incision along the Langer's line encircling the external opening. The skin flaps are raised.
+ A probe may be passed gently through the tract for identification during operation.
+ The tract is dissected upward by incising the platysma. At the level of the upper border of the thyroid cartilage the deep fascia is incised and the tract is dissected higher up to the bifurcation of the common carotid artery.
+ A second skin incision along the Langer's line is made higher up at the neck at the level of upper border of thyroid cartilage and the already dissected tract is delivered up through this second incision. The tract is then dissected off from the constrictor muscles of pharynx where it lies superficial to the stylopharyngeus muscle and glossopharyngeal nerve but lying deep to the hypoglossal nerve and the stylomandibular ligament.

The internal orifice of the tract is located on the anterior aspect of the posterior pillar of the fauces just behind the tonsil. But more commonly the track ends blindly on lateral pharyngeal wall. The tract is dissected as high as possible ligated and excised.

Q. What is cervical auricle?

Ans. It is a cutaneous projection found in relation to the external orifice of branchial fistula.

Q. What is branchial cartilage?

Ans. It is a small piece of cartilage, which is connected to deep surface of a cutaneous dimple in relation to external orifice of a branchial fistula.

Q. What is branchiogenic carcinoma?

Ans. This is a rare tumor which arises from the remnants of branchial clefts.

◼ TUBERCULAR CERVICAL LYMPHADENITIS

Clinical Examination

See Page No. 382, Chapter 9.

History

+ Detailed history about the swellings in the neck
+ Onset, progress (usually involves upper deep cervical lymph nodes and progresses slowly)

- Any pain (usually painless, but pain may occur if there is rapid enlargement of the swelling or if there is secondary infection)
- Any history of sinus formation and discharge
- Swelling of other lymph nodes in the body
- Any systemic symptoms of weight loss, fever, night sweats, and pruritus [these symptoms may be found in tuberculosis, present in about 30% patients of Hodgkin's lymphoma and 10% patients of non-Hodgkin's lymphoma (NHL)]
- Any past history of similar swelling in the neck
- Any past history of pulmonary tuberculosis.

Examination—Inspection/Palpation

- *Local examination of the neck:* Which levels of lymph nodes are enlarged?
- Temperature (usually the temperature is normal. Even if abscess has formed the temperature may be normal, so called a cold abscess).
- Tenderness (usually nontender, if the abscess is tense the swelling may become tender).
- Size, shape, surface, margin, and consistency (usually firm in feel, may feel soft if an abscess has formed, in lymphomas lymph nodes are soft rubbery in feel).
- Discrete or matted (tubercular lymph nodes are usually matted, in lymphomas the lymph nodes may be discrete).
- Skin over the swelling may be normal, if an abscess has formed the overlying skin may appear reddish purple. If abscess ruptures a sinus may form with an undermining edge.
- *Fluctuation*: If an abscess has formed the swelling may become fluctuant.
- Examination of the drainage area to exclude the presence of any infective focus or any malignant lesion.
- Examine the scalp, face, ears, lips, cheek, gum, tongue, oropharynx, floor of mouth, parotid, submandibular, and thyroid gland.
- *Examine other lymph node sites*: Axilla, epitrochlear, inguinal, and popliteal group to assess any other lymph node enlargement.
- Examine the breast.
- Examination of abdomen (for hepatosplenomegaly or any other mass in abdomen) and genitalia.
- Examination of nasopharynx and larynx with a mirror.
- *Examination of chest*: To exclude pulmonary tuberculosis.

Q. What is your case? (Summary of a case of tubercular cervical lymphadenitis)

Ans. This 50-year-old lady presented with multiple swellings in the right side of the neck for last 8 months. She first noticed the swelling in the right supraclavicular region, afterwards further swelling appeared in the right side of the neck. Three months back one swelling started discharging pus for about 15 days and then was healed with treatment. History of irregular fever for last 8 months, fever is more towards the evening, and complains of excessive sweating at night. Patient also complains of loss of appetite and mild weight loss for the same duration (Fig. 11.13).

On examination: There is mild pallor. Multiple cervical lymph nodes are palpable on the right side of the neck involving the supraclavicular (level V) and jugular group (level II, III, and IV) of lymph nodes. There are multiple palpable nodes at level I. The lymph nodes are nontender, firm in feel, matted together, free from the skin, and are mobile. There is a healed scar in the middle third of the posterior border of sternocleidomastoid. There are no other lymph node enlargements in the body. On abdominal examination there is no hepatosplenomegaly.

Q. What is your diagnosis?

Ans. This is a case of tubercular cervical lymphadenitis affecting the (level I, II, III, IV, and V) cervical lymph nodes on the right side.

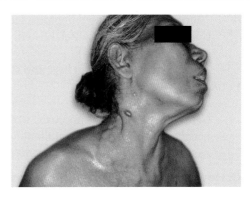

Fig. 11.13: Right-sided tubercular cervical lymphadenitis

Courtesy: Dr Amitava Sengupta, NRS Medical College, Kolkata

Q. What are the different lymph node groups in the neck?

Ans. Depending on the location of the lymph nodes in relation to the investing layer of deep cervical fascia the cervical lymph nodes may be:
- *Superficial*: Lymph nodes lying superficial to the investing layer of the deep cervical fascia.
- *Deep*: Lymph nodes lying deep to the investing layer of deep cervical fascia.

Q. What are the different levels of lymph nodes in the neck?

Ans. There are six levels of lymph nodes in the neck (*See* Page No. 18, Chapter 1).

Q. What is Virchow's gland?

Ans. The left supraclavicular lymph node lying between the two heads of sternocleidomastoid is called the Virchow's lymph node. This lymph node may be involved by metastasis from carcinoma stomach, testicular tumor, carcinoma esophagus, and bronchogenic carcinoma.

Q. How will you palpate the cervical lymph nodes?

Ans. *See* Page No. 19, Chapter 1.

Q. What are the differential diagnoses for chronic cervical lymphadenopathy?

Ans.
- *Chronic pyogenic lymphadenitis:* Firm, discrete, tender lymph nodes, and evidence of infection in the drainage area. Overlying skin may be erythematous.
- *Tubercular cervical lymphadenitis:*
  - Firm, matted lymph nodes
  - May be associated with a cold abscess
  - Tubercular sinus in the skin with undermined skin edge
  - General features of tuberculosis like irregular fever, anorexia, and weight loss.
- *Metastatic cervical lymph node:*
  - Hard, nontender, solitary or multiple lymph nodes, mobile or fixed.
  - Evidence of primary growth in the drainage area.
- *Hodgkin's lymphoma:*
  - Single or multiple sites of lymph node enlargement, discrete, rubbery lymph nodes, mobile, free from skin and underlying structures.

- There may be associated hepatosplenomegaly or other lymph node enlargements.
- General symptoms like Pel–Ebstein type of fever (fever for 7–14 days alternating with similar apyrexial period).
- Malaise, anorexia, weight loss, and sweating may be present.
- *Chronic lymphatic leukemia:*
  - Usually elderly patient.
  - General symptoms like anorexia, weight loss, and fever.
  - Localized or generalized lymphadenopathy, firm in feel, mobile, and nontender.
  - Associated hepatosplenomegaly may be present.

Q. How will you confirm your diagnosis?

Ans. A fine-needle aspiration cytology (FNAC) is a reliable investigation for diagnosis of tubercular lymphadenitis (95% accuracy).

Q. If fine-needle aspiration cytology (FNAC) is inconclusive what will you do?

Ans. An excisional biopsy of one of the lymph nodes will give an accurate diagnosis. The acid-fast bacilli (AFB) may be cultured from the biopsy specimen and the drug sensitivity may also be determined.

Q. What are the histological features of tubercular lymphadenitis?

Ans.
- Epithelioid granuloma
- Central caseous necrosis
- Presence of Langhans type of giant cells.

Q. What are the pathological changes in tubercular lymphadenitis?

Ans. There are four stages in the pathogenesis of tubercular lymphadenitis:
1. *Stage I (Stage of inflammation)* There is solid enlargement of the affected lymph node.
2. *Stage II (Stage of abscess formation)* With progress of inflammation the lymph node breaks down and liquefies and there is formation of pus. This pus initially remains deep to the deep fascia and it is difficult to elicit fluctuation at this stage.
3. *Stage III (Stage of collar stud abscess)* After a variable period the pus erodes through the deep fascia and pus accumulates under the lax superficial fascia. The two pockets of pus, one lying deep to the deep fascia and the other pocket lying in between the deep fascia and superficial fascia remains communicated through a rent in the deep fascia and forms a collar stud abscess.
4. *Stage IV (Stage of sinus formation)* If not treated properly the abscess enlarges further and the overlying skin becomes inflamed and ultimately gets eroded and discharges pus from underneath resulting in a tubercular sinus.

Q. What further investigation will you do?

Ans.
- Chest X-ray to exclude associated pulmonary tuberculosis
- Sputum for AFB on 3 days to exclude associated pulmonary tuberculosis
- Blood for Hb%, TLC, DLC, and erythrocyte sedimentation rate (ESR)
- Blood for sugar, urea, and creatinine.

Q. How will you treat patients with tubercular lymphadenitis?

Ans.

◆ The treatment is with administration of antitubercular drugs (ATDs).
◆ *Regime of antitubercular treatment:*
  – *Initial phase four drugs for 2–3 months:*
    - *Capsule rifampicin (R)—450–600 mg daily.*
    - *Tablet isoniazid (H)—300 mg daily.*
    - *Tablet ethambutol (Z)—1,000 mg daily.*
    - *Tablet pyrazinamide (P)—1,500 mg daily.*
  – *Subsequently two drugs for 4-6 months:*
    - Capsule rifampicin and tablet isoniazid (INH).

Q. What are the mechanism of actions and side effects of these drugs?

Ans.

◆ *Rifampicin*: Derived from *Streptomyces mediterranei*. This acts to inhibit bacterial ribonucleic acid (RNA) synthesis by interfering with deoxyribonucleic acid (DNA)-directed RNA polymerase. This is excreted in urine.
  – *Side effects*: Hepatotoxicity and flu-like syndrome.
◆ *Isoniazid*: This is a bactericidal drug that acts by inhibiting the synthesis of mycolic acid by affecting the enzyme mycolase synthetase. This is excreted by kidney.
  – *Side effects:* Peripheral neuropathy in patients treated with higher doses of INH. This is due to enhanced pyridoxine excretion and is prevented by daily administration of oral pyridoxine.
    - Hepatotoxicity in 10% of patients.
◆ *Ethambutol:* Ethambutol inhibits mycobacterial cell wall synthesis. This is excreted in urine.
  – *Side effects:* Rarely causes retrobulbar neuritis (changes in visual acuity and red-green color perception) and it should be discontinued if ocular changes occur.
◆ *Pyrazinamide:* It acts through inhibition of fatty acid synthase I of *Mycobacterium tuberculosis*. This is excreted in urine.
  – *Side effects:* Nausea and vomiting.

Q. What do you mean by directly observed therapy short course (DOTS) treatment regimen for tuberculosis?

Ans. This is called directly observed therapy short course (DOTS). This treatment protocol is followed under Revised National Tuberculosis Control Program (RNTCP). There are different categories of treatment under DOTS regime:

◆ *Category I treatment:*
  Indicated in:
  – New pulmonary tuberculosis.
  – New extrapulmonary tuberculosis.
  Intensive phase:
  – Rifampicin (R)—450–600 mg (10 mg/kg body weight)
  – Isoniazid (H)—600 mg (10–15 mg/kg body weight)

- – Ethambutol (E)—1,200 mg (30 mg/kg body weight)
- – Pyrazinamide (H)—1,500 mg (35 mg/kg body weight).

Administered thrice a week for 2 months.

Continuation phase:

- – Rifampicin and INH in same dose.
- – Administered thrice a week for 4 months.

◆ *Category II retreatment:*

Indicated in:

- – Patient with treatment failure with category I.
- – Defaulter (i.e. off ATD for >2 months after taking drugs for >1 month).

Intensive phase:

- – Rifampicin, INH, ethambutol, and pyrazinamide in same dose
- – Streptomycin—0.75 gram (15 mg/kg body weight)
- – Administered thrice a week for 2 months.

Continuation phase:

- – Rifampicin, INH, and ethambutol in same dose
- – Administered thrice a week for 5 months.

Q. What are second lines of antitubercular drugs?

Ans.

- ◆ *Capreomycin*—15 mg/kg intramuscular (IM)
- ◆ *Kanamycin*—15 mg/kg IM/intravenous (IV)
- ◆ *Amikacin*—15 mg/kg IM, IV
- ◆ *Cycloserine*—250–500 mg BID orally
- ◆ *Ethionamide*—250–500 mg/BID orally
- ◆ *Ciprofloxacin*—500–750 mg/BID orally
- ◆ *Ofloxacin*—300–400 mg/BID orally
- ◆ *Levofloxacin*—500–100 mg/OD orally
- ◆ *Gatifloxacin*—400 mg/OD orally
- ◆ *Moxifloxacin*—400 mg/OD orally
- ◆ *Aminosalicylic acid*—4 g/TID orally.

Q. How will you manage patient who does not respond to first-line antitubercular drugs (ATDs)?

Ans. Second-line antitubercular treatment may help these patients.

If the patient does not respond to second line of ATD treatment, I will consider modified radical neck dissection (MRND) to remove all the involved nodes. The material is to be sent for histopathological examination as well as culture and sensitivity examination. The drugs may be selected depending on the culture sensitivity report.

Q. How the lymph nodes are affected by tubercle bacilli?

Ans. The primary tubercular infection occurs in the tonsil and the infection spreads from there to the cervical lymph nodes. This primary lesion may heal and calcify. The viable bacilli may spread by bloodstream and may affect the distant site and the lymph nodes.

CASE—METASTATIC CERVICAL LYMPH NODE SWELLING WITH UNKNOWN PRIMARY

Q. What is your case? (Summary of a case of metastatic cervical lymph node)

Ans. This 50-year-old gentleman presented with a swelling in the left upper part of the neck for last 6 months. The swelling was small at the onset of about 1 cm in diameter but is rapidly growing in size for last 4 months. There is no history of pain over the swelling. No history of fever, cough, hemoptysis, or chest pain. No difficulty in swallowing or breathing. No history of alteration of voice. Patient complains of anorexia and weight loss for the same duration (Fig. 11.14).

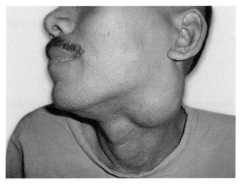

Fig. 11.14: Metastatic cervical lymph node involving the level II lymph nodes in the left side of the neck

Courtesy: Dr Soumya Mondal, IPGMER, Kolkata

On examination: There is a swelling in the left side of the neck lying partly deep to the sternocleidomastoid muscle at the level of the upper border of thyroid cartilage, 5 cm × 4 cm in size, smooth surface, well-defined margin, hard in consistency, and free from skin and the underlying structures. No other lymph nodes are palpable. There is no growth in oral cavity. Tongue is normal. Thyroid gland is not palpable.

So, this is likely to be metastatic carcinoma of the cervical lymph node.

Q. What are the other possibilities?

Ans.
- Tuberculous cervical lymphadenitis
- Chronic pyogenic lymphadenitis
- Lymphoma
- Chronic lymphatic leukemia.

Q. What are the different sites you have looked for to find out a primary lesion?

Ans.
- *Head and neck:*
  - Scalp and face
  - Lip and cheek
  - Floor of the mouth
  - Tongue
  - Nasal cavity
  - Nasopharynx
  - Larynx
  - Oropharynx
  - Thyroid
  - Salivary glands

- Hypopharynx
- Esophagus.
* *Other sites:*
  - Breast
  - Gastrointestinal (GI) tract
  - Testis.

Q. What are the tumor, node, and metastasis (TNM) classifications for head and neck carcinoma?

Ans. The tumor, node, and metastasis (TNM) classifications for head and neck carcinoma as well as its histologic grade and anatomic stage/prognostic groups are described in Tables 11.1 to 11.3.

Table 11.1: Tumor, node and metastasis (TNM) classifications for head and neck carcinoma	
Primary tumor (T)	
TX	Primary tumor cannot be assessed
T0	No evidence of primary tumor
Tis	Carcinoma in situ
T1	Tumor 2 cm or less in greatest dimension
T2	Tumor >2 cm but not more than 4 cm in greatest dimension
T3	Tumor >4 cm in greatest dimension
T4a	Moderately advanced local disease • *Lip:* Tumor invades through cortical bone, inferior alveolar nerve, floor of mouth, or skin of face • *Oral cavity:* Tumor invades adjacent structures (e.g. through cortical bone into deep extrinsic muscle of the tongue, maxillary sinus, or skin of face).
T4b	Very advanced local disease • Tumor invades masticator space, pterygoid plates, or skull base and/or encases internal carotid artery
Regional lymph nodes (N)	
NX	Regional nodes cannot be assessed
N0	No regional lymph node metastasis
N1	Metastasis in a single ipsilateral lymph node 3 cm or less in greatest dimension
N2	Metastasis in a single ipsilateral lymph node >3 cm but not more than 6 cm in greatest dimension; or in multiple ipsilateral lymph nodes, none >6 cm in greatest dimension; or in bilateral or contralateral lymph nodes, none >6 cm in greatest dimension
N2a	Metastasis in a single ipsilateral lymph node >3 cm but not more than 6 cm in greatest dimension
N2b	Metastasis in multiple ipsilateral lymph nodes, none >6 cm in greatest dimension
N2c	Metastasis in bilateral or contralateral lymph nodes, none >6 cm in greatest dimension
N3	Metastasis in a lymph node >6 cm in greatest dimension
Distant metastasis (M)	
M0	No distant metastasis
M1	Distant metastasis

Table 11.2: Histologic grade	
Histologic grade (G)	
GX	Grade cannot be assessed
G1	Well differentiated
G2	Moderately differentiated
G3	Poorly differentiated
G4	Undifferentiated

Table 11.3: Anatomic stage/prognostic groups			
Stage	*T*	*N*	*M*
0	Tis	N0	M0
I	T1	N0	M0
II	T2	N0	M0
III	T3	N0	M0
	T1	N1	M0
	T2	N1	M0
	T3	N1	M0
IVA	T4a	N0	M0
	T4a	N1	M0
	T1	N2	M0
	T2	N2	M0
	T3	N2	M0
	T4a	N2	M0
IVB	T any	N3	M0
	T4b	N any	M0
IVC	T any	N any	M1

The tumor, node, and metastasis (TNM) classifications of major salivary glands (parotid, submandibular, and sublingual) and its anatomic stage/prognostic groups are illustrated in Tables 11.4 and 11.5.

The tumor, node, and metastasis (TNM) classifications of mucosal melanoma and its anatomic stage/prognostic groups are given in Tables 11.6 and 11.7.

Table 11.4: Tumor, node and metastasis (TNM) classifications of major salivary glands (parotid, submandibular and sublingual)	
Primary tumor (T)	
TX	Primary tumor cannot be assessed
T0	No evidence of primary tumor
Tis	Carcinoma in situ
T1	Tumor ≤2 cm in greatest dimension without extraparenchymal extension (clinical or macroscopic evidence of invasion of the soft tissues, not microscopic evidence)
T2	Tumor >2 cm but not more than 4 cm in greatest dimension without extraparenchymal extension
T3	Tumor >4 cm and/or tumor having extraparenchymal extension
T4a	Moderately advanced disease • Tumor invades the skin, mandible, ear canal, and/or facial nerve
T4b	Very advanced disease • Tumor invades skull base and/or pterygoid plates and/or encases carotid artery
Regional lymph nodes (N)	
NX	Regional nodes cannot be assessed
N0	No regional lymph node metastasis
N1	Metastasis in a single ipsilateral lymph node ≤3 cm in greatest dimension
N2	Metastasis in a single ipsilateral lymph node >3 cm but not more than 6 cm in greatest dimension; or in multiple ipsilateral lymph nodes, none >6 cm in greatest dimension; or in bilateral or contra-lateral lymph nodes, none >6 cm in greatest dimension
N2a	Metastasis in a single ipsilateral lymph node >3 cm but not more than 6 cm in greatest dimension
N2b	Metastasis in multiple ipsilateral lymph nodes, none >6 cm in greatest dimension

Contd...

Contd...

N2c	Metastasis in bilateral or contralateral lymph nodes, none >6 cm in greatest dimension
N3	Metastasis in a lymph node >6 cm in greatest dimension
Distant metastasis (M)	
M0	No distant metastasis
M1	Distant metastasis

Table 11.5: Anatomic stage/prognostic groups

Stage	*T*	*N*	*M*
0	Tis	N0	M0
I	T1	N0	M0
II	T2	N0	M0
III	T3	N0	M0
	T1	N1	M0
	T2	N1	M0
	T3	N1	M0
IVA	T4a	N0	M0
	T4a	N1	M0
	T1	N2	M0
	T2	N2	M0
	T3	N2	M0
	T4a	N2	M0
IVB	T any	N3	M0
	T4b	N any	M0
IVC	T any	N any	M1

Table 11.6: Tumor, node and metastasis (TNM) classifications of mucosal melanoma

Primary tumor (T)	
TX	Primary tumor cannot be assessed
T3	Mucosal disease
T4a	Moderately advanced disease • Tumor involving deep soft tissue, cartilage, bone, or overlying skin
T4b	Very advanced disease • Tumor involving brain, dura, skull base, lower cranial nerves (IX, X, XI, XII), masticator space, carotid artery, prevertebral space, or mediastinal structures
Regional lymph nodes (N)	
NX	Regional lymph nodes cannot be assessed
N0	No regional lymph node metastases
N1	Regional lymph node metastases present
Distant metastasis (M)	
M0	No distant metastasis
M1	Distant metastasis

Table 11.7: Anatomic stage/prognostic groups			
Stage	*T*	*N*	*M*
III	T3	N0	M0
IVA	T4a	N0	M0
	T3	N1	M0
	T4a	N1	M0
IVB	T4b	N any	M0
IVC	T any	N any	M1

Q. What are the characteristics of a metastatic cervical lymph node?

Ans.
* Usually occurs in elderly individual (>50 years). Metastatic lymph node from thyroid carcinoma may occur at an earlier age
* Usually presents with progressively increasing painless neck lump
* Enlarged lymph nodes are firm or hard in feel
* Nodes may infiltrate the deeper structures and may become fixed
* May present with symptoms referable to the primary lesion
* Ulcer in the tongue or oral cavity
* Hoarseness of voice in laryngeal lesion
* Dysphagia in esophageal lesion
* Cough, hemoptysis, or breathlessness—due to chest lesion
* Pain in abdomen, dyspepsia—due to abdominal lesion
* Examination of the drainage site may reveal a primary lesion.

Q. How will you treat this patient?

Ans.
* I will do a FNAC from the swelling
* I will do an ear-nose-throat (ENT) examination and if a growth is found I will take biopsy from the growth
* Baseline workup.

Q. If the fine-needle aspiration cytology (FNAC) of the lymph nodes shows that it is metastatic squamous cell carcinoma what will you do?

Ans. A thorough clinical examination of the possible primary sites in the scalp, face, mouth, cheek, lips, nasopharynx, and larynx to detect any primary lesion.

Q. If the clinical examination is noncontributory what investigations will you suggest?

Ans.
* If clinical examination is noncontributory patient should undergo triple endoscopy—laryngoscopy, bronchoscopy, and upper GI endoscopy for detection of primary tumor.
* If no tumor is found blind biopsy from nasopharynx, pyriform fossa, base of tongue, and tonsil should be done in the same sitting.

Q. In spite of all investigation the primary tumor could not be found. What should be the treatment strategy?

Ans. I will proceed with radical neck dissection (level I to level VI) and postoperative irradiation of the possible primary sites.

Q. When will you give radiotherapy to the neck following radical neck dissection?

Ans.
◆ If the node is larger than 3 cm, there is extracapsular spread of the tumor, multiple nodes are involved, and a postoperative radiotherapy to the neck is indicated.
◆ N2a, N2b, and N3 neck should receive postoperative radiotherapy.

Q. What may be the alternative option?

Ans. Alternatively irradiation of the lymph node field and the possible primary sites may cause regression of the lymph node disease. If the lymph node remains persistent a MRND may be considered later.

Q. If the fine-needle aspiration cytology (FNAC) revealed metastatic adenocarcinoma. How will you proceed?

Ans. The primary sites like thyroid, salivary glands, lungs, and GI tract should be investigated to find out any primary site of carcinoma in these organs.
    Treatment of the primary lesion if it is found.
    A radical neck dissection is done in thyroid and the salivary gland carcinomas.

Q. What is the follow-up protocol?

Ans. These patients should be regularly followed-up. In 30% of cases the primary growth becomes obvious afterwards in follow-up.

Q. How will you manage bilateral neck node metastasis?

Ans. Metastasis to bilateral neck nodes implies a very bad prognosis with 5-years survival of only 5%.
    Earlier staged radical neck dissection was advised. Simultaneous bilateral radical neck dissection is followed more recently. However, the mortality and morbidity of bilateral neck dissection is significant. Surgery, however, does not alter the natural history of the disease.

Q. How will you manage fixed node (or nodes more than 6 cm in diameter) in the neck?

Ans. These nodes are usually fixed to the underlying structures or to the skin. If the nodes are fixed to the underlying important structures like carotid sheath, larynx, trachea, and esophagus then surgery is contraindicated. If the nodes are fixed to the overlying skin only it can be excised with the adherent skin, the defect being covered with skin flap.
    Patient needs postoperative radiotherapy.

Q. What are the different types of neck dissection?

Ans.
◆ *Classical radical neck node dissection:* This includes removal of all lymph node groups from level I to level VI.

In addition to this the internal jugular vein, sternomastoid muscle, and the spinal accessory nerve are sacrificed.

◆ *Modified radical neck dissection:* The lymph node dissection is same as in radical neck dissection. One or more of the structures like accessory nerve, sternomastoid muscle, and internal jugular vein are preserved.

Modified radical neck dissection may be:

– *Type 1*: Spinal accessory nerve is preserved.

– *Type 2*: Spinal accessory nerve and internal jugular vein are preserved.

– *Type 3*: Spinal accessory nerve, internal jugular vein, and sternomastoid muscles are all preserved.

◆ *Selective neck dissection:* One or more of the major lymph node groups are removed with preservation of the remaining lymph node groups along with preservation of sternomastoid muscle, accessory nerve, and internal jugular vein.

◆ *Supraomohyoid neck dissection:* Involves dissection of level I, II, and III groups of lymph nodes. The lower limit of the dissection is the superior belly of omohyoid where it crosses the internal jugular vein.

◆ *Anterior compartment neck dissection:* Involves dissection of level VI or anterior compartment lymph nodes.

■ MALIGNANT LYMPHOMA

Clinical Examination

See Tubercular Lymphadenitis, Page No. 501.

Q. What is your case? (Summary of a case of malignant lymphoma)

Ans. This 45-year-old gentleman presented with multiple swellings in both sides of the neck for last 9 months. Initially there was a single swelling on the left upper part of the neck which was about 2 cm in size at the onset. Afterwards this swelling gradually increases in size and patient noticed appearance of multiple swellings in both sides of the neck. The swellings were slowly increasing in size from the onset but for last 3 months they are growing rapidly. No pain over the swellings. No difficulty in swallowing, no dyspnea. Patient complains of anorexia, weight loss, and excessive sweating for the same duration. He also complains of fever

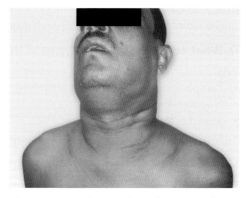

Fig. 11.15: Malignant lymphoma involving bilateral cervical lymph nodes

Courtesy: Dr Rajat Subhra Morel, IPGMER, Kolkata

for last 6 months. Fever persists for 5–7 days and there is alternate period of pyrexia and apyrexia during this period at an interval of 5–7 days. Patient has no other complaints (Fig. 11.15).

On examination: Patient is anemic. On local examination there are multiple enlarged lymph nodes in both sides of the neck involving all the levels of lymph node. There are multiple enlarged lymph nodes varying in size between 2 cm and 4 cm in diameter. The nodes are discrete, smooth surface, rubbery in feel, mobile, and free from skin and underlying structures. There are no other palpable lymph nodes in the axilla, groin, or abdomen. Abdominal examination is normal, no hepatosplenomegaly. No evidence of superior mediastinal syndrome.

Q. What is your diagnosis?

Ans. This is a case of bilateral cervical lymphadenopathy probably due to Hodgkin's lymphoma.

Q. How do you ascertain that patient has no superior mediastinal syndrome?

Ans. Patient does not complain of dyspnea, difficulty in swallowing, or swelling of the face. On local examination there are no engorged veins in the neck, no puffiness of face. Pemberton's sign is negative.

Q. How will you proceed to manage this patient?

Ans. As there is suspicion of lymphoma, I will consider excision biopsy of one of the significant lymph node for definite diagnosis of the type and grade of lymphoma which cannot be ascertained on FNAC.

Q. What are the histological features of lymphoma?

Ans. There may be a central area of necrosis. There are various types of cells which are predominantly lymphocytes. In addition there are eosinophils, plasma cells, reticulum cells, and characteristic Reed–Sternberg giant cells.

Q. What are the characteristics of Reed–Sternberg giant cells?

Ans. These are characteristic giant cells found in lymphoma. This is a large cell with two large nuclei which are mirror image of each other. Owl eye appearance.

Q. What are the histologic types of Hodgkin's disease?

Ans.
* Lymphocyte predominance. Most favorable histology
* Nodular sclerosis
* Mixed cellularity
* Lymphocyte depletion. Most unfavorable histology.

Q. What investigations will you suggest for staging the disease?

Ans.
* *Detailed clinical history:* Enquire about fever, night sweats, pruritus, and weight loss.
* *Complete physical examination:* Examination of regional lymph nodes and abdominal examination for hepatosplenomegaly
* Complete hemogram
* Chest X-ray, if chest X-ray shows some abnormalities. Computed tomography (CT) scan of chest is indicated
* Ultrasonography of abdomen. If abnormality is found in USG, CT scan of abdomen in selected cases.

Q. Would you like to do a bone marrow biopsy?

Ans. In stage IA or IIA a bone marrow biopsy is not essential. In advanced disease a bone marrow biopsy is indicated.

Q. What is the role of staging laparotomy in Hodgkin's lymphoma?

Ans. Earlier staging laparotomy was done routinely. With advent of helical CT scan and magnetic resonance imaging (MRI) scan staging laparotomy is no longer practiced in view of increased morbidity of the routine laparotomy.

Q. How do you stage lymphoma?

Ans. Lymphoma can be staged by Cotswolds modification of the Ann Arbor staging system (Table 11.8).

Table 11.8: Staging of lymphoma by Cotswolds modification of the Ann Arbor staging system	
Stage	*Area of involvement*
I	Single lymph node group
II	Multiple lymph node groups on same side of diaphragm
III	Multiple lymph node groups on both sides of diaphragm
IV	Multiple extranodal sites or lymph nodes and extranodal disease
X	Bulk >10 cm
E	Extranodal extension or single, isolated site of extranodal disease
A/B	B symptoms: Weight loss >10%, fever, and drenching night sweats

Sites are denoted by: Lymph nodes (N), liver (H), spleen (S), lung (L), bone (O), skin (D), and marrow (M).

Q. What do you mean by A and B groups in staging?

Ans.

◆ A denotes asymptomatic patients
◆ B denotes patients having:
  – Weight loss more than 10% in last 6 months
  – Unexplained fever more than 38°C
  – Night sweats.

Q. How will you treat this patient?

Ans. This patient has involvement of cervical lymph nodes on both sides.

If staging investigation reveals that the disease is confined only to the cervical lymph nodes (stage II) I will treat this patient with wide field megavoltage radiotherapy. The radiotherapy is given as a wide mantle field in a dose of 3,000–4,000 cGy over a 4-weeks period.

Patient should be kept under regular follow-up.

Q. What is the area of irradiation for Hodgkin's disease?

Ans. Stage I and stage II disease is highly sensitive to radiotherapy (Fig. 11.16).

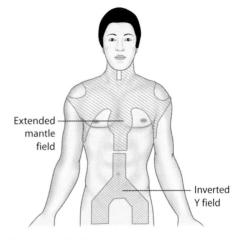

Fig. 11.16: Field of radiotherapy for lymphoma.

- *For disease confined to the cervical node or axillary or mediastinal nodes*—extended mantle radiotherapy is indicated.
- *For disease in the subdiaphragmatic nodes*—an inverted Y field of radiation is recommended.

Q. How will you treat recurrent disease following radiotherapy?

Ans. Most of the relapses occur within 2 years of radiotherapy. The recurrent disease is treated with combination chemotherapy.

Combination chemotherapy using adriamycin, bleomycin, vinblastine, and dacarbazine (ABVD) or mechlorethamine, vincristine, prednisone, and procarbazine (MOPP) regimen.

Q. What is the treatment for stage III and stage IV disease?

Ans. The treatment is primarily by combination chemotherapy.

Q. What is the standard chemotherapy regime for Hodgkin's lymphoma?

Ans. A combination chemotherapy using ABVD is very effective in Hodgkin's lymphoma.
- *A: Adriamycin (doxorubicin)*—25 mg/sq. meter IV on days 1 and 15.
- *B: Bleomycin*—10 mg/sq. meter on days 1 and 15.
- *V: Vinblastine*—6 mg/sq. meter on days 1 and 15.
- *D: Dacarbazine* (DTIC)—150 mg/sq. meter on days 1–5.

Repeat every 28 days for six cycles.

Q. What is mechlorethamine, vincristine, prednisone, and procarbazine (MOPP) regimen of chemotherapy?

Ans. This is also a standard chemotherapy for Hodgkin's lymphoma.
- *M: Mechlorethamine*—6 mg/sq. meter on days 1 and 8.
- *O: Oncovin (vincristine)*—1.4 mg/sq. meter (not more than 2.5 mg) IV on days 1 and 8.
- *P: Procarbazine*—100 mg/sq. meter orally on days 1–14.
- *P: Prednisolone*—40 mg/sq. meter orally on days 1–14.

Repeat every 28 days for six cycles.

Q. What are the follow-up protocols for Hodgkin's lymphoma?

Ans. Most of the relapse occurs within 2 years.
- *First year*—every 2 months
- *Second year*—every 3 months
- *Third year*—every 4 months
- *Fourth year*—every 6 months.
  Thereafter yearly follow-up.

In each follow-up visit—detailed clinical history and examination, hemogram. Other investigations depending on the symptoms and any findings on the clinical examination.

Q. What are the side effects of chemotherapy?

Ans. The important side effects are:
- Varying degrees of neutropenia and/or thrombocytopenia and anemia due to bone marrow suppression.
- Vincristine causes peripheral as well as autonomic neuropathies.
- Immunosuppression leading to increased susceptibility of infection with tuberculosis, cytomegalovirus, or other viruses.

Q. How will you treat superior mediastinal syndrome?

Ans.
* Confirmation of diagnosis by lymph node biopsy, mediastinoscopy, or thoracoscopy.
* If patient has respiratory distress urgent treatment with corticosteroid or radiotherapy may provide relief of symptoms.

Q. What are the characteristics of non-Hodgkin's lymphoma?

Ans.
* Non-Hodgkin's lymphoma is a heterogeneous group of tumors of the immune system.
* Majority of the patients presents with painless enlargement of one or more lymph node groups. Occasionally extranodal site may be the primary site of the disease. This may include GI tract, tracheobronchial tree, central and peripheral nervous system, skin, orbit thyroid, etc.
* Poorly differentiated type is usually disseminated at presentation with involvement of bone marrow and hepatic involvement.
* Involvement of Waldeyer's ring, retroperitoneal nodes, epitrochlear nodes, inguinal nodes, and popliteal nodes are more commonly seen in NHL.
* Bone marrow involvement is more common in NHL.

Q. What are the different types of non-Hodgkin's lymphoma (NHL)?

Ans. The different types of NHL include:
* *Low-grade NHL:*
  - Small lymphocytic type.
  - Follicular predominantly small cell type.
  - Follicular mixed cell type.
* *Intermediate-grade NHL:*
  - Follicular predominantly large cell type.
  - Diffuse—small cell, large cell, or mixed type.
* *High-grade NHL:*
  - Large cell immunoblastic.
  - Lymphoblastic.
  - Burkitt's lymphoma.

Q. What is the chemotherapy regimen for non-Hodgkin's lymphoma (NHL)?

Ans. Most patients with NHL have advanced disease at presentation. CHOP is a standard chemotherapy regimen for different types of NHL.
* *C*—Cyclophosphamide 750 mg/sq. meter IV on day 1.
* *H*—Doxorubicin 50 mg/sq. meter IV on day 1.
* *O*—Oncovin (vincristine) 1.4 mg/sq. meter IV on day 1 (not more than 2 mg).
* *P*—Prednisolone 100 mg orally for days 1–5.
Repeat every 21 days for at least six cycles.

Q. What are the alternative regimens for non-Hodgkin's lymphoma (NHL) treatment?

Ans.
* CVP: Cyclophosphamide, vincristine, and prednisone.
* COPP: Cyclophosphamide, vinblastine, procarbazine, and prednisone.
* COP: Cyclophosphamide, mitoxantrone, vincristine, and prednisone.

■ CERVICAL RIB

Clinical Examination

See Page No. 382, Chapter 9.

History

* *Pain*: Duration, onset, site of pain, radiation of pain, character of pain, and relation of pain with exercise.
* Pain due to nerve compression occurs along the distribution of C8 and T1 segments.
* Pain due to vascular compression occurs during exercise when the patient uses the upper limbs during working and gets relief with rest.
* *Other symptoms due to nerve compression*: Tingling, numbness and weakness, and wasting of the small muscles of the hand.
* *Other symptoms due to ischemia*: Ischemic ulcer or gangrene—onset, site progress, and type of gangrene—dry or moist.
* Any swelling in the supraclavicular fossa (patient with cervical rib may present with a swelling in supraclavicular fossa).

Examination—Inspection/Palpation

* Examine the swelling in supraclavicular fossa
* Examine the gangrenous area
* *Neurological examination of the upper limb:* Motor and sensory system
* Examination of peripheral pulses
* Adson's test.

Summary of a Case of Cervical Rib

This 60-year-old gentleman presented with a swelling in the right side of the neck for last 15 years. He complains of dull aching pain in the right upper limb for last 3 years, the pain is aggravated while the patient uses his right upper limb. Patient complains of acute onset of pain in the right middle finger about 1 month back. Following the onset of pain patient noticed gradual onset of black discoloration of the tip of the right middle finger and afterwards the black discoloration has extended up to the middle of the right middle finger. Patient is not a known hypertensive or diabetic. No history suggestive of ischemic heart disease. Patient has no other systemic complaints (Fig. 11.17).

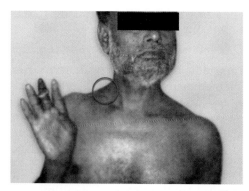

Fig. 11.17: Right cervical rib with ischemic gangrene of the right middle finger

Courtesy: Dr A Lakra, IPGMER, Kolkata

On examination: There is a bony hard swelling in the right supraclavicular region 3 cm × 2 cm, surface smooth, nontender, overlying skin normal, and the swelling is fixed. There is a dry gangrene involving the right middle finger. The gangrene has extended up to the middle of middle finger and there is a line of demarcation between the gangrenous and the healthy area.

There are signs of ischemia in the right upper limb. The temperature of the right hand and forearm is less than the left side, there is loss of hair in the distal forearm on the right side, and the nails are brittle on the right side.

The right radial, ulnar, brachial, axillary, and the subclavian pulses are absent. Other peripheral pulses are normal.

Q. What is your diagnosis?

Ans. This is a case of right-sided cervical rib with ischemic gangrene of the right middle finger with evidence of peripheral ischemia in the upper limb.

Q. What are the other possibilities in this patient?

Ans.
* Ischemic gangrene of the right middle finger due to diabetes mellitus
* Atherosclerotic peripheral vascular disease with ischemic gangrene of the right middle finger
* Embolic gangrene
* Ischemic gangrene of the right middle finger due to collagen vascular disease.

Q. What investigations will you do in this patient?

Ans.
* An X-ray of cervical spine to detect cervical rib or to ascertain the nature of bony swelling palpated in the neck.
* As there is vascular compression symptoms and ischemic gangrene, I will do a duplex scanning of the right upper limb vessels to assess the vascular supply of the upper limb. The duplex scanning may demonstrate the site of occlusion of the vessels and any thrombus if present may be visible.
* Other routine workup:
  - Blood for complete hemogram
  - Blood for postprandial (PP) sugar
  - Lipid profile
  - Chest X-ray
  - Electrocardiogram (ECG).

Q. How will you treat this patient?

Ans.
* This patient has a cervical rib with occlusion of right subclavian artery and ischemic gangrene of the right index finger
* I will consider extraperiosteal excision of the cervical rib
* For thrombotic occlusion of subclavian artery—a vascular bypass graft is required between the proximal subclavian artery and the axillary artery
* The gangrenous finger needs a ray amputation.

Q. What is the incidence of cervical rib?

Ans. Approximately 0.5% of people has cervical rib. In 50% cases, this is unilateral and more commonly found on the right side.

Q. What are the different varieties of cervical rib?

Ans. The cervical rib arising from the transverse process of the 7th cervical vertebra may be (Figs 11.18A to D):

* A complete rib articulating with manubrium sterni or the first rib (Fig. 11.18A).
* The rib may be incomplete and the free end expands into a bony mass (Fig. 11.18B).
* The rib is incomplete but the free end is connected to first rib by fibrous band (Fig. 11.18C).
* There is no bony rib but a fibrous band may pass from the transverse process of the 7th cervical vertebra to the first rib (Fig. 11.18D).

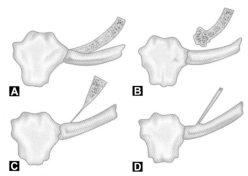

Figs 11.18A to D: Types of cervical rib

Subclavian vessels and the lower trunk of brachial plexus may be compressed by this fibrous cord.

Q. What is the consequence of the presence of a cervical rib?

Ans. At the exit from the neck the brachial plexus and subclavian artery passes through a narrow triangle (scalene triangle) bounded by scalenus anterior in front, scalenus medius behind, and first rib forms the base of the triangle. When the cervical rib is present the base of the triangle is raised by the height of one vertebra and the subclavian artery and first thoracic nerve (or the lower trunk of brachial plexus) is angulated or compressed (Fig. 11.19).

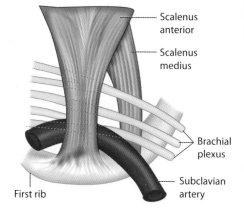

Fig. 11.19: Scalene triangle

Q. What are the changes in the artery?

Ans. The artery may become constricted due to angulation and there is a poststenotic dilatation for 2–3 cm beyond the constriction. There may be a thrombus formation in the artery in the poststenotic dilated segment or in the constricted segment and a portion of the thrombus may be dislodged as emboli and may cause gangrene at the tip of finger. The thrombus may extend proximally and when this involves the vertebral artery origin the vertebrobasilar insufficiency may occur (Fig. 11.20).

Q. What are the effects of nerve compression?

Ans. The first thoracic nerve or lower trunk of brachial plexus is angulated and compressed against the cervical rib. There will be tingling and numbness along the distribution of 8th cervical and 1st dorsal nerve.

Q. Cervical rib is a congenital condition, how do you explain presentation at a late age?

Ans. In majority of patient the cervical rib may remain asymptomatic throughout life. With age there is gradual saging of shoulder girdle (due to some atrophy of the shoulder muscles) and this may aggravate the angulation of the subclavian vessels and the 1st dorsal nerve.

There may be associated spondylotic changes.

Q. What is Adson's test?

Ans. This is a test to detect subclavian artery compression.

Patient seated and the radial pulse is felt with the arm in abducted position. The patient is then asked to extend the neck, take a deep breath, and turn his head towards the same side (Fig. 11.21).

If there is obliteration or diminution of the radial pulse the sign is positive.

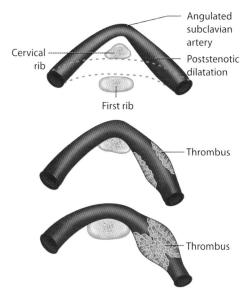

Fig. 11.20: Changes in the artery

Q. How does the patients of cervical rib usually presents?

Ans.

* May present with swelling in the neck.
* May present with pain, tingling and numbness, and sensory loss along the distribution of C8 and T1 segments. The pain is brought on by the use of the arm and gets aggravated when the arm is raised above the head and the pain is relieved by rest.
* Motor weakness and wasting of the small muscles of hand (supplied by C8 and T1 nerve segments).

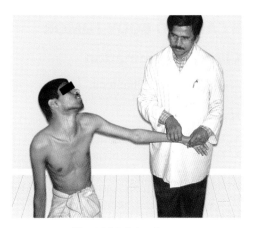

Fig. 11.21: Adson's test

* Vasomotor symptoms like coldness of fingers, cyanosis, trophic changes, ulceration, and gangrene may occur in the fingers.

Q. What are the differential diagnoses for patients presenting with cervical rib?

Ans.

* Cervical spondylosis
* Carpal tunnel syndrome
* Syringomyelia
* Motor neuron disease
* Pancoast tumor

* Atherosclerotic peripheral vascular disease
* Raynaud's disease.

Q. What is the treatment for cervical rib with mild symptoms?

Ans.

* In patient with mild symptom a conservative treatment is to be tried first. Exclude other causes of the presenting symptom.
* Shoulder girdle exercise to strengthen the shoulder muscle to reduce the tendency for the shoulder girdle to drop which aggravates the symptoms.
* Analgesics [nonsteroidal anti-inflammatory drug (NSAID)] for relief of pain.

Q. What is the operative treatment for cervical rib?

Ans.

* Extraperiosteal resection of the cervical rib.
* Sometimes excision of the rib alone does not cause relief of symptoms.
* Division of scalenus anterior muscle is required for relief of symptoms.
* If vasomotor symptoms are predominant a cervical sympathectomy is also required. This involves removal of the lower half of the stellate ganglion and second and third thoracic ganglia.

■ CAROTID BODY TUMOR

Clinical Examination

See Page No. 381, Chapter 9.

History

* Detail history about the swelling.
* Onset and progress of the swelling (carotid body tumors are very slow growing and develops over many years).
* Any swelling on the opposite side (carotid body tumor may be bilateral).
* Any pain (usually painless).
* Any history of syncopal attack (rarely the tumor may cause compression of the carotid artery and there may be history of transient ischemic attacks).

Examination—Inspection/Palpation

* Swelling (palpate gently—pressure over the swelling may precipitate a syncopal attack).
* Site (usually located at the upper part of the neck near the carotid bifurcation at the anterior border of the sternocleidomastoid muscle at the level of the upper border of the thyroid cartilage).
* Size (variable, may be as small as 2 cm and may be around 10 cm in diameter).
* Shape (usually spherical).
* Surface (usually smooth, may sometimes be irregular).
* Consistency (usually firm or hard in feel).
* Pulsation (usually swelling is pulsatile because of its close relation to the common carotid artery).

- *Mobility*: Better mobile form side to side than above downwards.
- Relation with the sternocleidomastoid muscle (on contracting the muscle), the swelling becomes less prominent—suggesting that the swelling lies deep to the sternocleidomastoid muscle.

Q. What is your case? (Summary of a case of carotid body tumor)

Ans. This 50-year-old lady presented with a swelling in the upper part of the neck in the left side for last 2 years which is growing very slowly in size. She gives history of two bouts of fainting attacks in last 1 year, the last attack was 3 months back (Fig. 11.22).

On examination: There is a firm swelling in the left lateral side of the neck at the level of upper border of the thyroid cartilage at the anterior border of sternocleidomastoid. The swelling is globular about 2 cm in diameter, the margins are

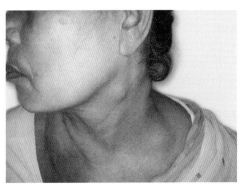

Fig. 11.22: Carotid body tumor on the left side
Courtesy: Dr Subhra Ganguly, IPGMER, Kolkata

well defined, surface is smooth, nontender, free from skin and underlying structure and readily mobile from side to side, but up and down mobility is slightly restricted, the swelling is pulsatile (transmitted pulsation of the common carotid artery), and the swelling is situated at the region of the bifurcation of common carotid artery. There are no palpable lymph nodes in the neck.

Q. What is your diagnosis?

Ans. This is a case of carotid body tumor on the left side.

Q. What else this swelling could be?

Ans.
- Koch's lymphadenitis
- Metastatic lymph node
- Carotid artery aneurysm
- Sternomastoid tumor
- Solitary thyroid nodule at the level of thyroid cartilage.

Q. Why there is fainting attack in patient with carotid body tumor?

Ans. This is due to impairment of cerebral circulation. As the tumor grows it compress the common or internal carotid artery and this may be aggravated in certain postures resulting in transient syncopal attack.

Q. How will you treat this patient?

Ans. I would like to do a duplex scanning and a carotid angiography to assess the relation of the swelling with the carotid artery.

Q. What do you find in carotid angiogram in such patients?

Ans. Carotid artery may be displaced or there may be splaying of carotid fork. There may be presence of an abnormal mass of new vessels. Angiography may differentiate the swelling from the aneurysm.

Q. Would you like to do a fine-needle aspiration cytology (FNAC) or biopsy?

Ans. When clinical diagnosis is carotid body tumor—FNAC or open biopsy is contraindicated, as this is a very vascular tumor and any attempted FNAC or biopsy may result in bleeding.

Q. How will you treat this patient?

Ans.

* I will consider excision of this tumor.
* In some cases it can be dissected off from the carotid artery and excised.
* In other cases when the tumor is large and adherent to carotid fork—then a segment of carotid artery is to be excised along with the tumor.
* Before excision of the tumor a stent is inserted into the carotid artery so that the cerebral circulation is maintained to prevent cerebral damage. After excision a bypass graft between the common carotid artery and internal carotid artery is required.

Q. What are the complications of surgery?

Ans. The most important complication of surgery is impairment of cerebral blood supply resulting in contralateral hemiplegia. This can be avoided by inserting a stent from common carotid artery to the internal carotid artery during excision of the tumor along with a segment of common carotid artery.

Q. You have explored the mass with the diagnosis of a lymph node enlargement and found it to be a carotid body tumor. What will you do?

Ans. If the operation was attempted under local anesthesia the procedure should be stopped immediately. For proper management the operation is to be planned jointly with the help of a vascular surgeon.

Q. What will happen if the common carotid artery is ligated?

Ans. This will result in contralateral hemiplegia.

Q. What is carotid body tumor pathologically?

Ans.

* Carotid body tumor is regarded as nonchromaffin paraganglioma.
* These tumors are regarded as benign but there is chance of local recurrence following excision and rarely these tumors may metastasize.
* It is hard and whitish yellow in color.
* It is a well-encapsulated tumor with yellowish orange cut surface with dense fibrous septa.
* The cells of carotid body tumors are not hormonally active.

Q. What are the histological features of carotid body tumor?

Ans.

* Solid masses of cells resembling chief cells.
* The cells may slow pleomorphic nucleus.
* The cells may stain black chromic acid.

Q. What is carotid body?

Ans. Carotid body is a flat brownish nodule situated in the adventitial coat of common carotid artery at or just below its bifurcation.

Two types of cells are present in the carotid body:
1. Chief cells containing granules of catecholamines.
2. Supporting cells having long processes embedded in the adjacent capillaries.

Q. What is carotid body hyperplasia?

Ans. People living in high altitudes are exposed to chronic hypoxia. In such individuals there is proliferation of these chemoreceptors cell leading to carotid body hyperplasia. The carotid body is one of the chemoreceptor organ of the body.

Q. What are the other chemoreceptor apparatus in our body?

Ans.

* *Aortic bodies:* Aortic bodies are situated at the points of origin of left coronary, innominate artery, bifurcation of pulmonary artery, or in the arch of the aorta.
* *Glomus jugulare:* Lies in relation to the bulb of the internal jugular vein.
* *Glomus intravagale:* Lies in relation to ganglion nodosum of the vagus nerve.
* *Other paragangliomas* lying in relation to glossopharyngeal nerve, femoral artery, small bowel mesentery, and the retroperitoneum (Fig. 11.23).

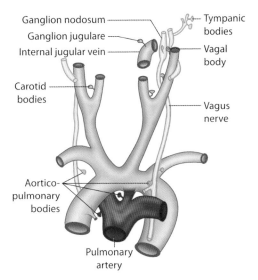

Fig. 11.23: Different chemoreceptor organs

Q. What are the functions of this chemoreceptor apparatus?

Ans. The different chemoreceptor apparatus of the body are sensitive to hypoxia and pH changes in the body and helps in autoregulation of circulation and respiration.

Q. What should be the management strategy for a carotid body tumor in an elderly patient with comorbid medical disease?

Ans. This tumor is very slow growing and may be asymptomatic. So, in elderly and enfeebled patient can be observed without active intervention.

■ PHARYNGEAL POUCH

Clinical Examination

See Page No. 382, Chapter 9.

History

* Detail history of swelling.
* Swelling in the neck (in early phase there may be no apparent swelling in the neck, in long-standing case swelling becomes visible on one side of the neck).
* History of regurgitation of food into the mouth (usually no acid or bile is present in the regurgitated food).
* Any history of cough or choking (regurgitation of food at night may cause bouts of coughing and choking).
* Any history of dysphagia (in long-standing case dysphagia may occur). Patient swallows some amount of food and when the pouch fills up and presses on the esophagus, resulting in dysphagia.
* Any gurgling sound in the neck (particularly occurring on compression of the cervical swelling).

Examination—Inspection/Palpation

* Site (swelling usually lies behind the sternocleidomastoid muscle and below the level of thyroid cartilage).
* Size, shape, surface, and margin (size is variable, surface is usually smooth, and margins are usually indistinct).
* *Compressibility:* The swelling may be emptied by compression. This may result in regurgitation of food into the mouth and the swelling may disappear. The swelling may refill during the next meal.
* Percussion over the swelling—usually resonant.
* Relation of the swelling with sternocleidomastoid muscle on contraction of the muscle the swelling becomes less prominent—suggesting that the swelling lies deep to the sternocleidomastoid muscle.
* Examination of chest to exclude—lung collapse, pneumonia, or lung abscess.

Q. What is your case? (Summary of a case of pharyngeal pouch)

Ans. This 60-year-old gentleman presented with a swelling on the right lateral side of the neck for last 3 years gradually increasing in size. Patient complains of a sensation of a foreign body in the throat. Patient also complains of occasional regurgitation of food into the mouth. He occasionally c/o gurgling sound in the neck during swallowing.

On examination: There is a soft cystic swelling 4.5 × 2.5 cm in size on the right lateral side of the neck. The swelling lies behind the sternocleidomastoid muscle at the lower border of the thyroid cartilage. The surface is smooth but the margins are not well defined. The swelling is compressible and can be emptied completely. Fluctuation is positive but transillumination is negative.

Q. What is your diagnosis?

Ans. This is a case of pharyngeal pouch on the right side of the neck.

Q. What are the other possibilities?

Ans.
* Cold abscess in the neck
* Dermoid cyst

+ Hemangioma
+ Lymphatic cyst
+ Branchial cyst.

Q. How will you confirm your diagnosis?

Ans.
+ The diagnosis may be confirmed by a barium swallow X-ray.
+ Small amount of barium is given and the examination is done under fluoroscopic control.
+ There is filling of the pouch by barium and the pouch can cause lateral compression of the esophagus.
+ On compression of the swelling barium may be emptied from the pouch into the esophagus.

Q. Would you like to do an esophagoscopy?

Ans. If the diverticulum is demonstrated in barium swallow study an esophagoscopy is not required. During esophagoscopy if the scope enters into the pouch unknowingly it may result in perforation and mediastinitis.

Q. How will you treat this patient?

Ans. As the pouch is symptomatic and large I will consider excision of the pouch and cricopharyngeal myotomy.

Q. What are the indications of surgery in pharyngeal pouch?

Ans.
+ Patient with progressive symptoms.
+ Disordered upper esophageal sphincter mechanism resulting in dysphagia.

Q. How will you identify the pouch during operation?

Ans. After induction of anesthesia an endoscope identifies the pouch and a nasogastric tube is passed through the esophagus. The pharyngeal pouch may be packed with acriflavine soaked ribbon gauge for better identification during surgery.

Q. Why do you want to do a cricopharyngeal myotomy?

Ans. One explanation for the development of pharyngeal pouch is incoordinate contraction of the two parts of the inferior constrictor muscle. Normally when the thyropharyngeus part of the inferior constrictor muscle contracts the cricopharyngeus muscle relaxes thereby allowing food to pass distally. Due to neuromuscular incoordination both the thyropharyngeus and cricopharyngeus muscle may contract simultaneously. As a result there is a rise of intrapharyngeal pressure and the mucous membrane bulges out through a weakness at the junction of thyropharyngeus and the cricopharyngeus muscle at the posterior midline. This area of weakness is called Killian's dehiscence. There is hypertrophy of cricopharyngeus muscle.

So, the myotomy of cricopharyngeus muscle and circular muscle fibers of the upper esophagus forming the upper esophageal sphincter mechanism is required to prevent subsequent development of a pharyngeal pouch and for relief of dysphagia.

Q. What are the complications of this operation?

Ans.
- Wound infection
- Mediastinitis
- Pharyngeal fistula
- Upper esophageal stenosis.

Q. What is the alternative technique for tackling the pharyngeal pouch?

Ans. An endoscopic stapling device divides the anterior wall of the pharyngeal pouch and the posterior wall of the pharynx and at the same time staples the divided pharyngeal wall. This division also allows a full cricopharyngeal myotomy.

Q. What is pharyngeal pouch?

Ans. It is a pulsion diverticulum of the pharynx where there is herniation of the pharyngeal mucosa through the Killian's dehiscence (Fig. 11.24).

Q. What is Killian's dehiscence?

Ans. The inferior constrictor muscle has two parts:
1. *Thyropharyngeus muscle:* Fanning out obliquely from the thyroid cartilage and meeting the corresponding muscle of the opposite side in the midline.
2. *Cricopharyngeus muscle:* Horizontal fibers attached anteriorly to the cricoid cartilage and meeting in the posterior midline with the fiber from the opposite side.

On the posterior aspect of the pharyngeal wall and in between these two heads of inferior constrictor there is a potential area of weakness called Killian's dehiscence. There may be a depression at this site called pharyngeal dimple.

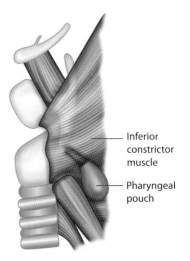

Inferior constrictor muscle

Pharyngeal pouch

Fig. 11.24: Pharyngeal pouch

Q. What are the characteristics of these two parts of inferior constrictor muscle?

Ans. Their arrangement and functions are different.

The fibers of the thyropharyngeus muscle are arranged obliquely arising from the oblique line in the lamina of the thyroid cartilage and are inserted posteriorly in the fibrous median raphe meeting the same fibers from the opposite side. The nerve supply is from pharyngeal plexus carrying fibers of cranial accessory nerve.

The thyropharyngeus muscle helps in propulsion of food downward during deglutition.

Cricopharyngeus muscle fibers are disposed horizontally and arises from the side of the cricoid cartilage and posteriorly becomes continuous with the same muscle arising on the opposite side from cricoid cartilage. There is no median raphe.

Cricopharyngeus is supplied by recurrent laryngeal nerve and the external laryngeal nerve.

During deglutition when the thyropharyngeus contracts the cricopharyngeus relaxes thereby helping downward propulsion of swallowed food. Cricopharyngeus muscle has a sphincteric action and remains normally in tonic contraction except during the act of deglutition when it relaxes and food is pushed down (Fig. 11.25).

Q. Why is the pharyngeal pouch seen in the lateral side of the neck?

Ans. The pharyngeal pouch starts in the middle in posterior pharyngeal wall but as the swelling expands it meets the resistance of the vertebral column and deviates laterally on either side usually to the left side of the neck.

Q. What are the different stages in the development of a pharyngeal pouch?

Ans. The pharyngeal pouch starts as a small diverticulum in the posterior midline and then enlarges further to produce a visible swelling on the lateral side of the neck. There are three stages in the development of a pharyngeal pouch.

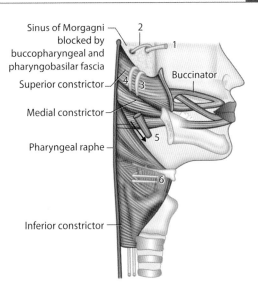

Fig. 11.25: Arrangement of constrictor muscles of pharynx

Q. What are the characteristics of stage I pharyngeal pouch?

Ans.
- Small diverticulum
- Pointing towards the vertebral column
- Asymptomatic
- Incidentally diagnosed during barium swallow examination
- Occasionally may have a sensation of foreign body in the throat.

Q. What are the characteristics of stage II pharyngeal pouch?

Ans. Diverticulum becomes:
- Larger and globular
- Mouth of the pouch is vertical
- Regurgitation of undigested food after a variable time of meals and more so when turning from one side to the other
- Sense of suffocation and violent bouts of cough may occur.

Q. What are the characteristics of stage III pharyngeal pouch?

Ans.
- The diverticulum becomes larger and usually points to the lateral side of the neck and the opening of the pouch becomes horizontal.
- May compress esophagus causing dysphagia.
- Gurgling sound in the neck during swallowing as the food materials enters into the pouch.
- Loss of weight and cachexia due to starvation.
- Aspiration pneumonia and lung abscess may be the presenting symptom.

Salivary Gland

Clinical Examination (*See* Page No. 382, Chapter 9)

History

- Detailed history about the swelling.
- Onset, progress (mixed parotid tumor is a usually slow growing tumor and may present over months or years).
- Any history of rapid increase in size (rapid increase in size following long years of slow growth suggest malignant change in a preexisting benign tumor).
- Rapid increase in size from the onset usually suggests a malignant tumor.
- Any variation of the size of the swelling with eating (in salivary ductal calculi the gland may swell during eating and the swelling may diminish in size in between meals).
- Any history of pain during eating and increase in size of the swelling (in ductal calculi there is dull aching pain over the swelling during eating and the pain disappears when the swelling diminishes in size).
- Any history of purulent discharge from the ductal opening in the mouth (parotid duct opens in the vestibule of the mouth opposite the crown of upper second molar tooth, submandibular duct opens in the floor of mouth on either side of frenulum linguae).
- Any history suggestive of facial nerve palsy.
  - Any asymmetry of face.
  - Difficulty in closing the eyes.
  - Difficulty in chewing food (food may collect in the vestibule of the mouth due to weakness of buccinator muscle which pushes the food from the vestibule of the mouth into the oral cavity during chewing).
  - Any drooling of saliva from the angle of the mouth.

Local Examination

Examination of Neck—Inspection/Palpation

- Inspections
- *Swelling*: Position and extent (parotid gland is situated in the parotid region, submandibular gland lies in submandibular triangle).

- Shape and size (variable, may be spherical or irregular in shape).
- Surface and margin (in benign tumor surface is usually smooth; in malignant tumors surface may become irregular).
- Skin over the swelling.
- Consistency (usually firm in feel. In adenolymphoma the consistency is typically soft and cystic and may show positive fluctuation).
- *Mobility*: Test for fixity to skin and to the underlying structures (benign tumor are usually mobile—free from skin and underlying structure. In advanced malignancy the swelling may be fixed to the skin or underlying structures).
- *Examination of deep part of the parotid gland*:
  – Inspect the oral cavity, enlargement of the deep part of the gland will push the tonsil and the pillar of the fauces toward the midline.
  – Palpation of the deep part of the parotid gland by bidigital palpation—keeping one finger in the tonsillar fossa and the other finger in the upper part of the neck behind the ramus of the mandible.
- Examination of the deep part of the submandibular gland.
  Palpated bidigitally keeping one finger in the floor of the mouth in between the alveolus and lateral margin of tongue and other finger in the submandibular triangle.
- Examination for facial nerve palsy.
- Examination of cervical lymph node.
- Examination of other salivary glands.
- Test temporomandibular joint movement.

▌MIXED PAROTID TUMOR

Q. What is your case? (Summary of a case of mixed parotid tumor)

Ans. This 45-year-old lady presented with a swelling in the right side of the upper part of the neck below the ear lobule for last 8 years, which is increasing very slowly ever since. No pain over the swelling, no history suggestive of facial nerve paralysis. There are no other swellings in the neck (Fig. 12.1).

On examination: There is a firm swelling in the right parotid region 6 cm × 4 cm in size, surface is smooth, margins are well defined and rounded, free from the skin and underlying structures. The deep lobe of the parotid gland is not enlarged. There is no evidence of facial nerve palsy. There are no palpable lymph nodes in the neck.

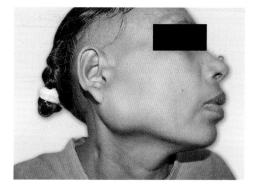

Fig. 12.1: Mixed parotid tumor involving the right side

Courtesy: Dr Ajay Kumar, IPGME and R, Kolkata

Q. What is your diagnosis?

Ans. This is a case of mixed parotid tumor on the right side.

Q. Why do you say this is a parotid swelling?

Ans. The swelling is situated in the parotid region. The ear lobule is pushed upward and swelling has filled the furrow in between the posterior border of the mandible and the mastoid process.

Q. Why do you say this is mixed parotid tumor?

Ans. History and clinical examination suggests this to be a benign tumor and mixed parotid tumor is the most common benign tumor of the parotid gland. So this likely to be mixed parotid tumor.

Q. How do you palpate the parotid gland?

Ans. The parotid swelling is situated in front and behind the ear lobule and fills the furrow between the ramus of the mandible and the mastoid process. The superficial lobe of the parotid gland is palpated with palmar aspect of the fingers (Fig. 12.2).

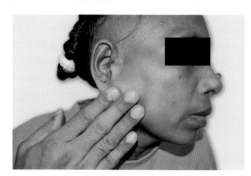

Fig. 12.2: Palpation of the superficial lobe of parotid gland

Q. Where do you find the parotid duct orifice?

Ans. The orifice of the parotid duct (Stensen's duct) is inspected on the buccal aspect of the cheek opposite the upper second molar tooth (Fig. 12.3).

Q. How will you palpate the parotid duct?

Ans. The parotid duct is palpated as it lies on the masseter muscle by a finger rolling across the masseter muscle as the patient clinches his teeth to make the muscle taut (Fig. 12.4A). The terminal part of the duct is palpated bidigitally between the index finger inside the mouth and the thumb over the cheek (Fig. 12.4B).

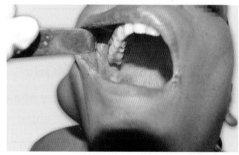

Fig. 12.3: Inspection of parotid duct orifice at the vestibule of mouth opposite second upper molar tooth

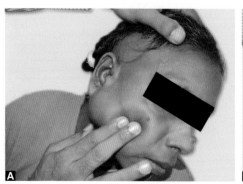
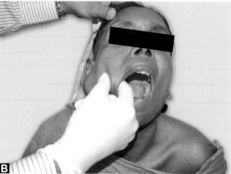

Figs 12.4A and B: (A) Palpation of right parotid duct by rolling fingers over the masseter muscle; (B) Bidigital palpation of the right parotid duct

Q. How will you palpate the deep part of the parotid gland?

Ans. By bidigital palpation with one finger inside the mouth against the tonsillar fossa and the other finger outside in the parotid region (Fig. 12.5).

Q. What are the symptoms of facial nerve palsy?

Ans. In patients with parotid tumor the branches or the trunk of the facial nerve may be affected.

* Patient may have difficulty in closing the eyes due to paralysis of the orbicularis oculi.
* Patient may have difficulty in chewing of food as the food gets accumulated in the vestibule of the mouth due to paralysis of buccinator muscle.
* Patient complains of deviation of angle of mouth while talking, laughing, difficulty in lip movement, whistle blowing due to paralysis of orbicularis oris.

Q. How do you test for facial nerve palsy?

Ans.

Orbicularis oculi: Steady the head of patient. Ask the patient to close his eyes. Failure of closure of eyelids suggests paralysis of orbicularis oris. If the patient can close his eye try to open the eyelids with your fingers. If it can be opened easily, it suggests weakness of the orbicularis oculi (Fig. 12.6).

Frontal belly of occipitofrontalis: Ask the patient to look up toward the roof. Normally, there are furrows in the forehead. Absence of these furrows indicates paralysis of frontal belly of occipitofrontalis (Fig. 12.7).

Corrugator supercilii: Ask the patient to frown. There is appearance of corrugation in the forehead. Absence of these corrugations suggests paralysis of corrugator supercilii (Fig. 12.8).

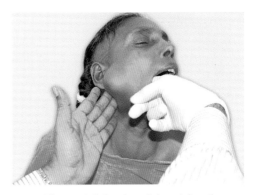

Fig. 12.5: Palpation of deep lobe of parotid gland

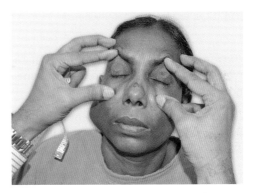

Fig. 12.6: Testing for orbicularis oculi

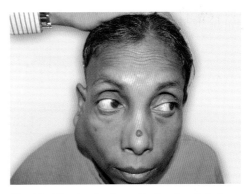

Fig. 12.7: Testing for frontal belly of occipitofrontalis by asking the patient to look up and look for appearance of transverse furrows in forehead

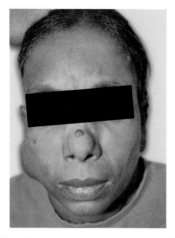

Fig. 12.8: Test for corrugator supercili

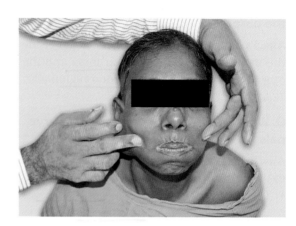

Fig. 12.9: Test for buccinator muscle

Buccinator muscle: Ask the patient to blow with the mouth closed and feel the tone of the buccinator (Fig. 12.9).

Orbicularis oris: Ask the patient to blow whistle. Failure indicates paralysis of orbicularis oris (Fig. 12.10).

Levator anguli oris: Ask the patient to show his teeth. Paralysis of levator anguli oris causes deviation of angle of mouth toward the opposite side (Fig. 12.11).

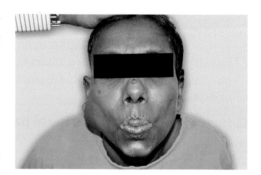

Fig. 12.10: Test for orbicularis oris

Platysma: Ask the patient to stretch her neck. The contracted platysma muscle stands out. Paralysis of platysma causes loss of contraction (Fig. 12.12).

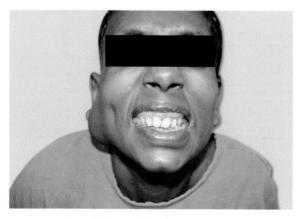

Fig. 12.11: Test for levator anguli oris

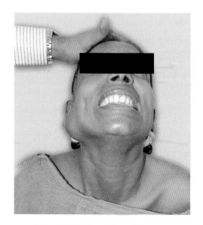

Fig. 12.12: Test for platysma

Q. What are the other possibilities?

+ Adenolymphoma of the parotid gland
+ Chronic sialadenitis
+ Carcinoma of parotid gland
+ Cervical lymphadenopathy due to tuberculous lesion or metastasis of lymphoma
+ Lipoma
+ Fibroma
+ Rhabdomyosarcoma.

Q. How will you treat this patient?

Ans.
+ I will do fine needle aspiration cytology (FNAC) from the swelling.
+ If report is benign, I will do baseline workup to assess fitness of patient for anesthesia and surgery.
+ I will consider superficial parotidectomy in this patient.

Q. Can FNAC cause tumor cell implantation in the track?

Ans. Earlier, FNAC was contraindicated in parotid tumor for fear of implantation of tumor cells into the tract. However, evidence suggests that a FNAC using 18-G needle does not cause implantation of viable tumor cells in the needle tract.

Q. Would you like to do an incisional biopsy?

Ans. Incisional biopsy is not indicated in parotid tumors as there is chance of tumor cell implantation and parotid fistula. If incisional biopsy is done in cases of mixed parotid tumor then there is breach of the thin capsule and tumor burst into the surrounding normal tissue and may result in local recurrence.

Q. What is superficial parotidectomy?

Ans. Removal of superficial part of the parotid gland along with the tumor is called superficial parotidectomy. The superficial part of the parotid gland lies superficial to faciovenous plane.

Q. What is the incision for superficial parotidectomy?

Ans. The incision starts below the zygomatic process just in front of the tragus then curves round the ear lobule and descend downward along the anterior border of the upper third of the sternocleidomastoid muscle (Fig. 12.13).

Q. Describe the steps of superficial parotidectomy.

Ans. *See* Operative Surgery Section, Page No. 1133, 1134, Chapter 22

Q. How will you identify the facial nerve trunk during operation?

Ans. After incising the deep cervical fascia, the lower pole of the parotid gland is dissected and lifted up.

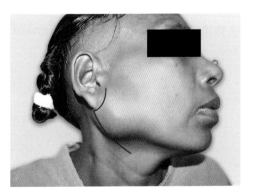

Fig. 12.13: Incision for superficial parotidectomy

The digastric muscle is dissected up to its origin. The junction of the bony and cartilaginous part of the external auditory canal is delineated. The styloid process is palpated. The facial nerve emerges at this point through the stylomastoid foramen.

Q. What are the branches of facial nerve?

Ans. The facial nerve emerges from the stylomastoid foramen and enters the posteromedial surface of the parotid gland. It initially divides into an upper division (zygomaticofacial) and a lower division (cervicofacial). Within the gland the nerve branches and rejoins to form a plexus within the parotid gland (known as pes anserinus).

The nerve branches then emerges from the upper pole, anterior border and the lower pole of the parotid gland. These branches are (Fig. 12.14):

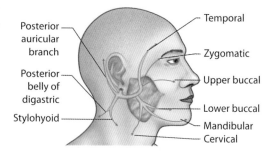

Fig. 12.14: Branches of facial nerve

- Temporal
- Zygomatic
- Upper buccal
- Lower buccal
- Mandibular
- Cervical.

Q. What is mixed parotid tumor?

Ans.
- This is a benign tumor of parotid gland.
- This is called pleomorphic salivary adenoma because there is pleomorphic appearance of this tumor.
- Epithelial cells proliferate in strands and may form a duct like structure.
- Other cell may proliferate in sheets.
- In some parts, a hyaline material may be present which separate the cell producing appearance of cartilage.
- Mucoid material may occur at one part giving a cystic appearance of the tumor.
- The adenoma may compress the peripheral normal glandular tissue producing a pseudocapsule.
- The tumor cells may penetrate this tumor capsule with multiple finger-like processes all around so that simple enucleation of the adenoma may leave behind these finger-like extensions of the tumor resulting in local recurrence.

Q. Which features suggest malignant change in a mixed parotid tumor?

Ans.
- Sudden or rapid increase in the swelling which was so long, growing very slowly
- The swelling become painful
- The swelling become hard
- The swelling become fixed to the skin and underlying structures
- Concomitant facial nerve palsy
- Surface ulceration of skin
- Presence of prominent veins over the swelling

- If the tumor has infiltrated the capsule, it may cause restriction of movement of temporomandibular joint
- Cervical lymph nodes may become enlarged.

Q. Why mixed parotid tumor recurs after excision?

Ans. The mixed parotid tumor has finger-like extension into the normal gland through the pseudocapsule formed by the normal gland substance. If the tumor is simply enucleated, these finger-like extensions will be left behind and will result in local recurrence.

Q. What are the different tumors in salivary gland?

Ans. The international classifications of salivary tumors are:
1. *Epithelial tumors*
   - *Adenomas*:
     - Pleomorphic adenomas
     - Adenolymphoma—Warthin tumor
     - Oxyphilic adenoma
     - Monomorphic adenomas
   - *Carcinomas*:
     - Acinic cell carcinoma
     - Mucoepidermoid carcinomas
     - Adenoid cystic carcinoma
     - Adenocarcinoma
     - Squamous cell carcinoma
     - Undifferentiated carcinoma
     - Carcinoma superimposed on a pleomorphic adenoma
2. *Nonepithelial tumors*:
   - Hemangioma
   - Lymphangioma
   - Neurofibroma
   - Neurilemmoma
3. Malignant lymphoma
4. Unclassified and allied condition.

Q. What are the parts of parotid gland?

Ans. Parotid gland is divided into superficial and deep parts by the faciovenous plane.

Q. What is the boundary of parotid region?

Ans. The parotid region is bounded (Fig. 12.15):
- Anteriorly—by the posterior border of mandible.
- Posteriorly—by the mastoid process and the attached sternocleidomastoid muscle.
- Below—by the posterior belly of digastric.
- Above—by the zygomatic arch.

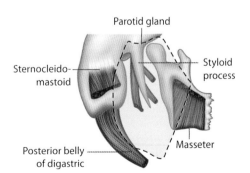

Fig. 12.15: Boundary of parotid region

Q. What is the disposition of parotid fascia?

Ans. The investing layer of deep cervical fascia splits at lower pole of parotid gland and invest the gland. This is called the false capsule of the gland. The superficial layer of this fascia gets attached above to the zygomatic arch and it prolong over the masseter muscle as masseteric fascia. The deep layer of the parotid fascia gets attached to the tympanic plate, the styloid process and the attached muscle. This deeper layer gets thickened to form the stylohyoid ligament.

Q. What is the disposition of parotid duct?

Ans. The parotid emerges from the deep part of the gland lying deep to behind the angle of the mandible. It runs forward through the gland substance receiving intralobular ducts. The main duct emerge at the anterior border of the gland and runs over the masseter muscle and then pierces the buccinator muscle runs in the submucus plane for some distance and open into a papillae in the vestibule of the mouth opposite the upper second molar tooth. Length of the parotid duct is about 5 cm.

Q. Which vein lies within the parotid gland?

Ans. The retromandibular vein formed by joining of maxillary vein and the superficial temporal vein enters the substance of the gland and joins the plexus of veins in the substance of the gland. As the retromandibular vein exits from the gland, it divides into anterior and posterior divisions.

Anterior division of retromandibular vein joins with the anterior facial vein to form the common facial vein.

Posterior division of retromandibular veins joins with the posterior auricular vein to form the external jugular vein.

Q. Which arteries lie in relation to the parotid gland?

Ans. The external carotid as it goes up pierces the posteromedial surface of the parotid gland and divides into its terminal branches—superficial temporal and maxillary artery. The posterior auricular artery may emerge from the external carotid artery within the substance of the gland and runs laterally and emerges from the posteromedial surface of the gland. The maxillary artery runs on the anteromedial surface of the gland and then passes deep to the neck of the mandible. The superficial temporal gives off transverse facial artery within the substance of the gland and then ascend and appear at the upper pole of the gland.

Q. What is the disposition of artery, veins, and nerves within the substance of the parotid gland?

Ans. The arteries lie in the deepest plane. next are the veins and the facial nerve lies at the most superficial plane. The nerves and the veins form a faciovenous plane and divide the parotid gland into superficial and deep part.

Q. Apart from facial nerve what other nerves lies in relation to the parotid gland?

Ans.

- *Auriculotemporal nerve*: It is a branch of mandibular division of trigeminal nerve, which comes in relation to the upper part of the parotid gland and supplies secretomotor fibers to the parotid gland.
- *Great auricular nerve*: It does not enter the substance of the gland but lies on the superficial fascia supplying the area near the angle of the mandible and may be injured during approach to the parotid gland.

Q. What is Frey's syndrome?

Ans. This is a condition of gustatory sweating and flushing in the parotid region following parotidectomy and may occur in more than 50% of patients.

Q. How do you explain development of this syndrome?

Ans. This follows injury to auriculotemporal nerve during surgery of parotid gland or temporomandibular joint, or may follow accidental injury to the parotid gland or temporomandibular joint.

Following injury to auriculotemporal nerve, the postganglionic parasympathetic fiber from the otic ganglion reroutes to the sympathetic nerve from the superior cervical ganglion destined to supply the cutaneous vessels and sweat gland of the skin in the parotid region.

Q. How will you manage Frey's syndrome?

Ans.
- Surgical intervention is not helpful
- Patient manages to live with this as there may be spontaneous recovery in some cases
- Some local antiperspirant may help.

Q. How do secretomotor fibers reach the parotid gland?

Ans. Secretomotor preganglionic fibers from inferior salivary nucleus → glossopharyngeal nerve → tympanic branch → tympanic plexus → lesser superficial petrosal nerve → otic ganglion → postganglionic fibers → joins auriculotemporal branch of mandibular division of trigeminal nerve → parotid gland.

■ ADENOLYMPHOMA

Q. What is your case? (Summary of a case of adenolymphoma)

Ans. This 45-year-old gentleman presented with a swelling in lower part of the right parotid region for last 3 years which is slowly increasing in size. No pain over the swelling, no symptoms suggestive of facial nerve palsy.

On examination: There is a soft cystic swelling lying between the ramus of mandible and mastoid process which is fluctuant but not transilluminant. The surface is smooth, free from skin and underlying structures. There are no palpable lymph nodes in the neck.

Q. What is your diagnosis?

Ans. This is a case of adenolymphoma involving the lower pole of right parotid gland.

Q. What are the other possibilities?

Ans.
- Mixed parotid tumor
- Parotid cyst
- Lipoma
- Neurofibroma
- Chronic cervical lymphadenitis.

Q. What is adenolymphoma?

Ans. This is a benign tumor of parotid salivary gland. This is composed of multiple cystic spaces lined by a single layered epithelium. The epithelium is composed of columnar cells and they may form papillary projections into these spaces. The stroma contains lymphoid tissue. The adenolymphoma does not undergo malignant change.

Q. How will you manage this patient?

Ans. Clinically, this appears to be a benign tumor:
* I will do a FNAC from the swelling for confirmation of diagnosis
* I will do superficial parotidectomy in this patient.

Q. How will you differentiate a mixed parotid tumor and adenolymphoma?

Ans. These can be differentiated by ^{99m}Tc scan. Adenolymphoma takes up the ^{99m}Tc and appear as hot spots whereas other neoplasms of parotid do not take up ^{99m}Tc and appear as cold spots.

Q. What is the common age group of the patient affected by adenolymphoma?

Ans. Elderly patient with the mean age of 60 years are usually affected.

Q. What is the sex incidence?

Ans. Adenolymphoma occurs more commonly in males. Male:Female (4:1).

■ CARCINOMA PAROTID GLAND

Clinical Examination (*See* Page No. 382, Chapter 9)

History

* *Swelling*: Onset and progress (a rapidly increasing swelling from the onset or recent rapid increase of a preexisting benign swelling).
* History of facial nerve palsy (inability to close the eyes, asymmetry of face, drooling of saliva from angle of mouth, difficulty in chewing).
* Any other swelling in the neck (cervical lymph nodes may be enlarged).

Examination—Inspection/Palpation

* Details about the swelling
* Site and extent
* Skin over the swelling, if infiltrated may appear reddish blue. Temperature over the swelling may be higher
* Tenderness (usually nontender)
* Surface is irregular
* Consistency is hard
* Mobility (may become fixed to the skin and the underlying structures and becomes immobile).
* Examination of cervical lymph nodes (cervical lymph nodes may become enlarged and palpable).
  Test movement of temporomandibular joint, if gross infiltration is there, the temporomandibular joint movement may be restricted.

Q. What is your case? (Summary of a case of carcinoma parotid gland)

Ans. This 40-year-old lady presented with a swelling in right upper part of the neck for last 4 year. The swelling was about 3 cm in size at the onset, afterward initially the swelling was increasing slowly in size but, for last 8 months, there is rapid increase in size of the swelling to attain the present large size. She complains of dull aching pain over the swelling for last 3 months. Patient says that she could not close her right eye completely for last 2 months and has difficulty in chewing, as the food tend to accumulate between the right side of the cheek and the gum. She complained of an ulcer over the swelling 6 months back which healed with conservative treatment. Patient does not complain of any other swelling in the neck (Fig. 12.16).

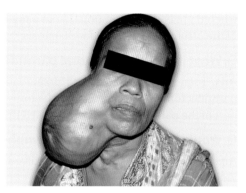

Fig. 12.16: Carcinoma right parotid gland

Courtesy: Prof Pradip Kumar Gupta, MGM Medical College, Kishangunj, Bihar

On examination: General survey is essentially normal. On local examination, there is a swelling in the right parotid region, elliptical in shape and 20 cm × 15 cm in size, surface lobulated, margins rounded, hard in consistency, slightly tender. There is skin fixity at the center of the swelling, but the remaining skin over the swelling is free. The swelling is mobile but is slightly fixed to the underlying masseter muscle. The deep part of the gland is not palpable. Testing of facial nerve reveals a lower motor neuron type of facial palsy on the right side. There are no palpable lymph nodes in the neck.

Q. What is your diagnosis?

Ans. This is a case of carcinoma right parotid gland with facial nerve palsy.

Q. What are the malignant tumors of the parotid gland?

Ans. There are different types of malignant parotid tumors.

Acinic cell carcinoma and mucoepidermoid carcinoma are considered as low-grade carcinoma histologically and clinically it behaves less aggressively.

Adenocarcinoma, adenoid cystic carcinoma, squamous cell carcinoma, and undifferentiated carcinoma are all aggressive tumors and carry a poor prognosis in spite of radical treatment.

Q. How will you treat this patient?

Ans.
- I will do a FNAC from the swelling to confirm my diagnosis.
- Computed tomography (CT) scan of the parotid region to assess the tumor extent.
- Baseline workup to assess fitness of patient for anesthesia and surgery.
- Radical parotidectomy is the treatment of choice in this patient. As the facial nerve is already involved, the facial nerve has to be sacrificed.
- The facial nerve may be grafted in the same sitting using great auricular nerve.

Q. When will you consider incisional biopsy in parotid carcinoma?

Ans. Incisional biopsy is contraindicated in parotid tumor. Incisional biopsy is only justified when there is skin ulceration due to a malignant parotid tumor when biopsy from the margin of the ulcer will be helpful for diagnosis.

Q. What is conservative total parotidectomy?

Ans. Total parotidectomy with preservation of the facial nerve is called conservative total parotidectomy. Superficial parotidectomy is done first preserving the facial nerve. The deep part of the parotid gland is then excised preserving the facial nerve branches.

Q. Would you like to do a neck lymph node dissection?

Ans. As the lymph nodes are not involved, I will not do a prophylactic neck dissection in this patient.

Q. Will you consider postoperative radiotherapy?

Ans. Parotid tumors are said to be radioresistant, but this is not always true. Routine postoperative radiotherapy is indicated in patients of parotid carcinoma following radical surgery. This has beneficial effect of lowering the incidence of local recurrence.

Q. When will you consider radical lymph node dissection?

Ans. Carcinoma parotid with lymph node metastasis needs radical parotidectomy along with radical lymph node dissection of neck.

Q. If the parotid tumor has involved the local structures, how will you manage?

Ans. As the tumor is relatively radioresistant, radical surgery is the treatment of choice.

For malignant tumors involving skin, facial nerve, mandible, and neck lymph nodes:

* *Radical surgery:* Radical parotidectomy with a wide margin (1 cm), hemimandibulectomy along with radical neck dissection in continuity and postoperative radical radiotherapy is the optimal treatment.
* If the tumor has involved the internal carotid artery, resection is contraindicated as it will result in hemiplegia.

Q. How will you manage facial nerve injury or involvement during operation?

Ans.
* When nerve is divided inadvertently, it may be sutured.
* If a segment of nerve is sacrificed during radical surgery, primary grafting by using great auricular nerve or and hypoglossal nerve may be done. Hypoglossal nerve may be transposed for anastomosis to the peripheral branches of facial nerve.
* Alternatively, fascial slings may be used to support facial tissue and mask the deformities due to facial nerve palsy.

Q. How will you manage a patient with inoperable tumor?

Ans. If the tumor is fixed to the underlying structures and is irremovable, palliative treatment with radical radiotherapy is advisable.

Q. What is the role of chemotherapy in parotid carcinoma?

Ans. Chemotherapy has very limited role in parotid carcinoma. Chemotherapy has been tried in advanced inoperable disease. A combination of methotrexate and 5-fluorouracil has been used with some success.

Q. What are the characteristics of adenoid cystic carcinoma?

Ans. Adenoid cystic carcinomas are extremely slow growing tumors but there is relentless perineural spread along the cranial nerve and into the brain. It may invade the medullary bone for many centimeters or traverse the periosteum before inducing significant bone resorption.

Thus tumors of adenoid cystic carcinoma are more extensive than the clinical sign or radiographic appearance suggest.

Q. How will you treat patients with adenoid cystic carcinoma?

Ans. Radical parotidectomy followed by radical postoperative radiotherapy. The radiotherapy should include the skull base in order to control the perineural tumor extension.

Q. What are the characteristics of mucoepidermoid tumor?

Ans.
* Composed of epidermoid cells in sheets. There are clefts and cystic spaces lined by mucus secreting cells.
* Varying speed of growth
* Mostly slow growing and invade local tissue to a limited degree and occasionally metastasize to lymph node, lungs or skin.

Q. What are the characteristics of acinic cell tumor?

Ans.
* Mainly involves the parotid gland
* Cell resembles those of serous acini
* Slow growing may invade the local structures
* Usually soft cystic in feel.

Q. What are the relative incidences of tumors in different salivary gland?

Ans.
* 75% tumors in parotid gland:
  – 85% benign—80% pleomorphic adenomas
  – 15% malignant
* 10% tumors in submandibular salivary gland:
  – 65% benign—95% pleomorphic adenoma
  – 35% malignant
* 15% tumors in minor salivary glands including sublingual gland:
  – 50% benign—almost all are pleomorphic adenoma
  – 50% malignant
  Tumors in sublingual gland are commonly malignant.

Q. What is TNM classification of parotid (salivary gland) carcinoma?

Ans. TNM classification of parotid (salivary gland) carcinoma has been shown in Table 12.1.

Table 12.1: TNM classification of parotid (salivary gland) carcinoma	
Primary tumor (T)	
TX	Primary tumor cannot be assessed
T0	No evidence of primary tumor
Tis	Carcinoma in situ
T1	Tumor ≤ 2 cm in greatest dimension without extraparenchymal extension
T2	Tumor > 2 cm but not > 4 cm in greatest dimension without extraparenchymal extension
T3	Tumor > 4 cm and/or tumor has extraparenchymal extension
T4a	Moderately advanced disease: • Tumor invades the skin, mandible, ear canal, and/or facial nerve
T4b	Very advanced disease: • Tumor invades skull base and/or pterygoid plates and/or encases carotid artery
Regional lymph nodes (N)	
NX	Regional nodes cannot be assessed
N0	No regional lymph node metastasis
N1	Metastasis in a single ipsilateral lymph node, ≤ 3 cm in greatest dimension
N2	Metastasis in a single ipsilateral lymph node > 3 cm but not > 6 cm in greatest dimension; or in multiple ipsilateral lymph nodes, none > 6 cm in greatest dimension; or in bilateral or contralateral lymph nodes, none > 6 cm in greatest dimension
N2a	Metastasis in a single ipsilateral lymph node > 3 cm but not > 6 cm in greatest dimension
N2b	Metastasis in multiple ipsilateral lymph nodes, none > 6 cm in greatest dimension
N2c	Metastasis in bilateral or contralateral lymph nodes, none > 6 cm in greatest dimension
N3	Metastasis in a lymph node > 6 cm in greatest dimension
Distant metastasis (M)	
M0	No distant metastasis
M1	Distant metastasis

Anatomic stage/prognostic group

Stage	T	N	M
0	Tis	N0	M0
I	T1	N0	M0
II	T2	N0	M0
III	T3	N0	M0
	T1	N1	M0
	T2	N1	M0
	T3	N1	M0
IVA	T4a	N0	M0
	T4a	N1	M0
	T1	N2	M0
	T2	N2	M0
	T3	N2	M0
	T4a	N2	M0
IVB	T Any	N3	M0
	T4b	N Any	M0
IVC	T Any	N Any	M1

Q. What is dumbbell parotid tumor?

Ans. Tumor arising from the deep part of the parotid gland enlarges medially passing between the styloid process and mandible to present as a swelling of the soft palate on the lateral wall of the pharynx behind the posterior pillar of tonsil.

This tumor with the component in the neck and the lateral pharyngeal bulge is called the dumbbell parotid tumor.

Q. How will you approach the deep lobe of the parotid gland?

Ans. Approach is by a standard parotidectomy incision.
* A formal superficial parotidectomy is done with preservation of facial nerve branches.
* The facial nerve branches are mobilized and lifted in nylon slings.
* The deep part of the gland is then dissected all around and removed. It is easy to dissect the deep lobe by finger or a sharp dissection with scissors.
* Only rarely, it is necessary to do a mandibulectomy to gain access to the deep lobe.

Q. How will you identify facial nerve during surgery?

Ans. There are some anatomical landmarks which lead to identification of facial nerve during surgery.
* The nerve lies at the junction of cartilaginous and bony part of external auditory canal.
* There is a palpable groove between the bony external auditory meatus and the mastoid process which is filled with fibro-fatty tissue. the facial nerve lies deep in this groove.

- The posterior belly of digastric muscle is inserted into the mastoid process just behind the stylomastoid foramen. By dissection at the medial border of the posterior belly of digastric near its insertion, facial nerve may be identified.
- The styloid process itself can be palpated superficial to the stylomastoid foramen and nerve is identified just lateral to the styloid process.

Q. What is the incidence of transient facial nerve palsy following parotidectomy?

Ans. Temporary facial nerve palsy due to neuropraxia may occur in up to 30% cases but usually recovers within 6 weeks.

Q. What will happen if great auricular nerve is injured during parotidectomy?

Ans. This results in an area of anesthesia around the angle of mandible and ear lobule. This is troublesome in female who finds it difficult to wear ear rings. Spontaneous recovery may occur in 18 months.

■ CHRONIC SIALADENITIS OF LEFT SUBMANDIBULAR SALIVARY GLAND DUE TO CALCULUS IN SUBMANDIBULAR DUCT

Clinical Examination (*See* Page No. 381, Chapter 9)

History

- *Swelling*: Onset and progress (swelling in the submandibular region, appears just before and during eating, the swelling gradually disappears in between meals. In long standing cases the swelling becomes persistent and aggravates during intake of meals).
- Pain (usually a dull aching pain over the swelling, appears during the meals when the gland swells and pain disappears when the swelling subsides).
- Any history of relief of symptoms (stone may pass out and the symptoms may disappear and may reoccur again once the stone reforms).
- Any history of discharge of purulent saliva in the floor of mouth.

Examination—Inspection/Palpation

- *Swelling*: Position (usually lies in the submandibular triangle below the horizontal ramus of the mandible).
- Tenderness (usually tender during the meals when the gland is enlarged or if the gland is infected).
- Size, shape, surface, margins (usually 3–5 cm in diameter, globular swelling, smooth surface or the surface may appear bosselated. The anterior, posterior and the inferior margins are distinct and well palpable. The upper margin is lying between the mandible and the mylohyoid is not well palpable).
- Consistency (usually firm in feel).
- Mobility (usually free from the skin and the underlying structures and so it freely mobile).
- Palpation of the deep part of the submandibular gland (by bidigital examination with one index finger on the floor of the mouth and the other index finger over the mylohyoid muscle).
- Examination of cervical lymph nodes (cervical lymph nodes are usually not palpable).

Q. What is your case? (Summary of a case of chronic sialadenitis due to calculus in the submandibular duct).

Ans. This 25-year-old male patient presented with a swelling in left submandibular region for last 6 months. The swelling gets aggravated in size and becomes painful during intake of meals and after few hours the swelling gets reduced. Initially the swelling used to disappear in between meals but for last 3 months patient noticed the swelling is persistent and gets aggravated during intake of meals (Fig. 12.17).

On examination: A swelling is palpable in left submandibular region. The swelling is slightly tender, surface is smooth, and all the margins are palpable and rounded, firm in consistency, free from skin and underlying structures. The swelling is bidigitally palpable. A stone is palpable in the left submandibular duct at the floor of mouth.

So this is a case of left sided chronic submandibular sialadenitis due to a calculus in left submandibular duct.

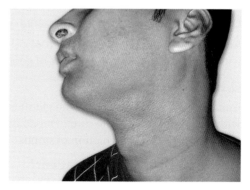

Fig. 12.17: Chronic sialadenitis involving left submandibular gland due to calculus in left submandibular duct

Courtesy: Dr Asish Gupta, IPGME and R, Kolkata

Q. How will you do a bidigital palpation of submandibular salivary gland?

Ans. One index finger is inserted inside the floor of the mouth between the undersurface of the tongue, inner surface of the alveolus and the other index finger is kept below the mandible in submandibular region (Fig. 12.18).

An enlarged submandibular gland is bidigitally palpable.

By bidigital palpation the stone in submandibular duct may be palpated. Enlarged submandibular lymph node is not bidigitally palpable.

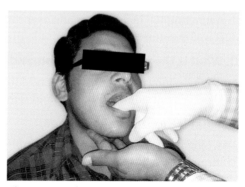

Fig. 12.18: Bidigital palpation of submandibular salivary gland

Q. What is the relative incidence of calculi in salivary glands?

Ans.
* 80% in submandibular gland
* 10% in parotid gland
* 7% in sublingual gland
* 3% in other minor salivary gland.

Q. Why stone formation is more common in submandibular duct?

Ans.
* The secretion of submandibular gland is more mucus and viscid.

- Submandibular duct has a long curved course. The duct opens in the floor of the mouth at a little higher level than the level of the submandibular gland itself. Because of this upward course, there may be stasis of saliva in the submandibular duct resulting in precipitation of calcium salts.

Q. What is the composition of salivary calculi?

Ans. Salivary calculi are composed of calcium magnesium phosphate and carbonate along with some organic matter. Because of good calcium content the stone is radiopaque.

Q. How does the stone form?

Ans. Chronic inflammation of the gland or papillary stenosis results in retention of secretion within the gland or in the duct. Deposition of calcium salts on the nidus of a degenerated epithelium results in formation of stone.

Q. How will you treat this patient?

Ans.
- I will take an X-ray of floor of mouth (intraoral occlusal view) to look for any radiopaque calculus in the line of submandibular duct.
- When the stone is lying in the submandibular duct in the floor of the mouth anterior to the point where it is crossed by lingual nerve (at the level of second molar tooth), removal of the stone from the duct is curative. A suture is passed around the duct proximal to the site of stone so that it does not slip backward.

  A longitudinal incision is made over the duct wall and stone extracted. The opening in the duct wall is sutured with the mucosa in the floor of the mouth for free drainage of saliva.

Q. What is the indication of submandibular gland excision?

Ans. When stone is present in the gland substance and gland is the seat of chronic inflammation then excision of submandibular gland is the treatment of choice.

Q. What is Sjögren's syndrome?

Ans. Sjögren's syndrome is an autoimmune disease characterized by progressive lymphocytic infiltration of salivary and lacrimal glands resulting in xerostomia and keratoconjunctivitis sicca. There may be symmetrical enlargement of all the salivary glands, lacrimal glands and there may be systemic manifestation of generalized arthritis (rheumatoid type), scleroderma polyarteritis nodosa.

Q. What are the characteristics of malignant lymphoma of salivary gland?

Ans.
- May arise from the lymph node lying on the surface of the gland
- May arise within parenchyma of the gland
- May arise as complication of HIV diseases, benign lymphoepithelial disease or in Sjögren's syndrome
- Common in late age sixth to seventh decade
- Presents with painless swelling
- 90% occurs in parotid.

Q. How will you treat parotid lymphoma?

Ans.

- When confined to parotid gland—total parotidectomy followed by radiotherapy.
- When spread beyond the gland—polychemotherapy.

■ CARCINOMA OF SUBMANDIBULAR SALIVARY GLAND

Clinical Examination (*See* Page No. 382, Chapter 9)

Q. What is your case? (Summary of a case of carcinoma of submandibular salivary gland)

Ans. This 50-year-old gentleman presented with a swelling in upper part of lateral side of neck on the left side for last 6 months. The swelling is rapidly increasing in size since the onset and attained the present large size. Patient complains of pain over the swelling for last 3 months. There are no other swellings in the neck (Fig. 12.19).

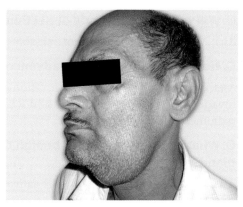

Fig. 12.19: Carcinoma of left submandibular gland
Courtesy: Dr Dushmanta Burman, IPGME and R, Kolkata

On examination: There is a swelling in left submandibular triangle 7 cm × 5 cm in size. The swelling is nontender, hard in feel, surface is irregular, margins are rounded, mobile, and free from skin and underlying structures. The swelling is bidigitally palpable. There is no lymph node enlargement in the neck.

Q. What is your diagnosis?

Ans. This is a case of carcinoma in left submandibular salivary gland without any lymph node metastasis.

Q. What are the other possibilities?

Ans.

- Mixed tumor involving the submandibular salivary gland
- Submandibular lymph node enlargement due to Koch's infection
- Metastatic submandibular lymph node
- Malignant lymphoma.

Q. How will you confirm your diagnosis?

Ans. I would like to confirm my diagnosis by doing a FNAC.

Q. Do you like to do a CT scan?

Ans.

- As the tumor is palpable all around, a CT scan will not give further information; hence CT scan is not essential in this patient.
- If the swelling is large and the deeper extent is not palpable a CT scan can delineate the deeper extent of the mass.

Q. How will you treat this patient?

Ans. I will consider total excision of the left submandibular gland followed by postoperative radiotherapy.

Q. Will you do lymph node dissection?

Ans. As the lymph nodes are not palpable prophylactic lymph node dissection is not indicated.

Q. How will you treat locally advanced disease?

Ans. A radical surgery with total excision of submandibular gland, with sacrifice of structures invaded by the tumor along with block dissection of lymph node. Postoperative radical radiotherapy is also required.

Q. What is the treatment for benign tumor (adenoma) of submandibular salivary gland?

Ans. Excision of the submandibular salivary gland is the optimal treatment.

Q. Which nerves are at risk for injury during excision of submandibular salivary gland?

Ans. A number of nerves are at risk for injury during submandibular gland excision.

- The mandibular branch of facial nerve, which supplies orbicularis oris and other muscles of the lip. To avoid injury to this nerve skin, incision is made at least 3 cm below the lower border of mandible.
- The lingual nerve runs close to the submandibular gland as it gives secretomotor supply to the submandibular gland. The lingual nerve hooks around the submandibular duct. It is important to identify the lingual nerve during dissection of deep part of the gland.
- The hypoglossal nerve lies deeply in the deep part of the gland on the hyoglossus muscle and the hypoglossal nerve is identified during dissection of the deep part of the gland.
- Cervical branch of facial nerve which supplies the platysma crosses the lateral surface of the superficial part of the gland.

Q. What are the anatomical parts of submandibular gland?

Ans. The submandibular gland situated in the submandibular triangle is divided into superficial and deep part by the mylohyoid muscle.

- The deep part of the gland lies between the mylohyoid and hyoglossus muscle.
- The superficial part of the gland lies on mylohyoid, hyoglossus and the middle constrictor muscle of pharynx.

Q. Which artery lies in relation to the submandibular gland?

Ans. The facial artery runs in close relation to the submandibular gland. It runs on the medial aspect of the superficial lobe and then arches along its superior border and then ascends in the face curving around the lower border of mandible.

Q. Where does the submandibular duct end?

Ans. The submandibular duct emerges from the deep part of the gland. The duct runs in the floor of the mouth along the side of tongue and opens in the sublingual papilla on either side of frenum. The sublingual salivary gland lies just lateral to the submandibular duct.

Q. How do the secretomotor fibers reach the submandibular salivary glands?

Ans. Preganglionic fibers from superior salivary nucleus → facial nerve → chorda tympani nerve → lingual nerve → submandibular ganglion → postganglionic fibers → reaches submandibular and sublingual salivary gland.

▌PAROTID FISTULA

Q. What is your case? (Summary of a case of parotid fistula)

Ans. This 30-year-old gentleman presented with watery discharge from the left parotid region for last 3 months. The discharge is more during eating. Patient had a swelling in the same region 3-and-half months back. The swelling was very painful and was associated with fever. Patient underwent incision and drainage operation 7 days after the onset of the swelling. Following the operation the swelling disappeared, but the patient complained of watery discharge from the site of incision.

On examination: There is a cruciate scar in right parotid region and there is watery discharge from a small opening situated near the upper part of the left side of the neck. The parotid gland is not palpable.

Q. What is your diagnosis?

Ans. This is a case of parotid fistula on left side following incision and drainage of parotid abscess.

Q. What are the other causes of parotid fistula?

Ans.
◆ Congenital parotid fistula
◆ Following penetrating injury to the parotid gland
◆ Following superficial parotidectomy.

Q. What are the types of parotid fistula?

Ans. It may be:
◆ *Gland fistula*: Where there is fistula from the gland parenchyma. Fistula discharge minimal.
◆ *Duct fistula*: Where there is a fistulous opening into a major duct. Discharge is profuse.

Q. How will you treat the patient?

Ans.

- I will do a fistulogram to assess the fistulous tract, whether duct or gland fistula. As this patient is having discharge from the fistula tract, initially I will give hyoscine bromide (15 mg) one tablet twice daily. This will reduce the salivary secretion.
- If there is no stenosis or obstruction of the parotid duct, some parotid fistula particularly the gland fistula closes spontaneously.
- If there is stenosis at the terminal part of the parotid duct, a papillotomy may allow good drainage and fistula may heal spontaneously.

Q. If the fistula is from the main duct, how will you treat the patient?

Ans. The duct may be reconstructed by Newman and Seabrock's operation.

Q. If the reconstruction of the duct fails, what will you do?

Ans. Total parotidectomy with preservation of facial nerve will be curative.

Mouth and Oral Cavity

■ CLINICAL EXAMINATION

Clinical examination of patient presenting with cleft lip and palate.

History

* History of split in lip, palate, or both since birth.
* Any difficulty in feeding? How is the infant fed? Any nasal regurgitation? (cleft lip does not usually cause difficulty in feeding, cleft palate patient has difficulty in sucking)
* Any difficulty in speech? If so, which alphabets? Any nasal intonation?
* Any nasal deformity?
* Any defect in dentition?
* Any respiratory complaints—cough and breathlessness?

Examination

For cleft lip:
* Assess the type of cleft lip:
  – Incomplete—when the cleft in the lip does not extend into the nasal floor.
  – Complete—when the cleft in the lip extends into the nasal floor.
  – Unilateral cleft lip—when the cleft is on one side of philtrum.
  – Bilateral cleft lip—when the cleft occurs on both sides of the philtrum and philtrum lies free in the midline hanging from the nasal floor.
* Examine the alae nasi—in complete cleft lip, the ala nasi is flattened on that side. Septal cartilage may be deviated to the opposite side.
* Assess the length of columella—in bilateral complete cleft lip, the columella may be short.
* Look for any problems with alignment of teeth. The teeth underlying the cleft may be protruding.
* Examine the palate for presence of any associated cleft palate (see below for cleft palate).
* If the child can utter words—assess the pronunciation—child may have difficulty in pronunciation of consonants requiring closure of the lips, e.g. B, P, V, M, etc.

- Look for any other associated congenital anomalies:
  - Undescended testis
  - Hypospadias or epispadias
  - Cardiac anomalies
  - Vertebral anomalies
  - Anorectal anomalies.

Examination for Cleft Palate:

- Ask the patient to open the mouth and assess the type of cleft palate.
- Whether involves soft palate, hard palate, or both.
- Different types may be:
  - Cleft of soft palate only
  - Cleft of both soft and hard palate up to its junction with the premaxilla.
  - Cleft of both soft and hard palate and cleft extending to one side of premaxilla.
  - Cleft, both soft and hard palate, extending on both sides of the premaxilla—the premaxilla lies freely.
- Assess whether the nasal septum lies freely (complete cleft palate) or the nasal septum is attached to one side of the hard palate (incomplete cleft palate).
- Any defect in dentition.
- Examine the lip for any associated cleft lip.
- Assess any speech defect—nasal intonation is usual.
- Assess any difficulty in swallowing or drinking.
- Any evidence of chronic ear infection—look for any discharge from ear.
- Look for any other congenital anomalies.

■ CLEFT LIP

Q. What is your case?

Ans.

- This is a case of left-sided incomplete cleft lip in a 7-month male child (Fig. 13.1).
- This is a case of left-sided complete cleft lip with complete cleft of hard and soft palate (Fig. 13.2).

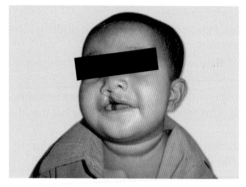

Fig. 13.1: Unilateral incomplete cleft lip on the right side

Courtesy: Prof Sasanka Sekhar Chatterjee, IPGME and R, Kolkata

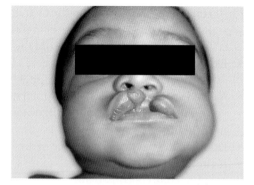

Fig. 13.2: Left-sided complete unilateral cleft lip

Courtesy: Prof Sasanka Sekhar Chatterjee, IPGME and R, Kolkata

The diagnosis should include:
* Laterality, i.e. unilateral or bilateral
* Complete or incomplete
* Age of the child
* Any associated cleft lip.

Q. What is central cleft lip?

Ans. This is a very rare congenital defect, where the cleft of the lip is central and forms due to failure of fusion of two globular processes (Fig. 13.3).

Q. What is lateral cleft lip?

Ans. This is the common type of cleft lip where there is cleft of the lip on one or both side between the philtrum and the lateral part of the upper lip. Lateral cleft may be unilateral or bilateral. In bilateral cleft lip, the philtrum hangs freely (Figs 13.4A to C).

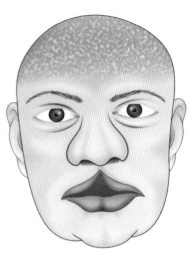

Fig. 13.3: Central cleft lip

Q. What is unilateral cleft lip?

Ans. There is cleft of the lip on one side between the philtrum and the lateral part of the upper lip (Figs 13.4A and B).

Q. What is bilateral cleft lip?

Ans. When there is cleft of the lip on either side of the philtrum and lateral parts of the lip (Fig. 13.4C).

Q. What is incomplete cleft lip?

Ans. Unilateral cleft is characterized by varying degrees of vertical separation of the lip but the nasal slit is intact. There may be associated nasal deformity (Fig. 13.4B).

Q. What is complete cleft lip?

Ans. Cleft lip extending up to the nostril is called complete cleft lip (Fig. 13.4A).

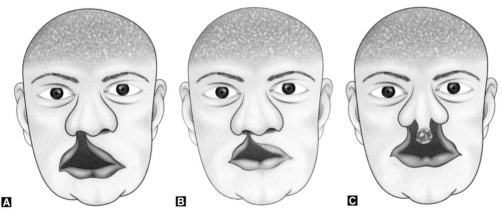

Figs 13.4A to C: (A) Unilateral complete cleft lip; (B) Unilateral incomplete cleft lip; (C) Bilateral complete cleft lip

Q. What is simple cleft lip?

Ans. Cleft lip alone is called simple cleft lip.

Q. What is compound cleft lip?

Ans. Cleft lip associated with cleft of the alveolus is called compound cleft lip.

Q. What is complicated cleft lip?

Ans. Cleft lip associated with a cleft in the posterior hard palate is called complicated cleft lip.

Q. What are the usual problems in patients with cleft lip?

Ans.

* *Cosmetic*—in patients with incomplete cleft lip the only problem is cosmetic
* *Difficulty in sucking breast milk*—particularly in patients with combined cleft lip and palate
* *Defective dentition*—alveolus may protrude through the cleft lip gap resulting in defective dental alignment
* *Defective speech*—particularly in pronunciation of some letters requiring labial closure, e.g. B, F, P, V, etc.

Q. What is the distribution of muscles in lips?

Ans. Three muscular rings constitute the muscles in the lips and face (Fig. 13.5). These are called muscular rings of Delaire.

* *Nasolabial muscles*:
    - Transverse nasalis
    - Levator labii superioris alaeque nasi
    - Levator labii superioris.
* *Bilabial muscles*:
    - Orbicularis oris (oblique head—upper lip)
    - Orbicularis oris (horizontal head—upper lip)
    - Orbicularis oris (horizontal head—lower lip).

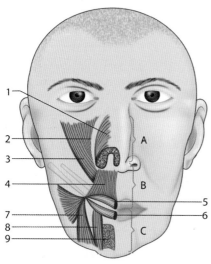

Fig. 13.5: Muscles of lip; A—nasolabial muscles (1–3): 1. Transverse nasalis, 2. Levator labii superioris alaeque nasi, 3. Levator labii superioris. B—bilabial muscles (4–6): 4. Orbicularis oris (oblique head), upper lip, 5. Orbicularis oris (horizontal head), upper lip, 6. Orbicularis oris, lower lip. C—labiomental muscles (7–9): 7. Depressor angulioris, 8. Depressor labii inferioris, 9. Mentalis.

* *Labiomental muscles*:
  - Depressor anguli oris
  - Depressor labii inferioris
  - Mentalis.

Q. What are the abnormalities of lip muscles in unilateral cleft lip?

Ans. Nasolabial and bilabial muscles are disrupted on one side. This results in an asymmetrical deformity involving external nasal cartilage, nasal septum, and anterior maxilla (premaxilla). These deformities cause displacement of nasal skin on to the lip and retraction of labial skin (Fig. 13.6).

Q. What are the abnormalities of lip muscles in bilateral cleft lip?

Ans.
* In bilateral cleft lip, the deformity in muscles is more pronounced but is symmetrical.
* The two superior muscular rings are disrupted on both sides.
* There is lack of nasolabial muscle continuity resulting in flaring of nose, a protruding premaxilla and an area of skin in the front of premaxilla (prolabium), which is devoid of muscle (Fig. 13.7).

Q. How do you classify associated nasal deformity in cleft lip?

Ans. The associated nasal deformity may be classified as:
* *Mild*: Wide alar base but normal alar contour
* *Moderate*: Wide alar base with either a depressed dome or alar crease
* *Severe*: Wide alar base, a deep alar crease, and an under projecting alar dome.

Q. How the lips develop?

Ans. The lips and palate develop by fusion of a number of structures.
* Around 6th week of intrauterine life, the first branchial arch contributes to the formation of maxillary and mandibular prominences on either side. The frontonasal prominence is formed by the proliferation of the mesenchyme, which is ventral to the forebrain. The primitive stomodeum is bounded cranially by the frontonasal process and on either side by the paired maxillary and mandibular processes.
* The two olfactory pits on either side divide the frontonasal process into lateral and medial nasal process. The medial nasal process bifurcates and forms two globular processes.

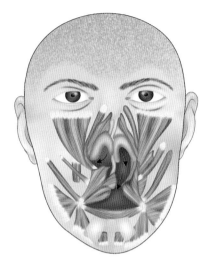

Fig. 13.6: Muscular defect in unilateral cleft lip

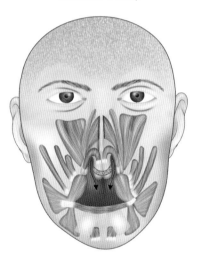

Fig. 13.7: Muscular defect in bilateral cleft

- The two maxillary processes continue to grow medially and fuse with the lateral nasal and medial nasal processes.
- Fusion of the medial nasal, lateral nasal, and maxillary prominences produces continuity between the nose, upper lip, and the palate.
- The medial nasal process (globular processes) forms the philtrum and Cupid's bow region of the upper lip, the nasal tip, the premaxilla and the primary palate, and the nasal septum.
- The lateral nasal processes form the ala nasi
- Merging of the paired mandibular processes produces the lower jaw, lower lip, lower cheek, and chin regions of the face
- The maxillary prominence accounts for the development of the major portion of the upper lip excluding the philtrum and the upper cheek regions.

Q. How do the upper lips develop?

Ans. The central part of the upper lip (philtrum and the Cupid's bow) develops from the fusion of two globular processes.

The lateral parts of the upper lip develop from maxillary process, which fuses with the medial nasal process.

Q. How do the lower lips develop?

Ans. The lower lip develops by merging of the mandibular processes of two sides.

Q. What are the etiological factors for development of cleft lip and palate?

Ans.
- *Hereditary factor*—sex-linked recessive inheritance in 15% of cases
- *Nutritional* deficiency during pregnancy—particularly vitamin A and B deficiencies
- *Rubella* infection during pregnancy
- *Teratogenic drugs*—steroid, phenytoin, and diazepam are associated with increased incidence of cleft lip and palate
- *Threatened* abortion may be associated with congenital malformation
- *Radiation* exposure during pregnancy
- *Maternal* age—late pregnancy
- *Maternal* diabetes mellitus
- *Consanguineous* marriage
- *Some* syndromes are associated with cleft lip and palate, e.g.
- *Pierre Robin's syndrome*—cleft palate, retrognathia, and a posteriorly displaced tongue.
- Other syndromes associated with cleft lip and palate include:
- *Down's* syndrome
- *Apert's* syndrome
- *Treacher-Collins* syndrome
- *Stickler* syndrome
- *Shprintzen* syndrome.

Q. How can you diagnose cleft lip antenatally?

Ans.
- Unilateral or bilateral cleft lip may be diagnosed by ultrasound scan after 18 weeks of gestation.
- Reassurance of mother is essential with such a defect.
- Cleft palate cannot be diagnosed in antenatal period.

Q. What are the aims of surgery in cleft lip?

Ans. Proper cleft lip surgery should achieve:
- Good cosmetic appearance of lip, nose, and face
- Normal dentition
- Normal speech
- Normal facial growth.

Q. How will you treat this patient with unilateral cleft lip?

Ans.
- I will prepare this patient for surgery. Hb% level should be more than 10 gm%.
- I will repair this cleft by Millard's rotation—advancement flap technique.

Q. What are the principles of operation in cleft lip?

Ans.
- The normal shape and symmetry of the lips have to be restored.
- The vertical length from the floor of the nose to the vermillion border of lip should be maintained.
- Accurate apposition of margins is essential for proper healing.
- Vermillion border of the lip should be constructed well.
- Cupid's bow should be intact.
- Integrity of orbicularis oris should be maintained by proper suturing of muscle layer to have a good oral sphincter.
- Associated deformity of the nose should be corrected.

Q. What is Millard's operation?

Ans. The Millard's rotation–advancement flap involves advancement of a lateral flap into the upper portion of the lip combined with a downward rotation of the medial segment (Fig. 13.8).

This technique preserves both the Cupid's bow and the philtral dimple and has the additional advantage of placing the tension of closure under the alar base, thereby reducing the alar flare and promoting better molding of alveolar process.

The vertical length from the alar base to the Cupid's bow peak on the noncleft side determines the length of the normal philtrum and is also used to describe the length of the rotation flap and the advancement flap.

The rotation flap is marked as a gentle convexity following the cleft margin to the columellar base. This length equals the vertical lip length and the length of the advancement flap.

The advancement flap is cut free of the nostril and leaving a full complement of muscle underneath the ala. The muscle underneath the ala base is also mobilized from fibrous connection in the lower nasal cartilages.

The orbicularis muscle is dissected free of the skin and mucosa. The nasolabial muscles are sutured to the premaxilla with nonabsorbable suture. Oblique muscle of the orbicularis oris are sutured to the base of anterior nasal spine and the nasal septum. The repair of the muscle is completed by suturing the horizontal fibers of orbicularis oris with absorbable suture to the opposite horizontal fibers to form a functioning oral sphincter.

The cleft margins are pared on both rotation and advancement flap. The undermining is less extensive in the medial rotation flap. The skin is closed with simple interrupted 5-0 nylon

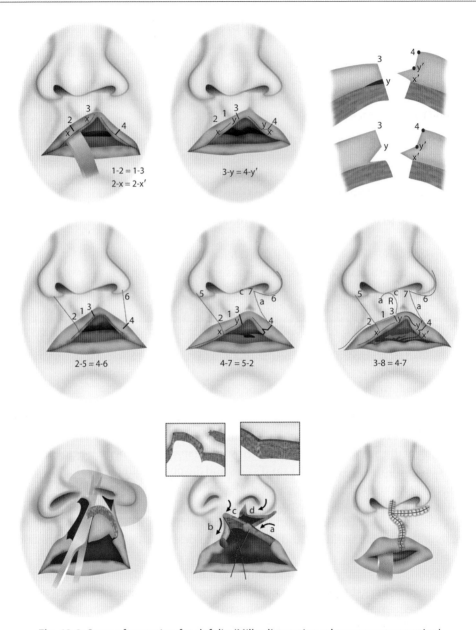

Fig. 13.8: Steps of operation for cleft lip (Millard's rotation advancement operation)

sutures. The dry mucosa is sutured similarly with 5-0 nylon sutures. The wet mucosa is closed with interrupted 4-0 chromic catgut sutures.

Nasal reconstruction with suturing of the nasolabial muscles with the alar base. Nasal skin closure about the nasal sill using a C-flap.

Q. What are the advantages of Millard's repair?

- This repair creates a normal Cupid's bow
- A normal looking philtrum is achieved
- The action of rotation and advancement aid in the nasal correction
- Well performed procedure gives an aesthetic result
- Secondary procedure, if required, may be done easily.

Q. What are the techniques for correction of nasal deformity?

Ans.
- A unilateral short columella is lengthened with a C-flap.
- Deviation and distortion of the septum are corrected during presurgical orthodontics.
- Flaring of the alar cartilages is corrected by an alar cinch procedure.

Q. What are the other techniques for repair of cleft lip?

Ans.
- *Straight line repair*: This is applicable for very small clefts (microform cleft lip).
- *Delaire's technique*: A form of Z-plasty with proper reconstruction of muscles of the lip.
- *LeMesurier technique*: Repair involves using a lateral quadrilateral flap. The quadrilateral flap from the cleft side is inset into a releasing incision on the noncleft side.
- *Tennison's repair*: This is a form of Z-plasty of the cleft edges.
- *Mirault-Blair technique*: The lip length on the cleft side is lengthened by using a lateral triangular flap from the cleft side.

Q. What is the ideal age for repair of isolated cleft lip?

Ans. Although debate remains, the recommended age for repair of isolated cleft lip is 10–12 weeks.

Q. What anesthesia will you prefer for this operation?

Ans. This is done under general anesthesia with endotracheal intubation. Infiltration of the lip 0.5% lignocaine with 1:200,000 adrenaline is helpful to minimize bleeding.

Q. How will you take care in postoperative period?

Ans.
- The child hands are splinted to prevent pulling of sutures
- Liquid diet may be started on the same day
- Suture line is cleaned with povidone–iodine solution and an ointment containing polymyxin-bacitracin is applied.
- Stitches are removed on 5th or 6th postoperative day.
- Normal diet is started from 9th or 10th postoperative day.

■ BILATERAL CLEFT LIP

Q. What is the deformity in a bilateral incomplete cleft lip?

Ans. In bilateral incomplete cleft lip, the cleft involves only the lip. The premaxilla is intact with a normal or near normal nose.

Q. What is the deformity in a bilateral complete cleft lip?

Ans.

* The cleft involves the lip on either side of the philtrum (Fig. 13.9).
* The premaxilla is protruded, as it is not reined back by its attachment to the lateral palatal shelves.
* The nasal tip is flat and broad. The alae are spread wide. The cartilaginous columella is very short or absent.
* The central prolabium forms a wide short disk, which hangs directly from the nasal tip skin, is devoid of muscle.
* No philtrum and no Cupid's bow.

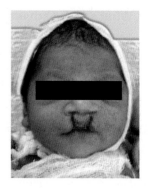

Fig. 13.9: Newborn child with bilateral complete cleft lip

Courtesy: Dr Kalyani Saha Basu, NRS Medical College, Kolkata

Q. How will you manage a patient with bilateral incomplete cleft lip?

Ans. I will consider repair of the bilateral cleft lip in one stage. The standard technique of repair is Millard's rotation-advancement technique (Fig. 13.10).

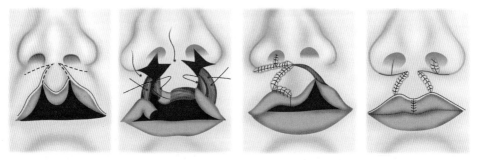

Fig. 13.10: Millard's rotation-advancement technique for repair of bilateral cleft lip

Q. How will you repair complete cleft lip (along with cleft of the palate)?

Ans. The protruding premaxilla, associated nasal deformity, the wide prolabium deficient of muscles poses special problems in bilateral complete cleft lip repair. In bilateral cleft lip, the alar cartilages have failed to reach the nasal tip and stretch the columella. The alar cartilages are flared.

The definitive surgical repair is preceded by orthodontic treatment (Fig. 13.11). The objective of presurgical orthodontic treatment is to lengthen the columella, reposition the nasal cartilages toward the tip, and align the alveolar segments. The first stage of this orthodontic treatment involves repositioning of the everted premaxilla into the space between the lateral alveolar segments using a progressive modification of an intraoral acrylic plate in conjunction with elastic bands hat are adhered to the cheeks. In the second stage, the nasal stents are built from the anterior rim of the oral plate and enter into the nasal aperture. This provides support and gives shape to the dome of the alar cartilages in the neonatal period. A horizontal prolabial band is attached to the two nasal stents that depresses the columellar base. An adhesive tape is applied to the prolabium pulled down and adhered to the inferior surface of the molding plate. Each functional component of the appliance is gradually modified by the clinician to mold the soft and hard tissues toward the desired form.

When the presurgical phase of treatment is coordinated with primary surgical repair, the outcome is better.

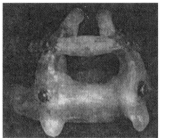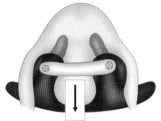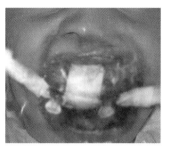

Fig. 13.11: Orthodontic appliance for preoperative molding of cleft lip and palate

The surgical treatment involves one stage repair of:
- Alveolar repair by gingivoperiosteoplasty—once the premaxilla is kept on good alignment by maxillary orthodontics.
- Lip repair using a narrow central prolabial flap.
- Nasal repair with retrograde dissection and suturing of the domes of the ala in the midline.
- The palate repair should be done as a second stage operation at the age of 1–1½ years.

Q. What is gingivoperiosteoplasty?

Ans. Presurgical orthodontic treatment may bring the protruding premaxilla in good alignment with the lateral hard palate. Small incisions are then made on the gingival periosteum on either side of the cleft. The gingival periosteum is then mobilized on either side. The nasal floor of the gingival periosteum is sutured. The labial and the palatal gingival periosteum are then sutured. If the cleft segments are close together, bone formation occurs across the cleft.

Q. When do you require bone grafting for cleft of the primary palate?

Ans. If the premaxillary segment is aligned well by presurgical orthodontics, a properly performed gingivoperiosteoplasty may obviate the need for bone grafting. But after gingivoperiosteoplasty, if there is a wide gap then this area needs to be grafted with a bone as a secondary procedure.

■ CLEFT PALATE

Terminologies associated with cleft of the palate:
- Primary palate
- Secondary palate
- Incomplete cleft palate
- Complete cleft palate.

Q. What is primary palate?

Ans. The palate has two distinct parts. The anterior triangular part is the premaxilla or the primary palate. This lies anterior to the incisive foramen. This constitutes the anterior triangular part of the hard palate and the alveolus. There may be cleft unilaterally or bilaterally.

Q. What is secondary palate?

Ans. The secondary palate is the remainder of the palate lying behind the incisive foramen. This consists of anterior part, which is the hard palate proper, and the posterior part which is called the soft palate.

Q. What is incomplete cleft palate?

Ans. There is cleft of the hard palate but it remains attached to the nasal septum and the vomer. This type of cleft is typed as incomplete cleft palate.

Q. What is complete cleft palate?

Ans. When the nasal septum and vomer are completely separated from the palatine processes then the cleft is typed as a complete cleft palate.

Q. What is submucus cleft of the palate?

Ans. This is not an overt cleft of the palate. The levator muscles fail to fuse completely in the midline usually leading to velopharyngeal incompetence. A notch can be palpated at the posterior end of the hard palate.

Q. What is your case?

Ans. The diagnosis may be stated as follows:
* This is a case of cleft of the soft palate.

Or

* This is a case of cleft of the soft and hard palate with intact premaxilla (Fig. 13.12).

Or

* This is a case of cleft of the soft palate, hard palate, and unilateral cleft of the premaxilla and the alveolus.

Or

* This is a case of complete cleft palate involving the soft palate, hard palate, and the premaxilla.

Or

* This is a case of bilateral cleft lip with complete cleft of the hard and soft palate, and cleft of alveolus (Fig. 13.13).
* Diagnosis will depend on the history and the findings on examination.

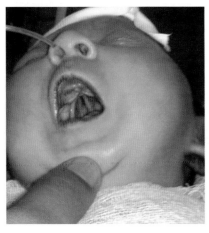

Fig. 13.12: Cleft of secondary palate in a newborn child

Courtesy: Dr Kalyani Saha Basu, NRS Medical College, Kolkata

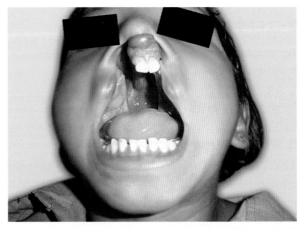

Fig. 13.13: Bilateral complete cleft lip with bilateral complete cleft palate

Courtesy: Prof Sasanka Sekhar Chatterjee, IPGME and R, Kolkata

Q. What is LAHSHAL system of cleft lip and cleft palate classification?

Ans. LASH: Type of cleft can be categorized by alphabets:
* L—cleft lip
* A—cleft of alveolus
* S—cleft of soft palate
* H—cleft of hard palate.

Incomplete cleft designated by small letter—lash.
* *LAHSHAL*: Complete bilateral cleft of lip, alveolus, hard, and soft palate.
* *lahSh*: Incomplete unilateral cleft lip, alveolus, a complete cleft of soft palate extending partly on to hard palate on both sides (Fig. 13.14).

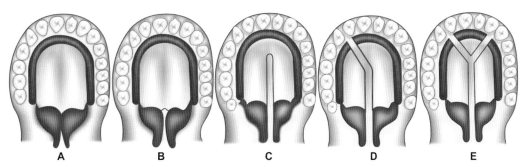

Fig. 13.14: Types of cleft palate. (a) Incomplete cleft of soft palate; (b) Complete cleft of soft palate; (c) Cleft of soft palate and secondary palate; (d) Cleft of soft palate and unilateral cleft of hard palate; (e) Cleft of soft palate and complete cleft of hard palate

Q. How does the palate develop?

Ans. The premaxilla or the primary palate develops from the median nasal process, which also forms the alveolus and the philtral part of the upper lip.

The secondary palate is formed by fusion of two palatine processes developing from the maxillary processes on either side.

These three parts fuse before backwards.

Q. How do you explain development of cleft palate?

Ans.
* Failure of fusion of two palatine processes developing from maxillary process leads to development of the cleft of the secondary palate.
* Failure of fusion of palatine processes with the median nasal process (premaxilla) leads to development of cleft of the alveolus and the cleft of the primary palate.

Q. What are the problems in patients with cleft palate?

Ans.
* *Difficulty in suction*:
  - Defective closure of oral cavity due to cleft palate results in defective suction.
  - Need spoon feeding or maxillary orthodontic appliances.
* *Defective hearing*:
  - Eustachian tube dysfunction may result in otitis media.
  - There may be associated sensorineural and conductive hearing loss.

- *Defective speech*:
  - For proper pronunciation of palatal consonants, velopharyngeal competence is essential. Cleft palate, involving the hard and soft palate, results in velopharyngeal incompetence as the soft palate fails to close the nasopharyngeal isthmus during pronunciation of palatal consonants, thus produces hypernasal quality of speech.
- *Defective dentition*:
  - Dental abnormalities may be found in patients with cleft lip and palate
  - Abnormalities include delayed tooth development and delayed eruption
  - Number of teeth may be altered—hypodontia or hyperdontia.
  - A protruding premaxilla results in gross malalignment of the teeth.
- *Repeated respiratory* tract infection may occur.
- *Cosmetic defect.*

Q. What are the causes of ear problems in patients with cleft palate?

Ans. The levator veli palatini and the tensor veli palatini muscles are inserted into the Eustachian tube and are probably responsible for the competence of the tube in preventing reflux of fluid from the nasopharynx into the middle ear through the Eustachian tube. In patients with cleft palate, there is reflux of fluid into the middle ear through the Eustachian tube resulting in otitis media.

Treatment consists of myringotomy, evacuation of fluid, and insertion of a Grommet's tube.

Q. How will you feed the child with a cleft palate?

Ans. Most children born with cleft palate have normal sucking motions, but the child could not build up adequate suction. The child can swallow normally. The child should be held in a head-up position at about 45° and fed with a bottle fitted with a long nipple. The nipple should not deliver too much milk at a time otherwise the child may be choked. The baby may swallow more air and needs burping to get rid of the swallowed air.

Q. What is orthodontic management?

Ans.
- Regular dental examination
- Repair of associated cleft lip by 6 months
- Appropriate repair of cleft palate in 12–15 months time
- Obturator placement.

Q. What are the muscles in soft palate?

Ans. In normal soft palate, the muscles are oriented transversely with no significant attachment to hard palate. There are five different muscles in soft palate, which function in a coordinated fashion to close the velopharyngeal isthmus.

In the cleft of soft palate, the muscle fibers are oriented in an anteroposterior direction and are inserted into the posterior edge of hard palate.

The muscles of the soft palate include tensor palati, levator palati, palatopharyngeus, palatoglossus, and musculus uvulae (Fig. 13.15).

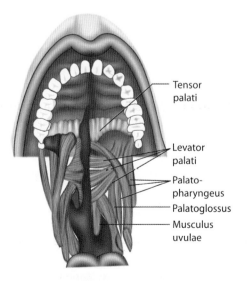

Fig. 13.15: Muscles of soft palate

Tensor palati

Levator palati

Palato-pharyngeus

Palatoglossus

Musculus uvulae

Q. What is the peculiarity of fibromucosa lining of the hard palate?

Ans. The fibromucosa lining of the hard palate is divided into three zones:

1. The central palatal fibromucosa—This area is very thin and lies directly below the floor of the nose. In complete cleft palate, the central palatal vault is absent and palatal fibromucosa is reduced in size.
2. The maxillary fibromucosa, lining the remainder of the hard palate, is thick and contains the greater palatine neurovascular bundle.
3. The gingival fibromucosa lies more laterally lining the alveolus adjacent to the teeth.

Q. What is the timing of surgery for cleft lip and cleft palate?

Ans. Delaire recommends following timing for surgery:

Cleft lip alone:
- Unilateral (5–6 months)
- Bilateral (4–5 months) (one-stage repair).

Cleft palate alone:
- Soft palate only (6 months)
- Soft + hard palate (two-stage operation):
  - Soft palate (6 months)
  - Hard palate (12–15 months).

Cleft lip and palate:
- Unilateral (two-stage operation):
  - Cleft lip + soft palate (5–6 months)
  - Hard palate + alveolus (12–15 months).
- Bilateral (two-stage operation):
  - Cleft lip + soft palate (4–5 months)
  - Hard palate + alveolus (12–15 months).

Q. What preoperative preparation will you do?

Ans.
- Hemoglobin estimation (hemoglobin level should be more than 10%)
- Throat swab for culture sensitivity
- The child should be habituated to spoon feeding
- Half unit of blood should be kept ready for operation.

Q. What are the principles of operation for cleft palate?

Ans.
- Mobilization and reconstruction of the aberrant soft palate musculature
- Closure of the hard palate cleft by minimal dissection and minimum scar formation.

Q. What operation will you do?

Ans.
- I will repair cleft palate by Wardill–Kilner–Veau four-flap technique. This is a form of V-Y advancement of mucoperiosteum of the hard palate and achieves anteroposterior lengthening (Fig. 13.16).
- Vertical incisions are made on the central palatine fibromucosa on either side of the cleft palate. The nasal and oral layers of the fibromucosa are mobilized.

- Lateral longitudinal release incisions are made on either side at the junction of the hard palate and the alveolus. At the anterior end, this incision is made continuous with the medial incision.
- The muscular attachment of the soft palate is detached from the hard palate and is sutured with the palatal muscles of the opposite side. The soft palate should be mobilized well, so that it causes good closure of the nasopharyngeal isthmus for production of proper speech. For adequate mobilization of the soft palate, the pterygoid hamulus needs to be broken.
- The cleft is repaired in two layers. The nasal side of the fibromucosa is sutured as first layer. The oral side of the fibromucosa is sutured as second layer.
- The greater palatine vessels need to be preserved.

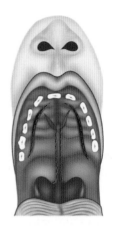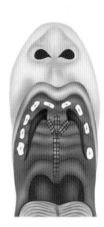

Fig. 13.16: Wardill–Kilner–Veau four flap technique for repair of cleft palate

Q. What is two-stage operation for cleft palate?

Ans. Earlier, two-stage operation was preferred for repair of cleft palate.
- Soft palate repaired at 6 months
- Hard palate repaired at 12–15 months.

Q. What is pharyngoplasty?

Ans. It is the reconstruction of the nasopharyngeal isthmus, which is made narrow by surgical procedure.

Q. How will you manage residual speech problem after cleft palate surgery?

Ans. With minor or inconsistent incompetence speech therapy alone may be successful in improving speech. In some cases, a secondary operation may be necessary. With minimal incompetence, a palatal lengthening operation may be sufficient. In other cases, pharyngoplasty with advancement of posterior pharyngeal wall may be done for relief of velopharyngeal incompetence.

■ ORAL LEUKOPLAKIA

Q. What is your case?

Ans. This is a case of leukoplakia involving both lips/buccal aspect of cheek/floor of mouth/tongue.

Q. What is leukoplakia?

Ans. World Health Organization (WHO) has defined leukoplakia as any white patch or plaque that cannot be characterized clinically or pathologically as any other disease.

Q. What are the common sites of leukoplakic change?

Ans.
- Oral cavity

- Tongue
- Lips
- Larynx
- Penis
- Vulva
- Other cutaneous or mucus lined areas.

Q. What are the characteristics of a leukoplakic patch?

Ans.
- Circumscribed area of white plaque.
- Surface is smooth, or may be traversed by cracks or fissure.
- Color may be white, yellowish, or grayish.
- Some lesions are homogeneous, others may be nodular on an erythematous base.
- Surrounding induration of the white plaque suggests malignant change.

Q. Which types of leukoplakia are more prone to undergo malignant change?

Ans.
- Speckled or nodular leukoplakic patch
- Leukoplakia of long duration
- Leukoplakia in elderly patient (70–89 years) has more chance of malignant change than in younger patients
- Leukoplakia on floor of mouth and tongue has a higher incidence of malignant change.

Q. What are the possible etiological factors for development of leukoplakia?

Ans.
- Smoking or chewing tobacco is the most important factor.
- Alcohol intakes have been found to be associated with increased incidence of leukoplakia.
- Chronic irritation due to ill-fitting denture or a sharp tooth may lead to leukoplakic change.

Q. What are the histological characteristics of a leukoplakic patch?

Ans.
- Hyperplasia of superficial epithelium with hyperkeratosis
- Swelling and vacuolation of cells in the middle layer
- Hyperplasia of cells in the basal layer
- There may be dyskeratosis.

Q. How will you manage this patient?

Ans.
- Patient should be asked to stop smoking and chewing tobacco. Alcohol intake should also be forbidden. If there is a sharp tooth causing chronic irritation, extraction of the offending tooth is to be done.
- With stoppage of smoking the leukoplakic patch may disappear in 1 year in 60% of cases.

Q. What is the indication of biopsy of a leukoplakic patch?

Ans.
- Simple leukoplakic patch need only regular follow-up and surgical biopsy is not required.

• Leukoplakic patch with an area of induration, cracks, fissure or surface ulceration, or adjacent erythroplakia, requires surgical biopsy to exclude malignant change in the leukoplakic change.

Q. What are the indications for excision of a leukoplakic patch?

Ans.

• Leukoplakic patch with suspicion of malignant change.
• Leukoplakic patch with histological features of severe epithelial dysplasia.
   The leukoplakic patch is removed either by surgical excision or by carbon dioxide laser excision.

Q. How will you manage the area of defect after excision of the leukoplakic patch?

Ans.

• *For smaller lesion*: The small defect may be closed by mobilization of the flap.
• *For larger lesion*: The large defect may be covered with split skin grafting or is left for epithelialization.

Q. What will you do when you find mild-to-moderate epithelial dysplasia?

Ans. These patients can be followed up at every 4-month intervals. The offending agent is withdrawn. If the patch shows signs of regression, it can be observed. If the lesion progresses or shows signs suspicious of malignancy, the lesion should be excised.

Q. What is erythroplakia?

Ans. Erythroplakia is defined as a lesion in oral mucosa presenting with red velvety plaque with irregular outline clearly demarcated from the normal epithelium and cannot be characterized clinically or pathologically as any other recognizable condition. In some cases, erythroplakia may be associated with adjacent leukoplakia.

Q. What is the incidence of malignant change in erythroplakia?

Ans. The erythroplakic patches are premalignant lesion and chance of development of malignant change is 17 times higher than the similar risk in leukoplakia. The erythroplakic patch may show areas of epithelial dysplasia and carcinoma in situ change.

Q. How will you treat erythroplakic patch?

Ans. In view of high risk of malignancy, an erythroplakic patch requires excision either by surgery or by carbon dioxide laser.

■ CARCINOMA OF TONGUE

Clinical Examination (*See* Page No. 382, Chapter 9)

History

• History of swelling or ulcer in the tongue
• Duration, onset, and progress
• Any pain in the tongue
• Any pain in ear
• History of excessive salivation or foul smelling discharge from the mouth

- Difficulty in chewing or swallowing
- Difficulty in speech
- Any swelling in the neck (cervical lymph nodes may be enlarged)
- Past history of venereal disease
- Any teeth trouble, whether using denture or not
- Any history of traumatic ulcer in the tongue
- Any history of smoking, chewing tobacco, or history of alcohol intake.

Examination—Inspection/Palpation

- Assess extent of mouth opening (in oral cancer the mouth opening may be restricted due to infiltration of growth into the infratemporal fossa or by involvement of temporomandibular joint).
- Any facial deformity.
- Examination of ulcer:
  - Site (common on the lateral border of anterior two-thirds of tongue)
  - Size and shape (usually an ovoid ulcer size variable 1–5 cm)
  - Margins (usually raised and everted margin)
  - Floor (usually covered by grayish slough)
  - Base (usually indurated base)
  - Any extension of the ulcer to the floor of mouth or gum (alveolar margin) ascertained by palpation.
- Assess movement of tongue (tongue movement may be restricted).
- Examine the different levels of cervical lymph nodes.

Q. What is your case? (Summary of a case of carcinoma of tongue)

Ans. This 60-year-old gentleman presented with an ulcer in right lateral margin of tongue for last 1 year. The ulcer was initially small in size, but for last 6 months, it increased in size to attain the present size. Patient complains of excessive salivation for last 6 months, also complains of dull aching pain in the local site, but does not complain of any swelling in the neck. Patient is a chronic smoker and is also in the habit of chewing tobacco for last 8 years.

On examination: There is a 1.5 × 1.5 cm ulcer in the right lateral margin of tongue. The margin is everted, the base is indurated and the floor of the ulcer is covered with a necrotic slough. Movements of the tongue are normal. The ulcer is not adherent to mandible. The cervical lymph nodes are not palpable.

Q. What is your diagnosis?

Ans. This is a case of ulcerative type of carcinoma tongue on the right lateral aspect of the anterior two-thirds of the tongue without any lymph node metastasis (Fig. 13.17).

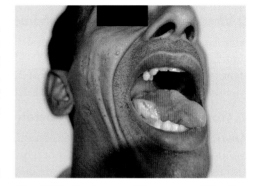

Fig. 13.17: Carcinoma of tongue involving the anterior two-thirds of right lateral margin

Courtesy: Dr Debarchan Ghosh, IPGME and R, Kolkata

Q. What is the differential diagnosis for an ulcerative lesion in tongue?

Ans.

- *Traumatic ulcer*: Usually follows chronic irritation by a sharp tooth or a denture.
- *Tubercular ulcer*: Ulcer with an undermined edges. Floor covered with a pale granulation tissue. May be associated with tuberculosis elsewhere in the body.
- *Infective ulcer*: Due to nonspecific bacterial infection.
- *Syphilitic ulcer*: Very rare nowadays. Painless punched out ulcer, floor covered with a wash leather slough.
- *Aphthous ulcer*: Usually multiple and shallow painful ulcers.

Q. How will you manage this case?

Ans.

- I will like to confirm my diagnosis by taking an incisional biopsy from the margin of the ulcer
- X-ray of mandible to exclude bony involvement (orthopantomogram—OPG)
- Indirect laryngoscopy to exclude lesion in posterior third of tongue
- Chest X-ray to exclude chest metastasis
- Baseline investigations—complete hemogram, blood sugar, urea, and creatinine.
- Electrocardiogram (ECG)
- Maintenance of oral hygiene by antiseptic mouth wash.

Q. What precaution should you take while taking an incisional biopsy?

Ans.

- The biopsy should be taken from the most suspicious area and should include some normal adjacent mucosa.
- The biopsy should not be taken from the necrotic or infected area, as the result may be fallacious.

Q. How will you treat this patient?

Ans. I will consider surgical treatment in this patient. My plan is to do a right hemiglossectomy along with elective lymph node dissection on right side removing the level I, II, III (supraomohyoid node dissection).

Q. Would you like to do hemimandibulectomy in this patient?

Ans. The lesion is confined to the lateral margin of the tongue and has not infiltrated into the floor of the mouth or the mandible, so I will not consider hemimandibulectomy in this patient. If the lesion has infiltrated into the floor of the mouth or if the lymph nodes are involved requiring modified radical neck dissection (MRND) then concomitant hemimandibulectomy is required.

Q. Would you like to give postoperative radiotherapy?

Ans. If the lines of resection are free of tumor and the tumor is well-differentiated postoperative radiotherapy to the primary site is not required. Patient should be kept under regular follow up and if there is recurrence, it may be treated with radiotherapy.

Postoperative radiotherapy is indicated when:

- If primary lesion is large
- Poor grade tumor
- The resection lines are involved with tumor

+ If there are two or more involved nodes with extracapsular extension postoperative radiotherapy to the neck is required.

Q. What is the role of prophylactic irradiation of the neck?

Ans. There is good evidence that elective irradiation of the N0 neck with 40 Gray is of same benefit as elective node dissection and carries less morbidity.

Q. What are the predisposing factors for development of carcinoma tongue?

Ans.
+ Long-standing traumatic ulcer
+ Leukoplakia
+ Chronic irritation—smoking, spirits, and spices
+ Syphilitic glossitis
+ Chronic superficial glossitis
+ Erythroplakia
+ Plummer–Vinson syndrome
+ Papilloma.

Q. What is the relative site distribution of carcinoma tongue?

Ans.
+ Posterior one-third—25% (Fig. 13.18)
+ Anterior two-thirds—75%
  – Lateral margin—50%
  – Dorsum—5%
  – Tip—10%
  – Ventral surface—10%.

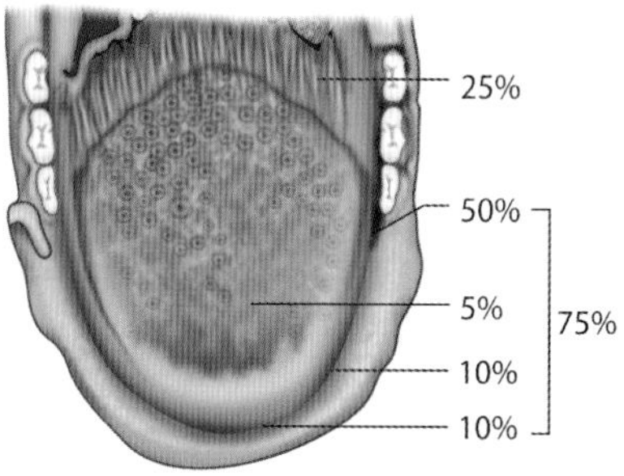

Fig. 13.18: Site distribution of carcinoma tongue

Q. What are the gross types of carcinoma tongue?

Ans.
+ *Ulcerative type*:
  – Ulcer initially superficial
  – Later on, a typical ulcer with irregular everted margin with indurated base and floor covered with necrotic tissues and bleeds to touch.
+ *Exophytic or papillary type*:
  – Papillary tumor with a broad and indurated base
  – Papillary lesion with a central ulceration.
+ *Nodular type*:
  – Presents as a submucous nodule, which may ulcerate later on.
+ *Fissure type*:
  – Presents as an ulcer in the depths of a fissure.

Q. What are the histological types of carcinoma tongue?

Ans. The histological types of carcinoma tongue may be:
+ Squamous cell carcinoma is the most common
+ Basal cell carcinoma
+ Adenocarcinoma rare
+ Malignant melanoma.

Q. Why there is speech problem in patients with carcinoma tongue?

Ans. The growth may cause deeper infiltration of the muscles of tongue and floor of the mouth resulting in restriction of tongue movement and difficulty in articulation.

Q. How does carcinoma tongue spread?

Ans.
- *Direct spread or local spread*:
  - Floor of mouth, mandible, tonsil, and epiglottis.
- *Lymphatic spread*:
  - Both by lymphatic permeation and lymphatic emboli
  - May metastasize to submental (level IA), submandibular (level IB), and jugulodigastric (level II) and jugulo-omohyoid (level III) lymph nodes.
- *Blood spread*:
  - Rare route of spread
  - May metastasize to lungs, liver, and bones.

Q. What is tumor/node/metastasis (TNM) classification of oral carcinomas?

Ans.

T—Primary tumor:
- *Tx*: Primary tumor cannot be assessed
- *T0*: No evidence of primary tumor
- *Tis*: Tumor in situ
- *T1*: Tumor less than or equal to 2 cm in greatest dimension
- *T2*: Tumor more than 2 cm but less than 4 cm in greatest dimension
- *T3*: Tumor more than 4 cm in greatest dimension
- *T4*: Tumor invading adjacent structures (Table 13.1).

N—Lymph node status:
- *Nx*: Regional lymph nodes cannot be assessed
- *N0*: No regional lymph node metastasis
- *N1*: Metastasis in a single ipsilateral lymph node (<3 cm)
- *N2*:
  - *N2a*: Metastasis in a single ipsilateral lymph node (>3 cm but <6 cm)
  - *N2b*: Metastasis in multiple ipsilateral lymph nodes (none > 6 cm)
  - *N2c*: Metastasis in bilateral lymph nodes or contralateral lymph nodes none more than 6 cm.
- *N3*: Metastasis to lymph nodes more than 6 cm in diameter.

Table 13.1: Tumor invading in oral carcinoma	
Region	*Tumor invasion*
T4a (lip)	Tumor invades through cortical bone, inferior alveolar ner ve, floor of mouth, or skin (chin or nose)
T4a (oral cavity)	Tumor invades through cortical bone, into deep/extrinsic muscle of tongue (genioglossus, hyoglossus, palatoglossus, and styloglossus), maxillary sinus, or skin of face
T4b (lip and oral cavity)	Tumor invades masticator space, pterygoid plates, or skull base; or encases internal carotid artery

M—Metastasis
* *Mx*: Distant metastasis cannot be assessed
* *M0*: No distant metastasis
* *M1*: Distant metastasis present.

Q. What is TNM stage grouping for oral carcinomas?

Ans.

Stage 0	TIS	N0	M0
Stage I	T1	N0	M0
Stage II	T2	N0	M0
Stage III	T1/T2	N1	M0
	T3	N0/N1	M0
Stage IVA	T1/T2/T3	N2	M0
Stage IVB	Any T	N3	M0
	T4	Any N	M0
Stage IVC	Any T	Any N	M1

Q. What structures will you remove in radical neck dissection?

Ans. The standard RND as described by Crile in 1906 involves removal of:
* All levels of lymph nodes (level I to level VI)
* Sternocleidomastoid and omohyoid muscle
* Internal jugular vein
* Spinal accessory nerve and cervical plexus of nerves
* Submandibular salivary gland and tail of parotid gland
* All intervening lymphoareolar tissues.
* Removes all the lymph nodes as in radical node dissection.

Q. What structures will you preserve in modified radical node dissection?

Ans.
* Preserve any one of the nonlymphatic structures removed in RND-spinal accessory nerve, internal jugular vein, and sternocleidomastoid muscle.
* *Type I*: Spinal accessory nerve is preserved.
* *Type II*: Spinal accessory nerve and internal jugular veins are preserved.
* *Type III*: Spinal accessory nerve, internal jugular vein, and sternocleidomastoid muscle are preserved.

Q. What is functional neck dissection?

Ans.
* A variation of MRND where group of lymph nodes from level I to level VI are removed.
* All nonlymphatic structures are preserved.

Q. What do you mean by elective neck dissection?

Ans.
* Involves removal of cervical lymph nodes considered to be at high risk for metastasis from a given primary site. The extent of elective dissection depends on the type of primary lesion.
* Selective lymph node dissection is usually performed in N0 neck.

Q. What is the role of radiotherapy in treatment of N0 neck?

Ans.

- Radiotherapy is an effective modality of treatment of N0 neck when the lymph nodes are not clinically palpable.
- Results of surgery and radiotherapy are comparable.
- If the primary lesion is treated by radiotherapy, the neck nodes may be irradiated electively.

Q. How does the lymphatics of tongue drains?

Ans.

- There is a rich plexus of lymphatics in the tongue.
- The lymphatics from the tip may drain into the submental lymph nodes on either side.
- The lympahatics from the lateral margin and undersurface of the anterior two-thirds of the tongue drains into the submental (level IA), submandibular (level IB), jugulodigastric (level II), and jugulo-omohyoid (level III) group of lymph nodes.
- The level II lymph nodes are the most commonly involved nodes in metastasis from carcinoma tongue. The level I and level III nodes are also at high risk for metastasis from carcinoma tongue.
- In patients with N0 nodes, dissection of level I, level II, and level III nodes (supraomohyoid lymph nodes) is sufficient to assess the lymph node status in patients with squamous cell carcinoma of tongue.

Q. What are different lymph nodes in the neck?

Ans. The cervical lymph nodes are situated either superficial or deep to the deep-cervical fascia, and so grouped as superficial or deep-cervical lymph nodes.

The cervical lymph node groups are also described as seven levels of lymph nodes:

- *Level I*: Submental (IA) and submandibular (IB) lymph nodes
- *Level II*, Level III and level IV lymph nodes lying in relation to the upper, middle, and lower thirds of the internal jugular vein
- *Level V*: Lymph nodes lying in the posterior triangle of the neck
- *Level VI*: Pre- or paralaryngeal and pre- or paratracheal lymph nodes
- *Level VII*: Anterior mediastinal lymph nodes.

Q. What is the cause of ear pain in patient with carcinoma tongue?

Ans. It is usually a referred pain. There is infiltration of the lingual nerve and the pain is referred via the auriculotemporal nerve, which is also a branch of mandibular division of trigeminal nerve.

Q. What is the cause of excessive salivation in patients with carcinoma tongue?

Ans. Often patients of carcinoma tongue presents with excessive salivation. This is either due to excessive secretion of saliva due to an irritative lesion in the tongue or due to difficulty in swallowing of saliva due to restriction of tongue movement as a consequence of infiltration into the floor of the mouth.

Q. What is the treatment of choice for early carcinomatous lesion in tongue?

Ans. Early carcinomatous lesion of tongue less than 1 cm is best treated by surgical excision with 1 cm margin of excision all around.

Q. What is the treatment of choice for intermediate lesion?

Ans. For intermediate stage of the disease, the outcome of surgery and radiotherapy is comparable.

Q. How will you manage the defect following excision of tongue?

Ans. If less than one-third of tongue is excised, formal reconstruction is not required.

The area following excision is fulgurated and allowed to granulate and epithelialize spontaneously.

Alternatively, the area can be covered with split skin graft.

- If a hemiglossectomy or two-thirds tongue is resected—reconstruction may be done with a free radial forearm flap with microvascular anastomosis.
- For a very large volume defects following total glossectomy for a deep infiltrating lesion with resection extending up to the hyoid bone needs more bulky flaps to fill the dead space.
- A pectoralis major myocutaneous flap is the best in such situation.

Q. How will you manage a patient with a growth in the posterior third of the tongue?

Ans. Carcinoma involving the posterior third of the tongue is usually advanced at the time of diagnosis, and is best treated with radiotherapy.

Q. What may be the cause of lymph node enlargement in patient with carcinoma tongue?

Ans. The lymph node enlargement is either due to infection or metastasis. A course of broad-spectrum antibiotics is given for 2 weeks. The infective lymph nodes will regress. A fine-needle aspiration cytology (FNAC) will confirm the metastatic disease.

Q. If lymph nodes are not involved clinically, how will you treat the lymph node in patients with carcinoma tongue, carcinoma lip, and carcinoma of the floor of the mouth (N0)?

Ans. The management of clinically impalpable node in this clinical situation is controversial. There are proponents for prophylactic neck dissection when the lymph nodes are not clinically palpable. The justification for a prophylactic neck dissection is:

- Incidence of histological positive node in case of clinical N0 ranges between 25% and 65%.
- By waiting for lymph nodes to become clinically palpable leads to a worse prognosis. Survival rates are lowered in patient who presents with subsequent lymph node metastasis.
- Some patients fail to attend for regular follow up and often present subsequently with extensive nodal metastasis.
- Prophylactic neck dissection carries negligible morbidity and mortality.
- Retrospective reviews confirmed that patients undergoing prophylactic neck dissection have a better survival rate.
- High-recurrence rate following block dissection for extensive nodal disease.
- Failure to control nodal disease is a frequent cause of death.

In N0 node, a supraomohyoid block dissection is sufficient.

Q. What are the points against prophylactic neck dissection?

Ans.

- Incidence of histologically positive node in prophylactic block dissection exceeds the incidence of subsequent clinical nodal metastasis. Some micrometastases in lymph nodes possibly are destroyed by body's own defense mechanism.

- The primary tumor may recur or a second primary may develop and metastasis to dissected neck makes subsequent management difficult.
- Block dissection of neck has considerable morbidity and some mortality.
- There is no prospectively controlled trial to support the argument that prophylactic neck dissection does improve the prognosis.

Q. How will you treat a patient of carcinoma tongue with mobile lymph nodal metastasis (N1, N2)?

Ans.

- Patient with carcinoma tongue and oral carcinoma often has bilateral lymph node metastasis
- An RND on the ipsilateral side and a supraomohyoid dissection on the other side are indicated. Internal jugular vein on one side should be spared.

Q. What are the indications of radiotherapy?

Ans.

- Postoperative radiotherapy is indicated when:
  - There are multiple lymph nodes metastasis on histology
  - There is extracapsular extension of the tumor.
- Locally, advanced primary lesion not amenable to surgical treatment, then both the primary lesion and the lymph node metastasis may be treated by irradiation.
- If the patient is unfit for surgery, the lymph nodal metastasis may be treated with radical radiotherapy.

Q. How will you treat a patient of carcinoma tongue with lymph nodes metastasis, which are fixed (N3)?

Ans.

- Large fixed lymph nodes metastasis are often associated with advanced primary disease with a poor prognosis.
- Most cases are treated by irradiation both for the primary disease and the lymph node metastasis.
- A course of preoperative radiotherapy may render the fixed nodes in the neck to become mobile and may be amenable to RND.

Q. A patient of carcinoma tongue treated with surgical excision came with metastatic lymph nodes in the neck in follow up. How will you manage?

Ans.

- A detailed clinical examination to exclude local recurrence and metastatic disease in other sites
- FNAC from the lymph nodes
- Radical neck dissection is the treatment of choice. Postoperative radiotherapy, if there are multiple lymph nodes metastasis or if there is extracapsular extension.

Q. What are the different techniques for administration of radiotherapy?

Ans. Radiotherapy may be administered by:

- Brachytherapy with implantation of radium needle, radioactive tantalum wires, or iridium-192 wires. This can deliver very high dose of radiation locally.

The radium needles are kept for 9–10 days.
- *Teletherapy*: External beam radiation with a telecobalt or linear accelerator.

Q. What are the causes of death in patients with carcinoma tongue?

Ans. Advanced disease leads to death by:
- Hemorrhage from the primary growth or hemorrhage from erosion of carotid artery or internal jugular vein by a metastatic lymph node.
- Asphyxia resulting from growth in the tongue or huge lymph node metastasis blocking the upper air passage. Edema of the glottis may aggravate the airway obstruction.
- Aspiration bronchopneumonia
- Starvation and malignant cachexia.

■ CARCINOMA OF LIP

Clinical Examination

See Carcinoma of Tongue, Page No. 570.

Q. What is your case? (Summary of a case of carcinoma of lip)

Ans. This 65-year-old man presented with an ulcer in his both upper and lower lip for last 3 years. Initially, the ulcer was about 1 cm in size and started in the lower lip near the angle. The ulcer was increasing slowly in size for last 2.5 years. But for last 6 months, the ulcer is increasing rapidly in size and has spread to the adjacent area and the ulcer has involved the upper lip and the left angle of the mouth. Patient is in the habit of chewing tobacco (Fig. 13.19).

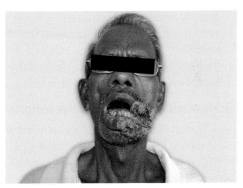

Fig. 13.19: Carcinoma of lip
Courtesy: Prof SS Chatterjee, IPGME and R, Kolkata

On examination: There is a large ulcerative lesion involving both the upper and lower lip extending up to the left angle of the mouth. The margin of the ulcer is rolled out and everted. The floor is covered with necrotic granulation tissue and the base of the ulcer is indurated. There are multiple enlarged palpable cervical lymph nodes in the submental and submandibular group (level I) in the left side of the neck.

Q. What is your diagnosis?

Ans. This is a case of carcinoma of lower lip extending up to the left angle of mouth and upper lip with left-sided cervical lymph node metastasis.

Q. In which lip, carcinoma is more common?

Ans.
- This is the most common in vermilion border of upper lip—80%.
- In commissural region—15%.
- In lower lip—5%.

Q. How will you treat this patient?

Ans. I would like to confirm my diagnosis by taking an incision biopsy from the margin of the ulcer. If malignancy is confirmed, I will consider surgical treatment.

As the lesion is very large, I will consider wide excision of the growth with 2 cm clear margin and primary reconstruction of the defect and modified RND on the left side.

Q. How will you reconstruct the defect?

Ans. Surgical resection will create a large area of full thickness defect of mucosa, muscle, and skin. Restoration of function will require replacement of internal lining and external skin coverage. The reconstruction may be done by a pectoralis major myocutaneous flap for internal lining and a deltopectoral skin flap for external skin coverage.

Q. What are the other methods for the reconstruction of defects after excision of lips or cheek?

Ans. The defect may also be covered by:

◆ The forehead flap based on superficial temporal artery for inner lining and deltopectoral flap for external skin coverage.
◆ Latissimus dorsi myocutaneous flap folded on itself for both inner lining and outer skin coverage.
◆ The recent trend in reconstruction is by free microvascular flap transfer. A radial forearm flap based on radial artery may be used for both inner lining and outer skin coverage.

Q. How will you treat smaller lesions?

Ans. Lesion in the lip up to 2 cm—can be excised in V-shaped manner comprising full thickness of lip taking 1 cm—margin on either side.

The residual defect is reconstructed by approximating and suturing the cut margin in three layers—mucosa-to-mucosa, muscle-to-muscle, and skin-to-skin. Initially, the lip may appear tight but subsequently improves.

Q. How else smaller defects may be reconstructed?

Ans.

◆ *For central defect in the lower lip*:
  – *Mini facelift of Jonathan*: This consists of symmetrical bilateral flaps from the lower third of the face in a stepladder pattern. This gives good cosmetic result.
◆ *For more lateral defects in upper or lower lip or in commissure*:
  – *Fries universal technique of reconstruction*: In this technique, full thickness lateral facial flaps are developed following full thickness incision in the cheek parallel to the branches of the facial nerve.

These flaps are then advanced into the lip defect. The pedicle is divided after 3 weeks.
For larger defects:

◆ Deltopectoral flap for reconstruction
◆ Free flap transfer for reconstruction.

Q. In ultraviolet radiation-induced carcinoma lip there are also actinic changes in the rest of the lip. How will you manage?

Ans. In such case, in addition to the resection of the primary tumor, total lip shave is to be done.

The resection is reconstructed either by advancing labial or buccal mucosal flap or by an anteriorly based tongue flap.

Q. How will you manage clinically noninvolved nodes?

Ans. There has been controversy regarding elective lymph node dissection.

For primary lesion in the central part of the lower lip with N0 nodes—elective bilateral supraomohyoid block dissection (removal of level I, II, and level III) of lymph nodes is recommended.

For lateral lesion—elective ipsilateral supraomohyoid block dissection is recommended.

Q. How will you manage clinically involved lymph nodes?

Ans. For unilateral involvement, a unilateral modified RND is recommended.

If there is bilateral involvement, a bilateral modified radical lymph node dissection is recommended.

Fixed lymph nodes are inoperable. A course of neoadjuvant chemotherapy may cause regression of the lymph node enlargement. If the lymph nodes become mobile, a modified radical lymph node dissection may be done.

Q. When will you consider excision of mandible?

Ans.
- If the bones are not involved, bony resection is not indicated.
- If the mandible is involved, a segmental resection of mandible is required.
- If 2 cm segment of mandible can be retained close to the chin then bony reconstruction of mandible is not essential.

Q. How mandible may be reconstructed after excision?

Ans. After hemimandibulectomy, reconstruction may be done by:
- Rib graft
- Fibular bone graft
- Radial forearm flap along with a segment of radius.

Q. What is precancerous lesion of lip?

Ans.
- Leukoplakia
- Oral lichen planus
- Discoid lupus erythematosus
- Erythroplakia
- Sideropenic dysphagia
- Chronic hyperplastic candidiasis.

Q. What are the gross types of carcinoma lip?

Ans. Gross lesion may be:
- *Ulcerative*
- *Nodular*
- *A warty papillary* lesion
- *Infiltrative* lesion.

Q. What are the histological types of carcinoma lip?

Ans.

* Majority are squamous cell carcinomas
* Rarely basal cell carcinoma
* Adenocarcinoma is also very rare
* Malignant melanoma.

Q. How does carcinoma lip spreads?

Ans.

* *Direct spread*: It spreads laterally and may infiltrate deeply and may involve the floor of mouth, mandible, and maxilla.
* *Lymphatic spread*:
  - *From lower lip*: Submental, submandibular group, and then to jugulodigastric nodes
  - *From upper lip*: Preauricular, submandibular, and jugulodigastric node
  - *From commissural region*: Lymphatics drain along with lymphatics from both upper and lower lips.
* Blood spread is extremely rare.

Q. In which case of carcinoma, lip surgery is preferred to radiotherapy?

Ans.

* No facilities for radiotherapy
* In cases of bulky tumor
* Recurrence after radiotherapy
* Carcinoma lip involving the jaw
* Carcinoma supervening on a leukoplakic patch
* Carcinoma supervening on a syphilitic sore
* Carcinoma invading the floor of mouth and the mandible.

■ CARCINOMA OF CHEEK

Q. What is your case? (Summary of a case of carcinoma of cheek)

Ans. This 45-year-old lady presented with an ulcer on the inner part of cheek on the left side for last 6 months. Initially, it was about 1 cm in size but the ulcer is increasing in size for last 3 months and has extended to involve the adjacent area of the left side of the cheek. Patient complains of dull aching pain over the local site. Patient has habit of chewing tobacco for last 20 years (Fig. 13.20).

On examination: There is an ulcer on the inner aspect of the left cheek 3.5 cm × 3.5 cm in size, margins are raised and everted. There is induration at the margin. The floor of the ulcer is covered by necrotic granulation tissue. The ulcer has infiltrated up to the skin. Cervical lymph nodes are not palpable.

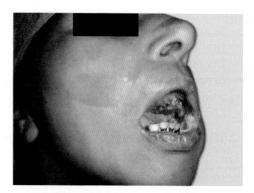

Fig. 13.20: Carcinoma of cheek

Courtesy: Dr Bijay Majumdar, IPGME and R, Kolkata

Q. What is your diagnosis?

Ans. This is a case of carcinoma of cheek involving the left side without any clinical evidence of lymph node metastasis.

Q. What is the extent of cheek or buccal mucosa?

Ans. The buccal mucosa extends from the upper alveolar ridge to lower alveolar ridge and from the commissure anteriorly to the mandibular ramus and the retromolar region, posteriorly.

Q. What are the gross types of carcinoma cheek?

Ans.
* Exophytic or proliferative lesion
* Ulcerative lesion
* Verrucous carcinoma.

Q. What are the characteristics of proliferative lesion?

Ans.
* Exophytic lesion projects into the oral cavity
* Infiltrate adjacent tissue early.

Q. What are the characteristics of ulcerating lesion?

Ans.
* A typical malignant ulcer with everted margin
* The ulcer may infiltrate the overlying skin and may fungate outside with multiple sinuses.

Q. What are the features of verrucous carcinoma?

Ans.
* Very slow growing superficial proliferative lesion
* Minimal deep muscle invasion and induration
* This may present as a white velvety lesion
* Behaves as a low-grade squamous cell carcinoma
* Lymph node metastasis is late.

Q. How will you manage this patient?

Ans. I will confirm my diagnosis by incisional biopsy, from the junction of healthy tissue and tumor.

Q. What surgery will you consider in this patient?

Ans. As the lesion is large and has involved the full thickness of cheek, I will consider full thickness excision of cheek with primary reconstruction of the defect.

Q. How will you reconstruct the defect?

Ans.
* For more extensive lesion extending posteriorly to the retromolar area, wide excision with primary reconstruction is advisable.

A free radial forearm flap adapts very well and remains soft and mobile posteriorly.

If free flap transfer is not appropriate then other flaps may be used.

For small intraoral defect up to 3 cm—buccal fat pad may be used for reconstruction. This well-vascularized flap may be left raw for spontaneous epithelialization. This may be used for reconstruction of defect involving maxilla, hard palate, soft palate, cheek, and retromolar area.

For larger defects at these sites, the buccal fat pad flap may be combined with temporalis muscle flap.

Q. Why forehead flap is not used commonly nowadays?

Ans. Forehead flap based on superficial temporal artery can provide good coverage of defect in the most areas of the face. But it produces a deformity at donor site and it requires a two-stage procedure.

Q. How will you manage lymph node in carcinoma of cheek?

Ans.
* *No lymph node involvement*: Elective lymph node dissection is not recommended.
* *Lymph nodes are involved*: A radical lymph node dissection is indicated.

Q. How will you manage smaller defect following excision of carcinoma of cheek?

Ans.
* For smaller defect tongue flap, palatal mucoperiosteal flap or buccal fat pad has been used with success.
* Platysma myocutaneous flap may be used for reconstruction of superficial defect.

Q. What is the role of radiotherapy in carcinoma of cheek?

Ans. Squamous cell carcinoma of cheek is radiosensitive.

In early cases without lymph node metastasis—radiotherapy either with interstitial radiation or by external beam radiation is effective in carcinoma of cheek and provides comparable results as surgery.

■ CARCINOMA OF THE FLOOR OF MOUTH

Q. What is your case? (Summary of a case of carcinoma of the floor of mouth)

Ans. This 55-year-old gentleman presented with an ulcer in the floor of the mouth on right side for last 8 months. Initially, the ulcer was about 1 cm in size at the onset, but for last 2 months the ulcer is gradually increasing in size and has reached up to the lower jaw. Patient complains of excessive salivation, difficulty in chewing food, and offensive smell in the mouth. Patient also complains of swelling in the right side of neck for last 3 months. There is complain of dull aching pain at the site of ulcer, aggravated during chewing of food.

On examination: There is an ulcer in right side of floor of mouth 2 cm × 1.5 cm. The ulcer has raised margin, floor is covered by necrotic granulation tissue. The ulcer has involved the lateral margin of tongue medially and the lower alveolus laterally. There are multiple significant lymph node enlargements in the submandibular group. The lymph nodes are firm in consistency free from the skin and mobile.

Q. What is your diagnosis?

Ans. This is a case of carcinoma of the floor of mouth on the right side involving the adjacent body of mandible with metastasis to the right submandibular lymph nodes (level IB).

Q. How will you manage this patient?

Ans.
* I would like to confirm my diagnosis by taking an incision biopsy from the margin of the ulcer along with a rim of normal tissue.
* FNAC from the enlarged cervical lymph node
* An OPG of mandible to look for any bony involvement
* Baseline investigations to assess patient fitness for anesthesia and surgery.

Q. What surgery will you plan for this patient?

Ans. As the lesion has involved the margin of the tongue and there is involvement of mandible with lymph node enlargement, I will consider surgical treatment in this patient.

Excision of the ulcerating lesion along with hemiglossectomy and hemimandibulectomy with modified RND of right side with primary reconstruction of the defect so created.

Mandibular reconstruction is done by using a vascularized fibular bone graft.

Q. How else can mandible be reconstructed?

Ans.
* By using a rib as a bone graft
* By nail and plate.

Q. How will you treat small tumor in the floor of mouth?

Ans.
* Small tumor in floor of mouth not infiltrating into the tongue or gingiva may be simply treated by excision with 1 cm margin.
* The residual defect may be left as such to granulate or defect may be fulgurated with diathermy.
The defect can be covered using a bilateral nasolabial flaps turned into the floor of the mouth.

Q. How will you gain access to the tumor in floor of mouth?

Ans. The access is best gained through midline lip split and a midline or lateral mandibulotomy.

Q. How will you tackle lymph node in carcinoma floor of mouth?

Ans.
* In carcinoma, floor of mouth lymph node involvement is common.
* In N0 stage—a prophylactic supraomohyoid block dissection in continuity with the primary growth is done.
When significant lymph nodes are present and is mobile—an RND is to be done en-bloc.

For fixed lymph nodes—neoadjuvant chemotherapy—if lymph nodes become mobile, RND may be considered. Alternatively, fixed neck nodes may be treated with palliative radiotherapy.

Q. What is marginal mandibular resection?

Ans. Partial resection of mandible from lingula to the mental foramen is preserving the lower margin of the mandible.

Q. Which area denotes the floor of the mouth?

Ans. The floor of the mouth is a U-shaped area between the lower surface of the tongue and the lower alveolus.

Q. How will you manage carcinoma of floor of the mouth infiltrating into the mandible?

Ans.
* A wide excision with segmental mandibular resection and radical lymph node dissection, if lymph nodes are involved.
* If lymph nodes are not involved, an elective bilateral supraomohyoid block dissection is recommended.
* Postoperative adjuvant radiotherapy is required.

■ CARCINOMA OF HARD PALATE AND THE UPPER ALVEOLUS

Q. What is your case? (Summary of a case of carcinoma of hard palate and the upper alveolus)

Ans. This 60-year-old gentleman presented with a proliferative lesion in the roof of mouth for last 6 months, which is gradually increasing in size.

On examination: There is a 2 cm × 2 cm proliferative lesion over the mucosa of hard palate confined to the left. The growth has invaded up to the left upper alveolar margin.

There are no palpable lymph nodes in the neck.

Q. What is your diagnosis?

Ans. This is a case of carcinoma of hard palate involving the upper alveolar margin.

Q. What are the histological types of carcinoma in hard palate?

Ans.
* Squamous cell carcinoma is the most common arising from the squamous epithelial lining of hard palate
* Adenocarcinoma arising from minor salivary glands.

Q. How will you manage this patient?

Ans.
* I would like to confirm my diagnosis by an incisional biopsy.
* X-ray (OPG) to look for any invasion into the maxilla.

Q. What surgery will you plan for this patient?

Ans. In majority of patients, squamous carcinoma involving the upper gum or the hard palate arises from maxillary antrum.
* The tumor confined to the floor of the antrum, upper alveolus, or the hard palate requires partial maxillectomy.

- The tumor involving the whole of antrum needs total maxillectomy.
- The tumor extending more posteriorly into the infratemporal fossa or base of the skull—requires a more extensive procedure. A combined anteroposterior or lateral facial approach is required for such wide resection.
- Adjuvant postoperative radiotherapy is required.

Q. How will you do reconstruction after maxillectomy?

Ans.
- Obwegeser technique of reconstruction by using a split rib graft.
- Reconstruction by temporalis muscle flap.

■ DENTAL CYST

Clinical EXAMINATION

History

- History of swelling—onset and progress (usually slow growing swelling)
- Site (dental cysts are more common in upper jaw)
- Any dental pain (dental cyst often develops in relation tom a caries tooth).

Examination

- Examination of the swelling
- Site and extent
- Size and shape (size is variable, usually globular)
- Surface and margin (usually smooth surface and well-defined rounded margins)
- Consistency (bony hard in feel)
- Examination of teeth—look for any caries.

Q. What is your case? (Summary of a case of dental cyst)

Ans. This 20-year-old boy presented with painless slow growing swelling in the right half of lower jaw for last 6 months. He complains of occasional pain in that region for the same duration.

On examination: There is a swelling in the right half of the lower jaw nontender/tender (if secondary infected), hard in consistency, immobile, and free from skin. The upper second molar tooth is showing caries.

Q. What is your diagnosis?

Ans. This is a case of dental cyst in the lower jaw in relation to the right lower second molar tooth.

Q. How will you manage this patient?

Ans. I will advise X-ray of the local part or OPG.

Q. What is the X-ray finding in dental cyst?

Ans. There is a circular radiolucent area in relation to the root of a normally erupted tooth. The margin of the radiolucent area may be sclerotic.

Q. How will you treat?

Ans.

- Treatment is complete excision of the cyst through an intraoral approach.
- The carious tooth is extracted.

A curved incision is made on the mucoperiosteum over the maximum convexity of the swelling. The mucoperiosteal flaps are raised. An opening is made in the thin bony shell lining the cyst. The cyst content is then scooped out along with the epithelial debris and the epithelial lining of the cyst wall.

Q. How to manage the residual cavity?

Ans. The cavity may be obliterated by:

- Packing with bone chips or pushing in of soft tissue and the cut margin of the mucoperiosteum is sutured over it.
- If the cyst is large, it may be marsupialized. The cyst contents are scooped out.

The mucoperiosteal flaps are then sutured to the margin of the cyst.

Q. How does the dental cyst develop?

Ans. The dental cyst develops at the apices of a carious tooth with necrotic pulp. The chronic irritation due to infection stimulates the epithelial cells to proliferate. Subsequently, there is degeneration of these epithelial cells leading to formation of a cyst. The cyst is lined by stratified squamous epithelium. The cyst enlarges slowly and causes resorption of adjacent bone and leads to expansion of jaw.

It left untreated, they can become large, involving the greater part of the body of the mandible. In the maxilla, the cyst may enlarge to fill the maxillary antrum.

Q. What are the contents of a dental cyst?

Ans. The cyst contains epithelial debris mainly, which may be semisolid or fluid. There may be cholesterol crystal and foreign body giant cells.

■ DENTIGEROUS CYST

Q. What is your case? (Summary of a case of dentigerous cyst)

Ans. This 30-year-old gentleman presented with a swelling in left half of lower jaw for last 2 years, gradually increasing in size. There is no pain over the swelling.

On examination: There is a swelling in the left half of the mandible, nontender, hard in consistency, and immobile. The left lower-third molar tooth has not erupted.

Q. What is your diagnosis?

Ans. This is a case of dentigerous cyst in left half of the body of mandible in relation to an unerupted third molar tooth.

Q. How does the dentigerous cyst develop?

Ans. Dentigerous cyst arises from the sequestrated enamel epithelium from the surface of the crown of an unerupted tooth. This sequestrated epithelium proliferates and there is also accumulation of fluid within the cyst. The cyst is lined by stratified squamous epithelium and there is a fibrous sheath outside the epithelial lining. Like dental cyst, the cyst contains epithelial debris, cholesterol, and foreign body giant cells. The cyst also contains an unerupted tooth, which may lie free in the cyst cavity or may remain embedded in the wall of the cyst and the crown protrudes into the cavity of the cyst.

Q. How will you treat the patient?

Ans. I will advise OPG of mandible.

- The X-ray will show a cystic lesion in relation to an unerupted tooth. The cyst may be unilocular or there may be soap bubble appearance of the cyst due to pseudotrabeculation in larger cyst.
- The treatment is same as dental cyst. (*see* Page No. 588).

Q. What is the differential diagnosis for a bony jaw swelling?

Ans.

- *Dental cyst*: Usually found in relation to a carious tooth.
- *Dentigerous cyst*: Usually found in relation to an unerupted tooth slowly growing.
- *Solitary bone cyst*: Slowly growing bony swelling more come in lower jaw.
- *Monostotic fibrous dysplasia*: Slowly increasing bony swelling in adolescence. Enlargement may slow down once skeletal growth is complete.
- Ossifying fibroma.
- Giant cell granuloma or brown tumor of hyperparathyroidism.
- Adamantinoma.
- *Aneurysmal bone cyst*: A variety of giant cell granuloma of bone.
- Osteoma.
- Osteoclastoma.
- Osteosarcoma.

■ AMELOBLASTOMA OR ADAMANTINOMA

Q. What is your case? (Summary of a case of ameloblastoma or adamantinoma)

Ans. This 35-year-old lady presented with a swelling in right half of mandible for last 3 years, slow-growing with no pain over the swelling. Patient states that the teeth overlying the swelling got loose spontaneously and fell down over last 6 months (Fig. 13.21).

On examination: There is a bony hard swelling in the right half of mandible extending from the angle of the mandible to the adjacent part of the body of mandible. There is expansion mainly of the outer cortex of the bone and the swelling is more prominent outward than on the inner aspect. There is malalignment and malocclusion of teeth due to the swelling. The molar teeth overlying the swelling are absent.

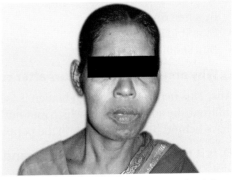

Fig. 13.21: Adamantinoma involving the right half of the mandible

Courtesy: Dr Asif Ayaz, IPGME and R, Kolkata

Q. What is your diagnosis?

Ans. This is a case of adamantinoma involving the right half of the mandible arising from the ramus and part of the body.

Q. What is ameloblastoma?

Ans. This is a benign neoplasm arising from the ameloblasts, which are the enamel forming cells of the tooth. Some believes that this is a variant of basal cell carcinoma, which arises from the primitive ectodermal epithelium of the stomodeum.

Q. What are the pathological features of ameloblastoma?

Ans. Ameloblastomas are benign tumors arising from the odontogenic epithelium. This is a slowly growing tumor and there is a tendency for local recurrence following removal by curettage. Most ameloblastomas occur in the mandible near the angle and ramus of the mandible and may extend into the coronoid process.

The lesion may be a solid soft tissue tumor or there may be areas of cystic degeneration and a multiloculated cyst is formed with trabeculae in-between.

Histologically, there are sheets or nests of ameloblastic cells lying in a connective tissue stroma. The ameloblastic cells comprise a peripheral columnar or cuboidal cells and a central core of stellate reticulum like cells with large-vacuolated cytoplasm.

Q. How will you treat this patient?

Ans.
- I will advise an OPG of mandible.
- In ameloblastoma, there will be an expanding bony lesion in the mandible with more expansion of the outer cortex. There is soap bubble or honeycomb appearance due to bony trabeculae inside.
- The tumor has involved the angle of mandible up to the lower border.
- The optimum treatment would be excision of the tumor along with 1 cm healthy margin of the mandible.

Q. How will you bridge the bony gap after local excision of tumor or following hemimandibulectomy?

Ans.
- By a free rib graft
- By a fibular bone graft
- By a stainless steel plate.

Q. Why ameloblastoma recurs after curettage?

Ans. This neoplasm although benign is locally invasive within the medullary bone. This may infiltrate the adjacent bone, which may not be apparent to the naked eye. Simple curettage may leave behind rim of the tumor in the periphery and may result in local recurrence.

Q. Is it possible to conserve the mandible?

Ans.
- Curettage and bone grafting is not advisable, as it is associated with high chance of recurrence.
- If the lower border of mandible is not affected, the tumor may be excised leaving behind the lower border of the mandible intact to maintain the continuity of the jaw.

Q. When will you consider hemimandibulectomy?

Ans.

* If the tumor is large and involve almost the whole of one-half mandible then hemimandibulectomy will be required.
* If the tumor recurs after local excision then hemimandibulectomy is indicated.

Q. What is the role of radiotherapy in ameloblastoma?

Ans. The tumor is radioresistant, so radiotherapy has no role in treatment.

■ OSTEOMYELITIS OF JAW

Q. What is your case? (Summary of a case of osteomyelitis of jaw)

Ans. This 30-year-old gentleman presented with discharge of pus through a sinus in the left side of lower jaw for last 6 months. Patient also complains of occasional discharge of whitish bony spicules through this sinus opening. Patient had history of pain and swelling in the left half of lower jaw 6 months back associated with throbbing pain and fever. The swelling resolved with discharge of pus externally. Since then patient is having these problems of discharge of pus and bone chips through the sinus opening.

On examination: There is a cutaneous sinus opening on the left half of the lower jaw at the level of second molar tooth. The sinus opening is fixed to the underlying mandible and on squeezing there is some discharge of pus through this opening. There is thickening of the left half of the body of mandible.

Submandibular lymph node on the left side is palpable and tender.

Q. What is your diagnosis?

Ans. This is a case of chronic osteomyelitis involving the left half of mandible.

Q. Why mandible is commonly affected by osteomyelitis?

Ans. The lower jaw has tenuous blood supply, which may be further jeopardized by infection or trauma leading to necrosis of the bone.

Q. What are the sources of infection?

Ans.

* Spread of infection from pulp abscess of tooth
* Spread of infection from alveolar abscess
* Compound fracture of the jaw—Infection from oral cavity
* Hematogenous spread of infection.

Q. What is the pathogenesis of chronic osteomyelitis of mandible?

Ans. Chronic osteomyelitis of mandible is usually a sequela of acute osteomyelitis. During the phase of acute osteomyelitis, there is swelling in the mandible which is associated with throbbing pain and fever. If not treated at this stage, the pus may penetrate the cortex of the mandible and lift the periosteum. The pus may reach the surface and discharge through a sinus in the skin. Once the pus is discharged, the disease enters a less painful chronic phase. Thrombosis of intraosseous blood vessels results in infarction of the bone. The periosteum lays down new bones known as involucrum. The infarcted bone forms the sequestrum. The infecting organism remains at the site, as the antibiotic and body's own defense mechanism cannot reach the dead bone.

Q. How will you treat this patient?

Ans.

- I will advise a local X-ray or OPG. X-ray may reveal periosteal reaction, sequestrum may be seen. A cavity may be seen in the body of the mandible.
- Pus sent for culture and sensitivity.
- A combination of amoxicillin and flucloxacillin is effective and may be required to be continued for 4–6 weeks. Subsequently, the antibiotic therapy may be changed depending on the culture sensitivity report.
- If a sequestrum has already formed, surgical treatment is required.
- A suitable incision is made in the skin over the most dependent part of the mandible. Saucerization is done by removing the involucrum and the sequestrum is removed. The cavity is lightly packed with gauze. Suitable antibiotic is continued in the perioperative period.

▌EPULIS

Q. What is your case? (Summary of a case of epulis)

Ans. This 30-year-old gentleman presented with a swelling in the upper gum on the external side for last 6 months and is slowly growing in size. Patient complains of a painful cavity in the upper left lateral incisor for last 1 year.

On examination: There is a firm, nontender sessile swelling in the upper gum on the external aspect lying in the region of the upper left incisor teeth. The adjacent mucous membrane in the gum is healthy. There is evidence of caries in the upper left lateral incisor tooth. The cervical lymph nodes are not palpable.

Q. What is your diagnosis?

Ans. This is a case of fibrous epulis in the upper jaw in the region of upper left incisor teeth.

Q. What is epulis?

Ans. Any discrete lump on the gum is loosely termed as epulis.

Q. What is a fibrous epulis?

Ans. Fibrous epulis is a localized inflammatory hyperplasia of the gum.

Q. How does fibrous epulis develop?

Ans. This localized inflammatory hyperplasia occurs due to local irritation from a sharp margin of a caries tooth or from a subgingival calculus. It may arise from an interdental papilla.

Q. What are the histological features of fibrous epulis?

Ans. The fibrous epulis consists of cellular and vascular connective tissue.

Q. How will you treat this patient?

Ans.
* I will advise for an OPG of the maxilla to look for any bony lesion.
* I will consider local excision of the swelling with a wedge of gingiva and local gingival recontouring.
* The source of chronic irritation like a caries tooth needs to be dealt with at the same time, otherwise the epulis will recur.

Q. What is a false epulis?

Ans. This is a mass of granulation tissue formed around a carious tooth or at the site of irritation by a denture.

Q. What are the characteristics of pregnancy epulis?

Ans.
* In response to local irritation by a caries tooth, a pedunculated mass appears as an enlargement of interdental papilla, which grows rapidly partly due to hormonal changes of pregnancy. This remains soft, pink and vascular, and readily bleeds on touch. This is a form of granulomatous epulis.
* These pregnancy epulis usually regresses after the childbirth.
* If bleeding is troublesome, the mass may be excised with a diathermy and at the same time the local irritation factor is dealt with.

Q. What is a carcinomatous epulis?

Ans. This is actually a squamous cell carcinoma arising from the mucosa of the alveolar margin. The lesion may become ulcerated with a typical rolled out (everted) edge of a malignant ulcer.

Q. What are the different types of epulis?

Ans. Epulis may be:
* Benign epulis:
  – Fibrous
  – Granulomatous
  – Giant cell.
* Malignant epulis:
  – Carcinomatous
  – Sarcomatous.

Breast, Hernias and Abdominal Wall

Chapter

14

▌CARCINOMA IN MALE BREAST

Clinical Examination

(*See* Page No. 381, Chapter 9)

History

- History of swelling—onset and progress
- Any pain in the breast
- Any skin changes noticed by the patient
- Any history of retraction of nipple and areola
- Any swelling in the axilla, neck, or opposite breast
- Any history of loss of appetite, loss of weight, and any history of jaundice
- Any chest pain, cough, and hemoptysis. Any history of breathlessness
- Any history of recent onset of backache, aches, and pains in the limbs or any bony swelling
- Any history of headache, mental changes, loss of consciousness, convulsion, and weakness of any of the limbs.

Examination

- *Inspection*:
  - Position and symmetry of both breasts
  - Nipple and areola (any discharge, retraction, cracks, fissure, or ulcer)
    Any swelling in the breast—site and extent/size and shape/surface and margin
  - Skin over the breast and the swelling (color change, peaud'orange, ulcer, or satellite nodules)
  - Lift arm above the head and assess any change—any skin dimpling or alteration of position of nipple.
- *Palpation*:
  - Palpate the breast with the palmar surface of the fingers
  - Palpate the normal breast first
  - Palpation of the swelling—temperature/tenderness/site and extent/size and shape/surface and margin/consistency

- Any skin tethering (ascertained by moving the lump and note whether any skin dimple appears on the skin).
- Any skin fixity—try to lift the skin from the underlying lump—skin may be free or fixed to the underlying lump
- Test for fixity to chest wall
- Test for fixity of the lump to the underlying pectoralis major muscle or to serratus anterior muscle
- Palpation of axillary lymph nodes and supraclavicular lymph nodes.

Q. What is your case? (Summary of a case of carcinoma in male breast)

Ans. This 55-year-old gentleman presented with a swelling in his right breast for last 1 year. The swelling was about 2 cm in size at the onset and was increasing in size slowly, since the onset for about 9 months. But for last 3 months, the swelling is rapidly increasing in size and there is ulceration over the swelling for last 2 months. The ulcer was about 1cm at the onset and increasing in size since then. There is discharge of serous fluid from the ulcer site. Patient also complains gradual destruction of the right nipple. He complains of dull aching pain over the swelling for last 2 months. He also complains of a swelling in his right axilla from last 3 months, which was about 1 cm at the onset and is gradually increasing size. Patient has no other systemic complaints (Fig. 14.1).

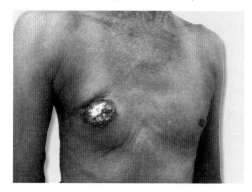

Fig. 14.1: Carcinoma of right breast in male
Courtesy: Prof Diptendra Kumar Sarkar, IPGME and R, Kolkata

On examination: The right breast is enlarged and asymmetric in comparison to left breast. The nipple is pushed outward and upward, there is destruction of areolar area. there is a swelling in the right breast 6 cm × 5 cm, occupying all the quadrants of the breast, spherical in shape, surface is irregular, and margins are well defined. the swelling is firm in consistency, mobile, fixed to the overlying skin, and underlying pectoral muscle, but not to chest wall. There is an ulcer overlying the tumor involving the areolar area—3 cm in diameter circular in shape, margins are raised and floor is covered with necrotic tissue. A single lymph node is palpable in the right axilla, which is firm in consistency and is mobile.

Q. What is your diagnosis?

Ans. This is a case of carcinoma of right breast in a male patient aged 55 years T4bN1M0.

Q. What are the risk factors for development of male breast cancer?

Ans.
- Gynecomastia
- Klinefelter's syndrome—associated with testicular atrophy
- Mutation in *BRCA2* gene is associated with increased risk of breast cancer in males.

Q. Why disease is more advanced in male patient at presentation?

Ans. The breast is small in size. As the tumor grows, there is early invasion of the growth into the skin and the underlying pectoral muscles or chest wall.

Q. How will you manage this patient?

Ans. I would like to confirm my diagnosis by doing an ultrasonography (USG) of both breast and a trucut biopsy from the breast lump.

Other investigations will include:

* Chest X-ray posteroanterior (PA) VIEW
* Electrocardiogram (ECG)
* Complete hemogram
* Liver function test (LFT)
* USG of abdomen
* As the disease is local advanced, a whole body bone scanning is required.

Q. How will you treat this patient?

Ans. Modified radical mastectomy followed by adjuvant therapy.

Q. What adjuvant therapy you will plan for this patient?

Ans. In view of large tumor and lymph node metastasis for locoregional treatment, I will give postoperative radiotherapy to the breast flap and lymph node fields in the supraclavicular and internal thoracic chain. If adequate axillary dissection is done, axillary irradiation is not required except when there is extracapsular spread of the tumor.

If axillary lymph node shows metastasis postoperative chemotherapy with either CMF (cyclophosphamide, methotrexate, 5-fluorouracil) or CAF (cyclophosphamide, adriamycin, 5-fluorouracil) is to be considered.

Q. What is the role of hormone therapy in male breast cancer?

Ans. About 70–80% male breast cancer is estrogen receptor positive and about 65% is progesterone receptor positive. Hormone therapy is effective in such cases.

* *First-line hormone therapy*: Orchidectomy or tamoxifen therapy.
* *Second-line therapy*: Analogues (goserelin) or aromatase inhibitors (anastrozole or letrozole).

■ BILATERAL GYNECOMASTIA

Clinical Examination

See Page No. 382, Chapter 9.

History

* Age (in patient between 10 years and 20 years majority are idiopathic. In elderly patient, usually secondary to some cause)
* Onset and progress of enlargement of the breast—unilateral or bilateral
* Any history of pain (usually painless)

- Any history of liver disease (hepatitis), renal disease, and mumps orchitis
- Any history of drug intake like estrogens (given for prostatic carcinoma), diuretics, digitalis, steroids, and tranquilizers. These drugs may cause gynecomastia.

Examination—Inspection/Palpation

- Unilateral or bilateral enlargement
- Degree of enlargement—mild, moderate, or severe (in severe type may resemble female breast).
- Feel the breast disk.
- Hard (commonly found in young boys) or soft enlargement (usually found in elderly patients commonly due to drug therapy).
- The skin over the breast, nipple, and areola. These are usually normal.
- Examine the axillary lymph nodes (axillary lymph nodes are not enlarged).
- Examine abdomen for hepatic enlargement.
- Examine chest to exclude any lung lesion.
- Examine both testes (testicular atrophy or estrogen secreting testicular tumor may be associated with gynecomastia).

Q. What is your case? (Summary of a case of bilateral gynecomastia)

Ans. This 12-year-old boy presented with gradually increasing swelling of his both breasts for last 2 years. No history of rapid increase in size of the swelling, no discharge from the nipple. Patient has no other complaints (Fig. 14.2).

on examination: There is symmetrical enlargement of both breasts. Nipple and areola appears normal. On palpation, the firm breast disk palpable on both sides, which is mobile, free from skin, and the underlying pectoral muscle. Abdominal and chest examination is normal. Both the testes are normally palpable.

Q. What is your diagnosis?

Ans. This is a case of bilateral gynecomastia.

Q. What is idiopathic gynecomastia?

Ans. Gynecomastia may be secondary to some causes, when no cause could be discerned from history, clinical examination, and investigation then it can be regarded as idiopathic gynecomastia.

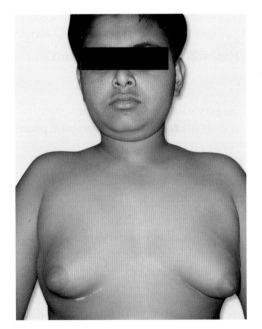

Fig. 14.2: Bilateral gynecomastia in a 12-year-old male child

Courtesy: Prof Biswanath Mukhopadhyay, NRS Medical College, Kolkata

Q. What is gynecomastia?

Ans. Enlargement of the male breast is called gynecomastia.

Q. What is physiological gynecomastia?

Ans. Teenage boys achieving puberty and the elderly men (senescence) may have physiological enlargement of breast.

Q. What are the important causes of gynecomastia?

Ans.

- *Secondary to some drug therapy:*
  - Digoxin
  - Spironolactone
  - Anabolic steroid or estrogens.
- *Secondary to some underlying disease:*
  - Testicular tumors
  - Testicular atrophy (due to mumps orchitis or leprosy)
  - Chronic liver disease
  - Klinefelter's syndrome
  - Bronchial carcinoma
  - Adrenocortical carcinoma
  - Chronic renal failure
  - Thyrotoxicosis.

Q. How will you treat this patient?

Ans.

- Reassurance
- Surgery—for cosmetic reason.
  - Subcutaneous mastectomy with preservation of nipple and areola.

▊ FIBROADENOMA BREAST

Q. What is your case? (Summary of a case of fibroadenoma of breast)

Ans. This 20-year-old girl presented with a swelling in her right breast for last 3 years. The swelling was 1 cm in size at the onset and the swelling is increasing very slowly in size over last 3 years. There is no history of rapid increase in size of the swelling. No discharge from the nipple. No other complaint is there.

On examination: There is a swelling in the upper–outer quadrant of right breast, globular in shape 2 cm × 2 cm smooth surface, well-defined rounded margins, firm in consistency, free from the skin, and is very much mobile in relation to the breast tissue, the swelling is slipping under finger when pressed. No other swelling in the breast. No palpable lymph nodes in the axilla.

Q. What is your diagnosis?

Ans. This is a case of fibroadenoma in right breast located at the upper–outer quadrant.

Q. What is fibroadenoma?

Ans. This is a benign breast disease containing both fibrous and glandular tissue. This is not a true tumor and has been regarded as one spectrum of aberrations of normal development and involution (ANDI).

Q. What is the natural history of fibroadenomas?

Ans. The fibroadenomas are very slow-growing lesions. It has been observed that majority of the fibroadenomas regress spontaneously over years.

Q. How will you manage this patient?

Ans.
* I would advise an ultrasonography of breast to assess the lump.
* A fine-needle aspiration cytology (FNAC) may confirm the diagnosis of fibroadenoma.
* As the lesion is small, I will wait and watch and do regular follow up, as majority of fibroadenomas may regress spontaneously.

Q. When you will consider surgical treatment?

Ans. Excision of the fibroadenoma is indicated:
* Fibroadenoma larger than 4 cm in size.
* When the tumor is increasing in size at follow up.
* Patient is apprehensive and wants to get the tumor removed.
* In patient with age more than 30 years.
* When there is suspicion of malignancy.

Q. What operation will you do?

Ans. Emulative of fibroadenoma—approach is usually through a circumareolar or submammary incision. The incision is deepened and an incision is made over the capsule and the tumor is enucleated leaving behind the capsule.

Q. What are the pathological types of fibroadenoma?

Ans. Depending on the relative preponderance of the fibrous and the glandular tissue two types of fibroadenomas are described:
* *Pericanalicular type (hard fibroadenoma)*—the proliferation of fibrous tissue is more than the glandular element. The tumor may feel firm and is freely mobile within the breast tissue.
* *Intracanalicular type (soft fibroadenoma)*—proliferation of glandular tissue is more preponderant than the fibrous tissue and the lump may appear soft in feel.

Q. What do you mean by giant fibroadenoma?

Ans. Fibroadenomas more than 5 cm in diameter are called giant fibroadenomas.

▇ CYSTOSARCOMA PHYLLODES OR PHYLLODES TUMOR IN BREAST

Characteristics of Phyllodes Tumor

* These tumors increase in size rapidly and may attain very large size and occupy the whole breast (Fig. 14.3).

* The lump is soft in feel, surface may be lobulated, mobile, free from the skin, and the underlying pectoral muscle.
* The skin may appear shiny and there may be dilated veins in the skin, in late stages, there may be pressure necrosis of the overlying skin resulting in an ulcer.
* Histologically, the phyllodes tumor shows a picture intermediate between a benign histology and a sarcoma like appearance. There are more cellularity, pleomorphism, and mitotic activity.
* Following excision there is increased chance of local recurrence.

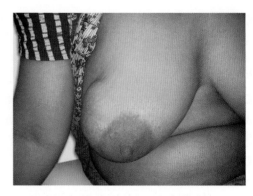

Fig. 14.3: Cystosarcoma phyllodes
Courtesy: Dr Kallol Roy, IPGME and R, Kolkata

Q. How will you treat patients with cystosarcoma phyllodes?

Ans.

* A phyllodes tumor should be excised with a margin of normal tissue.
* Patient presenting with recurrent phyllodes tumor is to be treated with simple mastectomy.

■ CONGENITAL HERNIA

Clinical Examination

See Page No. 382, Chapter 9.

History

* History of the swelling—onset (usually from birth), progress of the swelling
* Site of the swelling—in the groin or in both groin and scrotum
* Progress of the swelling and what happens to the swelling when the child strains (coughing and crying) or when the child is lying in the bed—a hernial swelling gets aggravated on straining and reduces or disappears on lying down.
* Any pain over the swelling
* Any history of irreducibility of the swelling
* Any history suggestive of acute intestinal obstruction associated with irreducibility of the swelling—pain abdomen, vomiting, absolute constipation, and abdominal distension
* Any history of chronic straining factors like—chronic cough, constipation, or difficulty in passing urine.

Examination—Inspection/Palpation

* *Swelling*—Site and extent (congenital hernia usually extends up to the bottom of the scrotum)/size and shape/surface and margin/consistency
* Expansile impulse on cough
* Whether it is possible to get above the swelling (swelling is scrotal or inguinoscrotal?)
* *Reducibility*—An uncomplicated hernia is reducible

◆ *Deep ring occlusion test*—Congenital hernia occurs through the deep ring. a deep-ring occlusion test is not required in examination of congenital hernia as inguinal canal is not developed in infants.
◆ Assess the content of the hernia sac—omentum or intestine
  – Doughy feel, dull note on percussion and absent bowel sounds will suggest omentocele.
  – Soft elastic feel, reduction with gurgling sound, resonant percussion note, and presence of bowel sound will suggest enterocele.

Q. What is your case? (Summary of a case of congenital hernia)

Ans. Patient's mother states that this 10-month-old male child has swelling in left inguinoscrotal region since birth, and since then the swelling is gradually increasing in size. The swelling increases when the child sits, crawls, and strains. The swelling disappears when the child lies down (Fig. 14.4).

On examination, there is a left-sided inguinoscrotal swelling showing expansile impulse on cough. The swelling is reducible and there is gurgling sound during reduction.

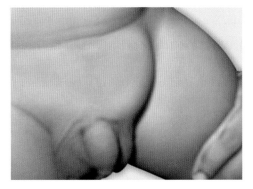

Fig. 14.4: Left-sided congenital hernia in a 10-month-old male child

Courtesy: Dr Kalyani Saha Basu, NRS Medical College, Kolkata

Q. What is your diagnosis?

Ans. This is case of left-sided congenital hernia in a 10-months-old male child, content is intestine.

Q. How is the inguinal canal in children?

Ans. In newborn, the inguinal canal does not develop and superficial and deep inguinal rings lie close to each other. By 2 years, the deep ring moves laterally and proper inguinal canal can be identified.

Q. What is the basic defect in congenital hernia?

Ans. The basic defect in congenital hernia is the failure of obliteration of processus vaginalis. The inguinal canal structure and mechanism remain intact.

Q. Why early operation is indicated in infants?

Ans. Early operation is indicated in infants particularly those below 6 months of age because of high chance of strangulation.

Q. What operation will you do?

Ans. The surgical treatment will be herniotomy.

Q. What is the difference in technique in older children?

Ans. In child more then 2 years of age, the external and internal ring become widely separated, so that direct dissection is no longer possible.

In these cases, skin incision is made slightly laterally over the internal inguinal ring. The skin and superficial fascia is incised. The external oblique aponeurosis is incised and inguinal canal exposed—the external ring is not opened.

The cremasteric fascia and internal spermatic fascia is incised and sac dissected free from the cord structures. The sac is clamped across and the distal part of the sac transected and kept open. The proximal part of the sac is dissected up to the deep ring and tackled as described above.

Q. Describe the steps of herniotomy for congenital hernia?

Ans. *See* operative Surgery, Section, Page No. 1084, 1085, Chapter 22.

Q. What are the indications of herniorrhaphy in children?

Ans.
* Children with high risk of recurrent hernia should have a formal herniorrhaphy.
* These include:
    - Children who underwent ventriculoperitoneal shunt.
    - Patient on continuous ambulatory peritoneal dialysis.
    - Malnutrition.
    - Growth failure.
    - Patient with connective tissue disorder as in Ehlers–Danlos syndrome and Marfan's syndrome.

Q. What is the chance of developing hernia on opposite side?

Ans. About 10% of children on follow up develop contralateral hernia.

Q. What is the incidence of patent processus vaginalis on the contralateral side?

Ans.
* Patent processus vaginalis may be present on opposite side of hernia in 100% of cases up to 1 week after birth.
* By the age of 2 years, only 25% has patent processus vaginalis.
* However, all patients with patent processus vaginalis do not develop hernia.
* Only 5–10% patient will develop hernia on the contralateral side.
* So, routine exploration of the opposite side is not advisable.

Q. Do you like to do routine contralateral exploration in congenital hernia?

Ans.
* Earlier, it was done routinely in children with unilateral hernia.
* But different series showed only 5–10% chance of developing hernia on contralateral side.
* So, routine contralateral exploration is not required.

■ UMBILICAL HERNIA

Q. What is your diagnosis?

Ans. This is a case of uncomplicated umbilical hernia in a female child aged 4 years (Fig. 14.5).

Q. What is your case? (Summary of a case of umbilical hernia)

Ans. This 4-year-old female child presented with a swelling in her umbilicus since birth. The swelling is increasing in size since then. The swelling gets aggravated by strenuous activities like walking, running, and crying and the swelling gets spontaneously reduced on lying down. No pain over the swelling and there is no history of irreducibility.

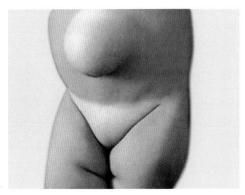

Fig. 14.5: Umbilical hernia

Courtesy: Prof BN Mukhopadhyay, NRS Medical College and Hospital, Kolkata

On examination: The umbilicus is stretched and everted due to a swelling in the umbilicus. The swelling shows expansile on cough and the swelling gets reduced spontaneously on lying down. There is a gurgling sound during reduction of the swelling. A gap of about 2 cm is palpable in the umbilical cicatrix.

Q. What is your diagnosis?

Ans. This is a case of uncomplicated umbilical hernia in a female child aged 4 years.

Q. What is umbilical hernia?

Ans. This is a herniation through a weak umbilical cicatrix, which fails to close after birth.

Q. How will you manage this patient?

Ans. There is a wide gap and the child is 4-year-old, so this hernia is unlikely to close spontaneously, so I will consider surgical treatment.
* I will do some investigations to assess her fitness for anesthesia.
* Blood for Hb% total leukocyte count (TLC), differential leukocyte count (DLC), and erythrocyte sedimentation rate (ESR)
* Urine examination
* Chest X-ray.

Q. What operation will you do?

Ans. I will do an anatomical repair.
* A curved incision is made below the umbilicus with convexity downward and the anterior rectus sheath is exposed.
* The skin flap is raised above and the hernial sac is dissected free.
* The hernial sac is opened and the contents reduced.
* The redundant sac is excised and the hernial sac is closed at the neck.
* The gap in the linea alba is approximated by interrupted absorbable suture.
* The skin is closed with interrupted monofilament polyamide sutures (Fig. 14.6).

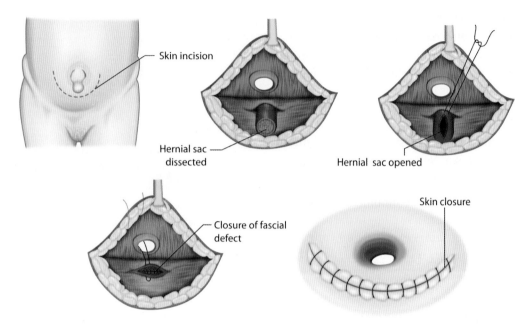

Fig. 14.6: Repair of umbilical hernia

Q. What is exomphalos?

Ans. Exomphalos is a rare congenital hernia occurring through the umbilicus and is due to failure of all or part of the midgut to return into the peritoneal cavity (Fig. 14.7).

Q. What are the linings of an exomphalos sac?

Ans. The sac covering the exomphalos may rupture during birth. The unruptured sac is transparent and is lined by outer amniotic membrane and the inner peritoneum.

Q. What is exomphalos minor?

Ans. When the umbilical defect is less than 4 cm, this is called exomphalos minor. This is also termed as herniation of the umbilical cord and a loop of small gut may remain in the sac and may be injured, if umbilical cord is ligated and divided in the usual way. The umbilical cord is attached to the summit of the sac.

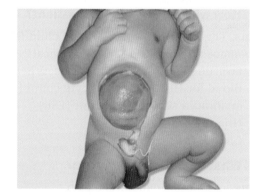

Fig. 14.7: Exomphalos major

Courtesy: Prof BN Mukhopadhyay, NRS Medical College and Hospital, Kolkata

Q. How will you treat exomphalos minor?

Ans. These small defects may be closed spontaneously soon after birth.

Q. What is exomphalos major?

Ans. When the fascial defect is more than 4 cm, this is called exomphalos major. The sac contains a large part of the small intestine and a part of the large intestine. The liver, spleen, and pancreas may be seen through the transparent membrane.

Q. When will you consider nonoperative therapy?

Ans. Premature infants with large defect are unlikely to withstand major operation, so a nonoperative treatment is indicated in such situation. The intact sac is painted daily with 2% mercurochrome lotion. An eschar forms over the sac and granulation tissue grows from the periphery. The subsequent ventral hernia is repaired at a later date when the child is fit for a major surgery (months to years later).

Q. What are the operative techniques for management of exomphalos major?

Ans. There are number of techniques for closure of the defect:

- *Skin flap closure*: The skin is freed from the fascial edges and undermined laterally. The skin margins are then apposed in the midline, if necessary, by release incisions in the flanks. The remaining ventral hernia is repaired at a later date.
- *Primary closure*: The skin is dissected away from the fascial margin. The intestine is decompressed both proximally and distally. The abdominal wall is stretched in all the quadrants manually. The herniated viscera are then replaced into the abdominal cavity and the fascial defect apposed in the midline. Care should be taken to monitor development of abdominal compartment syndrome.
- *Staged repair*: The skin margin is freed from the fascial attachments and a PTFE (polytetrafluoroethylene) mesh is sutured circumferentially in the margin of the fascial gap. The mesh is opened daily under aseptic condition and the viscera underneath is inspected and the mesh is tied again at a reduced level. This is continued daily till the fascial margins are lying closer. Once this is achieved, the fascial margins are apposed with interrupted sutures and the skin closed over the gap.

■ PARAUMBILICAL HERNIA IN ADULTS

Q. What is your case? (Summary of a case of paraumbilical hernia)

Ans. This 45-year-old gentleman presented with a swelling around the umbilicus for last 3 years. The swelling was small about 2 cm in size at the onset but for last 3 years the swelling is gradually increasing in size and attained the present size. The swelling increases in size during walking and during strenuous activities and reduces in size on lying down. Patient complains of dull aching pain over the swelling for last 6 months. Patient underwent open cholecystectomy 5 years back. No other complaints are there (Fig. 14.8).

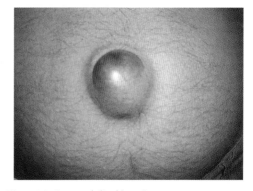

Fig. 14.8: Paraumbilical hernia
Courtesy: Dr Nilanjan Panda, RG Kar Medical College, Kolkata

On examination: On local examination, there is a swelling in the umbilical region. The whole umbilicus is stretched and thinned out. The swelling shows expansile impulse on cough. The swelling is reducible on lying down position and with slight manipulation of the contents. There is gurgling sound during reduction of the contents of the swelling. A gap of about 4 cm is palpable in the linea alba.

Q. What is your diagnosis?

Ans. This is a case of paraumbilical hernia.

Q. Why do you say this is a paraumbilical and not an umbilical hernia?

Ans. In adults, this hernia does not occur through the umbilical scar but occurs through the linea alba either above or below the umbilicus.

Q. What are the usual contents in a paraumbilical hernia?

Ans. The greater omentum is the most common contents. Apart from this small intestine, transverse colon or the urinary bladder may be a content of paraumbilical hernia.

Q. Why paraumbilical hernia is more common in females?

Ans. Increasing obesity, weakness of the abdominal muscles due to repeated pregnancy may be an etiological factor for development of a paraumbilical hernia in females.

Q. What are the complications of paraumbilical hernia?

Ans.
- *Irreducibility*: This may be due to the narrow neck of the sac or may be due to the adhesions of the contents within the sac.
- *Obstruction*: Intestinal obstruction may be due to adhesion of the gut within the sac or constriction of the gut at the neck of the sac.
- *Strangulation*: Unrelieved obstruction may lead to strangulation.
- *Intertrigo*: Obese patient with large hernia may have intertrigo. Ulceration in skin in-between redundant skin fold.

Q. How will you manage this patient?

Ans.
- *Weight reduction*: This is one of the important aspects before operation. Obese or overweight patients have more postoperative complication.
- Baseline workup to assess fitness for anesthesia.
- USG of abdomen to exclude any associated intra-abdominal pathology.

Q. What operation you will do in this case?

Ans. As the defect is large (4 cm in this patient), I will consider repair of this hernia with preperitoneal mesh placement.
- A transverse elliptical incision is made around the umbilicus.
- The skin and the subcutaneous tissue are dissected off from the rectus sheath to expose the neck of the sac.

* The hernial sac is opened at the neck and the contents are returned into the abdomen.
* If there are adhesions within the sac, the adhesions are lysed.
* The redundant sac is excised and the neck of the sac is closed with absorbable suture.
* A preperitoneal space is created by dissecting between the peritoneum and the posterior rectus sheath.
* A polypropylene mesh is placed in the preperitoneal space. The mesh should cover about 4 cm area all around the gap.
* The mesh is fixed to the anterior rectus sheath by interrupted sutures.
* The margins of the anterior rectus sheath are apposed in front of the mesh by nonabsorbable sutures.
* A suction drain is kept in the preperitoneal space.
* The skin is closed with interrupted monofilament polyamide sutures.

Q. What is anatomical repair?

Ans.
* If the defect is small (<3 cm) then an anatomical repair is feasible.
* The sac and its contents are tackled as above.
* The neck of the sac is closed with running absorbable suture.
* The margin of the fascial defect is apposed with interrupted nonabsorbable suture.
* Skin closed in usual way.

Q. How will you diagnose strangulation in a paraumbilical hernia?

Ans. Patient will present with irreducibility of the hernial mass and features of acute intestinal obstruction (pain abdomen, distension, vomiting, and absolute constipation). The pain may be severe.

On examination, there will be tachycardia, dehydration, and patient may be toxic.

Local examination will show that the hernial mass is irreducible and there will be both tenderness and rebound tenderness over the hernial mass. There is associated abdominal distension. Hyperperistaltic bowel sounds may be audible on auscultation.

Q. How will you manage strangulated paraumbilical hernia?

Ans. Resuscitation of patient with:
* Intravenous fluid
* Nasogastric aspiration
* Antibiotics
* Urinary catheterization
* Operation as soon as possible.

The hernial sac is exposed as described above. The hernial sac is opened at the fundus to drain the toxic fluid. The gangrenous content is exposed. If small intestine is gangrenous resection, anastomosis is done. If large gut is gangrenous, the gangrenous segment is excised and the segment is brought out as colostomy and a mucous fistula. The neck of the sac is widened and a formal hernia repair is deferred.

■ EPIGASTRIC HERNIA

Q. What is your case? (Summary of a case of epigastric hernia)

Ans. This 50-year-old gentleman presented with a swelling in middle of the upper part of the abdomen for last 2 years. The swelling was 1 cm in size when the patient first noticed it 2 years back. Afterwards, the swelling is increasing slowly in size over this period. Swelling gets aggravated in size after strenuous activities and the swelling diminishes in size after patient takes rest. Patient complains of dull aching pain over the swelling for last 1 year. Patient experiences pain more toward the evening after strenuous activities and gets relief from pain with rest. Patient has no other complaints (Fig. 14.9).

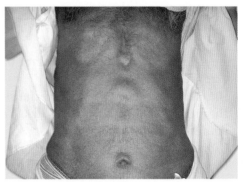

Fig. 14.9: Epigastric hernia

Courtesy: Dr Rajkumar Singh Mohapatra, IPGME and R, Kolkata

On examination: There is a swelling in the midline about 6 cm below the xiphoid, globular swelling, 2 cm in diameter, free from the skin, and slight expansile impulse on cough. The swelling is partially reducible and the gap in the linea alba cannot be felt clearly. Abdominal examination is normal.

Q. What is your diagnosis?

Ans. This is a case of epigastric hernia.

Q. What is epigastric hernia?

Ans. Herniation through the linea alba anywhere between the xiphoid and the umbilicus is called an epigastric hernia.

Q. What is false epigastric hernia?

Ans. When there is protrusion of only extraperitoneal fatty tissue through the linea alba without any peritoneal pouch then it is called a false epigastric hernia.

Q. What is true epigastric hernia?

Ans. With protrusion of the extraperitoneal fat, a pouch of peritoneum may follow. When the epigastric hernia contains a peritoneal sac then it is called a true epigastric hernia.

Q. What are the usual contents of a true epigastric hernia?

Ans. Usually, the sac is very small and does not contain any viscus. The sac is either empty or may contain only omentum.

Q. What may be the cause of pain in patients with epigastric hernia?

Ans.

* Usually, the epigastric hernias are asymptomatic.

- The patient may have dull aching pain over the swelling due to traction on the parietal peritoneum.
- The pain may also be due to strangulation of the contained omentum.
- The pain may be due to associated underlying peptic ulcer or gallstone disease.

Q. How will you manage this patient?

Ans. As the patient is having pain over the swelling and there is definite epigastric hernia, I will consider surgical treatment.

I will advise for:

- An upper gastrointestinal (GI) endoscopy to exclude an underlying peptic ulcer disease.
- A USG to exclude an underlying gallstone disease.
- Baseline investigation to assess patient fitness for anesthesia.

Q. What operation will you do?

Ans. I will do an anatomical repair of the defect.
- The operation is usually done under general anesthesia.
- A transverse incision is made over the swelling.
- The skin and subcutaneous tissue are dissected off from the anterior rectus sheath.
- The hernial mass is dissected all around the gap in the linea alba.
- The hernial sac is opened and any content is reduced.
- The neck of the hernial sac is closed with absorbable suture.
- The fascial defect in the linea alba is closed with interrupted nonabsorbable polypropylene suture.

    If the defect is large (>4 cm), a polypropylene mesh is placed in the preperitoneal space and the fascial defect closed in front of the mesh with nonabsorbable polypropylene suture.

▌FEMORAL HERNIA

Q. What is your case? (Summary of a case of femoral hernia)

Ans. This 30-year-old lady presented with a swelling in her right groin for last 1 year, which gradually increasing in size. The swelling appears when the patient walks and does strenuous activities and reduces in size and sometimes disappears on lying down (Fig. 14.10).

On examination, there is a swelling in right groin. The swelling shows an expansile impulse on coughing. The swelling lies below and lateral to pubic tubercle and is reducible.

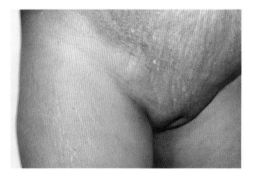

Fig. 14.10: Right-sided femoral hernia

Courtesy: Dr Somak Krishna Biswas, NRS Medical College, Kolkata

Q. What is the incidence of femoral hernia?

Ans. Abut 20% of hernia in women and 5% of hernia in men are femoral hernia.

Q. Through which anatomical defect femoral hernia emerges?

Ans. The hernia emerges through the Hesselbach's triangle and then finds its way out through the femoral ring into the femoral canal and descends into the thigh through the saphenous opening.

Q. What is the boundary of femoral canal (Figs 14.11A and B)?

Ans.
+ Femoral canal is a tunnel about 1.25 cm long and 1.25 cm wide at its base.
+ This is the most medial compartment of the femoral sheath.
+ This extends from femoral ring above to the saphenous opening below.
+ Laterally separated from the femoral vein by a septum.
+ The femoral canal is closed above by septum crurale and below by cribriform fascia.

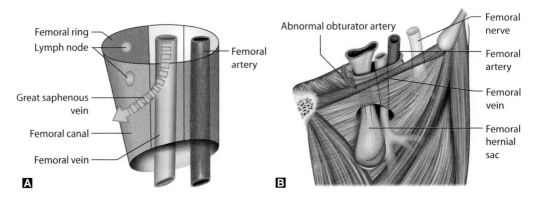

Figs 14.11A and B: Boundaries of femoral sheath

Q. What are the contents of femoral canal?

Ans. It contains a deep inguinal lymph node (Cloquet's lymph node) and lymphatics and loose areolar tissue.

Q. What is the boundary of femoral ring?

Ans.
+ *Anteriorly*: Inguinal ligament
+ *Posteriorly*: Cooper's ligament, pubic bone, and fascia covering pectineus
+ *Medially*: Lacunar ligament
+ *Laterally*: By a septum separating the femoral vein.

Q. What is the differential diagnosis of a femoral hernia?

Ans.
+ Inguinal hernia

* Saphena varix
* An enlarged Cloquet's node (conditions associated, i.e. enlargement of cloquet's node)
* Lipoma
* Femoral aneurysm
* Psoas abscess pointing into the thigh
* An enlarged iliopsoas bursa
* Rupture of abductor longus
* Hydrocele of a femoral hernia sac.

Q. What is Laugier's femoral hernia?

Ans.
* It is the hernia through a gap in the lacunar ligament.
* Unusually, medially placed femoral hernia
* High chance of strangulation.

Q. What is Narath's femoral hernia?

Ans.
* Hernia lies hidden behind the femoral vessels.
* Occurs in patient with congenital dislocation of hip due to lateral displacement of psoas muscle.

Q. What is Cloquet's hernia?

Ans.
* Here the hernial sac lies behind the fascia covering pectineus muscle.
* High chance of strangulation.

Q. Why femoral hernia may develop following repair of inguinal hernia?

Ans. In repairs of inguinal hernia, which involve apposition of conjoint tendon and fascia transversalis to inguinal ligament, there may be tension on the fascia transversalis and it may pull up the inguinal ligament, thereby causing weakness of tissues of the femoral canal leading to herniation.

However, it may also be true that femoral hernia was missed during first operation.

Q. Why femoral hernia needs early operation?

Ans. The incidence of strangulation in femoral hernia is very high. About 30–45% of femoral hernia may undergo strangulation in 2 years' time. The narrow and its tight femoral ring predispose to strangulation.

Q. What are the sites of constriction in strangulated femoral hernia?

Ans. The site of constriction may be at:
* Lacunar ligament
* Neck of the sac.

Q. How a patient of femoral hernia may present?

Ans. May present in the OPD:
* Lump in groin.

May present in the ER:

* Acute intestinal obstruction
* Strangulated hernia with pain, vomiting, tender, and irreducible swelling in groin.

Q. What operation will you do?

Ans. I will consider mesh repair of femoral hernia for this patient.

Q. What is the technique of repair for a femoral hernia?

Ans.

* The inguinal canal is exposed by a standard inguinal incision.
* The femoral hernia sac is dissected and the content reduced and the neck of the hernial sac is ligated and the redundant sac is excised.
* The femoral ring is closed by one or two interrupted polypropylene suture apposing the inguinal ligament to the Cooper's ligament.
* A polypropylene mesh is then placed (15 cm × 7.5 cm) to reinforce the posterior wall of the inguinal canal.
* The mesh is then fixed below to the Cooper's ligament medially and inguinal ligament laterally.
* Above the mesh is fixed to the conjoint tendon.
* Medially, the mesh is fixed to the lateral border of the rectus sheath and laterally the mesh is split to accommodate the round ligament or spermatic cord.
* The external oblique aponeurosis is apposed in front of the mesh.
* Skin is apposed with interrupted monofilament polyamide sutures.

Q. What is the technique of McVay or Cooper's ligament repair for femoral hernia?

Ans.

* The operation is done under regional anesthesia.
* Groin crease incision above and parallel to the inguinal ligament.
* External oblique aponeurosis incised in the same line.
* Fascia transversalis incised medial to inferior epigastric vessels. The hernial sac is seen emerging through the femoral ring.
* The hernial sac is dissected from below the inguinal ligament and the sac delivered through the femoral ring.
* The hernial sac is opened and the contents of hernial sac reduced.
* The neck of the sac is ligated and redundant sac excised.
* The repair involves:
  - interrupted suture of polypropylene between the conjoint tendon and Cooper's ligament medially.
  - In the middle 1–2 interrupted suture of polypropylene apposes inguinal ligament to Cooper ligament thereby closing the femoral ring.
  - Laterally, the conjoint tendon is apposed to inguinal ligament with interrupted polypropylene suture.
  - This type of repair closes the myopectineal orifice of Fruchaud.

Q. What is low repair for femoral hernia?

Ans.

* Femoral hernia may be tackled by a low operation (Lockwood technique).

- The incision is located in the medial aspect of the thigh below the inguinal ligament centering over the femoral canal.
- The subcutaneous fat is incised to expose the hernial sac.
- The hernial mass is dissected all around the inguinal ligament, Cooper's ligament, and the neck of the hernial sac is delineated by gauge dissection. The sac is dissected beyond its neck up to the fundus.
- The sac is opened, contents inspected, and reduced into the peritoneal cavity. Neck of the sac may be digitally dilated to facilitate reduction. If the neck of the sac is very tight—lacunar ligament may need to be incised to facilitate reduction of hernial content. Abnormal obturator artery is to be taken care of while incising the lacunar ligament.
- The sac is ligated by transfixation at the neck and redundant sac is excised.
- The margin of the femoral ring is well delineated.

The repair is done with 2-0 polypropylene suture apposing the inguinal ligament to Cooper's ligament with few interrupted suture or by a purse string suture closing the femoral ring.

■ LUMBAR HERNIA

Q. What is your case? (Summary of a case of lumbar hernia)

Ans. This 30-year-old gentleman presented with a swelling in the upper part of the left loin for last 2 years. The swelling was about 2 cm in size at the onset but for last 2 years, it is gradually increasing in size to attain the present size of about 5 cm. The swelling appears only on standing, walking, and on strenuous activities and disappears spontaneously on lying down position. Patient complains of occasional dull aching pain over the swelling for last 1 year (Fig. 14.12).

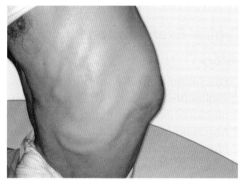

Fig. 14.12: Left-sided lumbar hernia through superior lumbar triangle

Courtesy: Dr Sarvesh Gupta, IPGME and R, Kolkata

On examination: With the patient standing, there is a swelling in the left loin just below the 12th rib. There is expansile impulse on cough over the swelling. The swelling is easily reducible on lying down. A gap is felt in the region superior lumbar triangle.

Q. What is your diagnosis?

Ans. This is a case of left lumbar hernia through superior lumbar triangle.

Q. What is the boundary of the inferior lumbar triangle?

Ans. The inferior lumbar triangle of Petit is bounded:
- *Below*—by the iliac crest
- *Medially*—by the latissimus dorsi
- *Laterally*—by the external oblique muscle.

Q. What is the boundary of the superior lumbar triangle?

Ans. The superior lumbar triangle is bounded:
- *Above*—by the 12th rib
- *Medially*—by the sacrospinalis muscle
- *Laterally*—by the posterior border of the internal oblique muscle.

Q. What are the other possibilities of such a swelling?

Ans.
- Lipoma
- Neurofibroma
- A cold abscess.

Q. How will you treat this patient?

Ans. As there is a tendency for this hernia to increase in size with time, I will consider surgical treatment. It is difficult to close the gap by apposing the local tissue. So, a repair using a polypropylene mesh is preferred.

■ PERSISTENT VITELLOINTESTINAL DUCT

Clinical Examination

History

- Discharge from the umbilicus. Duration, quantity, and type of discharge [in patent vitellointestinal duct (VID), mother usually complains of feculent discharge through the umbilicus since birth].
- Any mass protruding through the umbilicus (in patent VID, a reddish mucosal tag may protrude through the umbilicus).

Examination—Inspection/Palpation

- Assess the type of discharge
- Examination of the umbilicus to look for any protruding mucosal tag
- Look for any other congenital anomalies.

Q. What is your case? (Summary of a case of persistent vitellointestinal duct)

Ans. This 1-year-old male child presented with mucous and occasional feculent discharge through the umbilicus since birth. Mother also says that there is a reddish mass protruding from the umbilicus for last 6 months (Fig. 14.13).

On examination: There is slight feculent discharge through the umbilicus. A reddish mucous membrane is seen prolapsing through the umbilicus.

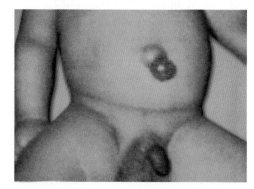

Fig. 14.13: Persistent vitellointestinal duct

Courtesy: Dr BN Mukhopadhyay, NRS Medical College, Kolkata

Q. What is your case?

Ans. This is a case of fecal fistula due to persistent VID.

Q. What is vitellointestinal duct?

Ans. This is a tubular diverticulum, which extends from the midgut to the extraembryonic part of the yolk sac. During normal development, the VID disappears.

Q. What are the different abnormalities of vitellointestinal duct?

Ans. The VID may show following developmental abnormalities:
* *Patent VID*: The VID persists completely and leads to a fecal fistula (Fig. 14.14A).
* *Raspberry tumor or umbilical adenoma*: The major part of the VID disappears except a small part near the umbilicus. The mucous lining of the distal part of the VID at the umbilicus gives rise to a raspberry tumor (Fig. 14.14B).
* *Enterocystoma*: The proximal and the distal part of the VID disappear but the intervening part remains patent. This unobliterated intermediate part of VID gives rise to cystic swelling known as enterocystoma (Fig. 14.14C).
* *Meckel's diverticulum*: The proximal end of the VID remains patent and the rest disappears. This leads to formation of Meckel's diverticulum (Fig. 14.14D). The tip of the Meckel's diverticulum may be free or may remain attached to the umbilicus by a fibrous cord, which is the obliterated distal part of the VID (Fig. 14.14D).
* *Fibrous cord*: The lumen of the VID gets obliterated, but it persists as a fibrous cord running between the ileum and the umbilicus. This fibrous band may cause intestinal obstruction (Fig. 14.14E).

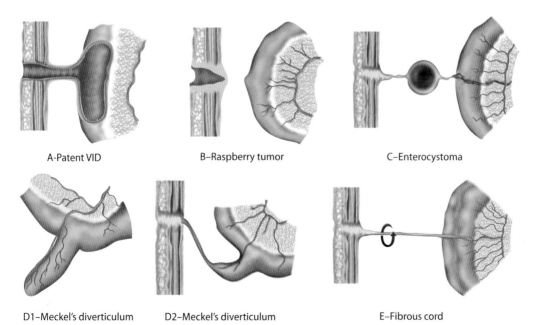

A-Patent VID   B–Raspberry tumor   C–Enterocystoma

D1–Meckel's diverticulum   D2–Meckel's diverticulum   E–Fibrous cord

Figs 14.14A to E: Different abnormalities of vitellointestinal duct

Q. How will you manage this patient?

Ans. I would like to do a fistulogram to confirm that the tract is continuous with the intestine.
* I will do baseline investigations (complete hemogram, blood sugar, urea, creatinine, and a chest X-ray).
* I will go for an umbilectomy with total excision of the VID with a wedge of ileum and end-to-end anastomosis of the cut margin of the ileum.

Q. What are the other causes of fecal discharge through the umbilicus?

Ans. Fecal fistula through the umbilicus may result due to:
* Abdominal tuberculosis
* Crohn's disease
* *Neoplastic disease*: Carcinoma colon or small gut infiltrating the umbilicus
* Intra-abdominal abscess may point to the umbilicus resulting in fecal fistula.

■ UMBILICAL ADENOMA OR RASPBERRY TUMOR

Q. What is your case? (Summary of a case of umbilical adenoma or raspberry tumor)

Ans. This 10-year-old male child presented with a swelling in the umbilicus for last 6 months. The swelling is static and has not grown in size since onset. Patient complains of slight mucus discharge from the umbilicus for the same duration. He has no other complaints.

On examination: There is a soft pinkish mass in the umbilicus 1 cm × 1 cm, there is mucus discharge from this mass and bleeds on touch. No other mass is palpable in the abdomen.

Q. What is your diagnosis?

Ans. This is a case of raspberry tumor of umbilicus.

Q. What is raspberry tumor?

Ans. This is not actually a neoplastic lesion. This results from the unobliterated distal portion of the VID. The mucosa of the unobliterated distal part of the VID near the umbilicus prolapses through the umbilicus and gives the appearance of a raspberry like tumor.

Q. What other condition may be associated with this?

Ans. Raspberry tumor may be associated with presence of Meckel's diverticulum.

Q. How will you investigate for presence of Meckel's diverticulum?

Ans.
* Barium meal follow through examination or small-bowel enema examination
* 99mTC scan.

Q. How will you treat this patient?

Ans. I will consider umbilectomy and excision of the raspberry tumor.

Q. Would you like to do routine laparotomy?

Ans. Some surgeon advocate routine laparotomy to excise associated Meckel's diverticulum.

Laparotomy has to be done in patients where there is presence of a Meckel's diverticulum for excision of the associated Meckel's diverticulum.

Q. What is endometrioma?

Ans. This is a condition where there is presence of ectopic endometrial glands in the umbilicus. This appears as a fleshy mass in the umbilicus, which becomes painful and discharges blood during each menstrual cycle. This may be associated with endometriomas in ovary or uterus.

Q. What is the treatment for endometrioma?

Ans. Umbilectomy with excision of the endometrioma.
   If associated with endometriosis of uterus and ovary, Danazol therapy may help.

■ URACHAL FISTULA

Q. What is your case? (Summary of a case of urachal fistula)

Ans. This 8-year-old male child presented with intermittent watery discharge from the umbilicus for last 2 years. The discharge smells of urine. Patient has no other complaints.
   On examination, there is uriniferous discharge from the umbilicus. External genitalia is normal. No lump is palpable in the abdomen.

Q. What is your diagnosis?

Ans. This is a case of urinary fistula due to patent urachus in a boy of 8 years of age.

Q. What is allantois?

Ans. Allantois is a diverticulum found in embryo, which passes through the umbilicus from the cloaca to the placenta.

Q. What happens to the allantois?

Ans. The allantois forms the bladder except the trigonal area. The part of the allantois from the apex of the urinary bladder to the umbilicus forms the urachus. The urachus also disappears during development into a fibrous cord and forms the median umbilical ligament.

Q. How does urachal fistula develop?

Ans. The urachus instead of obliteration may remain patent leading to formation of a urachal fistula. A patent urachus may not result in urinary fistula unless there is an associated bladder outlet or urethral obstruction.

Q. Why patient usually presents in late age?

Ans. The patent urachus does not result in urinary fistula in all cases. The urinary fistula is manifested only when there is an associated lower urinary tract obstruction like, e.g. posterior urethral valve, stricture urethra, bladder neck obstruction, or prostatic enlargement.

Q. What is urachal cyst?

Ans. Urachal cyst develops due to persistence of the central portion of the urachus and presents as a cystic swelling in the hypogastrium.

Q. How will you manage this patient of urachal fistula?

Ans.

* Before excision of the urachal fistula is considered any associated lower urinary tract obstruction needs to be excluded.
* A USG of kidneys, ureters, and bladder (KUB) region will reveal any back pressure changes in the urinary bladder, ureter, or the kidneys due to distal obstruction.
* An intravenous urography with voiding cystourethrography will diagnose any associated posterior urethral valve.

Q. If there is associated posterior urethral valve, what will you do?

Ans. Cystoscopic fulguration of the posterior urethral valve will relieve the urethral obstruction. This may result in spontaneous closure of the urachal fistula.

Q. If the urachal fistula is persistent, how will you treat?

Ans. Umbilectomy with excision of the urachus up to the apex of the urinary bladder. The apex of the bladder is to be repaired with polyglycolic acid suture.

■ DESMOID TUMOR IN THE LOWER ABDOMINAL WALL

Summary of a Case of Desmoid Tumor in the Lower Abdominal Wall

This 45-year-old lady presented with a swelling in her lower abdomen for last 2 years. The swelling was initially increasing slowly in size, but for last 6 months, the swelling is increasing rapidly to attain the present size. He complains of dull aching pain over the swelling for last 6 months. Patient has no other complaints.

On examination: There is a swelling in the umbilical, hypogastric, and right iliac fossa region, the swelling is parietal as evidenced by rising test, firm in feel, the surface is irregular, margins are well defined and rounded, the swelling is mobile from side to side and slightly from above downward, the swelling is free from the overlying skin. Liver and spleen are not palpable and there is no other mass in the abdomen.

Q. What is your diagnosis?

Ans. This is a case of desmoid tumor in the lower abdominal wall.

Q. What is desmoid tumor?

Ans. This is a benign tumor arising from the musculoaponeurotic structures of the rectus sheath. Although grouped as benign, the tumor has high potential of local recurrence following excision. This tumor is commonly found in the infraumbilical abdominal wall, but may also arise from the musculoaponeurotic structures in the region of shoulder, thigh, buttocks, and chest.

Q. How will you treat this patient?

Ans. I will advise a USG of the abdomen to ascertain the nature of the swelling.

* Routine preoperative workup
* I will consider wide excision of the tumor with a 2.5 cm margin of healthy tissue. The defect of the abdominal wall is made good by placement of a PROLENE mesh.

Q. Why such wide excision is necessary?

Ans. Desmoid tumors have notorious tendency for local recurrence following excision. So, a wide margin of excision is necessary to reduce the incidence of local recurrence.

Q. What are the pathological features of desmoid tumors?

Ans.
+ A slow growing benign fibroma
+ Nonencapsulated and locally invasive
+ Histologically consists of mature fibrous tissue
+ There are multinucleated plasmodial masses resembling foreign body giant cells
+ May undergo myxomatous degeneration
+ Unlike fibroma at other sites, it does not undergo sarcomatous change.

Q. What are the important etiological factors for development of desmoid tumor?

Ans.
+ 80% cases occurs in multiparous women
+ May occur in previous abdominal scars
+ Trauma due to repeated pregnancy, or a small hematoma of abdominal wall may be an etiological factor
+ Desmoid tumor may be associated with familial polyposis coli (Gardner's syndrome).

Genitalia and Urethra

▪ VAGINAL HYDROCELE

Clinical Examination

See Page No. 382, Chapter 9.

History

- History about the swelling—onset and progress (insidious onset and grows very slowly in size)
- Any history of alteration of the size of the swelling with straining and lying down (a vaginal hydrocele does not show any alteration in size)
- Any pain (a vaginal hydrocele is usually painless except in secondary hydrocele when patient may have pain in the scrotum due to trauma or infection)
- Any history of painful micturition—may be found in patient with secondary hydrocele associated with epididymo-orchitis
- Any history of general symptoms—such as anorexia, weight loss, chest pain, cough, or hemoptysis in patient with scrotal swelling due to testicular tumor.

Examination

- *Inspection*:
  - Position and extent
  - Size and shape
  - Surface and margin
  - Skin over the swelling
  - Position of pains
  - Any cough in pulse.
- *Palpation*:
  - *Swelling*—site and extent (swelling confined to the scrotum)
  - Temperature or tenderness.
- Get above the swelling—possible to get above the swelling—suggesting this to be a scrotal swelling.
- Size (variable)/shape (globular)/surface (smooth)/margin (well defined all around)/ consistency (soft cystic in feel).
- Fluctuation (positive) and transillumination (positive).

♦ Palpation of testis and epididymis (in vagina hydrocele, the testis and epididymis are not palpable separately).

♦ In suspected testicular tumor—examine abdomen and neck for enlarged Virchow's lymph node.

Summary of a Case of Vaginal Hydrocele

This 50-year-old gentleman presented with a swelling in both side of the scrotum for last 3 years. The swelling is slowly increasing in size. There is no history of alteration in size of the swelling during standing, walking, with strenuous activities or on lying down. There is no pain over the swelling and patient has no other complaints (Fig. 15.1).

On examination: On inspection, there is swelling on both side of the scrotum. The swelling does not show expansile impulse on cough. On palpation, it is possible to get above the swelling. The swelling is soft cystic in feel, surface is smooth, margins are rounded, nontender, fluctuation is positive, transillumination is also positive, no palpable expansile impulse on cough is present, and dull on percussion. The testis cannot be felt separately from the swelling.

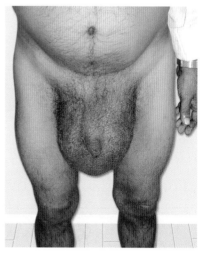

Fig. 15.1: Bilateral vaginal hydrocele

Courtesy: Dr Sidhartha Bhattacharya, IPGMER Kolkata

Q. What is your diagnosis?

Ans. This is a case of bilateral vaginal hydrocele.

Q. What are the other possibilities?

Ans.
♦ Hematocele
♦ Chylocele
♦ Testicular tumor
♦ Epididymal cyst
♦ Inguinal hernia
♦ Encysted hydrocele of the cord
♦ Filariasis of scrotum.

Q. How will you demonstrate that it is possible to get above the swelling (Fig. 15.2)?

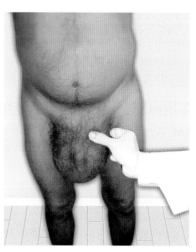

Fig. 15.2: Demonstration that it is possible to get above the swelling

Ans. Palpate the swelling at the scrotum.

Bring the finger at the root of scrotum and palpate. If at the root of the scrotum swelling is not palpable and the spermatic cord can be palpated easily then inference is possible to get above the swelling. In scrotal swelling, it is possible to get above the swelling

Q. How will you test for fluctuation?

Ans. The swelling is held at the upper pole in-between the thumb and the index finger of one hand to make the swelling tense. These are watching fingers. The thumb and index finger of

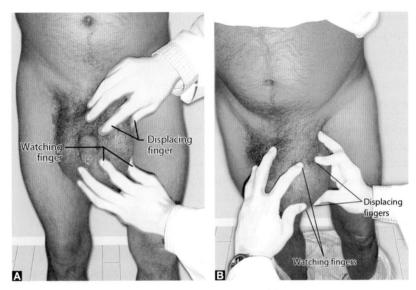

Figs 15.3A and B: Demonstration of fluctuation

the other hand are placed apart at the lower pole of the swelling. These are displacing fingers. The swelling is now pressed at the lower pole between the thumb and the index finger. The fingers at the upper pole will be lifted up due to the pressure exerted at the lower pole. This test is repeated at right angle to the previous axis. If the watching fingers are lifted up at both axes then the fluctuation is said to be positive (Figs 15.3A and B).

The can also be tested by placing only the index finger of one hand at the upper pole as the watching finger and index finger of the other hand as displacing finger at the lower pole.

Q. How will you demonstrate transillumination?

Ans. A roll of black paper is placed on one side of the swelling and light is thrown from a torch light from the other side of the swelling. If transillumination is positive, a red glow will be seen in the swelling.

The light should not be thrown from the back of the swelling, as the testis will come on the way.

Transillumination is positive in vaginal hydrocele-containing clear fluid. If the scrotal skin or the hydrocele sac is very thick transillumination may be negative (Fig. 15.4).

Q. How will you treat this patient?

Ans. This is moderate-sized hydrocele on both sides and is causing discomfort for the patient, so I will consider surgical treatment.

I will do baseline preoperative workup.

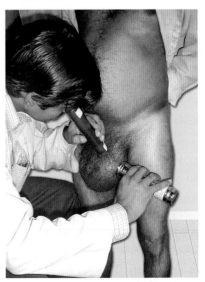

Fig. 15.4: Transillumination test

Q. What operation you will do?

Ans. I will do bilateral eversion of sac.

Q. Describe the steps of eversion of sac?

Ans. *See* Operative Surgery, Section, Page No. 1142, Chapter 22.

Q. What is Lord's operation for hydrocele?

Ans. In this procedure after incision in the tunica vaginalis sac, the fluid is drained and the testis delivered from the tunica vaginalis sac. The cut margin of the tunica vaginalis is then plicated with interrupted suture. As these sutures are tied, the tunica vaginalis sac becomes bunched up at the periphery of the testis. The testis with the plicated tunica vaginalis sac is then placed in the dartos pouch. Scrotal incision is then closed (Fig. 15.5).

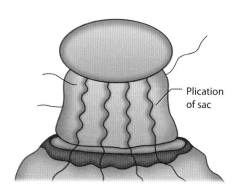

Plication of sac

Fig. 15.5: Lord's operation

Q. Would you like to put a drain-following hydrocele operation?

Ans. If the hemostasis is good, no drain is required. If there is some oozing, a drain is kept in the dartos pouch to prevent formation of a hematoma.

Q. What are indications of excision of the tunica vaginalis sac?

Ans. The excision of redundant tunica vaginalis sac is considered when the sac is large and very thick and may be indicated in:
- Hematocele
- Chylocele
- Infected hydrocele.

The hydrocele fluid is drained by incising the tunica vaginalis sac. The redundant tunica vaginalis sac is excised leaving a margin of 2 cm around the testis. The bleeding from the cut margin of the sac is controlled either by diathermy or by continuous interlocking suture. A scrotal drain is required to be kept to prevent formation of a hematoma.

Q. What is the role of tapping for relief of hydrocele?

Ans. Tapping is not a favorable method of treatment. But tapping may be considered when:
- Surgery cannot be done for some medical problems.
- Patient is not willing to undergo surgery.
- For appearing in a medical test for a job—provides rapid relief without operation.
   Tapping, however, does not cure the condition and is always associated with recurrence.

Q. What is the role of sclerotherapy in hydrocele?

Ans. Tapping of hydrocele fluid and instillation of sclerosant have been tried as a modality of treatment for hydrocele.

The hydrocele fluid is drained by tapping. A sclerosant solution polidocanol or sodium tetradecyl sulfate or tetracycline is injected into the tunica vaginalis sac and compression bandage is applied for 4 weeks. The instilled sclerosant results in a sterile inflammation and fibrosis with obliteration of tunica vaginalis sac.

Q. What are the complications of tapping?

Ans.
- Infection
- Bleeding—hematocele
- Injury to testis
- Recurrence.

Q. What is hydrocele?

Ans. Hydrocele is a condition of collection of fluid in the tunica vaginalis sac.

Q. What is primary hydrocele?

Ans. When there is no obvious cause to explain collection of fluid in tunica vaginalis sac.

Q. How does primary hydrocele develop?

Ans. There may be collection of fluid in the tunica vaginalis due to:
- Excessive secretion of fluid within the tunica vaginalis sac—as in secondary hydrocele
- Defective absorption of the secreted fluid—most primary hydrocele is due to this
- Due to defective lymphatic drainage of the scrotal structures
- Peritoneal fluid may reach the patent processus vaginalis leading to a congenital hydrocele.

Q. What is secondary hydrocele?

Ans. When there is collection of fluid in tunica vaginalis sac secondary to some disease of testis or the epididymis. Secondary hydrocele is usually small and lax.

Secondary hydrocele may be secondary to epididymo-orchitis, testicular tumor, torsion or trauma.

Q. What is the explanation for development of hydrocele following inguinal herniorrhaphy?

Ans. One of the explanations is probably due to interruption of lymphatics draining the scrotal contents following herniorrhaphy.

Q. What is hydrocele of the hernial sac?

Ans. This is one of the complications of an inguinal hernia. If the neck of the hernial sac is plugged with omentum then there may be collection of fluid in the distal part of the sac resulting in hydrocele of the hernial sac.

Q. What is chylocele?

Ans. Hydrocele resulting from lymphatic obstruction of the scrotal contents leads to development of chylocele. One of the lymphatic varix may rupture and discharge chyle into the tunica vaginalis sac. This is usually secondary to filarial epididymo-orchitis.

The fluid contains liquid fat, which is rich in cholesterol.

Q. What is hematocele?

Ans. Hemorrhage into the tunica vaginalis sac may occur due to:
- Tapping of hydrocele
- Trauma to the testis.

Q. What are the different types of hydrocele?

Ans. There are different types of hydrocele depending on the extent of fluid collection in the processus vaginalis sac (Figs 15.6A to G).

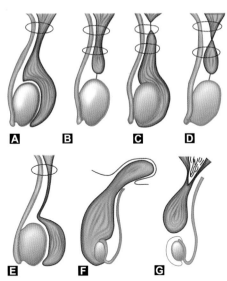

Figs 15.6A to G: Types of hydrocele

- *Congenital hydrocele*: When the whole of processus vaginalis is patent and there is accumulation of fluid within the processus vaginalis sac. The hydrocele sac communicates with the peritoneal cavity through the deep ring. So, this is also known as communicating hydrocele. The swelling is inguinoscrotal, soft, cystic, fluctuant, and also transilluminant.
- *Funicular hydrocele*: When there is collection of fluid in the patent processus vaginalis extending from the deep inguinal ring to the upper pole of the testis then it is called a funicular type of hydrocele.
- *Infantile hydrocele*: There is collection of fluid in the processus vaginalis sac, which extends from the tunica vaginalis of the testis up into the inguinal canal and extends up to but not beyond the deep inguinal ring.
- *Encysted hydrocele of the cord*: When there is accumulation of fluid in the intermediate segment of the processus vaginalis then it is called encysted hydrocele of the cord.
- *Vaginal hydrocele*: When there is accumulation of fluid in the tunica vaginalis sac then it is called vaginal hydrocele. The swelling is scrotal, soft cystic, fluctuant, and transilluminant.
- *Bilocular hydrocele or hydrocele en bisac*: There is accumulation of fluid in the tunica vaginalis sac in the scrotum and there is prolongation of the tunica vaginalis sac into the inguinal canal either deep to the skin or between the muscle layers. There are two loculi, one lying in the scrotum and another in the inguinal canal, which shows cross-fluctuation.
- *Hydrocele of the hernial sac*: There is accumulation of fluid in the distal part of the hernial sac.

Q. How to treat congenital hydrocele?

Ans. The treatment of congenital hydrocele is same as congenital hernia. Herniotomy through an inguinal approach.

Q. What are the characteristics of fluid?

Ans. The fluid is usually amber colored. It contains inorganic salts, traces of albumin and fibrinogen. Long-standing fluid may contain cholesterol and tyrosine crystals. Because of the fibrinogen content the hydrocele fluid clots in contact with blood.

Q. What investigation you will do to exclude an underlying testicular enlargement associated with?

Ans. An ultrasonographic examination of the scrotum using a 7.5 mm probe can delineate the anatomy of testis.

Q. What are the complications of hydrocele?

Ans. The hydrocele, if untreated, may be treated:

- Infection—pyocele
- Trauma—hematocele
- Atrophy of testis
- Rupture
- Calcification of the sac
- Hernia of the sac.

■ ENCYSTED HYDROCELE OF THE CORD

Clinical Examination

See Page No. 382, Chapter 9.

History

- About the swelling (see before).
- Any pain.

Local Examination—Inspection/Palpation

- Detailed examination of the swelling.
- Site, size, shape, surface (a swelling in relation to the spermatic cord and smooth surface).
- Expansile impulse on cough (absent).
- Consistency, fluctuation (swelling is soft cystic in feel and fluctuation is positive).
- Transillumination (transillumination is positive).
- Mobility (mobile from side to side and above downwards).
- Traction test (traction on the testis results in restriction of movement of the swelling).

Q. What is your case? (Summary of a case of encysted of the cord)

Ans. This 30-year-old gentleman presented with a swelling in upper part of left side of the scrotum for last 2 years. The swelling is slowly increasing in size and there is no alteration in size of the swelling with strenuous activities or lying down (Fig. 15.7).

On examination: There is a swelling in relation to the left spermatic cord. The swelling is elongated, soft-cystic in feel, fluctuation, and transillumination tests are positive. There is no expansile impulse on cough, the swelling is mobile from side to side and from above downward, on traction on the testis, the mobility of the swelling becomes restricted.

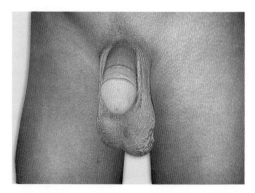

Fig. 15.7: Encysted hydrocele of the cord on the left side

Courtesy: Dr PK Sarkar, IPGMER, Kolkata

Q. What is your diagnosis?

Ans. This is a case of left-sided encysted hydrocele of the cord.

Q. What is traction test?

Ans. In cases of an encysted of the cord when the testis is pulled downwards gently, the swelling moves downwards and becomes less mobile, as the swelling is fixed to the spermatic cord (Fig. 15.8).

Q. What are the other possibilities?

Ans. The important other possibilities are:
- Cyst of the epididymis
- Spermatocele
- Lipoma of the cord
- Varicocele
- Lymphangioma of the cord.

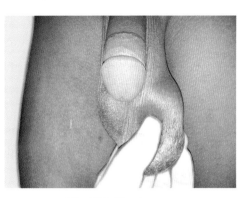

Fig. 15.8: Traction test

Q. How will you treat this patient?

Ans. I will advise baseline investigations and consider excision of the encysted hydrocele of the cord under local anesthesia.

Q. What is encysted hydrocele of the cord?

Ans. This is a condition where there is collection of fluid in unobliterated intermediate portion of the processus vaginalis. The swelling may be situated in the inguinal, inguinoscrotal, or scrotal region.

■ CYST OF EPIDIDYMIS

Q. What is your case? (Summary of a case of epididymal cyst)

Ans. This 45-year-old gentleman presented with a swelling in right side of the scrotum for last 3 years, which is increasing very slowly in size. There is no pain over the swelling.

On examination: There is a soft cystic swelling in relation to the head of the right epididymis. The swelling has a lobulated surface and feels like a bunch of grapes. Testis can be felt separately from the swelling. The swelling is brilliantly transilluminant.

Q. What is your diagnosis?

Ans. This is a case of right-sided epididymal cyst.

Q. What are the other possibilities?

- Spermatocele
- Cyst of the appendix of the testis (cyst of Morgagni)
- Encysted hydrocele of the cord
- Epididymo-orchitis.

Q. How will you treat this patient?

Ans. As the cyst is large, I will consider excision of the cyst under local anesthesia.

Q. What is the problem of excision of epididymal cyst?

Ans. Excision of the epididymal cyst will result in blockage of the sperm conducting epididymis of that side.

Q. Where from epididymal cyst arises?

Ans. Epididymal cyst arises due to cystic degeneration of the epididymis.

Q. What is spermatocele?

Ans. Spermatocele is a unilocular retention cyst developing from some portion of the epididymis usually the head of the epididymis.

Q. What are the characteristics of spermatocele?

Ans.
* Lies in the head of the epididymis above and behind the upper pole of the testis.
* Soft cystic in feel and fluctuation is positive.
* Transillumination poorly positive, as it contains barley water like fluid.

Q. How will you treat spermatocele?

Ans.
* *Small cyst*: Wait and watch
* *Large cyst*: Aspiration, or complete excision through scrotal route.

Q. What is the appearance of fluid in cyst of epididymis and spermatocele?

Ans.
* Cyst of epididymis—crystal clear fluid
* Spermatocele—barley water-like fluid.

■ VARICOCELE

Clinical Examination

See Page No. 382, Chapter 9.

History
* *History of swelling*—onset and progress of the swelling (insidious onset of swelling in the scrotum with history of gradual increase in size).
* What happens on straining and on lying down (the swelling appears on standing and disappears on lying down).
* Any pain (there may be a sensation of dragging pain or ache in the scrotum).
* Any history of subfertility (in married individual enquire about history of infertility).
* Any pain abdomen, abdominal mass, or hematuria (triad of presentation of renal cell carcinoma—left-sided varicocele is common in patient with left-sided renal cell carcinoma).

Examination—Inspection/Palpation

- Examination in standing position.
- *Swelling*—site and extent, size (dilated tortuous veins are palpable above the upper pole of testis in relation to the spermatic cord and feels like a bag of worms).
- *Impulse on cough*—no expansile impulse on cough is palpable.
- *Reducibility*—on lying down, the dilated veins gets emptied.
- Assess the testicular size (in long-standing varicocele, the testicular volume may be reduced in size in comparison to the normal testis).

Q. What is your case? (Summary of a case of varicocele)

Ans. This 30-year-old gentleman presented with a swelling in the left side of the scrotum for last 4 years. The swelling started in the lower part of the scrotum and subsequently the swelling is slowly increasing in size and grown up to the root of the scrotum. The swelling disappears on lying down position and reappears on standing and walking. Patient complains of dull aching pain in the left side of the scrotum for last 6 months, the pain is more toward the evening when the swelling enlarges in size. There is no pain abdomen and no urinary complaints (Fig. 15.9).

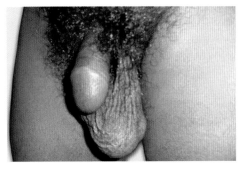

Fig. 15.9: Left-sided varicocele

Courtesy: Dr Subhamitra Chowdhury, IPGMER, Kolkata

On examination: A mass of dilated vein feeling like a bag of worms is palpable on the left side of the scrotum along the left spermatic cord extending from the upper pole of the testis up to the superficial inguinal ring. No expansile impulse on cough is palpable, instead a thrill is palpable. On lying down and on elevation of the scrotum, the swelling disappears. On asking the patient to stand up, the dilated vein reappeared. The left testicular volume is smaller than the right one. Abdominal examination is normal.

Q. What is your diagnosis?

Ans. This is a case of varicocele on left side.

Q. Apart from examination of swelling, what else you have to look for?

Ans. As left-sided varicocele may be secondary to renal cell carcinoma on the left side, so it is necessary to examine the abdomen to rule out any mass.

Q. What is bow sign?

Ans. The varicocele mass is held between index and middle finger and the thumb and the patient is asked to bow down—the tension within the pampiniform plexus of veins becomes appreciably less and the varicocele gets reduced in size. Bowing position cuts off the continuity of the blood inside the varicocele and the testicular vein.

Q. What are the other possibilities?

Ans.
- Inguinal hernia
- Congenital hydrocele

- Encysted hydrocele of the cord
- Lipoma of the cord
- Epididymal cyst
- Vaginal hydrocele.

Q. Which veins form the pampiniform plexus?

Ans. The pampiniform plexus are the bunch of veins draining the testis, epididymis, vas deferens, and the cremaster muscle.

Q. How the pampiniform plexus ends?

Ans. Anastomosing veins from the testis, epididymis, vas deferens, and the cremaster muscle gives rise to a plexus of veins at upper pole of the testis, which are about 15–25 in number. As the vein ascends, it reduces to 12–15 in number. At the level of the superficial inguinal ring, the number of vein becomes 4–5. At the level of deep inguinal ring, the veins are reduced to 2 in number. The two veins ascend in the retroperitoneum and join to from a single vein, which on right side ends at the inferior vena cava obliquely and on left side ends at the left renal vein at right angle. Near the termination, the testicular vein is provided with a valve. There is communication between the cremasteric veins and the veins draining the vas, which provides alternative path of venous drainage from the testis. The cremasteric veins drain into the inferior epigastric veins (Fig. 15.10).

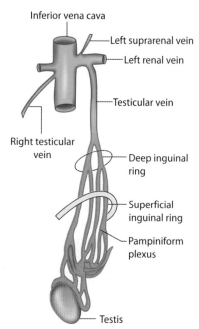

Fig. 15.10: Pampiniform plexus

Q. What is varicocele?

Ans. This is a condition of dilatation and tortuosity of pampiniform plexus of veins of the spermatic cord.

Q. What are the types of varicocele?

Ans. There are two types of varicocele:
1. Primary
2. Secondary.

Q. What is primary varicocele?

Ans. In 95% cases, no cause for varicocele could be found. This is called primary varicoccle.

Q. What is secondary varicocele?

Ans. When the varicocele is secondary to obstruction of testicular vein then it is called secondary varicocele. The obstruction of the testicular vein may bc duc to retroperitoneal tumor or kidney tumor.

Q. What ancillary investigation is helpful for confirmation of diagnosis of varicocele?

Ans. Color Doppler study is helpful for diagnosis of varicocele. The diagnosis is made when two to three veins of 3 mm or greater in size are found or there is enlargement of veins on standing and reflux on Valsalva maneuver.

Q. Why varicocele is common on left side?

Ans. 90% cases of varicocele are found on the left side. The important cause for this left preponderance is:
* The left testicular vein joins the left renal vein at right angle.
* The left testicular vein joins the left renal vein, which drains into the inferior vena cava 8–10 cm more cranial than the right testicular vein, as a result, the left testicular vein has an 8–10 cm greater pressure head than the right testicular vein.
* Left testicular vein is longer, as left testis lies at a lower level and left renal vein lie at a higher level. Hence, longer column of blood in left testicular vein exerting more pressure in left pampiniform plexus.
* Left testicular vein is liable to be compressed by loaded pelvic colon, as it ascends behind the left colon.
* The left renal vein may be sandwiched between the abdominal aorta and superior mesenteric artery and compression of the left renal vein may lead to varicocele.
* Left testicular artery may arch over the left renal vein and may cause compression of the renal vein and testicular vein leading to varicocele.
* In carcinoma of left kidney, the tumor may grow along the renal vein causing obstruction of left testicular vein leading to varicocele.

Q. Which factors are responsible for development of primary varicocele?

Ans. Varicocele formation usually is caused by:
* Increased venous pressure in the left renal vein.
* Incompetent valves of the testicular vein.

Q. How scrotal temperature is kept lower?

Ans. For normal spermatogenesis, the scrotal temperature is kept 2.5°C lower than the core temperature. The pampiniform plexus encircles the testicular artery, as it supplies the testis. There is effective countercurrent heat exchange mechanism that permits the arterial blood to be cooled from intra-abdominal temperature to the cooler temperature found in the scrotum.

Q. What are the effects of varicocele on testicular function?

Ans. Varicocele is one of the important causes of male infertility. There is adverse effect on spermatogenesis. The pathophysiology of testicular dysfunction due to following mechanisms:
* *Hyperthermia*: Presence of varicosities impedes the countercurrent heat exchange mechanism. Increased scrotal temperature inhibits spermatogenesis.
* *Intratesticular hyperperfusion injury*: Abnormal elevation of microvascular blood flow and increased intratesticular temperature increases the metabolic activity and depletes the intracellular glycogen store and induces testicular parenchymal injury.
* *Hypoxia*.
* *Local testicular hormonal imbalance*: Leydig cell dysfunction in patients with varicocele may be caused by diminished intratesticular testosterone.
* *Unilateral varicocele* may show bilateral finding of decreased spermatogenesis, maturation arrest, and tubular thickening.

Q. What are the different grades of varicocele?

Ans. Depending on the physical finding, there are three grades of varicocele.
* *Grade I*: Small varicocele, which is palpable only when patient performs Valsalva maneuver (expiration against a closed glottis).
* *Grade II*: Moderate sized. Easily palpable varicocele without Valsalva maneuver.
* *Grad III*: Large varicocele visible through the scrotal skin.

Q. What is the effect of varicocele on testicular volume?

Ans. One of the important effects of varicocele is loss of testicular volume. So, assessment of testicular volume is essential in evaluation of varicocele patient. The testicular volume may be measured by using an orchidometer, which is like a calliper.

Q. Do all varicoceles need treatment?

Ans. Majority of the varicoceles are diagnosed as an incidental finding. Grade I varicocele does not require active management.

Grade II and grade III varicoceles need treatment when associated with:
* Subfertility and infertility
* Testicular volume loss greater than 2 mL in comparison to the normal side
* Pain and discomfort
* Cosmetic problems.

Q. How surgery is helpful in varicocele?

Ans.
* The stagnation of blood in the pampiniform plexus is prevented.
* The spermatogenesis may return to normal.
* The testicular volume may return to normal.

Q. How will you treat this patient?

Ans. This patient has grade III varicocele and is associated with loss of testicular volume and pain and discomfort. I will consider surgical treatment in this case.

Q. What operation will you do in this patient?

Ans. I will do Palomo's operation in this patient.

Q. What is Palomo's operation?

Ans.
* This is a technique of high ligation of testicular vein.
* This is usually done under regional anesthesia.
* An oblique incision is made 3 cm above the level of deep inguinal ring. After incising the skin, subcutaneous tissue, external oblique muscle and aponeurosis, internal oblique and transversus abdominis muscle, the retroperitoneum is exposed. Testicular vein is dissected in retroperitoneum lateral to external iliac artery. The testicular vein is then ligated and divided.

Q. What will happen, if testicular artery is ligated high up by mistake?

Ans. If testicular artery is ligated inadvertently during Palomo's operation—then the testis usually does not suffer from ischemic injury, as it will get its supply by way of anastomosis with the artery to the vas, which is a branch of superior vesical artery and anastomosis with cremasteric artery, which is a branch of inferior epigastric artery. But in different studies, it was shown that there is 20–30% chance of testicular atrophy.

Q. How the venous drainage of testis will be maintained after Palomo's operation?

Ans. The venous drainage of testis will be maintained by anastomosis of pampiniform plexus with the cremasteric veins and the veins draining the vas.

Q. What is laparoscopic Palomo's operation?

Ans. Ligation of the testicular vein in the retroperitoneum may be done by laparoscopic technique by using a transperitoneal approach.

Q. What is triangle of Doom?

Ans. It is a landmark in laparoscopic approach for varicocele or hernia. This is a triangular area bounded by the vas deferens medially, testicular vessels laterally, and the line joining these two structures above. The external iliac vessels run through this triangle (Fig. 15.11).

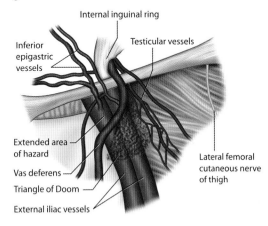

Fig. 15.11: Triangle of Doom

Q. What is inguinal operation for varicocele?

Ans. Inguinal ligation is an alternative procedure for varicocele.

Through a groin incision—the spermatic cord is exposed and cremasteric muscle and fascia is incised. The testicular artery is identified, if necessary by using a Doppler ultrasound probe. The vas deferens and the vessels supplying the vas are separated from the main mass of dilated veins. Two pairs of clamps are applied proximally and distally at a gap of 5 cm and the intervening segment of veins are excised. The two clamps are then approximated and ligated. This removes the main mass of dilated vein and also shortens the cord. At the completion of operation only the testicular artery, lymphatics and the vas deferens with its vessels remain.

Q. What else may be the approach for ligation of varicocele?

Ans. This may be done by a scrotal approach. But scrotal approach is not usually favored, as the dilated veins are more numerous here and there is increased chance of scrotal hematoma formation.

Q. How interventional radiography may help in management of varicocele?

Ans. Transvenous occlusion is one modality of treatment for varicocele. Access is gained through the femoral vein and testicular vein is cannulated. Therapeutic embolization is done by using detachable balloons or steel coils, which causes occlusion of testicular vein.

Q How does surgery help?

Ans. Surgical treatment of varicocele will help to not increase any further damage to the testicular function. The testicular volume may return to normal and the spermatogenesis may return to normal.

Q. What are the complications of varicocele operation?

Ans.

- *Hydrocele*: This is due to lymphatic obstruction.
- *Testicular artery injury*: There is 10–20% chance of testicular atrophy. In children, the incidence of testicular atrophy is less than in adults.
- Recurrence of varicocele.

■ UNDESCENDED TESTIS

Clinical Examination

History

- Absence of testis in the scrotum—one side or both side.
- *Duration*—whether since birth or it was present in the scrotum at birth and subsequently not present in the scrotum (retractile testis or atrophic testis).
- Any swelling present in the line of normal descent of testis—in the loin, right iliac fossa, or inguinal canal.
- Any swelling present at the sites of location of ectopic testis—in thigh, root of penis, perineum, and in subinguinal pouch.
- Any pain over the swelling (pain may be due to the trauma or torsion of an undescended testis).
- Any swelling in the groin, which comes up on straining and disappears on lying down (suggestive of an associated inguinal hernia—which may be present with undescended testis).
- In patient with bilateral undescended testes—enquire about appearance of secondary sex characters and infertility (in aged patients).

Examination—Inspection/Palpation

- *Look at the scrotum*—whether well developed or ill developed on one or both sides (in undescended and ectopic testis the scrotum is ill developed, whereas in retractile testis, the scrotum is well developed).
- *Palpate along the normal line of descent*—from lumbar region to the region of deep-inguinal ring, inguinal canal, superficial inguinal ring, and root of the scrotum to ascertain the presence of undescended testis at these sites.
- *Palpate at the sites of ectopic location of testis for any swelling at*—root of penis, thigh, perineum, and inguinal canal at subinguinal pouch.
- *Examine inguinal canal for any swelling*—any expansile impulse on cough over that swelling, whether the swelling is reducible or not (reducible swelling with expansile on cough suggests associated inguinal hernia).
- If testis is palpable at the inguinal canal, try to manipulate the testis into the scrotum—in retractile testis, it can be brought down to the bottom of the scrotum. If the testis cannot be brought down to the scrotum—this is likely to be ectopic or undescended testis.
- Look for any other congenital anomalies.

Q. What is your case? (Summary of a case of undescended testis)

Ans. This 10-year-old male child presented with history of absence of left testis in the scrotum since birth. Patient noticed a small swelling in left groin for last 2 years. The swelling appears when the child stands up, walks, and strains, the swelling disappears on lying down (Fig. 15.12).

On examination: The right scrotal sac is well formed and the right testis is well seen and palpable. The left hemiscrotum is ill-formed and the left testis is not palpable in the left scrotal sac.

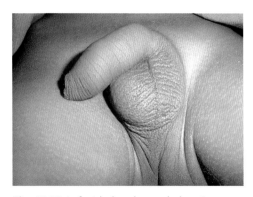

Fig. 15.12: Left-sided undescended testis

Courtesy: Dr Kalyani Saha Basu, NRS Medical College, Kolkata

The testis is also not palpable in the inguinal canal or in other ectopic sites like near the root of the penis, perineum, and thigh. On standing, a swelling is found which is confined to the left inguinal canal, there is an expansile impulse on cough over the swelling and the swelling reduces easily on lying down.

Q. What is your diagnosis?

Ans. This is a case of left-sided undescended testis, testis is impalpable in the inguinal canal and there is an associated left-sided inguinal hernia.

Give a complete diagnosis:

- Unilateral or bilateral undescended testis.
- Whether testis is palpable or impalpable, if palpable at what site?
- Presence of any associated inguinal hernia.

Q. How will you proceed to manage this patient?

Ans.

- In this child, as the testis is impalpable, I would suggest ultrasonography (USG) of groin, pelvis, and retroperitoneal area to localize the testis.
- I will advise baseline investigations to assess patient fitness for general anesthesia and surgery.

Q. What is the limitation of ultrasonography?

Ans. Ultrasonography is a cheap and noninvasive investigation; but in majority, it cannot localize the testis, if it is intra-abdominal.

Q. How else impalpable testis may be localized?

- Computed tomography (CT) scan and magnetic resonance imaging (MRI) are not very reliable investigations for localization of impalpable testis.
- Diagnostic laparoscopy is now the standard method of localization of impalpable testis.

Q. What may be the findings in diagnostic laparoscopy?

Ans. After induction of pneumoperitoneum, the telescope attached to the camera is inserted through a subumbilical incision.

- The deep ring can be seen clearly.
- Associated hernia can be seen.
- If cord structures (vas deferens and the testicular vessels) are seen emerging from the deep ring then the testis has descended through the deep inguinal ring into the inguinal canal.
- If no cord structure is seen emerging through the deep ring then the testis is intra-abdominal.
- If a blind ending vas is found, it may be a testicular agenesis or vanishing testis.

Q. How will you treat this patient?

Ans.
- If the testis is localized by USG then I will do orchidopexy.
- If the testis is not localized by USG, I will do diagnostic laparoscopy and orchidopexy.

Q. What are the principles of orchidopexy?

Ans.
- Good mobilization of the spermatic cord.
- Fixation of testis in the scrotum without tension.
- Repair of associated hernia.

Q. How does orchidopexy help the patient?

Ans.
- Psychological satisfaction of having both the testes in the scrotum.
- Maximizes the prospect of normal spermatogenesis.
- Reduces the risk of torsion.
- Associated inguinal hernia is repaired.
- Minimizes the risk of tumor development and diagnosis can be done early.

Q. What is the ideal time for orchidopexy?

Ans.
- In majority of undescended testis, the testis descends into the scrotum by 3 months of age except in premature infants where it descends by 1 year of age.
- Earlier, it was said that the ideal time for operation is 5–6 years.
- But current consensus is that the ideal time for orchidopexy is 0.5–1 year.

Q. What are the steps of orchidopexy?

Ans.
- Operation is done under general anesthesia.
- A groin incision is made parallel to the inguinal ligament (Fig. 15.13A).
- The external oblique aponeurosis is incised in the same line and the inguinal canal is exposed (Figs 15.13B and C).
- Herniotomy is done for an associated inguinal hernia.
- The spermatic cord and the testis are mobilized, so that these can be easily brought down to the bottom of the scrotum (Fig. 15.13D).
- A finger is passed into the scrotum from the inguinal incision and the scrotum is stretched (Fig. 15.13E).

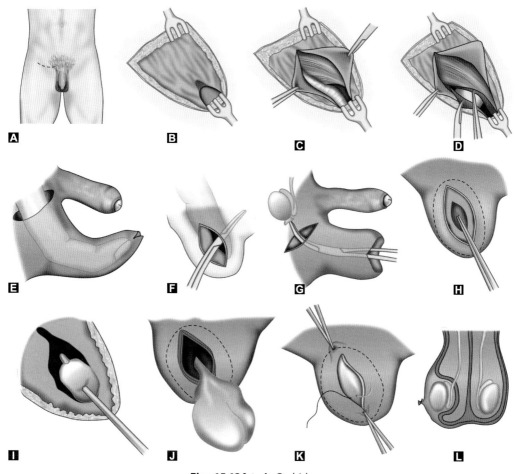

Figs 15.13A to L: Orchidopexy

- About 2.5-cm long incision is made over the scrotum and a subdartos pouch is created by dissecting between the scrotal skin and the dartos muscle (Fig. 15.13F). The testis is brought down into the subdartos pouch by making small incision in the dartos muscle (Figs 15.13G to I).
- The testis is then placed in the subdartos pouch. Skin closed over it (Figs 15.13J to L). If good mobilization is done, no fixation is required.

Q. What are the other techniques of anchoring the testis in the scrotum?

Ans. There are a number of other techniques for fixing the testis to the scrotum.
- *Ladd and gross technique*:
  - Scrotal sac on the side is enlarged by finger dissection.
  - Testis is mobilized well and placed in the scrotal sac. The neck of the scrotal sac is narrowed around the cord. The testis is anchored to the thigh by passing a stitch through the tunica albuginea, which is brought out through the scrotal skin and thread is anchored to the thigh over a rubber tube. This suture is removed after 10–14 days.

- *Ombredanne's technique*: The mobilized testis is placed in the opposite scrotal sac by passing it through the media septum of the scrotum.
- *Keetley-Torek technique*: Testis is mobilized well and it is placed into a pocket on the medial aspect of the thigh in-between the skin and fascia lata. Testis is brought out through the scrotal skin and placed on the medial aspect of thigh. Margins of scrotal and thigh incisions are apposed. This is maintained for 3–6 months after which the scrotal sac is separated from the thigh.

Q. While trying to bring the testis by mobilization then adequate length cannot be gained, what will you do?

Ans. If the testis and the spermatic cord cannot be mobilized well, one of the following procedures may be undertaken:

- The fascia transversalis is incised medially and the cord structures are dissected high up in the retroperitoneum, this may allow some gain in length.
- Division of the inferior epigastric vessel may allow medial displacement of the cord and the spermatic cord takes a more direct course and thereby gains some more length.
- *Two-stage orchidopexy*: The testis and the spermatic cord are mobilized as much as possible and testis is kept in the inguinal canal in first stage of the operation.

After 3–6 months, the testis and spermatic cord is further mobilized and brought down to the scrotum in a second-stage operation.

- *Fowler-Stephens procedure*:
  - One of the factors hindering mobilization is the short length of the testicular vessels. In Fowler-Stephens procedure, the testicular vessels are divided high up and this provides very good mobilization and the testis could be mobilized well and brought down into the scrotum. The blood supply to the testis is maintained by artery to the vas and cremasteric vessels.
- *Silbar procedure*: Orchidopexy by microvascular anastomosis.

Testis is mobilized well. The testicular vessels are divided and the testis placed in the scrotal pouch. The testicular artery is anastomosed to inferior epigastric artery and testicular vein is anastomosed to the inferior epigastric vein.

Q. When will you consider orchidectomy in undescended testis?

Ans.

- If there is complication, e.g. torsion or tumor, orchidectomy is necessary.
- If the testis is atrophic and is unlikely to function.
- If the testis cannot be mobilized to a sufficient length in spite of all maneuvers.

Q. What is the role of hormonal treatment in undescended testis?

Ans. Two types of hormones have been used—exogenous human chorionic gonadotropin (hCG) given by injection and gonadotropin-releasing hormone (GnRH), or luteinizing hormone-releasing hormone (LHRH) given as a nasal spray. Success has been claimed in patients with canalicular testis or retractile testis.

A typical treatment schedule is hCG 1,500 IU/m^2 given by intramuscular (IM) injection twice a week for 4 weeks or GnRH 1.2 mg/day as nasal spray for 4 weeks.

Overall efficacy of 20% has been claimed with hormonal treatment. So, surgery is the gold standard of treatment for undescended testis.

Q. In which situation, hormonal treatment is not indicated?

Ans. Hormonal treatment is not indicated in patients with ectopic testis, when associated with a hernia and who has undergone earlier inguinal surgery.

Q. What are the side effects of hormonal therapy?

Ans. The side effects include:
* Increased rugosity and pigmentation of the scrotum
* Increase size of the penis and development of pubic hair.

Q. Where from testis develops?

Ans. The testis develops from the genital ridge on the medial aspect of mesonephros in the retroperitoneum during 4–6 weeks of gestation. The developing testis in this site is attached to posterior abdominal wall by a fold of peritoneum called meso-orchium through which testicular vessels and nerve enter the testis. The primordial germ cells located at the caudal wall of the embryonic yolk sac migrate to the genital ridge via the dorsal mesentery. Interstitial cells are derived from the mesonephros. The gubernaculum develops in the 7th week of intrauterine life extends from the developing gonad in the retroperitoneum to the developing scrotum.

Q. Where from vas deferens develops?

Ans. The mesonephros disappears but the mesonephric duct persists and becomes the epididymis and vas deferens.

Q. Which factors help in descent of testis?

Ans. There are three phases of testicular descent:
1. Transabdominal
2. Transinguinal
3. Extracanalicular.

A number of factors are responsible for descent of testis to the scrotum from the lumbar region:
* *Endocrine factors*:
  - A normal hypothalamic–pituitary–gonadal axis is essential for testicular descent to occur.
  - Androgens (testosterone and dihydrotestosterone). Deficiency of these hormones or androgen insensitivity is associated with failure of transinguinal phase of descent of testis and in such cases, the undescended testis is mostly found deep to the deep ring.
  - Mullerian inhibiting substance (MIS) secreted by the fetal Sertoli cells is important for testicular descent. Deficiency of MIS is associated with cryptorchidism.
* *Pull of gubernaculum*—which is a fibromesoblastic tissue attached to the lower pole of the testis. Earlier, it was said that the gubernaculum lower end reaches up to the scrotum, which pulls the testis into the scrotum. Subsequently, it is shown that gubernaculum has no firm attachment into the scrotum. Testicular descent is a complex process mediated by both mechanical and hormonal factors.
* Increased intra-abdominal pressure hastens descent of testis.
* Differential growth of abdominal wall in relation to gubernaculum.

Q. What is processus vaginalis?

Ans. Before testis descends into the inguinal canal, a fold of peritoneum descends into the scrotum—this fold of peritoneum is called the processus vaginalis. Later on, the major part of the processus vaginalis disappears except the most distal part which forms the tunica vaginalis, which encircles the testis.

Q. What is the incidence of undescended testis?

Ans. Cryptorchidism is one of the most common congenital anomalies accounting for 3% of full-term male newborns. By 1 year after birth, majority of these testes descend to the scrotum and the incidence at 1 year of age is 1%.

Q. Which factors hinder testicular descent?

Ans.

- Short vas deferens
- Short testicular vessels
- Retroperitoneal adhesions
- Adhesion at deep inguinal ring
- Inefficient pull by gubernaculum testis
- Defective hormonal stimulation
- Defective development of testis.

Q. What is the chronology of testicular descent?

Ans. Testis develops at the level of L1 vertebra in the retroperitoneum at the 2nd month of intrauterine life.

- During 2nd–3rd month, it traverses the retroperitoneum and reaches right iliac fossa at the end of 3rd month.
- Reaches the deep inguinal ring by 7th month of intrauterine life.
- It traverses the inguinal canal between 7th and 9th month.
- It reaches the bottom of the scrotum at the end of 9th month (Fig. 15.14).

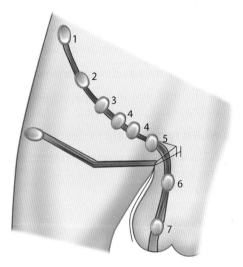

Fig. 15.14: Chronology of testicular descent

Q. Which changes occur in an undescended testis?

- An undescended testis is exposed to higher temperature of abdomen, which hinders proper spermatogenesis.
- The histopathological hallmark of cryptorchidism are apparent between 1 years and 2 years of age and include decreased number of Leydig and Sertoli cells, reduced number of germ cells and defective spermatogenesis.
- After 6 years, testicular growth is retarded and the testis becomes hypoplastic.
- The seminiferous tubule starts degenerating at 6 years of age and by 16 years, there is gross destruction of seminiferous tubules and spermatogenesis is grossly impaired.

Q. What is the effect on fertility in undescended testis?

Ans. Untreated bilateral undescended testis is usually associated with sterility. In unilateral undescended testis, infertility is usually not a problem but this may also be associated with subfertility due to defective spermatogenesis in the normally descended testis.

Q. What does an impalpable testis implies?

Ans. The term impalpable testis implies that the testis cannot be detected on physical examination and therefore it may be:
* Absent (agenesis or vanishing)
* Atrophic
* Intra-abdominal
* Missed on clinical examination.

Q. How will you evaluate a patient with bilateral impalpable testis?

Ans.
* A detail history.
* A clinical examination and palpation along the route of normal descent and also the ectopic sites of testis.
* If basal gonadotropin level particularly follicle-stimulating hormone (FSH) level is high in a prepubescent boy then it indicates bilateral anorchia.
* If basal gonadotropin levels are normal hCG stimulation test is to be done. If following injection of hCG there is no rise of testosterone level then it indicates bilateral anorchia.
* Ultrasonography of groin and abdomen.
* Diagnostic laparoscopy useful for localization of impalpable testis.

Q. What is ectopic testis?

Ans. It is one form of maldescent of testis, where testis has deviated from the normal route of descent and lies in a site other than the scrotum.

Q. Where an ectopic testis may lie?

Ans. An ectopic testis may lie at (Fig. 15.15):
* Suprapubic region at root of penis (A)
* Perineum (B)
* Femoral triangle (C)
* Opposite scrotal sac (D)
* Superficial inguinal pouch, which is a space between the external oblique aponeurosis and fascia of Scarpa (E).

Q. What are tails of Lockwood?

Ans. Lockwood has explained location of ectopic testis by describing five tails of gubernaculum of testis. The tails are (Fig. 15.16):
* Scrotal tail
* Pubic tail
* Perineal tail

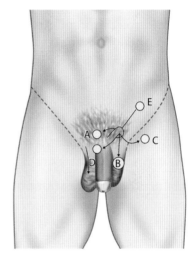

Fig. 15.15: Location of ectopic testis. (A) Pubic; (B) Perineum; (C) Femoral triangle; (D) Opposite stratum; (E) Superficial inguinal pouch

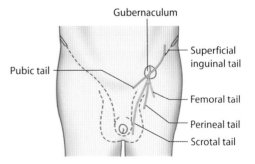

Fig. 15.16: Tails of Lockwood

- Femoral tail
- Superficial inguinal tail.
   Differential growth of any of these tails may lead to deviation of the testis to an ectopic site.

Q. What is retractile testis?

Ans. The retractile testis is one which is withdrawn out of the scrotum by an active cremasteric reflex but can be easily brought down into an orthotopic position within the scrotum and remains thereafter the traction is withdrawn.

Q. How will you differentiate an ectopic testis and retractile testis in superficial inguinal pouch?

Ans.
- A retractile testis was in the scrotum at birth and then drawn up by reflex.
- The scrotum is well formed in retractile testis.
- The testis can be manipulated down to the scrotum in retractile testis.
- The retractile testis is normally developed.

Q. How will you differentiate an ectopic testis in superficial inguinal pouch from an undescended inguinal testis?

Ans. By leg raising test, the abdominal muscles are made taut. The ectopic testis lying superficial to the external oblique aponeurosis becomes more prominent whereas the undescended testis lying deep to the external oblique aponeurosis becomes less prominent.

Q. What is emergent testis?

Ans. Testis lies in the inguinal canal and may sometimes project beyond the superficial inguinal ring but again slips back into the inguinal canal.

Q. What are the complications of undescended testis?

Ans.
- Testicular atrophy
- Liable to repeated trauma
- Undescended testis is more liable to develop torsion due to long mesorchium
- 10% of testicular tumors occur in undescended testis
- Subfertility or infertility
- Associated hernia—a patent processus vaginalis is found in 90% patient of undescended testis.

Q. What is the risk of malignancy in undescended testis?

Ans. Undescended testis has 40 times greater risk of developing tumors than in normally descended testis. The risk has been said to be 1 in 20 in abdominal testis and 1 in 80 in inguinal testis.

Q. Which type of tumor is more common in undescended testis?

Ans. The most common tumor that develops in an undescended testis is seminoma. Other types of tumor that may develop in an undescended testis include—embryonal carcinoma (teratocarcinoma and choriocarcinoma).

Q. Does orchidopexy reduce the chance of malignancy?

Ans. This is controversial. There is emerging evidence that prepubescent orchidopexy lessens the risk to some extent. Orchidopexy also allows thorough examination and earlier detection, if a tumor develops.

■ FILARIAL SCROTUM AND RAMHORN PENIS

Clinical Examination

See Page No. 382, Chapter 9.

History

- *History of swelling*—onset and progress area of involvement—scrotum, penis, or both.
- Any pain over the swelling.
- *Any history of lymphatic discharge*—sometimes vesicles may form in the scrotum, which may result in lymphorrhea.
- Swelling in other parts of body—lymphedema of upper or lower limb.
- Any past history of filarial infection—pain, fever, and swelling of the groin lymph nodes.

Examination—Inspection/Palpation

- *Swelling*—site and extent/size and shape/surface and margin/consistency.
- *Skin of scrotum and the penis*—thickening of skin with nonpitting edema. The glans penis may be buried due to the gross thickening of penile skin.
- Examine inguinal lymph nodes—may be enlarged.
- Examine other areas and the limbs for any lymphedema.

Q. What is your case? (Summary of a case of elephantiasis of scrotum with Ramhorn penis)

Ans. This 50-year-old gentleman presented with gradually progressive thickening and swelling of skin of scrotum and penis for last 5 years. Patient also complains of occasional watery discharge from the skin of the scrotum. There is history of recurrent attacks of fever with chill and rigor and pain in the groin and scrotum for last 3 years (Fig. 15.17).

On examination: There is enormous thickening of skin overlying the scrotum and penis. The skin is rough and there is nodular thickening of the skin and the whole of the penis is buried under the thickened skin. The skin of the scrotum is similarly rough and there is nodular thickening. It is difficult to palpate the testis epididymis and the spermatic cord.

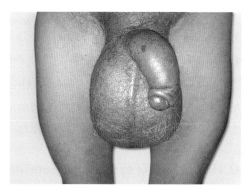

Fig. 15.17: Elephantiasis of scrotum with Rams horn penis

Courtesy: Dr A Acharya, IPGMER, Kolkata

Q. What is your diagnosis?

Ans. This is a case of elephantiasis of scrotum with Ramhorn penis.

Q. How will you manage this patient?

* I would like to exclude active filariasis by blood examination for microfilaria. Usually, a nocturnal blood smear is taken for diagnosis of microfilaria.
* *Complete hemogram*: Differential count may show eosinophilia.
* *Other routine workup*: Blood urea, creatinine, liver function test, chest X-ray, and electrocardiography (ECG).
* If active filariasis is present, medical treatment is initiated with diethylcarbamazine citrate 100 mg thrice daily for 3 weeks (6 mg/kg/day for 3 weeks).
* Alternatively, a single dose of ivermectin and albendazole may be effective for treatment of active filarial disease.
* There may be secondary skin infection.
* A course of antibiotics like tablet ciprofloxacin 500 mg twice daily for 7 days.
* This lymphedema with gross disfigurement of scrotum and penis is unlikely to reverse, so I will consider surgical treatment for this patient.

Q. What operation are you planning for this patient?

Ans.
* I will consider excision of thickened hypertrophied skin of both scrotum and penis.
* There may be some normal skin near the root of the scrotum, which may be retained.
* Sometimes, the preputial skin may be normal and may be retained and may be used to cover the raw penile surface. However, in this case, the preputial skin is also thickened and needs to be sacrificed.
* After excision of the skin of the penis, it is covered with split skin graft. If preputial skin is normal, it may be used for the coverage.
* If some amount of scrotal skin is normal then it is retained and mobilized. If there is associated hydrocele, then eversion of sac is to be done. The exposed testis is covered with mobilized scrotal skin.
* If scrotal skin is completely excised then the testes may be placed in a subcutaneous pocket on the medial side of the thigh.
* Alternatively, the raw scrotum may be covered with a split thickness skin grafting.
* An indwelling Foley catheter is inserted to prevent contamination of the wound during urination.

Q. How is filariasis caused?

Ans. Filariasis is caused by a parasite *Wuchereria bancrofti*. This is a viviparous nematode.

Q. Who are the definitive and intermediate host?

Ans. Man is the definitive host and mosquito is the intermediate host for continuation of life cycle of the parasite.

Q. How is the life cycle of the parasite continued?

Ans.
* Adult worm of *Wuchereria*, both male and female lives in the lymphatic system of human being.
* The male and female worms mate in the lymphatic system.

* After sporulation, the female worm dies and liberates large number of microfilaria.
* These microfilariae enter into systemic circulation more commonly at night.
* When a mosquito bites a man, along with blood it sucks the microfilaria.
* These microfilariae undergo several changes in the gut of mosquito and get matured.
* These mature microfilariae reenter into human being by the bite of mosquito.
* These mature microfilariae enter the lymph node through the lymphatics.
* These mature microfilariae then develop into an adult worm and the cycle continues.

Q. What are the pathological effects of filarial infection?

Ans. The adult worm liberates some toxins. These toxins and the adult worm by its mechanical effect cause lymphangitis and lymphadenitis.

Recurrent attacks of lymphangitis cause lymphatic obstruction due to occlusion of lymphatic vessels and the lymph nodes.

This obstruction is due to both occlusions of the lymph vessels due to proliferation of endothelium of lymph vessels and also due to fibrosis around the lymphatic vessels.

Q. What are the causes of lymphatic obstruction in filariasis?

Ans. The lymphatic obstruction may be due to the adult worm (living or dead) causing mechanical blockage of the lymph nodes and the lymph vessels. The toxins liberated by the adult worm and the microfilaria can block the lymphatic channels due to sclerosing lymphangitis.

Q. What are the sequelae of lymphatic obstruction?

Ans.

* Lymphatic obstruction causes dilatation and tortuosity of lymphatic system. Subsequently because of sclerosing lymphangitis there is occlusion of these lymphatic vessels.
* As a result of the lymphatic obstruction, the interstitial fluid rich in protein cannot return via the lymphatic system and there is stagnation of interstitial fluid rich in protein. The colloidal osmotic pressure in the interstitial fluid increases and this results in increased filtration of fluid across the capillary membrane. This results in swelling of the subcutaneous tissues and the part becomes swollen, which pits on pressure. With recurrent attacks, the swelling increases further due to overgrowth of connective tissue as the result of accumulation of protein-rich fluid in the tissues. The subcutaneous tissue is replaced by fibrous tissue and the lymph logged gelatinous tissue, which does not pit on pressure. The skin also becomes enormously thickened and hyperkeratotic. There may be lymph-filled vesicles on the surface of the skin, which may rupture resulting in discharge of lymph. The skin surface may become rugose and there may be warty growths on the surface of the skin.

Q. How complement fixation test will help in diagnosis of filariasis?

Ans. Complement fixation may be positive in majority of patients. A positive complement test indicates a past or present filarial infection.

Q. Apart from elephantiasis of scrotum and penis, which other sites may be affected by filariasis?

Ans.

* Filarial epididymo-orchitis
* Chylocele

+ Lymphangiectasia of lymph vessel of spermatic cord
+ Elephantiasis of lower limb
+ Elephantiasis of vulva and breast.

Q. Why filariasis is more common in lower limb and scrotum?

Ans. Microfilaria and adult filarial worm have special predilection for lymphatics of the inguinal region for reasons unknown, so filariasis of these parts are more common.

■ PHIMOSIS

Clinical Examination

History

+ Inability to retract the preputial skin beyond the corona glandis—enquires whether from birth (congenital phimosis) or developed in adult life (acquired or secondary phimosis).
+ Any history of ballooning of prepuce during micturition, any difficulty in passing urine (in severe preputial orifice stenosis may present with acute retention of urine).
+ Any pain.
+ Any purulent discharge from the preputial orifice (suggests balanitis).
+ In adult, any discomfort during erection and sexual intercourse.
+ In adult, enquire about diabetes (prone to recurrent balanoposthitis and development of secondary phimosis).

Examination—Inspection/Palpation

+ Look at the preputial orifice (usually preputial orifice is small).
+ Look at the preputial skin—in congenital phimosis, the preputial skin may be unduly long.
+ Try to retract the preputial skin beyond the glans penis (in phimosis, it is not possible to retract the preputial skin beyond the corona glandis).
+ In adult with secondary phimosis—palpate the glans penis and the body of the penis to exclude a growth in the penis.
+ In suspected case of carcinoma penis—examine the inguinal lymph nodes.

Q. What is your case? (Summary of a case of phimosis)

Ans. This 14-year-old male child presented with complaint of inability to retract the prepuce beyond the glans penis since his birth. Patient has noticed gradual whitish discoloration of preputial skin for last 2 years. Patient has no other complaint (Fig. 15.18).

On examination: The preputial skin shows leukoplakic changes and the skin cannot be retracted behind the glans. The glans penis on palpation appears normal.

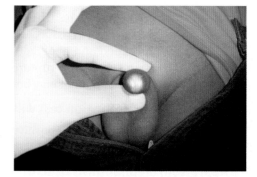

Fig. 15.18: Phimosis—the preputial skin cannot be retracted. Note the leukoplakic change in the preputial skin

Courtesy: Dr Sohabrata Mukherjee, Calcutta National Medical College, Kolkata

Q. What is your diagnosis?

Ans. This is a case of congenital phimosis with leukoplakia of prepuce.

Q. What is phimosis?

Ans. Phimosis is a condition when the preputial skin could not be retracted beyond the corona glandis.

Q. What is physiological phimosis?

Ans. At birth, normally the preputial skin is adherent to the glans penis. During the first 3–4 years as the penis grows, epithelial debris (smegma) accumulates under the prepuce and gradually separates the prepuce from the glans. By 3 years of age, 90% of foreskin can be retracted.

Q. How these patients usually present?

Ans.

- Difficulty in retracting the skin of prepuce beyond the corona glandis.
- In case with very small preputial orifice, the prepuce may blow up during micturition.
- Associated balanitis or balanoposthitis may cause pain and purulent discharge.

Q. How will you treat this patient?

Ans.

- I will do baseline investigations.
- I will do circumcision.

Q. Describe the steps of circumcision.

Ans. *See* Operative Surgery Section, Page No. 1143, Chapter 22.

Q. What is preputioplasty?

Ans. This is a technique of enlarging the preputial orifice. In phimosis, the pathology is usually a tight ring at the distal end of the prepuce. In preputioplasty, the preputial orifice is enlarged by incising the tight preputial ring vertically and stitching it up horizontally.

The foreskin is retracted back over the body of the penis and the tight preputial ring stands out. The tight ring is incised vertically and the incision is closed transversely with interrupted chromic catgut sutures. By this, tight ring of preputial skin including the preputial orifice is enlarged, so that the foreskin can now be retracted easily over the glans penis (Figs 15.19A to C).

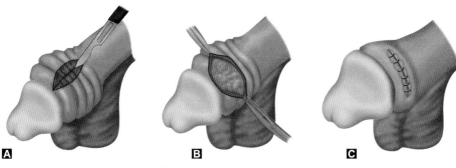

A   **B**   **C**

Figs 15.19A to C: Preputioplasty

Q. What is paraphimosis?

Ans. This is a condition where preputial skin is suddenly retracted beyond the corona glandis and forms a constricting ring at this site and it cannot be pulled forward leading to edema and swelling of glans penis. The preputial skin also becomes edematous.

The constricting ring causes venous congestion and further aggravates the swelling and can cause gangrene of glans penis.

Q. How will you treat paraphimosis?

Ans.

- Squeeze the edematous foreskin of the penis between the thumb and index finger, so that the fluid is squeezed into the shaft of the penis. Slide the preputial skin forward and at the same time push the glans penis back. This may cause reduction of paraphimosis (Figs 15.20A to D).
- If constricting ring is too tight, a dorsal slit may be required to relieve the paraphimosis (Fig. 15.20E).
- Alternatively inject hyaluronidase with xylocaine into the foreskin. This will reduce the edema of the foreskin and may help in reduction.

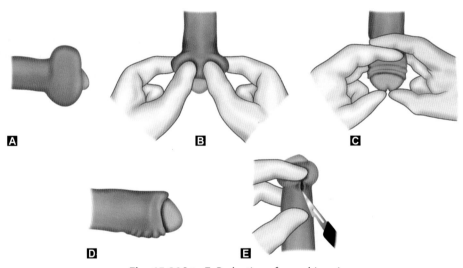

Figs 15.20A to E: Reduction of paraphimosis

Q. What are the complications of phimosis?

Ans.

- Recurrent balanitis and balanoposthitis.
- Paraphimosis.
- Preputial stenosis may cause ballooning of preputial skin and may cause chronic retention of urine.
- Retained smegma may form calculi in the preputial sac.
- Chronic urinary retention may cause back pressure changes in bladder, ureter, and kidneys.

◆ Carcinomatous change. Phimosis with recurrent balanoposthitis is a premalignant lesion. Retained smegma may also cause chronic irritation leading to carcinomatous change.

Q. What is circumcision by Guillotine method?

Ans.

◆ This is the method of circumcision used in children.
◆ The preputial adhesion with the glans penis is separated. The preputial skin is stretched beyond the glans and held by a clamp and the redundant preputial skin is excised.
◆ The cut margin of the prepuce is approximated by interrupted atraumatic chromic catgut sutures.

Q. What are the complications of circumcision?

Ans.

◆ Bleeding
◆ Wound infection
◆ Removal of too much skin or too little skin
◆ Injury to glans penis and urethra
◆ Thermal or laser injury to the penis, if these are used during circumcision.

Q. What is secondary phimosis?

Ans. The prepuce was normal and it was possible to retract, it beyond the corona glandis earlier. When, afterward due to some local disease, the prepuce cannot be retracted beyond the corona glandis then it is called secondary phimosis. Secondary phimosis may be due to:

◆ Recurrent balanoposthitis causing adhesion of prepuce to the glans penis.
◆ Repeated injury to prepuce due to forcible retraction may cause ulceration of the prepuce, fibrosis, and secondary phimosis.
◆ Underlying carcinoma of the glans penis.

Q. What are the indications of circumcision?

Ans.

In infants and children:

◆ On religious ground
◆ Phimosis with recurrent attacks of balanitis or balanoposthitis.

In adults:

◆ Difficulty in retraction of the preputial skin during intercourse
◆ For an abnormally tight frenulum
◆ Recurrent balanitis
◆ Sometimes prior to radiotherapy for carcinoma penis.

Q. What is Plastibell technique for circumcision?

Ans.

◆ This is a technique for circumcision. The foreskin is retracted after freeing the adhesion. The Plastibell is then slipped into place over the glans penis.
◆ The foreskin is ligated over the groove of the bell and redundant skin is cut away.
◆ The plastibell ring separates by 5th postoperative day.

■ PEYRONIE'S DISEASES

Q. What is your case? (summary of a case of Peyronie's diseases)

Ans. This 55-year-old gentleman presented with a hard area in right lateral side of the body of penis for last 2 years, which is gradually increasing in size over this period. Patient complains of pain during erection of penis. Patient also noticed bending of the penis to the side of hard mass during erection. Patient has no other complaint.

On examination: On inspection, there is no obvious deformity. On palpation, there are two areas of induration involving the right corpora cavernosa. Apart from these areas of induration, the rest of the corpora are normally elastic.

Q. What is your diagnosis?

Ans. This is a case of Peyronie's disease of the penis.

Q. What are the causes of Peyronie's disease?

Ans.
* Exact cause is unknown
* Past history of trauma may cause injury to the septal insertion of tunica albuginea. This causes extravasation of blood and fibrinogen gets activated. This leads to formation of a thrombus. The blood components activate a number of factors, which leads to local fibrosis.

Q. What is the natural history of this disease?

Ans.
* There are two phases in the natural history of this disease.
* The first phase is the active phase, which is associated with painful erection and changing deformity of the penis.
* This is followed by a quiescent secondary phase, which is characterized by stabilizing of the deformity. Painful erection disappears, but there is development of painless deformity.

Q. What are the usual presentations of patients with Peyronie's disease?

Ans. The presenting symptom may be:
* Penile pain with erection
* Penile deformity
* Penile shortening
* Notice of a plaque or an indurated area in the penis
* Erectile dysfunction.

Q. What investigation may help in this patient?

Ans. Duplex Doppler ultrasound study may help in some patient. This may show abnormalities in peak systolic velocity, end diastolic velocity, and resistive index.

Q. How will you treat this patient?

Ans.
* There is no effective treatment for this condition.
* Reassurance of the patient is the most important aspect.

* Some drugs are said to be helpful.
* Surgery in selected cases.

Q. Which drugs are effective in Peyronie's disease?

Ans.

* Vitamin E in a dose of 800–1,000 mg has some beneficial effect.
* Potaba (potassium aminobenzoate) 12 g/day in divided doses.
* Tamoxifen 20 mg twice daily.
* Terfenadine and fexofenadine—nonspecific antihistaminic drug.
* Colchicine and corticosteroid have also been used.
* Intralesional injection of verapamil. A course of injection consist of 12 injection (10 mg each) given once in every 2 weeks.

Q. What operation may help the patient?

Ans. Surgical treatment may help the patient when the disease is stable and mature. Many operations have been described:

* *Fitzpatrick's operation*: Involves excision and plication of the corpora of penis opposite the Peyronie's lesion. This procedure counteracts the effects of the inelastic lesion by shortening the opposite more compliant aspect of the corpora cavernosa.
* *Gelbard's operation*: This operation involves multiple incisions over the fibrous plaque and bridging the gap with a compliant tissue like temporal fascia.
* *Lockhart's operation*: The fibrous plaque is excised and the corporotomy defect is covered by a tunica vaginalis flap based on dartos and cremaster.
* *Devine and Horton's operation*: This operation involves excision of the fibrous plaque and closure of the corporotomy defect by using a dermal flap.
  The approach is through a circumferential incision and the plaque is reached by degloving the penis by retraction of the penile skin toward the base.

Q. What is the role of penile prosthesis?

Ans. Erectile dysfunction associated with Peyronie's disease may be treated with suitable penile prosthesis.

■ CARCINOMA PENIS

Clinical Examination

See Page No. 382, Chapter 9.

History

* Age of onset (usually middle age and elderly patients are affected, and may also affect younger age group).
* History about the lump or ulcer—onset and progress.
* Any history of purulent or foul-smelling discharge.
* Any history of development of secondary phimosis (patient, who was earlier able to retract the preputial skin beyond the corona glandis, cannot do so after the appearance of the mass in the penis).

◆ Any difficulty in passing urine (usually patient with carcinoma penis does not have difficulty in passing urine).

◆ Any history of swelling in either groin (suggestive of lymph node metastasis).

Examination—Inspection/Palpation

◆ Examine the prepuce for phimosis. Try to retract the preputial skin beyond the corona glandis.

◆ Note any discharge form the preputial orifice.

◆ Examine the proliferative growth or the ulcer over the penis—site and extent, size and shape, surface and margins. If ulcer—size, shape, margin, edge, floor, and base.

◆ Extent of involvement in the body of the penis—appreciated by presence of induration—assesses the extent of involvement of shaft and assesses the length of uninvolved shaft.

◆ Examination of inguinal lymph nodes—number of nodes involved—any tenderness, size, surface, and consistency. Mobility—any skin fixity or fixity to deeper structures.

◆ Examine abdomen for any pelvic or para-aortic lymph node enlargement.

Q. What is your case? (Summary of a case of carcinoma of penis)

Ans. This 60-year-old gentleman presented with an ulcer in the glans penis for last 10 months. The ulcer was initially about 1 cm in size at the onset but for last 10 months, this ulcerating lesion was increasing in size and involved almost the whole of glans penis. Patient complains of a foul-smelling discharge from the ulcer site and occasional bleeding from the lesion. Patient has no difficulty in passing urine. He complains swelling in the left groin for last 4 months. Initially he noticed a single swelling 4 months back. Afterwards, he has noticed multiple swellings in the left groin, which are also slowly increasing in size (Fig. 15.21).

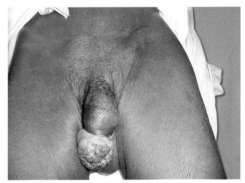

Fig. 15.21: Carcinoma of penis with metastasis to left inguinal lymph node metastasis

Courtesy: Dr Vivek Sharma, IPGMER, Kolkata

On examination: On local examination, there is an ulceroproliferative lesion involving almost the whole of the glans penis. The ulcer margin is rolled out and everted, the floor is covered by a necrotic tissue, the base is indurated, and the growth is firm in consistency. The shaft of the penis is normal. There is phimosis. There are multiple enlarged lymph nodes in the left inguinal region. The lymph nodes are nontender, mobile, and firm in feel. There are no palpable lymph nodes in the right inguinal region.

Q. What is your diagnosis?

Ans. This is a case of carcinoma penis involving the glans penis with left inguinal lymph node metastasis.

The alternative case may be:

◆ This is a case of a carcinoma penis without any clinical evidence of lymph node metastasis in the groin.

Q. What are the important aspects of examination in this patient?

Ans.
◆ The penile lesion is assessed to ascertain the size of the lesion, location, and involvement of the penile body.
◆ Inspection of the base of the penis and scrotum is necessary to rule out extension into these areas.
◆ Rectal examination to rule out a pelvic mass.
◆ Examination of both groins to rule out inguinal lymph node enlargement.

Q. What are the other possibilities?

Ans.
◆ Condyloma acuminata
◆ Buschke–Löwenstein tumor
◆ Balanitis xerotica obliterans
◆ Tuberculosis.

Q. How will you manage this patient?

Ans. I would like to confirm my diagnosis by taking an incisional biopsy from penile lesion from the periphery of the lesion from its junction with the normal tissue.

Microscopic examination will assess depth of invasion, presence of vascular invasion, and histological grade of the lesion. Vascular invasion of the tumor has significant prognostic importance.

Q. What is the problem of taking a biopsy from the center of the lesion?

Ans. If a biopsy is taken from the center of the lesion, it may show only necrotic tissue and no tumor tissue may be seen, so biopsy may be inconclusive.

Q. What further investigation you would like to do?

Ans. I would like to do some investigation to stage the disease:
◆ Chest X-ray
◆ Computed tomography (CT) scan of abdomen to assess lymph node enlargement in the pelvis, as the inguinal lymph nodes are palpable
◆ Baseline workup in all patients:
  – Complete hemogram
  – Blood for sugar, urea, and creatinine
  – Electrocardiography
  – Urine routine examination and culture sensitivity.

Q. How will you treat this patient?

Ans.
◆ Once biopsy proved, I will consider definitive treatment. The lesion has involved whole of glans penis and involved up to the corona glandis. The growth has not involved the shaft of the penis.
◆ I will do partial amputation of penis. The proximal line of resection should be 2 cm proximal to the proximal margin of the growth.

Q. What do you remove in partial amputation?

Ans.

- In partial amputation of the penis, a part of the penis is with a 2 cm margin proximal to the proximal margin of the tumor is resected.
- A long-ventral skin flap is raised. The corpora cavernosa is divided at the proposed line of resection and is over run with sutures. The corpus spongiosum is also divided, and the corpus spongiosum with the urethra is brought out through an opening in the ventral skin flap. The opening in the corpus spongiosum is enlarged by a lateral cut, and the mucous membrane of the urethra is sutured with the skin and a neourethra is formed on the ventral aspect of the penis.

Q. If the biopsy report revealed an anaplastic carcinoma, what will you do?

Ans. Anaplastic carcinoma has poor prognosis and progresses rapidly. The optimum surgical treatment in such cases should be total amputation.

Q. If the growth involves the body of the penis, what surgery will you plan?

Ans.

- If the growth involves the body of the penis and if the resection with a 2-cm margin leaves behind a good segment of the penis then a partial amputation of penis may be done.
- If the growth has involved a large segment of the body of the penis and a resection with 2 cm margin is not possible then a total amputation should be considered.

Q. What structures would you remove in total amputation of penis?

Ans.

- The two corpora cavernosa with ischiocavernosus muscle are excised up to their origin from the ischiopubic rami.
- The corpus spongiosum along with the penile and glandular part of the urethra is excised keeping 1.5–2.0 cm margin projecting beyond the perineal membrane. The urethral opening is brought out through a separate incision in the perineum behind the scrotum and a perineal urethrostomy is done.

Q. What do palpable groin nodes signify?

Ans. In 50% cases, the enlarged nodes are due to infection. Persistent lymphadenopathy after treatment of primary lesion and 2 weeks of antibiotic therapy are most often due to metastasis.

Q. How will you treat lymph nodes?

Ans.

- The palpable lymph nodes in the groin are clinically significant. I will advise fine-needle aspiration cytology (FNAC) of the groin nodes. If FNAC is negative, I will administer antibiotics and keep the patient under surveillance.
- If the lymph nodes are positive, patient should undergo inguinopelvic lymph node dissection on the affected side and a superficial inguinal lymph node dissection on the other side. The pelvic node clearance is indicated when there are more than two inguinal node metastases and when the Cloquet lymph node is metastatic.

Q. How will you treat nonpalpable lymph nodes?

Ans. There has been controversy regarding the management of noninvolved inguinal lymph nodes. Prophylactic lymphadenectomy is not indicated in all cases.

Carcinoma in situ (TIS), T1 tumors, grade 1, and grade 2 tumors have less than 10% chance of lymph node metastasis, so these patients should be kept on regular follow up and once the lymph node becomes palpable in follow up, FNAC confirmation and a therapeutic lymphadenectomy are indicated.

T2, T3, and T4 tumors, grade 3 tumors, tumors with vascular invasion have greater than 50% chance of lymph node metastasis. In these situations, sentinel lymph node biopsy is indicated to assess the status of groin nodes.

Q. What is a sentinel lymph node?

Ans. A sentinel node is one, which is the site of first lymphatic drainage from a lesion.

Q. What is the role of sentinel lymph node biopsy in carcinoma penis?

Ans.
+ Sentinel lymph node biopsy has been established as a standard procedure in carcinoma penis.
+ Sentinel lymph node mapping and biopsy may be done in a number of ways.
+ Isosulfan blue is injected into the lesion in the penis and inguinal exploration is done. The sentinel lymph node is identified by the bluish color, which has received lymphatic flow from the lesion. The lymph node is excised and histopathological examination is done.
+ If the sentinel lymph node is positive, an inguinopelvic lymph node dissection is done.
+ The sentinel lymph node may also be identified by injecting a radiocolloid into the lesion and by using a gamma probe, and the sentinel node is identified by localizing the lymph node, which has taken up the radioactive material.

Q. What should be the extent of dissection in prophylactic lymphadenectomy?

Ans. The lymphatics of penis drain freely on either side.

So, for prophylactic lymphadenectomy, a bilateral superficial inguinal lymph node dissection is done. The material is subjected to frozen section. If a positive node is found, a formal inguinopelvic node dissection is done on that side (removal of deep inguinal lymph nodes and the pelvic lymph nodes).

Q. If patient presented with mobile inguinal lymph node, how will you treat?

Ans.
+ The enlarged lymph node may be infective or metastatic.
+ Patient is given a course of antibiotic and if the lymph nodes are infective, they will disappear.
+ If the lymph nodes are persistent, I will do a FNAC from the lymph node.
+ If FNAC is positive, I will consider inguinopelvic lymph node dissection on the involved side and a superficial inguinal lymph node dissection on the other side.

Q. Why a pelvic lymph node dissection is required?

Ans. The penile metastasis spreads in a sequential fashion superficial inguinal lymph nodes, deep inguinal lymph nodes, and pelvic lymph nodes.

When multiple inguinal lymph nodes are involved, there is high chance of pelvic lymph nodes being involved, so a concomitant pelvic node dissection is indicated. The status of pelvic lymph node is a very good prognostic marker and if pelvic nodes are shown positive after dissection, patient should be given adjuvant chemotherapy.

Q. If the involved lymph node is fixed, how will you treat?

Ans. The fixed lymph nodes are inoperable. Patient should be given a course of neoadjuvant chemotherapy with taxanes + cisplatinum and 5-fluorouracil. If the lymph nodes become mobile, palliative inguinopelvic lymph node dissection may be considered.

Q. What is the role of radiotherapy in treatment of primary lesion?

Ans. Radiotherapy is effective in treatment of primary lesion under certain circumstances:
- Small lesion less than 3 cm
- Superficial lesion confined to glans penis
- Young patient presenting with small lesion
- Patient refusing surgery
- Carcinoma in situ
- Advanced inoperable disease for palliation.

Q. How will you administer radiotherapy to primary lesion in carcinoma penis?

Ans. Radiotherapy may be delivered by:
- Implantation of radioactive tantalum wire delivering a dose of 6,000 cGy in 5–7 days.
- By radium mold applicator applied around the penis, which is worn either continuously or intermittently delivering a dose of 6,000 cGy in 7–10 days.
- External beam radiation using a linear accelerator delivering a dose of 5,000–6,000 cGy in 3–5 weeks.

Q. What is the role of chemotherapy in carcinoma penis?

Ans. The role of systemic chemotherapy is limited in carcinoma penis.

In patients with more than 1 lymph node metastasis on histology after inguinopelvic lymph node dissection adjuvant chemotherapy is indicated.

Three cycles of chemotherapy with cisplatinum and 5-fluorouracil are effective and improve survival. In advanced disease, combination chemotherapy has shown some response. Different chemotherapy regimens are:
- *VBM*: Vincristine (1 mg), bleomycin (15 mg), and methotrexate (30 mg)—12 weekly courses.
- *PMB*: Cisplatinum (100 mg/m^2), methotrexate (25 mg/m^2), and bleomycin (10 mg/m^2)—six cycles every 3 weeks.
- *MPB*: Methotrexate (200 mg/m^2), leucovorin (25 mg), cisplatinum (20 m/m^2), and bleomycin (10 mg/m^2)—four cycles every 4 weeks.
- Topical 5-fluorouracil has been tried carcinoma in situ.

Q. If the primary tumor is small and confined to prepuce only and has not involved the glans penis, what may be the optimum treatment?

Ans. In such a situation, circumcision may be adequate treatment. Regular follow up to detect any local recurrence or lymph node metastasis.

Q. What is the follow-up protocol for carcinoma penis patient?

Ans. For initial 2 years, follow up at interval of 3–6 months and yearly for 5 years. Clinical examination, if required, USG and FNAC of lymph nodes.

Q. What are the premalignant lesions in the penis?

Ans. Premalignant lesions in penis are:
* Cutaneous horn
* Leukoplakia of the glans penis
* Long-standing genital warts
* Balanitis xerotica obliterans
* Erythroplasia of Queyrat or Bowen's disease—carcinoma in situ
* Paget's disease of the penis.

Some factors contribute to increased incidence of carcinoma of penis:
* *Chronic balanoposthitis*: Recurrent balanoposthitis is associated with higher incidence of carcinoma of penis.
* *Phimosis*: Chronic irritation due to retained smegma has been ascribed to one of the etiological factor. In Jews, who are circumscribed at birth has virtually least incidence of carcinoma penis.

Q. Why circumcision at puberty does not reduce the incidence of carcinoma of penis?

Ans. This is suggested that the critical period for exposure to certain etiological agents may have already occurred at puberty rendering later circumcision relatively ineffective for prevention of penile cancer.

Q. What are the gross types of carcinoma penis?

Ans. *See* Surgical Pathology Section, Page No. 926, Chapter 18.

Q. What are the microscopic types of carcinoma penis?

Ans. *See* Surgical Pathology Section, Page No. 927, Chapter 18.

Q. How does carcinoma penis spread?

Ans. *See* Surgical Pathology Section, Page No. 927, Chapter 18.

Q. What is the TNM classification of carcinoma penis?

Ans. T categories:
* *TX:* Primary tumor cannot be assessed.
* *T0:* No evidence of primary tumor.
* *Tis:* Carcinoma in situ called "*erythroplasia of Queyrat*" when it occurs on the glans of the penis. Called "*Bowen disease*" when it occurs on the shaft of the penis.
* *Ta:* Verrucous (wart-like) carcinoma that is only in the top layers of skin (*noninvasive*)
* *T1:* The tumor has grown into the *subepithelial connective tissue.*
  - *T1a:* The tumor has grown into the subepithelial connective tissue, but it has not grown into blood or lymph vessels. The cancer is of grade 1 or 2.
  - *T1b:* The tumor has grown into the subepithelial connective tissue and has either grown into blood and lymph vessels or it is of high-grade (grade 3 or 4).

- *T2:* The tumor has grown into the corpus spongiosum or corpora cavernosum.
- *T3:* The tumor has grown into the urethra.
- *T4:* The tumor has grown into the adjacent structures—scrotum, pubic bone, or prostate.

N categories:

- *NX*: Nearby lymph nodes cannot be assessed.
- *N0:* No spread to lymph nodes.
- *N1:* Spread to the single *inguinal lymph node.*
- *N2:* Spread to multiple inguinal lymph node—unilateral or bilateral.
- *N3:* Spread to lymph nodes in the pelvis and/or extracapsular extension of lymph nodes spread.

M categories:

- *M0:* The cancer has not spread to distant organs or tissues.
- *M1:* Distant metastasis such as lymph nodes outside of the pelvis, lungs, or liver.

Stage grouping:

Once the T, N, and M categories have been assigned, this information is combined to assign an overall stage from 0 to IV. This is known as *stage grouping*.

- *Stage 0*: Tis or Ta, N0, M0
- *Stage I*: T1a, N0, M0
- *Stage II*: Any of the following:
  - *T1b, N0, M0*
    OR
  - *T2, N0, M0*
    OR
  - *T3, N0, M0*
- *Stage IIIa*: T1 to T3, N1, M0
- *Stage IIIb*: T1 to T3, N2, M0
- *Stage IV*: Any of the following:
  - T4, any N M0
    OR
  - *Any T, N3, M0*
    OR
  - *Any T, any N, M1.*

Q. What is Jackson staging of carcinoma penis?

Ans.

- *Stage I*: Tumor confined to glans penis or prepuce or both.
- *Stage II*: Tumor invasion into shaft of the penis (corpora cavernosa and spongiosum).
- *Stage III*: Tumor with metastasis to inguinal lymph nodes, which are mobile.
- *Stage IV*: Tumor invades adjacent structures, scrotum pubic bone, or prostate, fixed (inoperable) inguinal lymph node metastasis.

Q. How do the lymphatics from the penis are drained?

Ans.

◆ The lymphatics of the prepuce form a connecting network that joins with the lymphatics of the shaft of the penis and these lymphatics drain into the superficial inguinal lymph nodes.

◆ The lymphatics from the glans penis join with the lymphatics draining the corporal bodies and they form a collar of connecting channels at the base of the penis, and drain into the superficial inguinal lymph nodes. Some lymphatics from the glans may directly drain into the deep inguinal lymph nodes.

◆ The superficial inguinal lymph nodes drain into the deep inguinal lymph nodes and from there drain into the external iliac, internal iliac, and obturator lymph nodes (Fig. 15.22).

◆ The penile lymphatics usually drain into both inguinal areas.

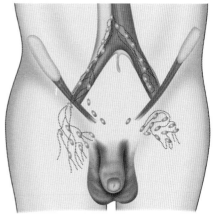
Fig. 15.22: Lymphatic drainage of penis

Q. What are the anatomical parts of penis?

Ans. The penis consists of:

◆ Root of the penis formed by two crura attached to the ischiopubic rami and the bulb of the penis attached to the perineal membrane.

◆ Body or shaft of penis formed by two corpora cavernosa and the corpus spongiosum containing the penile part of the urethra.

◆ Tip or glans penis is the expanded part of the corpus spongiosum and contains the terminal part of the urethra and the external urethral meatus (Fig. 15.23).

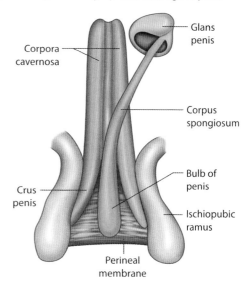
Fig. 15.23: Anatomical parts of penis

Q. What are the arterial supplies of the penis?

Ans.

◆ Artery to the bulb of penis.

◆ Deep artery to the penis one on either side pierces the crura of the penis and runs along the corpora cavernosa.

◆ Dorsal artery of the penis runs along the dorsal aspect of the penis and gives off circumferential branches.

Q. What are the veins draining the penis?

Ans.

◆ The deep dorsal vein of the penis runs deep to the dartos fascia and passes below the symphysis pubis and drains into the prostatic venous plexus.

• The superficial dorsal vein of the penis runs superficial to the dartos fascia at the root of penis. This vein divides and forms the superficial external pudendal vein and drains into the great saphenous vein near its termination.

Q. What is secondary carcinoma of penis?

Ans. Secondary carcinoma of the penis is very rare and may be due to secondary spread from prostate rectum or urinary bladder.

The spread may either be direct, lymphatic, or retrograde venous spread along the deep dorsal vein of the penis.

Q. What is Buschke–Löwenstein tumor of penis?

Ans. Buschke–Löwenstein tumor is a form of verrucous carcinoma. It is a locally destructive invasive lesion; it displaces, invades, and destroys adjacent structure by compression. It does not spread to lymph node and there is no potential for distant metastasis.

Q. How will you treat Buschke–Löwenstein tumor?

Ans.
• Small lesion may require local excision with a healthy margin.
• Large lesion may require partial amputation of penis.

Q. What is erythroplasia of Queyrat of the penis?

Ans. This is a carcinoma in situ involving the penis. The lesion consists of a red, velvety, well-marginated lesion of the glans penis and may resemble long-standing balanitis. After a variable time, this may progress to invasive carcinoma.

Q. How will you manage?

Ans.
• Incisional biopsy from the lesion to exclude underlying invasive carcinoma.
• Local 5-fluorouracil ointment application may help.
• Small noninvasive lesion may be treated with local excision that preserves penile anatomy and function.

■ HYPOSPADIAS

Clinical Examination

History
• Where is the urethral orifice located?
• Any difficulty in micturition?
• Any bending of the penis?
• Any other complaint?

Examination—Inspection/Palpation
• Assess the type of hypospadias—classified depending on the location of external urethral meatus.

- Any chordee?
- Assess the size of the penis (usually the penis is hypoplastic).
- Look at the prepuce—usually there is a dorsal hood of skin and deficient ventral skin.
- Look at the urethral meatus—normal or stenosed.
- Examine both testes—whether normally descended or not.
- Examine the scrotum—in perineal hypospadias, the scrotum may be bifid.
- Look for any other congenital anomalies.

Q. What is your case? (Summary of a case of hypospadias)

Ans. This 2-year-old male child presented with urethral orifice on the undersurface of the penis since birth. Patient has difficulty in passing urine and the stream is narrow and the patient soils his under clothes while passing urine (Figs 15.24A and B).

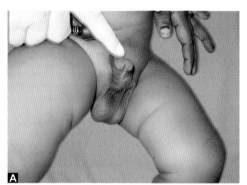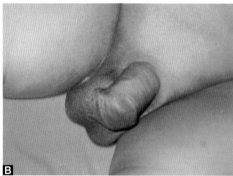

Figs 15.24A and B: (A) Distal penile type of hypospadias. Note the proximal location of urethral meatus and deficient ventral preputial skin; (B) Note the dorsal hood of preputial skin in same patient

Courtesy: Dr Kalyani Saha Basu, NRS Medical College, Kolkata

On examination: The penis appears hypoplastic. The external urethral orifice is situated on the undersurface of the penis near the distal part of the body. The distal part of the penis is bent downward due to the presence of a chordee. There is a dorsal hood of preputial skin and deficient ventral aspect of preputial skin. There are no other congenital anomalies.

Q. What is your diagnosis?

Ans. This is a case of distal penile type of hypospadias with meatal stenosis in a boy of 2 years age.

Q. What else you have looked for in this patient?

Ans.
- I have looked for the testes in this patient they are normally descended. Undescended testes may be associated with hypospadias.
- Inguinal hernia or congenital hydrocele may be associated. I have looked for this in this patient.
- Associated pinhole meatus may cause chronic retention of urine and there may be associated hydronephrosis. These are also to be looked for.

Q. What is hypospadias?

Ans. Hypospadias is defined classically as association of three anatomic and developmental anomalies of the penis:

1. An abnormal ventral opening of the urethral meatus, which may be located anywhere from the ventral aspect of the glans penis to the perineum.
2. An abnormal ventral curvature of the penis—chordee.
3. An abnormal distribution of the foreskin with a hood presents dorsally and deficient foreskin ventrally.
   The second and the third criteria may not be present in all cases.

Q. What are the different types of hypospadias?

Ans. Depending on the location of external urethral meatus, the hypospadias may be classified into (Fig. 15.25):

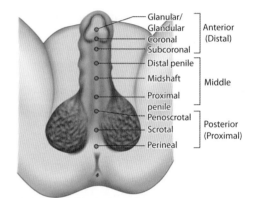

Fig. 15.25: Different types of hypospadias depending on location

* *Anterior hypospadias*—most common 50%. This includes:
    – *Glandular*—external urethral meatus on the undersurface of glans penis
    – *Coronal*—external urethral meatus at corona glandis
    – *Subcoronal*—external urethral meatus at the junction of corona glandis and body of penis.
* *Middle hypospadias*—30%. This includes:
    – *Distal penile*—external urethral meatus on the undersurface of the distal shaft of penis
    – Midshaft penile
    – Proximal penile.
* *Posterior (proximal) hypospadias*—20%. This includes:
    – *Penoscrotal*—external urethral meatus at the junction of penile shaft and scrotum
    – *Scrotal*—external urethral meatus on the undersurface of penis between the two halves of the scrotum.
    – *Perineal*—external urethral meatus at the perineum. This is associated with bifid scrotum.

Q. What are the problems in patients with hypospadias?

Ans.
* *Abnormal location of external urethral meatus*: Often the external urethral meatus is stenosed. There may be narrowing of stream. Ventral location of meatus may cause wetting of underclothes during micturition.
* *Chordee*: Distal to the external urethral orifice; there is a fibrous band, which causes bending of penis ventrally, which becomes more pronounced on erection.
* *Abnormal preputial skin*: The prepuce is deficient in its ventral aspect and there is hood of prepuce on dorsal aspect.
* Perineal type of hypospadias may be associated with undescended testis and ambiguous genitalia.
* Infertility is often associated in patients with posterior hypospadias.
* Due to chordee, there may be difficulty in sexual activity.

Q. How does normal urethra develop?

Ans. Development of urethra begins at 4th week of intrauterine life. The urethral plate develops as an outgrowth from the walls of the cloaca and urogenital sinus, and appears as a thickening on the anterior wall of the endodermal cloaca.

A urethral groove is formed by the development of the urethral folds on the ventral aspect of the phallic portion of the urogenital sinus on either side of the urethral plate. The roof of the primary urethral groove disintegrates and forms the definitive urethral groove.

In male fetus, as the testis develops and the Leydig cells start functioning, the urethral folds begin to fuse ventrally in the midline to form the urethra.

The distal portion of the glandular urethra is formed by lamellar ingrowth of the surface epithelium (ectodermal origin), which grows toward the distal extent of the urethral plate. This part of the urethra is lined by the ectoderm. The part of the urethra developing from the urogenital sinus is lined by endoderm.

Q. Which factors are responsible for development of hypospadias?

Ans.

- *Endocrine factors*: Deficiency of testosterone or dihydrotestosterone during development, or androgen insensitivity syndrome may result in failure of development of urethra leading to development of hypospadias. Maternal progesterone therapy during early pregnancy is associated with high incidence of hypospadias.
- *Enzyme deficiency*: Deficiency of 3-beta hydroxysteroid dehydrogenase enzyme is associated with incomplete masculine development and hypospadias. This enzyme is required for synthesis of almost all biologically active steroid hormones.
- Local tissue failure and arrested development leads to hypospadias.

Q. What investigations you would like to do?

Ans.

- Blood for hemogram
- Ultrasonography of kidney, ureter, and bladder (KUB) region
- Voiding cystourethrogram in selected cases.

Q. What are the aims of operation in hypospadias?

Ans.

- To provide an external urethral meatus at the tip of glans penis, i.e. at its normal site.
- To correct chordee, so that penis remains straight during erection.
- To correct any associated meatal stenosis for proper urinary flow.
- To provide a cosmetically good-looking penis.

Q. What is the ideal age for operation for hypospadias?

Ans. Earlier, it was said that the ideal time for repair of hypospadias is between 4 years and 6 years. With improvement of pediatric anesthesia and techniques in surgery, the consensus now is to repair the hypospadias between 6 months and 1 year of age.

Q. How will you manage this patient?

Ans. This is a distal penile type of hypospadias with a chordee and associated meatal stenosis. So, I will plan for a one-stage operation for repair of this hypospadias.

Q. What are the principles of hypospadias repair?

Ans. The hypospadias repair involves:
- *Orthoplasty*—attention to penile curvature and its correction (chordee correction).
- *Urethroplasty*—construction of a neourethra.
- *Meatoplasty and glanuloplasty*—enlargement of the meatal stenosis and reconstruction of the glans penis.

   In patient with distal hypospadias with mild or moderate chordee, this can be done as a one-stage procedure.

Q. How the degree of penile curvature is assessed?

Ans. The curvature is assessed during erection of penis. Intraoperatively injection of normal saline or PGE1 injection into the corpora cavernosa will provide an artificial erection and will help to assess the degree of penile curvature.

Q. What is chordee?

Ans. The chordee may be due to short penile skin ventrally or a disparity in length of tunica albuginea resulting in ventral curvature of the penis.

Q. How will you do chordee correction (orthoplasty)?

Ans.
Heineke–Mikulicz technique: After a degloving incision on the penis, the shorter concave surface of the penis is exposed. Several transverse incisions in the tunica are closed longitudinally to achieve lengthening of the concave aspect of the penis (Figs 15.26A to D).

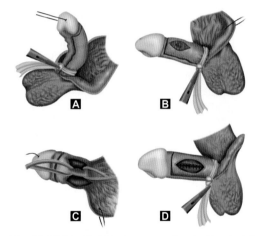

Q. How else the chordee may be corrected?

Ans.
- *Tunica albuginea plication (Baskin and Duckett):* A degloving incision is

Figs 15.26A to D: Chordee correction (orthoplasty)

made over the penis. Parallel incisions, approximately 1 cm in length, are made bilaterally on the anterolateral surface of the tunica albuginea, directly opposite the point of maximal penile curvature. The outer edges of the parallel incisions are sutured with interrupted 4-0 polydioxanone suture (PDS). This buries the intervening strip of tunica albuginea and shortens the disproportionately long-corporal surface, thus correcting the opposite penile curvature.
- *Dermal graft (Devine and Horton):* This is ideal for short phallus with severe penile curvature. A transverse incision is made at the site of maximal curvature (concavity) and the dermal graft is anastomosed to the edges of the corporal defect, thereby correcting the chordee.

Q. How will you do urethroplasty?

Ans. There are numerous techniques for reconstruction of the urethra and bringing the external urethral meatus to the tip of glans penis.

This is a distal type of penile hypospadias, so I will consider transverse preputial island flap (TPIF) technique of urethroplasty in this patient.

Q. How will you do urethroplasty in distal penile hypospadias?

Ans. In distal penile type of hypospadias, there are various types of island flap urethroplasty. TPIF or Duckett's technique is a good technique for construction of a neourethra.

This employs preputial skin for formation of a tubularized neourethra. The inner prepuce with its vascular pedicle forms the inner lining of the island flap and the longitudinally split outer prepuce forms the skin cover.

Traction suture is applied in the glans and the prepuce. A ventral midline longitudinal incision is marked from the urethral meatus to the circumcising incision. The skin is incised and the penile shaft is degloved, and the penis is assessed for curvature.

Curvature of the penis is corrected by a ventral orthoplasty technique.

After orthoplasty, a transversely oriented rectangle of preputial skin is marked at a length equal to the distance of the urethral meatus up to the tip of glans penis and 15 mm in width.

After dissection from the outer layer of the prepuce, the pedicle inner prepuce is tubularized over a 6 Fr silastic catheter to form the neourethra.

This neourethra is transferred to the ventrum of the penis on a tension-free pedicle.

A small circular incision is marked in the glans penis at the site of proposed neomeatus. A core of glans penis is excised to achieve sufficient channel caliber. The proximal anastomosis is performed with interrupted suture. The distal extent of the neourethra is then passed through the glans channel and the meatus is trimmed and then fixed to the glans with interrupted polyglactin sutures.

This neourethra is covered by a vascularized tunica vaginalis flap. The degloved penis is then covered with the penile skin (Figs 15.27A to J).

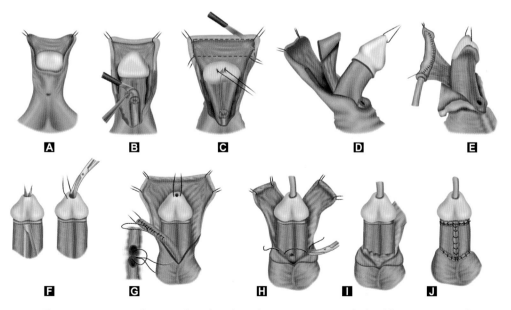

Figs 15.27A to J: Technique of urethroplasty (transverse preputial island flap repair—TPIF)

Q. What is Asopa's technique of urethroplasty?

Ans. Asopa also described a similar operation of tubularized preputial skin for construction of a neourethra. The inner prepuce from the tubularized neourethra and the attached outer prepuce form skin cover.

Q. What is glanuloplasty?

Ans. Glanuloplasty is required as an adjunct to tubularized skin graft urethroplasty. The technique of glanuloplasty involves extensive dissection of the glans penis with the development of a midline, and anteriorly based flap of glans epithelium. The tubularized neourethra is brought out through this glans incision and the neomeatus is constructed at the tip of the glans penis.

Q. How will you treat glandular hypospadias?

Ans. Glandular hypospadias, if not associated with meatal stenosis, does not require active treatment, as it does not interfere with normal functions.

Q. What are the complications of hypospadias repair?

Ans.
+ Bleeding and hematoma
+ Meatal stenosis
+ Urethrocutaneous fistula
+ Urethral stricture
+ Urethral diverticulum
+ Wound infection
+ Breakdown of repair.

Q. When will you consider a two-stage repair?

Ans. Majority of the hypospadias may be managed with a single stage repair. In the setting of scrotal or perineal hypospadias with short penis or severe chordee, a two-stage procedure is preferred.
1. In the first stage, orthoplasty is performed and the prepuce is repositioned ventrally.
2. At a second stage, operation after 6 months a neourethra is constructed using either local flaps or a tubularized flap.

▉ ECTOPIA VESICAE

Q. What is your case? (Summary of a case of ectopia vesicae)

Ans. This 5-year-old male child presented with continuous dribbling of urine since birth. The child's mother says that he was borne with deformity of external genitalia and absence of lower part of abdominal wall and exposed raw area from where the urine is dribbling continuously. Complaint of occasional fever, difficulty in walking and walks with a limp, occasional bleeding from the raw surface in the abdominal wall often due to friction of the worn clothes (Fig. 15.28).

On examination: There is deficiency of the infraumbilical part of the anterior abdominal wall and the anterior wall of the bladder is deficient. The posterior wall of the bladder is exposed. The trigonal area is visible and the ureteric orifices are seen on either side from where there is dribbling of urine. The umbilicus is absent. A gap can be felt in the infraumbilical part of the anterior abdominal wall through which the bladder is protruding. The penis is hypoplastic and there is complete epispadias, which extends up to the neck of bladder. There is no associated hernia. Patient walks with a waddling gait.

Q. What is your diagnosis?

Ans. This is a case of ectopia vesicae in a 5-year-old female child.

Q. How do you explain this congenital anomaly?

Ans. The cloacal membrane is a bilaminar membrane situated at the caudal end of the germinal disk. Mesenchymal ingrowth from the primitive node between the ectodermal and endodermal layers of the cloacal membrane results in development of lower abdominal muscles and the pelvic bones. Failure of this mesenchymal growth results in deficient growth of the infraumbilical abdominal wall. The defective cloacal membrane is subject to premature rupture. Depending on the extent of the infraumbilical defect and the stage of development during which the rupture occurs, bladder exstrophy, cloacal exstrophy, or epispadias results (Figs 15.29A to E).

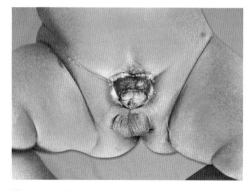

Fig. 15.28: Ectopia vesicae

Courtesy: Prof BN Mukhopadhyay, NRS Medical College and Hospital, Kolkata

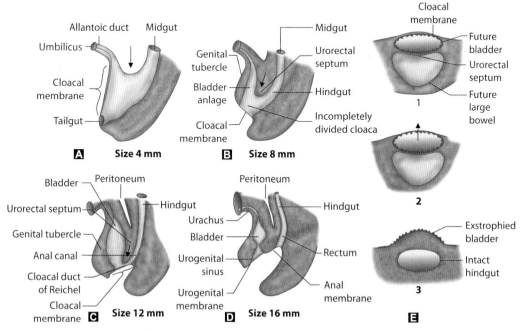

Figs 15.29A to E: Development of urinary bladder

Q. What may be the associated defects in cases with ectopia vesicae?

Ans. There may be associated anomalies of the urinary tract, genital tract, musculoskeletal system, and intestinal tract.

- *Skeletal defects*: Widening of symphysis pubis, shortening of pubic bones, and malrotation of the iliac bones.
- *Abdominal wall defects*: Deficient infraumbilical abdominal wall and associated inguinal hernias in 80% cases.
- *Anorectal defects*: Perineum is short and broad, and the anus is situated more anteriorly.

Defects of levator ani, puborectalis, and external sphincter may result in anal incontinence and rectal prolapse.

- *Male genital defects*: The penis is short, and broad penis due to widening of symphysis pubis and short corpora cavernosa and epispadias.
- *Female genital defects*: Vagina is short, vaginal orifice may be stenotic, clitoris is bifid, labia and clitoris are divergent.
- *Urinary defects*: The exposed bladder mucosa may appear normal. However, metaplastic changes may occur in the bladder mucosa. Vesicoureteric reflux is usual. Horseshoe kidney, unilateral agenesis, and megaureter may all be associated.

Q. What are the problems in patient with exstrophy of bladder?

Ans.
- Urinary incontinence with constant dribbling of urine from the exposed bladder wall.
- Vesicoureteric reflux and recurrent urinary tract infection.
- Squamous metaplasia and neoplastic change.
- Renal failure in long-standing cases.
- Cosmetic problems.
- Associated skeletal defects—gait problems.

Q. How will you manage this patient?

Ans. Routine workup to assess patient's fitness for general anesthesia.

I will consider staged repair of the exstrophy of the bladder.

- *Stage I*: Combined bladder closure, iliac osteotomy, abdominal wall closure, and posterior urethral closure.
- *Stage II*: Repair of epispadias and urethral reconstruction.
- *Stage III*: Continence and antireflux procedure.

Q. What will you achieve in stage-I operation?

Ans. The first stage of the operation may be done as early as 4–6 months of age.

- *Bladder closure*: An appropriate plane is entered just above the umbilicus and a plane is established between the rectus fascia and the bladder. The peritoneum is reflected off from the dome of the bladder. The dissection is continued caudally up to the urogenital diaphragm. The bladder wall is closed. A suprapubic cystostomy catheter is kept.
- *Iliac osteotomy and pubic symphysis closure*: An iliac osteotomy is done. Pressure over the greater trochanters allows easy approximation of the pubic bones in the midline. Horizontal mattress sutures are placed in the pubis and tied with a knot away from the neourethra.

Q. What will you achieve in stage-II operation?

Ans. Epispadias repair and urethroplasty may be done at 6 months of age. This involves correction of dorsal chordee, urethral reconstruction by tubularization of urethral plate.

Q. What will you do in stage-III operation?

Ans. This is usually done at 4–5 years of age. The basic premise is to create a mucosa-lined tube inside a muscular funnel that narrows from its junction with floor of the bladder that extends caudally into the urethra.

Vesicoureteric reflux is very common. Reimplantation of the ureter into the bladder is required to correct the reflux.

Q. When will you consider urinary diversion in patients with ectopia vesicae?

Ans. Not all patients with ectopia vesicae are candidates for bladder reconstruction. Urinary diversion is indicated in:

* Very small bladder that is not suitable for closure
* Associated hydronephrosis
* Failure of initial closure with a small remaining bladder
* Failed continence surgery.

Q. What are the types of urinary diversion procedure?

Ans.
* *Ureterosigmoidostomy*: Implantation of the ureters into the sigmoid colon. This form of diversion is not suitable in patients with anal incontinence.
* *Problems of ureterosigmoidostomy*:
  – Recurrent pyelonephritis
  – Rectal incontinence
  – Hyperchloremic acidosis
  – Ureteral obstruction
  – Delayed development of malignancy.

Urinary diversion by implanting ureters into an isolated loop of ileum (ileal conduit) or sigmoid colon.

■ TESTICULAR TUMOR

Clinical Examination

See Page No. 382, Chapter 9.

History

* Age of the patient (teratoma usually occurs between 20 years and 30 years of age and seminomas occur at an age between 30 years and 40 years).
* *History about the swelling*: Onset, progress, and any history of injury (often the swelling is first noticed following history of an injury which may be mild). However, there is no definite relation between the injury and onset of the disease.

- Any pain over the swelling (testicular tumors are usually painless to start with or there may dragging pain in the scrotum, sometimes there may be acute pain resembling acute epididymo-orchitis).
- Any swelling in the abdomen or neck (para-aortic lymph node or Virchow lymph node enlargement).
- Any history of swelling in the legs (due to venous or lymphatic obstruction).
- Any history of loss of appetite, weight or generalized weakness, jaundice, cough, hemoptysis, and chest pain (suggestive of metastatic disease).
- Any history of undescended testis or orchidopexy in childhood.
- Any history of gynecomastia (some testicular tumor may secrete estrogen).

Examination—Inspection/Palpation

- *Examination of the swelling*: Possible to get above the swelling—suggesting a scrotal swelling.
- Site and extent, size and shape, surface and margin, and consistency.
- Assess testicular sensation (press the swelling) and assess whether testicular sensation is preserved or not (in testicular tumor, testicular sensation is lost early).
- Examination of the spermatic cord.
- Examination of abdomen—for any mass, palpate liver, and spleen.

Q. What is your case? (Summary of a case of testicular tumor)

Ans. This 32-year-old gentleman presented with a swelling in the right side of the scrotum for last 6 months. The swelling was gradually increasing in size at the onset for about 2 months, but for last 4 months, the swelling is rapidly increasing in size to attain the present large size. There is no alteration in size of the swelling during his daily activities. Patient does not complain of any swelling in the groin, abdomen, and neck. Patient complains of a sensation of heaviness in his right side of the scrotum.

On examination: There is a right-sided scrotal swelling, as it is possible to get above the swelling. The swelling is globular in shape, firm in feel, irreducible and there is loss of testicular sensation. The right spermatic cord is normal. The left testis and the spermatic cord are normal. Abdominal examination is normal.

Q. What is your diagnosis?

Ans. This is a case of right-sided testicular tumor.

Q. What are the other possibilities?

Ans.
- Epididymo-orchitis
- Vaginal hydrocele
- Old hematocele

Q. How will you proceed to manage this patient?

Ans. I will suggest some investigations:
- Complete hemogram, liver function test, urea, and electrolytes.
- Ultrasonography of scrotum to ascertain the nature of the swelling.

- Blood for serum alpha-fetoprotein (AFP), lactate dehydrogenase, and beta-human chorionic gonadotropin (beta-hCG).
- A chest X-ray to look for any chest metastasis.
- A CT scan of abdomen to assess any retroperitoneal lymphadenopathy or intra-abdominal metastasis.

Q. What treatment will you consider?

Ans. I will plan for high-inguinal orchidectomy—orchidectomy is to be done through the inguinal approach. An inguinal incision is made. The skin and subcutaneous tissue is cut. The external oblique aponeurosis is incised and the spermatic cord is exposed. A vascular clamp is applied to the spermatic cord. The testicular tumor is mobilized from the scrotum and delivered into the wound. The spermatic cord is divided in-between clamps as high as possible in the inguinal canal. The testis along with the spermatic cord is excised (Figs 15.30A and B).

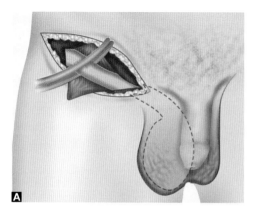 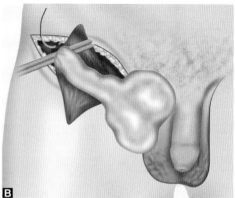

Figs 15.30A and B: High-inguinal orchidectomy

Q. How will you plan further treatment?

Ans. The subsequent treatment will depend on the histopathology report and stage of the disease.

Q. What are the important testicular tumors?

Ans. Depending on the predominant cellular types, testicular tumors are classified as:
- Seminomas
- Teratomas
- Mixed seminoma and teratoma
- Interstitial cell tumors
- Lymphomas.

Q. Why FNAC is not done in testicular tumor?

Ans. If a FNAC is done through the scrotal skin then there is chance of seedling of tumor cells in the scrotal skin and this opens a separate avenue of spread of tumor cells to the inguinal lymph nodes.

Q. What are the TNM staging for testicular tumors?

Ans. The TNM staging system is based on four key pieces of information:
1. *T—Primary tumor*
2. *N—Lymph nodes*
3. *M—Distant metastasis*
4. *S—serum* levels of tumor markers.

Primary tumor (T):

- *TX*: The primary tumor cannot be assessed.
- *T0*: There is no evidence of primary tumor.
- *Tis*: Carcinoma in situ (noninvasive cancer cells).
- *T1*: Tumor confined to testis and epididymis:
  - No vascular/lymphatic invasion
  - May invade tunica albuginea but not to tunica vaginalis.
- *T2*: Tumor confined to testis and epididymis:
  - Vascular/lymphatic invasion
  - May invade up to tunica vaginalis.
- *T3*: The tumor invades the spermatic cord with or without vascular/lymphatic invasion.
- *T4:* The tumor invading into the scrotal skin with or without vascular/lymphatic invasion.

Regional lymph nodes (N):

- *NX*: Regional lymph nodes cannot be assessed.
- *N0*: No spread to regional lymph nodes.
- *N1*: Single or multiple lymph node metastasis, none larger than 2 cm
- *N2*: Single or multiple lymph node metastasis that is larger than 2 cm but is not greater than 5 cm
- *N3*: Lymph node metatstasis with at least one lymph node greater than 5 cm.

If the lymph nodes were taken out during surgery, there is a slightly different classification:

Distant metastasis (M)

- *M0*: There is no distant metastasis.
- *M1*: Distant metastasis is present:
  - *M1a*: The tumor has metastasized to distant lymph nodes or to the lung.
  - *M1b:* The tumor has metastasized to other organs, such as the liver, brain, or bone.

Serum tumor markers (S)

For staging, serum levels of tumor markers are measured after the testicle containing the cancer has been removed with surgery (Table 15.1).

Stage grouping

Once the T, N, M, and S categories have been determined, they are combined in a process called "stage grouping" to assign an overall stage (using Roman numerals and letters) (Table 15.2).

Table 15.1: Staging of serum tumor markers

	LDH (lactate dehydrogenase) (U/L)	HCG (human chorionic gonado-trophic hormone) (mIU/mL)	AFP(alpha fetoprotein) (ng/mL)
SX	Marker studies not available or not done.		
S0	Normal	Normal	Normal
S1	<1.5 × normal	<5,000	<1,000
S2	1.5–10 × normal	5,000–50,000	1,000–10,000
S3	>10 × normal	>50,000	>10,000

Table 15.2: Stage grouping

Stage	T	N	M	S
Stage 0	Tis (in situ)	N0	M0	S0
Stage I	T1-T4	N0	M0	SX
Stage IA	T1	N0	M0	S0
Stage IB	T2-T4	N0	M0	S0
Stage IS	Any T	N0	M0	S1-S3
Stage II	Any T	N1-N3	M0	SX
Stage IIA	Any T	N1	M0	S0-S1
Stage IIB	Any T	N2	M0	S0-S1
Stage IIC	Any T	N3	M0	S0-S1
Stage III	Any T	Any N	M1	SX
Stage IIIA	Any T	Any N	M1a	S0-S1
Stage IIIB	Any T	N1-N3	M0	S2
	Any T	Any N	M1a	S2
Stage IIIC	Any T	N1-N3	M0	S3
	Any T	Any N	M1a	S3
	Any T	Any N	M1b	Any S

Q. What are the implications of serum markers?

Ans.

- Serum markers AFP and beta-hCG are elevated in patients with nonseminomatous germ cell tumors. Both markers may be elevated in 40% of patients and one of the markers may be elevated in 90% patients.
- Human chorionic gonadotropin may be elevated in some cases of seminomas. Elevation of AFP always indicates the presence of a teratomatous element.

Serum markers are also useful for follow-up. Rising concentration of these serum markers in follow-up indicate active metastases, long before the disease becomes obvious on clinical and radiological examination.

Q. If the biopsy report of the excised specimen is pure seminoma, how will you plan further treatment?

Ans. Details staging investigations:

* Abdominal and pelvic CT scan
* Chest CT scan when there is positive finding in abdominal CT or chest X-ray
* Repeat serum markers—beta hCG, LDH, and AFP
* Brain MRI and bone scan in selected cases.

Subsequent treatment depends on the stage of the disease:

Stage I:

* Postoperative radiotherapy to the para-aortic and pelvic nodes. Scrotal irradiation is not required unless the scrotal skin is breached. The dose of radiotherapy is 30–36 Gy.
* The alternative strategy keeps the patient under follow up and treatment initiated when the nodes appear.

Stage II:

* Treated with adjuvant radiotherapy to the retroperitoneum.
* In high-risk stage II disease—primary chemotherapy with EP (etoposide and cisplatin) or BEP (bleomycin, etoposide, and cisplatin).

Stage III: Primary chemotherapy with EP or BEP.

Q. How will you plan further treatment in stage II and stage III disease after primary chemotherapy?

Ans. Investigations:

* Abdominal and pelvic CT scan
* Chest CT scan
* Serum marker study.

Subsequent treatment will depend on investigation findings:

* No residual mass or residual mass less than or equal to 3 cm and normal serum markers—patient is kept under follow up.
* Residual mass more than 3 cm and normal markers—positron emission tomography (PET) CT scan.
* If PET CT scan is negative—patient kept under follow up.
* If PET CT scan is positive—consider retroperitoneal lymph node dissection (RPLND) or second-line chemotherapy.
* Progressive disease—consider second-line chemotherapy.

Q. If the biopsy report is teratoma, how will you plan further treatment?

Ans.

- *Stage I*:
  - Patient with negative tumor marker may be kept under follow up or patient can undergo nerve-sparing RPLND.
  - If there is progressive disease, treatment with chemotherapy or RPLND is done.
  - Patient with positive tumor markers is given combination chemotherapy till the tumor markers become negative.
- *Stage II*: Nerve-sparing RPLND or primary chemotherapy with EP or BEP 3–4 cycles. After chemotherapy, if there is residual disease—RPLND.
- *Stage III*: Primary chemotherapy with EP or BEP 3–4 cycles. If tumor markers become normal and there is residual disease in the retroperitoneum, RPLND is to be done. Persistent tumor marker may require further cycles of chemotherapy.

Q. What is the standard chemotherapy regimen for testicular tumors?

Ans. A combination of cisplatin and etoposide (EP) or a combination of BEP is effective in testicular tumor. Three to four cycles of chemotherapy is given. The response rate is around 90%.

Q. What are the important etiological factors for development of testicular tumors?

Ans.

- Cryptorchidism
- Fetal exposure to maternal estrogens
- Trauma
- Viral (mumps) orchitis.

Q. How does the testicular tumor spread?

Ans. *See* Surgical Pathology Section, Page No. 925, Chapter 18.

Q. What is the correlation between cryptorchidism and malignancy?

Ans.

- In large series of testicular tumor, about 10% are associated with cryptorchidism.
- The relative risk of testicular cancer in patients with cryptorchidism is 3–14 times than the normal expected incidence.
- Between 5% and 10% of patients with a history of cryptorchidism may develop malignancy in the contralateral normally descended testis.
- Orchidopexy does not prevent carcinogenesis, but rather allows early diagnosis by surveillance.

Surgical Problems

1. **A 30-year-male patient, sustained road traffic accident and brought to emergency with severe multiple trauma. How will you proceed to manage?**

OR

A 30-year-male patient has been brought to emergency in an unconscious state following a road traffic accident. How will you proceed to manage?

Q. What is prehospital care?

Ans. Management of a trauma victim starts at the injury site. The management at the site of injury is by BTLS (basic trauma and life support). The components of BTLS are:

* Assess and control the scene of accident for the safety of the patient and the prehospital caregiver
* Control external hemorrhage with direct pressure
* Stabilize the spine
* Clear the airway and provide oxygen supplementation
* Extricate the patient
* Splint the long-bone fracture.

Q. What is field triage?

Ans. When there is mass casualty, the trauma victim needs to be screened at the scene of accident and decision is to be taken for shifting these patients to next level of trauma care center. Critically injured patient is to be directly shifted to a level I trauma care center or to a level II trauma care center, is if the level I trauma care center > 30 minutes travel.

Q. Which factors are taken into consideration for field triage of trauma victim?

Ans. Different factors are taken into consideration for triage of trauma victim at the scene of accident and decision for shifting the patient to a higher level of trauma care center.

Physiologic criteria:
* *Glasgow Coma Scale*: Less than 14
* *Systolic blood pressure*: Less than 90 mm Hg
* *Respiratory rate*: Less than 10 or more than 29.

Anatomic criteria:
* Penetrating injuries
* Flail chest
* Two or more long bone fracture
* Pelvic fracture
* Traumatic amputation of a limb
* Degloving injury
* Open or depressed skull fracture
* Paralysis.

Mechanism of injury:
* *Falls* from > 20-feet high
* High-risk automobile crash
* Death of other victim in same accident.

Other considerations:
* *Age of the patient*: More than 55 years
* Patient on anticoagulant therapy
* Patient with end-stage renal disease
* Pregnancy more than 20 weeks.

Q. What is the guideline for declaration of death at the scene of accident?
Ans.

For penetrating injures:
* Prehospital cardiopulmonary resuscitation (CPR) for 15 minutes with no signs of life
* Asystole without pericardial tamponade.

For blunt trauma:
* Prehospital CPR more than 10 minutes with no signs of life
* Asystole.

Q. How to proceed for management on arrival to emergency room (ER)?
Ans. Management of road traffic accident victim is by ATLS (Advanced Trauma and Life Support) approach, which includes:
* Primary survey and resuscitation
* Secondary survey
* Definitive care.

Q. What are the components of primary survey and resuscitation?
Ans. The elements of primary survey are (ABCDE):

- *A*: Maintenance of airway with cervical spine control
- *B*: Maintenance of breathing and ventilation
- *C*: Maintenance of circulation and control of hemorrhage
- *D*: Assessment of dysfunction of central nervous system
- *E*: Exposure in a controlled environment. Remove all clothing and look for any obvious external injury. If environment is too cold, cover the patient with a blanket to avoid hypothermia.

Q. How will you maintain airway?

Ans. Assessments of airway to exclude any airway obstruction are:
- Maintenance of airway with cervical spine control achieved by:
  - Sucking of airway to clear blood, foreign body, secretions, vomitus by a "two finger" sweep and suction under vision
  - Chin lift or jaw-thrust maneuvers to prevent tongue falling back
  - Passing an oropharyngeal airway tube to prevent tongue falling back
  - Endotracheal cuffed tube intubation, if above measures fail
  - Some cases may require—emergency needle cricothyrotomy
  - Emergency tracheostomy in selected cases when above measures fails.
- During all these maneuvers, cervical spine is immobilized in neutral position by neck brace, sand bags or forehead tape. Avoid hyperextension of the neck.

Q. How will you manage breathing?

Ans.
- *Assessment of breathing by:*
  - Expose neck and chest and determine the rate and depth of respiration
  - Inspect and palpate the neck and chest for any tracheal deviation, any restriction of chest movement and any signs of local injury
  - Percuss chest for presence of dullness or hyperresonance
  - Auscultate chest bilaterally.
- *Maintenance of breathing and oxygenation is achieved by:*
  - Ventilate with a bag-valve mask device
  - Administer high concentration of oxygen
  - If endotracheal tube is inserted, consider mechanical ventilation
  - Alleviate tension pneumothorax by needle thoracostomy
  - Seal an open pneumothorax
  - Connect the patient to a pulse oximeter.

Q. How will you maintain circulation?

Ans. Maintenance of circulation and hemorrhage control is achieved by:
- *Initial assessment for signs of shock:*
  - Pulse
  - Blood pressure (BP)
  - Capillary filling
  - Temperature of extremities
  - Look for any external bleeding and control it by external pressure and bandaging
  - Identify potential source of internal bleeding.

- *Management*:
  - In presence of shock, vascular access by cannulating peripheral vein with 14 Fr intravenous (IV) cannula
  - In infants less than 6 years, intraosseous infusion after cannula is placed in the medullary cavity of a long bone
  - Blood is drawn for blood grouping and cross-matching
  - *Baseline laboratory investigations*—hemogram, blood sugar, urea, creatinine and serum electrolytes, and coagulation profile
  - For an adult, 1–2 liters of Ringer's solution is recommended as initial fluid challenge
  - Control external bleeding by pressure and bandaging
  - Consider presence of internal hemorrhage and need for early surgical intervention.

Q. How pulse may correlate with blood pressure?

Ans. In general:
- Palpable radial pulse—systolic BP more than 80 mm Hg
- Palpable femoral pulse—systolic BP more than 70 mm Hg
- Palpable carotid pulse—systolic BP more than 60 mm Hg.

Q. What should be the endpoint of initial resuscitation?

Ans. The endpoint of initial resuscitation would be:
- Systolic BP more than 90 mm Hg
- Heart rate less than 120 beats/min
- Central venous pressure (CVP) more than or equal to 10 cm of H_2O
- Hemoglobin (Hb) level more than or equal to 10 gm%.

Q. What life-threatening injuries should be looked for immediately?

Ans. Some life-threatening injuries should be looked for and taken care of at this stage before one proceeds for secondary survey.
- Tension pneumothorax is diagnosed by:
  - Cyanosis
  - Severe respiratory distress
  - Tracheal and apex beat shifting to opposite side
  - Decreased chest movement
  - Hyperresonant percussion note
  - Absent breath sound on the side of injury.
- Tension pneumothorax may be relieved by:
  - Needle thoracocentesis at the second intercostal space (ICS) in the midclavicular line and followed by tube thoracostomy.
- Open pneumothorax (sucking wounds) is managed immediately by an occlusive dressing on three sides. After tube thoracostomy the dressing is sealed on the fourth side.
- Massive hemothorax is diagnosed by:
  - Features of shock
  - Mediastinal shift (trachea and apex beat) to the opposite side
  - Decreased chest movement
  - Dull percussion note
  - Absent breath sounds.

* Management is by:
  – Resuscitation with IV fluids
  – Tube thoracostomy.
* Major flail chest with pulmonary contusion may be life-threatening. Endotracheal intubation with ventilatory support may be life-saving.
* Cardiac tamponade may be life-threatening and is usually suspected in patient with penetrating chest injury. Diagnosed by:
  – Increased jugular venous pressure (JVP)
  – Pulsus paradoxus
  – Muffled heart sounds
  – Cardiac tamponade may be relieved by needle pericardiocentesis.

Q. How will assess dysfunction of nervous system?

Ans. Initial assessment of dysfunction of central nervous system is done as:
* A—Alert
* V—Respond to voice
* P—Respond to pain
* U—Unresponsive.

Assessment of pupil—normal, dilated, or constricted. Comparison of two sides and reaction to light.

More detail assessment of nervous system is done in secondary survey.
* E—Exposure in a controlled environment.

The remaining clothing is removed and any other obvious injury assessed.

If the environment is too cold, cover the patient with a blanket to avoid hypothermia.

Q. What are the components of secondary survey?

Ans. The subsequent management depends on the response of the patient to primary survey and resuscitation. If the patient has responded well and in whom no life-threatening condition is found a detail secondary survey is done.

If the patient does not respond well and there is continuous bleeding, patient should be shifted to operation theater for definitive management.

There may be transient response with subsequent deterioration and patient needs to be transferred to a critical care unit.

The secondary survey comprises:
* Detail history
* Head-to-foot examination
* Relevant investigations.

History:

History from the patient, if he is conscious and if unconscious obtain, history from the relatives or attendant who has accompanied the patient.
* History about the mechanism of injury.
* Any history of death of other persons due to accident usually indicates a serious accident.
* Any history of loss of consciousness and any lucid interval.
* Any history of vomiting.

* Any bleeding or cerebrospinal fluid (CSF) discharge from the ear, nose and throat.
* Any history of convulsion or weakness of any of the limbs.
* Any history of chest pain, cough, hemoptysis, or breathlessness.
* Any history of pain abdomen.
* Any history of retention of urine, bleeding per urethra, or hematuria.
* Any obvious swelling/pain/difficulty in movement of extremities.
* Any past medical illness, e.g. diabetes, epilepsy, asthma, heart disease, steroid, or anticoagulant therapy.
* Time interval between last feed and injury has a bearing with aspiration during surgery.

Detailed head-to-foot examination:

* *Head*:
  - Any external injury—bruising, laceration, or fracture
  - Assessment of Glasgow coma scale
  - Look for CSF leakage through nostrils, or ears
  - Pupillary reflexes
  - Any focal neurological deficit.
* *Face*:
  - Any foreign body in eyes, perforation, or subconjunctival hemorrhage
  - Bleeding or CSF discharge from ear, nose, or throat
  - Look for any fracture of mandible, maxilla, or nasal bone
  - Any foreign body, broken teeth in mouth
  - Look for any threat to airway.
* *Neck and spine*:
  - Log roll the patient to look for any swelling/bruise around the spine
  - Examine for any sensory and motor deficit in the extremities.

Examination of chest:

* *Inspection*:
  - Respiratory rate
  - Symmetry of chest
  - Chest wall contusion—any bruise or laceration or open wounds
  - Paradoxical respiration (flail chest)
  - Stove in chest (indented segment)
  - Movement of chest.
* *Palpation*:
  - Mediastinal shift—position of trachea and apex beat
  - Tenderness (over the rib)
  - Palpable crepitus (surgical emphysema)
  - Movement of chest.
* *Percussion*:
  - Normal resonance
  - Hyperresonance (pneumothorax)
  - Dullness on percussion (hemothorax).

♦ *Auscultation*:
  – Breath sound present or absent
  – Any added sound.

Examination of abdomen:

♦ *Inspection*:
  – Inspect the anterior and posterior abdominal wall for any evidence of external injury—any bruising or abrasion
  – Distension of abdomen
  – Bruise or ecchymosis around umbilicus/flanks/left hypochondrium
  – Any obvious bleeding
  – Movement of abdomen—normal/restricted
  – London sign (London sign is presence of imprint of clothing or a vehicle wheel on the abdominal wall and usually indicates a severe underlying injury).
♦ *Palpation*:
  – Temperature
  – Tenderness—suggests inflammation/hemoperitoneum
  – Any muscle guard or rigidity—suggests underlying peritonitis
  – Any rebound tenderness
  – Palpation of liver/spleen/kidneys
  – Hematoma or clots around liver, spleen, kidney—tender enlargement.
♦ *Percussion*:
  – Obliteration of liver dullness—suggests perforation of hollow viscera
  – Hepatic/splenic dullness
  – Shifting dullness for assessing presence of free fluid in abdomen.
♦ *Auscultation*:
  – Bowel sounds—normal/silent.

Examination of the pelvis:

♦ Inspect perineum for any contusion, hematoma, or laceration
♦ Look for any rectal or urethral bleeding
♦ To exclude pelvic injury clinically—palpate all bones (iliac bone and the sacrum)
♦ Compress pelvis—side-to-side and anteroposteriorly (AP) for presence of any tenderness
♦ *Per rectal examination*—assess integrity of rectum, any bone fragment projecting into the rectum. Position of the prostate
♦ *Per vaginal examination*—any blood in the vaginal vault. Any vaginal, laceration.

Examination of the extremities:

♦ Inspect both the upper and lower extremities:
  – Any evidence of blunt or penetrating injury
  – Any bruise, abrasion or laceration, hematoma or deformity.
♦ Palpate the extremities—for any tenderness, local crepitus and abnormal movement suggestive of fracture.
♦ Palpate all peripheral pulses—present or absent.
♦ Assess for any neurological deficit in the limbs.

Q. What investigations will you suggest in a polytrauma patient?

Ans.

♦ *Baseline investigations*:
  – Hematological—blood Hb%, packed cell volume (PCV), total leukocyte count (TLC) and differential leukocyte count (DLC)
  – Biochemical—blood sugar, urea and creatinine
  – Chest X-ray
  – Electrocardiogram (ECG).
  Further investigations will depend on the type of injury ascertained on clinical examination.
♦ *In suspected cases of head injury*:
  – X-ray of skull
  – X-ray of cervical spine—AP and lateral view
  – Computed tomography (CT) scan of brain.
♦ In facial injury—CT scan of face/X-ray of facial bones.
♦ In suspected chest injury:
  – Chest X-ray
  – CT scan of chest
  – Arterial blood gas (ABG) analysis.
♦ In suspected case of abdominal injury:
  – Urine examination to exclude hematuria
  – Ultrasonography (USG) of abdomen
  – CT scan of abdomen in selected cases
  – DPL—diagnostic peritoneal lavage in selected cases
  – Diagnostic laparoscopy.
♦ In injury to extremities:
  – X-ray of the relevant part
  – Angiography in cases with suspected major vessel injury.
♦ In suspected spinal injury:
  – X-ray of spine.
  – Magnetic resonance imaging (MRI) of spine.

Q. Why initial hemoglobin level is not a reliable marker of blood loss?

Ans. The initial Hb level may be misleading either because the patient has not been received adequate volume of fluid lost or there has not been sufficient time for influx of fluid from interstitial fluid to intravascular space. Hb level estimation again after volume resuscitation will be more informative. A drop of Hb greater than 2gm% will be a ground for concern.

Q. How will you plan for definitive treatment?

Ans. Further care plan is decided depending on findings of clinical examination and investigations.

The plan for definitive treatment includes:

♦ General care
♦ Resuscitation from shock

- O_2 inhalation
- Intravenous fluid
- Catheterization
- *Sympathomimetic drug*: In hypovolemic shock—dopamine, and dobutamine in selected cases
- Monitoring of pulse, BP, respiration and central venous pressure
- Specific management depends on the type of injury. See individual injuries.

2. A 40-year-male patient sustained road traffic accident and brought to emergency room with suspicion of head injury. How will you proceed to manage?

Ans. The initial management of patient with head injury will be as per ATLS protocol. This will include:
- Primary survey and resuscitation (*See* Page No. 678)
- Secondary survey
- Definitive management.

Q. How will you assess level of consciousness in a patient with head injury?

Ans. This is done by Glasgow coma scale. This needs to be recorded hourly to monitor any deterioration during the period of observation. The Glasgow coma scale involves evaluation of following:
- *Eye opening (E)*:
  - Spontaneously—4
  - To speech—3
  - To pain—2
  - Nil—1.
- *Best motor response (M)*:
  - Obeys commands—6
  - Localizes pain—5
  - Withdraws to pain—4
  - Abnormal flexion—3
  - Extension to pain—2
  - No response—1.
- *Best verbal response (V)*:
  - Oriented—5
  - Confused and disoriented—4
  - Inappropriate words—3
  - Incomprehensible sounds—2
  - No response—1.

There is a total score of 15.

- Score of 11–15 indicates good prognosis
- Score of 7–10 indicates intermediate prognosis
- Score of < 7 indicates poor prognosis.

Q. What is cerebral concussion?

Ans. This is a condition of temporary dysfunction of brain without any structural damage following head injury. The manifestations are transient and usually resolve after a variable period. The manifestations include:

- Transient loss of consciousness
- Transient loss of memory
- Autonomic dysfunction like bradycardia, hypotension, and sweating.

Q. What are the features of cerebral contusion?

Ans. This is a more severe degree of brain injury manifested by areas of hemorrhage in the brain parenchyma but without any surface laceration. There is neurological deficit that persists longer than 24 hours. There may be associated cerebral edema and defects in blood-brain barrier.

Contusion may resolve after a variable time along with associated neurological deficit or the neurological deficit may be persistent.

Q. What is cerebral laceration?

Ans. This is a severe degree of brain injury associated with a breach in the surface parenchyma. The tearing of brain surface may be due to skull fracture or due to shearing forces. There is tearing of pia and arachnoid mater and there may be associated intracerebral hemorrhage.

Focal neurological deficit is present, which may be permanent.

Q. What is diffuse axonal injury?

Ans. This is the condition of shearing of axons at the white and gray matter interface due to severe acceleration and deceleration force. No obvious structural damage may be evident on the surface.

The manifestations may be mild confusion, coma, or even death due to diffuse axonal injury involving the brainstem.

Q. What investigations will you suggest in patients with head injury?

Ans.

- Baseline investigations
- Special investigations:
  - X-ray of skull—AP and lateral view
  - Plain X-ray may show fracture, foreign bodies, or air in the cranial cavity.
- X-ray of cervical spine—AP and lateral view. May show fracture and dislocation
- CT scan brain. The indications of CT scan in head injury are:
  - History of loss of consciousness or patient is unconscious
  - Patient has disturbance of memory
  - Presence of neurological deficit
  - CSF leakage
  - Pupillary asymmetry
  - Penetrating injury.

- CT scan may show:
  - Skull fracture
  - Intracranial hematomas (intracerebral, subdural, or extradural)
  - Midline shift
  - Cerebral edema
  - Cerebral contusion.

Sometimes CT scan immediately after injury may be normal and hematoma develops hours after the injury. So, serial CT scan may be required in patients who are deteriorating during observation.

Q. What is extradural hematoma?

Ans. Collection of blood between the cranial bones and the dura mater is called extradural hematoma.

The extradural hematoma causes increase in intracranial pressure, distortion and herniation of brain with compression of brainstem. The source of bleeding may be:

- Rupture of the middle meningeal artery due to fracture of the temporal bone
- Fracture bone edges
- Tearing of dural venous sinuses.

Q. What are the features of extradural hematoma?

Ans. Patients with extradural hematoma may present in a number of ways:
- *Classical type*:
  - Deterioration in level of consciousness with or without lucid interval
  - Pupillary changes
  - Contralateral hemiplegia
  - Lucid interval is absent when patient has associated primary brain injury.
- *Subacute or chronic type*: Slow collection of hematoma.
  - Lucid interval is prolonged to days or weeks
  - During this period, patient is irritable, confused and has headache.
- *Hyperacute type*:
  - Lucid interval is short
  - Patient is extremely restless, talkative and violent, but remains conscious
  - Afterwards within an hour or so patient lapses into deep coma and may die rapidly.

Q. What investigations may help in diagnosis of extradural hematoma (EDH)?

Ans.
- *Plain X-ray of skull*: It may demonstrate skull fracture.
- *CT scan of brain*:
  - Appears as a biconvex or planoconvex zone of increased density adjacent to the inner table of the skull
  - There may be midline shift.

Q. How will you treat EDH?

Ans.

- If the EDH is localized by CT scan, a burr hole is to make at the appropriate site.
- This is done under general anesthesia with endotracheal intubation. In desperate situation, this can be done under local anesthesia.
- The burr hole is made at the appropriate site. Once the burr hole is made, the hematoma bulges out. The burr hole enlarged by either doing a craniectomy or raising a bone flap with multiple burr holes. The hematoma is evacuated, the source of bleeding is looked for and the bleeding point controlled with diathermy or suture ligation.
- The dura is opened only if there is associated underlying subdural hematoma (SDH).
- The dura mater is then hitched up all around the margins of the bony defect with atraumatic stitches passing through the dura mater and the adjacent pericranium.
- Bone flap is replaced and the scalp wound is closed.
- Postoperative care to prevent metabolic, respiratory and infective complications.

Q. When will you consider exploratory burr hole without CT scan?

Ans.

- In desperate situation with rapid neurological deterioration, urgent operation may be considered without CT scan.
- Exploratory burr hole is done toward the side of fracture, as this is the most likely side of EDH. If there is no fracture, a burr hole is done toward the side of first dilated pupil.

A temporal burr hole is done first. If this is negative, a frontal and parietal burr hole is done next. If there is no clot in any of these sites, the same procedure is done on the opposite side.

Q. What are the features of subdural hematoma?

Ans. The diagnosis of SDH is often difficult and needs a high degree of suspicion for clinical diagnosis.

- Patient may become unconscious from the time of injury or there may be gradual deterioration of level of consciousness or rarely there may be a lucid interval.
- Patient may become increasingly restless.
- There may be focal or generalized convulsion.
- There may be true localizing signs—ipsilateral dilated nonreacting pupil or contralateral motor weakness.
- The false localizing signs include—contralateral pupillary dilatation and ipsilateral motor weakness due to Kernohan's notch.

Q. What investigations may help in diagnosis of SDH?

Ans.

- Plain X-ray of skull—may show skull fracture.
- *CT scan of brain*: Acute SDH appears a hyperdense crescentic-shaped lesion that follows the curvature of the brain.
- *Angiography*: Indicated when facility for CT scan is not there. An acute SDH produces an avascular space between the vascularized brain and the skull.
- Exploratory burr hole.

Q. How will you treat acute subdural hematoma?

Ans.
- Initial resuscitation.
- When the symptoms of acute SDH develop rapidly exploratory burr holes may be considered immediately without CT scan or angiography.
- Exploratory burr holes are done at temporal, frontal and parietal regions. Once dura is opened, fresh blood or blood clot escapes. The burr hole should be extended by wide craniectomy centered over the hematoma. The underlying contused brain parenchyma may need debridement. Proper hemostasis should be achieved at the end of operation. Hitch stitches are given between the dura mater and the adjacent pericranial tissues. Once the clot is evacuated, the source of bleeding is sought for and the bleeding point controlled with diathermy or suture. Bone flap is replaced and scalp wound closed.
- If the evolution of symptoms is slower, a CT scan is to be done to localize the hematoma and the placement of burr hole is planned accordingly.
- Postoperatively, patient is nursed in an intensive therapy unit with the head slightly elevated.
- Maintain airway and, if necessary, mechanical ventilation may be required.
- Treatment of cerebral edema with mannitol or diuretics.

3. **A person sustained chest injury following a road traffic accident and presented at emergency room with severe respiratory distress. How will you manage?**

Ans. The management of this patient will be as per ATLS protocol of management, which includes:
- Primary survey and resuscitation
- Secondary survey (*See* Page No. 681)
- Definitive treatment.

Before proceeding to secondary survey I will like to exclude life-threatening injuries like:
- *Tension pneumothorax*:
  - If tension pneumothorax is present, relieve it by inserting wide-bore needle in second ICS.
- *Massive hemothorax*—relieves by inserting a chest drainage tube.
- *Open pneumothorax*—managed immediately by an occlusive dressing sealing three sides and keeping one side open. Once chest tube is inserted, the wound is sealed on all sides.
- *Cardiac tamponade*:
  - If cardiac tamponade is present, needle cardiocentesis is to be done by inserting a wide-bore needle to the left of xiphisternum.

  After stabilization of the patient, a detail secondary survey is done.

History:
  - Nature of trauma, other symptoms like chest pain, hemoptysis and angina like pain
  - Symptoms due to injury to other regions.

Examination:

A detail examination from head to foot—see above.

- *Detail chest examination*:
  - *Inspection*:
    - Respiratory rate
    - Symmetry of chest
    - Chest wall contusion—any bruise or laceration or open wounds
    - Paradoxical respiration (flail chest)
    - Stove in chest (indented segment)
    - Movement of chest.
  - *Palpation*:
    - *Mediastinal shift*—position of trachea and apex beat
    - Tenderness (over the rib)
    - Palpable crepitus (surgical emphysema)
    - Movement of chest.
  - *Percussion*:
    - Normal resonance
    - Hyper-resonance (pneumothorax)
    - Dullness on percussion (hemothorax).
  - *Auscultation*:
    - Breath sound present or absent
    - Any added sound.

Q. What investigation would you suggest for evaluation of chest injury?

Ans.
- Baseline investigations
- Chest X-ray—PA view.

A simple chest X-ray may show rib fracture, pneumothorax, or hemothorax.

- Contrast-enhanced computed tomography (CECT) scan in selected cases—useful in diagnosis of tracheobronchial and esophageal injuries
- CT angiography—for definite diagnosis of aortic and great vessel injuries
- Arterial blood gas analysis
- Other investigations, if patient has other associated injury.

Q. What is the implication of first rib fracture?

Ans. First rib fracture is usually due to a severe violence. When first rib fracture is diagnosed, further investigations are required to exclude associated vascular or brachial plexus injury.

Q. What are the implications of lower rib fracture?

Ans. When there is fracture of 8th to 12th rib, further investigations are required to exclude liver, spleen, or kidney injury.

Q. How will you diagnose rib fracture?

Ans. The diagnosis of rib fracture is based on:
- Pain-aggravated on deep inspiration
- Splinting of chest wall during inspiration
- Prevention of adequate cough

* Tenderness on AP and lateral compression
* Routine chest X-ray may diagnose rib fracture.

Q. How will you treat isolated rib fracture?

Ans. Isolated rib fracture without underlying lung injury may be treated by:
* *Analgesics*—nonsteroidal anti-inflammatory drugs like diclofenac or aceclofenac
* Intercostal nerve block
* Respiratory physiotherapy
* There is no role of strapping of chest wall.

Q. How will you diagnose traumatic hemothorax?

Ans. Traumatic hemothorax is suggested by:
* Presence of shock
* Respiratory distress
* Chest pain
* Mediastinal shift to opposite side
* Restricted movement of hemithorax on affected side
* Dull percussion note
* Absent breath sounds.
The diagnosis is confirmed by a chest X-ray.

Q. What is the source of bleeding in traumatic hemothorax?

Ans.
* In most cases, bleeding is due to injury of intercostal vessels.
* Bleeding may be due to laceration of underlying lung.
* Rarely, major vessel injury.

Q. How will you treat traumatic hemothorax?

Ans. In traumatic hemothorax, the drainage of accumulated blood is essential as:
* Blood is a good culture media and infection of accumulated blood may lead to empyema.
* Accumulated blood may result in fibrosis.
Hemothorax requires drainage by insertion of a chest tube.

Q. What are the indications of thoracotomy in traumatic hemothorax?

Ans. Thoracotomy is indicated in following situations:
* Massive bleeding more than 1 liter of blood drains on insertion of chest tube.
* Brisk bleeding—bleeding more than 100 mL every 15 minutes for 1 hour.
* Continuous bleeding—bleeding more than 200 mL per hour over 3 hours.
* Associated major airway injury requiring thoracotomy.
  A posterolateral thoracotomy is done. The bleeding vessel identified and secured by ligation. Chest closed by placing an intercostal tube drain.

Q. How will you diagnose traumatic pneumothorax?

Ans. Traumatic pneumothorax is suggested by:
* Respiratory distress
* Mediastinal shift to opposite side

- Diminished movement of the hemithorax on affected side
- Hyperresonant percussion note on the affected side of the hemithorax
- Absent breath sounds.

Q. How will you treat traumatic pneumothorax?

Ans.

- *Tension pneumothorax*:
  - Immediate relief at emergency by inserting a wide-bore needle at second ICS at midclavicular line
  - Subsequently, a chest drainage tube is to be inserted through the second ICS or through the triangle of safety.
- Massive pneumothorax with collapsed lung needs intercostal tube drainage.
- Small pneumothorax with a partially expanded lungs may be treated with:
  - Analgesic
  - Chest physiotherapy
  - Antibiotics.

Q. What are the indications of thoracotomy in cases with traumatic pneumothorax?

Ans.

- Continuing air leak for more than 7 days
- Massive air leak suggesting major airway injury
- Associated lung contusion.

Q. What is tension pneumothorax?

Ans. A tension pneumothorax develops when "one-way valve" air leak occurs through the lung or chest wall. Air is forced into the pleural cavity without any route of exit. There is complete collapse of the affected lung and there is shift of mediastinum to the opposite side, compressing the opposite lung.

There is also decrease of venous return to the heart.

The tension pneumothorax is clinically diagnosed by:

- Chest pain
- Respiratory distress and air hunger
- Increased JVP
- Mediastinal shifting ascertained by shifting of trachea and apex beat to the opposite side
- Tachycardia and hypotension
- Hyperresonant percussion note
- Unilateral absence of breath sounds.

Q. How will you manage tension pneumothorax?

Ans. This is a life-threatening condition and requires immediate relief by inserting a wide-bore needle through the second ICS at the midclavicular line.

Subsequently, a tube thoracostomy is required by placement of a chest drainage tube through the fifth ICS at the triangle of safety.

Q. How cardiac tamponade may occur following trauma?

Ans. Cardiac tamponade usually occurs following penetrating chest trauma. However, cardiac tamponade may also occur following high-speed blunt trauma.

Accumulation of even 15–20 mL of blood in pericardial cavity may result in features of shock due to inadequate cardiac filling.

Q. How will you diagnose cardiac tamponade?

Ans.
- History of penetrating or high-speed blunt to the central chest
- Beck's triad:
  - Hypotension
  - Distended neck veins
  - Muffled heart sounds
- Pulsus paradoxus
- Kussmaul's sign—raised JVP during inspiration.

Q. What investigations help in diagnosis?

Ans.
- Chest X-ray—globular heart
- ECG—low-voltage complexes
- Focused abdominal sonogram for trauma (FAST)—fluid in pericardial cavity.

Treatment:
- Pericardiocentesis
- Thoracotomy and percardiotomy and tackling of injured vessels.

Q. What is flail chest?

Ans. When more than two ribs are fractured at two or more places on one side of the chest or on either side of the sternum then a segment of the chest wall may lie separated from the rest of the chest wall and this flail segment moves paradoxically during respiration. There is disruption of the stability and normal respiratory mechanics of the rib cage.

Q. Why there is paradoxical movement of the flail segment?

Ans. Inspiration is an active process—the intercostal muscles contract, the diaphragm descends, there is expansion of the chest cavity resulting in negative intrathoracic pressure, and air is drawn in. During expiration, which is a passive process, the chest wall recoils and air is exhaled out.

The flail segment of the chest wall lies loose from the rest of the rib cage. During inspiration, the flail segment does not move outward along with the rest of the chest wall instead the flail segment is drawn inwards due to the negative intrathoracic pressure. During expiration, the chest recoils and this results in a positive intrathoracic pressure, so the flail segment is pushed outwards. This reverse movement of the flail segment during the phases of respiration is called paradoxical movement of the flail segment.

As the flail segment is drawn inwards during inspiration, this prevents expansion of the underlying lung, interfering with gaseous exchange in that segment of lung and results in a right to left shunt leading to hypoxemia.

Q. What is central flail chest?

Ans. When there is fracture of ribs on either side of the sternum resulting in a flail segment of sternum is called central flail chest or sternal flail chest.

Q. What is lateral flail chest?

Ans. When there is fracture of multiple ribs on one side resulting in a flail segment on one side of the chest is called a lateral flail chest.

Q. What is minor flail chest?

Ans. If the flail segment is small and does not interfere with respiration and does not cause alteration of ABG analysis, it is called a minor flail chest.

Q. How will you manage minor flail chest?

Ans.

- Patient should be treated in an intensive therapy unit
- Analgesics
- Respiratory physiotherapy and incentive spirometry
- Serial ABG analysis.

    Patient usually gets stabilized in 2–3 weeks. Some cases may require ventilatory support, if there is deterioration and if there is development of hypoxemia.

Q. What is major flail chest?

Ans. The flail segment is large and interferes with respiration resulting in alteration of blood gas analysis reading to hypoxemia and hypercarbia.

Q. How will you manage major flail chest?

Ans.

- Patient should be treated in an intensive therapy unit.
- Patient needs intermittent positive pressure ventilation (IPPV) for about 2–3 weeks.
- The flail segment gets stabilized in 2–3 weeks time.
- General care:
    - Intermittent suction
    - Care of skin
    - Antibiotics
    - Bowel and bladder care
    - Maintenance of nutrition.
- Routine fixation of flail segment is not required. However, if there are other underlying injuries requiring thoracotomy, the flail segment can be fixed simultaneously.

Q. What is sucking wound in the chest?

Ans. A penetrating injury in the chest wall through the pleura is called a sucking wound in the chest. The underlying lung collapses, as air moves in through the open wound during inspiration and air moves out of the pleural cavity through the wound during expiration. This results in inadequate ventilation of the underlying lung resulting in a right-to-left shunt leading to hypoxemia and hypercarbia.

Q. How will you manage a sucking wound of the chest?

Ans. The wound is sealed with an occlusive dressing, which is taped on three sides and kept open on one side to allow expulsion of air from the pleural cavity but prevents sucking in of air into the pleural cavity.
* It is necessary to exclude underlying injury to lungs, heart, or major vessels.
* The wound is repaired and a chest drainage tube is inserted.

Q. What is stove in chest?

Ans. Fracture of multiple ribs at one point may cause indentation of a segment of chest wall without showing any paradoxical movement, this is called stove in chest.

4. **A 30-year-male patient sustained a road traffic accident presented with pain abdomen in emergency room with suspicion of abdominal injury. How will you proceed to manage this patient?**

Ans. I will follow ATLS protocol of management, which includes:
* Primary survey and resuscitation
* Secondary survey
* Definitive treatment.
  Life-threatening injuries like tension pneumothorax and cardiac tamponade should be excluded and appropriate measures taken.
  When patient is stable, I will proceed with secondary survey.
The secondary survey will include:
* *History*:
  – Details of the nature of the injury and time of injury.
  – In case of vehicular accident—enquire about the type of impact—frontal, lateral side swipe, rear impact, or roll over.
  – In penetrating injury—type of weapon used and the time of injury.
  – *Details about pain abdomen*: Site—localized or generalized, character of pain, any shifting or radiation, aggravating, or relieving factors.
  – Any episode of vomiting and its details.
  – Any history of hematemesis.
  – Any swelling in the abdomen.
  – Any history suggestive of renal injuries—hematuria/pain or swelling in the loin.
  – Any other injury in other parts of the body.
  – Any history of past medical illness—diabetes, hypertension, and current medications—steroid, antidiabetic drugs, or anticoagulants.

Examination of the patient: A detail head-to-foot examination is to be done:
* Examination of head, face, neck, chest, and extremities.

A detailed examination of abdomen:
* *Inspection*:
  – Inspect the anterior and posterior abdominal wall and the lower chest for any external injury—bruising or ecchymosis
  – Distension of abdomen

- Bruise or ecchymosis around umbilicus/flanks/left hypochondrium
- Any obvious bleeding
- Movement of abdomen—normal/restricted
- London sign (London sign is presence of imprint of clothing or a vehicle wheel on the abdominal wall and usually indicates a severe underlying injury).
- *Palpation*:
  - Temperature
  - Tenderness—suggests inflammation/hemoperitoneum
  - Hematoma or clots around liver, spleen, kidney—tender enlargement.
- *Percussion*:
  - Obliteration of liver dullness—suggest perforation of hollow viscera
  - Hepatic/splenic dullness
  - Free fluid in abdomen detected by shifting dullness.
- *Auscultation*:
  - Bowel sounds—normal/silent.
- Per rectal examination (per-vaginal examination in female patient).
- Examination of pelvis and perineum.

Investigations suggested:

- Once the patient is stable, relevant investigations should be done.

Apart from baseline investigations, the specific investigations include:

- Chest X-ray (PA view) may show:
  - Free gas under diaphragm
  - Rib injuries
  - Splenic injury—indicated by:
    - Homogenous opacity on left side of upper abdomen
    - Hematoma may compress or push fundal gas shadow
    - Elevation of left dome of diaphragm
    - Fracture ribs on left side of chest.
- Straight X-ray of abdomen (erect posture) may show:
  - Ground-glass appearance—in hemoperitoneum
  - Renal outline enlarged—in renal injuries/perinephric hematoma
  - Psoas shadow obliterated in hemoperitoneum
  - Homogenous opacity on right side—liver injury
  - Homogenous opacity on left side—splenic injury
  - Bony injury like vertebral fracture and pelvic fracture.
- X-ray of pelvis—for any fracture.
- Focused abdominal sonogram for trauma:
  - This is a rapid USG examination with four areas being scanned at the initial investigation
  - Scanning over the xiphisternal area to exclude pericardial collection causing cardiac tamponade
  - Scanning over the right and left upper quadrant to exclude fluid in hepatorenal pouch of Morrison and left subphrenic space
  - Scanning in the pelvis to exclude free fluid in the pelvic cavity.

- Diagnostic peritoneal lavage:
  - A method for diagnosing intraperitoneal injuries by infusing a liter of normal saline into peritoneal sac and analyzing the returning fluid.
- Contrast-enhanced CT scan of abdomen in selected cases—particularly solid visceral injury or retroperitoneal injury.
- Single shot IV urography in suspected cases of renal injury.
- Ascending urethrography in suspected case of urethral injury.
- Retrograde cystography in suspected case of bladder injury.
- Diagnostic laparoscopy.

Q. What is extended FAST (eFAST) examination?

Ans. Extended FAST (eFAST) involves additional examination of:
- Pleural movement to exclude pneumothorax
- Assessment of pleural cavity to exclude hemothorax.

Q. How diagnostic peritoneal lavage is done?

Ans.
- Patient supine
- Nasogastric tube and Foley's catheterization
- Antiseptic dressing and draping of subumbilical area
- The subumbilical area is infiltrated with 1% lignocaine
- A 1-cm vertical skin incision is made in the subumbilical region
- The incision is carried down to the linea alba and the peritoneum is incised
- A 16-Fr Ryle's tube is inserted into the peritoneal cavity toward the pelvis
- If more than 10 mL of blood is aspirated, DPL is said to be positive
- If no blood is aspirated, 1 liter of normal saline is infused through the catheter into the peritoneal cavity
- The patient is turned to right, left, and head up and down, so that the fluid is distributed throughout the whole peritoneal cavity
- The saline bottle is lowered to the ground and the infused normal saline retrieved by siphonage. About 75% of infused fluid should be retrieved.
- The fluid is examined:
  - Macroscopically (for presence of blood, bile, or undigested food particles)
  - Microscopically [for red blood cell (RBC) and white blood cell (WBC)]
  - Biochemically (for amylase and alkaline phosphatase).

Q. What are the criteria to decide that DPL is positive?

Ans. The criteria are as follows:
- *Aspirate the catheter*: If there is more than 10 ml blood or intestinal contents—DPL is positive.
- *Lavage fluid*: Criteria for a positive DPL are:
  - RBC—more than 100,000/mm^3
  - WBC—more than 10,000/mm^3
  - Lavage fluid amylase—more than 20 IU/L, and alkaline phosphatase more than 3 IU/L
  - Lavage fluid containing bile
  - Lavage fluid containing undigested food particles and bacteria.

Q. What are the limitations of DPL?

Ans. The limitations of DPL are as follows:
- This is an invasive investigation.
- DPL could not identify the source of bleeding.

  As most solid organ injury with hemoperitoneum is managed conservatively, so the specificity of DPL for operative intervention is low.

Treatment of blunt abdominal trauma:

The treatment of abdominal injury comprises:
- Resuscitation of shock
- Definitive management—depending on the type of injury.

Q. When will you consider immediate laparotomy in patients with blunt trauma abdomen?

Ans. Urgent laparotomy is indicated in following situations:
- Overt features of peritonitis or massive hemoperitoneum
- Diagnostic peritoneal lavage is positive and patient is hemodynamically unstable.
- Hemodynamically unstable patient with equivocal DPL
- Hemodynamically unstable patient—CT scan abdomen showing major solid visceral injury
- Chest X-ray showing free gas under diaphragm suggesting perforation of a hollow viscus.

Q. What incision will you prefer for laparotomy in abdominal trauma?

Ans. A midline incision is preferred for exploration. Provide good exposure for majority of the abdominal contents. If required may be extended and may be continued up as a median sternotomy.

Q. How will you do laparotomy in blunt trauma abdomen?

Ans. Once peritoneal cavity is entered by a midline incision, the exploration of the abdomen is done in a systematic manner.
- The aim is to reduce blood loss, reduce contamination, prevent iatrogenic injury, and prompt identification of site of injury.
- The small bowel is delivered out of the abdomen and gross blood evacuated.
- Packs are placed in right upper quadrant, left upper quadrant, and both lower quadrant.
- Blood pressure may drop once the abdomen is opened and this maneuver is done.
- Allow anesthetist to manage this BP drop.
- Once the patient is stabilized, the exploration of the abdomen starts.
- The whole of small gut is delivered out of the abdomen.
- The packs around the liver and spleen are kept. The other packs are removed sequentially and any blood evacuated and any bleeding site controlled by a clamp and ligature.
- The gastrointestinal (GI) tract is examined in an orderly fashion. The anterior surface of the stomach is examined from esophagogastric junction to the pylorus. The posterior aspect of the stomach is examined by entering the lesser sac after division of greater omentum. At the same time, examine the anterior surface of the pancreas.
- In suspected duodenal injury—kocherize the duodenum and C loop of duodenum examined. At the same time, examine the head of the pancreas.

- The examination of the small intestine starts at the duodenojejunal flexure and the whole small intestine is examined up to the ileocecal valve. Both side of the small intestine and the mesentery are properly inspected.
- The colon is inspected from the cecum to ascending colon, transverse colon, descending colon, sigmoid colon, and the rectum.
- Finally, the packs around the liver and spleen are removed sequentially and bleeding points are localized and managed.
- After exploration of the peritoneal cavity, the retroperitoneum needs to be explored for any suspected injuries.
- The retroperitoneum is divided into number of zones as follows:
  - *Zone 1*—central zone—bounded laterally by the kidneys and above up to the diaphragm and below up to the bifurcation of the aorta
  - *Zone 2*—comprises the lateral area of the retroperitoneum on either side, which extends from the kidneys to the paracolic gutter
  - *Zone 3*—the area of the pelvis.
- The need for exploration of the retroperitoneal hematoma will be one which is expanding and is pulsatile.
- The pelvis is examined for rectal and urogenital injury.
- The whole process of inspection may be repeated.

5. **A man has sustained blunt trauma abdomen and has the suspicion of splenic injury. How will you manage?**

Ans. The initial management is as described for abdominal trauma:
- Primary survey and resuscitation
- Secondary survey—details history, examination, and relevant investigations
- Definitive management.

Q. What are the types of splenic injury?

Ans. Types of splenic injury:
- Subcapsular hematoma
- Laceration of spleen
- Polar tear
- Avulsion of splenic pedicle.

Q. What are the different clinical presentations of splenic injury?

Ans. Patient may present with:
- Classical features of splenic injuries:
  - Seen in case with severe injuries and polar tear.
- *Silent*:
  - History of abdominal trauma with impact on left upper quadrant
  - There may be slight pain abdomen with no other symptoms and signs
  - The splenic injury is diagnosed by USG.
- *Delayed rupture of spleen*:
  - Seen in subcapsular hematoma when there is mild left hypochondriac pain with no symptoms or signs at initial presentation and the injury is often missed.

After 7–14 days, the hematoma grows and ruptures—patient presents with symptoms and signs of intraperitoneal hemorrhage.

Q. What are the classical features of major splenic trauma?

Ans. The manifestations of splenic trauma may be:

- *General symptoms and signs of internal hemorrhage:*
  - Pallor
  - Tachycardia
  - Hypotension
  - Restlessness
  - Sweating
  - Deep and sighing respiration
  - Cold and clammy extremities
  - Collapsed veins.
- *Abdominal symptoms and signs of splenic rupture:*
  - There may be cutaneous bruising in the left upper quadrant of abdomen
  - Increasing left upper abdominal pain and tenderness
  - Increasing left upper abdominal rigidity
  - Increasing abdominal distension
  - Diminished or absent bowel sounds
  - Kehr's sign may be present—elevation of the foot end of the bed causes pain in the left shoulder
  - Ballance's sign—fixed dullness in the left flank due to clotted blood around the spleen and shifting dullness in the right flank due to unclotted blood in the peritoneal cavity.

Q. Which investigations may help in diagnosis of splenic trauma?

Ans.

- *Complete hemogram:* Initially Hb percentage may be normal for 6 hours, as hemodilution does not occur. Leukocytosis may be present.
- Straight X-ray of abdomen with both domes of diaphragm, findings may be:
  - Increase in splenic shadow with haziness
  - Obliteration of left psoas shadow
  - There may be indentation of fundic gas shadow
  - Left colonic gas shadow is displaced downwards
  - Free fluid between gas-filled intestinal coils
  - Associated rib fractures on left side
  - Elevation of left dome of diaphragm
  - Basal pleural effusion on left side.
- Ultrasonography of abdomen is investigation of choice. It can diagnose:
  - Small tear
  - Subcapsular hematoma
  - Free blood in peritoneal cavity.
- CT scan of abdomen, if USG is inconclusive and there is strong suspicion of injury. CT scan of abdomen is done for diagnosis of small tear.
- Diagnostic peritoneal lavage:
  - Positive in splenic trauma with intraperitoneal hemorrhage.

Q. What are the grades of splenic injury?

Ans. These are as follows:
* *Grade I:*
  - *Hematoma*—subcapsular, nonexpanding, and less than 10% surface area
  - *Laceration*—capsular tear, nonbleeding, and less than 1 cm parenchymal depth.
* *Grade II:*
  - *Hematoma*—subcapsular, nonexpanding, and 10–50% surface area
  - *Intraparenchymal hematoma*—nonexpanding and less than 5 cm in diameter
  - *Laceration*—capsular tear, active bleeding, 1–3 cm parenchymal depth, and not involving a trabecular vessel.
* *Grade III:*
  - *Hematoma*—subcapsular more than 50% surface area or expanding. Ruptured subcapsular hematoma with active bleeding
  - *Intraparenchymal hematoma* more than 5 cm or expanding
  - *Laceration*—more than 3 cm parenchymal depth or involving trabecular vessels.
* *Grade IV:*
  - *Hematoma*—ruptured intraparenchymal hematoma with active bleeding
  - *Laceration*—laceration involving segmental or hilar vessel with major devascularization (>25% of spleen).
* *Grade V:*
  - *Laceration*—completely shattered spleen
  - *Vascular*—hilar vascular injury with complete devascularization of spleen.

Q. How will you treat subcapsular hematoma of spleen?

Ans. If there is no other injuries requiring laparotomy, the subcapsular hematoma of spleen may be managed successfully with conservative treatment.
* Patient should be treated in an intensive therapy unit
* Adequate fluid replacement—IV/orally, if no vomiting
* Parenteral antibiotics
* Blood requisitioned and reserved
* Intensive monitoring is the most important part of conservative management
* *Clinically*: Pulse, BP, and respiration should be checked every hour
* *Laboratory*: Serial hematocrit
* *Radiological*: Serial USG (every 24 hours).
   If the patient is stable, hematoma is not increasing and shows signs of regression conservative treatment may be continued.
   If the hematoma is expanding and there is evidence of free intraperitoneal rupture, immediate laparotomy should be done.

Q. What are the indications of conservative treatment in splenic trauma?

Ans. Nonoperative management (NOM) of splenic injuries is well established. Conservative treatment may be offered in:
* Hemodynamically stable patients
* No overt symptoms and signs of peritonitis
* There are no other indications for laparotomy may be offered conservative treatment.

Q. What are the situations where conservative treatment may fail?

Ans.
- High-grade injuries
- Large hemoperitoneum
- Contrast extravasation
- Pseudoaneurysm.

Q. What are the indications of laparotomy in splenic trauma?

Ans. The indications are:
- Severe degree of splenic injury with symptoms and signs of intraperitoneal hemorrhage
- Minor splenic injury associated with other intra-abdominal injury requiring laparotomy
- Failure of conservative treatment of splenic injury.

Q. How will you manage splenic injury on exploratory laparotomy?

Ans. Earlier the dictum for treatment of splenic injury was splenectomy. In view of serious postsplenectomy complications, the recent trend is to conserve spleen unless the organ is extensively shattered and bleeding is uncontrollable.
- *Small capsular tear:*
  - Control bleeding with local hemostatic agent like oxidized regenerated cellulose (surgical) or fibrin glue
  - If it fails splenorrhaphy, the bleeding from the splenic tear may be controlled with a series of mattress suture
  - Polar tear may be managed with partial splenectomy.
- *Extensive laceration or avulsion of splenic pedicle*—splenectomy is to be done.

If splenectomy is done, a portion of the spleen (six pieces of 40 × 40 × 3 mm) may be reimplanted within the leaf of greater omentum (splenic slice graft).

Q. How will you mobilize the spleen during emergency splenectomy?

Ans. To ensure repair or removal of spleen (partial or total) the spleen should be mobilized well, so that it can be brought out of the abdominal incision without tension.

An incision is made along the white line of Toldt along the left colic flexure and the incision is taken up along the lateral border of the spleen cephalad up to the esophagus. The spleen along with the pancreas is mobilized medially by dividing the leinorenal ligament. Any bleeding from the splenic vessels may be controlled by manual compression at the hilum of the spleen till the spleen is mobilized and brought out of the abdominal wound.

Once the spleen is mobilized, the spleen may be repaired or splenectomy done by dividing the splenic vessels.

Q. What are the complications of splenectomy?

Ans. The complications are:
- *Bleeding*—loosening ligature of splenic vessels, and bleeding from a missed short gastric artery or from the surface of the repaired spleen
- Left basal atelectasis
- Pleural effusion
- Gastric fistula due to greater curvature injury while ligating short-gastric vessels

- Pancreatic fistula due to damage to tail of pancreas
- Thrombocytosis is the rule following splenectomy. There is risk of thrombosis, if the platelet count goes above 1,000,000/mm³ and patients need prophylaxis against thrombosis with unfractionated heparin or low-molecular weight heparin (LMWH)
- *Subphrenic abscess*—may need percutaneous drainage
- Overwhelming postsplenectomy infection (OPSI).

Spleen is the crucial site for production of opsonin and properdin that helps in phagocytosis of encapsulated bacteria. Following splenectomy the most common form of OPSI is pneumococcal or meningococcal septicemia. In addition, infection with *Haemophilus influenzae* is also common.

Diagnosis of OPSI:
- Infection starts insidiously, but rapidly develops into a fulminant infection
- Fever, vomiting, dehydration, and circulatory collapse may occur
- Hemogram—shows leukocytosis
- Blood culture may show the organisms.

Treatment of OPSI:
- Intravenous fluid
- Broad spectrum parenteral antibiotics.

Prophylaxis against OPSI:
- Antibiotic prophylaxis using—penicillin, erythromycin, or amoxicillin and co-amoxiclav combination
- Vaccination against *Pneumococcus* and *H. influenzae*—one dose in the immediate preoperative period and needs to be repeated every 10 years.

6. **A 40-year-male patient presented to emergency with blunt trauma abdomen. He is suspected to have sustained liver injury. How will you manage?**

Ans. Only a major violence usually leads to liver injury as it is well protected and in 80% of cases of liver injury associated other intra-abdominal injuries are present.

General management is same as for management of blunt trauma abdomen.
- Primary survey involves maintenance of airway, breathing, and circulation.
- Secondary survey includes details history, clinical examination, and relevant investigations.
- Definitive management depends on the type of liver injury and presence of other associated injuries.

Q. What are the grades of liver injury?

Ans. These are:
- *Grade I:*
  - *Hematoma*: Subcapsular, nonexpanding hematoma less than 10% surface area
  - *Laceration*: Capsular tear, nonbleeding less than 1 cm of parenchymal depth.
- *Grade II:*
  - *Hematoma*: Subcapsular, nonexpanding hematoma, 10–50% surface area. Intraparenchymal hematoma, nonexpanding less than 10 cm in diameter
  - *Laceration*: Capsular tear, active bleeding, and 1–3 cm parenchymal depth.

- *Grade III*:
  - *Hematoma*: Subcapsular hematoma more than 50% surface area or expanding, ruptured hematoma with active bleeding. Intraparenchymal hematoma more than 10 cm in diameter or expanding.
  - *Laceration*: Parenchymal laceration more than 3 cm depth.
- *Grade IV*:
  - *Hematoma*: Ruptured intraparenchymal hematoma with active bleeding
  - *Laceration*: Parenchymal disruption involving 25–75% of hepatic lobe or 1–3 couinaud segment within a single lobe.
- *Grade V*:
  - *Hematoma/laceration*: Parenchymal disruption involving more than 75% of hepatic lobe or more than 3 couinaud segment in one lobe
  - Injuries of major hepatic veins or juxtahepatic vena cava.
- *Grade VI*:
  - *Vascular injury*: Hepatic avulsion.

Q. How will you diagnose liver injury?

Ans.

- Severe crushing injury in the right lower chest with fracture ribs or to the right upper quadrant of abdomen may be associated with liver injury
- Penetrating or missile injury in the right upper quadrant
- Symptoms and signs are similar to splenic injury except that the pain and rigidity will be in the right upper quadrant of abdomen.

Investigations for diagnosis of liver trauma:

- *FAST: The initial investigation for all trauma patients is FAST*. FAST-positive patient with hemodynamic instability and patient with penetrating injury with FAST positive should undergo urgent laparotomy
- *CECT scan:* FAST-positive patient with hemodynamic stability should undergo CECT scan. The CT scan is helpful for diagnosis of solid organ injury and may accurately grade the injury
- Diagnostic peritoneal lavage—largely replaced by FAST
- Baseline hemogram.

Q. What are the indications of conservative treatment of hepatic injuries?

Ans. Patients with grade III or higher should be admitted in surgical intensive care unit.

- In majority of hepatic injuries bleeding stops spontaneously
- Majority—about 80% of hepatic injuries are now treated by nonoperative means (NOM)
- Patient hemodynamically stable on admission
- Achievement of hemodynamic stability with a modest volume of IV fluid
- Neurologically stable patient
- Not requiring excessive blood transfusion for hepatic injury
- No other injury, which requires laparotomy.

Conservative treatment of hepatic injury includes:

- Intravenous fluids infusion
- Blood transfusion, if required
- Analgesics

* Antibiotics
* Intensive monitoring every hour:
  - Pulse, BP, respiration, and abdominal signs
  - Serial contrast CT scan or ultrasonography to assess the progress of hematoma or to assess continuing bleed. Free contrast in and around the liver indicates continuous bleed.

Q. What are the indications of surgery for hepatic trauma?

Ans. These are:
* Laparotomy is indicated for persistent or recurrent bleeding
* Shocked patient with a distended or distending abdomen
* Temporary response to IV fluid followed by hemodynamic instability
* Failure of conservative treatment due to ongoing or recurrent bleeding
* Associated injury requiring laparotomy
* Penetrating abdominal injury with peritoneal penetration and hemodynamic instability
* Patient with contrast extravasation into the peritoneal cavity on CT scan may require laparotomy.

Q. On exploratory laparotomy and evacuation of hemoperitoneum, a minor liver injury is found which is not bleeding. What to do?

Ans. The strategy in such situation is not to explore the hematoma.

Q. On exploration there is minor liver injury, which is actively bleeding, what to do?

Ans. The strategy in such situation is to compress the fracture and maintain the compression for 20 minutes. If the bleeding stops, the fracture sites should not be opened.

Q. How will you achieve temporary control bleeding from hepatic injury?

Ans. The temporary control of bleeding may be achieved by:
* Manual compression by laparotomy pads
* Perihepatic packing—by laparotomy pads
* Pringle maneuver—by finger compression or by applying a vascular clamp.

Q. In which situation, perihepatic packing cannot control bleeding?

Ans. Following packing if the bleeding is continuing then bleeding may occur from hepatic artery, portal vein, or retrohepatic inferior vena cava (IVC).

Q. What may be the sequelae of perihepatic packing?

Ans. Although perihepatic packing may control bleeding, there may be some ill effects of packing:
* Excessive packing may compress the IVC resulting in decrease of venous return and cardiac output
* Hypovolemic patient may not tolerate the resultant decrease in cardiac output
* Excessive packing may splint the diaphragm higher up and may reduce tidal volume.

Q. How long Pringle maneuver may be continued?

Ans. For Pringle maneuver, the lesser omentum is opened up and a long vascular clamp is applied from the left side occluding all the portal structures.

The Pringle maneuver may be continued for a warm ischemia time of 30 minutes. Another alternative is to apply clamp for 15 minutes and release intermittently for 5 minutes.

Q. If Pringle maneuver could not control the bleeding, what may be the site of injury?

Ans. Effective Pringle maneuver controls bleeding from hepatic artery and portal vein. If bleeding continues with Pringle maneuver, the bleeding may be either form hepatic venous injury or juxtaheaptic IVC.

Q. How bleeding from inferior vena cava injury may be managed?

Ans. Bleeding from juxtahepatic vena cava may be controlled with perihepatic packing. If not controlled with packing, complex intervention is required. Hepatic vascular isolation may be achieved with venovenous bypass.

Clamps are applied at superior vena cava and suprahepatic vena cava.

An 18-Fr catheter is placed in the IVC via the femoral vein and 12-Fr catheter is placed into the superior mesenteric vein via the inferior mesenteric vein. A 22-Fr catheter is placed into the internal jugular vein. A centrifugal pump delivers the blood from IVC and portal venous system to the internal jugular vein. Pringle maneuver is achieved by applying a vascular clamp at epiploic foramen occluding the hepatic artery and portal vein.

All these techniques are associated with high-operative mortality.

Q. How interventional radiology may help?

Ans. If there is massive bleeding for the liver injury, damage control surgery by perihepatic packing may be done. Patient is shifted to radiology suite. Bleeding from arterial injury may be controlled by embolization. In venous injuries, stents may be placed to bridge the injury site.

Q. What should be the operative strategy in patients with major liver injury and active bleeding, which could not be controlled by compression?

Ans.
- When compression fails to stop the bleeding then inflow occlusion is done by applying a noncrushing clamp in the hepatoduodenal ligament to occlude the hepatic artery and portal vein.
- If bleeding is controlled with inflow occlusion, then the possible source of bleeding is either hepatic artery or portal vein branches. Intermittent release of the clamp will allow to identify the site of bleeding, which may then be suture ligated. Direct suturing requires a good view into the depths of the injury.
- If bleeding could not be controlled by suturing, perihepatic packing would be the most prudent approach as a damage control measure. Patient is returned to ITU and re-explored after 24–36 hours when he is hemodynamically stable.
- On re-exploration, the pack is removed and bleeding reassessed.
  - There may be no bleeding and no evidence of necrosis or bile leaks. No resection is required in such situations.
  - The bleeding may stop, but there may be nonviable or macerated liver tissue, which requires debridement or nonanatomic resection.
  - If bleeding recurs on pack removal, decision is to be taken whether to repack or to do definitive procedure. If the patient's condition is stable nonanatomical or segmental liver resection may be done by an experienced surgeon.
  - If bleeding is not controlled by inflow occlusion then the likely source of bleeding is either hepatic vein or intrahepatic IVC injury.

Q. What is the role of hepatic resection in hepatic trauma?

Ans. In major hepatic trauma when other measures—packing, suture ligation fails hepatic resection may be considered. Only experienced surgeon may embark on major procedure like hepatic resection.

Nonanatomic resection removes the injured portion of the liver that is peripheral to the fracture line and the bleeding from the raw surface is controlled with suturing, or local hemostatic agents—argon beam laser, surgical, or fibrin glue.

Anatomic resection—right, left lobectomy, or segmentectomy is major procedure and is associated with increased mortality and morbidity and should be ventured by only experienced hepatobiliary surgeons.

Q. How will you manage subcapsular hematoma on exploration?

Ans.
* A small subcapsular hematoma should not be explored and left as such
* An expanding subcapsular hematoma or a large subcapsular hematoma, which is compressing the liver, needs to be explored. The large surface area of bleeding is difficult to control. The bleeding may be controlled with:
  - Application of local hemostatic agents
  - Suturing
  - Hepatic artery embolization or ligation.

Q. What is the role of angioembolization in liver trauma?

Ans. With advent of interventional radiology, some liver trauma patient may be managed with angioembolization.

Patient with bleeding requiring transfusion of 4 units of blood in 4 hours or 6 units of blood in 24 hours should undergo hepatic angiography and angioembolization.

Contrast extravasation on CT scan is also a candidate for hepatic artery embolization.

Q. Why there is coagulopathy in liver trauma?

Ans. Major liver trauma is often associated with coagulopathy:
* Dilutional effect of massive transfusion on platelets and coagulation factors
* Liver synthesizes procoagulants and anticoagulants and liver trauma combined with ischemia from hypotension and inflow occlusion has deleterious effect on hemostatic function and may lead to coagulopathy.

Q. What are the complications following hepatic trauma?

Ans. The complications are:
* *Deranged liver function test*—bilirubin, transaminase, alkaline phosphatase, and gamma-glutamyltransferase (GGT) level may raise. Serum albumin level may fall.
* External biliary fistula may occur due to minor or major ductal injury. Endoscopic retrograde cholangiopancreatography (ERCP) and stenting may allow healing. Development of delayed biliary stricture may require appropriate surgery at a later date.
* Hemobilia is a rare complication. Hepatic artery angiography and selective embolization may help.
* Subphrenic abscess and septicemia.
* Pulmonary complications.
* Multisystem organ failure.

7. **A 40-year-male patient has been admitted with blunt trauma abdomen and there is suspicion of pancreaticoduodenal injury. How will you manage?**

Ans. General management is same as described earlier.

Q. What are the important causes of pancreatic injury?

Ans.
- Road traffic accident
- Steering wheel injury
- Fall from height
- Hit by a bicycle handle or motorcycle handle
- Direct blow to epigastrium
- Penetrating injury.

Q. Why pancreatic injury is common at the neck?

Ans. When there is compression injury of the abdomen, the pancreas is compressed against the vertebral column and is commonly injured at the neck.

Q. What are the types of pancreatic trauma?

Ans. There are four types of pancreatic injuries as per Lucas classification:
- *Type I*: Minor contusion (small hematoma) with minimal parenchymal damage. Main Pancreatic duct intact.
- *Type II*: Major contusion, laceration, or transection, confined to body and tail of pancreas with or without ductal disruption.
- *Type III*: Major contusion, laceration, or transection involving head of pancreas with or without ductal disruption.
- *Type IV*: Combined pancreaticoduodenal injury.
  - A—duodenal injury with minor pancreatic injury
  - B—duodenal injury with severe pancreatic injury with duct disruption.

Q. What is AAST (American Association for the Surgery of Trauma) grading for pancreaticoduodenal injury?

Ans. *Pancreatic injury*:
- *Grade I*: Small hematoma, superficial laceration of pancreatic parenchyma, and no ductal disruption.
- *Grade II*: Large hematoma or major laceration without tissue loss, and no ductal disruption.
- *Grade III*: Ductal disruption or parenchymal laceration with ductal injury.
- *Grade IV*: Proximal laceration or parenchymal laceration involving the ampulla.
- *Grade V*: Massive disruption of the pancreatic head.

Duodenal injury:
- *Grade I*: Single segment hematoma and partial thickness laceration without perforation.
- *Grade II*: Multiple segment hematoma and laceration involving less than 50% circumference.
- *Grade III*: 50–75% disruption of second part of duodenum or 50–100% disruption of first, third, or fourth part of duodenum.

♦ *Grade IV*: 75–100% disruption of second part of duodenum or rupture of ampulla or distal common bile duct (CBD).
♦ *Grade V*: Massive duodenal and pancreatic injury and devascularization of duodenum.

Q. How will you diagnose pancreaticoduodenal trauma?

Ans.

♦ Diagnosis is very difficult, as there are no specific symptoms and signs of pancreatic injury. High index of suspicion is important for diagnosis of pancreatic injury.
♦ More than 80% cases are diagnosed during laparotomy for some other injuries.
♦ In patients without pressing need for laparotomy, diagnosis of pancreatic injury is suspected under the following circumstances:
  – History of impact in the upper abdomen.
  – Pain abdomen initially localized to upper abdomen later becoming generalized.
  – Abdominal wall bruising in the upper abdomen with a pattern of a solid object.
  – Unexpected deterioration 24–48 hours after admission in a previously stable patient.

Q. Which investigations are helpful for diagnosis of pancreaticoduodenal injury?

Ans. These are:

♦ Elevated serum amylase level
♦ USG is not very reliable for diagnosis of pancreatic trauma
♦ CT scan may show:
  – Fluid collection around the pancreas
  – Retroperitoneal hematoma or fluid
  – Intrapancreatic hematoma
  – Thickened renal fascia
  – May show fracture of the body or neck of pancreas
  – Magnetic resonance cholangiopancreatography (MRCP) or ERCP in selected cases may demonstrate duct disruption.

Q. What are CT findings in duodenal injury?

Ans.

♦ Presence of retroperitoneal air
♦ Contrast extravasation
♦ Adjacent fat stranding
♦ Duodenal wall thickening.

Q. What is the importance of repeat CT scan study for pancreaticoduodenal injury?

Ans. Often the initial CT scan done immediately after trauma may not reveal the changes found in pancreaticoduodenal injury. If the index of suspicion for pancreaticoduodenal injury is high a repeat CT scan should be done after 48 hours.

Q. What is the importance of serum amylase level?

Ans. Elevation of serum amylase level abdominal trauma is not diagnostic of pancreaticoduodenal injury. But high-serum amylase level is an indication of further investigation to exclude pancreaticoduodenal injury.

Q. How pancreatic ductal disruption may be diagnosed?

Ans. In suspected cases—ERCP or intraoperative pancreatogram may show extravasation of contrast material suggesting pancreatic ductal disruption.

MRCP is also emerging as a modality of investigation for diagnosis of ductal disruption.

Q. During laparotomy for abdominal trauma, peripancreatic hematoma is found. What should be done?

Ans. Peripancreatic hematoma even if small needs to be explored. The whole pancreas needs to be explored. The lesser sac is entered by opening the greater omentum. The right colic flexure is mobilized downwards to expose the duodenum and the head of the pancreas. The duodenum with the head of the pancreas is kocherized. The peritoneum at the lower border of the pancreas is incised to the left of superior mesenteric vessels and the posterior surface of the pancreas is examined.

Q. While doing laparotomy for other condition, when will you do complete assessment of duodenum and pancreas for any injury?

Ans. Thorough duodenal and pancreatic assessment for trauma should be done under following circumstances:
- Central retroperitoneal hematoma
- Pancreatic edema or peripancreatic fluid collection
- Fat saponification
- Retroperitoneal bile staining.

Q. How will you assess duodenum and pancreas for any injury on exploration?

Ans. For thorough assessment of the duodenum and pancreas, a full right visceral rotation is required. Kocherization of duodenum is done and duodenum with head of the pancreas is lifted medially. The right colon along with the terminal ileum is mobilized medially. The lesser sac is entered by dividing the gastrocolic ligament. The whole of the pancreas and duodenum may now be examined.

For assessment of the tail of the pancreas, the spleen along with the left colic flexure is mobilized medially by dividing the lienorenal ligament. This maneuver allows palpation of the posterior surface of the body of the pancreas.

Q. What is the strategy for treatment of pancreaticoduodenal injury?

Ans. When pancreaticoduodenal injury is associated with other life-threatening injury then principle of damage control surgery should be applied. Complex repair in a hemodynamically unstable patient is not worthwhile as it may be associated high rate of anastomotic failure. In first stage control, the bleeding and contamination and shift patient to ICU. Once the condition is stabilized patient is re-explored after 24–48 hours.

Q. What are the different options for surgical treatment of duodenal injury?

- Duodenal hematoma—one option is to explore, the hematoma incising the seromuscular coat.
- However, most hematomas resolve on conservative treatment.
- *Duodenal laceration*:
  - Simple closure after freshening the margin. The repair should be tension free and vascularity should be adequate. This is the most common repair done for duodenal injury

- In D1 injuries, if after debridement primary closure is not possible—Billroth I or Billroth II reconstruction may be done
- In D2 injuries, resection and primary anastomosis. If primary anastomosis is not possible Roux en Y duodenojejunostomy
- In D3 and D4 injuries, when primary repair is not possible—resection with primary anastomosis or Roux en Y duodenojejunostomy is to be done
- Whipple's pancreaticoduodenectomy is rarely indicated for complex pancreaticoduodenal injury.

Q. What adjunctive procedure is done along with duodenal injury repair?

Ans. Duodenal injury repair has the risk of leak and may result in fistula particularly following repair of high-grade injury. Some adjunctive procedure is recommended to overcome this problem. The concept is to divert the gastric, and the pancreaticobiliary flow from the site of duodenal repair.

- *Triple tube decompression*: Tube gastrostomy, tube duodenostomy, and a tube jejunostomy to divert flow away from the repair. This is now replaced by pyloric exclusion procedure
- *Pyloric exclusion procedure*: Repair of the duodenal injury, closure of pylorus from inside by a purse string suture using a nonabsorbable suture, and a gastrojejunostomy. Biliary drainage by inserting a tube in the bile duct, vagotomy and a feeding jejunostomy may also be added to this procedure. The pylorus eventually opens up after 2 weeks to 2 months and gastrojejunostomy also becomes nonfunctional.

Q. What are the indications of nonoperative treatment of duodenal injury?

Ans. The indications are:

- Grade I and Grade II injuries may be managed with conservative treatment
- Hemodynamically stable patient without features of peritonitis
- No associated injuries requiring urgent laparotomy
- Duodenal hematomas causing gastric outlet obstruction
- Endoscopic injury of duodenum.

Q. What are the indications of conservative treatment of pancreatic injury?

Ans. The indications of conservative treatment of pancreatic injury are:

- Hemodynamically stable patient with Grade I and Grade II injuries
- Patient needs close monitoring
- Conservative treatment may fail due to complications of pancreatic injury or associated missed which requires laparotomy.

Q. What are the options of surgical treatment of pancreatic injury?

Ans.

- *External drainage and hemostasis*: When laparotomy done for other indications and grade I or grade II pancreatic injury is found, the treatment is external drainage. The surface parenchymal laceration need not be sutured. A suction drain is placed in the lesser sac. The drain is removed when the fluid amylase becomes normal.
- *Distal pancreatectomy*: Distal parenchymal laceration with disruption of main pancreatic duct is best treated by distal pancreatectomy with or without conservation of spleen. The proximal

pancreatic stump is managed by suturing the pancreatic duct separately and closure of the proximal cut end of the pancreatic parenchyma by interrupted suture.

- *Extended distal pancreatectomy*: Injuries involving the pancreatic head with ductal disruption may be managed with an extended distal pancreatectomy. The proximal part of the gland closed with suture. If there is concern about very little residual pancreatic tissue, the proximal end may be suture closed and the healthy distal pancreatic tissue may be conserved and a Roux-en-y pancreaticojejunostomy may be done with the distal stump.
- *Damage control surgery*: Gross proximal pancreatic injury with a hemodynamically unstable patient with hypothermia, coagulopathy, and acidosis is best managed by damage control surgery. Wide external drainage achieved by placement of closed suction drain. Patient shifted to ICU and once stabilized by 24–48 hours, re-exploration is done for resection or reconstruction. Postoperative ERCP and pancreatic duct stenting may be an option.
- *Whipple pancreaticoduodenectomy*: In complex pancreaticoduodenal injury, rarely Whipple's operation may be required.

Q. What should be the optimal surgical treatment for different grades of pancreatic trauma?

Ans. *Grade I and grade II injuries (constitute about 75% of pancreatic injury)*: Minor contusion, hematoma, and parenchymal laceration without ductal injury:

- Best managed by achieving hemostasis external drainage by placement of drains
- Complete transection of the neck of pancreas is best treated with distal pancreatectomy.

Grade III injury—distal parenchymal laceration with ductal injury:

- Best managed by distal pancreatectomy with or without distal pancreatectomy.

Grade IV injuries: *Laceration of pancreatic head with ductal injury*:

- Pancreatic head injury is an extremely challenging situation. Pancreatic head injury with ductal disruption but intact ampulla and duodenum:
  - Extended distal pancreatectomy and suture closure of proximal pancreatic duct and pancreatic parenchyma at residual head of pancreas
  - Debridement of pancreatic tear. Closure of the proximal pancreatic duct and parenchymal closure of pancreatic head. The distal pancreas at body may be anastomosed to a Roux-en-Y loop of jejunum
  - Hemodynamically unstable patient with hypothermia acidosis is best managed with damage control surgery. Achieve hemostasis and place drains at the lesser sac.
  Re-exploration after 24–48 hours or alternatively consider ERCP and stenting of pancreatic duct.

Grade V injuries: *Combined pancreaticoduodenal injury or massive injury of pancreatic head*:

- Simple repair and external drainage with pyloric exclusion
- Pancreaticoduodenectomy (Whipple procedure) in selected cases
- In hemodynamically unstable patient, damage control surgery by external drainage and re-exploration after 24–48 hours.

Q. Following external drainage of pancreatic injury patient developed pancreatic fistula. How will you manage?

Ans.

* Pancreatic fistula is defined as measurable output in drain after 3rd postoperative day with fluid amylase 3 times the serum amylase level.
* Pancreatic fistula may develop in 25% of patients following external drainage for pancreatic injuries.
* Drainage between 100 mL and 300 mL should be allowed to continue with the drain left in place and majority of these fistulae close in 6–12-week time. The closure of the fistula may be hastened by a short course of octreotide for 5 days. The drain is removed when the fistula discharge becomes less than 30 mL per day and fluid amylase becomes normal. Premature removal of the drain may result in abscess formation.
* Drainage in excess of 300 mL per day is unlikely to close spontaneously. This is usually associated with major ductal disruption. If the fistula persists due to ductal disruption, this should be treated by internal drainage into a Roux-en-Y loop of jejunum.

Q. What are the complications of pancreaticoduodenal trauma?

Ans. There is high incidence of complications following pancreaticoduodenal injury. About 20–40% patients undergoing surgical treatment may have some postoperative complications.

* Duodenal fistula and stricture
* Pancreatic fistula
* Pancreatic abscess
* Pancreatitis
* Pancreatic pseudocyst
* Secondary hemorrhage
* Pancreatic exocrine insufficiency—steatorrhea
* Pancreatic endocrine deficiency—diabetes mellitus.

8. **A 40-year-male patient sustained abdominal trauma following a road traffic accident/assault and presented with pain in the right loin and hematuria. How will you manage?**

Ans. Gross hematuria following abdominal trauma indicates urinary tract injury. General management will be according to ATLS protocol of management:

* Primary survey and resuscitation
* Secondary survey
* Definitive management.

After primary survey and resuscitation, I will proceed with secondary survey. A detail history and clinical examination is essential for diagnosis of the nature of injury.

History:

* Detail history about type of injury and time of injury
* Hematuria—microscopic or gross hematuria. Progress—increasing or decreasing
* Pain—detail history about pain—site, character of pain, and radiation
* Any other symptoms due to associated injury.

General examination:

- To assess the degree of shock—pulse, BP, respiration, and temperature
- An examination from head to foot to exclude any other associated injury.

Local examination of abdomen:

- *Inspection*—perinephric ecchymosis or bruising, abdominal distension, and any swelling in the loin
- *Palpation*—muscle guard, or rigidity, tenderness, or any mass in the loin
- *Percussion*—free fluid in abdomen ascertained by shifting dullness, and obliteration of liver dullness suggesting free gas under the domes of diaphragm
- *Auscultation*—bowel sounds may be absent in patients with hemoperitoneum or peritonitis
- *Per rectal examination*—any fluid collection or tenderness in the pelvis.

Q. What investigations are helpful for diagnosis of renal trauma?

Ans. The investigations are as follows:

- Urine examination for gross or microscopic hematuria
- A contrast enhanced CT scan is the investigation of choice:
  - The grade of injury may be accurately diagnosed by CECT scan
  - Assess functional status of the affected and the contralateral kidney
  - Extent of injury
  - Extravasation of the contrast
  - Vascular injuries
  - Other associated injuries.
- A single-shot IV urography is very helpful, if there is no facility for CT scan:
  - Demonstrate the normal functioning opposite kidney
  - Functional status of the injured kidney, any dye extravasation.
- Ultrasonography of abdomen:
  - Demonstrate opposite normal kidney
  - Assessment of the injured kidney—enlargement, cortical tear, or perinephric hematoma.

Q. What are the grades of renal injury?

Ans. The types of renal injury depending on the severity are:

- *Grade I*: Subcapsular nonexpanding hematoma without parenchymal laceration
- *Grade II:* Cortical laceration less than 1 cm of parenchymal depth, no urinary extravasation, and contained perirenal hematoma
- *Grade III:* Cortical laceration more than 1 cm depth, no urinary extravasation
- *Grade IV:* Parenchymal laceration extending through the cortex, medulla, and collecting ductal system with urinary extravasation. Injury to main renal artery and vein with contained hemorrhage
- *Grade V*: Shattered kidney, avulsion of renal pedicle.

Q. What are the indications of conservative treatment for renal injuries?

Ans. 90–95% of renal injuries can be managed conservatively.

- Patient hemodynamically stable
- Hematuria is decreasing

- Perinephric hematoma not increasing
- No extravasation of contrast in CT scan.

The components of conservative treatment are:
- Bed rest
- Intravenous fluid and blood transfusion
- Analgesics
- Antibiotics
- Monitoring of patient—pulse, BP, serial urine examination, and perinephric hematoma assessment.

Q. What is the management for grade I and grade II renal injury?

Ans. These patients are usually hemodynamically stable. May present with gross or microscopic hematuria. The mainstay of treatment is conservative. Observe and continue bed rest till the urine is clear.

Q. What is the management for grade III, grade IV, and grade V renal injury?

Ans. Assess whether patient is hemodynamically stable or not and whether patient requires laparotomy for other injuries.

Hemodynamically unstable patient: Patient having expanding or pulsatile hematoma vascular grade IV injury in a solitary kidney or bilateral grade IV and V injury. Perform single-shot IV urography and perform exploratory laparotomy.

The aim of surgical treatment will be reconstruction of all renal units. In shattered kidney, where reconstruction is not possible and patient is exsanguinating from other injuries consider nephrectomy.

Hemodynamically stable patient: CECT scan with delayed films to grade the injury.

No associated injury requiring laparotomy:
- Conservative treatment for renal injury
- Intensive monitoring at ICU
- Bed rest till hematuria is present
- Observe for delayed bleeding
- In case of delayed bleeding—consider angiography and angioembolization
- If there is persistent urinary extravasation—consider ureteric stenting.

Laparotomy indicated for associated injury:
- Kidney injury explored
- Attempt reconstruction of renal units
- Nephrectomy in rare circumstances, as discussed above.

Q. What are the indications of exploration for renal trauma?

Ans. The indications of exploration for renal trauma are:
- *Absolute indications*:
  - Renal pedicle injury with persistent renal bleeding
  - Expanding or pulsatile perirenal hematoma.

- *Relative indications*:
  - Urinary extravasation
  - Nonviable tissue
  - Segmental arterial injury.

Q. How will you approach an injured kidney?

Ans. A transperitoneal approach is preferred to exclude other associated intra-abdominal injury and to have early control of the renal pedicle.

The renal pedicle is dissected and an umbilical tape passed around the renal vessels to control hemorrhage, once the Gerota's fascia is opened.

Q. What should be the extent of surgery for renal trauma?

Ans. The idea in renal trauma is to conserve as much renal tissue as possible.

In majority of cases, renorrhaphy is the treatment of choice except in grade V injury.

- *For renorrhaphy*:
  - The kidney is exposed completely
  - All nonviable tissues are debrided
  - Hemostasis obtained with chromic catgut sutures
  - Injured collecting system sutured
  - The cortical tear is repaired
  - The renal capsule is apposed.
- In cases with polar tear—a partial nephrectomy with removal of nonviable tissue, hemostasis, and closure of the collecting system. The raw area may be covered with an omental pedicle.
- Nephrectomy is reserved for:
  - Shattered kidney, which cannot be reconstructed
  - Renal injury along with other life-threatening injuries
  - Time taken for repair of renal injury will jeopardize the life of the patient in view of other injuries.

Q. What are the indications of nephrectomy in renal injuries?

Ans. Total nephrectomy is immediately indicated in extensive renal injuries when the patient's life would have been threatened by an attempted renal repair.

Grade V injuries with shattered kidney (nonreconstructible) may be treated by nephrectomy provided the other kidney is functioning normally.

Q. What are the complications of renal injury?

Ans. The complications are:
- Persistent urinary extravasation may result in an urinoma
- Infection of a perinephric hematoma—perinephric abscess
- Delayed bleeding
- Hypertension due to:
  - Renal vascular injury leading to stenosis of renal artery
  - Compression of renal parenchyma by the extravasated blood or urine
  - Post-traumatic arteriovenous fistula
  - Stimulation of renin angiotensin axis by relative renal ischemia.

9. **A male patient, aged 20 years, steps over a loose manhole cover. He falls only to be stopped by the edge of the everted manhole cover hitting him between his legs. Since then he is unable to pass urine. How will you manage?**

OR

A 20-year-male patient sustained pelvic injuries following a road traffic accident. Patient has been unable to pass urine since the accident. How will you proceed to manage?

Ans. If patient of road traffic accident management will be as per ATLS protocol:
- Primary survey and resuscitation
- Secondary survey
- Definitive management.

   If simple fall and hit by a manhole cover, it is usually a localized injury involving the bulbous urethra.

   In patient with pelvic fracture, usually the membranous urethra is ruptured.

Detailed history:
- About the nature of the accident
- Time of accident
- Whether passed urine or has the urge for passage of urine
- Any hematuria or bleeding per urethra
- Any swelling in the perineum
- Any symptoms related to other associated injuries.

General survey:
- To assess presence of shock, particularly in presence of fracture pelvis.

   A head-to-foot examination in patient with road traffic accident to exclude any associated injury.

Local examination:
- Any perianal hematoma
- Diffuse swelling in the perineum suggestive of extravasation
- Any bleeding per urethra.

Abdominal examination:
- To exclude any associated injury
- Tenderness in abdomen
- Free fluid in abdomen
- Urinary bladder full or not.

Per rectal examination:
- Position of prostate
- Fluid in rectovesical pouch.

Q. What is triad of urethral rupture?

Ans.
- Blood at the urethral meatus
- Inability to urinate
- Perianal hematoma.

Q. What are the types of urethral rupture and how will you differentiate?

Ans. Urethral rupture may be:
- Partial
- Complete.

It is difficult to differentiate a partial or complete rupture clinically. This may be diagnosed by retrograde cystourethrography.

In case of incomplete rupture, there is extravasation of the contrast, but some contrast passes into the bladder.

In complete rupture, there is extravasation of the contrast and no dye passes into the bladder.

Q. What are the grades of urethral injury?

Ans. The grades of urethral injury are as follows:
- *Grade I*: Contusion with blood at urethral meatus and normal urethrography
- *Grade II*: Stretch injury with elongation of urethra and normal urethrography
- *Grade III*: Partial rupture of urethra, extravasation at the site of injury, and urinary bladder visualized
- *Grade IV*: Complete transection with less than 2 cm urethral separation with extravasation of contrast on urethrography and urinary bladder not visualized
- *Grade V*: Complete transaction more than 2 cm urethral separation or extension into prostate or vagina.

Q. How will you treat a patient with suspected rupture urethra?

Ans.
- If rupture urethra is due to an associated fracture pelvis then patient will be in shock
- Resuscitation with IV fluid and blood transfusion
- If rupture urethra is suspected, patient is discouraged to pass urine
- A retrograde cystourethrogram is done to assess the type of urethral rupture
- If there is complete rupture of urethra:
  - A suprapubic cystostomy is done by percutaneous puncture
  - The definitive repair is planned after 3 months.
- In cases with incomplete rupture of urethra:
  - A gentle attempt is done to pass a 16-Fr Foley's catheter through the urethra. If the catheter can be passed successfully, patient is re-evaluated after 6–8 weeks
  - If urethral catheterization fails a suprapubic cystostomy is to be done by percutaneous puncture method.

Q. How will you evaluate the patient for definitive repair?

Ans. A descending cystourethrogram or a pericatheter ascending urethrogram is done to assess development of any urethral stricture and distance of the urethral defect.

Q. How will you treat traumatic urethral stricture?

Ans. The defect at the rupture site is bridged by scar tissue. The urethral stricture may be managed by:

+ *Endoscopic internal urethrotomy*—suitable for short-segment urethral stricture
+ Open surgical repair of urethral stricture:
  - Anastomotic urethroplasty is the procedure of choice
  - The site of the urethral scarring is approached through a perineal approach
  - The two ends are dissected and the scar tissue is excised
  - The ends are spatulated and an end-to-end anastomosis is done
  - An indwelling Foley's catheter is kept for 2 weeks.

10. A 25-year-female patient sustained severe burn injury. How will you manage?

Q. What measures you will take at the site of accident?

Ans. When seen at the scene of accident:

+ Remove her from source of heat to avoid further injury
+ Maintain airway—as victim may sustain respiratory tract burn due to inhalation of smoke or flame—maintenance of airway and breathing is essential before sending the patient to hospital
+ Start an IV line and start Ringer's lactate fluid infusion before sending her to hospital
+ If flame burn, there is a role of cold water lavage. Irrigating with copious amount of cold water or cold water sponging help in minimizing the depth of tissue damage due to the excessive temperature
+ Transport quickly to hospital.

On arrival at ER:

+ Like trauma management, primary survey and resuscitation is the first step by ABCDEF.
  - *A*: Maintenance of airway
  - *B*: Maintenance of breathing
  - *C*: Maintenance of circulation
  - *D*: Assessment of disability
  - *E*: Exposure in a controlled environment
  - *F*: Fluid resuscitation.
+ *Secondary survey*: A detailed history and a head-to-foot examination:
  - Detail history
  - About the mechanism of burn injury—flame burn or scald
  - Duration of contact
  - Time of accident
  - Pain
  - Respiratory distress
  - Any other injury
  - Any associated medical illness.

Examination:

+ Assess the surface area of burn by following the rule of 9

♦ Assess the depth of burn—superficial or deep burns

♦ Features of other injury, as patient might fall after sustaining burn.

So, a thorough head-to-foot examination is essential.

Q. How will assess the amount of burn area (Fig. 16.1)?

Ans. In adult, this is by following the rule of 9.

♦ Head and neck—9%

♦ Front of chest and abdomen—18%

♦ Back of chest and abdomen—18%

♦ Upper limbs—9% + 9%

♦ Lower limbs—18% + 18%

♦ Perineum—1%.

In children (Fig. 16.2):

♦ Head and neck—20%

♦ Upper limbs—9% + 9%

♦ Chest and abdomen—Front: 18% and Back: 18%

♦ Lower limbs—13% + 13%.

Q. What are the gradings for depth of burns?

Ans. Depending on the depth of burn, this may be:

♦ *First-degree burn:*
  – Involves only the epidermis—No blister, only erythema
  – Heals in 3–4 days by peeling off of the epidermis.

♦ *Second-degree burn may be:*
  – *Superficial dermal burn:*
    - Involves the upper layer of the dermis
    - Forms blisters and on removal of blisters, wound is pink, wet, sensitive, and blanches on pressure
    - Heals in 3 weeks by epithelialization.
  – *Deep dermal burn:*
    - Involves the reticular layer of the dermis
    - Forms blisters and on removal of the blister the wound is white, dry, and capillary refilling occurs slowly or absent
    - Heals in 3–9 weeks with scarring.

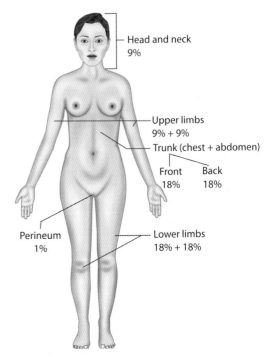

Fig. 16.1: Assessment of burn area in adult

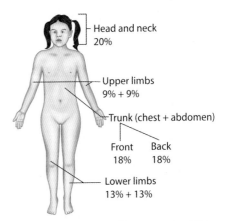

Fig. 16.2: Assessment of burn area in children

- *Third-degree burn or full thickness burn*:
  - Involves all the layers of the dermis
  - No blisters. The wound may be white, cherry red, or black and is leathery firm in feel, insensitive, and does not blanch on pressure
  - All epithelial elements are destroyed, and there is no potential for healing by epithelialization.
- *Fourth-degree burn*:
  - Involves all the layers of the skin, subcutaneous fat, and the variable amount of deeper structures
  - The wound is covered by a thick eschar.

Alternatively, the burns may also be classified as:
- *Superficial burn*—includes the first degree and the superficial dermal burns.
- *Deep burn*—involves the second degree deep dermal, third degree or full thickness burns, and the fourth degree burns.

Q. What are the different zones in a burn wound?

Ans. Jackson described three zones of a burn wound:
- *Zone of coagulation*: The central area of burn, most severely damaged, and cells undergo coagulative necrosis. This tissue needs debridement.
- *Zone of stasis*: Surrounding the area of coagulation necrosis is the zone of stasis where there is vasoconstriction and ischemia. Tissue in this zone is usually viable may become necrotic due to infection, edema, or decreased perfusion. With good wound care tissue in the zone of stasis remains viable.
- *Zone of hyperemia*: The outermost zone is the zone of hyperemia characterized by vasodilatation. Vasodilatation is due to release of local inflammatory mediators. The tissue in this area is viable.

Q. How will you assess depth of burns?

Ans. The depth of burns may be assessed by:
- Clinical observation of the wound as mentioned above
- Superficial burns are sensitive and are painful on pin-prick, whereas the deep burns are insensitive
- Assessment of blood flow by Doppler, or fluorescence in fluorometry, or thermography or MRI.

Q. What are the criteria for referring a burn patient to a specialized burn care unit?

Ans. Followings are the American burn association criteria for referral of a burn patient to a specialized burn care unit:
- Partial thickness burn of more than 10% of total body surface area
- Third-degree burns
- Electrical burns
- Chemical burns
- Inhalational injury
- Burn injury with pre-existing comorbid medical illness
- Burns with concomitant trauma.

Q. What are the causes of burns shock?

Ans.
- *Hypovolemic shock*—increased capillary permeability due to burn injury causes exudation of fluid out of the intravascular compartment and there is marked increase in extracellular fluid. The maximum fluid shift occurs in the first 8–12 hours. The decrease in intravascular volume is the most important aspect of burns shock
- *Psychogenic shock*—due to severe pain
- *Septicemic shock*—due to secondary infection of the burn wound.

Q. How will you treat burn shock?

Ans.
- Treatment of hypovolemic shock due to burn is managed primarily with IV fluid administration. The fluid is required to replace the intravascular fluid loss
- Relief of pain with IV narcotic analgesics
- Suitable antibiotics for infection.

Q. How will you calculate the amount of fluid required for resuscitation?

Ans. The amount of fluid required depends on the area of burn and weight of the patient. There are various formulae for calculating the fluid required.
- *Modified Parkland formula*:
  - Lactated Ringer's solution 4 mL/kg% burn in 24 hours
  - 50% of fluid in first 8 hours and rest 50% in next 16 hours
  - Idea of volume replacement is to maintain adequate tissue perfusion
  - The adequacy of fluid replacement may be assessed by monitoring:
    - Pulse
    - Blood pressure
    - Urinary output. A urinary output of 50 mL/h (or 0.5–1 mL/kg body wt/h) indicate adequate hydration.
- An alternative regime for fluid replacement is to infuse Ringer's lactate 1 L/h.
- Check vitals, pulse, BP, and monitor urine output
- The rate of fluid replacement is adjusted to maintain a urinary output of 30–50 mL/h.

Q. How do you plan fluid therapy in the postresuscitation period?

Ans. Intravenous fluid therapy in the postresuscitation period involves replacement of evaporative fluid loss in addition to maintenance fluid. Glucose in water or Ringer's solution or colloids are required to maintain the circulatory fluid volume.

Amount of fluid required is:
- 1,500 mL/m^2 of body surface + evaporative fluid loss.

Evaporative fluid loss in burn patient is equal to:
- 25 × % of burn × m^2 of body surface.
  This fluid may be given intravenously or by enteral route, if the patient can take orally.

Q. What are the choices of fluid used for management of burns shock?

Ans.

◆ *Lactated Ringer's solution*: A crystalloid solution like lactated Ringer's solution is the ideal fluid required for initial resuscitation. However, in major burns resuscitation with only crystalloid results in hypoproteinemia and causes aggravation of edema. Patients with less than 40% burn may be managed with only crystalloid infusion.

◆ *Hypertonic saline*: Hypertonic salt solution (240 mEq of sodium/L) is being used with increasing frequency. Patient can be resuscitated with less amount of fluid and in turn less edema. The serum sodium level should be monitored and once the serum sodium level exceeds 160 mEq/L the hypertonic saline infusion should be stopped and lactated Ringer's solution should be used. In patients with more than 40% burn, associated pulmonary injury and in elderly patient hypertonic saline may be used for resuscitation in first 8 hours followed by infusion of lactate Ringer's solution.

◆ *Colloid solution*: Earlier colloid solution was used more frequently to increase the plasma colloidal osmotic pressure. But, it has been observed that proteins are no more effective than crystalloid solution in maintaining intravascular volume in first 24 hours. Colloid should be added to the resuscitation fluid after 8–12 hours in the form of 5% albumin or plasma.

◆ *Dextran solution*: Dextran is a colloid consisting of glucose molecules that has been polymerized into chains to form polysaccharides. Dextran with molecular weight of 40,000 is referred to as low-molecular weight dextran and has been used in burns shock, as it improves the microcirculation.

Q. How will you manage the burn wound?

Ans. The burn wound management depends on the degree of burn.

◆ *First-degree burn or epidermal burns*:
  - No dressing and topical antibiotics are required. Soothing moisturizing lotion application. This heals in 3–7 days time.
◆ *Second-degree burn*:
  - Superficial dermal burns usually heal by epithelialization by 2–3 weeks.
  - The wound needs to be dressed with topical antibiotics to prevent infection and layered padded dressing applied—paraffin gauze, and a thick layer of gauze.
  - The burns in the face and neck are usually treated by exposure method with application of topical antibiotics and keeping the area open.
◆ *Deep dermal burns, third-degree burns, and fourth-degree burns*:
  - Do not heal by epithelialization and may heal by granulation with gross scarring. There are two options for surgical treatment of deep burns:
    - *Early operation—tangential excision and skin grafting*: Surgical management of the burn wound has now become more aggressive. Following resuscitation of burn wound operative debridement is planned early. Tangential excision of the burn wound is done till a bleeding dermal bed or subcutaneous tissue is reached and the area covered with split skin graft. The skin graft may be meshed to cover a larger area of the defect. The healing process may be expedited by this method.

- *Delayed operation*: The burn wound is dressed and time is allowed for spontaneous separation of the slough and once the wound starts granulating, the area is covered with split skin grafting.

  The advantage is avoidance of early operation, but the disadvantage is there is scarring following skin grafting of the granulating wound.
- In deep burns with exposed structures like bones, nerves, tendon, and vessels after debridement needs to be covered with skin flaps rather than split skin grafts.

Q. If patient's own skin is not available for grafting what may be done?

Ans. In some situations, the burnt area to be excised may be larger than the autograft available from the donor sites. The remaining areas may be covered with biologic dressings. The biologic dressings have following benefits:

- Provide a physical barrier
- Control water–vapor transmission from the surface of the wound
- Prevent desiccation and maceration of the tissue
- Resist microbial invasion into the depth of the tissue.

The donor site re-epithelializes in 2-week time and donor site may be reharvested for skin grafting by serially removing the biologic dressing.

Q. What are the different skin substitutes for wound coverage?

Ans. Different skin substitutes are available for wound coverage:

- *Integra*: This is bilayer membrane, outer layer is a silastic film and the inner layer consists of a porous matrix of fibers derived from bovine collagen and a single layer of chondroitin 6-sulfate. Integra should be applied on a viable noninfected wound.

  There is ingrowth of fibroblast and endothelial cells into the dermal matrix provided. Once the neodermis is formed the silastic membrane may be removed and the wound may be covered by autogenous split-thickness skin grafts.
- *AlloDerm*: This is an acellular dermal matrix produced from human cadaveric skin. The cadaveric skin is freed from all cellular component and the decellular matrix is the freeze dried. The AlloDerm is reconstituted by soaking in crystalloid solution and may be used for wound coverage along with a split-thickness autograft.
- *TransCyte*: This is produced by incorporating neonatal fibroblast into a synthetic dressing of silastic attached to a nylon mesh, which is coated with porcine peptides obtained from type I collagen. The silastic layer provides a temporary impermeable barrier and the fibroblast-impregnated nylon mesh acts as a dermal component.
- *Dermagraft*: This consists of human neonatal fibroblast incorporated into a polyglactin mesh scaffold. This can be used for burn wound coverage along with split-thickness skin graft.

Q. What are the roles of antibiotics in burn injury?

Ans. Infection remains an important problem in burn injury management. There is controversy about routine use of prophylactic antibiotics in burn injury. The routine administration of broad spectrum antibiotics may result in emergence of resistant strains of organisms.

Varied organisms may colonize the burn wound. The common organisms are *Streptococci, Staphylococci, Pseudomonas,* and *Escherichia coli*.

Infection may be treated by topical antibiotics.

Invasive infection is suggested by cellulitis, fever, and positive blood culture. This needs treatment with broad-spectrum parenteral antibiotics.

Q. What are the different topical antibiotics used for burn wound treatment?

Ans. Different topical microbial agents are used for burn wound care:

- *Silver sulfadiazine*—has broad-spectrum coverage including antipseudomonal activity, commonly used. Does not penetrate eschar, so no systemic absorption occurs. May cause leukopenia.
- *Nanocrystalline silver*—nanocrystalline silver provides sustained release of elemental silver having broad spectrum of activity. Nanocrystalline silver-coated dressings are available and are being used with success.
- *Silver nitrate*—provides broad spectrum of activity. Penetrates eschar poorly. May cause methemoglobinemia.
- *Mupirocin*—active against methicillin-resistant *Staphylococcus aureus* (MRSA). Has poor Gram-negative activity.
- *Mafenide acetate*—broad-spectrum activity including anticlostridial activity. Penetrates eschar easily.
- *Povidone iodine*—has broad spectrum of activity.

Q. How will you achieve tetanus prophylaxis in burn wound?

Ans. Burn wound is a tetanus-prone wound. The recommendations for tetanus prophylaxis for wound are:

- Patient is immunized and last booster dose within 5 years—nothing is required
- Patient is immunized and last booster dose between 5 years and 10 years—1 booster dose of injection tetanus toxoid
- Patient not immunized, immunization status unknown or last booster dose more than 10 years:
  - Injection tetanus toxoid
  - Injection human tetanus globulin (250 units)—at two different sites.

Q. How will you prevent stress ulcers (Curling's ulcer)?

Ans. In major burn injury, patient may develop stress ulcer, which may manifest with upper GI hemorrhage.

The stress ulcer may be prevented by using:

- H_2 blockers (Ranitidine or famotidine)
- Proton-pump inhibitor (Omeprazole or pantoprazole)
- Sucralfate.

Q. What are the special problems with circumferential burns?

Ans.

- Circumferential burns of the extremities and the trunk pose special problems
- Circumferential deep burns of the extremities with swelling beneath the unyielding eschar may result in distal ischemia in the fingers and toes
- To prevent permanent damage due to ischemia, escharotomy extending up to the deep fascia must be performed early

- Circumferential burns of the chest and abdomen may restrict ventilation. This may be relieved by longitudinal escharotomies
- The escharotomy may be done without general anesthesia.

11. A 30-year-female patient has come to emergency with acute pain in right upper quadrant of abdomen. How will you proceed to manage?

Ans. The important causes of acute pain in right upper quadrant of abdomen include:
- Acute cholecystitis
- Acute cholangitis
- Acute pancreatitis
- Acute peptic ulcer
- Peptic ulcer perforation
- Liver abscess
- Acute retrocecal appendicitis
- Acute intestinal obstruction
- Right-sided renal colic
- Acute right-sided pyelonephritis
- Acute myocardial infarction
- Basal pneumonia
- Empyema thoracis.

Q. What are the nonsurgical causes of acute pain abdomen?

Ans. Important causes of nonsurgical acute pain abdomen include:
- Acute myocardial infarction
- Basal pneumonia
- Acute intermittent porphyria
- Sickle cell disease
- Diabetes mellitus
- Acute epilepsy.

For rational management, a detailed history, physical examination, and some relevant investigations are required. Treatment will depend on the underlying cause.

- *History will include:*
  - *Detail history of pain*: Onset, site at onset, duration, progress, radiation of pain, character of pain, relation with food, aggravating and relieving factors, similar episodes of pain earlier
  - Associated symptoms like:
    - *Nausea and vomiting*: If vomiting is present, enquire about—duration, frequency (times/day), relation with pain and food intake
    - *Character of vomitus*—amount, sour/bitter (bile is bitter); contents; color (yellow/green/coffee ground/frank red)
  - History of jaundice, fever, loss of appetite, and loss of weight
  - History of sensation of fullness of abdomen after meals, heartburn, and belching Bowel habit and any alteration of bowel habits
  - Urinary habits like frequency, burning sensation, and history of hematuria

- – Other symptoms like chest pain, cough, hemoptysis, and breathlessness
- – *Details menstrual history*: Any history of missed periods
- – History of past illness: About similar attacks of pain in the past. History of peptic ulcer disease. White discharge P/V and any mass in abdomen.
- ◆ *Physical examination*:
  - – *General survey*:
    - - Look for features of shock
      - » Pulse (tachycardia, feeble pulse)
      - » Blood pressure (hypotension)
      - » Cold and clammy extremities
      - » Dry tongue and collapsed veins.
  - – Look for nutrition, jaundice, pallor, and temperature.
- ◆ *Local examination of abdomen*:
  - – *Inspection*:
    - - Look for any fullness or distension
    - - Any restriction of movement of right upper quadrant of abdomen or whole of abdomen
    - - Any visible peristalsis
    - - Any ecchymosis around the umbilicus (Cullen's sign) or in the loin (Gray Turner's sign)
    - - Look at the hernial sites to rule out any hernia
    - - Presence of any lump and detail examination of the lump.
  - – *Palpation*:
    - - Look for tenderness, rebound tenderness
    - - Muscle guard and rigidity
    - - Look for Murphy's sign (elicited in acute cholecystitis)
    - - Rovsing's sign, psoas sign, obturator sign (elicited in acute appendicitis)
    - - Any palpable mass—gallbladder may be palpable in acute cholecystitis or empyema gallbladder
    - - If a lump is palpable, details examination of the lump—whether parietal, intra-abdominal, or retroperitoneal, position and extent of the lump in different regions of the abdomen, size, shape, surface, margin, consistency, mobility, whether bimanually palpable, and ballotable
    - - Palpation of liver, spleen, and kidneys.
  - – *Percussion*:
    - - Look for general note of the abdomen and evidence of free fluid in abdomen by eliciting fluid thrill or shifting dullness (suggests perforative peritonitis)
    - - Obliteration of liver dullness found in perforative peritonitis
    - - Delineate the upper border of liver and spleen by percussion
    - - Intercostal tenderness during percussion may be found in liver abscess.
  - – *Auscultation*:
    - - *Peristaltic sounds*—present or absent. Any audible bruit or venous hum
    - - *Per rectal and per vaginal examination*—to exclude any pelvic mass, pelvic collection, or tenderness.
- ◆ *Systemic examination*:
  - – Examination of respiratory system to exclude basal pneumonia or empyema thoracis
  - – Examination of cardiovascular system (CVS) to exclude acute myocardial infarction.

- *Investigations*:
  - *Complete hemogram*—leukocytosis in acute inflammatory conditions
  - *Urine analysis*—WBC with or without RBC in urine suggests acute urinary tract infection (UTI). Retrocecal appendicitis lying in contact with ureter may cause minor pyuria
  - *Serum amylase and lipase*—elevated level suggests acute pancreatitis
  - *Liver function test*—in patients with suspected hepatic and biliary tract disease
  - *Chest X-ray PA view*—to rule out basal pneumonia and to look for free gas under the domes of diaphragm (found in hollow viscus perforation containing gas), e.g. peptic ulcer or gut perforation
  - *Staright X-ray abdomen*—to look for dilated loops of bowel and air–fluid levels
  - *Ultrasonography of abdomen*—helpful in hepatobiliary diseases, pancreatitis, appendicitis, and renal diseases
  - *CT scan of abdomen*—in selected cases
  - *MRCP in selected* case for diagnosis of choledocholithiasis
  - *Upper GI endoscopy* for diagnosis of peptic ulcer disease.
- *Treatment*—depends on the underlying cause:
  - If patient is in shock:
    - Resuscitation with IV fluids and monitoring of vital signs.
- Treatment of acute cholecystitis:
  - *Conservative treatment*:
    - Nothing per mouth
    - Nasogastric suction
    - Intravenous fluids
    - Analgesics (tramadol hydrochloride or pentazocine)
    - *Broad-spectrum antibiotics*: Second-generation or third-generation cephalosporin (Cefuroxime or ceftriaxone) with metronidazole administered parenterally
    - Monitoring of the patient (pulse, temperature, BP, respiration, fluid intake-output, symptomatic improvement, and improvement of abdominal findings)
    - Depending upon response to conservative treatment, further treatment is planned.
  - *If patient responds well*:
    - Discontinue nasogastric suction and IV fluids followed by fat-free diet and cholecystectomy after 6–8 weeks (interval cholecystectomy).
    - *Early cholecystectomy*: Assess fitness for anesthesia in same hospital admission and do cholecystectomy operation 2–3 days after the acute episode has subsided.
  - *Urgent exploratory laparotomy is indicated*:
    - When there is doubt in diagnosis
    - If patient does not respond well (within 48 hours) indicated by:
      » Persistent pain and vomiting
      » Persistent tachycardia and fever
      » Increasing tenderness and appearance of rebound tenderness.

Cholecystectomy may be done provided the surgeon is experienced, as the operation is very difficult. The gallbladder wall is friable, edematous, and there are lots of adhesions.

If anatomy is obscured and gallbladder wall is friable and patient's general condition is not good, simple cholecystostomy is to be done followed by cholecystectomy after 6–8 weeks.

* *Treatment of acute pancreatitis:*
  – *Conservative treatment:*
    - Nothing by mouth
    - Nasogastric suction
    - Intravenous fluid
    - Prophylactic antibiotics
    - Analgesics.
  Surgical treatment is indicated for complications such as phlegmon, pancreatic necrosis or pancreatic abscess, or pseudocyst.
* *Treatment of peptic ulcer disease:*
  – *Conservative treatment:*
    - Bland diet
    - *Antisecretory drugs:*
      » H_2 blockers—ranitidine/famotidine
      » Proton-pump inhibitors—omeprazole/pantoprazole/esomeprazole
      » *Sucralfate*—provides a protective covering over the ulcer and hastens healing
      » If *Helicobacter pylori* is demonstrated—anti *H. pylori* treatment.
  – *Surgical treatment:*
    - Failure of intensive medical treatment
    - Intractable symptom
    - Development of complications.
* *Perforated peptic ulcer:*
  – Resuscitation of shock with:
    - Intravenous fluid
    - Correction of fluid and electrolyte imbalance
    - Broad-spectrum antibiotics
    - Nasogastric suction.
* *Emergency exploratory laparotomy*—closure of peptic perforation and peritoneal toileting.

12. A 30-year-female patient presented with acute pain in right lower quadrant of abdomen. How will you proceed to manage?

Ans. Important causes of pain in the right lower quadrant of abdomen are:
* Acute appendicitis
* Acute typhlitis
* Meckel's diverticulitis
* Right-sided disturbed ectopic pregnancy
* Acute salpingitis
* Twisted right ovarian cyst
* Acute intestinal obstruction
* Ileocecal tuberculosis
* Acute Crohn's ileitis
* Perforated peptic ulcer
* Acute cholecystitis
* Acute pancreatitis
* Ureteric colic

+ Acute pyelonephritis
+ Psoas abscess.

For proper management, detail history, physical examination, and some relevant investigations are required.

The details of history, clinical examination, and investigations are same as described in right upper quadrant pain abdomen.

In acute appendicitis, classically pain starts around the umbilicus and shifts to the right iliac fossa. There is associated nausea, vomiting, and fever. Patient may have loss of appetite.

In female patient, exclude gynecological causes of pain—menstrual history, any bleeding per vagina.

On examination, the patient may have features of sepsis and shock.

Patient may be febrile.

Tenderness at McBurney's point: There may be positive Rovsing's sign, psoas sign, and rebound tenderness may be present.

If appendix is perforated, there may be generalized guarding and rigidity in abdomen.

Q. Which investigations are helpful for diagnosis of acute appendicitis?

Ans.

+ *Hemogram*—polymorphonuclear leukocytosis
+ *Urine for routine examination*—presence of pus cells and protein in urine—may be due to bladder irritation caused by a pelvic appendix or may indicate UTI.
+ C-reactive protein (CRP) may be elevated
+ *Ultrasonography*—sensitivity of 86% and specificity of 81% for diagnosis of acute appendicitis
+ *CECT scan of abdomen*—sensitivity of 94% and specificity of 95% for diagnosis of acute appendicitis
+ *In women of childbearing age*—urine for beta-human chorionic gonadotropin (β-hCG) to exclude ectopic pregnancy.

Treatment—depends on the underlying cause:
+ *Acute appendicitis*—emergency appendectomy is the standard-of-care for acute appendicitis
+ *Initial treatment*:
  – Nothing by mouth
  – Intravenous fluid
  – *Broad-spectrum antibiotics*—second-generation cephalosporin/aminoglycoside, and metronidazole
  – Analgesic.

Emergency appendectomy:

The operation should be preferably done within 24 hours of admission. The risk of perforation increases with time. After 36 hours, the risk of perforation is 16–36% and the risk increases by 5% for every 12 hours passed.
+ *Meckel's diverticulitis*: Meckelian diverticulectomy with a wedge of the ileum
+ *Acute intestinal obstruction*:
  – *Conservative treatment*:
    - Nothing by mouth
    - Nasogastric aspiration
    - Intravenous fluid resuscitation
    - Antibiotics

- Monitoring.
- *Indications of surgery*:
    - Failure of conservative treatment
    - Symptoms and signs of strangulation
    - Diagnosis uncertain.
- *Ureteric colic*:
    - Analgesics for pain relief—injection of diclofenac sodium may relieve the pain
        » Small stones less than 1 cm may pass out spontaneously
        » Stones more than 1 cm unlikely to pass spontaneously—extracorporeal shock wave lithotripsy (ESWL)/percutaneous nephrolithotomy (PCNL) or open surgery for removal of stone.
- *Acute pyelonephritis*:
    - Analgesics
    - *Antibiotics*—empiric antibiotic therapy followed by appropriate antibiotic depending on culture sensitivity of urine
    - Treatment of any underlying cause—stone or stricture.
- *Ectopic pregnancy*:
    - Resuscitation
    - Emergency laparotomy or laparoscopy and salpingectomy along with removal of the product of conceptus.

Q. What should be the preferred technique for appendectomy?

Ans. Currently, there has been debate regarding advantage of laparoscopic technique over open technique. In laparoscopic technique, there is less postoperative pain, better cosmetic result, and less postoperative wound infection. This is particularly useful when there is doubt in diagnosis.

Q. What should be the strategy when a normal appendix is found during operation?

Ans. When a normal appendix is found during either open or laparoscopic operation—the recommendation is to remove the normal appendix to avoid diagnostic confusion in future. There have been some studies where the normal appendix was not removed. In follow-up, 4–13% of such patients required appendectomy for recurrent abdominal pain. In one series, 58% of normal looking appendix shows histological features of inflammation. These studies suggest that the normal-looking appendix during operation should be removed.

13. **A 30-year-male patient presented with a lump in right iliac fossa for last 5 days following an acute attack of pain in right iliac fossa for last 1 week associated with fever and vomiting and clinically diagnosed as appendicular lump how to manage?**

OR

How will you manage a patient presenting with a lump in right iliac fossa?

Ans. Important causes of lump in right iliac fossa:
- *Parietal swelling*:
    - Lipoma

- Desmoid tumor
- Iliopsoas abscess pointing in the right iliac fossa.
- *Intra-abdominal swelling*:
  - Appendicular lump
  - Appendicular abscess
  - Ileocecal tuberculosis
  - Crohn's ileitis
  - Carcinoma cecum or ascending colon
  - Lymph node mass—Koch's or lymphoma
  - Hugely distended gallbladder.
- *Retroperitoneal swelling*:
  - Hydronephrosis or tumor in an unascended or dropped kidney
  - Retroperitoneal sarcoma
  - Iliopsoas abscess
  - Tumor in an undescended right testis.

If the patient presents with classic features of acute appendicitis and then presents with a lump in right iliac fossa, this is likely to be an appendicular lump.

For arriving at a diagnosis, a detail history, physical examination, and some relevant investigations are required.

- *History to include:*
  - Details history about the lump—onset progress, any history of rapid increase in size
  - Details history of pain abdomen, if present
  - Other associated symptoms—*See* Right Upper Quadrant Pain, Page No. 726.
- *A detail physical examination to include*:
  - General survey
  - Abdominal examination—*See* Right Upper Quadrant Pain, Page No. 726
  - Systemic examination.
- *Relevant investigation to ascertain the nature of the lump includes:*
  - Complete hemogram
  - Liver function test
  - Ultrasonography of abdomen to ascertain the nature of the lump (solid or cystic), and the organ from where the lump is arising. Examination of liver, spleen, kidneys, and lymph nodes
  - CT scan abdomen for evaluation of retroperitoneal lump
  - Colonoscopy for evaluation of suspected carcinoma cecum
  - Intravenous urography for evaluation of renal lesion.

Treatment will depend on the diagnosis.

Q. How is the appendicular lump formed?

Ans. Appendicular lump is a conglomerate consisting of inflamed appendix, adjacent terminal ileum, cecum, and the greater omentum.

Q. How to differentiate an appendicular lump and an appendicular abscess?

Ans.

- In a classical case, the appendicular lump forms around the 3rd day of acute attack of pain and develops into an abscess around 5th–10th days

- Pyrexia, aggravation of the local signs and a rising leukocyte count are indicators of abscess formation
- USG and CT scan may demonstrate pus within an appendicular lump.

Q. How will you plan management of appendicular lump?

Ans. If appendicular lump is palpable on admission conservative treatment (Ochsner–Sherren regimen) is the preferred treatment for following reasons:
- Immediate appendectomy is technically difficult
- There is increased chance of fecal fistula, postoperatively
- Operation may be done, if conservative treatment fails.

Q. What are the components of conservative treatment (Ochsner–Sherren regime) for appendicular lump?

Ans. These are:
- *For pain:* Nonsteroidal anti-inflammatory drugs (diclofenac or aceclofenac) or narcotic analgesics (injection pentazocine or pethidine)
- *For vomiting:* Stop oral fluids and nasogastric suction
- *Fluid administration:* IV fluids to maintain fluid electrolyte balance
  - If patient is not vomiting—oral fluids may be administered
- *Control infection:* Second- or third-generation cephalosporin (cefuroxime or ceftriaxone) along with metronidazole administered parenterally
- Alternatively, a combination of ampicillin + gentamicin + metronidazole may be given
- *Monitoring is the most important* component of conservative treatment:
  - Symptomatic improvement—pain and vomiting
  - Objective improvement:
    - Hourly monitoring of pulse, BP, and respiration
    - Monitoring of temperature 4 hourly
    - Tenderness in right iliac fossa
    - Progress of the lump (lump is to be marked).

If the patient responds well to conservative treatment, interval appendectomy should be considered after 6–8 weeks.

Q. What may be the outcome of conservative treatment of appendicular lump?

Ans. When the patient is kept on above management, one of the followings may happen.
- Lump may regress, pain decreases, pulse and temperature normalize:
  - Continue antibiotics for 7–10 days
  - Allow oral fluid and then food when patient has the desire to eat (4th–5th day)
  - Total disappearance of lump takes 6–8 weeks.
- Lump may increase in size, pain, and tenderness may increase, pulse rate may rise and there may be fever with chills and rigor—this indicates appendicular abscess formation.

Q. Patient is taken up for appendectomy and palpation of right iliac fossa under general anesthesia revealed a mass, what should be done?

Ans. If the symptoms has been present for few days (3–5 days) appendectomy should be performed as scheduled. In most of these cases, greater omentum is found loosely wrapped around an inflamed appendix. There is no evidence that appendectomy is associated with higher complication rate in such situation.

If the symptoms are present for a longer duration more than 7 days a firm lump is palpable it is preferable not to operate for fear of difficult, bloody, and dangerous operation, which may lead to increased risk of fecal fistula.

Q. How will you manage a case of appendicular abscess?

Ans.

- The patient may show features of septicemia
- Formation of pus is confirmed by USG or CT scan
- Resuscitation followed by drainage of abscess is the treatment of choice
  - Intravenous fluids
  - Nasogastric suction
  - Catheterization (for monitoring urine output)
  - Intravenous antibiotics—cefuroxime + metronidazole.
- *Steps of drainage of appendicular abscess:*
  - *Retrocecal/subcecal variety*—extraperitoneal drainage is to be done
  - General anesthesia with endotracheal intubation
  - *Rutherford Morrison incision*: This is a muscle cutting incision. Skin and external oblique incision like McBurney's incision. But the internal oblique and transversus abdominis muscles are cut in the same line of incision for better drainage
  - The abscess wall is incised and abscess drained without opening the peritoneum
  - A tube drain is inserted through separate stab wound and the main wound is closed in layers.
- Appendectomy at this stage is usually not done. But if appendix is lying free in abscess cavity, some surgeons prefer to do it.
  - *Pelvic appendix (leading to pelvic abscess)*: Points into rectum/vagina and may be drained by transrectal or transvaginal route
  - *For pre-ileal and post-ileal variety*: It is difficult to avoid the peritoneal cavity, so careful packing is to be done to isolate abscess from peritoneal cavity
  - *Percutaneous drainage*: With advent of interventional radiology appendicular abscess may be drained by placement of a tube into the abscess cavity under USG guidance.

Q. What is the rationality of interval appendectomy following conservative treatment of appendicular mass and appendicular abscess?

Ans.

- An elective appendectomy after 8–12 weeks is the norm.
- But it was conceded that in some cases, the appendix becomes a fibrotic cord and is unlikely to cause further problems.
- Many has questioned the routine use of interval appendectomy, since the recurrence rate of acute appendicitis is low ranging between 3% and 15% over a long follow-up period
- So, routine interval appendectomy is not advised following treatment of appendicular mass and abscess.
- This may be indicated in patient, who in the future may not have easy access to surgical facilities.
- However, cecal malignancy is to be excluded by barium enema or colonoscopic study.

14. **A 40-year-male patient who is a chronic alcoholic presented to emergency with acute pain in epigastrium since the previous night and later on become generalized. How will you proceed to manage the case?**

Ans. The most likely diagnosis in this patient is acute alcoholic pancreatitis. However, apart from this other possibilities for such pain are:
+ Acute perforated peptic ulcer
+ Acute exacerbation of chronic peptic ulcer
+ Acute gastritis
+ Acute cholecystitis
+ Relapsing chronic pancreatitis
+ Liver abscess.

Rarer cases:
+ Acute myocardial infarction
+ Basal pneumonia
+ Dissecting aneurysm of aorta.

To arrive at a diagnosis, a detailed history, physical examination, and some relevant investigations are required.

The approach of history taking, general survey, local examination, and systemic examination will be same as right upper quadrant pain.
+ *Family history*—history of familial pancreatitis
+ *Personal history*—details of alcohol intake, smoking, and dietary history.

Drugs, especially steroids aggravate pancreatitis, nonsteroidal anti-inflammatory drugs aggravate peptic ulcer disease or may be associated with peptic perforation.

Relevant investigations required are:
+ Complete blood count
+ Blood for sugar, urea, and creatinine
+ Serum amylase:
  – A value more than three times the normal is pointer for diagnosis of acute pancreatitis
  – Serum level rises early and may return to normal after 72 hours
  – Associated hyperlipidemia may interfere with serum level estimation.
+ *Serum lipase*:
  – Remains elevated in serum longer than serum amylase
  – Pancreas is the only source of lipase, so not elevated in extrapancreatic disorder.
+ Serum calcium
+ ECG
+ Straight X-ray of abdomen
+ chest X-ray—PA view
+ Ultrasonography of abdomen
+ *CECT scan abdomen*—if USG is inconclusive or in cases with pancreatitis developing complications
+ Upper GI endoscopy in suspected cases of gastritis or peptic ulcer disease.

Q. What are the important etiological factors for development of acute pancreatitis?

Ans. The important factors for development of acute pancreatitis are:

- *Gallstone disease*—most common cause of acute pancreatitis
- *Alcohol intake*—second most common cause of acute pancreatitis
- *Trauma*—usually blunt abdominal trauma may result in pancreatitis due to pancreatic contusion
- Hyperlipidemia
- *Post-ERCP*
- *Hyperparathyroidism*
- *Pancreas divisum*
- *Hereditary*
- *Infection*—mumps (paramyxovirus), Epstein-Barr virus, and cytomegalovirus
- *Autoimmune pancreatitis*—increased serum level of IgG4/IgG ratio
- *Drugs*—steroid, azathioprine, sulfonamides, nonsteroidal anti-inflammatory drugs, and diuretics
- *Scorpion bite*
- Alpha-1 antitrypsin deficiency
- *Idiopathic.*

Q. What is acute pancreatitis?

Ans. Acute pancreatitis is a nonbacterial inflammation of the pancreas associated with activation and interstitial liberation of its own enzymes resulting in cellular damage.

Clinically acute pancreatitis is characterized by acute abdominal pain, elevation of pancreatic enzymes in blood, and increased excretion of pancreatic enzymes in urine.

Q. What are the criteria for diagnosis of acute pancreatitis?

Ans. Diagnosis of acute pancreatitis is based on two of three following features:
1. Acute onset of upper abdominal pain characteristics of pain of pancreatic origin
2. Serum amylase and/or lipase level three times the normal level
3. Characteristics findings in CECT scan.

Q. How alcohol causes pancreatitis?

Ans. Alcohol can cause both acute and chronic pancreatitis.
- Alcohol causes spasm of sphincter of oddi leading to obstruction of flow of pancreatic juice
- Alcohol is a cellular metabolic poison and causes damage of parenchymal cells
- Alcohol causes precipitation of proteins and calcium in the pancreatic duct resulting in ductal obstruction
- Alcohol increases the permeability of the pancreatic duct to the enzymes, which leaks out into the surrounding tissues resulting in pancreatic damage
- Alcohol causes reduction of blood supply of the pancreas resulting in ischemic damage to the pancreas.

Q. How gallstones cause pancreatitis?

Ans.
- Transient obstruction of the pancreatic duct by a stone impacted in the ampulla of VATER
- Reflux of infected bile into the pancreatic duct causes activation of the pancreatic enzyme leading to pancreatitis.

Q. What is the usual presentation of patients with acute pancreatitis?

Ans.

- *Pain abdomen*—acute onset upper abdominal pain, severe in intensity, may radiate to back, chest, or flanks
- In rare occasion, may present without pain abdomen
- Nausea and vomiting
- May present with shock of unknown cause
- There may be past history of acute pancreatitis earlier, hyperlipidemia, hyperparathyroidism, ERCP, or history of cholecystectomy
- Physical examination may reveal evidence of shock—tachycardia and hypotension
- There may be signs of dehydration (sunken eyes, loss of skin turgor, and any icterus)
- Abdominal examination may reveal mild-to-moderate distension, tenderness in abdomen, muscle guard, and rigidity may be present mimicking perforative peritonitis
- Cullen's sign (ecchymosis around the umbilicus) and Grey Turner sign (ecchymosis in the flanks) although well described are rarely found
- Auscultation may reveal absent bowel sounds (due to paralytic ileus). Auscultation of chest may reveal absent bowel sounds at the lung base (due to sympathetic pleural effusion more commonly on the left side).

Q. What investigations are helpful for diagnosis?

Ans. Some laboratory and imaging tests are helpful for diagnosis of acute pancreatitis. These tests are also helpful for disease stratification.

- *Serum amylase and lipase*:
  - An elevation of these enzymes three times the normal is diagnostic of acute pancreatitis. Serum amylase may be cleared from the serum after 48 hours of onset of acute pancreatitis. Serum lipase may be cleared at the end of 96 hours. Currently, serum lipase level three times the normal is a considered a single test for diagnosis of acute pancreatitis (sensitivity—92%).
- A complete blood count
- Arterial blood gas and serum lactate
- Blood urea and creatinine helpful for assessment of systemic inflammatory response syndrome (SIRS) and organ dysfunction associated with acute pancreatitis
- Liver function test—(serum bilirubin, ALT, AST, and ALP) may be altered in patient with an impacted stone at ampulla of Vater. ALP three times the normal is usually suggestive of gallstone pancreatitis
- C-reactive protein levels over 15mg% is suggestive of necrotizing pancreatitis.

Imaging studies:

- *CECT scan*: Most important single test for diagnosis of acute pancreatitis also helpful for stratifying the severity (CTSI)
- *USG*: Useful for diagnosis of cholelithiasis and choledocholitiasis and biliary ductal dilatation
- *MRI and MRCP*: Helps in delineation of pancreatic necrosis and ductal anatomy may be well seen and helpful for better diagnosis of choledocholithiasis
- *Chest X ray*: May diagnose pleural effusion (a bad prognostic marker)
- *Endoscopic USG*: Most sensitive for diagnosis of cholelithiasis and choledocholithiasis.

Q. Why there is elevation of pancreatic enzymes (amylase and lipase) in serum in patients with acute pancreatitis?

Ans. There is release of these enzymes from the inflamed gland into the surrounding tissues and are absorbed into circulation resulting in increase of serum amylase and lipase level. However, the severity of pancreatitis does not correlate with the level of serum amylase.

Q. How could you explain normal serum amylase level in patients with acute pancreatitis?

Ans. As serum amylase is elevated in acute pancreatitis the urinary excretion of amylase increases and the serum level may return to normal after few days, as more amylase is excreted in urine.

Presence of associated hyperlipidemia may interfere with accurate estimation of serum amylase and may show false low values.

Q. Apart from acute pancreatitis, which other conditions may cause elevation of serum amylase and increase urinary excretion of amylase?

Ans.
* Perforated duodenal ulcer or small gut perforation
* Gangrenous cholecystitis
* Other intra-abdominal inflammatory conditions.

Q. What may be the findings in plain X-ray of abdomen in acute pancreatitis?

Ans.
* There may be a dilated loop of gut—jejunum or transverse colon adjacent to the inflamed pancreas. This is called a sentinel loop.
* Mild distension of ascending and transverse colon with an abrupt cut-off in the midline or to the left due to spasm of colon—"colon cut-off" sign.
* Ground glass appearance due to fluid collection in the abdomen.
* Radiopaque gallstones may be seen.

Q. How a chest X-ray helps in evaluation of a patient suspected of having acute pancreatitis?

Ans.
* There may be associated pleural effusion
* Demonstration of free gas under the diaphragm indicates perforative peritonitis rather than acute pancreatitis.

Q. How ultrasonography helps in evaluation of a patient with acute pancreatitis?

Ans.
* Ultrasound may show an edematous pancreas. There may be peripancreatic fluid collection.
* Pancreatic necrosis or pseudocyst may be demonstrated in USG.
* Serial USG may be helpful in following the course of acute pancreatitis and also to assess the progress of a pseudocyst.

Q. What is mild acute pancreatitis?

Ans. Acute pancreatitis without any evidence of organ failure.

(Modified Atlanta Definition)

Q. What is severe pancreatitis?

Ans. It is acute pancreatitis with persistent organ failure.

Q. What is intermediately severe pancreatitis?

Ans. Acute pancreatitis with transient organ failure, which gets corrected in 24–48 hours.

Q. What is acute fluid collection?

Ans. Collection of fluid around the pancreas, which is not walled off, which occurs early during the course of acute pancreatitis.

Q. What is pancreatic necrosis?

Ans. Nonviable pancreatic tissue demonstrated by CECT scan during the course of acute pancreatitis.

Q. What is pancreatic pseudocyst?

Ans. Fluid collection around the pancreas, which is properly walled off occurs late during the course of acute pancreatitis.

Q. What is walled off pancreatic necrosis?

Ans. Formation of a thick wall around the pancreatic necrosis and fluid collection is called walled off pancreatic necrosis.

Q. What is CT severity of acute pancreatitis?

Ans. CT severity index is calculated by adding scores of Balthazar grading and necrosis score (Table 16.1).

Table 16.1: Balthazar grading and score in acute pancreatitis in contrast-enhanced computed tomography (CECT) scan

Finding	CT grade	Score
Normal pancreas	A	0
Focal/diffuse enlargement	B	1
Mild heterogeneity		
Intrinsic and extrinsic pancreatic inflammatory changes	C	2
Prominent peripancreatic inflammatory changes	D	3
Multiple extrapancreatic fluid collection/abscess	E	4

(CT: computed tomography)

Q. What is necrosis score?

Ans. Necrosis defined as focal or diffuse area of diminished enhancement following contrast injection less than 50 Hounsfield units.

* No necrosis—0
* 33%—2
* 50%—4
* More than 50%—6
* CT severity index = Balthazar scoring + necrosis score: Ranges = 0–10.

Q. How to prognosticate acute pancreatitis?

Ans. The severity of acute pancreatitis may be prognosticated based on some scoring system taking into some clinical and laboratory data.

These include Ranson criteria, Glasgow score, and APACHE II (Acute Physiology and Chronic Health Evaluation II).

Both Glasgow score and Ranson criteria require data collection for 48 hours and have positive-predictive value of less than 50%.

APACHE II scoring can be done at any point of time. APACHE II score below 7 has 90% negative-predictive value, whereas score above 7 has positive-predictive value of 50%. Complexity of APACHE II scoring system hinders its general use clinically.

The severity of acute pancreatitis may also be assessed by taking into account the serum CRP and presence of SIRS.

C-reactive protein value of more than 15mg% within 72 hours of onset of acute pancreatitis is suggestive of severe acute pancreatitis.

Presence of SIRS (defined by presence of two or more of the following):

♦ *Pulse rate*: More than 90 beats/min
♦ *Rectal temperature*: More than 38°C or less than 36°C
♦ *WBC count*: More than 12,000/mm³ or less than 4,000/mm³
♦ *Respiratory rate*: More than 20 breaths/min or CO_2 tension less than 32 mm Hg.

Q. What are Ranson's criteria for predicting the severity of acute pancreatitis?

Ans. *On admission:*

♦ Age more than 55 years
♦ White blood cell count more than 16,000/mm³
♦ Blood glucose more than 200 mg%
♦ Serum lactate dehydrogenase (LDH) more than 350 IU/L
♦ Serum glutamic-oxaloacetic transaminase (SGOT) more than 250 IU/dL.

After 48 hours:

♦ Hematocrit drop more than 10%
♦ Blood urea nitrogen (BUN) rise more than 5 mg/dL
♦ Serum calcium less than 8 mg%
♦ Bicarbonate deficit more than 4 mEq/L
♦ Partial pressure of oxygen (PaO_2) less than 60 mm Hg
♦ Fluid sequestration more than 6 liter.

Q. How will you treat uncomplicated acute pancreatitis?

Ans. The mainstay of treatment is conservative.

♦ Nothing per mouth and nasogastric suction—till ileus improves
♦ Correction of fluid and electrolyte deficit with IV fluid
♦ Catheterization for monitoring urine output
♦ Maintenance of fluid intake—output chart
♦ Oxygen inhalation to correct arterial hypoxemia
♦ Hypocalcemia may develop—may need correction with IV calcium

* Hypomagnesemia may develop particularly in alcoholic patient—needs correction with IV magnesium
* *Prophylactic antibiotics*: There is no role of prophylactic antibiotics in mild pancreatitis. The risk of infection is greatest in patients having more than 30% pancreatic necrosis. The available data at present do not support use of antibiotics in patient with pancreatic necrosis. Antibiotics are indicated in patients with pancreatic necrosis having organ dysfunction and culture-proven sepsis. The antibiotics should be given for a defined period of time for 7–10 days.

Drug treatment:

* Gastric antisecretory drugs—ranitidine or omeprazole or pantoprazole
* Octreotide or somatostatin—reduces pancreatic secretion.

However, the efficacy of these drugs is not well established and is not recommended routinely.

* Monitoring of patient to assess response to the treatment.

Q. What are the indications of surgery in acute pancreatitis?

Ans.

* When the diagnosis is uncertain
* In gallstone pancreatitis—with persistent impaction of stone, which cannot be removed endoscopically
* Presence of infected pancreatic necrosis
* Pancreatic abscess.

Q. How will you treat gallstone pancreatitis due to a stone impacted at the ampulla of VATER?

Ans. The initial treatment is conservative and the majority of these patients respond to conservative treatment and the stone dislodges spontaneously and passes into the intestine.

If the stone remains impacted—indicated by elevated serum bilirubin, elevated alkaline phosphatase, and failure of response to conservative treatment—an ERCP with endoscopic sphincterotomy and stone retrieval may help in resolution of acute pancreatitis.

If endoscopic sphincterotomy is not feasible, open surgery may be considered.

Q. What is the role of ERCP in acute pancreatitis?

Ans. There is no role of early ERCP in patients with mild acute pancreatitis.

Early ERCP is indicated in patients with:

* Jaundice and associated cholangitis
* USG/MRCP demonstrating impacted stone in CBD.

Early ERCP preferably within 72 hours is indicated as ERCP at a later may be difficult due to edema and inflammation at the duodenum and ampulla.

Q. Laparotomy has been done for acute abdomen and diagnosed to have gallstone pancreatitis on exploration. What should be the optimum procedure?

Ans.

* If pancreatitis is mild-to-moderate in severity, cholecystectomy is to be done. An intraoperative cholangiogram is done and if CBD stone is found, choledocholithotomy and T-tube drainage are to be done.

◆ If pancreatitis is severe, cholecystostomy is done; and if CBD stone is present, the bile duct is decompressed with a T-tube. If a stone is impacted at the ampulla of vater, this is to be removed.

Q. What are the complications of acute pancreatitis?

Ans.
◆ *General complications:*
  - *Respiratory complications*—pleural effusion and adult respiratory distress syndrome
  - *Cardiovascular*—decreased myocardial contractility, ST, and T-wave changes in ECG
  - *Renal complications*—acute renal failure due to fluid and electrolyte deficits.
◆ *Local complications*:
  - *Acute fluid collection*—collection of fluid in the peripancreatic area, which is not walled off properly.
  - *Acute pseudocyst*—collection of fluid in the peripancreatic area, which is enclosed by granulation or fibrous tissue.
  - *Pancreatic necrosis*—a variable area of necrotic pancreatic tissue. If there is no infection, it is called sterile pancreatic necrosis. If infected results in infected pancreatic necrosis.
  - *Pancreatic abscess*—a localized collection of pus in the peripancreatic area with little or no pancreatic necrosis.
  - *Pancreatic ascites*—accumulation of peritoneal fluid rich in pancreatic enzyme usually associated with pancreatic duct disruption.

15. **A 40-year-male patient presented with acute pain in epigastrium, which later became generalized. On examination, there is cardboard-like rigidity and obliteration of liver dullness. How will you proceed to manage this case?**

Ans. The likely diagnosis is perforative peritonitis most commonly due to a perforated peptic ulcer. Other causes of pain are the same as mentioned in right upper quadrant pain (*See* Page No. 726).

The approach is same for right upper quadrant pain—details history and physical examination.

Investigations:
◆ Further investigation depends on the provisional diagnosis.
◆ In suspected perforated peptic ulcer a chest X-ray PA view in erect posture is done
  - If free gas under the diaphragm is demonstrated, no further special investigations are required
  - If patient cannot stand then an X-ray may be taken in left lateral decubitus—air will be seen over the liver shadow.
◆ Other investigations required are:
  - Complete hemogram
  - Blood sugar, urea, and creatinine
  - Serum electrolytes
  - An ECG should also be done.

Q. How patients with peptic perforation usually present?

Ans. *See* X-rays Section, Page No. 778, Chapter 17.

Q. How will you manage a patient presenting with peptic perforation?

Ans.
◆ *Resuscitation of patient with:*
 − Nothing per mouth
 − Nasogastric suction
 − Intravenous fluid
 − Catheterization
 − Maintain fluid balance chart
 − Broad-spectrum antibiotics
 − H$_2$ blockers—injection ranitidine or proton-pump inhibitor injection pantoprazole or omeprazole intravenously
 − Analgesics (pethidine)
 − Monitoring to assess response to treatment.
◆ *Early exploratory laparotomy following resuscitation:*
 − Simple closure of the perforation is the preferred treatment
 − The perforation is closed with interrupted suture using 2-0 polyglactin over an omental patch (Graham's patch)
 − Thorough peritoneal lavage should be done
 − A drain is to be placed in the hepatorenal pouch of Morrison.

Q. What is the role of laparoscopic surgery in peptic perforation?

Ans. There have been lots of reports in literature showing role of laparoscopy in closure of peptic perforation. Postoperative complications have been claimed to be less with laparoscopic surgery.

Q. What is Boey's score?

Ans. The Boey's score is used for risk stratification in patients undergoing repair of peptic perforation.

Boey's score is based on the following:
◆ Shock on admission (systolic BP <90 mm Hg)
◆ Severe medical illness (ASA III-IV)
◆ Late presentation (duration of symptoms >24 hours).

One point for each (Table 16.2).

Table 16.2: Postoperative mortality of Boey's score	
Boey's score	*Postoperative mortality*
0	1.5%
1	14.4%
2	32.1%
3	100%

Prognosis is also dependent on:
◆ Age of the patient
◆ The site of perforation
◆ Delay in treatment.

Other questions about peptic perforation—*See* X-rays Section, Page No. 777–779, Chapter 17.

16. **A 50-year-old male patient presented with pain in abdomen, vomiting, abdominal distension, and absolute constipation. How will you proceed to manage?**

Ans. The most likely diagnosis in such situation is acute intestinal obstruction. The important causes of intestinal obstruction include:

- Obstruction due to bands or adhesion, which is either congenital or postoperative
- External hernias
- Neoplastic—benign or malignant tumors of GI tract
- Volvulus
- Intussusception
- Strictures—due to tuberculosis or Crohn's disease
- Gallstone ileus
- Foreign bodies
- Radiation enteritis.

The approach for history and physical examination is same as in right upper quadrant pain.

- Details history about pain abdomen, vomiting, constipation, abdominal distension, and other associated symptoms
- History suggestive of external hernia—swelling in groin or around umbilicus
- *History of past illness*:
  - History of previous abdominal operation
  - History of tuberculosis (any history of chronic pain abdomen, history suggestive of subacute obstruction, and history of pulmonary tuberculosis)
  - History of recurrent subacute intestinal obstruction, which was relieved spontaneously.

General survey:

Look for features of shock—pulse and BP. Look for evidence of dehydration—dry tongue, loss of skin turgor, and oliguria.

Assess for presence of fever—pyrexia is not found in simple intestinal obstruction. Presence of fever may suggest onset of strangulation or perforation.

Hypothermia may be found in septic shock due to perforation or bacterial translocation.

Local examination of abdomen: (*See* Right Upper Quadrant Pain Abdomen, Page No. 726). Look specifically for:

- *Inspection*:
  - Abdominal distension—one of the most important features in obstruction
  - If it is present and central and flanks are not full, suggest small gut obstruction
  - If distension is mainly in flanks—suggest large gut obstruction
  - Visible peristalsis
    - If in central abdomen, and small peristaltic waves are seen in step-ladder pattern—suggest small gut obstruction
    - If large peristaltic waves are seen in upper abdomen passing from right to left or large peristaltic waves are seen in flanks—large gut obstruction
  - Scar mark of previous abdominal operation
  - Hernial sites—visible cough impulse.

- *Palpation*:
  - Presence of rebound tenderness suggests underlying gut strangulation
  - Growth/mass in abdomen may be palpable
  - *Hernial sites*—expansile cough impulse may be palpable. If hernia gets obstructed, it becomes irreducible and cough impulse is absent.
- *Percussion*:
  - To distinguish abdominal distension due to gas or fluid.
- *Auscultation*:
  - Hyperperistaltic sounds in intestinal obstruction
  - Silent/occasional metallic sounds in paralytic ileus.
- *Per rectal examination*:
  - Rectal growth may be felt
  - Apex of intussusception can be felt
  - Ballooning of rectum in acute intestinal obstruction
  - On removing, finger may get stained with blood and mucus (redcurrant jelly).
- Systemic examination
- *Investigations*:
  - Straight X-ray of abdomen in erect posture (for gas-fluid levels)
  - Straight X-ray of abdomen in supine posture—gas pattern in gut is better seen
    - Dilated jejunal loops are identified by central location, step-ladder pattern, and presence of valvulae conniventes. The ileal loops appear as characterless
    - May identify a calcified ectopic gallstone.
  - Chest X-ray PA view:
    - Exclude free gas under diaphragm
    - Pulmonary tuberculosis
    - Distant metastasis
  - *Complete hemogram*: Serial WBC count may help to identify a deteriorating patient. TLC may be normal or slightly raised. Increasing TLC may suggest underlying strangulation
  - *Serum urea* and *creatinine*
  - *Random blood sugar*
  - *Serum electrolytes*—GI losses may result in hyponatremia, hypochloremia, and hypokalemia
  - *If solid mass palpable*—USG/CT scan to delineate mass
  - *Contrast studies:*
    - Usually barium contrast studies are contraindicated in acute intestinal obstruction (as it aggravates it)
    - In small children having intussusception—a barium enema study is useful
      - » Because here, it has a diagnostic as well as therapeutic effect
      - » With the help of gravity, it will cause reduction of intussusceptions
- *Water-soluble contrast studies* in patients with adhesive small bowel obstruction has been claimed to be useful. The contrast is administered through the nasogastric tube and is followed by serial radiograph of the abdomen.
- Appearance of contrast in the cecum within 24 hours suggests that a nonoperative approach will be successful.

Q. What do you mean by adynamic obstruction or paralytic ileus?

Ans. Adynamic obstruction or paralytic ileus is caused by absent or disordered peristalsis.

Q. What are the important causes of adynamic obstruction?

Ans. Adynamic obstruction may occur in association with:
* Following GI surgery—manipulation of gut and release of inflammatory mediator release
* Anesthesia
* Systemic infection
* Dyselectrolytemia
* Some neurological disorder.

Q. What is mechanical obstruction?

Ans. In mechanical obstruction, there is physical obstruction at some point in the intestine and there is vigorous peristalsis in the proximal intestine to overcome the obstruction. The distal gut empties normally and ultimately collapses.

Q. Why the gut proximal to the point of obstruction dilates?

Ans. The bowel dilatations occur due to:
* *Swallowed air*: Oxygen is usually absorbed and the distension is mainly due to unabsorbed nitrogen.
* *The bacterial proliferation* in the proximal gut results in fermentation of undigested gut contents and results in accumulation of fermented gas.
* *Sequestration of intestinal fluid*: About 8–9 liters of fluid are secreted and reabsorbed within the gut. Due to obstruction and dilatation, there is increase interstitial pressure in the bowel wall impairing absorption of fluid from the gut lumen. This increased pressure in the gut wall results in further movement of fluid and electrolytes into the lumen of the gut.

Q. Why there is dehydration in intestinal obstruction?

Ans. A number of factors contribute to dehydration in intestinal obstruction:
* Vomiting
* Failure of oral intake
* Sequestration of fluid in intestinal lumen (third space loss).

Q. What is simple intestinal obstruction?

Ans. In simple obstruction, the blood supply of the intestine is not compromised.

Q. What is strangulation obstruction?

Ans. In strangulation obstruction, there is compromise of blood supply of the gut either because of venous congestion or arterial occlusion. As bowel gets distended, there is increased interstitial pressure in the bowel wall and this results in impairment of venous return and unrelieved this leads to arterial occlusion and infarction of the bowel.

Q. What do you mean by closed loop obstruction?

Ans. In closed loop obstruction, there is obstruction of a segment of bowel at two points. In closed loop obstruction, this segment of the gut dilates and may undergo strangulation and perforation before the proximal segment of gut dilates.

This type of obstruction occurs in external hernias, internal volvulus, and large gut obstruction with a competent ileocecal valve.

Q. What are the features of strangulation obstruction?

Ans.

* *Pain*: Colicky abdominal pain changes to constant, sharper, and localized pain
* Patient may become febrile
* On examination, there may be signs of peritonitis—muscle guard and rebound tenderness.

Treatment:

* For details of treatment of intestinal obstruction—*See* X-rays section, Page No. 787, Chapter 17.

17. **A 40-year-male patient underwent exploratory laparotomy for perforated peritonitis. On 7th postoperative day, there is serous discharge from the wound. How will you proceed to manage the situation?**

Ans. Serosanguinous discharge from the wound around 7th postoperative day usually suggest underlying burst abdomen.

For evaluation of this patient, I will take a detail history:

* Regarding the type of pathology for which he was operated
* The time gap between the onset of peritonitis and the operation
* The type of incision (midline or paramedian)
* Type of suture material used for closure of the incision
* Details of the postoperative course:
  - Any cough
  - Any evidence of postoperative intestinal obstruction (pain abdomen, abdominal distension, vomiting, and no passage of flatus or stool)
  - Any evidence of pus collection in the peritoneal cavity (pain abdomen and fever)
  - Any complain of a sensation of something being given away.

Physical examination to assess:

* Presence of shock—pulse, BP, and dehydration.

Local examination:

* Examination of the wound:
  - Assess the type of discharge
  - One or two stitches are removed to assess the underlying wound disruption
  - Look whether omentum or gut loops are seen protruding through the wound.
* Examination of the abdomen to exclude underlying intestinal obstruction—abdominal distension and visible peristalsis.

  If omentum and gut loops are protruding out of the wound, cover these with a sterile moist sheet.

Q. How will you treat abdominal wound dehiscence?

Ans.

- *Resuscitation*:
  - Intravenous fluid to correct fluid and electrolyte deficit
  - Nasogastric suction
  - Antibiotics.
- *Treatment of wound dehiscence*:
  - If there is evisceration:
    - Urgent exploratory laparotomy
    - The extruded gut and the omentum are washed with saline
    - Explore for any obstruction and measures for relief of obstruction (division of adhesive band, if present)
    - The extruded bowel is replaced into the abdomen
    - All layers of abdomen are approximated by interrupted through and through sutures (mass closure) using a monofilament polyamide sutures passed through soft rubber tubing.

The abdominal wall is supported by an abdominal corset.

Postoperative management:

- Intravenous fluid, nasogastric suction, and antibiotics are continued.
  - If there is no evisceration:
    - Patient may be treated nonoperatively
    - Sterile dressing
    - Abdominal binder
    - An incisional hernia is likely to develop, which is to be repaired at a later date.

Q. What is burst abdomen?

Ans. This is a condition of postoperative abdominal wound dehiscence, which usually occurs between 6th and 8th postoperative day.

Q. What is concealed burst abdomen?

Ans. In concealed burst abdomen, there is disruption of the deeper layers of the wound and the skin remains intact. The extruded omentum and the gut lie deep to the skin and are usually not seen, so this is called concealed burst abdomen.

Q. Which factors are important for development of a postoperative burst abdomen?

Ans.

- *General condition of the patient:*
  - Anemia
  - Jaundice
  - Hypoproteinemia
  - Malignant disease.
- *Type of operation*:
  - Operations for peritonitis
  - Operations on pancreas associated with postoperative complications of pancreatic fistula has higher incidence of burst abdomen.

- *Type of incision:*
  - The midline and vertical incision has higher incidence of wound dehiscence than the transverse incision.
- *Type of suture material:*
  - Closure of incision with absorbable suture has higher incidence of burst abdomen than when nonabsorbable sutures are used.
- *Method of closure:*
  - Mass closure of abdominal wound has lesser incidence of burst abdomen than when abdomen is closed in layers
  - Interrupted sutures have lesser incidence of burst abdomen than when continuous suture is applied.
- *Wound drainage:*
  - Insertion of drain through the incision is associated with higher incidence of wound dehiscence than when the drain is inserted through a separate stab wound.
- *Postoperative complications:*
  - Postoperative straining like—coughing, vomiting is associated with increased incidence of burst abdomen
  - Postoperative intestinal obstruction is one of the important factors for development of burst abdomen.

18. A patient underwent laparotomy for perforated appendicitis and developed fever on 3rd postoperative day. How will you manage this patient?

Ans. Important causes of fever on 3rd postoperative day:
- *Extra-abdominal causes*—responsible for postoperative fever in 60–80% of causes. The important causes are:
  - Urinary tract infection
  - Pulmonary complications—atelectasis, pneumonia, and effusion
  - Cardiac cause—infective endocarditis in patients with pre-existing valvular disease
  - Wound complications—cellulitis, abscess, and necrotizing fasciitis
  - Intravenous access site—thrombophlebitis, cellulitis, and septic phlebitis
  - Legs—deep vein thrombosis
  - Indwelling urinary catheter.
- *Intra-abdominal causes:*
  - Intra-abdominal sepsis—subphrenic abscess and pelvic abscess
  - Acute acalculous cholecystitis.

A detail history and physical examination will allow diagnosis in majority of patients. Some ancillary laboratory investigations are also helpful.

History will include:
- Any history of preoperative fever
- Details history about type of fever—continuous, intermittent, remittent, and whether associated with chills and rigor
- Any history of valvular heart disease or any prosthetic heart valve
- Any pre-existing lung disease, postoperative cough with expectoration, hemoptysis, and breathlessness

- Any pain and swelling along the IV access site and any purulent discharge
- Any pain and swelling in the wound and any purulent discharge from the wound
- Any pain abdomen, nausea vomiting or hematemesis, and melena
- Any pain and swelling in the legs.

A detail physical examination:

- General survey—look for temperature, pallor, and jaundice
- Examination of the wound:
    - Any induration
    - Discharge from the wound
    - Examination of abdomen:
        - Look for abdominal distension
        - Tenderness
        - Rebound tenderness
        - Any free fluid or localized collection of pus
        - Bowel sounds
    - Examination of respiratory system to exclude:
        - Lung collapse, consolidation, or
        - Pleural effusion
    - Examination of heart—look for any murmur
    - Examine the IV access site for any:
        - Induration
        - Cellulitis
        - Pus discharge
    - Examination of the leg to exclude deep venous thrombosis:
        - Swelling in leg
        - Tenderness in calf
        - Homan's sign
        - Moses' sign.

Relevant investigations for management:

- Complete hemogram—Hb%, TLC, and differential count
- Chest X-ray
- Urine for routine examination, culture, and sensitivity
- Blood culture
- Wound swab for culture and sensitivity
- Suspicion of infective endocarditis—echocardiography
- Suspicion of intra-abdominal sepsis—CT scan/USG
- Suspicion of acute acalculous cholecystitis—hepatobiliary iminodiacetic acid scanning (HIDA) scanning
- Suspicion of deep venous thrombosis—Doppler study/duplex scanning of venous system.

Treatment—depends on the underlying causes:

- *Pulmonary complications*:
    - Atelectasis—chest physiotherapy and bronchoscopic aspiration

- Pleural effusion—aspiration of pleural fluid. Culture sensitivity of the aspirate and appropriate antibiotics
- Pulmonary embolism—heparin.
- Wound complications—drainage, debridement, culture, and sensitivity of the pus and appropriate antibiotics.
- Infective endocarditis—blood culture and appropriate antibiotics
- Urinary tract infection—urine C/S and appropriate antibiotics
- Access site of complications—remove the catheter—send catheter tip for C/S and appropriate antibiotics
- Septic phlebitis—phlebectomy and drainage of pus
- Deep venous thrombosis—unfractionated heparin or low molecular weight heparin (LMWH)
- Intra-abdominal sepsis—USG/CT-guided aspiration of intra-abdominal pus at subphrenic space or pelvis. If fails open drainage
- Acute acalculous cholecystitis—cholecystectomy.

Q. What is pyrexia?

Ans. When core temperature is more than 38°C then patient is said to have pyrexia. The normal core temperature is 36–38°C.

Macrophages are activated by bacteria and endotoxin. These activated bacteria release a number of substances like interleukin-L, tumor necrosis factor, and interferon. These substances reset the hypothalamic thermoregulatory center to a higher level.

Q. What is malignant hyperpyrexia?

Ans. When patient has a core temperature of more than 40°C then it is called malignant hyperpyrexia. Malignant hyperpyrexia may be associated with acidosis, hypokalemia, coagulopathy, muscle rigidity, and circulatory collapse.

Q. How will you treat malignant hyperpyrexia?

Ans.
- *Reduce temperature*: Cool patient with alcohol sponges and ice
- *Correct acidosis*: Administer sodium bicarbonate (2 mEq/kg IV)
- Administer dantrolene (2.5 mg/kg IV stat the 1 mg/kg every 6 hours for 48 hours).

19. A 60-year-male patient presented with acute retention of urine in emergency. How will you manage?

Ans. Important causes of acute retention of urine in a 60-year male patient include:
- *Bladder outlet obstruction due to:*
  - Benign hyperplasia of prostate
  - Carcinoma of prostate
  - Prostatic abscess or prostatitis
  - Carcinoma of bladder
  - Bladder stone
  - Bladder neck muscular hypertrophy
  - Bladder neck fibrosis.

- *Urethral causes:*
  - Stricture
  - Calculus
  - Tumors
  - Urethritis.
- *Others:*
  - Rupture urethra following trauma
  - Meatal stenosis
  - Phimosis
  - Fecal impaction
  - Spinal injury
  - Postoperative especially after perianal operation
  - Following spinal anesthesia.

Drugs:

- Anticholinergics
- Antihypertensives
- Tricyclic antidepressants.

The management of this patient will include:

- Relief of retention
- Diagnosis of the cause of retention
- Treatment of the underlying cause.

Q. How will you evaluate this patient?

Ans. To come to a diagnosis detail history, clinical examination, and some relevant investigations are required.

I will take detail history about:

- *Onset of retention*—acute or acute on chronic. Any history of increase in frequency of micturition, nocturia, urgency, hesitancy, diminution of stream, burning sensation during micturition, purulent discharge, or passage of turbid urine. Any history of hematuria.
- Any lump in hypogastrium or loin.
- History of trauma or urethral instrumentation.
- History of operation or spinal anesthesia.
- *Drug history:* Some antihypertensive drugs (ganglion-blocking drugs), anticholinergic drugs or antidepressant drugs may cause retention.
- Any systemic symptoms due to underlying malignant disease—anorexia, asthenia, weight loss, and bone pain.

A detail physical examination:

- *General survey:*
  - To look for pallor, dehydration, and hypertension
  - Any features of uremia—hemorrhagic spots and acidotic breathing.
- Local examination of abdomen:
  - Tenderness in the renal angle, hypogastrium, or along the line of ureter. Any renal lump or bladder lump

- Per rectal examination for prostatic enlargement and if enlarged, feel of the gland
- Overlying rectal mucosa—free or fixed
- External genitalia—to exclude phimosis, meatal stenosis, induration, or scarring along the line of urethra. Any palpable stone or growth in penile part of urethra
- Before investigating further, if the bladder is full then the retention is to be relieved first.
- Conservative measures for relief of retention include:
  - Reassurance
  - Application of warmth on hypogastrium
  - Privacy
  - Sound of running tap may be helpful
  - Some antispasmodic drug may help.
- *Catheterization*:
  - If above conservative measures fail, the retention is to be relieved by catheterization under aseptic precaution. For acute on chronic retention an indwelling Foley's catheter is introduced and then patient is investigated to find out the cause of retention.
  - If Foley's catheter could not be passed, a stiff catheter like Gibbon's catheter may be tried.
- *Suprapubic cystostomy*: If catheterization fails, retention needs to be relieved by suprapubic cystostomy. Suprapubic cystostomy may be done by suprapubic puncture using a trocar or by open operation.

Q. Which investigations may help in diagnosis?

Ans. The special investigation will be guided by findings of history and physical examination.
- For evaluation of prostatic enlargement:
  - Ultrasonography of kidney ureter and bladder region
  - Transrectal ultrasonography
  - Urodynamics study
  - Serum prostate-specific antigen.
- For evaluation of bladder or urethral lesion:
  - Micturating cystourethrography
  - Cystoscopy and urethroscopy.

Q. How will you plan definitive treatment?

Ans. The definitive treatment depends on the cause of retention.
- *Benign enlargement of prostate:* Treatment may be:
  - *Drug treatment*: Two classes of drugs are used for treatment of bladder outlet obstruction.
    - *Alpha adrenergic blocking drugs (finasteride):* Inhibit contraction of smooth muscles of prostate
    - *5-alpha reductase inhibitor (terazosin)*: Inhibits conversion of testosterone to 5-dihydrotestosterone (5-DHT)
    - Tamsulosin hydrochloride is also effective in relieving symptoms due to benign prostatic hyperplasia (BPH)
  - Both these drugs improve flow rate and also cause shrinkage of the glands
  - Drug of treatment is indicated when:
    - Symptoms are mild
      - » Patient with severe symptoms but surgery cannot be done for medical problems

» These drugs are expensive and a significant number of patients require surgical treatment afterwards

» *Surgical treatment*: Transurethral resection of prostate or open prostatectomy.

- *Carcinoma of prostate*:
  - *Early stage (T1 and T2 tumors)*: Radical prostatectomy along with pelvic lymph node dissection
  - *Advance disease with urinary retention*: Transurethral resection of prostate followed by hormone therapy
  - *Radiotherapy*: Radical radiotherapy to prostatic bed and pelvic lymph node is an alternative option of treatment for localized disease. For disseminated disease radiotherapy has no role
  - *Hormone treatment*: Androgen ablation is indicated in patients with locally advanced or metastatic disease.
    - Androgen ablation by drugs:
      » Phosphorylated diethylstilbestrol (Honvan)
      » Progestogens—DepoProvera
      » Luteinizing hormone-releasing hormone (LHRH) agonist (Goserelin)—downregulates pituitary and suppresses LH production, thereby reducing serum testosterone concentration
      » Flutamide—blocks the androgen receptor
      » Cyproterone acetate blocks androgen receptor and also has some progestogenic effect
      » Androgen ablation by bilateral orchiectomy.

- *Treatment of urethral stricture*:
  - Urethral dilatation
  - Optical urethrotomy
  - Open urethroplasty.

- *Treatment of carcinoma of bladder*:
  - *Noninvasive tumors*:
    - Transurethral resection of bladder tumor followed by intravesical chemotherapy or immunotherapy
    - Intravesical chemotherapy with either mitomycin-C or Adriamycin or epirubicin weekly for 8–10 weeks
    - Intravesical immunotherapy with bacillus Calmette-Güerin (BCG) is also very effective
    - Radical cystectomy with diversion of urine is indicated in patients with multiple tumors and with extensive carcinoma in situ.
  - *Invasive tumors*:
    - Radical radiotherapy
    - *Surgery*: Partial cystectomy or radical cystectomy with ileal conduit
    - Adjuvant chemotherapy with methotrexate, vinblastine, adriamycin, and cisplatinum.

20. A 60-year-male patient presented with hematuria. How will you manage?

Ans. The important causes of hematuria are:

- *Renal:*
  - Tumor—carcinoma of kidney

- – Tuberculosis
- – Trauma
- – Calculus
- – Polycystic kidney
- – Medical cause—acute glomerulonephritis.
- ◆ *Renal pelvis and ureter*:
  - – Tumor—transitional cell carcinoma
  - – Calculus.
- ◆ *Urinary bladder*:
  - – Tumor—papilloma and papillary carcinoma
  - – Trauma
  - – Tuberculosis
  - – Acute cystitis
  - – Calculus.
- ◆ *Prostate*:
  - – Benign hyperplasia of prostate
  - – Carcinoma of prostate.
- ◆ *Urethra*:
  - – Tumor
  - – Granuloma
  - – Stone.
- ◆ *Systemic causes*:
  - – Drugs—analgesic and anticoagulant
  - – Blood dyscrasia.
- ◆ Subacute bacterial endocarditis
- ◆ Systemic lupus erythematosus (SLE)
- ◆ Pseudohematuria causes:
  - – Beetroot ingestion
  - – Rifampicin ingestion.

To come to a definite diagnosis, a detail history, clinical examination, and some relevant investigations are required.

Detail history includes:

- ◆ *History about hematuria*: Onset—progress whether blood is uniformly mixed with urine or blood is at the beginning of the act or occurs in later part of voiding. Any passage of clots.
- ◆ *Any history of pain*: Painless hematuria usually due to neoplastic lesion. Painful hematuria is typical of urinary calculi. Any renal or ureteric colic and hypogastric pain.
- ◆ *History suggestive of bladder outlet obstruction*: Hesitancy, urgency, frequency, and narrowing of stream.
- ◆ Any *history of urethral trauma.*
- ◆ Any *systemic symptoms like cough*, hemoptysis, or bone pain suggestive of metastasis.
- ◆ Any *history of drug intake like analgesics or anticoagulant.*

Physical examination:

- *General survey:* Look for pulse, BP, pallor, cachexia, and lymphadenopathy
- *Local examination of abdomen*: Any renal lump, palpable bladder in hypogastric region
- Per rectal examination to assess the prostatic size. Examination of external genitalia
- *Investigations*: The type of investigations to be done will be guided by the clinical examination
- Examination of urine:
  - Specific gravity, protein, sugar, blood, and ketone
  - Microscopic RBC and crystals
  - Exfoliative cytology
  - Acid-fast bacilli (AFB) smear and culture
  - Culture and sensitivity.
- *Renal function test*: Blood urea, creatinine, and creatinine clearance
- *Radiological*:
  - Straight X-ray kidney, ureter, and bladder (KUB)
  - Intravenous urography
  - Ultrasonography of abdomen
  - CT scan of abdomen
  - Renal arteriography
  - Transrectal USG
  - Urethrography
  - Cystography.
- Cystoscopic examination
- *Treatment*: Depends on the underlying cause
- Carcinoma of kidney:
  - *For operable tumors*: Radical nephrectomy. Radiotherapy and chemotherapy are not very effective. Cytokine interleukin-2 has shown promising results as adjuvant therapy.
  - For inoperable tumors, a preoperative course of radiotherapy followed by surgery may be possible.
- For renal pelvis tumor:
  - Nephroureterectomy is the optimum treatment.
- For renal and ureteric calculi:
  - Extracorporeal shock wave lithotripsy
  - Percutaneous nephrolithotomy
  - Open surgery—nephrolithotomy, pyelolithotomy, or ureterolithotomy.
- For bladder tumors: *See* Page No. 754.
- For prostatic enlargement: *See* Page No. 753.
- Renal trauma: *See* Page No. 714.

21. A 30-year-female patient presented with a solitary thyroid nodule. How will you manage?

Ans. To plan management, I will proceed as follows:
- Details history and clinical examination
- Relevant investigations
- Treatment depending on the cause.

History:

- *Details history about the swelling*: Duration, onset, progress of the swelling, size of the swelling at onset and the present size, any history of rapid increase in size of the swelling
- *Any history of pressure symptoms:* Dyspnea, dysphagia, and hoarseness of voice
- *Any history suggestive of hyper- or hypofunction of thyroid by enquiring about:*
  - Appetite and weight loss
  - Any history of diarrhea
  - Palpitation
  - Breathlessness
  - Anxiety
  - Sleep
  - Sweating
  - Cold/heat intolerance
  - Trembling
  - Any bulging of the eyes
  - Difficulty in vision
  - Menstrual history—any history of oligomenorrhea or menorrhagia.
- *Any history suggestive of metastasis in suspected cases of malignant thyroid nodule*:
  - Neck lymph nodes
  - Bone pain
  - Chest pain
  - Cough and hemoptysis
  - Headache
  - Abdominal pain and any mass in abdomen
  - Any history of jaundice.
- *Details physical examination*:
  - *General survey*:
    - Pulse especially sleeping pulse rate
    - Blood pressure
    - Jaundice
    - Neck lymph nodes.
  - Local examination of thyroid region:
    - Details about the swelling—site, size, shape, surface, margin, consistency, mobility of nodule, and movement with deglutition
    - *Carotid pulsation*: Berry's sign
    - Any thrill and bruit over the gland
    - Kocher's test.
  - Any retrosternal extension is ascertained by:
    - Any puffiness in the face, any engorged veins in the neck and chest wall
    - Palpating the lower border of the thyroid gland in the neck
    - Percussion over the manubrium sterni
    - Pemberton's sign.
  - Examination for toxic signs:
    - Pulse rate
    - Eye signs

- Tremor in tongue and hands
- Pretibial myxedema
- Thrill and bruit over the thyroid gland.
 – Systemic examination:
  - Abdominal examination
  - Skeletal system
  - Respiratory system
  - Cardiovascular system
  - Neurological system.
 – *Investigations*: I will suggest baseline investigations like—complete hemogram, blood for sugar, urea, and creatinine. Chest X-ray and ECG
 – Apart from baseline investigations, I will suggest following investigations:
  - *Thyroid profile*: T3, T4, and TSH
  - USG of thyroid region
  - USG-guided fine-needle aspiration cytology (FNAC) from the thyroid nodule
  - Soft tissue X-ray of the neck—AP and lateral view to look for any calcification and assess any tracheal compression
  - Indirect laryngoscopy to assess any vocal cord palsy.

With FNAC and USG of thyroid region, it is possible to ascertain the nature of the thyroid nodule in majority of cases and the treatment may be planned accordingly.

The following investigations are required in selected cases:

* Radionuclide scan of thyroid using ^{123}I or ^{131}I in cases with toxic thyroid nodule to ascertain whether the nodule is hyperfunctioning or not.
* CT scan of thyroid region in cases with suspected retrosternal prolongation.
* Thyroid autoantibodies in suspected cases of thyroiditis.
* Treatment will depend on the underlying cause:
 – *Colloid nodule*:
  - Wait and watch, if the nodule is small in size. May be treated with suppressive dose of L-thyroxine.
  - Hemithyroidectomy, if the nodules do not regress or show progressive increase.
 – *Solitary toxic nodule*: Hemithyroidectomy.
 – *Follicular adenoma:* Hemithyroidectomy.
 – *Follicular or papillary carcinoma*: Total thyroidectomy.

22. Patient underwent total thyroidectomy and on the same evening developed severe respiratory distress. How will you manage?

Ans. Important causes of respiratory distress after thyroidectomy are:
* Hemorrhage
* Laryngeal edema
* Bilateral recurrent laryngeal nerve palsy
* Tracheomalacia.

Unilateral or bilateral recurrent laryngeal nerve palsy may not cause immediate respiratory obstruction, but may contribute to development of respiratory obstruction, if there is associated laryngeal edema.

Q. How will you diagnose postoperative hemorrhage?

Ans. Diagnosis of hemorrhage may be done by:
* *Features of shock*—pallor, cold clammy extremities, tachycardia, and hypotension
* If a drain was inserted, assess the amount of blood in the drain. Excessive collection in the drain bag indicates continuing hemorrhage
* Remove dressing, and see if the stiches are under tension. Underlying hematoma is indicated by a swelling underneath the skin with tightness in the neck.

Q. How will you manage respiratory distress due to hemorrhage?

Ans. If the patient has respiratory distress due to a tension hematoma—few stitches are to be removed in the ward to relieve the compression.

Patient is to be shifted to the operation theater for re-exploration. Postoperative bleeding may be due to slippage of a ligature or bleeding from a thyroid remnant. The bleeding vessels need to be overrun by a suture. Wound resutured keeping a drain.

Blood transfusion may be required in cases with severe hemorrhage.

Q. How will you manage respiratory distress due to recurrent laryngeal nerve palsy?

Ans. Recurrent laryngeal nerve palsy may be unilateral or bilateral.

In unilateral recurrent laryngeal nerve palsy, there is usually no respiratory distress in the immediate postoperative period.

If both recurrent laryngeal nerves are damaged and patient has severe respiratory distress and stridor immediately after extubation—an immediate endotracheal intubation or tracheostomy is to be done.

Bilateral recurrent laryngeal nerve palsy, however, may not always cause respiratory obstruction.

If the cords lie in a cadaveric position, patient may not develop respiratory obstruction immediately, but if the patient develops laryngeal edema then respiratory obstruction may be obvious and patient might need intubation or tracheostomy.

If the cords lie in paramedian position, respiratory obstruction will become obvious immediately.

Q. How will you manage respiratory distress due to tracheomalacia?

Ans. In long-standing cases of large goiter, there may be tracheomalacia and following thyroidectomy and extubation there may be respiratory distress in the immediate postoperative period.

Patient will need immediate endotracheal intubation or tracheostomy.

23. A 30-year-male patient presented with dry gangrene of right great toe. How will you manage?

Ans. Important causes of gangrene in foot in this age group of patient:
* Buerger's disease
* Presenile atherosclerosis
* Embolic gangrene

- Infective gangrene
- Traumatic gangrene
- Diabetic foot
- Inflammatory arteritis.

For proper management, a detail history, physical examination, and some relevant investigations are required to come to a diagnosis and to plan treatment accordingly.

Detail history includes:

- History about the gangrene—onset (sudden or insidious) and progress of the gangrene
- Associated symptoms like—intermittent claudication—if present progress of claudication, any rest pain
- Any history of Raynaud's phenomenon—series of color changes on exposure to cold
  - Stage of pallor
  - Stage of local cyanosis
  - Stage of red engorgement
- Any history of superficial phlebitis—pain and redness along the course of veins
- Any history of trauma
- Any history of cardiac disease—chest pain on exertion, palpitation, breathlessness, and any history of transient ischemic attacks
- Any history of abdominal pain and impotency
- Detail history of smoking
- Any history of diabetes or hypertension.

A detail physical examination:

- General survey—any pallor, BP, and pulse.

Local examination of lower extremities:

- *Inspection*:
  - Any deformity
  - Condition of veins—well filled or empty, any discoloration along the veins
  - Evidence of peripheral ischemia of leg—shiny skin, loss of hair, brittle nails, ulcer, or gangrene
  - Examination of gangrenous area—dry or moist, site and extent, line of demarcation, and condition of area adjacent to the gangrene.
- *Palpation*:
  - Assess temperature of the limb and compare with the normal side
  - Any tenderness along the veins
  - Examination of the gangrenous area—site and extent of the gangrene, tenderness, and sensation
  - Examination of peripheral pulses—compare with the opposite side
    - Superficial temporal
    - Carotid
    - Subclavian
    - Axillary
    - Brachial

- Radial
- Ulnar
- Femoral
- Popliteal
- Posterior tibial
- Anterior tibial
- Dorsalis pedis
  - Some special tests:
    - Capillary filling time
    - Venous filling time
    - Buerger's test
    - Fuschig's test (cross leg test)—indirect method of testing popliteal artery pulse
◆ *Auscultation*: Over peripheral arteries for presence of any bruit
  – Examination for movement of joints
  – Examination of regional lymph nodes
  – Neurological examination:
    - Examination of motor system to assess any muscular paralysis
    - Examination of sensory system to assess any sensory deficit
    - Examination reflexes—jerks to ascertain the level of neurological lesion
  – Examination of regional lymph nodes.

Systemic examination:

◆ Examination of CVS
◆ Examination of abdomen
◆ Examination of respiratory system.

Investigations and treatment:

◆ Hemogram—Hb%, TLC, DLC, and erythrocyte sedimentation rate (ESR)
◆ Blood for fasting and postprandial (PP) sugar
◆ Serum urea and creatinine
◆ Complete lipid profile—triglyceride cholesterol, low-density lipoprotein (LDL), high-density lipoprotein (HDL), and very low-density lipoprotein (VLDL)
◆ Chest X-ray
◆ ECG
◆ Duplex study of peripheral vessels
◆ Arteriography in selected cases
◆ Local X-ray of gangrenous toe.

Treatment includes:

◆ Reassurance
◆ Stop smoking
◆ Control diabetes and hypertension, if any
◆ Dietary modification to control hyperlipidemia, if present
◆ Exercise to improve claudication distance

- *Drugs*: Pentoxifylline and cilostazol have some role. Vasodilator drugs have no role
- Care of gangrenous part:
  - Keep it dry—by dressing with dry antibiotic powder
  - Pus culture
  - Antibiotics.

For Buerger's disease:

- Indirect surgery in the form of lumbar sympathectomy may be tried
- Omentopexy may also be tried
- Conservative amputation of gangrenous toe.

For atherosclerosis:

- Direct arterial surgery has a role
- Transluminal angioplasty
- Atherectomy
- Intraluminal stents
- Vascular bypass graft.

24. **A-40-year-female patient presented with abnormal nipple discharge. How will you proceed to manage this patient?**

Ans. Important causes of abnormal nipple discharge include:
- *Abnormal milky*—hyperprolactinemia and hypothyroidism
- *Serous*—fibroadenosis and retention cyst
- *Brown*—fibroadenosis
- *Blood stained*—duct papilloma, duct carcinoma, and duct ectasia
- *Purulent*—infection.

   To come to a diagnosis to ascertain the underlying disease, a clinical examination and some relevant investigations are required.

Detail history is essential:

- Onset of discharge
- Duration
- Character of the discharge—milky, serous, brown, blood stained, or purulent
- Discharge from a single duct or from many ducts
- Any lump in the breast, if present its onset and progress
- Any pain in the breast or fever
- Any history of thyroid disease.

Examination of breast: By inspection and palpation.

- *Symmetry of breast*, any obvious swelling
- *Nipple and areola*—size, shape, any nipple retraction. Squeeze the nipple to inspect the character of the discharge and to ascertain discharge coming from a single or multiple ducts
- *Palpate breast* in all quadrants for any lump and if a lump is palpable, details of the lump—position and extent, size and shape, surface, margin, consistency, fixity to skin, breast tissue or underlying muscles, and the chest wall

- *Examination* of the lymph nodes in the axilla and the neck
- *Investigations*:
  - Examination of discharge—for blood, Gram stain, and Papanicolaou stain
  - Mammography
  - USG of breast
  - If a lump is palpable and trucut biopsy from the lump
  - If milky discharge—serum prolactin assay
  - Ductography
- *Treatment:* Depends on the underlying cause
  - *Fibroadenosis*—reassurance/evening primrose oil/danazol
  - Duct papilloma and duct ectasia—microdochectomy
  - If associated with underlying duct carcinoma—treatment depends on the stage of the disease.

25. A 40-year-female patient presented with a lump in her right breast. How will you manage?

Ans. The important causes of lump in breast in this age group may be due to:
- Benign neoplastic lesion:
  - Fibroadenoma breast
  - Duct papilloma.
- Malignant breast lesion:
  - Duct carcinoma
  - Lobular carcinoma.
- Non-neoplastic lesion:
  - Fibroadenosis of breast
  - Breast cyst
  - Galactocele
  - Duct ectasia
  - Tuberculosis of breast
  - Traumatic fat necrosis
  - Antibioma
  - Organized hematoma.

The management of a patient presenting with breast lump would include a detailed clinical evaluation and some relevant investigations and definitive treatment.

History about the lump—onset, size at the onset, progress, and any pain. Any other swelling in the opposite breast or axilla.

Other associated symptoms like anorexia, weakness, weight loss, bone pain, low backache, chest pain, cough, hemoptysis, any abdominal pain or swelling, and any history of jaundice.

Family history: History breast carcinoma or related carcinoma like colonic, gastric, or ovarian carcinoma in the family in earlier two to three generations.

Personal history: Detail of menstrual and obstetric history. Any history of oral pill or hormone replacement therapy.

Physical examination:

- Examination of breasts:
  - Shape and symmetry of breast
  - Nipple—position, size, shape, crack/ulcer, retraction, and discharge
  - Areola—size, shape, crack, ulcer, and fissure
  - Skin over the breast—scar, venous prominence, peaud'orange, nodule, ulcer, or cancer en cuirasse.
- Any swelling—site, size, shape, surface, margin, consistency, relation with breast tissue, fixity to skin, pectoral fascia, and chest wall.
- Examination of regional lymph nodes—axillary and cervical lymph nodes.

A detail systemic examination:

- Abdomen/respiratory system/CVS/nervous system and skeletal system
- Relevant investigations will include:
  - Blood—complete hemogram
  - Chest X-ray
- Biopsy from the lump:
  - Trucut biopsy from the breast lump
  - If biopsy diagnosis is a malignant lump, further investigations will be required to stage the disease
  - Liver function test
  - Ultrasonography/CT scan of abdomen
  - Whole body bone scanning in selected cases
  - CT scan of chest/brain in selected cases.

Treatment will depend on the diagnosis on the basis of clinical examination and investigations.

- *Fibroadenosis*—reassurance/evening primrose oil/danazol
- *Benign neoplastic lesion*:
  - *Fibroadenoma*—simple excision
  - *Duct papilloma*—microdochectomy
- *Carcinoma breast*—treatment depends on the stage of the disease
  - *Early carcinoma breast*:
    - Breast conservation surgery
    - Modified radical mastectomy
    - Adjuvant therapy—chemotherapy/radiotherapy and hormone therapy.
  - *Locally advanced carcinoma breast*:
    - if operable, modified radical mastectomy followed by adjuvant therapy
    - Inoperable locally advanced disease—neoadjuvant chemotherapy followed by simple mastectomy. Postoperative radiotherapy/hormone therapy
    - Breast-conserving surgery is selected cases after neoadjuvant chemotherapy
  - *Metastatic breast carcinoma*:
    - Systemic chemotherapy/hormone therapy
    - Simple mastectomy/radiotherapy to breast and axilla.

26.   **A 55-year-male patient underwent Whipple's operation. On 3rd postoperative day patient complained of swelling of both legs and fever.**

Q. What is the important cause of such situation?

Ans. This elderly patient having a malignant disease and probably having jaundice underwent major surgical intervention is at high-risk of developing deep venous thrombosis. The most likely cause of this situation is development of deep venous thrombosis.

Q. What may be the differential diagnosis?

Ans. Other causes of swelling in both lower limbs may be due to:
* Cellulitis
* Edema due to hypoalbuminemia
* Renal failure
* Congestive cardiac failure
* Ruptured Baker's cyst
* Calf muscle hematoma.

Q. What are the important clinical features of deep vein thrombosis?

Ans. In addition to the swelling of the legs and fever, the other important features are:
* Pain in legs
* Redness
* Dilatation of superficial veins in the leg
* Presence of calf tenderness
* Pain in the calf on dorsiflexion of the ankle (Homan's sign) is no longer regarded as a reliable sign of deep vein thrombosis
* In some patients, there may be no symptoms or signs in the legs and the patient may present with dyspnea due to pulmonary embolism.

Q. How will you confirm diagnosis of deep vein thrombosis?

Ans. The diagnosis of deep vein thrombosis is based on imaging investigations:
* Duplex USG is a noninvasive reliable way of diagnosing deep vein thrombosis. The imaged veins show intraluminal clot and the veins are noncompressible
* *Ascending phlebography*: If duplex sonography is not available, ascending phlebography is helpful for diagnosis.

Q. How will you treat deep venous thrombosis?

Ans. Once the diagnosis is made, patient should be started on IV heparin or LMWH.

The dose of heparin is adjusted depending on the body weight and by keeping activated partial thromboplastin time (aPTT) two and half times the normal. The heparin is continued for at least 5 days.

Patient is also started on oral anticoagulants (warfarin). Oral anticoagulants should be continued for at least 6 months.

The dose of warfarin is adjusted by prothrombin time keeping international normalized ratio (INR) between 2.5 and 3.5 times the normal control value.

Patient with thrombophilia should be given anticoagulant for life.

Q. What are the advantages of using low-molecular weight heparin?

Ans. Low-molecular weight heparin like enoxaparin, fraxiparine is being used as alternative to unfractionated heparin. The LMWH produces reliable anticoagulation without risk of hemorrhage and dose monitoring with blood tests are not required. Like heparin regime, oral anticoagulant should be started simultaneously and dose adjusted by INR.

Q. What is thrombolytic therapy?

Ans. In massive venous thrombosis, there may be impending venous gangrene in the limb. In such situation, rapid thrombolysis may be achieved by passing a catheter into the vein and infusing fibrinolytic agents like streptokinase or tissue plasminogen activator.

Q. What is venous thrombectomy?

Ans. In rare situation in cases with massive venous thrombosis, surgical removal of thrombus may be considered. A femoral venotomy is done and the blood clots are cleared using a Fogarty balloon catheter. However, the results of thrombectomy are not encouraging.

Q. Patient having deep vein thrombosis is at the risk of developing pulmonary embolism. How will you diagnose pulmonary embolism?

Ans. Pulmonary embolism is one of the serious complications of deep vein thrombosis.

Massive pulmonary embolism may cause complete occlusion of the pulmonary artery and may lead to sudden death.

Small emboli may cause occlusion of small peripheral pulmonary vascular bed causing pulmonary infarction. Patient may present with cough, breathlessness, and pleuritic type of chest pain.

Q. What investigations are helpful for diagnosis of pulmonary embolism?

Ans. The diagnosis may be confirmed by:
+ Contrast-enhanced CT scan of chest
+ Ventilation–perfusion scan.

Q. How will you treat pulmonary embolism?

Ans. Pulmonary embolism is a medical emergency. Once diagnosis is made, treatment started with IV unfractionated heparin or LMWH.

Fibrinolytic drugs may be infused into the pulmonary arteries in cases of massive pulmonary embolism.

Q. How will you prevent pulmonary embolism?

Ans. Some patients of deep vein thrombosis are at the risk of pulmonary embolism in spite of full anticoagulation. Pulmonary embolism may also occur in patient with silent deep vein thrombosis.

Pulmonary embolism may be prevented by insertion of IVC filter. This filter is usually inserted via the internal jugular or via femoral vein by interventional radiology. The dislodged blood clots are trapped in the IVC filter thereby preventing pulmonary embolism.

Q. What are the factors for development of deep vein thrombosis?

Ans. Virchow's triad is described as the factors responsible for development of deep venous thrombosis. This includes:

* *Changes in vessel*: The endothelium may be damaged by injury or inflammation.
* *Changes in blood flow*: Slowing of blood flow is an important factor for development of deep venous thrombosis. This may occur in patient confined to bed for prolonged period due to debilitating conditions. This may also occur in surgical patients during and after operations.
* *Alteration of blood viscosity*: Increased coagulability of blood may occur in some congenital condition (thrombophilia). Increased coagulability of blood may also occur after surgery or following infection.

Q. What is thrombophilia?

Ans. This is a congenital condition of increased susceptibility to deep vein thrombosis. This can occur in patients with deficiencies of antithrombin III, protein S and protein C, and factor V Leiden.

The deep vein thrombosis may occur in younger age. The milder form of the disease may present in later age.

Q. How do you classify surgical patient with respect to risk for development of deep vein thrombosis?

Ans. Hospitalized patients confined to bed and the surgical patients are at risk of developing deep vein thrombosis. Patients are classified as:

* High risk:
  - Age more than 40 years
  - Obesity
  - Associated comorbid conditions like diabetes and hypertension
  - Malignant disease
  - History of previous deep venous thrombosis
  - History of acute myocardial infarction
  - Prolonged preoperative confinement to bed
  - Undergoing major surgery lasting for more than 30 minutes
* Intermediate risk:
  - Age more than 40 years
  - Debilitating illness
  - Undergoing major surgery
  - No additional risk factors
* Low risk:
  - Age less than 40 years
  - Minor surgery
  - No additional risk factors.

Q. How will you provide prophylaxis against deep vein thrombosis?

Ans. All patients undergoing surgery are at the risk of developing deep venous thrombosis. The measures for prophylaxis will depend on the risk stratification.

* In low-risk patients, simple measures like early ambulation, active and passive exercise of lower limbs. No pharmacological therapy is required.

- In intermediate-risk patients in addition to above measures, use of graduated elastic stockinette or intermittent pneumatic compression device is effective in preventing deep vein thrombosis. In selected cases, pharmacological therapy is indicated
- In high-risk patients in addition to above measures, pharmacological therapy is indicated
- The pharmacologic therapy includes:
  - Low-dose heparin—5,000 iu subcutaneously thrice daily
  - Low-molecular weight heparin—enoxaparin, fraxiparine, etc. LMWH is preferred over heparin
  - Oral anticoagulants—heparin or LMWH is usually continued for about 5 days. Patient is started on oral anticoagulants 72 hours after surgery once the risk of bleeding is not there. The risk of deep vein thrombosis remains in postdischarge period, so prophylactic treatment should be continued in the postdischarge period with oral anticoagulant. The treatment with oral anticoagulant should be monitored with prothrombin time and INR should be kept between 2.5 and 3.5 times the normal.

27. **A 50-year-male patient underwent laparotomy for peptic perforation 7 days back. patient complains of pain and purulent discharge from the wound.**

Q. What may be the cause of such situation?

Ans. Pain at the local site and purulent discharge suggest development of wound infection.

Q. Which bacteria are commonly involved in wound infection?

Ans. Different bacteria may be responsible for development of wound infection. These include:

Gram-positive bacteria:

- *Streptococci*: Most important of these are beta-hemolytic *Streptococci*. *Streptococcus faecalis* and *Streptococcus pyogenes* are involved following colorectal surgery.
- *Staphylococci:* Most important organism causing wound infection. Most strains are beta-lactamase producers. Some are methicillin resistant and some methicillin-resistant strains are resistant to vancomycin.

Aerobic Gram-negative bacilli:

- Include *Escherichia coli, Klebsiella, Proteus species* and *Pseudomonas.* These are normal inhabitants in large bowel. Most of these organisms in combination with bacteroides cause wound infection.
- *Bacteroides*: Bacteroides fragilis is the most important organism in this group, a nonspore bearing strict anaerobe that is normally present in large bowel and vagina.

Q. What is Koch's postulate regarding infection?

Ans. The koch's postulate regarding infection:

- The organism must be found in considerable numbers at the site of infection.
- The organism should be grown in pure culture form the site of infective focus.
- The organism should be able to produce similar lesion when injected into another individual.

Q. What are the risk factors for postoperative wound infection?

Ans. The risk factors for postoperative wound infection include:
- Host factors:
  - local host defenses include:
    - an intact epithelium, which resists penetration by the microorganism
    - Flushing action of tears, urine, and cilia of tracheobronchial tree
    - Gastric pH, local immunity by secretion of IgA by intestinal epithelium.
- *Systemic host defense*: Once the microorganism invades, the body a complex system of defense mechanism comes into play to kill the invading microorganism. These include:
- *Cell-mediated immunity*: Polymorphonuclear leukocytes, tissue macrophages can phagocytose the invading microorganism and kill them.
- *Humoral immunity*: Antibodies against the invading organism, complement system, cytokines, leukotrienes, and other biologically inactive molecules may take part in killing the invading microorganisms.

The host defenses may be altered in:
- Malnutrition
- diabetes
- uremia
- jaundice
- immunosuppressed individuals (AIDS, steroid therapy, or other immunosuppressive therapy)
- Advanced malignancy
- Anemia
- Aostoperative patients
- Local wound factors:
  - Contaminated wounds
  - Presence of dead and devitalized tissue
  - Presence of foreign body in the wound
  - Local ischemia (due to shock or peripheral vascular disease)
- *Surgical technique*: It is an important determinant of wound infection
  - Gentle tissue handling
  - Removing all dead and devitalized tissue
  - Achieving adequate hemostasis
  - Optimal use of diathermy
  - Rational use of drains
  - Avoiding suturing under tension
  - May reduce the incidence of wound infection.

Q. How will you manage a patient having postoperative wound infection?

Ans. A thorough clinical assessment is required for proper management. This is important to differentiate whether patient is having minor or major wound infection and whether there is associated necrotizing soft tissue infection.

- Major wound infection:
  - Significant amount of pus discharge from the wound
  - May require drainage of pus
  - Systemic features like pyrexia, toxemia, and tachycardia
  - Leukocytosis indicating systemic infection
  - Hospital stay may be prolonged.
- Minor wound infection:
  - Minimal discharge of pus
  - No evidence of systemic sepsis.

Clinical evaluation will include a general assessment of patient including history regarding, fever, pain at the site of wound, and any discharge from the wound.

The local wound should be examined for any discharge, any underlying induration, any skin bullae, or overlying skin necrosis.

- *SIRS*: Systemic inflammatory response syndrome. Presence of any two of the following:
  - Hyperthermia (>38°C) or hypothermia (<36°C)
  - Tachycardia (>90/min) or tachypnea (>20/min)
  - White blood cell count more than 12,000/mm^3 or less than 4,000/mm3
- *Sepsis*: Presence of SIRS with a documented evidence of infection
- *Sepsis syndrome or severe sepsis*: Presence of sepsis with evidence of one more organ failure.
  - Respiratory failure—acute respiratory distress syndrome (ARDS)
  - Renal failure—acute tubular necrosis
  - Cardiovascular failure
  - Central nervous system failure.
- MODS—Multiorgan dysfunction syndrome (Criteria).
- MSOF—Multisystem organ failure (Criteria).
- Laboratory investigation will include TLC and DLC.

Few stitches from the wound may be removed and the pus drained. The pus is sent for culture sensitivity.

Patient is started on broad-spectrum antibiotics and the antibiotics should be changed later depending on the C/S report.

Q. What is superficial surgical site infection (SSSI)?

Ans. SSSI—superficial surgical site infection. Infection remained confined to the superficial layers of the wound.

Q. How do you classify wounds depending on wound contamination?

Ans. Surgical wounds are classified depending on the amount of contamination and risk of wound infection:

- Clean wounds (wound infection 1–3%):
  - Elective surgery where there is no breach of alimentary, respiratory, and genitourinary tracts
  - Wound is primarily closed
  - No drains in the wound
  - No inflammation and no break in asepsis.

- Clean and contaminated wounds (wound infection 3–4%):
  - There is controlled breach of alimentary, respiratory, or genitourinary tract
  - Drain in wound.
- Contaminated wounds (wound infection 8–10%):
  - Open and fresh traumatic wounds
  - Breach of genitourinary and biliary tree in presence of infected urine or infected bile
  - Gross spillage from alimentary tract.
- Dirty and infected wounds (wound infection 28–40%):
  - Traumatic wounds with retained dead and devitalized tissue and fecal contamination
  - Perforative peritonitis
  - Presence of pus during operation.

Q. What are the criteria for diagnosis of SSSI?

Ans. The criteria are as follows:
- Infection occurring within 30 days after operation
- Involves skin and subcutaneous tissue above the fascial layer
- Purulent discharge from the wound
- Organism is isolated from culture taken from the wound.

Q. What is the source of bacteria leading to wound infection?

Ans.
- *Endogenous:* The majority of the bacteria causing wound infection are derived from the endogenous source. These bacteria normally colonize the skin and mucosal surfaces. With altered host defense and altered pathogenicity of the microorganisms, these bacteria lead to wound infection.
- *Exogenous:* The bacteria for the hospital environment and the health personnel can infect the patient. This is also known as nosocomial infection.

Q. What do you mean by necrotizing soft tissue infection?

Ans. Necrotizing soft tissue infection is a type of deep wound infection when there is necrosis of deeper tissues of the wound. The necrotizing infection may involve the underlying fascia or the muscles. These infections are variously described as necrotizing fasciitis, bacterial synergistic gangrene, streptococcal gangrene, and clostridial myonecrosis.

Q. Which organisms are usually responsible for necrotizing soft tissue infection?

Ans. Most necrotizing infections are caused by mixed aerobic and anaerobic Gram-negative bacteria and Gram-positive bacteria.
- *Clostridia*: *Clostridium perfringens*, *Clostridium novyi*, and *Clostridium septicum* lead to extensive myonecrosis (gas gangrene)
- *Streptococcus pyogenes* can cause extensive tissue necrosis
- Halophilic marine *Vibrio* species may also cause extensive tissue necrosis.

Q. How will you diagnose necrotizing soft tissue infection?

Ans.
- Often the clinical manifestation may be subtle, overlying skin may be normal with evidence of only cellulitis

- There may be overlying skin necrosis or presence of bullae with evidence of underlying induration
- Presence of confusion and toxemia.

Q. How will you treat necrotizing soft tissue infection?

Ans.
- *Surgical treatment*: Adequate debridement of all necrotic tissue. The extent of necrosis may not be apparent at initial debridement. The wound should be inspected daily and repeated debridement may be necessary.
- *Antibiotics:* A Gram staining and culture sensitivity of the discharge should be sent. A broad-spectrum antibiotic should be started.
- *Hyperbaric oxygen therapy*: Patient is allowed to inhale oxygen in chamber having a pressure three times that of atmospheric pressure. Hyperbaric oxygen is effective in toxemia caused by *Clostridium* species. Hyperbaric oxygen therapy is not effective in soft tissue infection caused by nonclostridial organisms.

Q. What measures can prevent wound infection?

Ans. A number of factors are responsible for wound infection. The following measures may help to reduce the incidence of wound infection:
- Improvement of host resistance:
  - Correction of malnutrition and obesity
  - Control of diabetes mellitus
  - Abnormal physiologic states associated with cirrhosis, uremia should be corrected before surgery
  - Cessation of smoking before operation.
- Preoperative preparation:
  - *Preoperative hospital stay*—longer preoperative hospital stay is associated with higher rate of wound infection. Shorter hospital stay lowers the risk of colonization by methicillin-resistant and multiply-resistant microorganism.
  - *Preoperative shower*—preoperative shower with povidone iodine or chlorhexidine may reduce the incidence of wound infection.
  - *Hair removal*—hairs may be removed by clipping, use of depilatory agents, or shaving. Shaving may cause minute cuts, which may be the site of bacterial colonization. Incidence of wound infection is higher in shaving than when hairs are removed by clipping. Shaving at operation theater just before operation may reduce the bacterial colonization and the chance of wound infection is less.
  - *Skin preparation*—degerming of skin with antiseptic solution reduces the chance of wound infection. Antiseptic cleaning with a povidone iodine solution is adequate.
  - *Treatment of remote infection*—presence of remote infection may lead to higher incidence of wound infection. Elective surgery should be delayed till the remote infection is treated.
- Operating theater environment:
  - Operating room environment

- *Theater air*—filtration of operating theater air may reduce the airborne bacterial population in the operating room. Positive pressure inside the operating room will ensure no entry of unfiltered air inside the operating room. In most modern theater, laminar air flow system with high efficiency particulate filter provides the best operating room environment.
- *Health personnel*—there should be minimum number of health personnel inside the theater and the talking should also be minimized.
- *Instruments and drapes*—proper sterilization of operating instruments.
- *Handwashing*—handwashing with chlorhexidine or povidone iodine solution.
- *Gloves*—provide barrier to infection from healthcare personnel to the patient and from patient to healthcare personnel. Use of two pairs of gloves reduces further the likelihood of infection transmission.
- *Use of cap and mask*—prevents fall of skin scales and droplets from health personnel to patients. However, there is no evidence that use of cap and mask do reduce wound infection. However, cap and mask should still be used to prevent contact of patient blood with the health personnel.

Chapter

17

X-rays

■ INTRODUCTION

In practical examination, two types of X-rays are given—(1) plain or straight X-rays and (2) some contrast X-rays. The plain X-rays are taken without administering any contrast material.

When a plain X-ray is given, it is desirable that you describe the region included in the X-ray, e.g. this is a plain X-ray of abdomen with lower part of the chest and upper part of the pelvis showing.............. describe the abnormality.

The different contrast X-rays are taken after administering some contrast material. The different contrast X-rays are:

* Barium swallow
* Barium meal
* Barium enema
* Endoscopic retrograde cholangiopancreaticography
* T-tube cholangiogram
* Percutaneous transhepatic cholangiography
* Intravenous urography (IVU).

The contrast X-rays are usually taken in sequence in different times. When a contrast X-ray is given identify the type of contrast X-ray and note if the time is written. A contrast X-ray may be described as:

This is one of the skiagram from IVU series taken 10 minutes after injection of dye showing .... describe the details.

■ STRAIGHT X-RAY OF CHEST/ABDOMEN WITH FREE GAS UNDER BOTH DOMES OF DIAPHRAGM (FIGS 17.1 TO 17.3)

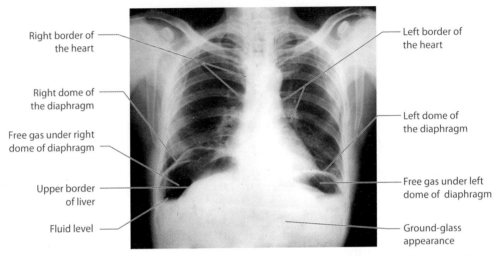

Fig. 17.1: This is a straight X-ray of chest along with upper part of abdomen showing free gas under both domes of the diaphragm and there is a ground-glass appearance in the abdomen

Courtesy: Prof Bitan Kumar Chattopadhyay, IPGME and R, Kolkata

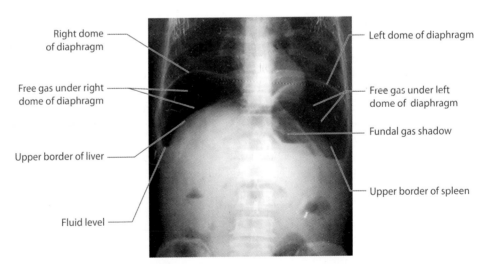

Fig. 17.2: Similar X-ray—Note huge amount of free gas under both domes of diaphragm

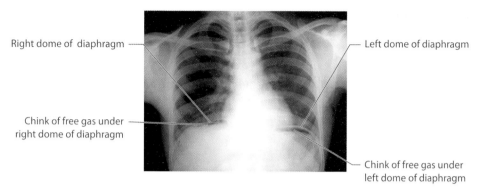

Right dome of diaphragm

Left dome of diaphragm

Chink of free gas under
right dome of diaphragm

Chink of free gas under
left dome of diaphragm

Fig. 17.3: Similar X-ray—Note chink of free gas under both domes of diaphragm

Q. What is this radiological appearance suggests?

Ans. This appearance is due to free gas and fluid in the peritoneal cavity.

Q. What are the causes of such X-ray appearance?

Ans.
- Perforation of hollow viscera containing gas:
  - Peptic ulcer perforation—gastric or duodenal
  - Perforation of malignant gastric ulcer
  - Small gut perforation due to typhoid ulcer, tubercular ulcer, and Crohn's disease
  - Large gut perforation due to tubular ulcer, Crohn's or ulcerative colitis.
    - Blunt trauma abdomen causing perforation or transaction of small or large gut.
- Penetrating injury abdomen causing peritoneal penetration—with or without underlying visceral injury.
- Bullet injury abdomen—with peritoneal penetration and with or without underlying hollow viscus injury.
- Following laparoscopic procedure or following abdominal operation—due to entrapment of carbon dioxide gas or air.
- Following tubal insufflation test for tubal patency.

Q. Why you do not find free gas under diaphragm in appendicular perforation?

Ans. Usually, obstructive type of appendicitis leads to perforation. The lumen of appendix contains very little amount of gas. So, there is no free gas under diaphragm in appendicular perforation. However, if there is perforation at the base of the appendix involving the cecal wall, there may be free gas under both domes of diaphragm.

Q. How do you explain the ground-glass appearance in X-ray?

Ans. The ground-glass appearance is due to fluid in peritoneal cavity. There may be air fluid level below the domes of diaphragm.

Q. Do you find free gas under the diaphragm in all cases of peptic perforation?

Ans. No. In 60–70% cases of peptic perforation, there will be free gas under the diaphragm, and in the remaining there may be no free gas under the diaphragm.

Q. How does a patient of peptic perforation will present to you in emergency?

Ans.

History:

- *Pain abdomen*—Acute onset of pain in right upper quadrant or in epigastric region, the pain then radiates along the right paracolic gutter toward the right iliac fossa and later on becomes generalized.
- There may be vomiting at the onset.
- Fever
- In late stage, there may be abdominal distension
- May have past history of peptic ulcer disease.

On examination: On general survey:

- Features of shock—tachycardia, hypotension, and dehydration.
- Patient may be febrile and toxic.

Abdominal examination:

- Restriction of movement of abdomen with respiration.
- There is muscle guard or rigidity all over abdomen.
- In late stage, there may be abdominal distension.
- Tenderness all over abdomen with maximal tenderness over the right hypochondriac region.
- On percussion, liver dullness may be obliterated and their may be evidence of free fluid in abdomen.
- On auscultation, bowel sounds may be absent.

Q. What are the stages in development of peritonitis in a case of peptic perforation?

Ans. There are three stages in development of peritonitis:

1. *Stage I: Stage of chemical peritonitis:*
   Immediately after perforation of peptic ulcer, the gastric contents escape into the peritoneal cavity and this results in a phase of chemical peritonitis, which lasts for about 2–4 hours.
   - During this stage, patient has acute pain abdomen, which starts in the right upper quadrant and then radiates along the right paracolic gutter and later on become generalized.
   - Features of shock—tachycardia and hypotension
   - Tenderness and muscle guard all over abdomen
   - There may be obliteration of liver dullness.
2. *Stage II: Stage of illusion or stage of peritoneal reaction:*
   Due to escape of gastric contents and peritoneal irritation, the peritoneum secretes excess amount of peritoneal fluid to dilute the chemical irritant:
   - During this phase, the pain may diminish
   - But all the signs are progressing—increasing tachycardia, hypotension, and dehydration
   - Generalized tenderness all over abdomen
   - Bowel sounds may be absent.

3. *Stage III: Stage of bacterial peritonitis—stage of abdominal distension*:
   Peritoneal cavity is next invaded by gut flora and leads to bacterial peritonitis. Paralytic ileus supervenes and the abdomen gets distended due to both peritoneal fluid and ileus.
   – Patient is critically ill, toxic, and dehydrated.
   – *Septicemic shock*—rapid feeble pulse, cold extremities, shallow respiration, and hypotension.
   – Abdomen is distended with generalized tenderness.
   – Bowel sounds are absent.

Q. How will you manage this patient?

Ans. As the patient has signs of peritonitis and plain X-ray has shown free gas under the both domes of diaphragm, the patient needs thorough clinical evaluation and some relevant investigations. I will resuscitate the patient and proceed for early laparotomy.

Q. What other investigations you will suggest?

Ans.
* Blood for Hb%, total leukocyte count (TLC), and differential leukocyte count (DLC). There may be polymorphonuclear leukocytosis.
* Blood for sugar, urea, and creatinine
* Chest X-ray
* Electrocardiogram (ECG)
* Blood for serum electrolytes.

Q. How will you resuscitate the patient?

Ans.
* Intravenous fluid—initially Ringer's solution to replace the fluid deficit
* Nasogastric tube insertion and aspiration
* Urinary catheterization to monitor urine output
* Broad spectrum antibiotic—A combination of broad-spectrum antibiotics:
  – Injection cefotaxime/ceftriaxone 1 g intravenous (IV) twice daily
  – Injection amikacin—500 mg IV twice daily
  – Injection metronidazole—500 mg IV thrice daily
* Injection ranitidine or injection omeprazole IV
* Monitoring of pulse/blood pressure (BP)/respiration/urinary output.

Q. What operation will you plan for this patient?

Ans.
* I will do exploratory laparotomy.
* The diagnosis of peptic ulcer perforation is confirmed.
* Simple closure of perforation with interrupted polyglactin suture with an omental patch (Graham's patch).
* Thorough peritoneal lavage.
* If it is a perforated gastric ulcer, a biopsy is to be taken from the ulcer margin to exclude malignancy.

Q. What are the steps of repair of peptic perforation?

Ans. *See* Operative Surgery Section, Page No. 1099, 1100, Chapter 22.

Q. On exploration of abdomen, no perforation is found in anterior wall of stomach or duodenum; what will you do?

Ans. If no perforation is found, the lesser sac is to be opened by dividing the greater omentum. The posterior wall of the stomach and duodenum is inspected for any perforation.

If no perforation is found in the posterior wall of the stomach or duodenum, thorough exploration of the abdomen is done to look for any perforation in the small intestine, large intestine, and appendix or in the rectum.

Q. Would you like to do definitive surgery for peptic ulcer during emergency laparotomy?

Ans. Definitive surgery for peptic ulcer disease may be done in certain situations:
* If patient presents early within 6 hours
* Peritoneal contamination is minimal
* General condition of the patient is good
* It is a chronic ulcer, which has perforated
* Surgeon is experienced.
  A definitive procedure like truncal vagotomy and gastrojejunostomy may be considered.

Q. A patient with blunt trauma abdomen has free gas under both domes of diaphragm. What does it signify?

Ans. Blunt trauma to abdomen may cause intestinal injury. There may be a simple perforation or traumatic transection of the gut.

The management involves resuscitation and exploratory laparotomy. The injured gut is repaired. If a segment of gut is devitalized, resection and anastomosis may be done.

Q. A patient with stab injury has a similar finding in X-ray. What does it signify?

Ans. A stab injury abdomen with free gas under diaphragm may be due to:
* Penetrating injury up to the peritoneum causing a breach in peritoneum without underlying visceral injury.
* Penetrating injury with peritoneal penetration and underlying visceral injury.

Q. What should be the management strategy for stab injury abdomen?

Ans. Routine laparotomy of all patients with stab injury results in large number of negative exploration. All stab wounds of abdomen do not breach the peritoneum. Stab injury causing peritoneal breach is associated with underlying visceral injury in about 50% of cases only. So, a selective approach for consideration of laparotomy is required.
* Stab injury abdomen with hypovolemic shock and symptoms, and signs of generalized peritonitis will require immediate laparotomy.
* Stab injury abdomen—No symptoms and signs of generalized peritonitis.
  - Chest X-ray—no free gas under diaphragm: Local wound exploration—no peritoneal breach—no further exploration is required.
  - Chest X-ray—free gas under diaphragm—indicates peritoneal penetration with or without underlying visceral injury.
    - Diagnostic peritoneal lavage:
      » If DPL positive—exploratory laparotomy
      » If DPL negative—local wound exploration.

■ PLAIN X-RAY OF ABDOMEN, MULTIPLE AIR FLUID LEVELS (FIGS 17.4 TO 17.6)

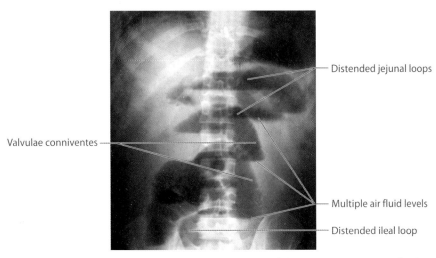

Fig. 17.4: This is a straight X-ray of abdomen with lower part of chest and upper part of pelvis taken in erect posture showing multiple air fluid levels. The distended gut loops are situated in the central part of the abdomen and are arranged in a stepladder fashion. The upper loops are showing presence of valvulae conniventes, which are closely packed and complete suggesting these to be distended jejunal loops. The distended gut loops in right iliac fossa region do not show presence of any valvulae conniventes and appear as characterless suggesting these to be distended ileal loops. This appearance is suggestive of acute small bowel obstruction

Courtesy: Dr QM Rahaman, Registrar, WBUHS, Kolkata

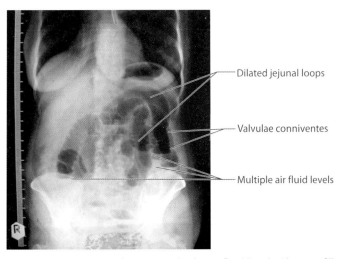

Fig. 17.5: Similar X-ray as in Figure 17.4 showing multiple air fluid levels. The gas-filled intestinal loops are central in location arranged in a stepladder fashion. Most of the distended loops do not valvulae conniventes and appear characterless, suggesting these to be distended ileal loops. This appearance is suggestive of acute small bowel obstruction

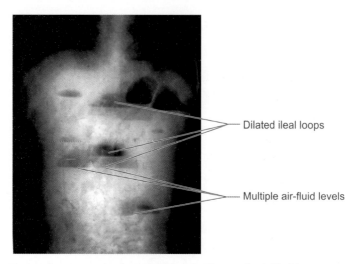

Dilated ileal loops

Multiple air-fluid levels

Fig. 17.6: Similar X-ray—showing multiple air fluid levels. The air–fluid-filled loops are central in location, arranged in a stepladder pattern. Note the characterless appearance (absence of valvulae conniventes) suggesting these to be ileal loops

Courtesy: Dr Partha Bhar, IPGME and R, Kolkata

Q. What is the diagnosis?

Ans. This is likely to be an X-ray of patient with small bowel obstruction.

Q. Why do you say these gas-filled loops are jejunal loops?

Ans. These gas-filled intestinal loops are likely to be jejunal loops because of following characteristics:
- These gas-filled loops are centrally located in the abdomen.
- They are arranged in a stepladder pattern.
- There are closely packed valvulae conniventes indicated by white lines in the gas-filled gut.

Q. What are the characteristics of gas-filled ileal loops?

Ans.
- These are also central in location and may have stepladder pattern of arrangement.
- But the valvulae conniventes, if present, are very sparse and incomplete.
- The gas-filled ileal loops are typically described as characterless.

Q. What are the characteristics of colonic gas shadows?

Ans. The characteristics of colonic gas shadows are:
- The colonic gas shadows are situated more peripherally.
- There are haustrations in the walls. These are incomplete mucosa folds in the walls placed at different levels.

Q. Which X-ray is important for evaluation of patient with acute intestinal obstruction?

Ans. A supine abdominal film gives better delineation of the gas-filled gut loop and an erect film is not required routinely.

Q. How many fluid levels in abdomen X-ray may be regarded as normal?

Ans. In adults, two inconstant fluid levels—one at duodenal cap another at terminal ileum—may be regarded as normal.

In infants, few fluid levels (2–4) in small gut may be regarded as normal.

Q. What are the important causes of small intestinal obstructions?

Ans.
- Causes in the wall of the intestine:
  - Inflammatory bowel disease—Crohn's and tuberculosis causing fibrous stricture in the wall.
  - Fibrous stricture in the wall secondary to trauma, ischemia, radiation, or intussusception.
  - Neoplastic lesion—benign or malignant tumors in the intestine.
- Causes in the lumen of the intestine:
  - Bezoars, gallstones, worms, or foreign body.
- Causes outside the wall of the intestine:
  - Postoperative adhesions or bands, hernias, internal volvulus, intussusception, infiltration by adjacent malignant lesions.

Q. What is the most common cause of small bowel obstruction?

Ans. Adhesion and bands are the most common cause of small bowel obstruction.

Q. How postoperative adhesions are formed?

Ans. Peritoneal injury may occur following operation, bacterial peritonitis, radiation, ischemic injury, foreign bodies, or some chemicals.

The peritoneal injury results in formation of inflammatory exudates in the peritoneum. These inflammatory exudates contain strands of fibrin. These fibrinous exudates get organized and there is invasion of fibroblast. These fibroblasts lay down collagen, which results in formation of permanent fibrous tissue.

However, the peritoneum possesses some fibrinolytic activity, which if not impaired may lyse the fibrin in the inflammatory exudates before organization and fibrosis takes place. The fibrinolytic activity of the peritoneum is impaired by peritoneal injury.

Q. How will you prevent intra-abdominal adhesions?

Ans.
- *Good surgical technique*: Minimize peritoneal injury by gentle handling, use of atraumatic instruments, and achieve good hemostasis.
- *Pharmacological agents*: Various agents has been used—Ringer's solution, hyaluronidase, dextran, anticoagulants, and streptokinase. However, the exact role of these substances has not been substantiated.
- Following newer substances has been used with variable success for preventing adhesion:
  - Intercreed—oxidized regenerated cellulose
  - Adept—4% icodextrin
  - Expanded pTFE (polytetrafluoroethylene) membrane
  - Seprafilm.

Q. What is the usual presentation of patient with acute intestinal obstruction?

Ans. The cardinal symptom of acute intestinal obstruction is:

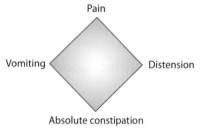

- *Abdominal pain*: Colicky abdominal pain, coinciding with the waves of peristalsis.
- *Vomiting*: More marked with proximal obstruction, less frequent but feculent in distal obstruction.
- *Abdominal distension*: The distension is more marked in distal obstruction than in proximal obstruction.
- *Absolute constipation*: No passage of flatus and feces. Some patients may pass flatus or feces at the onset of obstruction due to evacuation of the contents of the bowel distal to the point of obstruction.

However, constipation may not be a feature in following situations:

- Richter's hernia
- Gallstone ileus
- Intestinal obstruction associated with pelvic abscess
- Subacute intestinal obstruction.

Q. Which factors are responsible for distension of gut proximal to the site of obstruction?

Ans. The distension is produced by mainly two factors:
1. *Gas*: Swallowed air is mainly responsible for the distension. The main gas causing distension is nitrogen as the oxygen and carbon dioxide gets absorbed. There is overgrowth of both aerobic and anaerobic bacteria, which results in significant production of gas due to fermentation of the intestinal contents.
2. *Fluid*: Consequent to obstruction there is accumulation of fluid in the lumen of the gut. About 8–9 liters of fluid may be sequestrated in the lumen of the gut (third space loss). There is excessive secretion from the wall of the gut and the absorption of fluid from the lumen is also retarded.

Q. How the fluid and electrolyte deficits are caused?

Ans. The fluid and electrolyte deficits are caused by:
- Vomiting
- Reduced oral intake
- Defective absorption
- Sequestration of fluid in the lumen of gut.

Q. What are the volumes of different gastrointestinal (GI) secretions?

Ans.
- *Saliva*: 1–1.5 liters
- *Gastric juice*: 1.5–2.5 liters
- Bile—1 liter
- Pancreatic juice—1.5 liters
- Small intestinal juice—3 liters.

Q. How will you evaluate a patient with acute small intestinal obstruction?

Ans.
- Clinical evaluation by history and physical examination
- Details history about the abdominal pain, vomiting, abdominal distension, and obstipation
- Any history of previous abdominal surgery
- Any history of gallstone disease, inflammatory bowel disease, and any intra-abdominal malignant disease
- Any coexisting medical disease, hypertension, ischemic heart disease (IHD), diabetes mellitus, and respiratory disease
- On examination on general survey
- Features of shock—Tachycardia, dehydration, and hypotension
- Measurement of fever, toxemia—Signifies underlying strangulation of gut.

On abdominal examination:
- Abdominal distension
- Visible peristalsis
- There may be tenderness all over abdomen
- If rebound tenderness is present, it indicates underlying strangulation
- Bowel sound may be increased in initial phase, once strangulation sets in abdomen may be silent
- Rectal (P/R) examination may reveal ballooning of wrectum
- Finger may be smeared with blood or mucus
- In case of pseudo-obstruction, fecal scybala may be palpable.

Q. How will you manage this patient?

Ans. After history and clinical examination, it is necessary to decide whether patient has got an underlying strangulation of gut or not. If the patient has underlying strangulation of gut then early surgery is indicated after resuscitation of the patient.

Q. What other investigations are required for patient with acute intestinal obstruction?

Ans.
- Blood for Hb%, TLC, DLC, and erythrocyte sedimentation rate (ESR)
- Blood for sugar, urea, and creatinine
- Serum electrolyte—Na, K, Cl, and bicarbonate
- Serum amylase and lipase to exclude acute pancreatitis
- ECG
- Chest X-ray.

Q. What other imaging studies may be helpful?

Ans. In cases with clinical evidence of underlying gut strangulation, no further imaging investigations are required and patient should be prepared for laparotomy.

In cases with subacute obstruction:
- Oral contrast studies with barium or a water-soluble contrast (gastrografin) is helpful to:
  - Identify the site of obstruction
  - Demonstrate an intraluminal foreign body
  - Differentiate partial from complete obstruction.

- Computed tomography (CT) scan of abdomen is a very reliable investigation for evaluation of acute intestinal obstruction.
  - Any mass in abdomen may discern well—tumor and inflammatory mass (abscess).
  - Missed hernia may be diagnosed.
  - May distinguish subacute obstruction from paralytic ileus.
- Ultrasonography (USG) is not a very reliable investigation for evaluation of intestinal obstruction, as the distended gut interferes with USG examination.

Q. What do you mean by dynamic intestinal obstruction?

Ans. When there is mechanical obstruction of a segment of gut, the proximal intestine tries to overcome the obstruction by vigorous peristalsis. This is called dynamic obstruction.

Q. What is adynamic obstruction (paralytic ileus)?

Ans. In adynamic obstruction, the peristalsis is absent resulting in nonpropulsion of gut contents. In pseudo-obstruction, the peristalsis may be present in a nonpropulsive form.

Q. What do you mean by strangulation obstruction?

Ans. Intestinal obstruction with compromise of blood supply to the gut results in strangulating obstruction. The impairment of blood supply may be due to:

- Twisting of mesentery (volvulus)
- By massive distension of the bowel, which initially results in impairment of venous drainage, causing venous congestion and subsequent impairment of arterial supply, and resulting in gut infarction.
- External compression of the vessels due to hernia or adhesion bands.
- Primary obstruction of the mesenteric circulation (mesenteric vascular thrombosis).

Q. What are the pathophysiological changes in strangulation obstruction?

Ans.
- As the gut distends or there is compression of vessels, the venous return is compromised first.
- The increased capillary pressure in the gut wall results in extravasation of intravascular fluid and blood elements in the wall of the gut, in the lumen and outside the lumen of the gut.
- Subsequently, arterial occlusion sets in resulting in hemorrhagic infarction of the gut.
- There is translocation of bacteria and toxin through the wall of the gut into the systemic circulation.
- When there is massive loss of blood and the resultant toxemia may cause peripheral circulatory failure.

Q. What are the features of strangulation obstruction?

Ans.
- The pain, which was colicky, becomes continuous.
- Fever and toxemia
- Features of shock—Tachycardia and hypotension
- Abdominal tenderness, muscle guard, and rebound tenderness.
- A strangulated hernia is suggested by:
  - Irreducibility
  - Tense and tender swelling

- No impulse on cough
- There may be rebound tenderness
- Leukocytosis.

Q. What do you mean by closed loop obstruction?

Ans. A short segment of bowel is obstructed at a proximal and a distal point usually due to internal volvulus or by a tight ring at the hernial neck. The obstructed segment of the gut becomes hugely dilated and may result in strangulation or perforation before the proximal gut distension occurs.

Q. How will you treat patients with acute intestinal obstruction?

Ans. It is necessary to differentiate between simple obstruction and strangulation obstruction:
- In strangulation obstruction, resuscitation followed by early exploratory laparotomy
- In simple obstruction, the treatment is initially conservative. Resuscitation and monitoring of patient. Surgery is required when the conservative treatment fails.

Q. How will you resuscitate the patient?

Ans.
- Intravenous fluid—to correct the fluid and electrolyte deficit. Normal saline or Ringer's solution infusion.
- Nasogastric aspiration
- Prophylactic antibiotics
- Foley's catheterization to monitor urine output
- Monitoring of patient:
  - Symptomatic improvement—diminution of pain, vomiting, and abdominal distension. Passage of flatus and stool.
  - Observe the pulse, BP, respiration, temperature, and urinary output.

Q. What are the indications of surgery in acute intestinal obstruction?

Ans.
- Strangulation obstruction
- Failure of conservative treatment in simple obstruction
- When diagnosis is in doubt.

Q. What operation you will do in this patient?

Ans.
- I will do exploratory laparotomy.
- The cause of the obstruction diagnosed and dealt with accordingly.
- The distended bowel is to be decompressed.
- Assess the viability of the gut and if gangrenous—resection and anastomosis.

Q. How will you diagnose the site of obstruction on exploration?

Ans.
- Palpate the cecum. If cecum is collapsed, the obstruction is in the small intestine. If the cecum is dilated, the obstruction is in the distal large gut.
- Follow a collapsed segment of the gut from distal to the proximal end. The junction of the collapsed segment and dilated segment of the gut is the site of obstruction.

- In large gut obstruction, when the cecum is dilated, the obstruction lies distally. Palpate the sigmoid colon. If the sigmoid colon is collapsed, the obstruction is proximal to the sigmoid colon. If the sigmoid colon is also distended, the obstruction is in the rectum.

Q. While doing exploratory laparotomy, how will you ascertain the proximal and the distal small gut?

Ans. A loop of small bowel is held in the long axis of the body. A finger is passed deeply along the left side of the mesentery. If the finger is guided to the left iliac fossa or to the left side of the vertebra, the proximal end of the loop lies toward the thorax. If the finger is guided toward the right iliac fossa or to the right of the vertebral body then the loop is inverted and the proximal end of the gut lies toward the foot end.

Q. How will you differentiate a viable and nonviable segment of gut?

Ans. An obviously black, flaccid segment of gut is gangrenous and there will be no pulsation in the vessels in the mesentery.

When the gut is having doubtful viability with slight color change with very poor peristaltic wave and doubtful arterial pulsation then this segment of gut is covered with a hot moist pack and anesthetist is asked to give the patient 100% oxygen for about 10 minutes and the gut is reviewed. If the color becomes pink, the peristalsis returns and the arterial pulsation returns then that segment will be viable.

In doubtful cases, color Doppler study may demonstrate the blood flow and injection of IV fluorescent dye may help. The viable segment of the gut will fluoresces purple.

Q. How will you decompress the dilated segment of the gut?

Ans. The best way of decompression is retrograde decompression. The distended gut loop is milked off toward the proximal segment bringing the contents toward the stomach, which is then aspirated by using a wide-bore nasogastric tube.

Alternatively, the decompression may be done by an enterotomy and using a Savage's decompressor, but the risk of contamination is very high.

Large gut decompression may be done by inserting a needle obliquely through the tenia coli and suction under low pressure. The site of the needle puncture should be oversewn with a seromuscular suture using 3-0 polyglactin.

■ SIGMOID VOLVULUS (FIGS 17.7 AND 17.8)

Q. What is the likely diagnosis?

Ans. This is a typical X-ray appearance of sigmoid volvulus.

Q. What is Dahl Froment's sign?

Ans. In sigmoid volvulus, three distinct lines may be seen in plain X-ray of abdomen showing the dilated sigmoid gut loop. The two outer lines indicating the outer margins of the dilated gut loop and the intervening line formed by the two inner walls of the gut. All these three lines converge toward the pelvis. This is called Dahl Froment's sign.

Q. What are the predisposing factors for development of sigmoid volvulus?

Ans. The following factors are important for development of volvulus of sigmoid colon:
- Bands

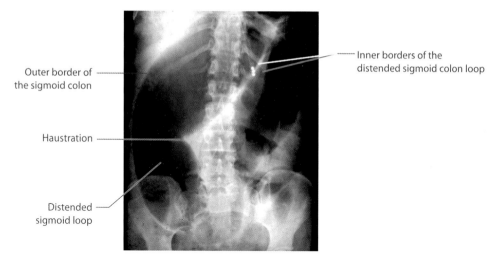

Outer border of the sigmoid colon

Inner borders of the distended sigmoid colon loop

Haustration

Distended sigmoid loop

Fig. 17.7: This is a straight X-ray of abdomen along with upper part of the pelvis taken in erect posture showing a hugely distended large gut loop extending from the pelvis to the upper abdomen. Two loops are distinctly seen with outer borders and an intervening wall formed by inner walls of the sigmoid colon. All these distended gut walls are seen converging toward the pelvis. This appearance is suggestive of large bowel obstruction due to sigmoid volvulus

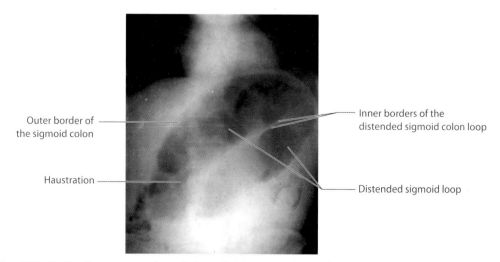

Outer border of the sigmoid colon

Inner borders of the distended sigmoid colon loop

Haustration

Distended sigmoid loop

Fig. 17.8: Similar X-ray omega-shaped distended large gut loop. All three lines converging toward the pelvis suggesting sigmoid volvulus (labeling)

- Long redundant sigmoid colon
- Long pelvic mesocolon
- Narrow attachment of pelvic mesocolon
- High residue diet and chronic constipation is also an important factor.

Q. What is volvulus?

Ans. Volvulus is an abnormal rotation of a segment of bowel around its narrow mesentery causing obstruction of its lumen and may subsequently lead to strangulation or gangrene. This is a form of closed loop obstruction. The rotation usually occurs in an anticlockwise direction.

A rotation of 180° is required for luminal obstruction and a rotation of 360° is required for vascular compromise.

Q. What is compound volvulus?

Ans. This is also known as ileosigmoid knotting. The ileum twist around the long sigmoid mesocolon and there may be gangrene in either ileum, sigmoid, or both.

Plain X-ray shows both distended ileal and sigmoid loops.

Q. What are the sites where volvulus may occur in the gastrointestinal tract?

Ans.
* Sigmoid colon
* Cecum
* Transverse colon
* Small intestine
* Stomach.

Q. What are the important causes of large gut obstruction?

Ans. The important causes of large gut obstruction are:
* Carcinoma colon
* Volvulus
* Stricture-tuberculosis, Crohn's disease, ischemic colitis, anastomotic and radiation-induced
* Hernias
* Fecal impaction
* Pseudo-obstruction (Ogilvie syndrome).

Q. What is the presentation of a patient with sigmoid volvulus?

Ans.
* Abdominal pain
* Distension
* Obstipation
* There may be similar history of pain and distension earlier.

Q. What are the features of strangulation obstruction?

Ans. *See* Page No. 786.

Q. Why ileocecal valve function is important in large bowel obstruction?

Ans. The clinical features of large bowel obstruction largely depend on the function of ileocecal valve.

A competent ileocecal valve allows only antegrade passage of feces and flatus into the cecum and this results in a closed loop obstruction of the segment of the colon between the valve and the site of obstructive lesion. The colon distends progressively and failure to relieve the obstruction results in further distension, increase in intracolonic pressure and ultimately ischemia and perforation of the wall of the cecum.

Cecum dilates more easily than other parts of the colon because of its larger diameter and thinner wall. A diameter of >12 cm in cecum suggests an impending perforation.

When the ileocecal valve is incompetent there will be distension of both small and large intestine, as there will be reflux of gas and fluid through the incompetent ileocecal valve.

Q. What may be the findings in a plain supine film of abdomen in large bowel obstruction?

Ans.
* Gas distended colon up to the point of obstruction
* Little or no gas in colon or rectum distal to the point of obstruction
* In closed loop obstruction, cecum may appear as large gas-filled gut in the right lower quadrant.

Q. Apart from plain X-ray of abdomen, what other investigations may help in sigmoid volvulus?

Ans. If the clinical evaluation of the patient reveals that there are signs of strangulation, no further imaging investigations are required.

If there are no signs of strangulation and the features are of subacute obstruction, the following investigations may be helpful:
* *Contrast enema*: A contrast enema using water-soluble contrast gastrografin may be done. The important findings in contrast enema may be:
  – In pseudo-obstruction—the dye flows freely into the cecum.
  – In sigmoid volvulus—bird's beak sign.
  – In neoplastic obstruction—a shouldered cut off sign.
  The contrast media is hyperosmolar and draws fluid into the lumen of the colon, softening the inspissated fecal matter and allowing it to pass through the obstruction thereby relieving the obstruction.
* *Ultrasonography of abdomen*—Not very helpful in diagnosis of large bowel obstruction. USG may provide information, if there is a palpable mass in abdomen, or if there is hepatic metastasis.
* *CT scan of abdomen*—Very useful in localizing the site of obstruction. The palpable mass may be delineated well and any invasion of bowel mass to the surrounding structures may be demonstrated. Lymph nodes and liver metastasis may be seen well. May also visualize small quantity of free gas in the peritoneal cavity.
* *CT colonography*—Provides a three-dimensional endoluminal image of the entire colon and can diagnose any intraluminal lesion better. Any synchronous tumor may be diagnosed.
* Magnetic resonance (*MR) colonography*—May provide information like CT colonography.

Q. What is bird's beak deformity?

Ans.
* The column of water soluble or barium contrast stops at the obstruction and tapers to a point. This is called bird's beak deformity.

Q. How will you manage this patient of sigmoid volvulus?

Ans. If strangulation is suspected and there are signs of peritoneal irritation—reduction should not be attempted and patient should undergo emergency laparotomy after resuscitation.

Q. What operation will you do?

Ans.
- Exploratory laparotomy and derotation of the volvulus.
- The condition of the gut is assessed:
  - If the gut is gangrenous, resection has to be done and if the patient's general condition is good, a primary anastomosis may be safely done.
- If patient's general condition is very poor, other options are:
  - *Hartmann's procedure*—the proximal end after resection is brought out as colostomy and the distal end of colon is closed, which is reanastomosed at a later date.
  - Proximal loop brought out as colostomy and distal loop brought out as a mucus fistula
- If the gut is viable, a primary resection anastomosis of the sigmoid colon may be safely done.

Q. If there are no signs of strangulation, what should be the management strategy?

Ans. Nonoperative decompression may be tried:
- Pushing a soft rubber catheter beyond the point of volvulus, if successful, decompression may occur.
- Decompression of the volvulus by passing a rigid sigmoidoscope beyond the point of volvulus.
- Decompression may also be achieved by passing a flexible sigmoidoscope beyond the point of volvulus.

Q. How will you manage sigmoid volvulus with symptoms and signs of strangulation?

Ans. If strangulation is suspected and there are signs of peritoneal irritation, reduction should not be attempted and patient should undergo emergency laparotomy after resuscitation.

Q. When you will not attempt sigmoidoscopic decompression?

Ans. Clinical evidence of strangulation, bloody discharge, and evidence of mucosal ischemia indicate strangulation—sigmoidoscopy should be terminated and the patient should undergo operation.

Q. What is the incidence of recurrence of volvulus following nonoperative decompression?

Ans. After nonoperative decompression, there is about 50–90% chance of recurrence of the volvulus.

Q. What should you do, if nonoperative decompression is successful?

Ans. As the chance of recurrent volvulus is high—patient should be prepared for elective sigmoid resection. Resection and primary anastomosis is the preferred treatment.

Q. What is the incidence of cecal volvulus?

Ans. 20% of colonic volvulus is due to cecal volvulus.

Q. Why does cecal volvulus occur?

Ans. This is due to abnormality in fixation of right colon to the retroperitoneum leading to a freely mobile cecum.

Q. What are the features of cecal volvulus?

Ans.
- Clinical features are like acute small gut obstruction
- Pain abdomen, nausea, vomiting, obstipation, or diarrhea are common
- There may be similar attacks in the past.

Q. What do you find in plain X-ray?

Ans. Kidney-shaped air-filled structure in left upper quadrant of abdomen with convexity, or loop toward left upper quadrant. The ileal loops may also be distended.

Q. What is the finding in water soluble contrast study?

Ans. The barium does not pass on to the cecum and the contrast tapers toward the site of obstruction—bird's beak deformity.

Q. How will you treat suspected cecal volvulus?

Ans. Exploratory laparotomy and derotation of the volvulus segment:
- If gut is gangrenous—resection with ileostomy and distal mucus fistula or primary ileocolic anastomosis
- If gut is not gangrenous—limited right hemicolectomy is the preferred treatment to prevent chance of recurrence.

Q. What other procedure may be done?

Ans.
- Cecopexy—Fixing the cecal wall to the parietal peritoneum in the right paracolic gutter
- Tube cecostomy through the abdominal wall, and wound complication rate is 15%
- Simple derotation only—however, there is 7–15% chance of recurrent volvulus
- Some authors recommended simple derotation, as adequate treatment.

Q. Why volvulus of transverse colon is rare?

Ans. The transverse colon does not undergo volvulus commonly, as it has a broad-based short mesentery.

Q. What is Ogilvie syndrome (or colonic pseudo-obstruction)?

Ans. This is a condition, when patient presents with clinical and radiological signs of large bowel obstruction, but without any apparent mechanical cause. If left untreated, there is chance of ischemic necrosis and perforation of the colon.

Q. How will you differentiate from mechanical obstruction?

Ans. A water-soluble contrast enema is helpful for diagnosis. In pseudo-obstruction, the dye passes freely into the cecum. In addition, the contrast may be therapeutic in decompression of the dilated colon.

Q. How will you manage pseudo-obstruction?

Ans.
Conservative treatment: The initial treatment is conservative. This includes:
- Decompression of the colon—By introducing a flatus tube or a flexible colonoscope. However, there is high incidence of recurrence.

♦ Pharmacological therapy—Motility-enhancing drugs like erythromycin and neostigmine has been found to be useful.

Surgical treatment: Surgical treatment is indicated when there are symptoms and signs of peritonitis due to perforation (or impending perforation), or there is failure of medical treatment.

♦ In presence of gangrene or perforation—Resection and exteriorization of the proximal segment is safe.

♦ In absence of gangrene or perforation—Tube cecostomy is ideal for decompression.

■ RADIOPAQUE GALLSTONE AND KIDNEY STONE (FIG. 17.9)

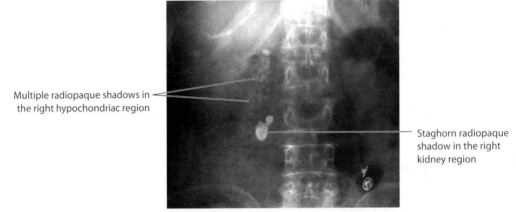

Multiple radiopaque shadows in the right hypochondriac region

Staghorn radiopaque shadow in the right kidney region

Fig. 17.9: This is a plain X-ray of abdomen with upper part of pelvis showing multiple radiopaque shadows in the right paravertebral region below the 12th rib, which appears closely packed. Apart from these, there is another dense staghorn type of radiopaque shadow in the right kidney region

Q. What is your diagnosis?

Ans. This appearance suggests radiopaque gallstones and kidney stone.

Q. What percentage of gallstone and kidney stones are radiopaque?

Ans. About 10% gallstones are radiopaque and about 90% kidney stones are radiopaque.

Q. What is the differential diagnosis of a radiopaque shadow in this region?

Ans.
♦ Kidney stone
♦ Gallstones
♦ Pancreatic calculi
♦ Foreign body
♦ Fecalith
♦ Phleboliths
♦ Calcified lymph node
♦ Calcified renal tuberculosis
♦ Calcified adrenal gland
♦ Chip fracture of a transverse process of vertebra or calcification of costal cartilage.

Q. How will you confirm your diagnosis?

Ans.

+ I will take a lateral view:
    - Gallstone lies anterior to the vertebral body
    - Kidney stone lies posterior to the vertebral body or overlaps the vertebral body
+ Confirmation will be by an USG.

Ultrasonography will show the gallbladder outline. The gallbladder wall thickness may be assessed and stone in the gallbladder will be confirmed by the presence echogenic mass inside the gallbladder, which casts acoustic shadows. The size of the common bile duct and presence of any stone in the bile duct may also be seen.

Kidney can be seen and its size may be measured. Cortex and medulla can be delineated. The pelvicalyceal system can be seen and presence of renal calculi may also be demonstrated by demonstrating the echogenic mass in the pelvicalyceal system showing acoustic shadows.

Q. What is limy bile?

Ans. When the gallbladder contains a mixture of calcium carbonate and calcium phosphate, which has a consistency of tooth paste. In plain X-ray, the gallbladder appears as a dense white shadow.

This occurs when there is gradual obstruction of the cystic duct or common bile duct. The bile contained within the gallbladder is absorbed and gallbladder epithelium secretes this white bile.

Q. What are the different types of gallstones?

Ans. *See* Surgical Pathology Section, Page No. 894–898, Chapter 18.

Q. What are the characteristics of cholesterol gallstones?

Ans. *See* Surgical Pathology Section, Page No. 894–898, Chapter 18.

Q. What are the characteristics, pigment stones?

Ans. *See* Surgical Pathology Section, Page No. 894–898, Chapter 18.

Q. What are the characteristics of mixed stones?

Ans. *See* Surgical Pathology Section, Page No. 894–898, Chapter 18.

Q. What is the composition of gallstone?

Ans. *See* Surgical Pathology Section, Page No. 894–898, Chapter 18.

Q. How does the cholesterol stone form?

Ans. *See* Surgical Pathology Section, Page No. 894–898, Chapter 18.

Q. How does the pigment stone form?

Ans. *See* Surgical Pathology Section, Page No. 894–898, Chapter 18.

Q. How patients with gallstone disease present?

Ans. *See* Surgical Pathology Section, Page No. 894–898, Chapter 18.

Q. What do you mean by silent or asymptomatic gallstones?

Ans. Gallstone is diagnosed in a patient in a routine health checkup or in the course of investigation for some other disease. Patient has no symptom pertaining to gallstones.

Q. What is the chance of such patients developing symptoms in follow-up?

Ans. Most of the series has shown that the chance of developing symptoms is around 10% in 5-year follow-up and 15–20% in 15-year follow-up.

Q. Do all patients with silent stone need treatment?

Ans. As the chance of developing symptoms in follow-up is not very high (10% in 5-year follow-up), routine cholecystectomy for all silent gallstones is not indicated.

Q. What are the indications of treatment for silent gallstones?

Ans.
- Elderly patients with diabetes mellitus
- Patients on immunosuppressive therapy or on dialysis
- Family history of carcinoma gallbladder or patient living in an area with high incidence of gallbladder carcinoma
- Large gallstones more than 2.5 cm
- Multiple small gallstones.

■ RADIOPAQUE KIDNEY STONES AND BLADDER STONE (FIGS 17.10 AND 17.11)

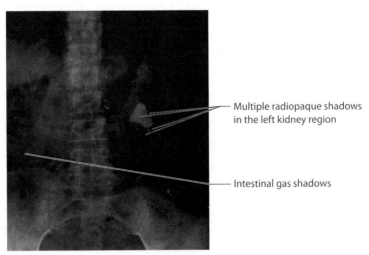

Multiple radiopaque shadows in the left kidney region

Intestinal gas shadows

Fig. 17.10: This is a plain X ray of kidney, ureter, and part of the bladder region showing multiple radiopaque shadows in the left kidney region

Courtesy: Dr Soumen Das, IPGME and R, Kolkata

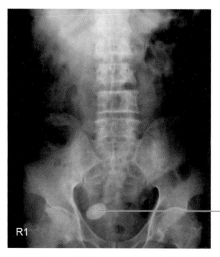

Oval radiopaque shadow in
the right side of the pelvis

R1

Fig. 17.11: This is plain X-ray of kidney, ureter, and bladder region showing an oval radiopaque shadow in the right-half of the pelvis

Courtesy: Dr Subhasis Saha, IPGME and R, Kolkata

Q. What are the possibilities of such X-ray appearance?

Ans. See above.

Q. How will you confirm your diagnosis?

Ans.

* Ultrasonography of kidney, ureter, and bladder (KUB) region will show the kidney, pelvicalyceal system, ureter, and the bladder region. Presence of calculi may be shown by an echogenic mass casting acoustic shadow.
* An IVU is also required to assess the functional status of the kidney.

Q. Which type of renal stones is radiopaque?

Ans.

* Oxalate stones
* Phosphate stones
* Cystine stones
* Xanthine stones.

Q. Which types of renal stones are radiolucent?

Ans. Uric acid and urate stones are radiolucent. If these stones are contaminated with calcium salts, they may be radiopaque.

Q. How the patients with renal stones present?

Ans.

* *Asymptomatic* stones seen on a routine X-ray or ultrasonography for some other reason.

- *Symptomatic*:
  - Fixed renal pain—dull aching constant pain in the loin or hypochondriac region
  - Renal or ureteric colic—acute, colicky pain starts in the loin and radiates to the groin. There may be associated nausea and vomiting and strangury
  - Hematuria—due to irritation by the stone
  - Pyuria—due to associated infection
  - May present with hydronephrosis or pyonephrosis.

Q. How renal stones are formed?

Ans. A number of factors are responsible for formation of renal stones:
- *Urinary infection*—Bacteria form the nidus for formation of renal stones. Some bacteria like proteus split urea and make the urine strongly alkaline. The inorganic phosphate compounds are less soluble in alkaline medium and result on formation of stones.
- *Urinary stasis*—Is associated with increased incidence of renal stones.
- *Vitamin A deficiency*—This may cause desquamation of urinary epithelium, which becomes the nidus for renal calculi.
- *Decreased urinary citrate*—Urinary citrate keeps the calcium phosphate in solution. Decreased urinary citrate may result in precipitation of calcium phosphate in urine.
- *Prolonged immobilization*—This causes demineralization of bones and increased excretion of calcium phosphate in urine and is associated with increased incidence of renal stones.
- *Hyperparathyroidism*—Increased parathormone in circulation causes hypercalcemia and hypercalciuria. There is gross demineralization of bones. Increased calcium in urine may result in increased incidence of renal stones.
- *Altered urinary solutes and colloids*—Dehydration results in increased concentration of urinary solutes and these may precipitate to form stones.
  Reduction of urinary colloids, which adsorb solutes or mucoproteins may result in formation of stones.
- *Randall's plaque*: The initial lesion is erosion at the tip of a renal papilla. Deposition of calcium salts on this erosion forms a calcified plaque (Randall's plaque). These minute plaques are carried by the lymphatics to the subendothelial region, where they accumulate. These microliths grow further by deposition of calcium salts.

Q. Why phosphate stones become very large before they produce any symptoms?

Ans. The phosphate calculi consisting of calcium phosphate and sometimes magnesium ammonium phosphate usually has smooth surface. The stone grows in alkaline urine. The bacteria in urine (Proteus species) split urea into ammonia and render the urine alkaline allowing further increase in size of this stone due to deposition of calcium phosphate.

Q. Why oxalate stones are commonly associated with hematuria?

Ans. Oxalate stones are irregular in shape and covered with sharp projections, which may cause recurrent bleeding. The stones get discolored by the pigments of altered blood.

Q. What are the complications of renal stones?

Ans.
- *Renal infection*—Acute pyelonephritis or pyonephrosis
- *Obstruction*—Hydronephrosis and hydroureter

* *Ureteral stricture*—Passage of stone may result in desquamation leading to fibrosis and stricture formation in ureter, calyces, or renal pelvis.
* *Chronic renal failure*—In bilateral calculi with associated infection or obstruction
* *Calculus anuria*
* *Epidermoid carcinoma*—Presence of stones in the renal pelvis may cause squamous metaplasia and squamous cell carcinoma of the renal pelvis.

Q. How the renal stones can be treated by nonoperative means?

Ans. *Extracorporeal shock wave lithotripsy* (ECSWL) is the modern method for nonoperative treatment of renal stones. The earlier generation of ECSWL machine requires the patient to be kept in a water bath. The newer generation of machines does not require a water bath. The ultrasound is focused on the stones, which result in fragmentation of the stones. These fragmented stones are cleared subsequently. However, these fragments may block the ureter or some of the fragments may be retained resulting in a recurrent calculus.

The success of treatment depends on the type of stone. Most oxalate and phosphate stones fragment well, but the hard stones like cystines and xanthine calculi do not fragment well and are difficult to treat by ECSWL.

Q. What is percutaneous nephrolithotomy (PCNL)?

Ans. This is minimally invasive technique for extraction of renal stones:
* A hollow needle is inserted percutaneously into the renal collecting system through the renal parenchyma.
* A guidewire is inserted through the needle and the needle is then withdrawn.
* Following the guidewire, the track is dilated using a series of dilators.
* The nephroscope is then inserted through this dilated tract.
* Smaller stones can be extracted under vision.
* The larger stone needs to be fragmented by an ultrasound or by an electrohydraulic probe.
* The fragmented pieces are removed through the nephroscope.

Q. What are the complications of PCNL?

Ans.
* Perforation of colon or pleura during placement of the needle
* Bleeding
* Perforation of the collecting system during insertion of the needle.

Q. What is the indication for open surgery for renal stones?

Ans. If there is no facility for ECSWL or PCNL or if these modalities fail, open surgery is indicated for removal of stones—nephrolithotomy or pyelolithotomy.

■ CANNONBALL METASTASIS

Q. What do you mean by a posteroanterior (PA) view chest X-ray?

Ans. Patient faces the X-ray film and X-ray exposure is done from the back (Fig. 17.12). The X-ray is done centering the T5 vertebra from a distance of 1.85 meter with 60–80 kV radiation.

In PA view, the heart shadow and lung fields are seen better.

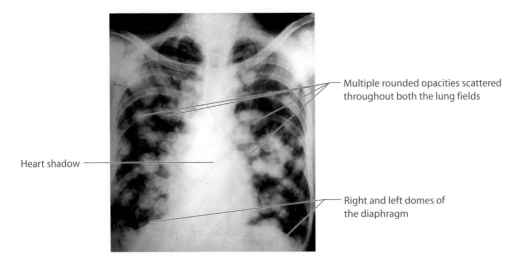

Multiple rounded opacities scattered throughout both the lung fields

Heart shadow

Right and left domes of the diaphragm

Fig. 17.12: This is a plain X-ray of chest posteroanterior (PA) view showing normal bony cage. The diaphragm domes are normal. There are multiple rounded opacities in both lung fields suggestive of cannonball metastasis in both lungs

Courtesy: Dr AG Ghosal, IPGME and R, Kolkata

Q. What do you mean by anteroposterior (AP) view of the chest X-ray?

Ans. The X-ray film is kept at the back and X-ray exposure is done from the front. Posterior chest wall is seen better and the vertebrae intervertebral disk space is seen better.

Q. What are the important things you look for in chest X-ray?

Ans.
- Bony cage—The ribs, vertebral body, and the transverse processes, clavicle, the manubrium sterni
- The trachea
- The cardiac shadow and assessment of cardiothoracic ratio
- The diaphragm—The dome level—Normally sixth rib anteriorly and tenth rib posteriorly, the costophrenic angle
- The lung fields—The bronchovascular markings
- The hilar region
- Below diaphragm—Free gas under the domes of diaphragm, dilated bowel loops, displacement of fundal gas shadow, interposition of colon between liver, and diaphragm (Chilaiditi's syndrome).

Q. What are Kerley's lines in Chest X-ray?

Ans. There are two types of Kerley's lines seen in chest X-rays:
1. *Kerley A lines*: These are 1–2 mm nonbranching lines radiating from the hilum, and 2–6 cm long. This is due to thickened interlobular septa.
2. *Kerley B lines*: These are transverse 1–2 mm nonbranching lines at lung bases perpendicular to the pleura, and 1–3 cm long. This is also due to thickened interlobular septa.

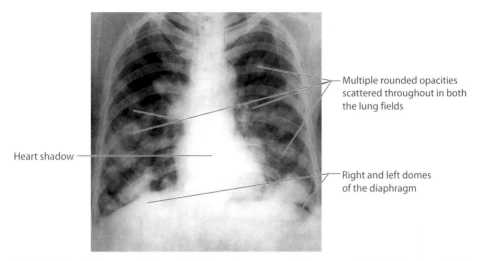

Multiple rounded opacities scattered throughout in both the lung fields

Heart shadow

Right and left domes of the diaphragm

Fig. 17.13: Similar X-ray as in Figure 17.12 showing cannonball metastasis in both the lung fields

Q. What are the important causes of cannonball shadows in chest X-ray?

Ans. This may be due to (Fig. 17.13):
* Metastasis
* Benign lesion:
    – Fungal infection—histoplasmosis, coccidioidomycosis, and aspergillosis
    – Parasitic infection—filarial infection and hydatid disease
    – Sarcoidosis
    – Wegener's granulomatosis
    – Rheumatoid nodules.

Q. What are the important primary sites, which can cause metastasis to the lungs?

Ans. The important primary sites are (PUBLIK-TS):
* Prostate
* Uterus and ovary
* Breast
* Lungs
* Intestine/Stomach
* Kidney
* Testis
* Thyroid
* Soft tissue sarcomas
* Osteosarcomas.

Q. What are the important causes of miliary shadows in chest X-ray?

Ans. Miliary shadows in chest X-ray may be due to:
* Miliary tuberculosis

- Tropical eosinophilia
- Metastatic—Particularly from thyroid carcinomas
- Fungal infections—Especially coccidioidomycosis and aspergillosis
- Occupational lung diseases—Asbestosis, byssinosis, and silicosis.

Q. How tumor metastasis to lungs may occur?

Ans. The different routes of spread of malignant tumors to lungs may be by:
- *Hematogenous spread*—Single tumor cell or multicellular cell aggregates reach through the circulation into the pulmonary vascular bed and may get attached to the capillary endothelium. The tumor cell proliferates and incites angiogenesis.
- *Lymphatic spread*—The tumor cell may reach larger lymphatic channel and then through thoracic duct may reach superior vena cava and thence to the pulmonary vascular bed. Extensive hilar lymph node involvement may cause retrograde spread of tumor cells into the pulmonary lymphatic bed.
- *Direct spread*—Primary tumors from esophagus, chest wall may involve the lungs by direct spread.
- *Intrabronchial spread*—Tumors from larynx, trachea, bronchi may spread to lungs by intrabronchial route through implantation of tumor cells.

Q. How can the chest metastasis be diagnosed?

Ans.
- *Asymptomatic:* Majority of lung metastasis is asymptomatic (90%). Diagnosed by routine chest X-ray.
- *Symptomatic*:
  - Cough, hemoptysis, and dyspnea
  - Features of collapse or pleural effusion
  - Superior mediastinal syndrome.
- *Investigations*:
  - Tumor markers for primary tumor may be elevated
  - Chest X-ray
  - CT scan of chest
  - Sputum cytology
  - Bronchoscopic examination
  - CT-guided fine-needle aspiration cytology (FNAC).

Q. How will you treat pulmonary metastasis?

Ans. Pulmonary metastasis usually indicates advance disease and treatment is mainly palliative:
- Treatment of the primary lesion
- For pulmonary lesion:
  - Chemotherapy
  - Hormone therapy
- Surgery—Metastasectomy or segmental lung resection.

Q. When will you consider surgical treatment for chest metastasis?

Ans. If there is multiple lung metastases or bilateral metastases, treatment is mainly palliative and surgery is not very helpful. Surgical treatment is helpful when:

- Primary tumor has been dealt with adequately and there is no evidence of local recurrence.
- Solitary lung metastasis is most suitable. Multiple lung metastasis confined to one lobe may also be considered for surgical resection.

■ SUBPHRENIC ABSCESS (FIG. 17.14)

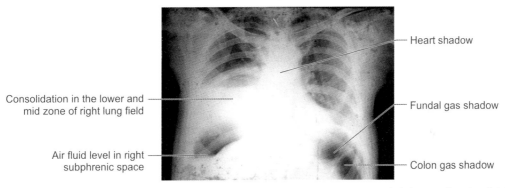

Fig. 17.14: This is a plain X-ray of chest posteroanterior (PA) view with upper part of abdomen showing fluid collection in the right subphrenic region with a horizontal air fluid level. There is a homogeneous opacity in the right lower zone of the lung field suggestive of consolidation of the right lower lobe of the lung. This appearance is suggestive of right-sided subphrenic abscess with consolidation of right lower lobe of lung

Courtesy: Dr PS Pal, BSMC, Bankura, West Bengal

Q. What are the subphrenic spaces?

Ans. The arrangement of the peritoneum results in formation of a number of spaces below the diaphragm. These are called subphrenic spaces.
- There are four intraperitoneal spaces and three extraperitoneal spaces.
- There are three subphrenic spaces on either side and one approximately in the midline.

Q. What are the boundaries of different subphrenic spaces (Fig. 17.15)?

Ans.

Intraperitoneal subphrenic spaces:
- Left anterior or superior intraperitoneal space (left subphrenic):
  - Bounded above by the diaphragm.
  - Bounded behind by the left triangular ligament, left lobe of the liver, lesser omentum (gastrohepatic omentum), and the anterior surface of the stomach.
  - To the right is the falciform ligament.
  - To the left are the gastrosplenic omentum, spleen, and the diaphragm.
- Left posterior or inferior intraperitoneal space (left subhepatic):
  - This is the "lesser sac".
  - Bounded anteriorly by gastrohepatic omentum, stomach, and the anterior leaf of the greater omentum.
  - Bounded posteriorly by the pancreas, transverse mesocolon, transverse colon, and the posterior leaf of the greater omentum.

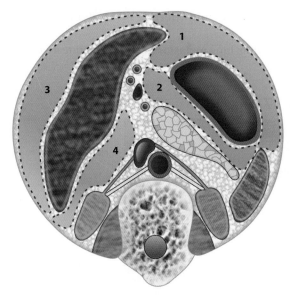

Fig. 17.15: Subphrenic spaces. (1) Left anterior or left superior intraperitoneal space (left subphrenic); (2) Left posterior or left inferior intraperitoneal space (lesser sac); (3) Right anterior or right superior intraperitoneal space (right subphrenic); (4) Right posterior or right inferior intraperitoneal space (hepatorenal pouch of Morison)

- Right anterior or superior intraperitoneal space (right subphrenic):
  - Lies between the right lobe of the liver and the diaphragm.
  - Bounded posteriorly by the anterior layer of coronary and the right triangular ligament.
  - Bounded to the left by the falciform ligament.
  - To the right, it is continuous with the right posterior intraperitoneal space.
- Right posterior or inferior intraperitoneal space (right subhepatic—hepatorenal pouch of Morison):
  - Lies between the right lobe of the liver and the diaphragm.
  - Bounded on the right by the right lobe of the liver and the diaphragm.
  - To the left, lies the foramen of Winslow above and the duodenum below.
  - Bounded in front by the liver and the gallbladder.
  - Bounded behind by the upper part of the kidney and the diaphragm.
  - Bounded above by the liver.
  - Bounded below by the hepatic flexure and the transverse colon.

Extraperitoneal subphrenic spaces:

- There are three extraperitoneal spaces.
- Right and left perinephric spaces are the right and left extraperitoneal spaces.
- The midline extraperitoneal space is the area corresponding to the bare area of the liver.

Q. What are the important causes of subphrenic abscess?

Ans. Subphrenic abscess may occur secondary to:
- Perforated gastric or duodenal ulcer

- Perforation of gallbladder
- Rupture of liver abscess
- Duodenal stump blow out
- Following appendicular perforation
- Intestinal perforation
- Operations on stomach, pancreas, and spleen or liver.

Q. What are the symptoms and signs of subphrenic pus collection?

Ans.

- *Symptoms*:
  - Nonspecific symptoms like—anorexia, sweating, and wasting
  - Fever with chills and rigor
  - Pain in the epigastrium or right hypochondriac region and there may be radiation of pain to the right shoulder
  - Toxemia and persistent hiccup.
- *Signs*:
  - High-grade pyrexia
  - Anterior abscess—abdominal tenderness may be present
  - Muscle guard and rigidity in abdomen
  - The mass may be palpable
  - Right side basal pneumonia.

Q. Which investigations help in diagnosis?

Ans.

- Hemogram—May reveal polymorphonuclear leukocytosis
- Chest X-ray PA view—May show the above classical features
- Ultrasonography and CT scan can accurately localize the abscess.

Q. How will you treat subphrenic abscess?

Ans.

- *Broad-spectrum antibiotics*: A combination of second- or third-generation cephalosporin (ceftriaxone or cefuroxime) + injection amikacin + injection metronidazole as empirical antibiotic therapy. Subsequent antibiotic choice will depend on the pus culture and sensitivity.
- Ultrasonography or CT scan-guided percutaneous aspiration of pus. A catheter may be placed into the abscess cavity percutaneously. The catheter may be used for irrigation of the abscess cavity and instillation of antibiotic.

Q. What is the surgical approach for drainage of subphrenic abscess?

Ans. Extraperitoneal drainage is the preferred treatment. The incision may be made over the site of maximal tenderness. The peritoneum is not opened. Approach may be through a subcostal incision.

Once the abscess cavity is entered, all the loculi need to be broken with the finger. All pus drained, the cavity irrigated with saline, and a drain is placed inside the cavity. The closure of the cavity is checked by doing cavitogram or by USG scanning.

■ ENDOSCOPIC RETROGRADE CHOLANGIOPANCREATOGRAPHY (FIGS 17.16 TO 17.18)

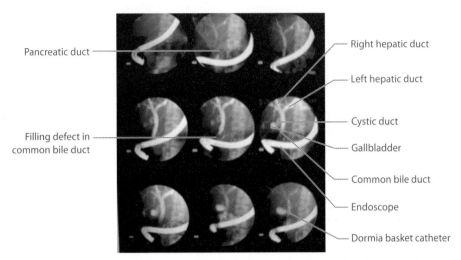

Fig. 17.16: This plate shows a series of pictures of endoscopic retrograde cholangiopancreaticography. The endoscope is in situ. The normal pancreatic duct is seen. The gallbladder is opacified and there are multiple filling defects in the gallbladder. The common bile duct is visualized well, appears dilated, and shows a radiolucent-filling defect in the lower end of the bile duct. In lower pictures, a Dormia basket catheter is seen and the bile duct stone has been extracted endoscopically

Courtesy: Dr GK Dhali, IPGME and R, Kolkata

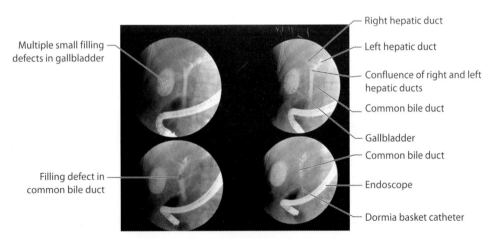

Fig. 17.17: This plate shows a series of pictures of endoscopic retrograde cholnagiography showing a dilated common bile duct and the hepatic duct with a rounded filling defect in the bile duct suggestive of a radiolucent bile duct stone. The cystic duct and the gallbladder are visualized well and there are multiple small rounded filling defects within the gallbladder suggestive of radiolucent gallstones. Dormia basket catheter is seen in lower two pictures and the bile duct stone has been extracted endoscopically. The pancreatic duct is not seen in these plates

Courtesy:Dr Kshaunish Das, IPGME and R, Kolkata

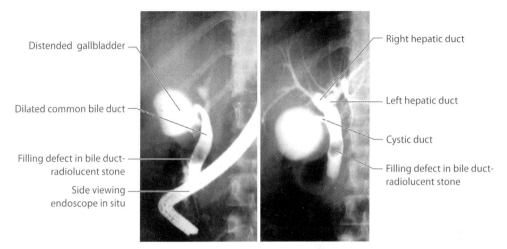

Fig. 17.18: These are two pictures from endoscopic retrograde cholangiopancreatography (ERCP) series. In first picture, endoscope is seen in situ. The gallbladder is opacified well. The common bile duct, hepatic duct, and intrahepatic biliary radicles are grossly dilated. There is a radiolucent filling defect in the bile duct suggestive radiolucent common bile duct stone. This is a diagnostic ERCP procedure, as no therapeutic intervention has been done

Courtesy: Dr Jayanta Dasgupta, IPGME and R, Kolkata

Q. How an endoscopic retrograde cholangiopancreatography (ERCP) is done?

Ans.
+ This is done in a gastroenterology unit with facility for X-ray and fluoroscopy.
+ A side viewing upper GI endoscope is used.
+ The procedure is done under sedation using midazolam or short IV anesthetic like propofol.
+ Patient is placed in prone position with head turned to the right side.
+ A mouth guard is inserted in-between the teeth, and the endoscope is inserted slowly.
+ The endoscope is inserted into the duodenum and the major papilla is localized on the posteromedial wall of the second part of the duodenum.
+ A cannula is inserted through the side channel of the endoscope and the cannula is inserted into the ampulla and then electively into the pancreatic duct and the bile duct.
+ The contrast (urografin 60%) is then injected through the cannula and pancreatogram and the cholangiogram is obtained.

Q. How do you know that the cannula has gone into the pancreatic duct or the bile duct?

Ans. This can be ascertained by following the direction in which the cannula is going. If the cannula goes obliquely across the vertebral body, it is most likely to go into the pancreatic duct. If the cannula has gone into the bile duct, it will be seen going vertically up along the side of the vertebral body.

Q. How will ascertain the ductal diameter during ERCP?

Ans. The adult endoscope is 13 mm, so the duct is compared with the endoscope diameter and its approximate dimension may be assessed.

Q. How will you extract stone from bile duct endoscopically?

Ans.

- This is achieved by endoscopic sphincterotomy and stone removal by using a Dormia basket catheter.
- Patient's prothrombin time should be more than 80%.
- Once ERCP is done and the stone is seen, the size of the stone is to be measured. Stones larger than 1.5 cm cannot be removed endoscopically by endoscopic sphincterotomy.
- An endoscopic sphincterotomy is done at 12 O'clock position by using an endoscopic papillotome and by passing diathermy current.
- A guidewire is passed through the side channel of endoscope beyond the stone.
- A Dormia basket catheter is introduced through the side channel of the endoscope over the guidewire into the bile duct in closed position beyond the stone. The Dormia basket is then opened and the stone is lodged within the basket. The basket is withdrawn and the stone is removed from the bile duct through the papilla. The stone can be left in the duodenum to be extruded with stool or may be retrieved outside along with the endoscope.

Q. What are the complications of ERCP?

Ans. ERCP may be associated with a number of complications:

- Cholangitis
- Acute pancreatitis
- Bleeding
- Duodenal injury.
  Other questions related to bile duct stones (see long case on choledocholithiasis).

■ WORM IN COMMON BILE DUCT (FIG. 17.19)

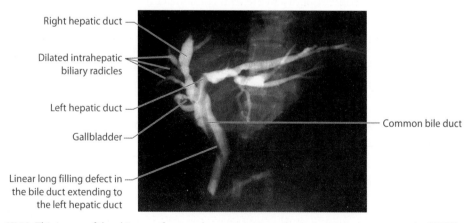

Fig. 17.19: This is one of the skiagram from endoscopic retrograde cholangiopancreatography (ERCP) series showing dilated bile duct and intrahepatic biliary radicles. There is a long linear filling defect in the bile duct suggestive of a round worm in the bile duct

Courtesy: Dr Abhijit Chodhury, IPGME and R, Kolkata

Q. How the worm has entered into the bile duct?

Ans. The worm *Ascaris lumbricoides* infests the intestine. The worm may find its way into the bile duct through the ampulla of Vater.

Q. What is the life cycle of Ascaris lumbricoides?

Ans. This is a nematode and the adult worm lives in the upper small intestine of human being. The worm may migrate into the biliary tree, esophagus, and the colon. The mature ova containing the larvae are excreted through the stool of infected individuals and contaminate the soil and vegetables.

The encysted larvae are ingested along with food or drinks. The cyst wall is digested by the gastric juice and the larvae are liberated in duodenum. The larvae invade through the wall of the intestine and enter into the portal circulation and reach the liver and thence to the systemic circulation. The larvae may also reach the systemic circulation via the intestinal lymphatics and the thoracic duct. The larvae get matured in the lungs and the pulmonary larvae are carried from the alveoli to the pharynx and then swallowed to reach the upper small intestine where they mature into adult worms.

Q. What are the consequences of worm in bile duct?

Ans.
* Majority of adult worms migrating into the bile duct die after few weeks.
* The dead worm may form a nidus for formation of primary bile duct stones—usually, pigment stones are formed.
* Spontaneous expulsion
* Secondary infection of the bile duct with *Escherichia coli* or other enteric organisms leading to suppurative cholangitis—pain abdomen, jaundice, fever with chills and rigor, and toxemia.
* Cholangiectatic liver abscess
* Empyema gallbladder
* Bile duct stricture.

Q. How do these patients usually present?

Ans.
* In stage of larval migration—systemic symptoms—rigors malaise, cough, and asthmatic attacks.
* Worms entering into the bile duct:
  – Episodes of epigastric pain
  – Recurrent attacks of cholangitis due to stone formation and secondary infection—biliary colic, fever with chills and rigor, and jaundice.
  – Cholangiectatic liver abscess—right upper quadrant pain abdomen, fever, and tender hepatomegaly.

Q. How will you manage a patient with worm in bile duct?

Ans.
* *Uncomplicated case*: Treatment with antispasmodic drugs may relax the sphincter of Oddi and may allow spontaneous expulsion of the worm into the duodenum and subsequent treatment with antihelminthic drug.
* Treatment of complications.
* Removal of worm by endoscopic sphincterotomy or by open operation—choledochotomy.

ENDOSCOPIC RETROGRADE CHOLANGIOPANCREATOGRAPHY— CHRONIC PANCREATITIS (FIGS 17.20 AND 17.21)

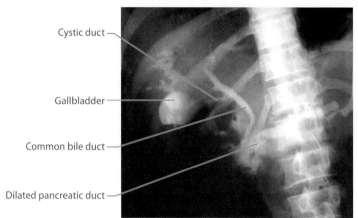

Cystic duct

Gallbladder

Common bile duct

Dilated pancreatic duct

Fig. 17.20: This is one of the skiagrams from endoscopic retrograde cholangiopancreaticography series showing normal bile duct. The gallbladder is also opacified. No filling defect is seen. The pancreatic duct is dilated, suggestive of chronic pancreatitis

Courtesy: Dr Sukanta Roy, SDLD, IPGME and R, Kolkata

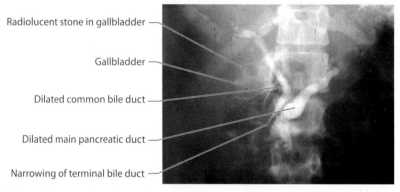

Radiolucent stone in gallbladder

Gallbladder

Dilated common bile duct

Dilated main pancreatic duct

Narrowing of terminal bile duct

Fig. 17.21: This is a skiagram of endoscopic retrograde cholangiopancreaticography (ERCP) showing dilated pancreatic duct. The common bile duct (CBD) is dilated and there is narrowing at the terminal part of the common bile duct. The gallbladder is opacified and there is a radiolucent filling defect in the lumen of the gallbladder. So, this is suggestive of chronic pancreatitis with CBD compression and cholelithiasis

Courtesy: Dr Sumit Sanyal, SDLD, IPGME and R, Kolkata

Q. How can you see these stones better?

Ans. Majority of the pancreatic stones are radiopaque, so are better seen in a plain X-ray of abdomen.

Q. How else you can visualize the pancreatic duct?

Ans.
* Magnetic resonance cholangiopancreatography (MRCP) is a very good method for visualization of the whole of pancreatic duct. This also visualizes the bile duct.

♦ CT scan of pancreas is also helpful in delineation of pancreatic duct. This also provides information about the pancreatic parenchyma.

Q. What is the normal dimension of pancreatic duct?

Ans.
♦ In the head region—5 mm
♦ In the body—3 mm
♦ In the tail—2 mm.

Q. What is chronic pancreatitis?

Ans. Chronic pancreatitis is characterized by irreversible progressive destruction of pancreatic parenchyma. Both the acinar cells and the islet cells show progressive destruction, which is replaced by fibrous tissue. The pancreatic duct may be dilated with focal areas of obstruction due to intraductal calculi or protein plugs.

Q. What is the most common cause of chronic pancreatitis?

Ans. Chronic alcoholism is the most common cause of chronic pancreatitis. Alcohol causes damage to the pancreas in a number of ways:
♦ Alcohol is a cellular metabolic poison and causes damage to both acinar and islet cells.
♦ Increase protein secretion in the pancreatic juice, which may block the pancreatic duct by these protein plugs.
♦ Alcohol increases the permeability of the pancreatic duct and the pancreatic enzyme leaks into the pancreatic parenchyma causing further parenchymatous damage.
♦ Alcohol can decrease the pancreatic blood flow and may thus cause ischemic damage to the pancreas.

Q. What are the other causes of chronic pancreatitis?

Ans.
♦ Pancreatic duct obstruction due to trauma and pancreatic cancer
♦ Hereditary pancreatitis
♦ Infantile malnutrition
♦ Autoimmune pancreatitis
♦ Idiopathic.

Q. What is pancreas divisum?

Ans. This is a congenital anomaly, which develops due to failure of the two embryonic pancreatic ductal systems to unite.

In this, the major pancreatic duct (duct of Wirsung) developing from the dorsal pancreatic bud is small and no more than 1–2 cm in length and opens into the major duodenal papilla.

The minor pancreatic duct (duct of Santorini) becomes the major ductal system of the pancreas and opens into the minor duodenal papilla.

The high incidence of recurrent pancreatitis in pancreas divisum is due to small papilla, where the main pancreatic duct is draining creating a relative stenosis at the site of drainage of main pancreatic duct.

Q. How does patient with chronic pancreatitis usually presents?

Ans.

◆ *Abdominal pain*: In 95% cases, principal symptom is pain.
   Pain is epigastric, may be episodic or continuous, cramping pain, may radiate to the back, sometimes there is acute exacerbation, may have some relief in sitting posture with knee flexed and with a pillow pressed on to the abdomen.
   – Variable weight loss both due to less food intake and due to malabsorption.
   – Insulin-dependent diabetes mellitus.
   – Steatorrhea—due to exocrine pancreatic insufficiency.

Q. What is the medical treatment for chronic pancreatitis?

Ans.

◆ *Diet*: A diet low in fat is helpful
◆ Stop alcohol
◆ Pancreatic enzyme supplementation
◆ Treatment of acute exacerbation—nil orally, IV fluid, analgesics, and prophylactic antibiotics
◆ Control of diabetes—requires insulin.

Q. Patients with chronic pancreatitis are more prone to hypoglycemic attacks when treated with insulin, why?

Ans. In chronic pancreatitis, there is associated glucagon deficiency, so the chance of hypoglycemia is more.

Q. What are the indications of surgery in chronic pancreatitis?

Ans.

◆ Pain-persistent severe pain, interfering with quality of life and daily activities, requiring large doses of analgesics
◆ Common bile duct obstruction
◆ Duodenal obstruction
◆ Colonic obstruction
◆ Suspicion of pancreatic cancer
◆ Complication of pseudocyst
◆ Portal vein obstruction causing portal hypertension.

Q. What surgery you will plan in this patient?

Ans. I will consider longitudinal pancreaticojejunostomy with a Roux-en-Y loop of jejunum and head coring (Frey's procedure).

Q. What are the indication for pancreatic resection—distal pancreatectomy or Whipple's operation in chronic pancreatitis?

Ans.

◆ Chronic pancreatitis with a normal duct diameter
◆ Failure of previous pancreaticojejunostomy
◆ Pathological change is confined to one part of the pancreas and the rest of the pancreas is normal.

■ T-TUBE CHOLANGIOGRAM (FIGS 17.22, 17.22A AND 17.23)

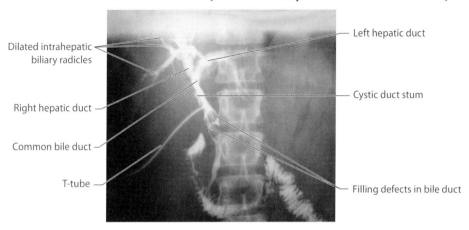

Dilated intrahepatic biliary radicles

Left hepatic duct

Right hepatic duct

Cystic duct stum

Common bile duct

T-tube

Filling defects in bile duct

Fig. 17.22: This is one of the skiagrams from T-tube cholangiogram series. The T-tube is seen in situ. The common bile duct, hepatic ducts, and the intrahepatic biliary radicles are dilated and there are two filling defects within the lumen of the bile duct. These are suggestive of residual radiolucent common bile duct stones. The dye has gone into the duodenum suggesting no obstruction in the terminal bile duct

Courtesy: Dr Suprya Ghatak, SDLD, IPGME and R, Kolkata

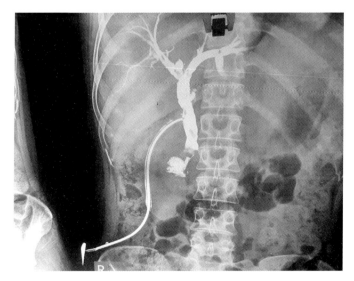

Fig. 17.22A: T-tube cholangiography. The T-tube is in situ. The intrahepatic biliary radicles, hepatic ducts and the common bile duct is dilated. There is filling defect at the lower end of the bile duct. This hs suggestive of a missed (residual) stone in the bile ductt

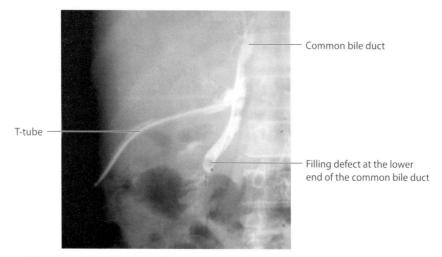

Common bile duct

T-tube

Filling defect at the lower
end of the common bile duct

Fig. 17.23: This is one of the skiagrams from T-tube cholangiogram series showing T-tube in situ. The bile duct is dilated and there is a radiolucent filling defect at the lower end of the bile duct. The dye, however, has reached the duodenum. This X-ray appearance is suggestive of residual stone in the bile duct following choledocholithotomy

Q. How T-tube cholangiography is done?

Ans.

* The postoperative T-tube cholangiography is done on 8th–10th postoperative day.
* The procedure is done under fluoroscopic control.
* The T-tube is clamped and cleaned with antiseptic solution.
* The T-tube is flushed slowly with 20 mL of normal saline.
* Urografin 60% is used as the contrast material. About 2–3 mL of contrast is then injected under fluoroscopic control and an X-ray exposure is taken.
* The flow of dye into the bile duct and duodenum can be seen.
* Further 4–5 mL of dye is injected. To see the hepatic ducts properly, an X-ray exposure is taken with the head end down.
* To see the lower end better, an X-ray exposure is taken with the head end-up position.

Q. How will you differentiate an air bubble from a filing defect due to a stone?

Ans. An air bubble in T-tube cholangiogram will appear as:
* Perfectly round
* Dense black-filling defect
* Air bubble goes up in head-up position and goes down with head-down position.
* A filling defect to a calculus is not denscly black, usually not completely round, and change direction opposite to the air bubble with change of posture, if the stone is impacted, there will be no change of position of the filling defect with change of posture.

Q. How will you manage this patient?

Ans. One of the stones is quite large, so this will not be suitable for mechanical flushing. I will consider endoscopic sphincterotomy and stone extraction by using a Dormia basket catheter.

Q. How can you avoid such a situation?

Ans. An intraoperative postexploratory cholangiogram may identify the residual stone on table and the stone may be removed.

Intraoperative choledochoscopy may also Visualize the residual stone and the stone may be removed.

Q. How mechanical flushing may help?

Ans. If the retained stone is small (<1 cm) then this can be managed by mechanical flushing with heparinized saline. The bile duct is irrigated with a heparinized saline (250 mL of normal saline mixed with 25,000 IU of heparin) by passing the fluid through the T-tube tract for consecutive 5 days.

An injection of hyoscine may relax the ampulla of Vater and may facilitate the expulsion of small stones.

Q. What is contact dissolution?

Ans. If the stone is a pure cholesterol one, contact dissolution by infusing monooctanoin or methyl terbutyl ether via the T-tube tract may be helpful.

Q. What is Burhenne technique for extraction of residual bile duct stones?

Ans. This technique, followed earlier, is not practiced nowadays.
- Patient is discharged home with the T-tube in situ, and a waiting period of 4–6 weeks allows the T-tube tract to get matured.
- The retained stone is extracted through the matured T-tube tract.
- The T-tube is removed and the T-tube tract is dilated under fluoroscopic control.
- A Dormia basket catheter is introduced through the T-tube tract into the bile duct and the stones may be removed.
- Alternatively, a choledoscope may be passed through the matured T-tube tract and the stones from the bile duct may be removed under vision.

Q. What is the role of extracorporeal shock wave lithotripsy?

Ans. Retained or recurrent bile duct stone may be fragmented by using extracorporeal shock wave lithotripsy. An endoscopic sphincterotomy may hasten expulsion of the fragmented stone.

Q. What are the other options for management of residual bile duct stones?

Ans. If the above measures fail, the options are:
- Laparoscopic choledocholithotomy
- Open choledocholithotomy.

Q. If the retained stone is detected after the removal of T-tube how will you manage?

Ans.
- Endoscopic sphincterotomy and stone extraction by a Dormia basket catheter introduced through the endoscope.
- Extracorporeal shock wave lithotripsy—if the stone is large, it may not be suitable for ECSWL. 50% patients need adjunctive procedure like endoscopic extraction, biliary lavage, and stenting.
- Percutaneous transhepatic route may be used to pass a cholangioscope to visualize the bile duct stones and removal by using Dormia basket catheter introduced through the cholangioscope.
- Laparoscopic or open choledocholithotomy.

■ BARIUM SWALLOW X-RAY OF ESOPHAGUS—ACHALASIA CARDIA (FIG. 17.24)

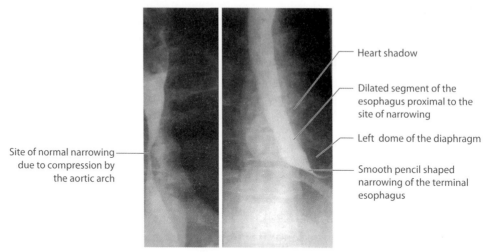

Heart shadow

Dilated segment of the esophagus proximal to the site of narrowing

Left dome of the diaphragm

Site of normal narrowing due to compression by the aortic arch

Smooth pencil shaped narrowing of the terminal esophagus

Fig. 17.24: This is one of the skiagrams from barium swallow X-ray of the esophagus showing a smooth pencil shaped narrowing at the lower end of the esophagus with dilatation of the esophagus proximal to this narrowing. This appearance is characteristic of achalasia cardia

Courtesy: Dr Swadapriya Basu, IPGME and R, Kolkata

Q. Why do you say this is due to achalasia and not carcinoma?

Ans. The narrowing is smooth and there is no irregularity in the mucosal lining, so this is likely to be achalasia.

Q. What is achalasia cardia?

Ans. This is a condition of failure of lower esophageal sphincter to relax due to loss of ganglion cells in the myenteric plexus.

Q. What are the important causes?

Ans.
* Congenital
* Infection with varicella zoster virus
* Infection with *Trypanosoma cruzi* (Chaga's disease).

Q. What are the changes in the esophagus?

Ans.
* Esophagus empties incompletely with retention of food and fluid in the dilated segment of the esophagus.
* The esophagus proximal to the site of narrowing becomes dilated and may become tortuous (sigmoid esophagus).
* The food residue in the esophagus may cause recurrent aspiration pneumonia.
* There is increased incidence of carcinoma in patients with achalasia cardia.

Q. What do you mean by pseudoachalasia?

Ans. This is an achalasia like disorder, which is usually caused by carcinoma at the cardia or extrinsic compression of the esophagus due to bronchogenic carcinoma or metastatic lymph node.

Q. How patient with achalasia usually presents?

Ans.
- Equal in both sexes
- Usually affects young adult and late middle age
- Retrosternal discomfort
- Dysphagia initially to liquids and later on to both solids and liquid. Often the swallowing may be improved by drinking liquids, eating in upright posture, breath holding, and often by Valsalva. These all increase the intraesophageal pressure, which helps to overcome the functional resistance at the gastroesophageal junction.
- Regurgitation of food and saliva into the mouth.
- Aspiration pneumonia and lung abscess
- Weight loss and anemia in advanced cases
- Chest pain and heart burn.

Q. What may be the endoscopic finding in achalasia cardia?

Ans.
- Dilated esophagus with food residue
- Smooth narrowing of the lower esophagus
- Endoscope can be negotiated easily into the stomach.

Q. How does manometry helps in diagnosis of achalasia cardia?

Ans.
- Resting esophageal pressure is increased.
- Increased pressure in the lower esophageal sphincter.
- Failure of lower esophageal sphincter to relax during swallowing.

Q. Which drugs are effective in achalasia cardia?

Ans. Calcium channel blocker like nifedipine is useful for relief of symptoms in achalasia cardia, but its use in long term is not very effective.

Q. What is the role of dilatation in achalasia cardia?

Ans. Wide dilatation may ameliorate symptoms in 75–85% cases. There is risk of perforation.

Q. What is the operative treatment for achalasia cardia?

Ans. Heller's cardiomyotomy is the standard surgical treatment for achalasia cardia. This may be done by an open operation or laparoscopically. This operation is effective in 90–100% cases.

The operation is done through a left thoracotomy or an upper midline incision. The lower esophagus is mobilized preserving the vagal trunks. This operation involves division of musculature of the lower end of the esophagus by anteriorly placed incision over the muscle coat till the mucosa bulges out. The distal limit of incision is up to the proximal stomach.

Q. What is the role of antireflux surgery along with Heller's operation?

Ans. Cardiomyotomy invariably destroys the lower esophageal sphincter and may result in reflux esophagitis. So, an antireflux procedure should be done along with Heller's operation. A loose or partial fundoplication should be done concomitantly during cardiomyotomy.

Q. What is the role of botulinum toxin?

Ans. Botulinum toxin has been used successfully in cases with achalasia cardia. The toxin is injected into the lower esophageal sphincter endoscopically.

Q. What is cricopharyngeal achalasia?

Ans. This is a condition of failure of relaxation of upper esophageal sphincter during swallowing.

Q. What is presbyesophagus or diffuse esophageal spasm?

Ans. This is a condition of uncoordinated contraction of the esophagus resulting in high intraesophageal pressure (400–500 mm Hg) and is associated with marked hypertrophy of circular muscle of the esophagus.

Q. What is the clinical manifestation of diffuse esophageal spasm?

Ans. Patient may present with dysphagia or chest pain.

Q. What is the typical finding in barium swallow X-ray?

Ans. The appearance in barium swallow is called corkscrew esophagus.

Q. What is the treatment for diffuse spasm of esophagus?

Ans.
- Esophageal dilatation
- Long esophageal myotomy—Extending from cardia to the aortic arch.

■ BARIUM SWALLOW—CARCINOMA OF ESOPHAGUS (FIGS 17.25 AND 17.26)

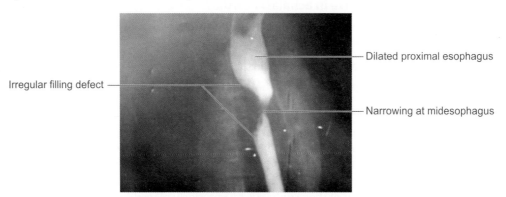

Irregular filling defect — Dilated proximal esophagus — Narrowing at midesophagus

Fig. 17.25: This is one of the skiagrams from barium swallow X-ray of esophagus showing an irregular filling at the midesophagus. There is dilatation of the proximal esophagus proximal to the site of narrowing. This appearance is suggestive of carcinoma of the midesophagus

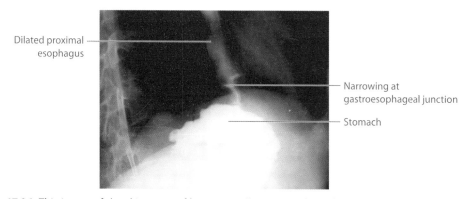

Dilated proximal esophagus

Narrowing at gastroesophageal junction

Stomach

Fig. 17.26: This is one of the skiagrams of barium swallow X-ray of esophagus and stomach showing an irregular narrowing at the level of gastroesophageal junction. This appearance is suggestive of carcinoma at the lower end of esophagus and gastroesophageal junction

Q. What is the usual presentation of patients with carcinoma esophagus?

Ans.

- Dysphagia initially to solids, later on to both solids and liquids
- Regurgitation of food
- Anorexia and weight loss
- Cough
- Pain indicates infiltration of tumor to the adjacent tissues
- Hoarseness of voice may indicate recurrent laryngeal nerve palsy
- Neck mass due to lymph node metastasis
- Hematemesis and melena.

Q. How will you confirm your diagnosis?

Ans.

- An upper GI endoscopy and biopsy from the lesion will confirm the diagnosis.
  If the diagnosis of carcinoma esophagus is confirmed, what further investigation will you do in this patient?
- Once diagnosis is confirmed the local extent of the growth may be assessed by:
  - Endoscopic USG
  - CT scan is useful for assessing local extent of the disease and also for detecting distant metastasis.

Q. How do you stage carcinoma esophagus depending on the above investigations?

Ans.

Primary tumor—T:

- T1—tumor invaded to the lamina propria and submucosa
- T2—tumor invaded to the muscularis propria
- T3—tumor extending to the adventitial coat
- T4—tumor extending to the adjacent structures.

Lymph nodes—N:

- N0—no regional lymph node metastasis
- N1—regional lymph node metastasis present.

Distant metastasis—M:

- M0—no distant metastasis
- M1—distant metastasis present.

  Endoscopic USG is very helpful to assess the primary tumor and lymph node spread. Computed tomography scan is helpful to delineate the lymph node and distant metastasis.

Q. What is the role of thoracoscopy or laparoscopy?

Ans. In suspected advanced disease, the minimally invasive surgery either by thoracoscopy or laparoscopy may help in assessment regarding the extent of the disease and may obviate the need for a thoracotomy or laparotomy.

Q. How does the carcinoma esophagus spread?

Ans.

- *Direct spread*: Spread both circumferentially and vertically. The submucosal spread vertically may form satellite nodules. The tumor may invade through the adventitia and involve the adjacent structures—trachea, lungs, and other mediastinal structures.
- *Lymphatic spread*: May spread to the regional lymph nodes.
- *Distant spread*: Via hematogenous spread to the liver, lungs, and bones. Involvement of celiac lymph node from a lesion of intrathoracic esophagus is regarded as distant metastasis rather than regional lymph node metastasis. Similarly, involvement of cervical lymph nodes from intrathoracic esophagus is regarded as distant metastasis.

Q. What are the predisposing factors for development of carcinoma esophagus?

Ans.

- *Dietary factors*—pickled vegetables, salted dry fish or meat, and high in nitrosamines.
- *Smoking*—both tobacco smoking and chewing.
- *Chronic alcohol intake*
- *Barrett's esophagus*
- *Lye stricture of esophagus*
- *Achalasia cardia*
- *Chronic esophagitis*
- *Hereditary*—tylosis et plantaris and palmaris.

Q. What is Barrett's esophagus?

Ans. This is a condition of columnar metaplasia of esophageal epithelium extending to more than 3 cm of distal esophagus in response to chronic gastroesophageal reflux. A progression from low-grade to high-grade dysplasia to adenocarcinoma is common.

Q. What are the histological types of carcinoma esophagus?

Ans.

- *Squamous cell carcinoma*—common in Asian and African population
- *Adenocarcinoma*—This is common in western countries and the incidence is increasing and approaches to about 60–70%.

Q. How will you treat a patient with carcinoma at the lower end of the esophagus?

Ans. If there is no evidence of distant metastasis, surgical treatment involves total esophagectomy with esophagogastric anastomosis at the neck.

Q. What is Ivor Lewis or Lewis Tanner approach for esophagectomy?

Ans. In this, first abdomen is opened through a midline incision and operability is assessed and stomach mobilized.

A right lateral thoracotomy is done and the whole esophagus mobilized up to the thoracic inlet and subtotal or total esophagectomy is done and an esophagogastric anastomosis is done in the thorax or neck.

Q. What is McKeown approach for esophagectomy?

Ans. This involves a three stage operation:
1. A midline abdominal incision for mobilization of the stomach
2. A right lateral thoracotomy for mobilization of the esophagus
3. A neck incision for proximal esophagus mobilization and an esophagogastric anastomosis at the neck.

Q. What may be the other approach?

Ans. A left thoracoabdominal incision may be used for mobilization of both stomach and the esophagus.

Q. What is transhiatal esophagectomy?

Ans. This is an alternative approach for total esophagectomy. Through a midline abdominal incision, the stomach is mobilized. The esophagus is mobilized by a transhiatal approach and no formal thoracotomy is done.

A neck incision is made and the proximal esophagus is mobilized. Total esophagectomy may be done by this approach. But lymph node dissection is not possible. Esophagogastric anastomosis is done in the neck.

Q. How reconstruction is done following esophageal resection?

Ans. Stomach, jejunum, and colon have been used for reconstruction following esophageal resection. Stomach is preferred for ease of mobilization and good blood supply of this organ.

Q. What is the role of radiotherapy in esophageal carcinoma?

Ans. Radical radiotherapy is effective in carcinoma esophagus particularly squamous cell carcinoma and may be an alternative to surgery in patient unfit for surgery.

However, postoperative or preoperative adjuvant radiotherapy does not improve survival.

Q. What is the role of chemotherapy in esophageal carcinoma?

Ans. Combination chemotherapy with cisplatin, mitomycin C, and 5-fluorouracil and bleomycin may offer worthwhile palliation in advanced disease.

Q. How will you offer palliation for dysphagia in advanced carcinoma of esophagus?

Ans. Relief of dysphagia may be done by:
- Endoscopic stenting by Celestin or Atkinson tube
- Use of self-expanding metallic stent
- Endoscopic laser treatment may be used to core a channel through the tumor

◆ Bipolar electrocautery and coagulation with tumor probes that uses heat to destroy the tumor cells and causes circumferential recanalization.
◆ Brachytherapy to deliver intralminal radiation.

■ BARIUM MEAL X-RAY—CHRONIC DUODENAL ULCER (FIG. 17.27)

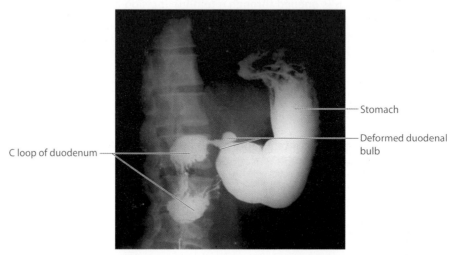

Fig. 17.27: This is one of the skiagrams of barium meal X-ray of stomach and duodenum. The stomach is seen normal. The duodenal cap is not well formed and there is an ulcer crater at the region of the duodenal cap. This appearance is suggestive of a deformed duodenal bulb due to chronic duodenal ulcer

Courtesy: Dr Subhendu Majhi, IPGME and R, Kolkata

■ BARIUM MEAL X-RAY—BENIGN GASTRIC ULCER (FIGS 17.28 AND 17.29)

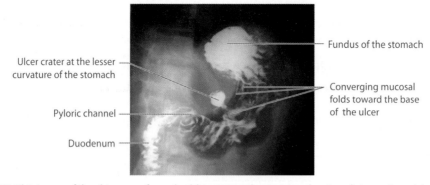

Fig. 17.28: This is one of the skiagrams from double-contrast barium meal series of stomach and duodenum showing an ulcer crater in the lesser curvature. Surrounding mucosal folds are seen converging toward the ulcer base. Double contrast has given a better delineation of mucosal pattern of stomach. So, this is a case of chronic gastric ulcer

Courtesy: Dr Soumya Mondal, IPGME and R, Kolkata

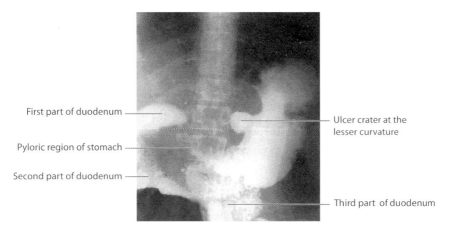

First part of duodenum

Pyloric region of stomach

Second part of duodenum

Ulcer crater at the lesser curvature

Third part of duodenum

Fig. 17.29: This is one of the skiagrams from the barium meal X-ray of stomach and duodenum series taken 30 minutes after ingestion of barium. There is a large ulcer crater at the lesser curvature. The duodenum is also visualized and appears normal. This appearance is suggestive of a chronic gastric ulcer

Courtesy: Dr Kamal Singh Kanwar, IPGME and R, Kolkata

Q. Why do you say this is a benign gastric ulcer?

Ans. This appearance is suggestive of a benign gastric ulcer. The radiological characteristics of benign ulcer are:

- Ulcers along the lesser curvatures are mostly benign.
- The ulcer crater projects beyond the lumen of the stomach.
- The mucosal folds converge toward the base of the ulcer.
- Benign ulcer is usually round or oval, whereas a malignant ulcer is irregular.
- Sometimes, a pencil thin-line of lucency may be found crossing the base of the ulcer. This is due to preserved gastric mucosa with undermining of underlying submucosa.

Q. How a double-contrast barium X-ray of stomach and duodenum is done?

Ans. Patient is given an injection of buscopan to delay the emptying of stomach. Patient is then given an effervescent tablet composed of calcium carbonate and an antifoaming agent. When this tablet is swallowed with water, it releases carbon dioxide. Patient is then given 150–200 mL of high-density barium. The double contrast study gives a very good delineation of mucosal pattern.

Q. What further investigations should be done before initiation of treatment?

Ans. An upper GI endoscopy and multiple biopsies from the ulcer are essential before initiation of treatment to exclude malignancy.

Q. What are the etiological factors for development of chronic gastric ulcer?

Ans. *See* Surgical Long Cases Section, Page No. 127–133, Chapter 3 and Surgical Pathology Section, Page No. 855-859, Chapter 18.

Q. How patients with chronic gastric ulcer present?

Ans. *See* Surgical Long Cases Section, Page No. 127–133, Chapter 3 and Surgical Pathology Section, Page No. 855-859, Chapter 18.

Q. What are the complications of gastric ulcer?

Ans. *See* Surgical Long Cases Section, Page No. 127–133, Chapter 3 and Surgical Pathology Section, Page No. 855-859, Chapter 18.

Q. What is the medical treatment for chronic gastric ulcer?

Ans. *See* Surgical Long Cases Section, Page No. 127–133, Chapter 3 and Surgical Pathology Section, Page No. 855-859, Chapter 18.

Q. What are the indications of surgery in chronic gastric ulcer?

Ans. *See* Surgical Long Cases Section, Page No. 127–133, Chapter 3 and Surgical Pathology Section, Page No. 855-859, Chapter 18.

Q. What are the options of surgical treatment for chronic gastric ulcer?

Ans. *See* Surgical Long Cases Section, Page No. 127–133, Chapter 3 and Surgical Pathology Section, Page No. 855-859, Chapter 18.

■ BARIUM MEAL X-RAY—CARCINOMA STOMACH (FIGS 17.30 AND 17.31)

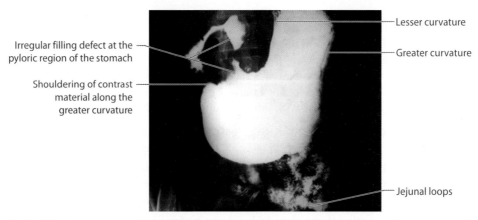

Fig. 17.30: This is one of the skiagrams from the barium meal series of stomach and duodenum taken 1 hour after ingestion of the barium. The picture shows a large irregular filling defect in the pyloric region of the stomach. There is shouldering of the contrast material along the greater curvature of the stomach. This appearance is suggestive of a proliferative growth in the pyloric region of the stomach. However, we should see other plates of the series to confirm that this filling defect is persistent

Courtesy: Dr Subhra Ganguly, IPGME and R, Kolkata

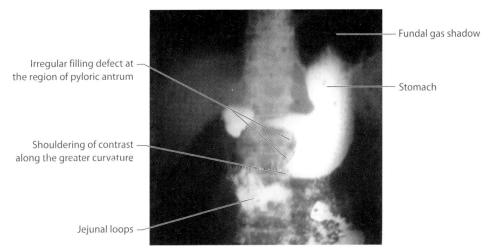

Fundal gas shadow

Irregular filling defect at the region of pyloric antrum

Stomach

Shouldering of contrast along the greater curvature

Jejunal loops

Fig. 17.31: This is one of the skiagrams from barium meal X-ray of stomach duodenum and part of the small intestine showing an irregular filling defect along the greater curvature in the pyloric antrum region. There is shouldering of the dye along the greater curvature. This appearance is suggestive of a proliferative mass in the pyloric region of stomach

Courtesy: Dr Saurav Das, IPGME and R, Kolkata

Q. What are the radiological characteristics of carcinoma stomach?

Ans.
* Mass lesion in the stomach
* The margin of the mass may exhibit a shouldering and forms an acute angle with the gastric wall.
* The pyloric antral region may be severely narrowed.

Q. What are the macroscopic types of gastric carcinoma?

Ans. The gross types of carcinoma stomach may be:
* Proliferative
* Ulcerative
* Infiltrating.

Q. What do you mean by early gastric carcinoma?

Ans. *See* Surgical Long Cases, Page No. 107–110, Chapter 3.

Q. What do you mean by advanced gastric carcinoma?

Ans. *See* Surgical Long Cases, Page No. 107–110, Chapter 3.

Q. How patients with gastric carcinoma usually presents?

Ans. *See* Surgical Long Cases, Page No. 107–110, Chapter 3.

Q. How will you confirm your diagnosis?

Ans. *See* Surgical Long Cases, Page No. 107–110, Chapter 3.

Q. What investigations will help in staging of carcinoma stomach?

Ans. *See* Surgical Long Cases, Page No. 107–110, Chapter 3.

Q. What operation you will do in patient with a growth in the pyloric antrum region?

Ans. *See* Surgical Long Cases, Page No. 107–110, Chapter 3.

■ BARIUM MEAL X-RAY—GASTRIC OUTLET OBSTRUCTION AND DUODENAL OBSTRUCTION (FIGS 17.32 TO 17.34)

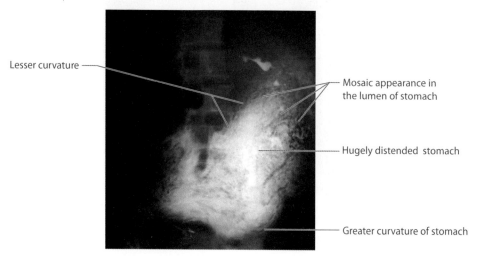

Fig. 17.32: This is one of the skiagrams from barium meal stomach series taken 8 hours after ingestion of barium. The stomach is hugely distended and there is a mosaic appearance due to admixture of barium with retained food particles in the stomach. The duodenum is not visualized yet. This appearance is suggestive of gastric outlet obstruction

Courtesy: Dr Amitava Sarkar, IPGME and R, Kolkata

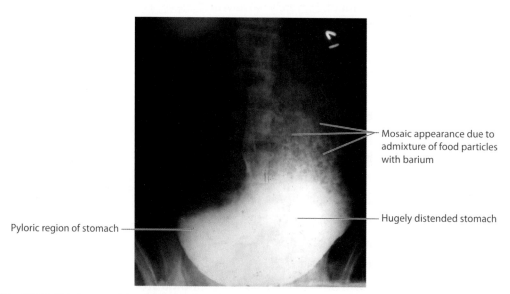

Fig. 17.33: This is one of the skiagrams from barium meal X-ray of stomach taken 8 hours after intake of contrast material. The stomach is hugely distended and there is a mosaic appearance due to admixture of the contrast with the retained food particles. The duodenum is not visualized. This appearance is suggestive of gastric outlet obstruction

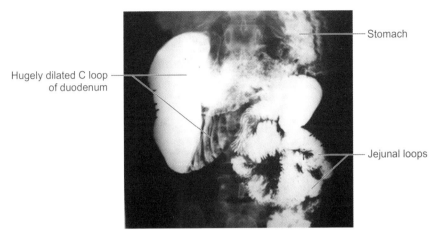

Fig. 17.34: This is one of the skiagrams from barium meal X-ray of stomach duodenum and small gut. There is gross dilatation of the 1st, 2nd, and 3rd part of the duodenum. The mucosal folds in the duodenum appeared prominent. This is a classic appearance of chronic duodenal ileus

Courtesy: Dr Thakur Thusu, IPGME and R, Kolkata

Q. What is the normal emptying time of stomach?

Ans. Following a meal normal gastric emptying time is 3–4 hours.

Q. What are the important causes of gastric outlet obstruction?

Ans.
- Causes in the lumen
- Causes in the wall
- Causes outside the wall.
  See Surgical Long Cases, Page No. 105, 106, Chapter 3.

Q. What may be the likely cause of gastric outlet obstruction in this X-ray?

Ans. The stomach is hugely distended. The duodenal bulb is not formed. So, this is likely to be due to chronic complication of chronic duodenal ulcer. In malignant obstruction, such huge distension is unlikely.

Q. What are the consequences of gastric outlet obstruction?

Ans.
- Anatomical effects—Proximal to the obstruction, the stomach dilates due to chronic retention of food materials.
- Biochemical changes—Hyponatremia, hypochloremia, hypokalemia, metabolic alkalosis, and dehydration.

Q. What is the usual presentation of a patient with gastric outlet obstruction?

Ans. *See* Surgical Long Cases, Page No. 103, Chapter 3.

Q. What are the biochemical changes in patient with gastric outlet obstruction presenting with vomiting?

Ans. *See* Surgical Long Cases, Page No. 106–108, Chapter 3.

Q. How will you correct those biochemical abnormalities?

Ans. *See* Surgical Long Cases, Page No. 106–108, Chapter 3.

Q. How will you treat a patient of gastric outlet obstruction due to chronic duodenal ulcer?

Ans. *See* Surgical Long Cases, Page No. 106–108, Chapter 3.

Chronic Duodenal Ileus

Q. What is chronic duodenal ileus?

Ans. This is a condition of duodenal obstruction due to compression by the superior mesenteric artery due to a narrow aortomesenteric angle. Normally, the retroperitoneal fat and lymphatic tissue act as cushion for duodenum.

Q. What else may be the cause for duodenal obstruction?

Ans.

* Ladd's band
* High insertion of ligament of Treitz
* Duodenal stricture
* Neoplastic lesion.

Q. What factors may aggravate duodenal ileus?

Ans.

* Sudden weight loss
* Confinement to bed particularly in a body cast.

Q. What is the presenting symptom of chronic duodenal ileus?

Ans.

* Early satiety
* Nausea and bilious vomiting
* Postprandial abdominal discomfort and pain
* Symptoms are often relieved in left lateral decubitus or knee chest position.

Q. How the diagnosis may be confirmed?

Ans.

* Contrast-enhanced computed tomography (CECT) scan abdomen may show the site of duodenal compression.
* Combined superior mesenteric angiography and barium study.

Q. What is the optimal treatment?

Ans.

* In acute presentation, treatment is usually conservative—improvement of nutrition if required by total parenteral nutrition. Motility-enhancing drugs—metoclopramide may help.
* In chronic duodenal ileus—requires surgical treatment.
  - Duodenojejunostomy will bypass the obstruction.

■ BARIUM MEAL FOLLOW-THROUGH—ILEOCECAL TUBERCULOSIS/JEJUNAL STRICTURE (FIGS 17.35 AND 17.36)

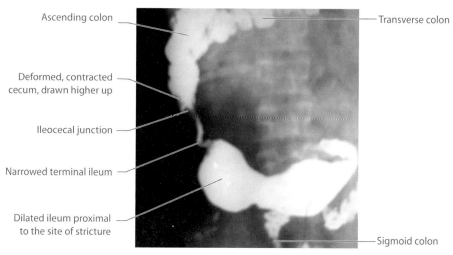

Ascending colon

Transverse colon

Deformed, contracted cecum, drawn higher up

Ileocecal junction

Narrowed terminal ileum

Dilated ileum proximal to the site of stricture

Sigmoid colon

Fig. 17.35: This is one of the skiagrams from the barium meal follow-through examination of small and large intestine series taken 8 hours after ingestion of the barium. There is gross narrowing of the terminal ileum, and the terminal ileum proximal to the narrowing is markedly dilated. The ileocecal junction is drawn higher up. The cecum is deformed with loss of normal distensibility and is also drawn higher up. This appearance is suggestive of ileocecal tuberculosis with stricture of terminal ileum

Courtesy: Dr AN Acharya, IPGME and R, Kolkata

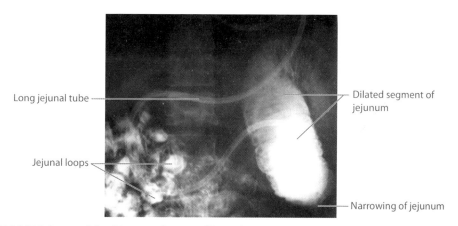

Long jejunal tube

Dilated segment of jejunum

Jejunal loops

Narrowing of jejunum

Fig. 17.36: This is one of the skiagrams from small bowel enema (enteroclysis) series showing a long jejunal tube in situ. A hugely distended loop of jejunum is seen with stenosis at the end of the dilated segment. This appearance is suggestive of a jejunal stricture

Q. Why do you say this is a jejunal loop?

Ans. The long tube is seen in this dilated loop. There are closely packed valvulae conniventes. So, this is a dilated jejunal loop.

Q. What are the important causes of small gut stricture?

Ans.

* Tuberculosis
* Crohn's disease
* Actinomycosis
* Primary carcinoma
* Lymphomas
* Carcinoid tumors
* Radiation enteritis
* Ischemic damage
* Intramural hemorrhage.

Q. How do tubercle bacilli infect the gut?

Ans. Tubercular infection may reach the gut by:

* Secondary to pulmonary tuberculosis due to swallowing of the bacilli.
* Ingestion of the bacilli with food.
* Hematogenous spread of the bacilli from a focus in the lung or lymph nodes.

Q. What are the types of ileocecal tuberculosis?

Ans. There are two types of ileocecal tuberculosis:

* Ulcerative
* Hyperplastic.

Q. What are the characteristics of ulcerative type of tuberculosis?

Ans. Multiple tubercular ulcer develops in terminal ileum. These ulcers are transversely placed and the overlying serosa is thickened and there may be tubercles on the serosal aspect.

Q. What is hyperplastic tuberculosis?

Ans. This is caused by ingestion of Mycobacterium with a high resistance to the organism. There is hyperplasia of the lymphoid follicles. There is gross thickening of the intestinal wall and there is narrowing of the lumen of intestine. The mesenteric lymph nodes may be involved and may show caseation.

Q. How patients with ileocecal tuberculosis usually present?

Ans.

* Recurrent attacks of lower abdominal pain
* Diarrhea
* Weight loss, anemia, and fever
* Mass in right iliac fossa
* Subacute intestinal obstruction—colicky pain, abdominal distension, vomiting, and constipation may occur.

Q. How will you treat patients with ileocecal tuberculosis?

Ans.

* Medical treatment—antitubercular drug treatment
    - Four drug regime—rifampicin, INH, ethambutol, and pyrazinamide for 2 months

- Followed by rifampicin and INH for next 4–6 months
- Alternatively may be treated with DOTS regimen.

Q. What are the indications for surgery?

Ans.

* If the patient shows symptoms and signs of subacute or acute intestinal obstruction, surgery is indicated
* Limited right hemicolectomy with ileoascending anastomosis is the optimum surgical treatment.

Q. What is Crohn's disease?

Ans. This is a chronic inflammatory disease of the GI tract, most commonly involving the ileum or colon. However, the disease may affect any part of the GIT.

Q. What are the possible etiological factors for development of Crohn's disease?

Ans.

* *Chronic infection*: There are some features of chronic infection in the pathology of Crohn's disease but no causative organisms have been identified.
* *Autoimmune disease* has been said to be one of the basis for this chronic inflammatory disease.

Q. Is Crohn's disease a premalignant lesion?

Ans. Crohn's disease is a premalignant lesion and predisposes to cancer but the chance is less than in ulcerative colitis.

Q. How patients with Crohn's disease usually present?

Ans.

* Chronic abdominal pain
* Chronic diarrhea
* Weight loss
* Intermittent fever
* Anemia
* Abdominal mass, particularly in right iliac fossa
* Signs and symptoms of acute intestinal obstruction or subacute intestinal obstruction
* Signs and symptoms of acute peritonitis due to perforation
* Perianal disease—anal fissure, perianal abscess, and fistula may be the presenting feature.

Q. What are the gross pathological changes in the gut in Crohn's disease?

Ans.

* Common site of involvement is ileum (60%) and colon (30%).
* May affect any part of GI tract from the mouth to the anus.
* The lesions are usually discontinuous—diseased areas separated by normal tissues—skip lesions.
* There is thickening of the wall of the gut due to transmural inflammation.
* There may be fibrous narrowing of a segment of a gut with proximal dilatation.
* There are multiple linear ulcerations in the mucosa with edema in-between the ulcer and this gives an appearance called cobble stone mucosa.

- There is thickening of the mesentery and there is fat wrapping over the gut wall.
- The mesenteric lymph nodes are enlarged.

Q. What are the histological features of Crohn's disease?

Ans.

- There is transmural inflammation of all the layers of the intestine with chronic inflammatory cell infiltrate.
- Noncaseating giant cell granuloma may be found in some patients.

Q. What is the medical treatment for Crohn's disease?

Ans.

- Corticosteroid—Oral corticosteroid in mild-to-moderate Crohn's disease.
- Parenteral corticosteroid is indicated in severe Crohn's disease.
- Sulfasalazine—Useful in mild-to-moderate Crohn's disease.
- *Immunosuppressive agent*: Azathioprine—reduces the dose of steroid.

Refractory disease:

- Monoclonal antibody—infliximab has shown marked response in complicated disease.
- Antibiotics—indicated when there are complications of abscess or fistula formation.

General treatment:

- Maintenance of nutrition
- Correction of anemia, hypoproteinemia, and electrolyte imbalance.

Q. What are the indications of surgery in Crohn's disease?

Ans. Surgery is usually indicated for complications like:

- Recurrent intestinal obstruction
- Perforation and fistula formation
- Failure of medical therapy
- Fulminant colitis
- Malignant change
- Perianal disease.

Q. What are the options of surgical treatment in Crohn's disease?

Ans. Surgical treatment involves resection of the grossly involved segment of the bowel responsible for the complication. Wide resection of the bowel is not indicated in Crohn's disease.

If there is normal looking bowel ends at the end of resection and there is no intra-abdominal sepsis, primary anastomosis may be done.

If there is significant intra-abdominal infection, a proximal ileostomy is to be done.

The options for surgical treatment are:

- Small segment ileal or colonic disease—segmental resection
- Ileocecal disease—ileocecal resection with ileoascending anastomosis
- Intra-abdominal abscess due to ileocccal disease—CT-guided percutaneous drainage of abscess. Once the abscess has settled—local resection of the gut.

♦ Colonic Crohn's disease—Surgery is indicated with shorter duration of symptoms. The extent of surgery will depend on the extent of the disease and the rectal involvement.
  – Total proctocolectomy with permanent ileostomy in advanced total colonic and rectal disease
  – Total abdominal colectomy with ileorectal anastomosis
  – Total abdominal colectomy with ileostomy and closure of rectal stump (Hartmann's procedure).
♦ Localized stricture—stricturoplasty.

■ BARIUM MEAL FOLLOW-THROUGH—RECURRENT APPENDICITIS (FIG. 17.37)

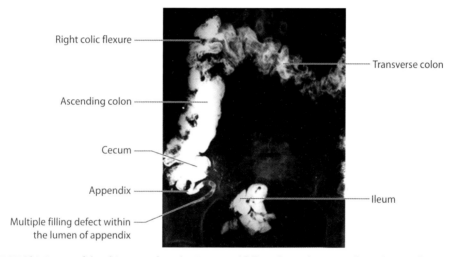

Fig. 17.37: This is one of the skiagrams from barium meal follow through series taken 5 hours after ingestion of barium, showing the ileocecal region and right-half of the colon. The appendix is visualized, but it shows multiple filling defects in the lumen suggestive of fecaliths. This appearance suggests a pathological appendix

Courtesy: Dr Shamita Chattarjee, Culcutta Medical College, Kolkata

Q. How are the fecaliths formed?

Ans. Fecaliths are formed by inspissated fecal matter, calcium phosphate, bacteria, and epithelial debris. The incidental finding of fecaliths in appendix is an indication for prophylactic appendectomy.

Q. What are the etiological factors for development of acute appendicitis?

Ans.
♦ *Bacterial infection*—There is usually a mixed growth of both aerobic and anaerobic organism.
♦ *Obstruction of the lumen* of the appendix by a fecalith, foreign body, or fibrous structure is an important predisposing factor.
♦ *Familial predisposition*.

Q. What is the classical presentation of a patient with acute appendicitis?

Ans.

- *Symptoms*:
  - Periumbilical colicky pain, which later shifts to the right iliac fossa. Coughing or sudden movement exacerbates the pain.
  - Fever—usually there is mild rise of temperature. In early stages, there may be no fever. High temperature (greater than 38.5°C) usually suggests other cause—mesenteric adenitis or urinary tract infection.
  - Nausea and vomiting.
- *Signs*:
  - Low-grade pyrexia
  - Muscle guarding in the right iliac fossa
  - Cutaneous hyperesthesia may be present in the right iliac fossa
  - Localized tenderness or rebound tenderness in the right iliac fossa
  - Rovsing's sign—deep palpation in left iliac fossa may cause pain in right iliac fossa.
  - *Psoas sign*—inflamed retrocecal appendix may cause psoas spasm and the patient will lie with the right hip flexed for relief of pain. Hyperextension of the right hip joint may induce abdominal pain.
  - Obturator sign (Zachary cope)—flexion and internal rotation of the right hip joint will cause pain in the hypogastrium—this is due to inflamed appendix lying over the obturatorinternus.

Q. What are the peculiarities of retrocecal appendicitis?

Ans.

- Classical pain in the periumbilical region and shifting to the right iliac fossa is usually absent. Pain may be felt in the loin.
- Tenderness in the right iliac fossa may be absent. Instead, there may be tenderness in the right loin.
- Psoas sign is usually present.

Q. What are the peculiarities of pelvic appendicitis?

Ans.

- Pain and tenderness may be elicited in the hypogastrium rather than in the right iliac fossa.
- Inflamed appendix in contact with rectum may cause diarrhea.
- Inflamed appendix in contact with bladder may cause frequency of micturition.
- Rectal examination may reveal tenderness in the pouch of Douglas, especially on the right side.

Q. What are the peculiarities of postileal appendicitis?

Ans.

- Classical pain is absent—Pain often felt to the right of umbilicus
- Diarrhea is an important feature, as the inflamed appendix lies in contact with the ileum.

Q. What laboratory investigations may help in diagnosis?

Ans. Apart from detail history and clinical examination, following laboratory investigations may help in diagnosis and may reduce the number of negative appendicectomy.
* Total and differential white blood cell (WBC) count-elevated count with polymorphonuclear leukocytosis.
* C-reactive peptide—Elevated in acute appendicitis.

Q. What are the roles of imaging investigations in acute appendicitis?

Ans.
* *Ultrasonography*—Effective in detection of distension of appendix, but cannot detect perforation. Interpretation is operator dependent. However, ultrasound is not superior to clinical examination in diagnosis of acute appendicitis.
* CT scan—Beneficial for evaluating patients with suspected recurrent or chronic appendicitis. CT scan has high positive-predictive value for diagnosis of acute appendicitis.

Q. How will you treat patients with acute appendicitis?

Ans. The ideal treatment is appendectomy.

Q. What is the role of conservative treatment for acute appendicitis?

Ans. A prospective study has demonstrated that 2 days of parenteral antibiotic therapy followed by 8 days of oral antibiotic was as effective as surgery for acute appendicitis. However, the recurrence rate of appendicitis requiring surgical intervention within 1 year was 35%. In view of the high recurrence rate, surgical treatment is preferred for treatment of acute appendicitis.

Q. What are the indications of appendectomy?

Ans.
* Acute appendicitis
* Recurrent appendicitis
* Mucocele of appendix
* Endometriosis of appendix
* Appendicular diverticulum
* Carcinoma of appendix involving the mucosa and not involving the base of appendix
* Small carcinoid tumor of appendix confined to tip or body of appendix.

Q. What are the techniques of appendectomy?
Ans.
* Open appendectomy
* Laparoscopic appendectomy.

Q. What are the incisions for open appendectomy?

* McBurney's gridiron incision
* Lanz's incision
* Midline incision
* Right paramedian incision.

Q. Describe the steps of appendectomy?

Ans. *See* Operative Surgery Section, Page No. 1107–1110, Chapter 22.

Q. What is retrograde appendectomy?

Ans. When the appendix is retrocecal, the tip may not be accessible easily. If the base is easily accessible a retrograde appendectomy is preferred in such situation.

The base of the appendix is dissected by passing a hemostatic forceps through the mesoappendix. The base of the appendix is crushed by a hemostatic forceps applied around the base of the appendix. The crushed base of the appendix is then ligated with 1–0 chromic catgut sutures. A hemostatic forceps is applied 5 mm distal to the ligature at the base of the appendix and the appendix is divided in-between. The mesoappendix is then held between the hemostatic forceps and divided and ligated from the base up to the tip. Once whole of the mesoappendix is ligated, the appendix becomes free and is removed.

Q. When you should not crush the base of appendix during appendectomy?

Ans.
- If the appendix is gangrenous
- If there is perforation at the base of the appendix
- If the base of appendix and the cecum is edematous.

Q. How many ports are required for laparoscopic appendectomy?

Ans. Three ports are required:
1. Infraumbilical 10 mm port—for telescope and the camera
2. One 5 mm port in the suprapubic area—left hand working port of surgeon. Alternatively, this port may be placed in the right iliac fossa.
3. One 10/5 mm port in left iliac fossa—right hand working port of surgeon.
   Management of appendicular lump and abscess—see surgical problems.
   Steps of appendectomy—see operative surgery section.

▮ BARIUM ENEMA—CARCINOMA COLON (FIGS 17.38 AND 17.39)

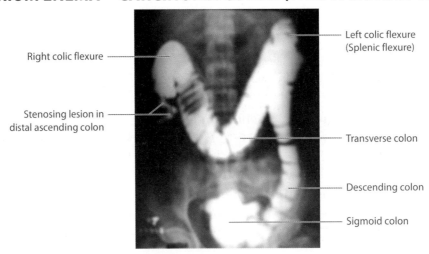

Right colic flexure

Left colic flexure (Splenic flexure)

Stenosing lesion in distal ascending colon

Transverse colon

Descending colon

Sigmoid colon

Fig. 17.38: This is one of the skiagrams from double-contrast barium enema series showing normal haustration and filling of the sigmoid, descending, and transverse colon. There is abrupt narrowing at the right colic flexure and a fine streak of barium is seen going down in the ascending colon. This appearance is suggestive of a stenosing lesion in the right colic flexure region, which may be due to carcinoma of right colic flexure

Courtesy: Dr Sushma Banerjee, IPGME and R, Kolkata

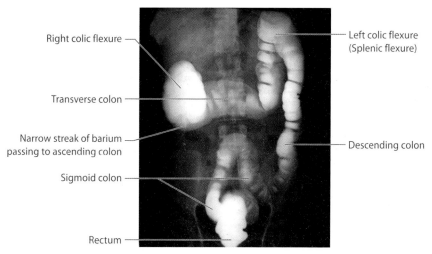

Right colic flexure

Transverse colon

Narrow streak of barium passing to ascending colon

Sigmoid colon

Rectum

Left colic flexure (Splenic flexure)

Descending colon

Fig. 17.39: This is one of the skiagrams from double-contrast barium enema series shown in normal left colon. There is abrupt narrowing of the contrast column at the right colic flexure with thin stream of the barium column going down the ascending colon. This appearance is suggestive of a stenosing lesion in the right colic flexure and the ascending colon may be due to carcinoma colon

Courtesy: Dr Rezaul Karim, IPGME and R, Kolkata

Q. What are the other possibilities of such a stenotic lesion?

Ans.
- Tuberculosis
- Crohn's disease
- Ischemic colitis
- Radiation enteritis
- Carcinoid tumor
- Lymphoma
- Anastomotic stricture.

Q. How will you prepare patient for barium enema examination?

Ans.
- Dietary restriction—liquid diet for 24 hours before the date of examination.
- Purgatives—osmotic purgatives for two consecutive nights before the date of examination
- Enema on the night before the examination.

Q. How will you do a double-contrast barium enema examination?

Ans.
- The examination involves three stages:
  1. Filling with barium
  2. Gas insufflation
  3. Radiography.

An injection of buscopan 20 mg is given intravenously to overcome any spasm in the colon. With the patient prone the barium suspension is introduced into the rectum and colon by using a catheter till the barium reaches the transverse colon.

Air (or carbon dioxide gas) is then insufflated gently to move the barium column further into the transverse colon.

By turning the patient to the left side up and head up the barium column is pushed into the right-half of the colon.

The barium from the rectum is then partially drained out.

Serial radiographs are then taken in different positions.

Q. What are the etiological factors for development of carcinoma colon?

Ans.

- *Diet:* High-dietary fiber is associated with low incidence of colonic cancer, whereas diet high in fat content is associated with high incidence of colonic cancer. High-fiber diet is associated with rapid evacuation due to short transit time thus allowing only a brief contact of carcinogens with the mucosa.
- *Genetic factors*:
  - *Familial adenomatous polyposis coli* is associated with colonic cancer and this is transmitted by an *adenomatous polyposis coli (APC)* gene.
  - Lynch syndrome I—hereditary nonpolyposis colorectal cancer:
    - Autosomal dominant inheritance
    - Early onset of colonic carcinoma
    - Frequent synchronous and metachronous cancer
    - High incidence of cancer in other sites like kidney, ureter, bladder, breast, ovary, endometrium, stomach, and small gut.
  - Lynch syndrome II—hereditary nonpolyposis colon cancer:
    - Both colonic and extracolonic manifestation of cancer.

Q. What are the macroscopic types of colonic carcinoma?

Ans. *See* Surgical Pathology Section, Page No. 879, 880, Chapter 18.

Q. How does colonic carcinoma spread?

Ans. *See* Surgical Pathology Section, Page No. 882, Chapter 18.

Q. How patients with right colonic carcinoma usually present?

Ans.

- *General symptoms*:
  - Anorexia
  - Weight loss
  - Anemia.
- *Bowel symptoms*:
  - Right lower quadrant abdominal pain
  - Abdominal mass
  - Melena
  - Diarrhea.
- *Advanced disease*:
  - Low backache
  - Cachexia
  - Jaundice
  - Ascites.

Q. How patients with left colonic carcinoma usually presents?

Ans.

+ General symptoms:
  - Anorexia
  - Weight loss
  - Anemia.
+ Bowel symptoms:
  - Alteration of bowel habit—increasing constipation
  - Passage of blood and mucus with stool
  - Left-sided abdominal pain and mass in abdomen
  - May present with acute or chronic obstruction.

Q. Apart from barium enema, what is the most important investigation for diagnosis of colonic carcinoma?

Ans. Colonoscopy and biopsy from the lesion.

Q. How will you assess the patient to decide about operability?

Ans.

+ Detail history and physical examination
+ Complete hemogram
+ Liver function test
+ CT scan of abdomen and pelvis
+ ECG
+ Chest X-ray.

Q. Why preoperative bowel preparation is required for colonic surgery?

Ans. Operation performed in unprepared colon is associated with high incidence of wound infection (about 40%). Mechanical gut preparation and parenteral antibiotic can reduce the wound infection rate to about 5%.

Q. How will you prepare gut for colonic surgery?

Ans. *See* Surgical Long Cases, Page No. 201, Chapter 3.

Q. What will be the extent of resection depending on the site of growth?

Ans.

+ Carcinoma cecum and ascending colon—Right hemicolectomy
+ Right colic flexure—Extended right hemicolectomy
+ Transverse colon—Extended right hemicolectomy or transverse colectomy
+ Descending colon—Left hemicolectomy
+ Sigmoid colon—Sigmoid colon resection or extended left hemicolectomy.

Q. How will you manage obstructing right colonic carcinoma?

Ans.

+ Right hemicolectomy and ileotransverse anastomosis are the preferred choice.
+ If growth is inoperable in view of local fixity, a bypass with ileotransverse anastomosis is to be done.

Q. How will you manage obstructing left colonic carcinoma?

Ans. Traditionally, the obstructing left-sided colonic carcinomas were managed in a:
* *Three-stage procedure*:
  – *First stage*: Exploratory laparotomy and colostomy for relief of obstruction.
  – *Second stage*: Resection of colon
  – *Third stage*: Closure of colostomy.

However, there has been change in concept of management of obstructing left colonic carcinoma:
* *Two-stage procedure*:
  – *First stage*—exploratory laparotomy, resection of the growth and colostomy with a mucus fistula or a Hartmann's type procedure.
  – *Second stage*—closure of colostomy or maintenance of continuity by anastomosis, if a Hartmann's type procedure was done earlier.
* *One-stage procedure*: If the patient's general condition is good, no evidence of peritonitis, a single-stage resection anastomosis has been shown to be safe, effective and comparable to staged procedure.

Q. What is the role of on-table colonic lavage?

Ans. In cases of left-sided colonic obstruction, resection and on-table lavage of colon allow primary anastomosis with least chance of anastomotic leakage.

Q. What is Duke's staging for carcinoma colon?

Ans.
* *Stage A*: Tumor in the bowel, but not beyond muscularis propria
* *Stage B*: Transmural invasion of bowel wall
* *Stage C*: Any degree of bowel wall invasion with lymph node metastasis:
  – C1—epicolic and paracolic nodes
  – C2—intermediate and proximal lymph nodes.

Q. What is Astler-Coller's modification for Dukes staging?

Ans.
* *Stage A*: Tumor confined to submucosa
* *Stage B*:
  – B1—tumors invading up to the muscularis propria
  – B2—transmural invasion of bowel wall
  – B3—lesion involving adjacent organs
* *Stage C*:
  – C1—lesion of B1 depth and lymph node metastasis
  – C2—lesion of B2 depth and lymph node metastasis
  – C3—lesion of B3 depth and lymph node metastasis
* *Stage D*: Presence of distant metastasis.

Q. What is tumor, node and metastasis (TNM) staging for carcinoma colon?

Ans.
* *Primary tumor (T)*:
  – T1—tumor invading submucosa
  – T2—invading muscularis propria

- T3—invades to the subserosa or to the paracolic tissue in areas not covered by serosa
- T4—invades through the serosa and/or involving the adjacent organs.
- *Regional lymph nodes (N0)*:
  - N0—no regional lymph nodes involved
  - N1—lymph node metastasis in one to three nodes
  - N2—lymph node metastasis in four or more nodes
  - N3—lymph node metastasis in central nodes.
- *Distant metastasis (M)*:
  - M0—no distant metastasis
  - M1—presence of distant metastasis.

Q. What is the role of carcinoembryonic antigen (CEA) estimation in colonic carcinoma?

Ans. *See* Surgical Long Cases, Page No. 201, Chapter 3.

Q. What is the role of adjuvant therapy in colonic carcinoma?

Ans. *See* Surgical Long Cases, Page No. 204–205, Chapter 3.

Q. What are the prognostic factors of colonic carcinoma?

Ans.
- *Stage of the tumor at diagnosis* is one of the very important prognostic factor
- *Degree of tumor differentiation*—5-year survival is better in patients with well-differentiated tumors
- *Lymph node involvement* is one of the determinants of 5-year survival
- *Lymphatic and blood vessel invasion* of the tumor is associated with poor prognosis
- *Obstructing and perforating carcinoma* of the colon are usually locally advanced diseases and are associated with poor prognosis
- *Age of the patient*—younger patient has poor prognosis. The disease is usually locally advanced at diagnosis and there is more incidence of poorly differentiated tumors in younger patients
- *Blood transfusion* in perioperative period is also a prognostic marker. Higher the transfusion poorer the prognosis.

Q. What is the follow-up protocol for colonic cancer?

Ans. The idea of follow-up is to detect local recurrence, metastatic disease, or a metachronous lesion.

Follow-up protocol includes:
- Clinical examination, fecal occult blood, complete blood count, and liver function test:
  - Every 3 months for first 3 years
  - Every 6 months for additional 2 years
  - Subsequently yearly follow-up
  - Blood for CEA every 8 weeks for 3 years and every 3 months for 2 more years
  - Colonoscopy yearly for 3 years and then every 2–3 years
  - Yearly chest X-rays.

■ INTRAVENOUS UROGRAPHY—HYDRONEPHROSIS (FIG. 17.40)

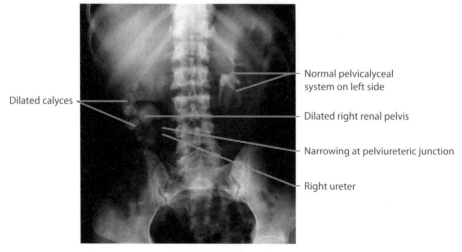

Normal pelvicalyceal system on left side

Dilated calyces

Dilated right renal pelvis

Narrowing at pelviureteric junction

Right ureter

Fig. 17.40: This is one of the skiagrams from intravenous urography series taken 25 minutes after injection of dye. The left kidney outline and pelvicalyceal system are seen normal. The right kidney outline is enlarged. There is gross dilatation of the right renal pelvis. The calcyces are dilated and clubbed. There is abrupt narrowing at the pelviureteric junction. This appearance is suggestive of unilateral hydronephrosis

Courtesy: Prof Sudip Ch Chakroborty, IPGME and R, Kolkata

Q. How will you prepare patient for intravenous urography study?

Ans.

- ◆ No fluid restriction is required.
- ◆ Patient should avoid solid food 6 hours before the procedure.
- ◆ Oral purgative and antiflatulent tablet—the night before the procedure.

Q. What contrast agents are used for IVU?

Ans. These are iodine-containing contrast agents:

- ◆ Ionic contrast like sodium diatrizoate or meglumine iothalamate
- ◆ Nonionic contrast like Omnipaque.

The dose required is 300 mg of iodine per kilogram of body weight. In well-hydrated patient, the dose may be increased to 600 mg iodine per kilogram body weight.

Q. How intravenous urography is done?

Ans.

- ◆ At first, a control X-ray of the KUB region is done to exclude any radiopaque calculi or any calcification in the KUB region.
- ◆ About 50 mL of contrast agent 76% urografin (sodium diatrizoate) is injected slowly intravenously and then serial radiographs are taken:
  - – 1-minute film will give a nephrogram phase.
  - – 5-minute film will show early filling of the pelvicalyceal system and the ureter may be visualized and any filling in the lower ureter may be seen well. In the delayed film, the lower ureter will be overlapped by the full bladder.

- If there is no obstruction, an abdominal compression is applied with a belt and exposure of renal area is taken at 10 minutes—the pelvicalyceal system is well visualized.
- Once the bladder gets filled in 10–15 minutes time, the oblique views are taken to look for any irregularity in the bladder wall.
- If an urethrogram is required, patient is asked to pass urine and a micturating cystourethrogram may be obtained in an oblique view.

Q. What is hydronephrosis?

Ans. This is a condition of aseptic dilatation of the collecting system of the kidney due to partial or intermittent complete obstruction.

Q. What are the grades of hydronephrosis?

Ans. There are four grades of hydronephrosis depending on the radiological findings:
1. *Grade-I*: Most minimal dilatation with slight blunting of calyceal fornices.
2. *Grade-II*: Enlargement and obvious blunting of the calyces, but intruding shadow of the papillae seen.
3. *Grade-III*: Rounding of the calyces with obliteration of the papilla shadow.
4. *Grade-IV*: Extreme calyceal ballooning.
   Renal parenchymal thinning is seen in grade-III and grade-IV hydronephrosis.

Q. What other investigations are helpful in evaluation of patients presenting with hydronephrosis?

Ans.
- *Ultrasonography*—Demonstrates pelvicaliectasis and thickness of renal parenchyma, but does not give any functional information.
- *Contrast CT scan*—Provides both anatomical and functional information.
- *Radionuclide ^{99m}Tc diethylenetriaminepentaacetic acid (DTPA) scanning*—Offers better functional information. Differential renal function may be assessed. Does not give better anatomical delineation than IVU or CT scan.
- *Retrograde pyelography*: If IVU, USG, and CT scan fail to localize the site of obstruction then retrograde pyelography is indicated, which helps to pinpoint the site of obstruction.

Q. What are the causes of unilateral hydronephrosis?

Ans. *See* Surgical Long Cases, Page No. 216–220, Chapter 4.

Q. What are the causes of bilateral hydronephrosis?

Ans. *See* Surgical Long Cases, Page No. 216–220, Chapter 4.

Q. How patients with hydronephrosis usually present?

Ans. *See* Surgical Long Cases, Page No. 216–220, Chapter 4.

Q. How will you manage hydronephrosis due to pelviureteric junction obstruction?

Ans. *See* Surgical Long Cases, Page No. 216–220, Chapter 4.

Q. What do you mean by dismembered pyeloplasty?

Ans. *See* Surgical Long Cases, Page No. 216–220, Chapter 4.

Q. What do you mean by nondismembered pyeloplasty?

Ans. *See* Surgical Long Cases, Page No. 216–220, Chapter 4.

■ INTRAVENOUS UROGRAPHY—CARCINOMA KIDNEY (FIGS 17.41 AND 17.42)

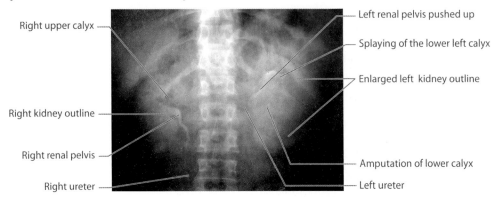

Fig. 17.41: This is one of the skiagrams from intravenous urography series taken 10 minutes after injection of dye. The right kidney outline and the pelvicalyceal system are seen normal. The left kidney outline is enlarged. There is distortion of the left pelvicalyceal system. The pelvis is pushed up. There is splaying (spider leg deformity) of the calyces. There is amputation of some of the calyces. This appearance is suggestive of carcinoma of the kidney

Courtesy: Dr Rajkumar Singh Mahapatra, IPGME and R, Kolkata

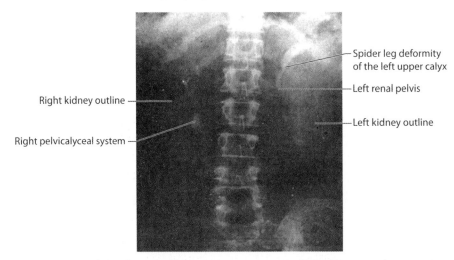

Fig. 17.42: This is one of the skiagrams from intravenous urography (IVU) series taken 10 minutes after injection of the contrast. The right kidney and the renal pelvis are normal. The left kidney outline is enlarged. The left renal pelvis is pushed up. There is splaying of the calyces (spider leg deformity) and also there is amputation of some calyces. This appearance is suggestive of carcinoma kidney

Courtesy: Dr Abhiram Majhi, CNMC, Kolkata

Q. How patients with carcinoma kidney usually presents?

Ans. *See* Surgical Long Cases, Page No. 220–223, Chapter 4.

Q. What further investigations are required for evaluation of a patient of carcinoma kidney?

Ans. *See* Surgical Long Cases, Page No. 220–223, Chapter 4.

Q. How will you treat a patient of carcinoma kidney?

Ans. *See* Surgical Long Cases, Page No. 220–223, Chapter 4.

■ X-RAY SKULL—SKULL BONE FRACTURE (FIGS 17.43 AND 17.44)

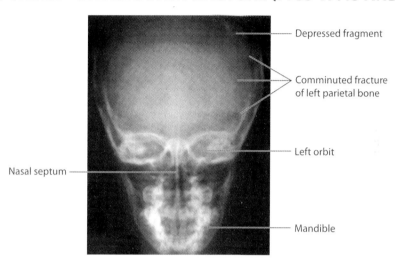

Fig. 17.43: This is a plain X-ray of skull anteroposterior (AP) view including both maxillae—mandible and the upper part of the neck showing a comminuted fracture involving the left parietal bone. One of the fracture fragments is seen depressed inward. This appearance is suggestive of comminuted depressed fracture of the left parietal bone

Courtesy: Dr Kaushik Ghosh, BIN/IPGME and R, Kolkata

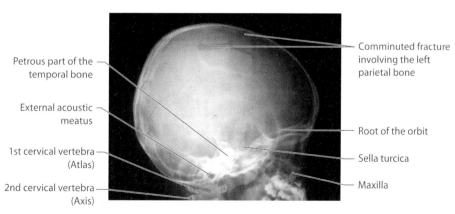

Fig. 17.44: This is a lateral view plain X-ray of the skull with part of maxilla showing a comminuted fracture is suggestive of depressed skull fracture involving the left parietal bone

Courtesy: Dr Kaushik Ghosh, BIN/IPGME and R, Kolkata

Q. How do you say whether fracture fragments are depressed or not?

Ans. In lateral view, it is not possible to comment whether the fracture fragments are depressed or not. The depressed fracture is better demonstrated in an AP view X-ray of skull where the depressed fragment of the skull is seen pushed inward.

Q. What is open depressed fracture?

Ans. If the skin and the pericraniums breached then it is an open or compound depressed fracture.

Q. What are the problems with depressed fracture?

Ans.
* Injury to the underlying dura and brain
* Mass effect due to inward displacement of the fracture fragment
* Risk of infection
* Cosmetic.

Q. What are the indications for elevating a depressed fragment?

Ans.
* Open depressed fracture
* Associated with underlying hematoma
* Sharp bony spicule when there is high chance of dural injury
* When there is mass effect
* When the depressed fragment lies over an important brain area—sensory or motor cortex.

Q. How will you treat depressed fracture?

Ans.
* *Primary management*: Resuscitation
* Treatment of the fracture:
  - A wide skin flap is raised surrounding the area of the fracture.
  - About 2–3 burr holes are made adjacent to the site of depressed fracture.
  - The burr hole is extended and the depressed fragment is elevated.
* A full course of parenteral antibiotics to prevent infection.

Q. How will you differentiate a suture line and a fracture?

Ans. Sutures are situated at certain anatomical landmarks at the junction of skull bones. The fractures may be situated anywhere in the skull bones.

Sutures have parallel-serrated margins, whereas the fracture line has smooth parallel margins.

Q. What is pond depressed fracture of skull?

Ans. This is usually found in children. There is a smooth depression of the cranial vault usually due to blunt trauma. This usually does not require active treatment.

Q. What is simple linear fracture of skull?

Ans. This is isolated fracture of skull bone without any displacement of the fracture fragment. This also does not require any active treatment.

Q. What are the features of anterior cranial fossa fracture?

Ans.

◆ Subconjunctival hemorrhage
◆ Anosmia
◆ Epistaxis
◆ Cerebrospinal fluid (CSF) rhinorrhea
◆ Rarely, caroticocavernous fistula.

Q. What are the features of middle cranial fossa fracture?

Ans.

◆ CSF otorrhea and rhinorrhea
◆ Hemotympanum
◆ Ossicular disruption of middle ear
◆ VII and VIII nerve palsy
◆ Battle's sign—ecchymosis over the mastoid region.

Q. How will you confirm that the watery discharge is CSF?

Ans. The fluid is analyzed for beta transferrin, presence of which confirms that the fluid is CSF.

Q. Extradural and subdural hematoma.

Ans. *See* Surgical Problems Section, Page No. 687–689, Chapter 16.

■ CHEST X-RAY—CHEST INJURY (FIG. 17.45)

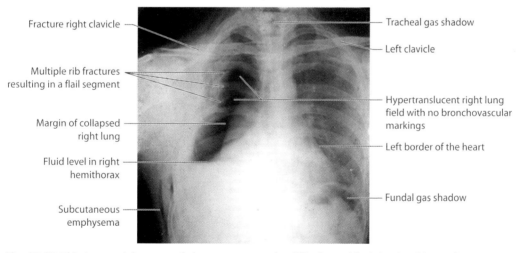

Fracture right clavicle

Multiple rib fractures resulting in a flail segment

Margin of collapsed right lung

Fluid level in right hemithorax

Subcutaneous emphysema

Tracheal gas shadow

Left clavicle

Hypertranslucent right lung field with no bronchovascular markings

Left border of the heart

Fundal gas shadow

Fig. 17.45: This is a straight x-ray of chest postroanterior (PA) view with right shoulder and upper part of abdomen showing multiple rib fractures on the right side involving 2nd, 3rd, 4th, 5th, and 6th rib at two points and the intervening fragment of the ribs are pushed inward. The right long field appears hypertranslucent. There is homogeneous opacity in the right hemithorax with a horizontal fluid level suggestive of hemopneumothorax. The margins of the collapsed right lung are seen. There is fracture involving the right clavicle. There is also evidence of subcutaneous emphysema. So, this x-ray appearance is suggestive of multiple rib fractures with flail chest with traumatic hemopneumothorax and fracture clavicle with subcutaneous emphysema.

Courtesy: Dr Sandip Roy, AMRI, Kolkata.

Q. How will you count ribs in chest X-ray?

Ans. The ribs are counted from the back starting with the first rib.

Q. Where is the margin of the collapsed lung?

Ans. The collapsed lung is seen as a dense shadow lateral to the heart shadow.

Q. How will you manage a patient presenting with major chest trauma?

Ans. Before going into detail evaluation of injury, I will first take measures to:
* Maintain his airway
* Breathing
* Circulation
* Exclude life-threatening situations like tension pneumothorax and cardiac tamponade.

Q. How will you maintain airway in a polytrauma patient?

Ans. *See* Surgical Problems Section, Page No. 679, Chapter 16.

Q. How will you maintain breathing in a polytrauma patient?

Ans. *See* Surgical Problems Section, Page No. 679, Chapter 16.

Q. How will you maintain circulation in a polytrauma patient?

Ans. *See* Surgical Problems Section, Page No. 679, 680, Chapter 16.

Q. How will you diagnose tension pneumothorax?

Ans.
* Severe respiratory distress
* Cyanosis
* Mediastinal shift (trachea and apex beat shifted to opposite side)
* Hyperresonant percussion note
* Absent breath sound.

Q. How will you relieve tension pneumothorax?

Ans. If tension pneumothorax is present, it should be relieved immediately by inserting a wide-bore needle in second intercostal space at the midclavicular line.

Q. How will you diagnose cardiac tamponade?

Ans. Cardiac tamponade is diagnosed by:
* Feeble, paradoxical pulse
* Increased jugular venous pressure
* Muffled heart sounds.

Q. How will you relieve cardiac tamponade?

Ans. If cardiac tamponade is present, it should be immediately relieved by needle cardiocentesis by inserting a wide-bore needle to left of xiphisternal junction into the pericardial cavity.

Q. What is flail chest?

Ans. When two or more ribs are fractured at two or more points then that segment of the chest lies loose from the rest of the rib cage and shows paradoxical movement during respiration. This is called flail chest.

Q. What is stove in chest?

Ans. There is fracture of multiple ribs at one point resulting in permanent indentation of a segment of chest wall without showing any paradoxical movement during respiration. This is called stove in chest.

Q. What is minor flail chest?

Ans. When the flail segment is small and does not result in any alteration in arterial blood gas analysis then it is called a minor flail chest.

Q. What is major flail chest?

Ans. When the flail segment is large and results in alteration of arterial blood gas analysis showing hypoxemia and hypercarbia.

Q. What is the treatment for an isolated rib fracture?

Ans.
* Analgesics
* May require intercostal nerve blockade
* Respiratory physiotherapy
* If there is associated traumatic pneumothorax or hemothorax appropriate treatment for that.

Q. How will you treat traumatic hemothorax? OR What is the indication of thoracotomy for management of hemothorax?

Ans.
* Massive bleeding—1 liter of blood drains on insertion of drainage tube
* Brisk bleeding—bleeding more than 100 mL every 15 minute
* Continuing bleeding—more than 200 mL/h over 3 hours
* Major airway injury, lung laceration.
   A posterolateral thoracotomy is performed and bleeding is stopped. Debridement of lung parenchyma and chest drain is inserted.

Q. What is the source of blood in traumatic hemothorax?

Ans.
* In most cases, it is due to injury of intercostal vessels
* Due to underlying lung laceration
* Rarely, major vessel injury.

Q. How will you treat traumatic pneumothorax?

Ans. Treatment depends on the type of pneumothorax:
* Tension pneumothorax—Immediate relief by insertion of a wide-bore needle in the second intercostal space at midclavicular line, followed by insertion of a chest drainage tube.
* Small pneumothorax:
   The lung is partially expanded:
   – Analgesics
   – Chest physiotherapy
   – Antibiotic.
* Massive pneumothorax with collapsed lung.

Intercostal tube drainage: The tube is inserted into the second intercostal space at the parasternal region.

Q. What are the indications of thoracotomy in traumatic pneumothorax?

Ans.
- Continuing air leak for more than 7 days
- Massive air leak
- Major airway injury
- Lung contusion.

Q. How will you treat patients with minor flail chest?

Ans.
- Managed by supportive measures but within an intensive therapy unit set up
- Analgesics
- Respiratory physiotherapy
- Antibiotics
- Serial arterial blood gas analysis
- Usually gets stabilized in 2–3 weeks
- Ventilatory support may be required in some cases, which develop hypoxemia.

Q. How will you treat patients with major flail chest?

Ans.
- Patient should be treated in an intensive therapy unit
- Intermittent positive pressure ventilation (IPPV). Patients usually require 2–3 weeks of ventilatory support for stabilization of the flail segment
- General care of patient is very essential
- Intermittent suction
- Care of skin
- Antibiotic
- Bowel and bladder care
- Nutritional care.

Q. What is the indication of fixation of flail segment?

Ans. Routine fixation of flail segment is not required. However, if there are other underlying injuries requiring thoracotomy, flail segment can be fixed simultaneously.

Q. What are the problems in patients with flail segment?

Ans.
- The flail segment lies loose from the rest of the rib cage.
- During inspiration, which is an active process, the chest expands and creates a negative intrathoracic pressure. As there is negative intrathoracic pressure, the flail segment is drawn inward during inspiration and during expiration, as the chest recoils and there is positive intrathoracic pressure, the flail segment is pushed outward resulting in paradoxical movement of the flail segment.

  This causes impairment of the gaseous exchange resulting in hypoxemia.

  The flail segment may cause underlying lung contusion or laceration and traumatic pneumothorax or hemothorax.

■ MAMMOGRAPHY

These is skiagram of mammography both mediolateral and craniocaudal views showing a dense mass in the right breast in the upper inner quadrant of the breast. The lump is having an irregular spiculated margin. The nipple appears retracted. This appearance is suggestive of a malignant mass in the right breast.

Q. What is mammography?

Ans. Mammography is a radiological investigation for diagnosis of breast lesion. It may be used for screening as well as diagnosis of breast cancer. The breast is compressed between two plates and internal picture (X-ray) of the breast is obtained. There is minimal exposure to the radiation dose.

Q. What is digital mammography?

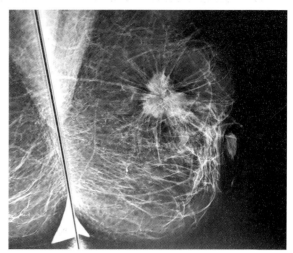

Fig. 17.46: Mammography picture craniocaudal view showing distortion of architecture of the breast and a hyoerdense mass in upper quadrant of the breast. The mass is having a spiculated margin with areas of calcification. The nipple appears retracted. This is most likely to be a malignant mass in the breast

Ans. Digital mammography is a newer modality of capturing the mammographic images. The computerized sensor collects the image instead of an X-ray film.

The CAD (computer-aided detection) software analyzes the images and any areas of concern are highlighted with markers on the screen. This can be useful in guiding the radiologist to check those areas more closely.

In digital mammography, the images are stored on a computer and may be read directly on a computer screen. Radiologists can enhance the images to get a better view of particular area.

The digital mammogram may detect a lesion otherwise undetectable in a film mammography. However, digital mammography is costlier than film mammography.

A study published in 2012 showed that digital mammography was better than film mammography at detecting "high-grade" ductal carcinoma in situ (DCIS).

Q. In which patient you will consider doing mammography?

Ans. Mammography is indicated in patient more than 35 years and woman having less dense breast. Woman with denser breasts, it is difficult to interpret the breast lesion on the background of dense breast tissue. So, premenopausal woman less than 35 years and woman with dense breast show a decreased mammographic sensitivity.

Ultrasound has been considered as an alternative to or supplementary to mammography for women with dense breasts because it can more effectively screen all of the breast tissue. However, ultrasound is not effective in detecting microcalcifications, which are an early sign of possible breast cancer. So, premenopausal woman less than 35 years should be offered USG for breast imaging.

Q. How is mammography done?

Ans. The patient is to undress above the waist. Avoid using powder or cream under the arm, which may interfere with the quality of the mammogram. Mammogram involves taking two views of each breast—(1) craniocaudal and (2) mediolateral. The breast is placed on the breast plate of the imaging machine the compression plate compresses the breast for few seconds. Compression allows better imaging of the breast tissue. Sometimes, this compression may be uncomfortable.

To avoid discomfort and pain during mammography, this investigation is avoided during the menstruation or 1 week prior to menstruation.

Q. What are the characteristics of a benign lesion on mammography?

Ans.

- Masses, which are round or oval
- Hypodense masses are most likely benign
- Margin of the mass are well defined and smooth
- Presence of macrocalcification.

Q. What are the characteristics of malignant lesion in mammography?

Ans.

- Architectural distortion of breast tissue
- Duct dilatation
- Dense stellate soft tissue mass, which is irregular in shape
- Margins of the mass are irregular or speculated (spiky projection)
- Microcalcification: In elderly patients, few microcalcifications may be normal
- Stippled calcification is characteristic
- Increased thickness of skin due to lymphedema
- Nipple retraction may be seen.

Q. What are the different types of calcifications on mammography?

Ans. Calcifications show up as white spots on a mammogram. This calcification may occur in two forms:

1. *Macrocalcifications*: Macrocalcifications tend to be large and coarse looking and are associated with aging. They are common in women over 50 and are present in a small percentage of younger women. Macrocalcification is usually not associated with cancer.
2. *Microcalcifications*: Groups of small calcifications huddled together are called clusters of microcalcifications. Microcalcifications are considered a sign of possible malignancy, even without a visible mass. The characteristics of the mass and associated microcalcification will dictate further diagnostic tests and possibly a biopsy for confirmation of the diagnosis.

Q. What is BI-RADS system of reporting of breast imaging?

Ans. The acronym BI-RADS stands for Breast Imaging Reporting and Data System and is proposed by American College of Radiology. This reporting system is applicable for USG, mammography, or MRI. This system is useful for standardization of reporting of breast cancer diagnosis. Other system is Nottingham classification.

Q. What is BI-RADS category for breast imaging reporting?

Ans.

- *BI-RADS category and definition:*
  - *BI-RADS 0:* Incomplete assessment. Further imaging or information is required, e.g. magnification, special mammographic views, and ultrasound
  - *BI-RADS I:* Negative. No masses, architectural distortion or suspicious calcifications present
  - *BI-RADS II:* Benign findings. Benign masses with characteristic appearance. No mammographic evidence of malignancy.
  - *BI-RADS III:* Probably *benign*, short interval follow-up study suggested.
  - *BI-RADS IV:* Suspicious mammographic abnormality of malignancy.
    - Biopsy should be considered for such a lesion.
    - These can be further classified as:
      - » *BI-RADS IVa:* Low level of suspicion for malignancy
      - » *BI-RADS IVb:* Intermediate suspicion for malignancy
      - » *BI-RADS IVc:* Moderate suspicion for malignancy.
  - *BI-RADS V:* There is a mammographic appearance, which is highly suggestive of malignancy. Biopsy of the lesion should be done.
  - *BI-RADS VI:* Known biopsy-proven malignancy.

Q. What is the risk of malignancy in different BI-RADS lesion?

- *BI-RADS III:* ~2%
- *BI-RADS IV:* ~30%[3]
- *BI-RADS V:* 95%.

Q. Is ultrasonography required after mammography?

Ans. X-ray mammograms are often followed up with ultrasound imaging to determine whether a lesion that appeared on a mammogram is a cyst or a solid mass. Ultrasound imaging may also be used to guide a needle into the abnormal tissue from which fluid or cells may be taken for histological examination.

Ultrasound imaging of the breast also evaluates some lumps that can be felt but that are difficult to see on a mammogram, especially in dense breasts.

In a study of 3,000 women who primarily had palpable lesions found that when ultrasound was used with standard mammography, 92% of breast cancers were detected. The specificity was 98%. In addition, when both imaging modalities excluded malignancy, the accuracy was 99% (i.e. false-negative result was 1%).

Q. How reliable is mammography for evaluation of breast malignancy?

Ans.

- *Sensitivity (true-positive):* 90%
- *False positive:* 10%
- *False negative:* 6–8%.

Q. What is false-negative mammogram?

Ans. A false-negative is when a mammogram is read as "negative" (i.e. no cancer) but other investigation revealed patient has cancer.

Q. What is false-positive mammogram?

Ans. A false-positive is when a mammogram is mistakenly interpreted as presence of cancer but other tests have revealed no cancer.

Q. What is the recommendation for screening mammography for detection of breast cancer?

Ans. In United States, the recommendation of American Cancer Society is to do screening mammography starting at the age of 45 years, once every year till the age of 55 years and afterward once in 2 years. This is continued till the woman is in good health and has a life expectancy of at least 10 years.

Q. What is the role of mammography following breast-conserving surgery?

Ans. Breast-conserving surgery (BCS) involves wide excision with a margin of normal breast tissue all around and adjuvant treatment with radiotherapy and chemotherapy. A baseline mammogram should be done 6 months after completion of treatment, which may be compared with the subsequent mammograms for any change. If reconstruction is done with muscle flap or implants, MRI is superior to mammography for follow-up imaging.

However, unaffected breast imaging may be done with mammography at follow-up.

Q. What is BSE?

Ans. BSE stands for breast self examination. This may be done monthly by all women over the age of 20. BSE may detect breast lumps and this is a great screening tool that can help in early detection of breast cancer.

Q. Is screening mammography is a risk factor for breast cancer?

Ans. There is no report of woman developing breast cancer due to screening mammography. Woman getting a mammogram every year from age of 40 years to 90 years would receive only around 10 rad of radiation exposure. Women getting treatment for breast cancer receive radiation up to 45–50 Gy. In screening mammography, the breast is being exposed to minimal dose of radiation, which can be a remote cause of cancer. The benefit of screening mammography outweighs the benefit of screening mammography for early detection of cancer.

Q. What is the advantage of mammogram over BSE?

Ans. Mammography may detect impalpable breast cancer by the typical appearance of the lesion detected on mammography and presence of microcalcification. The average size of a lump found by BSE is about the size of 2.5 cm and average size lump found by mammography is about 1 cm. The area of microcalcification may be the foci of cancer when no lump could be discerned.

Q. Is mammography helpful for diagnosis of male breast cancer?

Ans. Although incidence is less, men have breast cancer. Incidence of male breast cancer is 1%. Men presenting with breasts symptoms like pain, lump, or discharge will need evaluation by mammography.

The mass in the breast may be evaluated by a standard mammography.

Chapter 18

Surgical Pathology

■ BENIGN GASTRIC ULCER (FIG. 18.1)

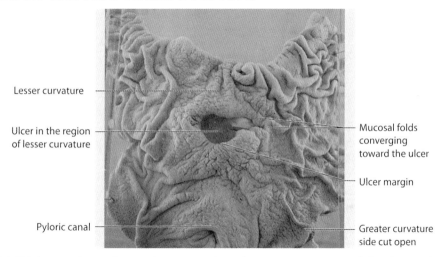

Lesser curvature

Ulcer in the region of lesser curvature

Mucosal folds converging toward the ulcer

Ulcer margin

Pyloric canal

Greater curvature side cut open

Fig. 18.1: This is a specimen of stomach cut open along the greater curvature and showing an ulcer in the region of the lesser curvature. The margins of the ulcer are well defined. There is convergence of mucosal folds toward the margin of the ulcer. So, this is a specimen of benign gastric ulcer

Q. Why do you say, this is a benign ulcer?

Ans.
- Ulcers along lesser curvature are more commonly benign.
- The margins of the ulcer are clear-cut and not everted.
- Surrounding gastric mucosal folds are converging toward the base of the ulcer. In malignant ulcer, these folds are effaced around the ulcer.

Q. What are the sites where peptic ulcer may occur?

Ans. Peptic ulcer occurs due to acid peptic digestion and may occur in sites exposed to acid and pepsin:
- *Stomach*: Majority occur near the lesser curvature.
- *Duodenum*: Most common in the first part. In Zollinger–Ellison syndrome (ZES), it may affect second and third part.

- *Lower end of esophagus*: Due to reflux esophagitis.
- *Meckel's diverticulum*: Due to presence of heterotopic gastric mucosa.
- Stoma of gastrojejunostomy toward the jejunum.

Q. Which factors are responsible for development of chronic gastric ulcer?

Ans. A number of factors are responsible for development of gastric ulcer:
- Diminished mucosal resistance due to some nutritional deficiencies predisposes the mucosa to acid peptic digestion and formation of ulcer.
- Nonsteroidal anti-inflammatory drugs and smoking are important etiological factors for development of peptic ulceration.
- *Antral stasis*: Antral stasis results in hyperchlorhydria due to increased gastrin release and is one of the factors for development of peptic ulceration.
- *Bile reflux*: Reflux of bile through the pylorus results in bile reflux gastritis, which predisposes to formation of gastric ulcer.
- *Helicobacter pylori infection*: One of the important etiological factors for development of peptic ulcers.

Q. How does *Helicobacter pylori* cause peptic ulcer?

Ans.
- *Helicobacter pylori* may colonize the gastric epithelium.
- *Helicobacter pylori* releases some cytotoxins, which induce gastritis and subsequent breakdown of surface epithelium resulting in ulceration.
- *Helicobacter pylori* also incites an inflammatory reaction resulting in accumulation of acute and chronic inflammatory cells in the gastric epithelium.
- *Helicobacter pylori* hydrolyzes urea and liberates ammonia, which is a strong alkali. This causes increased secretion of gastrin, which leads to hyperchlorhydria. This is one of the predisposing factors for development of duodenal ulcer.

Q. Does *Helicobacter pylori* normally colonize duodenum?

Ans.
- Normally *Helicobacter pylori* does not colonize duodenum.
- *Helicobacter pylori* colonization of stomach causes hyperacidity due to hypersecretion of gastric juice due to excessive gastrin release. The excess acid in the duodenum causes gastric metaplasia of duodenal epithelium.
- *Helicobacter pylori* can colonize gastric metaplasia duodenal epithelium and causes series of changes resulting in duodenal ulceration.

Q. Which part of the stomach is affected by chronic peptic ulcer?

Ans.
- About 95% of peptic ulcers in stomach are situated along the lesser curvature.
- In the pyloric region, 5 cm from the pylorus.
- The greater curvature, fundus, and cardia are rarely affected.

Q. What are the histopathological characteristics of a benign peptic ulcer?

Ans.
- There is destruction of the epithelial lining.

- At the margins, there is proliferation and downgrowth of the epithelial lining.
- There is variable destruction of muscular coat.
- The base of the ulcer is covered with granulation tissue.
- There is infiltration of both neutrophils and chronic inflammatory cells.
- The arteries show endarteritis obliterans changes.
- There is a zone of fibrous tissue at the base of the ulcer.
- The termination of the nerves may be seen in the fibrous tissue.

Q. Why benign ulcers are more common in the lesser curvature?

Ans. The lesser curvature and the adjacent part of the stomach constitute the principal food route or "magenstrasse" along which passes the bulk of the food entering the stomach. This area is subject to wear and tear, which explains increased incidence of ulcer in this site.

Q. What is the risk of malignant change in chronic peptic ulcer?

Ans. Chronic duodenal ulcer never turns malignant. Although extremely rare, a chronic gastric ulcer may turn malignant. Histologically, the appearance will be like a benign gastric ulcer with focal areas of malignant transformation. The incidence of such a malignant change has been quoted as 0.1%.

Q. What is ulcer cancer?

Ans. Patient is identified as having an ulcer in the stomach either endoscopically or radiologically, which on biopsy reveals malignancy.

Q. What do you mean by basal acid output (BAO) and how BAO is estimated?

Ans.
- BAO is defined as amount of acid secreted by the stomach in 1 hour under basal condition without any stimulation.
- Patient is kept fasting overnight for 12 hours. A Ryles tube is inserted in the morning and 12 hours night secretion of acid is aspirated and discarded.
- Next, gastric juice is collected by aspiration of Ryles tube every 15 minutes for 1 hour and the total acid in this 1 hour juice is estimated. This is BAO. Normal BAO is 5 mmol/L.

Q. What is peak acid output (PAO) and how will you estimate it?

Ans.
- This is the amount of acid secreted by stomach over 1 hour after maximal simulation.
- *Patient is kept fasting overnight*: Ryles tube is inserted at 8 AM, gastric juice is aspirated and the overnight secretion is discarded.
- Gastric juice is then collected every 15 minutes for 1 hour to estimate BAO.
- Injection pentagastrin (6 mg/kg of bodyweight) is injected and gastric juice is collected for every 15 minutes for next 1 hour.
- The mean acid secretion in two higher aliquot is calculated and amount of acid secreted in 1 hour is calculated, which gives PAO. Normal PAO is about 27 mmol/L.

Q. What do you mean by achlorhydria?

Ans. It can be defined as—when stomach cannot produce a juice with pH less than 7 even after maximal stimulation. Achlorhydria is found in 18% of patients with carcinoma of stomach.

Q. What happens in Zollinger–Ellison syndrome (ZES) with regard to secretory studies?

Ans.
* In ZES, there is hypergastrinemia and the parietal cells are maximally stimulated under basal condition.
* The BAO is more than 60 mmol/L.
* On further stimulation by injecting pentagastrin, there is no further rise of acid over the BAO level.

Q. What is the role of insulin test?

Ans. Insulin test was done earlier to assess completeness of vagotomy.

Q. Why insulin test is not done nowadays?

Ans. Insulin may cause fatal hypoglycemia. So, insulin test is replaced by chew-and-spit test.

Q. What is chew-and-spit test?

Ans.
* A Ryles tube is passed in empty stomach and the overnight juice is aspirated and discarded.
* Gastric juice collected for next 1 hour to calculate BAO.
* *Patient takes the food in the mouth*: Chew it and instead of swallowing spit it off.
* Gastric juice is collected for next 2 hours every 15 minutes and the mean acid level in each hour is calculated.
* *Early response*: If the test is positive in 1st hour.
* *Delayed response*: If the test is positive in 2nd hour.

Q. When do you call the test is positive?

Ans.
* *If basal sample was anacid*: A rise of 10 mmol/L is taken as positive.
* *If basal sample contains some acid*: A rise of 20 mmol/L is taken as positive.

Q. If the response is positive—what does it mean?

Ans.
* An early positive response suggests incomplete vagotomy. May be corrected by completion of vagotomy.
* Delayed positive response is usually due to antral gastrin release and may be corrected by antrectomy.

Q. How does patient with chronic gastric ulcer present?

Ans. *See* Surgical Long Cases, Page No. 131–133, Chapter 3.

Q. Why biopsy is required before initiating treatment of gastric ulcers?

Ans. Multiple biopsies (about 10) are required to exclude any malignancy. Modern antisecretory drugs may allow healing even of a malignant ulcer, but does not cure the malignancy. Hence, biopsy may be required even if the ulcer has healed if the symptoms persist.

Q. Medical management of chronic gastric ulcer

Ans. *See* Surgical Long Cases, Page No. 127–132, Chapter 3.

Q. Surgical management of chronic gastric ulcer.

Ans. *See* Surgical Long Cases, Page No. 127–132, Chapter 3.

■ PERFORATED BENIGN GASTRIC ULCER (FIG. 18.2)

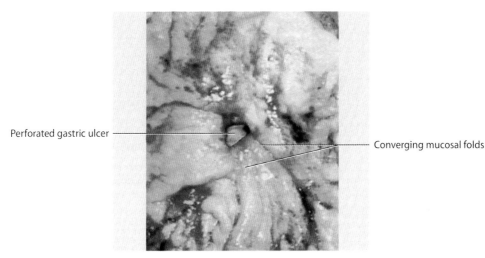

Perforated gastric ulcer

Converging mucosal folds

Fig. 18.2: This is a specimen of stomach cut open along the greater curvature showing an ulcer near the lesser curvature. The ulcer has penetrated the full thickness of stomach wall. There are converging mucosal folds toward the base of the ulcer. So, this is a case of perforated benign gastric ulcer

Q. Why do you say this is a benign ulcer?

Ans. *See* X-rays Section, Page No. 823, Chapter 17.

Q. What are the complications of peptic ulcer?

Ans.
- *Acute complications*: Perforation and hemorrhage.
- *Subacute complication*: Residual abscess.
- *Chronic complications*:
  - *Stenosis*: Pyloric stenosis/hour glass stomach.
  - Penetration into the pancreas or liver.
  - *Malignant change*: Rarely occurs in chronic gastric ulcer, but not in chronic duodenal ulcer.

Q. What are the pathological changes following perforation of a chronic peptic ulcer?

Ans. There are three stages in development of peritonitis following peptic perforation:
1. Stage of chemical peritonitis
2. Stage of peritoneal reaction or stage of illusion
3. Stage of bacterial peritonitis or stage of abdominal distension.

Q. Presentation, investigations, and management of peptic perforation.

Ans. *See* X-ray Section, Page No. 778, 779, Chapter 17.

■ CARCINOMA OF STOMACH (FIGS 18.3A TO G)

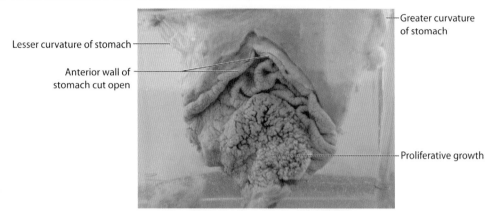

Lesser curvature of stomach

Anterior wall of
stomach cut open

Greater curvature
of stomach

Proliferative growth

Fig. 18.3A: This is a specimen of distal part of the stomach. One wall is cut open showing a proliferative growth in the pyloric region (the serosal side should be seen to look for any extension of the growth toward the serosal surface of the stomach). So, this is a specimen of proliferative type of carcinoma of stomach involving the pyloric region of stomach

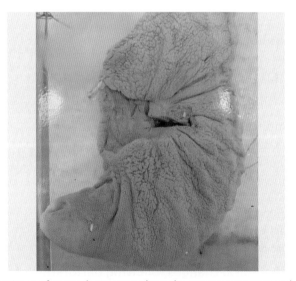

Fig. 18.3B: This is a specimen of stomach cut open along the greater curvature and showing an ulcerative lesion at the body of the stomach along the lesser curvature. The margin of the ulcer is rolled out and everted. There is flattening of the mucosal folds around the ulcer. So, this is a specimen of ulcerative type of carcinoma of stomach involving the body of the stomach

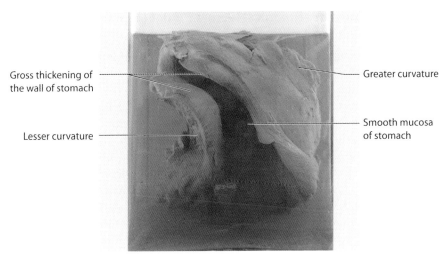

Fig. 18.3C: This is a specimen of stomach from which part of the anterior wall of the stomach is cut off. There is diffuse thickening of the whole of stomach. The capacity of the stomach is reduced to a great extent. The whole of the mucosal aspect appears smooth due to flattening of the mucosal fold. This appearance is suggestive of generalized linitis plastica of the stomach

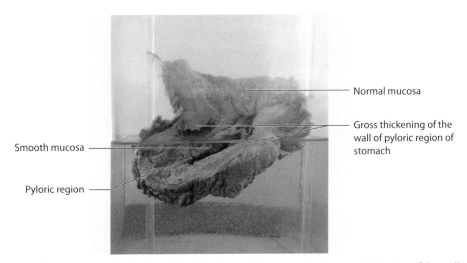

Fig. 18.3D: This is a specimen of a slice of the distal part of the stomach showing thickening of the wall of the stomach. There are white strands traversing the wall of the stomach. The mucosal aspect of the pyloric region appears smooth. The normal mucous membrane is seen more proximally. This appearance is suggestive of localized type of linitis plastica involving the pyloric region of the stomach

Q. What are the important etiological factors for development of carcinoma of stomach?

Ans. There are various factors causing gastric cancers. The important factors are:
* *Dietary factors*:
    - Gastritis due to ingestion of spirits is a predisposing factor.
    - Excessive salt intake and smoked food containing excessive amounts of nitrates are important etiological factors for development of carcinoma of stomach. Nitrates are converted into nitrites and N-nitrosamines, which are potent carcinogens.
    - Diet high in raw vegetables, vitamin C, and antioxidants may be protective.
* *Helicobacter pylori infection*: *Helicobacter pylori* causes gastritis, gastric atrophy, and intestinal metaplasia. These changes predispose to development of carcinoma of stomach. This mainly involves the body and distal stomach rather than the proximal part.
* *Following peptic ulcer surgery*: Patient who underwent partial gastrectomy, gastrojejunostomy, or pyloroplasty has increased risk of developing gastric cancer. Bile reflux gastritis following peptic ulcer surgery has been incriminated as the important factor.
* Pernicious anemia and atrophic gastritis are important predisposing factors.
* Cigarette smoking and alcohol are important factors.
* Gastric polyps are also rarely precursor of gastric cancer.
* *Ulcer cancer*: Rarely, benign gastric ulcer may undergo malignant change. The incidence is 0.1%.
* Genetic factors:
    - Mutations of HRas (also known as transforming protein p21) oncogene and overexpression of c-erb B_2 gene are incriminated in genesis of gastric cancers.
    - The adenomatous polyposis coli (APC) gene responsible for familial polyposis coli has also been incriminated in about 25% patients of cancer of stomach.
    - p53 is a tumor suppressor gene, but its role in gastric cancer is not clear.
    - Abnormalities in p53 tumor suppressor gene has been found in patients with intestinal metaplasia and in patients with advanced gastric cancers.
    - Hereditary nonpolyposis colorectal cancer (HNPCC) is associated with a genetic abnormality, which involves deficiency of a mismatch repair genes. There is increased incidence of gastric cancers in families of these patients.

Q. What is the relative site distribution of carcinoma of stomach?

Ans.
* Pyloric region—47%
* Body—23%
* Cardia—21%
* Fundus—2%
* Linitis plastica—7%.

Q. What is Lauren's classification for gastric cancer?

Ans. Two main types are described:

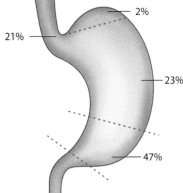

Fig. 18.3E: Distribution of carcinoma of stomach

1. *Type I: Intestinal type gastric cancer*—arises in site of intestinal metaplasia. Forms polypoid tumor or ulcer.
2. *Type II: Diffuse gastric cancer*—infiltrates deeply in stomach wall without producing obvious mass lesion.

Q. What are the macroscopic types of carcinoma of stomach?

Ans. There are four principal varieties of gastric cancer:
1. *Proliferative type*: This is a bulky cauliflower type of growth projecting into the lumen of the stomach.
2. *Ulcerative type*: This is the most common type of carcinoma of stomach. It arises most commonly in the pyloric antrum region toward the lesser curvature side. The ulcer has rolled out everted edges with surrounding induration.
3. *The colloid or mucoid type*: This is a rare variety and appears as a massive tumor of gelatinous appearance. Histologically, the cancer cells line the accumulation of colloid. The cells lining the tubular gland may also get distended with mucinous material.
4. *Linitis plastica*: This is also a rare variety of tumor. The tumor cells infiltrate the submucosa and subserosa and the muscle coat extensively without protruding into the lumen of the stomach. There is proliferation of fibrous tissue in the submucosa giving mother of pearl appearance. This may either be generalized or localized.
   – In generalized variety, the whole stomach is contracted and rigid. The mucosa may appear normal or there may be small superficial ulceration (Fig. 18.3C).
   – In localized variety, it usually involves the pyloric region of the stomach (Fig. 18.3D).

Q. What do you mean by early gastric cancer?

Ans. Gastric cancer confined to mucosa and submucosa irrespective of lymph node status (T1 Any N) is considered as early gastric cancer.
* However, when lymph nodes are involved with T1, it is then designated as early simulating advanced gastric cancer as prognosis is worse, once the lymph nodes are involved.

Q. What is Japanese classification for early gastric cancer?

Ans.
* *Type I*: Protruded (Fig. 18.3F)
* *Type II*: Superficial:
   – Elevated
   – Flat
   – Depressed
* *Type III*: Excavated.

Q. What is Bormann's classification for advanced gastric cancer?

Ans. Advanced gastric cancer extends beyond the submucous coat and involves the muscularis propria. Depending on the extent of involvement, advanced cancer is classified as type I to type IV (Fig. 18.3G).

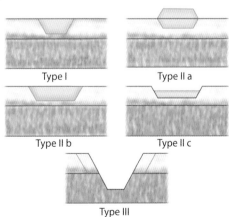

Fig. 18.3F: Japanese classification of "early gastric cancer"

Q. What are the histological types of carcinoma of stomach?

Ans.

- *Adenocarcinoma:* This is the most common type of carcinoma of stomach. The cells are either columnar or cuboidal. Mucinous or colloid degeneration may occur. There are two types of adenocarcinoma:
    1. *The intestinal type:* It is usually well differentiated, consisting of papillary, tubular, or glandular variants.
    2. *The diffuse type:* There is lack of organized gland formation and is usually poorly differentiated.
- *Squamous cell carcinoma:* This is common near the cardiac end and is usually an involvement from the lower end of esophagus.
- *Adenoacanthoma:* Mixed adenocarcinoma and squamous cell carcinoma.
- *Carcinoid tumor.*

Q. What are the prognostic factors in carcinoma of stomach?

Ans. The important prognostic factors are:
- *Tumor:* Depth of invasion.
- *Metastasis:* Metastasis to the lymph nodes or distant metastasis.
- Histological type and grading of tumor.

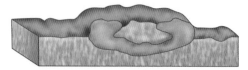

Type I

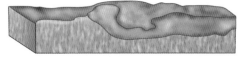

Type II

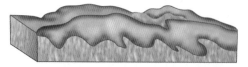

Type III

Type IV

Fig. 18.3G: Bormann's classification of "advanced gastric cancer"

Q. How does carcinoma of stomach spread?

Ans. Carcinoma of stomach spreads in different ways:
- *Direct spread:* Spread by continuity from mucosa to serosa. Involves adjacent part of stomach or extraserosal spread to adjacent structures—colon, pancreas and liver, esophagus, mesocolon, and rarely duodenum.
- *Lymphatic spread:* Occurs by permeation and embolization.
    - The first tier of lymph nodes involved is the perigastric nodes lying within 3 cm of the primary growth (lymph nodes station 1–6).
    - The next tier of lymph nodes is the nodes around the main and intermediate arterial trunk (lymph node stations 7–11).
    - The next tier of regional lymph node is lymph node station 12–18.
    - The lymphatic spread may occur to the left Virchow's gland in the neck via the thoracic duct.
    - Lymphatic spread may occur along the lymphatics in the falciform ligament leading to formation of subcutaneous nodule around the umbilicus.

- *Blood-borne spread*: Liver, lungs, and brain.
- *Transperitoneal spread*: Tumor cells may exfoliate and drop in the peritoneal cavity and may lodge on the surface of the ovary giving rise to Krukenberg's tumor. However, Krukenberg's tumor has now said to be due to retrograde lymphatic spread rather than transperitoneal spread.
- *Transluminal spread* may occur.
- *Transplantation*: During surgery, cancer cells may dislodge and implant at the sites of abdominal incisions.

Q. What is tumor, node, and metastasis (TNM) definition for carcinoma of stomach?

Ans. *See* Surgical Long Cases, Page No. 111–112, Chapter 3.

Q. What is the most important histological marker for development of gastric cancer?

Ans. Dysplasia is an important marker for development of gastric cancer. Dysplasia may be mild, moderate, or severe. Severe dysplasia is regarded as carcinoma in situ.

Q. How nitrates are related to development of gastric cancer?

Ans. Nitrates are converted into N-nitroso compounds in the stomach, which have been proved to be carcinogenic in animals. Reduction of nitrates to nitrite and combination of nitrite with amines to form nitrosamines are influenced by bacteria *Escherichia coli*.

Q. What are the different types of intestinal metaplasia?

Ans. There are three different types of intestinal metaplasia:
1. *Type I*:
   - Mature absorptive and goblet cells.
   - Goblet cells secrete sialomucin.
2. *Type II*: Absorptive cells in various stages of dedifferentiation.
3. *Type III*: Cell dedifferentiation is more marked.
   - Secrete predominantly sulfomucin.
   - Goblet cells secrete both sialomucin and sulfomucin.

Q. What are the common tumor markers in gastric cancers?

Ans. CEA, CA 19-9, CA 50, CA 12-5, and CA 72-4 are the important tumor markers to evaluate recurrence and prognosis. Most important is CA 72-4, which disappears with surgery and reappears with regional or distant recurrence.

■ ACUTE APPENDICITIS (FIGS 18.4A AND B)

Q. Why do you say, this is a specimen of appendix?

Ans. This is a cul–de–sac-like structure covered by a serous coat with a mesentery attached to one side. So, this is a specimen of appendix.

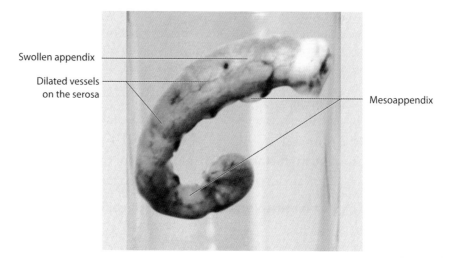

Swollen appendix

Dilated vessels on the serosa

Mesoappendix

Fig. 18.4A: This is a specimen of appendix, which is swollen. The serosal aspect of the appendix shows dilated vessels and there are fibrinous flakes over the serosal surface of the appendix. So, this is a specimen of acute appendicitis

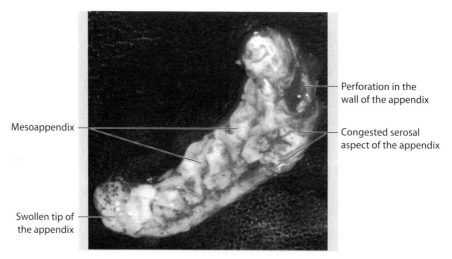

Perforation in the wall of the appendix

Mesoappendix

Congested serosal aspect of the appendix

Swollen tip of the appendix

Fig. 18.4B: This is a specimen of appendix, which is swollen, and there is congestion in the appendicular wall as well as in the mesoappendix. There is a perforation in the wall near the base of the appendix. So, this is a specimen of acute gangrenous appendicitis with perforation

Q. Why appendix is called abdominal tonsil?

Ans. Appendix is also called abdominal tonsil because of presence of abundant amount of lymphoid tissue.

Q. What are the important etiological factors for development of acute appendicitis?

Ans.

* *Bacterial infection*: Proliferation of mixed flora of aerobic, anaerobic, and *Bacteroides* causes appendicitis. The initiating event for this bacterial proliferation is not exactly known.

  The most common organism is *Escherichia coli*. Other organisms include *Enterococci*, *Bacteroides*, anaerobic *Streptococci*, and *Clostridia*.
* *Obstruction of the lumen of appendix*: This is usually held to be responsible for initiation of acute appendicitis. Obstruction of the appendix may be caused by:
  - Fecolith
  - Worms (*Oxyuris vermicularis*)
  - Foreign body
  - Fibrotic stricture in the wall of the appendix
  - *Tumor*: Carcinoma of cecum may obstruct the lumen of the appendix
  - Adhesion and kinks.
* *Dietary factors*: Low residue, high-protein diet is associated with increased incidence of acute appendicitis. This has been related to constipation because of such diet. The fecoliths may enter the appendix lumen and initiate an attack of appendicitis.
* *Familial*: There are some familial predispositions to the development of acute appendicitis. In most such cases, the location of the appendix is retrocecal.

Q. What are the pathological changes in acute appendicitis?

Ans.

* With bacterial proliferation, there is mucosal inflammation and lymphoid hyperplasia.
* Infection confined to the mucous membrane is called catarrhal appendicitis.
* Because of mucosal inflammation or other causes, the lumen of the appendix may become obstructed.
* Once there is obstruction of the lumen, there is accumulation of secretion within the lumen of the appendix.
* This causes obstruction of the lymphatic channel and causes edema and ulceration of the mucous membrane.
* Further progression will cause venous obstruction and ischemia of the appendix wall.
* This will cause translocation of bacteria through the wall.
* Thrombosis of the appendicular vessel will result in gangrenous appendicitis and free bacterial contamination of the peritoneal cavity.
* There may be perforation of the appendix at the tip or at the site of obstruction leading to formation of a localized appendicular abscess or generalized peritonitis.

Q. What are the microscopic features of acute appendicitis?

Ans.

* There may be necrosis and denudation of the mucous membrane at places.
* There is hyperplasia of lymphoid follicles.
* All the coats are congested and edematous.
* There is infiltration of acute inflammatory cells in all the coats.

Q. What are the sequelae of acute appendicitis?

Ans.

- *Resolution*: The inflammation may subside and resolution occurs with some scarring of appendix.
- *Appendicular lump*: Within 48–72 hours of inflammation, body tries to localize the inflammation. The greater omentum, terminal ileum, cecum, and appendix form a mass to localize the infection. This is called the appendicular lump.
- *Appendicular abscess*: Formation of pus within an appendicular lump, or localized collection of pus following perforation of appendix leads to formation of appendicular abscess.
- *Gangrenous appendicitis*: As the inflammation progresses, there may be thrombosis of vessels in the mesoappendix resulting in gangrenous change in the appendix.
- *Perforation*: Continuation of infection may result in perforation of the appendix. The most common site of perforation is the tip of appendix because of meager blood supply. The perforation may occur at the base or at the site of obstruction of the lumen of the appendix due to pressure necrosis.
- *Free perforation of the appendix into the peritoneal* cavity may result in generalized peritonitis.
- *Portal pyemia*
- *Septicemia*
- *Mucocele of appendix.*

Q. What are the risk factors for perforation of acute appendicitis?

Ans.

- Extremes of age
- Fecolith obstruction
- Pelvic appendix
- Diabetes mellitus
- Administration of purgative
- Immunosuppressed patients—chronic renal failure, steroid therapy.

Q. What is mucocele of appendix?

Ans. Mucocele of appendix is a condition where appendix is swollen with mucoid secretion due to occlusion of its lumen proximally.

The mucocele may rupture and the epithelial cells may be implanted on the peritoneal surface with formation of large mucoid mass. This condition is known as pseudomyxoma peritonei.

Q. What is the usual presentation of patient with acute appendicitis?

Ans. *See* Surgical Problems Section, Page No. 730, 731, Chapter 16.

Q. What investigation will you suggest for diagnosis?

Ans. *See* Surgical Problems Section, Page No. 730, 731, Chapter 16.

Q. Treatment of acute appendicitis.

Ans. *See* Surgical Problems Section, Page No. 730, 731, Chapter 16.

■ SMALL CUT STRICTURE (FIG. 18.5)

Q. What are the important causes of small gut stricture?

Ans.
- Tuberculosis
- Crohn's disease
- Actinomycosis
- Primary carcinoma
- Lymphomas
- Carcinoid tumors
- Radiation enteritis
- Ischemic damage
- Intramural hemorrhage
- Anastomotic stricture following surgery.

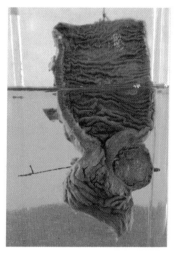

Fig. 18.5: This is a specimen of a segment of small intestine, and showing an area of circumferential narrowing due to fibrosis and gross thickening of the wall. The loop of the gut lying proximal to the stricture site is dilated. There is an enlarged lymph node toward the mesenteric side of the intestine. So, this is a specimen of small gut stricture probably due to tuberculosis

Q. What are the routes of infection in intestinal tuberculosis?

Ans.
- Ingestion of *Mycobacterium* with food or milk contaminated with bovine tubercle bacilli.
- Ingestion of *Mycobacterium* while swallowing sputum containing the bacilli.
- Hematogenous spread from a primary focus elsewhere in the body.

Q. What is the pathogenesis of tubercular stricture?

Ans.
- The tubercle bacilli lodge into the tubular glands of the intestinal mucosa and there is formation of inflammatory exudates.
- The bacilli are carried by the phagocytic cells into the submucous layer, wherein it forms tubercles, characterized by central area of caseation surrounded by lymphocytes, epithelioid cells, and Langhans type of giant cells.
- The adjacent tubercles coalesce and the inflammatory exudates over the mucosa breakdown result in mucosal ulceration. The serosa overlying the ulcer is thickened and congested and shows tubercles.
- These tubercular ulcers are placed circumferentially and with healing of these ulcers, there is fibrosis, which results in formation of stricture. These strictures may be single or multiple.

Q. What is tabes mesenterica?

Ans. The bacilli from the tubercular lesion are carried via the lymphatics to the mesenteric lymph nodes. A caseating granuloma is formed in the mesenteric lymph nodes. These enlarged lymph nodes in the mesentery are known as tabes mesenterica.

Q. What are the features of a tubercular ulcer?

Ans. The tubercular ulcers are placed circumferentially along the gut. The ulcers are shallow with undermined edges. The floor is covered with caseous material. There may be tubercles on the serosal aspect of the gut.

Q. What is hyperplastic tuberculosis?

Ans.

* This usually occurs in the ileocecal region. The disease starts in the cecum and may involve the ascending colon and the terminal ileum.
* This occurs due to ingestion of *Mycobacterium tuberculosis* in patients with high resistance to the organism.
* The organism lodges in the lymphoid follicles and excites a chronic inflammatory reaction.
* This chronic inflammation causes thickening of the intestinal wall resulting in narrowing of the lumen.
* Fibrosis is the outstanding pathological feature and caseation may occur rarely.
* The organism may spread to the mesenteric lymph nodes, wherein it forms a caseating granuloma.

Q. How do patients with intestinal tuberculosis usually present?

Ans.

* *General symptoms due to tuberculosis*: Anorexia, weight loss, irregular fever, and generalized weakness
* *Subacute intestinal obstruction*: Colicky abdominal pain, borborygmi, and abdominal distension after meals
* *Acute intestinal obstruction*: Pain abdomen, vomiting, abdominal distension, and absolute constipation
* *Steatorrhea* due to stasis and bacterial overgrowth
* *Palpable mass* in right iliac fossa.

Q. How will you confirm your diagnosis?

Ans.

* Chest X-ray to exclude associated pulmonary tuberculosis.
* Small bowel enema for diagnosis of stricture in the gut.
* Plain X-ray abdomen when patient presents with acute intestinal obstruction—multiple air fluid level.
* *Palpable lump in abdomen*: Ultrasonography (USG) or computed tomography (CT)-guided fine-needle aspiration cytology (FNAC).
* Immunological tests for tuberculosis.

Q. How will you treat abdominal tuberculosis?

Ans.

* *Patient presenting with intestinal obstruction*: Resuscitation followed by exploratory laparotomy.
* Stricture segment is managed either by stricturoplasty or by resection anastomosis. Patient needs full course of antitubercular chemotherapy.

♦ *Patient not having intestinal obstruction*: Antitubercular chemotherapy may cure the condition.

Q. Questions about Crohn's disease.

Ans. *See* X-rays Section, Page No. 831–833, Chapter 17.

◼ INTUSSUSCEPTION (FIGS 18.6A TO C)

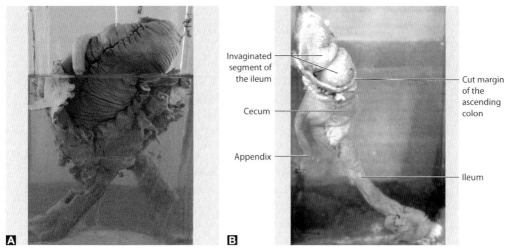

Figs 18.6A and B: This is a specimen of a part of the ileum, cecum, appendix, and ascending colon. The cecum and the ascending colon is cut open showing invagination of a portion of the ileum into the cecum and ascending colon. So, this is a specimen of ileocecocolic intussusception

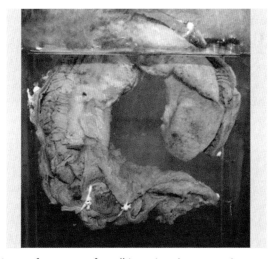

Fig. 18.6C: This is a specimen of segment of small intestine. A segment is cut open showing invagination of a segment of small intestine into the adjacent distal segment. The invaginated segment shows patchy gangrenous change. So, this is specimen of ileoileal intussusception with strangulation of the invaginated segment of the gut

Q. What is intussusception?

Ans. Intussusception is defined as invagination of one segment of gut into another immediately adjacent segment, usually proximal into the distal.

Q. What are the parts of intussusception?

Ans. The mass of intussusception consists of:
- The inner or entering tube
- The middle or the returning tube.
- The inner or entering tube and the middle or the returning tube together are called the intussusceptum.
- The outer tube or the sheath is known as intussuscipiens.
- The apex of the intussusception is the most distal advancing part of the intussusception where the entering and the returning layer become continuous.
- The neck of the intussusception is the junction of the entering layer and the outer sheath.
- As the intussusception progresses, the apex proceeds distally and the neck goes proximally.

Q. What are the etiological factors for development of intussusception?

Ans.
- About 75–95% incidence of intussusception in infants are idiopathic where no obvious cause is discernible.
- In older children and adults, intussusception may be secondary to:
  - *Benign tumors in the gut*—polyp, adenomas, leiomyoma, and submucous lipoma
  - *Malignant tumors*—carcinoma and leiomyosarcoma
  - Meckel's diverticulum
  - Intestinal tuberculosis
  - Henoch–Schonlein purpura.

Q. What is the pathogenesis of idiopathic intussusception in infants?

Ans.
- During weaning, there is alteration of bacterial flora in the intestine. This causes hyperplasia of Peyer's patches. This hyperplasia may also occur secondary to respiratory tract infection and is the initiating event for intussusception.
- The Peyer's patches project into the lumen of the intestine and with peristaltic movement, these may invaginate into the distal segment of the gut.
- The starting point of the intussusception becomes congested and swollen and constitutes a partial obstruction. In order to overcome this obstruction, continued peristaltic movement causes further progress of this invagination.
- Due to constriction at the neck of the intussusception, there is impairment of venous return and this causes congestion and further swelling. Blood exudes into the lumen of the gut.
- Subsequently, there is impairment of arterial supply and gangrenous change may set in, particularly in the inner layer.
- Sloughing and spontaneous resolution may occur rarely. The vitality of the outer tube is seldom impaired.

♦ If diagnosed late, the intussusception may progress and the apex of the intussusception may protrude through the anus.

Q. How does patient with intussusception usually present?

Ans. In idiopathic intussusception in infants, the presentation may be:
♦ Otherwise fit infants between 6 months and 9 months of age develop sudden onset of pain abdomen. The infant screams and draws up legs. The attack lasting for a few minutes recurs every 15 minutes and then becomes progressively severe.
♦ There may be facial pallor during pain.
♦ Vomiting may be absent at the onset, but later vomiting becomes predominant.
♦ At the onset, stool may be normal, but later there is passage of blood mixed with stool (red currant jelly).
♦ Abdominal examination may reveal a sausage-shaped mass with a concavity toward the umbilicus. The right iliac fossa may feel empty (the sign de Dance).
♦ On rectal examination, the finger may be smeared with red currant jelly. In advanced cases, the apex of the intussusception may be palpable in the rectum or it may protrude out of the anus.
♦ Later on, strangulation and perforation of the gut may occur. The abdomen may become distended and there may be tenderness all over abdomen with rebound tenderness.

Q. What investigations may help in diagnosis of intussusception?

Ans.
♦ Plain X-ray abdomen may show multiple air fluid levels. There may be no gas shadow in right iliac fossa in ileocolic intussusception.
♦ Barium enema study may be both diagnostic and therapeutic. It is helpful in diagnosis of ileocolic or colocolic intussusception. The contrast passes up to the apex of the intussusception and then goes around the middle layer giving a typical "claw sign".
♦ CT scan abdomen.

Q. How will you treat patient presenting with intussusception?

Ans.
♦ If there is no clinical evidence of strangulation, history is less than 48 hours.
  – Hydrostatic reduction with barium enema may be tried. Barium is inserted by gravity.
  – The barium column may cause gradual reduction of intussusception. Complete reduction is confirmed by passage of the barium into the terminal ileum.
♦ Operative reduction is indicated, if hydrostatic reduction has failed, or if there is evidence of underlying strangulation or perforation.
♦ Approach is by a transverse incision in infants and a midline incision in adult.
   Reduction is achieved by squeezing the most distal part of the mass toward the proximal part of the gut. The mass should not be pulled. Last part of the reduction is difficult and is achieved by squeezing the apex.
   If the mass of intussusceptions is gangrenous, resection and anastomosis are to be done.

Q. What is Cope's technique for reduction?

Ans. Sometime, there is adhesion near the neck of the intussusceptions. In difficult case, a finger may be gently inserted into the neck of the intussusceptions and adhesion may be separated. Subsequently, the mass is squeezed from the apex.

■ MECKEL'S DIVERTICULUM (FIG. 18.7)

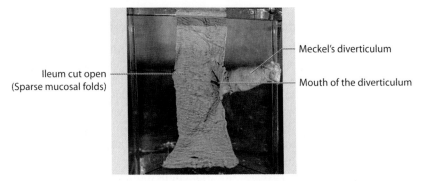

Ileum cut open
(Sparse mucosal folds)

Meckel's diverticulum

Mouth of the diverticulum

Fig. 18.7: This is a specimen of a segment of ileum cut open showing a diverticulum arising from it. The opening of the diverticulum is wide mouthed. So, this is a specimen of Meckel's diverticulum with a segment of ileum

Q. What is Meckel's diverticulum?

Ans. This is a congenital diverticulum arising from the terminal ileum and represents the proximal unobliterated portion of the vitellointestinal duct.

Q. What is the difference between a congenital (true) and acquired (false) diverticula of the intestine?

Ans. In congenital (true) diverticula, all the coats of the intestine from where they arise are present and have their own blood supply.

In acquired (false) diverticula, all the coats of the intestine are not present.

Q. What are the characteristics of Meckel's diverticulum?

Ans.
- Present in 2% of population.
- Situated in the terminal ileum in the antimesenteric border about 2 feet from the ileocecal valve.
- It is about 2 inches long.
- It has an independent blood supply, which arises from a terminal branch of superior mesenteric artery.
- The base is usually wide mouthed.

Q. What is the peculiarity of mucous membrane of Meckel's diverticulum?

Ans. The lining epithelium of Meckel's diverticulum is same as that of ileum in majority of cases. The diverticulum may contain heterotopic gastric, duodenal, colonic, or pancreatic tissue either singly or in combination.

Q. What is vitellointestinal duct (VID)?

Ans. Vitellointestinal duct is the connection between the midgut and the yolk sac of the embryo in early fetal life. During normal development, the vitellointestinal duct is converted to a fibrous cord and then disappears.

Q. What are the different abnormalities of vitellointestinal duct (VID)?

Ans.

- The vitellointestinal duct is obliterated but it persists as a fibrous cord, which connects the terminal ileum to the umbilicus. The band may predispose to volvulus or adhesive small bowel obstruction.
- The vitellointestinal duct may persist as a whole and gives rise to an omphaloenteric fistula (persistent vitellointestinal duct).
- The vitellointestinal duct may persist in its proximal part and the rest disappears. The unobliterated proximal part of the VID forms the Meckel's diverticulum. The distal part may, however, persist as a fibrous cord attaching the Meckel's diverticulum to the umbilicus.
- The VID may persist in its most distal part and the rest disappears. The unobliterated distal part of the VID forms an umbilical sinus.
- The VID may persist in its intermediate part and both proximal and distal parts disappear. The unobliterated intermediate part of the VID forms an enterocystoma.
- The proximal and the distal part may persist as a fibrous cord attaching the enterocystoma to the intestine and the umbilicus.

Q. What may be the associated congenital abnormalities in patients with Meckel's diverticulum?

Ans.

- Exomphalos
- Esophageal atresia
- Anorectal malformations
- Cardiovascular and nervous system anomalies.

Q. How does patient with Meckel's diverticula usually present?

Ans.

- *Asymptomatic*: Majority of cases are diagnosed incidentally during laparotomy for other reasons. Symptoms of Meckel's diverticulum are usually due to some complications.
- *The peptic group*: Due to presence of heterotopic gastric mucosa, chronic peptic ulcer may occur in the Meckel's diverticulum. Patient may present with chronic periumbilical pain, with severe hemorrhage, or symptoms and signs of peritonitis due to perforation of peptic ulcer in the Meckel's diverticulum.
- *The inflammatory group*: Acute inflammatory change may result in diverticulitis, gangrene, or perforation. The symptoms and signs resemble those of acute appendicitis.
- *The obstructive group*: Acute intestinal obstruction may occur due to intussusceptions, volvulus, or adhesion. Patient presents with pain abdomen, vomiting, constipation, and abdominal distension.
- *The umbilical group*: May present with an umbilical fistula or a granuloma.
- *Littre's hernia*: Meckel's diverticulum may be a content of inguinal or femoral hernia.

Q. Which investigations may help in diagnosis of Meckel's diverticulum?

Ans.

- Small bowel enema may delineate the diverticulum with the contrast.
- 99m pertechnetate scan is helpful for diagnosis of Meckel's diverticulum. A hot spot in the left lower abdomen suggests presence of Meckel's diverticulum. The uptake of radioactivity is due to presence of heterotopic gastric mucosa.

Q. How will you treat Meckel's diverticulum?

Ans.

- Symptomatic Meckel's diverticulum needs treatment.
- Meckelian diverticulectomy with a segment of small intestine is the ideal procedure.
- Incidentally discovered Meckel's diverticulum:
  - If Meckel's diverticulum is found during laparotomy for some other condition and provided the diverticulum is wide mouthed and the wall is not thickened, it should not be removed
  - Change of developing complication is only 1–2%. So, routine excision is not recommended.
  - If the wall is thickened and it is narrow mouthed—it should be removed.

Q. Why a segment of an ileum needs to be excised with the Meckel's diverticulum?

Ans. The heterotopic gastric or pancreatic tissue, if present, in the Meckel's diverticulum is found near the base. So, to include the heterotopic mucosa, a wedge of ileum needs to be excised.

◼ POLYPOSIS OF COLON (FIGS 18.8A TO C)

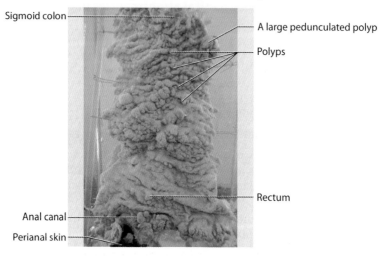

Fig. 18.8A: This is a specimen of anal canal, rectum, and part of the sigmoid colon, and showing a large number of small polyps projecting into the lumen. The intervening mucous membrane between the polyps appears normal. So, this is a specimen of polyposis colon, rectum, and anal canal

Q. What is a polyp?

Ans. Polyp is a tissue growth protruding from the mucous membrane into the lumen of the gastrointestinal (GI) tract.

Q. What are the different types of colonic polyps?

Ans.

- *Benign nonneoplastic polyp*:
  - *Hamartomatous polyp*: Juvenile polyps
  - Cronkhite–Canada syndrome
  - Peutz–Jeghers syndrome

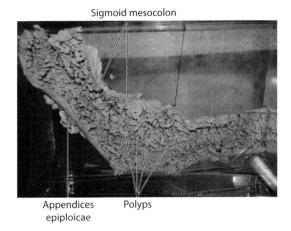

Fig. 18.8B: This is a specimen of colon showing innumerable polypoidal lesion within the lumen of the colon. The intervening mucosa appears normal. The serosal surface of the colon is also normal. So, this is a specimen of polyposis of colon

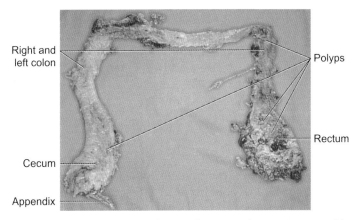

Fig. 18.8C: This is a specimen of whole colon along with rectum showing innumerable polypoidal lesion within the lumen of the colon. The intervening mucosa appears normal. The serosal surface of the colon is also normal. The appendix is also seen. So, this is a specimen of polyposis of colon and rectum

- – Inflammatory polyp
- – Hyperplastic polyp.
- ✦ *Benign neoplastic polyp*:
  - – Adenomatous polyp
  - – Familial adenomatous polyposis
  - – Gardner's syndrome
  - – Turcot's syndrome.

Q. What are the characteristics of familial adenomatous polyposis?

Ans.
- ✦ This is an inherited disorder transmitted by autosomal dominant trait.

* Genetic defect lies in the long arm of chromosome number 5 known as adenomatous polyposis coli (APC) gene.
* There are more than 100 polyps in the colon or any number of polyps in patients with family history of familial adenomatous polyposis.
* It appears in second decade of life but may appear earlier.
* If left untreated, the chance of malignant transformation is 100%.
* The mean age of cancer diagnosis is around 40 years.
* These are adenomatous polyps.

Q. What are the types of adenomatous polyps?

Ans. Adenomatous polyps may be of three types depending on the histological characteristics:
* *Tubular adenoma*: Most common type. Either pedunculated or sessile. Small tumors have smooth surface, while the larger tumors may be lobulated.
* *Villous adenoma*: These are usually sessile and have a velvety surface and there are finger like processes on the surface.
* *Tubulovillous adenoma*: Characteristics in-between the tubular and villous adenoma.

Q. How these patients usually present?

Ans. May present with:
* Bleeding per rectum.
* Lower abdominal pain.
* Mucus discharge.
* Diarrhea.
  Colonoscopy is helpful for evaluation.

Q. How will you screen family members of patients with familial adenomatous polyposis coli?

Ans.
* All family members should be examined at the age of 10 years, clinically, and with colonoscopy. Yearly colonoscopy should be done till the age of 20 years, as most of the patients develop these polyps by the age of 20 years.
  If there are no polyps at the age of 20 years, 5 yearly colonoscopy is to be done till the age of 50 years. If there are no polyps till the age of 50 years then the patient is unlikely to get the polyposis.
* Pigmented spots in the retina (CHIRPES) and tests for *familial adenomatous polyposis (FAP)* gene are also helpful for screening.

Q. How to manage patients of familial adenomatous polyposis coli?

Ans. Surgery is mandatory for these patients, as there is 100% chance of malignant transformation. Options for surgical treatment:
* *Total proctocolectomy with ileostomy*: Remove the whole gut susceptible for the disease. Patient, however, has a permanent ileostomy.
* *Total colectomy with fulguration of rectal polyp and ileorectal anastomosis*: Needs regular follow up, as the rectum is retained.
* *Proctocolectomy with ileoanal anastomosis* with *an ileal pouch reservoir*: Problems of pouchitis and other pouch-related complications will be there.

Q. What is Gardner's syndrome?

Ans.
- Familial APC along with some extracolonic manifestation.
- Osteomas, epidermoid cyst, and congenital hypertrophy of retinal pigment epithelium.
- Polyps of stomach and small intestine.
- Retroperitoneal fibrosis and desmoid tumor.

Q. What is Turcot's syndrome?

Ans. Familial APC with central nervous system tumors—medulloblastoma and glioblastoma. Transmitted by autosomal recessive gene.

Q. What are the characteristics of Peutz–Jeghers syndrome?

Ans.
- Transmitted by autosomal dominant gene.
- Gastrointestinal polyposis with melanin pigmentation of oral mucous membrane or melanin pigmentation in perianal region.
- Polyps may be present in the whole GI tract.
- These are hamartomatous polyps.
- Onset of symptoms is usually around the age of 10–30 years.
- Patient may present with GI bleeding, intestinal obstruction due to intussusceptions.
- May present with extraintestinal cancers involving the pancreas, breast, or ovaries.
- Surgery is usually conservative directed to the polyps-producing symptoms.

Q. What is Cronkhite–Canada syndrome?

Ans.
- Generalized GI polyposis mainly involving the stomach or colon.
- Cutaneous hyperpigmentation, alopecia, and nail dystrophy.
- Mean age of onset is around 60 years and is not linked genetically.

■ CARCINOMA OF COLON (FIGS 18.9A TO D)

Q. What are the macroscopic types of colonic carcinoma?

Ans. There are four macroscopic types of colonic carcinoma (Fig. 18.9C):
- *Type 1*: Annular
- *Type 2*: Tubular
- *Type 3*: Ulcerative
- *Type 4*: Proliferative or cauliflower.

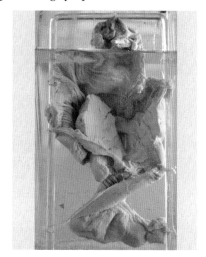

Fig. 18.9A: This is a specimen of cecum, appendix, and a part of the ascending colon. The cecum and the ascending colon is cut open showing an ulceroproliferative growth in the cecum. The serosal surface of the cecum is not invaded by the tumor. So, this is a specimen of carcinoma of cecum—ulceroproliferative type

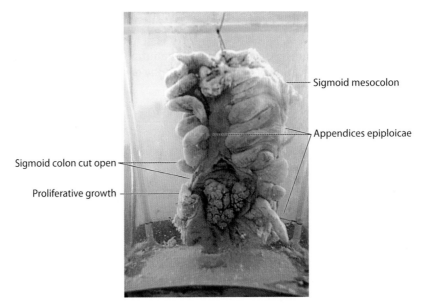

Fig. 18.9B: This is a specimen of sigmoid colon cut open along the antimesenteric border, showing a proliferative growth in the sigmoid colon. The serosal surface of the sigmoid colon is not invaded by the tumor. So, this is a specimen of carcinoma of sigmoid colon—proliferative type

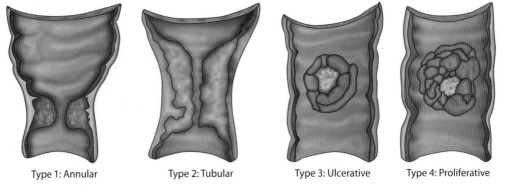

| Type 1: Annular | Type 2: Tubular | Type 3: Ulcerative | Type 4: Proliferative |

Fig. 18.9C: Different macroscopic types of colonic carcinoma

Q. What are the histological characteristics of carcinoma of colon?

Ans. This is an adenocarcinoma arising from the epithelium lining the mucous membrane or the crypts of Lieberkuhn. The histological features vary according to the degree of differentiation of the cells and the amount of fibrous stroma. Generally, the columnar cells are arranged in irregular acini, but sometimes the acinar arrangement is lacking and they lie in solid sheets interspersed with scanty areolar stroma.

The tumor may undergo colloid degeneration. The cells get filled with mucin and give the appearance of signet ring cells. This character is then reproduced in the metastases. The mucin may also be seen in interstitial space.

Q. What are the etiological factors for development of colonic carcinoma?

Ans.

- *Adenomatous polyp*: Sporadic or familial adenomatous polyposis is a premalignant lesion. The adenoma undergoes a series of changes leading to dysplasia and ultimately invasive carcinomas.
- *Genetic factors*:
  - *APC* gene responsible for familial adenomatous polyposis is also implicated in development of colonic carcinoma.
  - Hereditary nonpolyposis colon cancer (HNPCC) or Lynch syndrome is transmitted by HNPCC gene, which is transmitted as an autosomal dominant trait. There are two subtypes of Lynch syndrome:
    1. *Lynch syndrome I*: Early age of onset of carcinoma of colon. More commonly involves the right colon. May be associated with metachronous tumor in about 40% of cases.
    2. *Lynch syndrome II*: Family cancer syndrome. Colonic carcinoma may be associated with carcinoma involving the stomach, breast, endometrium, or ovarian cancer.
- *Dietary factors*: Diet rich in polyunsaturated or saturated fats have higher incidence of colonic carcinoma than diet-containing omega-3 and omega-6 monounsaturated fatty acids. High roughage-containing diet has lesser incidence of colonic carcinoma. This is due to decreased transit time of fecal matter, which allows lesser period of contact of the carcinogens with the gut mucosa.
- *Ulcerative colitis*: Long-standing ulcerative colitis is associated with higher incidence of colonic carcinoma. The risk increases by 1% per year after 10 years. So, the risk is about 10% at 20 years. Dysplasia is one of the markers for carcinomatous change in patients with ulcerative colitis.
- *Crohn's disease*: Long-standing Crohn's disease is also associated with higher incidence of colonic carcinoma.

Q. What is the relative site distribution of colorectal carcinoma?

Ans.

- Right colon—20% (Fig. 18.9D)
- Transverse colon—5%
- Left colon—35%
- Rectum and anal canal—40%.

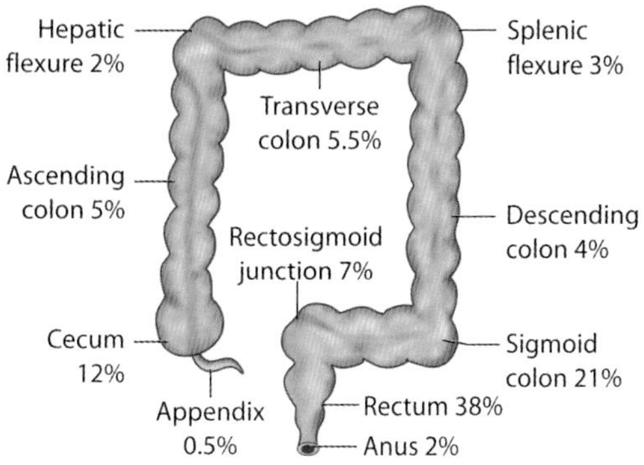

Q. What are the pathological effects of carcinoma of colon?

Ans.

Fig. 18.9D: Relative distribution of colorectal carcinoma

- The growth involving the right colon is usually of proliferative type. The tumor does not encircle the bowel and as the content of the right colon is usually liquid, obstruction does not supervene in right colonic growth until late.

  The only effects for long periods are anemia and cachexia aggravated by infection. The irritation from the tumor and the adjacent inflamed mucous membrane may lead to diarrhea with abundant mucus in stool.
- In left colon, the growth is usually stenosing type. In distal colon, as the lumen is of small caliber and the fecal content is solid, increasing constipation and gradual abdominal distension is common. Complete obstruction may be due to stenosis of the bowel or may be precipitated by impaction of fecal matter in the narrowed part. Obstruction may also occur due to intussusception.

- In progressive obstruction, the gut proximal to the growth becomes dilated. If the ileocecal valve is competent, maximal dilatation occurs in the cecum, which is distended by fluid fecal matter and gas. Cecal perforation may occur due to huge distension. Perforation of the cecum is especially likely to occur when the abdomen is opened and the colon is deprived of the support of the abdominal wall. Longitudinal splits may occur along the *Taenia coli*.
- Ulceration close to the site of cancer may cause infection of the retrocolic areolar tissues and may lead to intraperitoneal or extraperitoneal abscess.

Q. How does the carcinoma of colon spread?

Ans. There are various ways of spread of carcinoma of colon:
- *Direct spread*: Circumferential spread in the bowel wall. May spread vertically in the submucosa. Once it grows beyond the serosa, it invades the adjacent organs, tissues, lymphatics, and vessels in the mesentery.
- *Lymphatic spread*: Sequential spread to the different groups of lymph nodes.
  – Epicolic lymph nodes lying on the colonic wall.
  – Pericolic lymph nodes lying on the immediate vicinity of the colonic wall along the marginal artery.
  – Intermediate lymph nodes lying along the main arterial branches: Ileocolic, right colic, middle colic, left colic, and sigmoid arteries.
  – Main lymph nodes or the preaortic lymph nodes lying along the inferior or superior mesenteric vessels, as these vessels emerge from the aorta.
- *Blood spread*: Hematogenous spread may occur to the liver, lungs, brain, and bones.

Q. What is Dukes staging for carcinoma of colon?

Ans. *See* X-rays Section, Page No. 840, Chapter 17.

Q. What is Astler–Coller's modification of Dukes staging?

Ans. *See* Surgical Long Cases Section, Page No. 206, Chapter 3.

Q. What is the TNM classification for colonic cancer?

Ans. *See* Surgical Long Cases Section, Page No. 206–208, Chapter 3.

Q. What does L, V, or R in staging, denote?

Ans.
- *L*: Denotes invasion of lymphatic vessels.
  – L0—no lymphatic vessels involved
  – L1—lymphatic vessels involved.
- *V*: Denotes invasion of veins.
  – V0—no vessel invasion by the tumor
  – V1—tumor invading into the vessels.
- *R*: Denotes residual tumor following surgery.
  – R0—no residual tumor
  – R1—resection lines positive or residual tumor present.

Q. How does patient with right colonic carcinoma usually present?

Ans.
- More common in females

- May present with vague symptoms like—anemia, anorexia, and asthenia.
- May present with a lump
- Cecal carcinoma may present with symptoms and signs of acute appendicitis.
- May present with symptoms and signs of intestinal obstruction due to intussusception.
- May present with symptoms and signs of advanced disease—ascites, enlarged liver, metastasis to lungs, skin, brain, and bone.

Q. How does patient with left colonic carcinoma usually present?

Ans. Lesion in left colon is usually of stenosing variety and usually presents with:
- *Alteration of bowel habit*: Increasing constipation is the usual mode of presentation in stenosing lesion of left colon. Patient needs increasing doses of purgative for bowel evacuation, which may sometimes result in spurious diarrhea.
- Pain may be dull aching or colic due to obstructive lesion.
- May present with a lump
- May present with lower abdominal distension.

Q. Which investigations help in diagnosis of carcinoma of colon?

Ans.
- Colonoscopy and biopsy
- Double-contrast barium enema.

Q. Management of carcinoma of colon.

Ans. *See* Surgical Long Cases Section, Page No. 201–205, Chapter 3.

■ CARCINOMA OF RECTUM (FIGS 18.10A AND B)

Q. What are the macroscopic types of carcinoma of rectum?

Ans.
- Proliferative type
- Ulcerative type
- Annular or stenosing type
- Colloid carcinoma.

Q. What is adenoma carcinoma sequence?

Ans. Most rectal cancer starts is an adenoma. Due to series of genetic changes, the adenoma shows mild and later severe dysplasia and finally becomes a carcinoma. This is called adenoma carcinoma sequence.

Q. What are the microscopic types of carcinoma of rectum?

Ans.
- In majority, this is adenocarcinoma

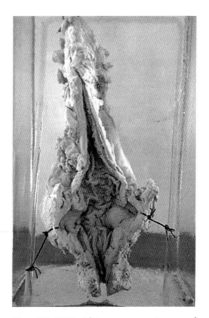

Fig. 18.10A: This is a specimen of anterior resection showing rectum and part of the sigmoid colon, which is cut open, and showing an annular growth involving the rectum. So, this is a specimen of carcinoma of rectum annular type

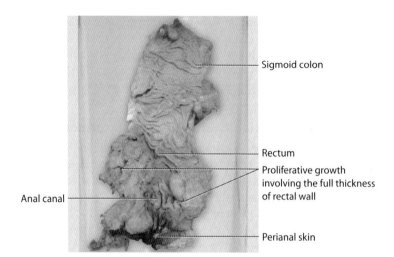

Labels on figure:
- Sigmoid colon
- Rectum
- Proliferative growth involving the full thickness of rectal wall
- Anal canal
- Perianal skin

Fig. 18.10B: This is a specimen of abdominoperineal resection of rectum showing anal canal, rectum, and part of the sigmoid colon, which is cut open, and showing a proliferative growth involving the distal rectum. So, this is a specimen of proliferative type of carcinoma of distal rectum

- In a few patients, the growth in lower third may be squamous cell carcinoma, which is likely to be an extension from anal carcinoma.
- Adenosquamous carcinoma
- Colloid carcinoma
- Malignant melanoma.

Q. What are the histological grades of carcinoma of rectum?

Ans. Depending on the degree of differentiation, carcinoma of rectum may be:
- Well-differentiated adenocarcinoma
- Moderately differentiated adenocarcinoma
- Anaplastic or highly undifferentiated adenocarcinoma.

Q. What is synchronous carcinoma?

Ans. In colorectal carcinoma, there may be two carcinomatous lesions at different segment of the rectum or colon. This is called synchronous carcinoma. Incidence is about 5%.

Q. What is metachronous carcinoma?

Ans. If a second tumor appears in the colorectum away from the site of anastomosis, 6 months after removal of primary tumor, then it is called a metachronous carcinoma. Incidence is about 10%.

Q. What are the etiological factors for development of rectal cancers?

Ans. *See* Carcinoma of Colon. Page No. 199, Chapter 3.

Q. How long does it take for a carcinomatous lesion to encircle the whole circumference of rectum?

Ans. The carcinoma of rectum spreads circumferentially around the rectal wall and it takes about 6 months to involve one quadrant of the circumference and it takes about 18 months to 2 years to involve the whole circumference of the rectum.

Q. How does carcinoma of rectum spread?

Ans.

* *Direct spread*:
  - Along the circumference of the wall of the rectum.
  - Infiltrates the wall of the rectum and as it goes beyond muscularis propria, it is limited by fascia propria (pelvic fascia). Later, it infiltrates the fascia propria and spreads to the adjacent structure.
  - Posteriorly, the growth involves the sacral plexus and the bony sacrum.
  - Anteriorly the growth may invade:
    - *In male*: Seminal vesicle, prostate, and urinary bladder.
    - *In female*: Vagina and uterus.
* *Lymphatic spread*:
  - Lymphatics from upper third of rectum drain to the nodes around the inferior mesenteric artery.
  - Lymphatics from middle third of rectum spread primarily upward to the inferior mesenteric nodes. Lymphatics may spread along the middle rectal artery to the internal iliac lymph nodes.
  - Lymphatics from lower third of the rectum spread primarily to the pararectal lymph nodes. Some lymphatics may spread upward to the inferior mesenteric nodes.
* *Hematogenous spread*:
  - Blood-borne spread is usually late. Anaplastic tumors may spread by hematogenous route to liver, lungs, brain, bones, and adrenals.
  - *Peritoneal dissemination*: Tumors in upper rectum may penetrate the peritoneal coat then spread by implantation.

Q. What is Dukes staging for carcinoma of rectum?

Ans. *See* X-rays Section 4, , Page No. 840, Chapter 17.

Q. What is TNM staging for rectal cancer?

Ans. *See* Surgical Long Cases Section, Page No. 206–208, Chapter 3.

Q. How patients with carcinoma of rectum usually present?

Ans.

* *Bleeding per rectum*: Most common symptoms. Painless bleeding, which resembles bleeding due to hemorrhoids.
* *Tenesmus*: Patient has a sense of incomplete evacuation. Patient goes to the toilet number of times, and has painful straining without passage of stool but may pass blood mixed with mucus.
* *Alteration of bowel habit*: In stenosing lesion, patient may have increasing constipation and may need to take increasing doses of purgative for evacuation.
* Patient with a proliferative growth in the ampulla of rectum may present with *early morning diarrhea*.
* *Pain*: Pain is usually a late symptom. A colicky lower abdominal pain may be due to a stenosing lesion causing subacute intestinal obstruction.

* *Low backache* may be due to advanced disease invading the sacral plexus. Invasion of the growth to the prostate or bladder may cause intense pelvic pain.
* *General symptoms due to metastatic disease*: Anorexia and weight loss.

Q. How will you achieve diagnosis in cases of suspected rectal carcinoma?

Ans.

* *Digital rectal examination*: In 90% of cases, the growth may be palpated by digital examination.
* Proctosigmoidoscopy and biopsy from the lesion.
* *Colonoscopy*: Visualization of the primary lesion, associated polyposis. Also excludes synchronous carcinoma.
* Double-contrast barium enema
* Ultrasonography and/or CT scan of abdomen magnetic resonance imaging (MRI) to ascertain any evidence of local spread and metastasis.
* Transrectal ultrasonography is helpful to delineate the tumor invasion into the rectal wall.

Q. What is sphincter saving operation for carcinoma of rectum?

Ans. For growth in upper two-thirds of the rectum, a sphincter saving operation is feasible. This involves resection of the rectum with adequate margin with colorectal anastomosis. A proximal margin of 5–7 cm and distal margin of 5 cm is required for adequate resection of rectal growth. A distal margin of 2 cm may be adequate in well-differentiated lesion.

* Either a stapled or hand sewn colorectal anastomosis may be done.
* Preoperative bowel preparation—*See* X-ray Section, Page No. 808, Chapter 17.

■ ULCERATIVE COLITIS (FIG. 18.11)

Q. Why these polyps are called pseudopolyps?

Ans. These mucosal lesions extending into the lumen of the colon are actually inflamed and edematous mucous membrane, so these are termed as pseudopolyps.

Q. What is ulcerative colitis?

Ans. Ulcerative colitis is a disease of unknown etiology, characterized by nonspecific inflammation of the colon with varying degrees of ulceration and with relapse and remissions.

Q. What is the usual progression of the disease?

Ans. The disease usually starts in the distal colon or rectum and spreads proximally

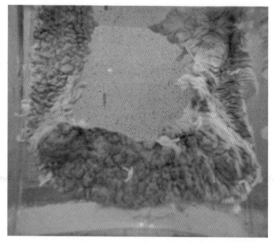

Fig. 18.11: This is a specimen of colon showing multiple small polyps involving almost the whole of the segment of the colon. The mucosa overlying the polyps is inflamed. The surrounding mucous membrane is also inflamed. There are small ulcerations in-between the polyps. So, this is a specimen of ulcerative colitis involving the whole of colon with pseudopolyp formation

from there toward the cecum and whole of the colon may be involved. When the ileocecal valve is incompetent, the terminal ileum may also be involved (backwash ileitis). The distal part shows more severe pathological changes than the proximal part. Unlike Crohn's disease, there are no skip areas.

Q. What are the etiological factors for development of ulcerative colitis?

Ans. The exact etiology is obscure.
+ Some bacterial or viral infection has been incriminated but not proved.
+ Autoimmune disease
+ Hypersensitivity to milk protein
+ Psychosomatic disorder.

Q. What are the gross changes in ulcerative colitis?

Ans. In early stages, the mucous membrane appears red and edematous and intensely hyperemic and bleeds on touch.
The ulcers are usually small and irregular, highly vascular, and are covered by a slough.
Pinpoint abscesses may be seen deep in the mucous membrane.

In later stage, the disease may involve the whole of colon.
+ The colon becomes thick walled and rigid and much smaller than its normal length and girth.
+ The mucous membrane appears bright red with purpuric hemorrhages.
+ The ulcers may be round or linear, usually of irregular shape, with undermined edges and floor covered with a necrotic tissue.
+ The ulcers sometimes may be very extensive.
+ The intervening mucosa is swollen and may form loose mucosal tags. These are called pseudopolyps.
+ The lymph nodes are usually not involved.

Q. What are the microscopic features of ulcerative colitis?

Ans.
+ There is extensive destruction of mucous membrane.
+ There is intense infiltration of mucous membrane with lymphocytes, plasma cells, and eosinophils.
+ Deeper in the mucous membrane there are collection of polymorphonuclear leukocytes, which may form crypt abscesses. These crypt abscesses rupture giving rise to the typical ulcers.

Q. How patients with ulcerative colitis usually presents?

Ans.
+ Most common mode of presentation is diarrhea, which is often watery and bloody.
+ Anemia, ill health, and hypoproteinemia are common.
+ Tenesmus—rectal discharge of blood or mucus is common when there is proctitis.
+ Fulminant colitis or toxic megacolon:
  - Patient is acutely ill.
  - Abdominal pain
  - Fever and tachycardia

– Leukocytosis
– Electrolyte imbalance
– Shock may occur.
• Perforation—once there is perforation—symptoms and signs of peritonitis are the presenting features.
• Malignant change:
– Stenosing lesion may present with subacute intestinal obstruction.
– Pain abdomen
– Abdominal distension.

Q. What is the extraintestinal manifestation of ulcerative colitis?

Ans.
• *Arthritis*:
– Polyarthritis involving knees, ankle, elbows, and wrist.
– Sacroiliitis and ankylosing spondylitis are also more common.
• *Skin lesion*:
– Erythema nodosum
– Pyoderma gangrenosum
– Aphthous ulceration.
• Sclerosing cholangitis and cholangiocarcinoma
• *Eye*—iritis and corneal ulceration.

Q. What are the grades of ulcerative colitis?

Ans. Depending on the severity of the disease:
• *Mild ulcerative colitis*:
– Less than four motions per day
– No systemic symptoms.
• *Moderate ulcerative colitis*:
– More than four motions per day
– Rectal bleeding more frequent than the mild form
– No systemic symptoms.
• *Severe ulcerative colitis*:
– More than four motions per day
– Rectal bleeding more frequent
– Systemic manifestations may be fever, weight loss, and hypoalbuminemia.

Q. Which investigations are helpful for diagnosis of ulcerative colitis?

Ans.
• Colonoscopy and biopsy
• Double-contrast barium enema. Loss of haustration, pipe stem-like colon, and pseudopolyposis revealed by filling defects.

Q. What is the medical treatment for ulcerative colitis?

Ans.
• Symptomatic treatment for diarrhea—diphenoxylate or loperamide may be used.
– Correction of fluid and electrolyte deficits
– Correction of hypoproteinemia and anemia.

* *Sulfasalazine and 5-aminosalicylic acid*: Effective in mild-to-moderate colitis. Given orally at a dose of 4 g/day. May be used as a retention enema in cases with proctitis.
* *Corticosteroid*—useful in acute flares of the disease and in chronic intractable disease.
* *Immunosuppressive*—azathioprine and 6-mercaptopurine have some beneficial effect in the short term.

Q. What are the indications of surgery in ulcerative colitis?

Ans.
* Inadequate response to medical therapy
* Extraintestinal manifestation
* Malnutrition and growth retardation
* Stricture and colorectal cancer
* Complication of hemorrhage and perforation
* Toxic colitis and megacolon
* Chronic-ill health.

Q. What are the different surgical procedures for ulcerative colitis?

Ans.
* Total proctocolectomy with ileoanal anastomosis (stapled or hand sewn)
* Total proctocolectomy and ileostomy or ileal pouch
* Subtotal colectomy with ileorectal anastomosis.

Q. What is the risk of cancer colon in ulcerative colitis?

Ans. Long-standing ulcerative colitis poses risk for development of carcinoma colon. The risk increases by 1% each year after 10 years. So that, at 20 years, the risk of developing cancer colon is 10%.

Carcinoma is more likely to occur when the whole colon is involved, earlier age of onset of the disease, and long duration of the disease.

■ HYDATID CYST (FIGS 18.12A TO C)

Q. Which parasite causes hydatid disease?

Ans.
* *Echinococcus granulosus*
* *Echinococcus multilocularis*.

Q. Who is the definitive host for the *Echinococcus*?

Ans. Definitive host is one who harbors the adult parasite. Dog is the definitive host for the *Echinococcus*.

Q. Who is the intermediate host for the *Echinococcus*?

Ans. Sheep is the intermediate host for the *Echinococcus*, as it harbors the larval forms of the parasite. Man is an incidental intermediate host.

Q. How does the man get the infection?

Ans. Man is an incidental host and gets infection by close contact with dogs or by eating raw vegetables contaminated with ova of the worm.

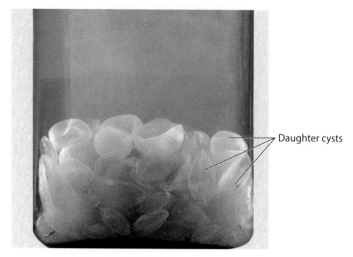

Fig. 18.12A: This is a jar containing large number of white laminated membrane of varying sizes. So, this is a specimen of daughter cysts of hydatid disease

Q. How does an adult *Echinococcus* look like?

Ans. Dog is the definitive host. It harbors the adult worm.

The adult worm consists of scolex and three or four segments. The last segment is gravid and contains numerous ova, on an average about 500 ova. The gravid segment gets detached and ova are shredded off with the stool of dogs.

Q. How is the lifecycle of worm continued?

Ans. Dog is the definitive host. Dogs are infected by feeding on offal of the infested sheep. In stomach of dog, the cyst wall gets digested and scolices are liberated. The scolices reach the small intestine and attach to the mucous membrane by its hooklets and develop into an adult worm. The last segment of the adult worm contains the mature ova and is shredded off with the stool.

The sheep swallows the ova while grazing in the field. As the ova are ingested by sheep, it reaches the stomach. The outer covering of the ovum is digested by the gastric juice and the hexacanth embryo is liberated. The embryo reaches the duodenum and burrows through the mucosa and reaches the liver via the portal circulation. After burrowing through the duodenum, the six hooklets are shredded off. Some embryos may pass out of the portal circulation and reaches

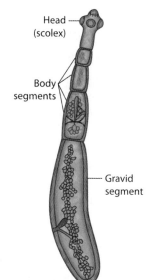

Fig. 18.12B: Adult worm of *Echinococcus granulosus*

the other organs via the systemic circulation. The hexacanth embryo develops into a hydatid cyst. The dogs get infected with these cysts while eating the offal of the sheep and the lifecycle is thus continued.

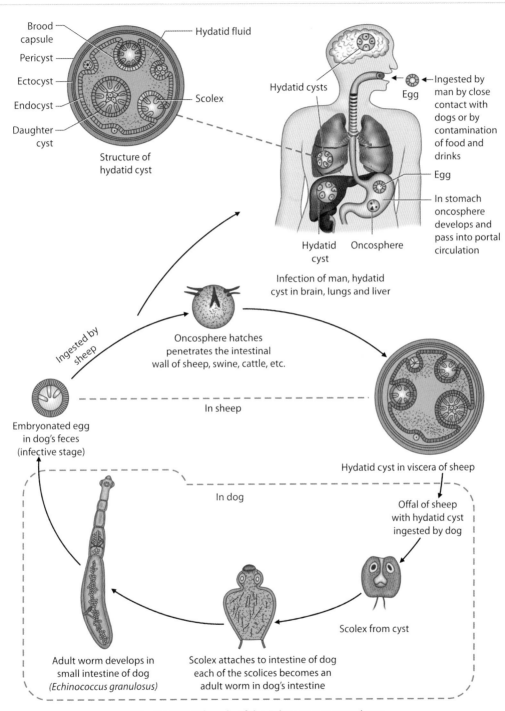

Brood capsule
Pericyst
Ectocyst
Endocyst
Daughter cyst
Hydatid fluid
Scolex

Structure of hydatid cyst

Hydatid cysts

Ingested by man by close contact with dogs or by contamination of food and drinks

Egg

Egg

In stomach oncosphere develops and pass into portal circulation

Hydatid cyst   Oncosphere

Infection of man, hydatid cyst in brain, lungs and liver

Oncosphere hatches penetrates the intestinal wall of sheep, swine, cattle, etc.

Ingested by sheep

In sheep

Embryonated egg in dog's feces (infective stage)

Hydatid cyst in viscera of sheep

In dog

Offal of sheep with hydatid cyst ingested by dog

Scolex from cyst

Adult worm develops in small intestine of dog (*Echinococcus granulosus*)

Scolex attaches to intestine of dog each of the scolices becomes an adult worm in dog's intestine

Fig. 18.12C: Lifecycle of the *Echinococcus granulosus*

Q. Which other animals can act as intermediate host?

Ans.

* Pig, horse, and cattle
* In some region, wolf and moose. Wolf can continue the cycle.

Q. How does a hydatid cyst develop in man?

Ans.

* Man is an incidental host and gets infection by ingesting ova of *Echinococcus* by close contact with dogs or by eating raw vegetables contaminated with ova.
* After the ovum is ingested, it first reaches the stomach. The acid in the stomach digests the outer shell of the ovum and a hexacanth embryo with six hooklets is liberated.
* The hexacanth embryo reaches the duodenum and burrows through the mucosa and enters the portal circulation and enters the liver. Liver is the first filter and in 80% case a cyst develops in liver. The hexacanth embryo may pass through portal circulation and reaches systemic circulation and disseminates in other organs like lungs, kidney, spleen, brain, etc.
* As the hexacanth embryo reaches the liver or other organs, the hooklets are shredded off and it is converted into a vesicle, which later develops into a hydatid cyst. The epithelial lining of the embryo forms the germinal epithelium.

Q. How do the different layers of the cyst develop?

Ans. The cyst has three layers:

1. *Endocyst*: The epithelial lining of the embryo forms the germinal epithelium and is known as the endocyst.
2. *Ectocyst*: The germinal epithelium secretes a white laminated membrane externally, which forms the ectocyst and protects the inner content of the cyst.
3. *Pericyst*: The liver tissue reacts to the formation of hydatid cyst by a fibrotic reaction at the periphery of the cyst, which forms the pericyst and it is derived from the liver.

Q. What are the functions of the endocyst?

Ans. The germinal epithelium lining the endocyst secretes:

1. *Externally*—the laminated membrane, which is a whitish elastic membrane, which contains the cyst structure and forms the ectocyst.
2. *Internally*—it secretes the hydatid fluid. In addition, the germinal epithelium forms pouching toward the lumen of the cyst, which develops into the brood capsules. The brood capsules are attached to the germinal epithelium by a pedicle. Within the brood capsules from its lining of germinal epithelium form the future scolices.

Q. How does the daughter cyst develop?

Ans. If the laminated membrane is damaged or disintegrated due to infection, the brood capsule gets detached from the germinal epithelium and grows into daughter cyst. In this case, the mother cyst ceases to exist and all the daughter cyst and hydatid fluid are confined by the pericyst.

Q. What is the characteristic of cyst formed by *Echinococcus multilocularis*?

Ans.

* The cysts formed by *Echinococcus multilocularis* are smaller, multiple, thin-walled cyst lacking a definite capsule.

- It is a spongy jelly like mass.
- Because of lack of capsule, the cyst grows and extends to a large area of the liver in a fashion like a malignant lesion.
- Liver function may be deranged by the expanding lesion in the liver or by local encasement or invasion of vascular, biliary, or lymphatic structures.
- The cysts formed by *Echinococcus multilocularis* is also known as malignant hydatid disease.

Q. What is the characteristic of hydatid fluid?

Ans. The hydatid fluid is secreted by the germinal epithelium and has following characteristics:
- It is crystal clear with a specific gravity of 1,005 to 1,009.
- It contains no albumin.
- It contains hydatid sand, which are detached scolices.

Q. What are the different layers of hydatid cyst?

Ans.
- *Pseudocyst or pericyst*: Outermost lining of the hydatid cyst consisting of fibrous tissue formed due to reaction of liver to the parasite, and grayish in color. It is blended with the liver tissue from which it is not separable.
- *Ectocyst*: It is the laminated membrane, which is white, elastic formed by germinal epithelium of the cyst.
- *Endocyst*: It is the germinal epithelium, which secretes externally the laminated membrane and internally the hydatid fluid and brood capsules.

Q. What is the usual presentation of hydatid cyst?

Ans.
- Asymptomatic in 75% cases
- An epigastric cystic lump is felt in relation to the liver
- Dull aching pain in right upper abdomen
- May present with some complications.

Q. What are the sequelae of hydatid cyst?

Ans.
- Cyst may gradually enlarge
- The parasite may die, fluid is absorbed, and the laminated membrane may calcify. A completely calcified cyst indicates a dead nonreactive cyst.
- May lead to some complications.

Q. What are the complications of hydatid cyst?

Ans. Hydatid cyst may lead to a number of complications:
- *Pressure effects*:
  - Pressure of cyst on bile duct—obstructive jaundice
  - Pressure of cyst on portal vein—portal hypertension.
- *Rupture*: It may rupture into:
  - Peritoneal cavity
  - Intestine or stomach—cyst content may be vomited out
  - Biliary tree—biliary colic, fever, and jaundice

- Pleural cavity—empyema
- Lungs—cyst content and bile may be coughed out.
 ♦ *Infection and suppuration*—pain, rigor, and fever.
 ♦ Anaphylactic shock due to rupture of the cyst.

■ GALLSTONE DISEASE (FIGS 18.13A TO E)

Q. What are the different types of gallstone?

Ans.
 ♦ Cholesterol stone
 ♦ Pigment stone
 ♦ Mixed stone.

Q. What are the characteristics of cholesterol gallstones?

Ans.
 ♦ Cholesterol stones are formed in the gallbladder
 ♦ The pure cholesterol stone is usually single (cholesterol solitaire) and may attain a large size and there are radiating crystalline appearance on cut section.
 ♦ These are radiolucent but cast an acoustic shadow in ultrasonography.

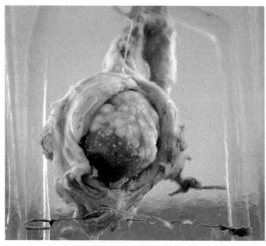

Fig. 18. 13A: This is a specimen of gallbladder, which is cut open, the gallbladder is shrunken in size, the wall appears whitish and thick, and the lumen contains a single stone. So, this is a specimen of chronic cholecystitis with cholelithiasis

Q. What are the characteristics of pigment gallstones?

Ans. There are two important types of pigment stones—black and brown pigment stones.

1. *Black pigment stones* are commonly found in patients with chronic hemolytic disease and are formed in the gallbladder. The black pigment stones are composed of bilirubin polymers and a matrix of organic material. These are usually multiple, small, dark green to black, and have a hard consistency.

   The black pigment stones are formed in the gallbladder containing a bile supersaturated with calcium bilirubinate. Some mucins MUC A and MUC C5 secreted by the peribiliary glands have been implicated in the development of black pigment stones.

2. *Brown pigment stones* are usually formed in the bile duct (primary bile duct stone) and are usually associated with biliary infection. In 98% cases, there is a nidus of bacteria in the center of the stone. Brown pigment stones contain calcium bilirubinate, calcium palmitate, and some amounts of cholesterol.

   Brown pigment stones are formed in the bile duct secondary to infection due to Gram-negative organisms like *E. coli* and *Bacteroides*. These bacteria elaborate beta glucuronidase, which causes hydrolysis of conjugated bilirubin to insoluble calcium bilirubinate.

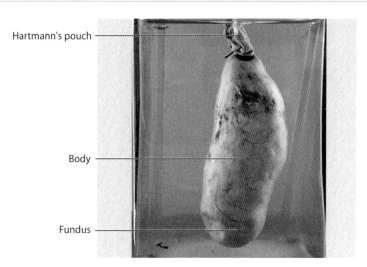

Fig. 18.13B: This is a specimen of gallbladder, which is distended in size. The gallbladder appears pale and there appears to be a stone near the neck of the gallbladder. So, this is a specimen of mucocele of gallbladder

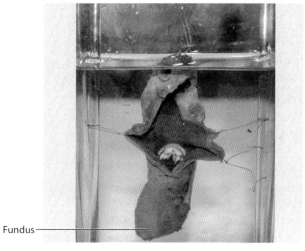

Fig. 18.13C: This is a specimen of gallbladder, which is distended in size. The wall of the gallbladder appears thick and shaggy and there are dilated vessels over the surface of the gallbladder. There is a stone in the lumen of the gallbladder. So, this is a specimen of empyema of gallbladder

Infestation of biliary tree with *Ascaris* and secondary infection is associated with increased incidence of brown pigment stones.

There may be formation of stones in both intrahepatic and extrahepatic bile ducts.

Q. What are the characteristics of mixed gallstones?

Ans. These are the most common stones that form in the gallbladder. The predominant component is cholesterol. In addition, it contains a protein matrix and variable amount of

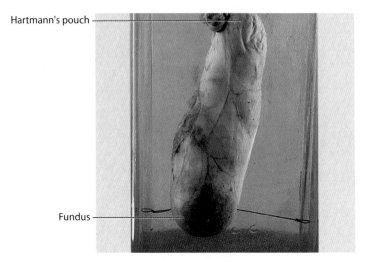

Hartmann's pouch

Fundus

Fig. 18.13D: This is a specimen of gallbladder, which is distended. The wall appears shaggy and congested. There is an area of black discoloration in the wall of the gallbladder near the fundus. So, this is a specimen of acute gangrenous cholecystitis

calcium carbonate and calcium palmitate and calcium bilirubinate. about 10% of these stones are radiopaque.

Q. Which factors are responsible for formation of gallstones?

Ans. The principal factors for formation of gallstones are:

* *Metabolic*—altered concentration of bile salts, lecithin, and cholesterol
* *Stasis* within the biliary tree
* *Infection* within the biliary tree
* *Alteration* of gallbladder epithelium
* *Hemolysis* leading to increased bile pigments in bile.

Q. How is the cholesterol stone formed?

Ans. A number of processes are involved in the formation of cholesterol gallstones.

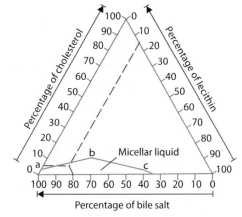

Fig. 18.13E: Cholesterol solubility in bile salt, a, b, and c denote normal solubility range of cholesterol in percentage of bile salts and lecithin.

* Supersaturation of bile with cholesterol due to altered concentration of bile salts, lecithin, and cholesterol. The normal ratio of concentration of bile salts + lecithin and cholesterol is 10:1.
* Cholesterol remains in solution in bile forming micelles with bile salts and lecithin. Some cholesterol also remains in solution by forming vesicles.
* In lithogenic bile, there is formation of abnormal high cholesterol containing vesicles. The cholesterol, which remained as micelles with bile salts and lecithin remains in solution.

- There is aggregation and fusion of cholesterol-containing vesicles. This leads to crystallization of cholesterol.
- This cholesterol monohydrate crystals remains as biliary sludge and is the precursor of stone.
- There is further deposition of cholesterol crystals in concentric layers leading to formation of stones.

Q. Which factors determine solubility of cholesterol in bile?

Ans. The solubility of cholesterol in bile depends on concentration of bile salts, phospholipid, and cholesterol in bile. Lecithin is the predominant phospholipid in bile and it is kept in solution as micelle by the bile salts. Cholesterol is also insoluble in aqueous solution but becomes soluble when incorporated into the lecithin bile salt micelle complex.

Q. When bile becomes supersaturated with cholesterol?

Ans. There is a critical relationship between the concentration of cholesterol, lecithin, and bile salts at which they remain in solution. The alteration of concentration of any of the components may lead to supersaturated bile with increased cholesterol concentration in relation to the bile salts and lecithin.

Q. In which form cholesterol remains in solution in bile?

Ans.
- About 30% cholesterol in bile remains as micelle with bile salts and lecithin
- Some cholesterol remains as vesicle with a bilayer of lipid, which can keep more cholesterol in solution than the micelle. Stability of these vesicles is said to be the key determinant in cholesterol saturation and precipitation.

Q. What is nucleation?

Ans. Nucleation is the process by which cholesterol monohydrate crystal forms and aggregates. A specific heat labile glycoprotein in cholesterol saturated bile induces vesicular aggregation and consequent stone growth.

Q. Which factors initiate cholesterol precipitation?

Ans. Following factors are implicated in precipitation of cholesterol:
- *Infection with bacteria or fungi*: Organisms have been recovered from gallstone.
- *Reflux of pancreatic fluid*—trypsin may disturb the colloidal balance. Pancreatic phospholipase may convert lecithin to toxic lysolecithin and leads to cholesterol supersaturation of bile.
- *Bile stasis due to hormonal effect and pregnancy* causes temporary cessation of bile flow into intestine and disturbs the enterohepatic circulation of bile salts. So, the bile salts and the lecithin concentration in the bile decrease resulting in cholesterol supersaturation of bile and precipitation may occur.
- *Worm infestation*.

Q. Which factors increases cholesterol secretion in bile?

Ans.
- Increasing age
- Women on oral contraceptive pills
- Obesity
- Drugs like clofibrate.

Q. What are the conditions causing reduced bile salts concentration in bile?

Ans.

- Estrogen
- Terminal ileal disease or resection interfering with enterohepatic circulation of bile salts
- Cholestyramine therapy.

Q. Why infection is important for development of gallstones?

Ans. Liver traps microorganisms from portal circulation and some microorganisms are excreted in bile. If the organisms find an appropriate nidus (cholesterol crystals and epithelial debris) they will persist and proliferate. The multiplication of the organisms may cause deconjugation and precipitation of bile salts, so that a mixed stone may form. Microorganisms have been recovered from the center of gallstones suggesting a role of these microorganisms in the development of gallstones.

Q. What is the composition of mixed stones?

Ans. Cholesterol is the main constituent. Other substances in a mixed stone include calcium bilirubinate, calcium phosphate, calcium carbonate, calcium palmitate, and protein.

Q. How chenodeoxycholic acid (CDCA) and ursodeoxycholic acid (UDCA) may prevent stone formation?

Ans. CDCA and UDCA may prevent cholesterol stone formation by:

- Replenishing bile acid pool
- Reduces cholesterol synthesis and secretion
- Supersaturated bile is converted into normal bile preventing stone formation.

Q. What may be the presentation of patients with gallstones?

Ans. Patients with gallstones may have varied presentation:

- *Stones remaining in the gallbladder*:
  - Silent stones—patient is asymptomatic and gallstones are detected in routine check up
  - Biliary colic
  - Acute cholecystitis and its sequelae—gangrene/perforation/local abscess/biliary peritonitis
  - Chronic cholecystitis
  - Mucocele of gallbladder
  - Empyema of gallbladder
  - Carcinoma of gallbladder.
- *Stones migrated into the bile duct*:
  - Obstructive jaundice
  - Recurrent cholangitis
  - Acute pancreatitis.
- *Stones migrated into the intestine*:
  - Gallstone ileus.

Q. Describe a classical attack of biliary colic.

Ans. Acute onset of pain in right upper quadrant of abdomen, severe spasmodic in nature, may radiate to back of chest or shoulder. Pain may last for few minutes to several hours. Pain is often precipitated by a fatty meal. Attacks of pain are usually self-limiting but recur in an unpredictable manner. Fever and leukocytosis are uncommon. Pain may occur in the epigastrium or rarely in the left upper quadrant of the abdomen.

Q. What are the pathological characteristics of chronic cholecystitis?

Ans.
* The gallbladder is shrunken, walls are thickened and pale in color.
* The mucous membrane often proliferates and projects into the lumen and forms deep clefts lined by epithelium. These clefts may project into the muscle coat and these forms Rokitansky–Aschoff's sinus.
* The muscle coat is atrophied and there is proliferation of fibrous tissue in the wall of the gallbladder.
* There is infiltration of chronic inflammatory cells in the wall of the gallbladder.

Q. What are the initiating events for acute cholecystitis?

Ans. Obstruction of the cystic duct by a stone or a tumor leads to distension of the gallbladder and the infection supervenes.

Q. What are the pathological features of acute cholecystitis?

Ans.
* The gallbladder is distended. The wall becomes thick and edematous. There may be exudation of pus within the lumen of the gallbladder. There may be dilated vessels over the wall of the gallbladder. Patchy gangrenous change may occur in the wall of the gallbladder.
* There may be ulceration in the mucous membrane.
* There is infiltration of acute inflammatory cells in the wall of the gallbladder.

Q. What are the common organisms causing acute cholecystitis?

Ans.
* Most common organism is *E. coli*
* Other organisms include nonhemolytic streptococci, *Proteus, Pseudomonas, Salmonella, Clostridium,* etc.

Q. What are the routes of infection in acute cholecystitis?

Ans.
* *Hematogenous*—infection reaches the gallbladder via the cystic artery.
* *Through bile*—enteric organisms gains entry into the portal circulation and filtered by the liver and excreted in bile and reaches the gallbladder.

Q. What are the sites of perforation in acute cholecystitis?

Ans.
* The perforation may occur at the fundus of the gallbladder or at the site of impaction of stone.

Q. What are the features of acute cholecystitis?

Ans. From history:

- *Pain*: Acute onset pain in right upper quadrant of abdomen. Severe spasmodic in nature with radiation to back or the right shoulder. Later on, pain becomes dull aching and constant and usually lasts longer than 24 hours.
- Marked nausea and vomiting
- Fever.

On examination:

- Tachycardia and jaundice may be present.
- Abdominal examination may reveal marked tenderness in right upper quadrant of abdomen or a vague mass may be palpable.

On blood examination:

- Leukocytosis is usually a feature.

Q. What are the sequelae of acute cholecystitis?

Ans.

- Resolution: Inflammation subsides and patient recovers.
- Gangrene: Infection may lead to gangrenous change in gallbladder manifested by increasing pain, toxemia, and appearance of rebound tenderness.
- Perforation of gallbladder: Perforation may be:
  - Localized—localized abscess formation manifested by severe pain, fever with chill and rigors, and extreme tenderness in right upper quadrant of abdomen.
  - Generalized perforation—leading to generalized biliary peritonitis manifested by generalized pain abdomen, muscle guard or rigidity, and extreme tenderness all over abdomen.
  - Perforation into a neighboring viscus most commonly duodenum, stomach, or colon.

Q. What is mucocele of gallbladder?

Ans. When there is obstruction to the cystic duct or the neck of the gallbladder by a stone or a growth then the contained bile in the gallbladder is absorbed by the gallbladder epithelium and is replaced by mucus secreted by the gallbladder epithelium. The content is usually a clear sterile fluid.

Q. What is empyema of gallbladder?

Ans. Gallbladder is filled with pus and may follow as a consequence of acute cholecystitis or as result of infection of a mucocele. In 50% cases, the continued pus is sterile.

Q. What is acalculous cholecystitis?

Ans. Acute or chronic inflammation of the gallbladder in absence of gallstone is known as acalculous cholecystitis.

Q. What are the predisposing factors for development of acalculous cholecystitis?

Ans.

- Critically-ill patients in intensive therapy unit
- Following major surgery, trauma, or burns.

Q. What is lithogenic bile?

Ans. In normal bile, the cholesterol, phospholipids, and bile salts remain in optimum concentration. This keeps the cholesterol in solution. Bile supersaturated with cholesterol is known as lithogenic bile, as this predisposes to gallstone formation.

Q. What do you mean by silent gallstone?

Ans. Incidentally found gallstones during examination for other pathology or in routine health check-up that does not produce symptoms are called silent gallstones.

Q. What is the incidence of silent gallstones?

Ans. In Western population, 10% of man and 20% of women have silent gallstones.

■ CHOLESTEROLOSIS OF GALLBLADDER (FIG. 18.14)

Q. What is the microscopic appearance of cholesterolosis?

Ans. The changes are confined to the mucous membrane. The mucous membrane is thrown into ridges and is filled with lipoid material. The lipoid material lies in large cells called "foamy cells" which phagocytose cholesterol.

There may be infiltration of mononuclear cells in the wall of the gallbladder.

Q. What is the pathogenesis of cholesterolosis of gallbladder?

Ans. The exact pathogenesis is not clear. In normal condition, the cholesterol from the bile is absorbed by the gallbladder epithelium and is transported back to circulation. Cholesterolosis may result either due to:

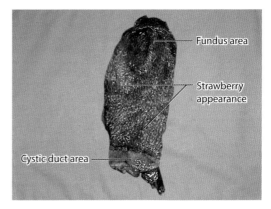

Fundus area

Strawberry appearance

Cystic duct area

Fig. 18.14: This is a specimen of gallbladder cut open showing yellowish mucous membrane. The mucous membrane is raised into ridges with clefts in-between giving an appearance like a strawberry. These changes do not extend into the cystic duct. Lipoid polyp may project into the lumen of the gallbladder. So, this is a specimen of cholesterolosis of gallbladder

- Increased absorption of cholesterol by the gallbladder epithelium due to high bile cholesterol content.
- Defective transport of the absorbed cholesterol, so that the absorbed cholesterol gets accumulated in the mucous membrane.

Q. What are the consequences of cholesterolosis of gallbladder?

Ans.
- Cholesterolosis renders the gallbladder liable to more infection.
- Cholesterolosis gallbladder may be associated with formation of cholesterol gallstones.
- Cholesterolosis is a premalignant condition and there is increased risk for development of carcinoma gallbladder.

Q. What is porcelain gallbladder?

Ans. There is deposition of calcium salts in the wall of the gallbladder. The gallbladder appears pale, smooth, and shiny like a porcelain.

Porcelain gallbladder is a premalignant condition. However, this is the being gallbladder.

Q. What investigations help in diagnosis of cholesterolosis of gallbladder?

Ans.

* Ultrasonography
* Oral cholecystography.

Q. How will you treat cholesterolosis of gallbladder?

Ans.

* Symptomatic patient—cholecystectomy
* Asymptomatic patient—prophylactic cholecystectomy, as it is a premalignant condition.

■ CARCINOMA GALLBLADDER (FIG. 18.15)

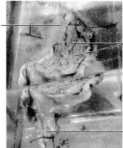

Fundus of gallbladder —
Proliferative growth in the fundus and body of gallbladder
Cystic duct area

Fig. 18.15: This is a specimen of gallbladder cut open showing thickened gallbladder wall. There is a proliferative growth at the fundus of the gallbladder extending to the body of gallbladder. So, this is a specimen of carcinoma gallbladder (proliferative type)

Q. What are the etiological risk factors for carcinoma of gallbladder?

Ans.

* Gallstone disease
* Choledochal cyst
* Porcelain gallbladder
* Anomalous pancreaticobiliary duct junction
* Gallbladder polyp more than 1 cm
* Adenomyomatosis of gallbladder
* Chronic typhoid carriers
* Carcinogens, e. g. nitrosamines.

Q. What is the relation between gallstone disease and carcinoma of gallbladder?

Ans.

* About 1–3% patients of gallstone disease may develop carcinoma of gallbladder
* About 65–90% patients with carcinoma of gallbladder have associated gallstone disease

◆ Risk of carcinoma of gallbladder is seven times more in patients with gallstone disease than in general population.

Q. What is the correlation between stone size and carcinoma of gallbladder?

Ans.
◆ Stone size 2–2.9 cm relative risk is 2.4
◆ Stone size more than 3 cm, relative risk is 10.7.

Q. How anomalous pancreaticobiliary duct junction (APBDJ) can cause carcinoma of gallbladder?

Ans.
◆ About 17% patients of carcinoma of gallbladder have associated APBDJ.
◆ Reflux of pancreatic juice into the bile duct and gallbladder—stasis of pancreatic juice into the biliary tree increased risk of carcinoma gallbladder.

Q. What is the sequence of changes in development of carcinoma gallbladder?

Ans.
◆ Normal epithelium → epithelial hyperplasia → metaplasia → dysplasia → carcinoma in situ → invasive carcinoma.

Q. What are the macroscopic types of carcinoma of gallbladder?

Ans.
◆ Mucosal plaques
◆ Polypoid or papillary
◆ Discrete thickening or scirrhous.

Q. What are the histological types of carcinoma of gallbladder?

Ans.
◆ Adenocarcinoma (80-95%)—papillary/tubular/mucinous
◆ Squamous cell carcinoma
◆ Adenosquamous carcinoma
◆ Rare types—carcinoid/undifferentiated.

Q. How does carcinoma gallbladder spread?

Ans.
◆ *Direct spread*: To adjacent liver, duodenum, bile duct, pancreas, hepatic flexure of colon, and right kidney
◆ *Lymphatic spread*: To pericholedochal, peripancreatic, and periduodenal lymph nodes
◆ *Blood spread*: Liver, lungs, and bones
◆ *Intraductal spread*: More common in papillary type
◆ Perineural spread.

Q. What is Nevin's staging for carcinoma of gallbladder?

Ans. *See* Surgical Long Cases Section, Page No. 175, Chapter 3.

Q. What is TNM definition for carcinoma of gallbladder?

Ans. *See* Surgical Long Cases Section, Page No. 175, 176. Chapter 3.

Q. What is TNM staging?

Ans. *See* Surgical Long Cases Section, Page No. 175, 176. Chapter 3.

Q. How the patient with carcinoma of gallbladder present?

Ans. Patient may present in different ways:
* *Symptoms and signs suggestive of acute cholecystitis.*
* *Symptoms and signs of chronic biliary tract disease*—right upper quadrant pain and jaundice.
* *General symptoms and signs suggestive of a malignant disease*—anorexia, weight loss, and generalized weakness.
* *Symptoms and signs suggestive of disease outside the biliary tract*—gastric outlet obstruction and GI bleeding.
* *Symptoms and signs suggestive of advanced malignant disease*—palpable gallbladder mass, hard nodular liver, and ascites.

Carcinoma of gallbladder is suspected in a patient who has long-standing history of gallstone disease in which a recent change in symptomatology and pain has occurred.

Q. Which tumor markers are important in carcinoma of gallbladder?

Ans. CEA and CA 19-9 may be elevated in carcinoma gallbladder. But these markers may be elevated in other GI malignancy.

■ POLYCYSTIC KIDNEY (FIG. 18.16)

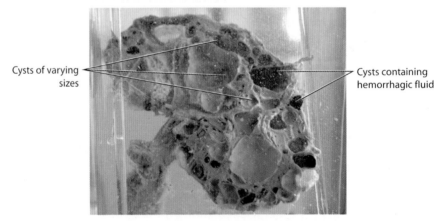

Cysts of varying sizes

Cysts containing hemorrhagic fluid

Fig. 18.16: This is a specimen of a kidney, which is enlarged in size, and showing multiple small cysts throughout the whole kidney. Some of the cysts contain hemorrhagic fluid. These cysts are not communicated with the pelvicalyceal system. So, this is a specimen of polycystic kidney

Q. What is the difference in appearance of hydronephrosis and polycystic kidneys?

Ans. In polycystic kidneys, there are varying sizes of cyst and these cysts do not communicate with the pelvicalyceal system.

In hydronephrosis, the cystic spaces in the kidney communicate with the pelvicalyceal system.

Q. How polycystic kidneys develop?

Ans. Polycystic kidneys develop due to congenital defects in development of kidneys. There is faulty development of the secretory and the collecting tubules of the kidneys. The functioning glomeruli with convoluted tubules fail to fuse with the collecting tubules leading to formation of the cysts.

Another explanation is, during development of the kidneys, the first generation of convoluted tubules gets detached from the collecting tubules and forms numerous cysts, which disappear normally with development. If these cysts from the first generation tubules persist, there is formation of polycystic kidneys.

Adult polycystic kidney disease is transmitted as an autosomal dominant trait.

Q. What are the pathological changes in polycystic kidneys?

Ans.
* *Gross*: The condition is almost always bilateral but may be more advanced on one side. The kidneys are usually enlarged and may be 3–4 times the normal size. The whole kidneys are studded with numerous cysts.
* On cut section, the cysts appear thin walled and do not communicate with the pelvicalyceal system. The contents of the cyst may be thin or thick, yellow or dark-brown hemorrhagic fluid.
* The intervening cortical tissue appears atrophic.
* *Microscopically*: The cysts are lined by epithelium, which may be flattened in large cysts but epithelium may be columnar in smaller cysts. The intervening renal tissue shows evidence of chronic interstitial nephritis.

Q. What may be the associated lesion in patients with polycystic kidney disease?

Ans.
* There may be polycystic disease involving the liver, pancreas, and spleen.
* There may be associated aneurysm in circle of Willis (Berry aneurysm).

Q. How patients with adult polycystic kidney disease usually presents?

Ans.
* *Asymptomatic*: This may be an incidental finding in course of investigations for other disease.
* *Renal lumps*: Usually patients present with bilateral renal lumps. Occasionally, lump may be palpable on one side only. Large renal lumps in fetus may be associated with obstructed labor.
* *Renal pain*: Fixed renal due to stretching of the renal capsule. Severe acute pain may occur due to hemorrhage in the cyst or due to an associated calculus.
* *Hematuria*: Recurrent hematuria is due to rupture of the cysts into the renal pelvis.
* *Infection*: Pyelonephritis is common and patient may have high fever with chills and rigor, renal pain, and pyuria.
* *Hypertension*: 70–75% of patients may have hypertension by the age of 20 years. Hypertension may be due to renal ischemia leading to increased secretion of renin or it may be due to a separate genetic factor.
* *Chronic renal failure*: In advanced cases, there is gradual deterioration of renal function. Anorexia, vomiting, fatigue, anemia, headache, and abdominal discomfort. Patient may pass large quantities of dilute urine or may ultimately develop anuria.

Q. What investigations may help in diagnosis?

Ans.
* Ultrasonography
* Intravenous urography.

Q. How will you treat polycystic renal disease?

Ans.
* Treatment of hypertension
* Treatment of associated anemia
* *Patient with end-stage renal failure*: Dialysis followed by bilateral nephrectomy and renal transplantation.

Q. What is the role of deroofing operation?

Ans. Deroofing operation (Rovsing's operation) is not very helpful in polycystic disease. Indicated only when the cyst causes pressure over the ureter. Ultrasound-guided aspiration may also decompress the cyst.

Q. What is infantile polycystic kidney?

Ans.
* Transmitted as an autosomal recessive trait
* Kidneys are hugely enlarged and may cause obstructed labor
* May be associated with cystic disease of other organs.

Q. What are the complications of polycystic kidneys?

Ans.
* Hematuria
* Anemia
* Hypertension
* Chronic renal failure
* Infection.

Questions related to renal stones—*See* X-rays Section, Page No. 796–799, Chapter 17.

■ HYDRONEPHROSIS (FIGS 18.17A AND B)

Q. What is hydronephrosis?

Ans. Hydronephrosis is an aseptic dilatation of pelvicalyceal system due to partial or intermittent culture obstruction to the outflow of urine.

Q. What are the important causes of unilateral hydronephrosis?

Ans. Obstruction to renal pelvis or ureter may cause unilateral hydronephrosis. The causes may be:
* *Congenital causes*:
  - Congenital ureteropelvic junction obstruction
  - Retrocaval ureter

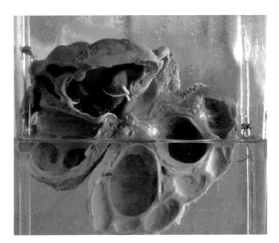

Fig. 18.17A: This is a specimen of cut section of a kidney with renal pelvis, which is cut open showing gross destruction of the cortex of the kidney with thinning of the cortex due to gross dilatation of the pelvicalyceal system. The pelvis is intrarenal and there is a large staghorn stone in the pelvis extending into the calyces. So, this is a specimen gross hydronephrosis of kidney associated with stone in the renal pelvis

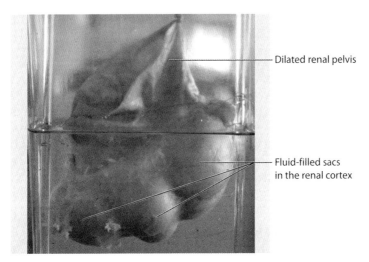

Dilated renal pelvis

Fluid-filled sacs
in the renal cortex

Fig. 18.17B: This is a specimen of kidney, which is grossly enlarged in size. The kidney substance is thinned out and there are dilated sacs in the substance of the kidney. The renal pelvis is also grossly dilated. So, this is a specimen of hydronephrosis of kidney

  – Ureterocele
  – Congenital ureteric stenosis
  – Aberrant renal vessel.
- *Acquired causes*:
  – *In the lumen*: Stones and sloughed papillary tumor.

- *In the wall*: Inflammatory stricture and postoperative stricture of ureter.
  - Transitional cell tumor in the renal pelvis or ureter
  - Transitional cell tumor in the bladder involving the ureteric orifice.
- *Outside the lumen*: Obstruction of the ureter secondary to carcinoma cervix, uterus, rectum, or colon.
  - Obstruction of the ureter by a retroperitoneal tumor or lymph node mass
  - Obstruction of ureter due to idiopathic retroperitoneal fibrosis.

Q. What are the important causes of bilateral hydronephrosis?

Ans. Above causes occurring bilaterally or obstruction from the level of bladder neck to the external urethral meatus. Important causes of lower urinary obstruction include:

- *Urethral obstruction*:
  - *Congenital*: Tight phimosis, pin hole meatus, and posterior urethral valve
  - *Acquired*: Inflammatory or post-traumatic urethral stricture
  - Benign hyperplasia of prostate and carcinoma prostate.
- *Bladder outflow obstruction*: Stone and bladder neck contracture.

Q. What are the pathological changes in hydronephrosis?

Ans.
- *Gross*: In early stage, the renal pelvis is dilated. There is broadening of major calyces and the cupping of the minor calyces may be lost. The kidney shows minimal change. There may be flattening of renal papillae.

  As the renal pelvis dilates further, the pelviureteric junction may not be the most dependent part. A valve like spur may develop between the dependent pelvis and the ureter.

  The changes also vary depending on whether the pelvis is intrarenal or extrarenal. When the pelvis is extrarenal, there is great dilatation of the pelvicalyceal system due to increased tension within the pelvicalyceal system. Later on, the kidney parenchyma atrophies gradually.

  When the pelvis is intrarenal, the minor and major calyces enlarge gradually at the expense of the kidney substance. The kidney becomes compressed and thinned out over the dilated calyces, so that a multiloculated sac, which resembles the shape of the kidney, is formed.
- *Microscopic*: The striking feature is great atrophy of renal tubules while the glomeruli remain comparatively intact. In late stages, the glomeruli also become fibrosed.

Q. What is the peculiarity of urine in the hydronephrotic sac?

Ans. The fluid in the hydronephrotic sac does not become stagnant but remains fresh. The formation of urine continues even in presence of partial or intermittent obstruction. As there is obstruction to the outflow, the reabsorption occurs through a number of accessory channels:

- *Pyelotubular backflow*—reabsorption through the tubular epithelium
- *Pyelovenous backflow*—reabsorption through the venous channels
- *Pyelolymphatic backflow*—reabsorption through the lymphatic network.

Q. How patients with hydronephrosis usually present?

Ans.
- *Renal lump*: This may present with a painless renal lump.
- *Pain:* Pain may be due to the underlying stone or inflammation—fixed renal pain, renal, or ureteric colic.

- *Dietl's crisis:* This is found in intermittent hydronephrosis. There is appearance of a lump in the loin with pain, the lump and pain disappears with passage of a large quantity of urine.
- *In bilateral hydronephrosis* may present with features of chronic renal failure.
- *If complicated with infection*—Pain, fever with chills and rigor, and pyuria.
- *Symptoms of bladder outlet obstruction*—Hesitancy, urgency, dribbling, and retention of urine.

Q. How will you evaluate a patient of hydronephrosis?

Ans. *See* Chapter 4, Page No. 217, 218.

Q. How will you treat a patient with hydronephrosis?

Ans. *See* Chapter 4, Page No. 218, 219.

Q. What are the complications of hydronephrosis?

Ans.
- Infection leading to pyonephrosis
- Formation of stones
- Hematuria
- Chronic renal failure.

■ CARCINOMA OF KIDNEY (HYPERNEPHROMA) (FIGS 18.18A AND B)

Q. What is this capsule around the tumor?

Ans. This is usually a pseudocapsule consisting of compressed renal tissue and fibrous tissue.

Q. What are the cells of origin of carcinoma kidney (renal cell carcinoma—RCC)?

Ans. All renal cell carcinomas are adenocarcinomas and are derived from renal tubular epithelial cells.

Q. What are the histological features of RCC?

Ans. The common type of RCC consists of clear or granular cells or a combination of both.
- The clear cells are typically round with abundant cytoplasm containing glycogen and cholesterol and the nucleus is small.
- The granular cells have an eosinophilic cytoplasm.
- The cells are disposed in sheets or in long columns bounded by delicate fibrous tissue.

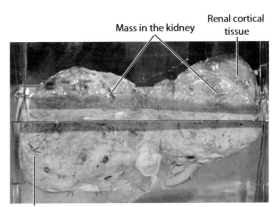

Fig. 18.18A: This is a specimen of kidney, which is cut open, and showing a large mass involving almost whole of the kidney except the lower pole. The mass is encapsulated and appears yellowish in color and there are areas of hemorrhage. There appears to be multiple lobules due to fibrous septae. The lower pole of the kidney is compressed. So, this is a specimen of carcinoma of kidney (hypernephroma)

◆ There is a network of delicate vascular sinusoid between sheets and acini of tumor cells.

Q. What is papillary renal cell carcinoma?

Ans. This is a variant of renal cell carcinoma. Microscopically, this consists of eosinophilic cells arranged in papillary or tubular fashion. The papillary tumors are usually less vascular and are often multicentric.

Q. What are the important etiological factors for development of renal cell carcinoma?

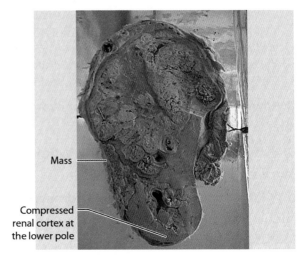

Mass

Compressed renal cortex at the lower pole

Fig. 18.18B: This is a specimen of a slice of kidney showing a similar growth

Ans. Exact etiological factors are unknown.

◆ *Smoking*: All forms of tobacco consumption have been implicated for increased risk of development of renal cell carcinoma.
◆ *Dietary factors*: Diet rich in fat and protein and low in fruits and vegetables have been associated with slight increase in risk for development of RCC.
◆ *Environmental factors* like workers in metal industries, coke oven workers, and asbestos workers have modest increase in risk for development of RCC.
◆ *Von Hippel–Lindau (VHL) disease*—Is the familial form of renal cell carcinoma.
  – Major manifestation of VHL includes:
    - Renal cell carcinoma
    - Pheochromocytoma
    - Retinal angiomas
    - Hemangioblastomas of brainstem, cerebellum, and spinal cord.
◆ *Patients with end-stage renal failure and cystic disease* of kidney have increased risk of development of RCC.

Q. How does the carcinoma kidney spread?

Ans. Initially, the tumor is confined to the kidney and may remain silent. The initial presentation may be due to metastasis.

◆ *Direct spread*: The tumor grows slowly at first. This may encroach into the pelvicalyceal system leading to hematuria. The tumor may grow along the lumen of the renal vein and may block the renal vein. The growth may extend by continuity to the inferior vena cava and right heart. Extension of the growth into the left renal vein may block the testicular vein leading to formation of left-sided varicocele.

The growth may invade the capsule and extends into the retroperitoneal tissue, duodenum, colon diaphragm, liver, and spleen.

- *Hematogenous spread*: Hematogenous spread occurs most commonly to the lungs and bones. Other sites of blood-borne metastasis are liver and brain. As the tumor grows along the renal vein, it may break as emboli and goes to systemic circulation.
- *Lymphatic spread*: Lymphatic spread is usually not common. Once the tumor invades the retroperitoneal tissues, it may spread to the retroperitoneal lymph nodes.

Q. What is Robson's staging for RCC?

Ans.
- *Stage I*: Tumor within the renal capsule.
- *Stage II*: Tumor invasion to perinephric fat (but confined to Gerota's fascia).
- *Stage III*: Tumor involvement to lymph nodes, renal vein, or vena cava.
- *Stage IV*: Tumor involving adjacent organs or distant metastasis.

Q. What is TNM staging for RCC?

Ans. *See* Surgical Long Cases Section, Page No. 224, Chapter 4.

Q. What are the prognostic factors of RCC?

Ans.
- *Pathologic stage of the disease:* Single most important prognostic factor.
  - Localized disease—5-year survival (70–90%)
  - Metastatic disease—5-year survival (15–20%).
- *Tumor size*: Small tumor less than 4 cm size has a better prognosis.
- *Tumor grade*: Well-differentiated tumor has better prognosis.

Q. What is the classical triad of presentation of carcinoma kidney?

Ans.
- Flank pain
- Gross hematuria
- Palpable flank mass.
  But this classical triad is not found in majority of patients.

Q. What is the atypical presentation of patient with carcinoma kidney?

Ans.
- *Persistent pyrexia* of unknown origin
- *Hypercalcemia*—Either due to osteolytic bone metastasis or due to secretion of parathormone-like substances from the tumor.
- *Hypertension*—Due to increased secretion of renin
- *Polycythemia*—Due to increased secretion of erythropoietin.
- *Hepatic dysfunction* also known as Stauffer's syndrome.
- *Nephrotic syndrome*
- *Constitutional symptoms* like anorexia, weight loss, and anemia
- *Symptoms due to metastasis*—Painful enlargement of bone, pathological fracture, persistent cough, or hemoptysis.

▌TUBERCULOSIS OF KIDNEY (FIG. 18.19)

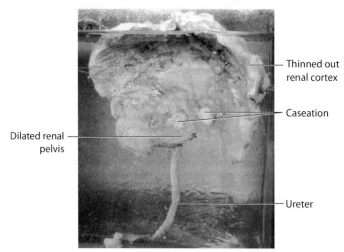

Thinned out renal cortex

Caseation

Dilated renal pelvis

Ureter

Fig. 18.19: This is a specimen of kidney and ureter, which is cut open showing gross destruction and thinning of renal cortex. There are multiple areas of accumulation of caseous material and there is associated evidence of dilatation of renal pelvicalyceal system. So, this is specimen of tuberculosis of kidney with hydronephrotic changes

Q. What is the mode of infection in urinary tuberculosis?

Ans. Tuberculosis of the urinary tract is usually secondary to a primary focus in other parts of the body either in lungs, GI tract, or bones. The infection reaches the kidney through hematogenous route.

Q. What is the pathogenesis of tuberculosis of kidney?

Ans. The organisms in the kidney settle in the blood vessel close to the glomeruli. A caseating granuloma develops, which consists of Langhans giant cells surrounded by lymphocytes and fibroblasts. A number of these tuberculous granulomas coalesce and form a tuberculous papillary ulcer. Mycobacteria and pus cells are discharged into urine. Untreated the lesion will enlarge and forms a tuberculous abscess.

The healing process results in fibrous tissue and calcium salts are deposited resulting in a classical calcified lesion. The fibrous tissue may cause stricture in the calyceal stem or at the pelviureteric junction. This results in formation of a tuberculous pyonephrosis, which may be confined to one pole or may involve the whole kidney.

The tuberculous abscess or pyonephrosis may point outward to form a perinephric abscess or it may involve the whole kidney. The whole kidney may be replaced by caseous material. Subsequent calcification may result in formation of pseudocalculi.

Both kidneys may be affected by miliary tuberculosis as part of generalized miliary tuberculosis.

Renal tuberculosis may be associated with tuberculous affection of ureter leading to formation of ureteric granulomas, ulcer and stricture. There will be dilatation of proximal ureter with hydronephrotic change in the kidney.

Urinary bladder may be affected by tuberculous lesion. The organisms reach the bladder through urine. The infection starts around the ureteric orifices, which become red, inflamed, and edematous. Tuberculous granuloma and ulcer form around the ureteric orifices. Fibrosis starts around the ureteric orifices, which contract producing a stricture. The ureteric orifice may be rigid and becomes dilated giving an appearance of golf hole. With severe involvement upward the whole bladder may become fibrosed with marked reduction of bladder capacity. This is called systolic bladder or thimble bladder.

Tuberculous infection may also involve the seminal vesicles, prostate, and the epididymis. Tuberculous epididymitis and affection of seminal vesicle and prostate is usually a blood-borne infection from a primary focus elsewhere in the body.

Q. What is the usual presentation of patients with tuberculosis of kidney?

Ans.

- *Frequency of urination*—Most common presenting symptom. Long-standing frequency of urination, initially at night and later during day as well.
- *Sterile pyuria*—Patient may pass opalescent urine but urine culture is sterile.
- *Hematuria*—Overt hematuria is present in about 10% of cases, but microscopic hematuria is present in about 50% of cases.
- *Painful micturition* due to cystitis.
- *Renal pain*—Dull aching pain in the loin may occur due to pyonephrosis.
- *Constitutional symptoms* like weight loss, anorexia, and evening pyrexia are common.

Q. What investigations may help in diagnosis?

Ans.

- *Urine analysis*—routine urine examination and culture may not reveal any organism.
  - Ziehl–Neelsen stain for acid fast bacilli (AFB) should be done at least on five occasions
  - Urine culture for AFB.
- Plain X ray abdomen—may reveal calcified kidney.
- Intravenous urography.
- Cystoscopy.
- Ultrasonography.
- Chest X-ray.

Q. How will you treat renal tuberculosis?

Ans.

- Antitubercular chemotherapy.
- *First-line drugs*: Four drugs for initial 2 months followed by two drugs for next 4 months.
- Rifampicin 450–600 mg + isoniazid 300 mg + ethambutol 15–25 mg/kg body weight + pyrazinamide 1,500 mg for initial 2 months followed by rifampicin 450–600 mg + isoniazid 300 mg for 4–6 months.

Q. What is the second line of antituberculous drugs?

Ans. Answer to be provided by the author.

Q. What are the side effects of antitubercular drug treatment?

Ans. See tuberculous lymphadenitis.

Q. What are the indications of nephrectomy in renal tuberculosis?

Ans.

+ Nonfunctioning kidney with or without calcification
+ Extensive disease involving the whole kidney
+ Extensive disease associated with hypertension and UPJ obstruction
+ Coexisting renal carcinoma.

Q. What are the indications of partial nephrectomy?

Ans.

+ Localized polar lesion that has failed to respond to a 6 weeks of chemotherapy. Area of calcification that is increasing and is threatening to destroy the whole kidney.

◼ PAPILLARY CARCINOMA OF URINARY BLADDER (FIG. 18.20)

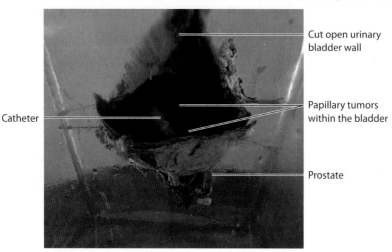

Cut open urinary bladder wall

Papillary tumors within the bladder

Catheter

Prostate

Fig. 18.20: This is a specimen of urinary bladder, which is cut open, and showing multiple papillary tumors with broad base projecting into the lumen of the urinary bladder. There is a catheter inside the bladder. So, this is a specimen of papillary carcinoma of urinary bladder

Q. Why do you say this is papillary carcinoma and not a benign papilloma of urinary bladder?

Ans. Papillary tumors of urinary bladder were earlier classified as papillomas (benign) and papillary carcinomas (malignant). Now most of the pathologists do not diagnose benign papillomas of the bladder. All papillary tumors are regarded as bladder cancer with varying grades of differentiation.

Q. What are the important etiological factors for development of bladder cancer?

Ans.

+ *Occupational exposure risk factors*—Beta-naphthylamine, 4-aminobiphenyl, benzidine, benzidine-derived azo dyes, ortho-toluidine, and methylenedianiline are important chemical carcinogens, which increase the risk of bladder cancer.

Occupations reported to be associated with increased risk of bladder cancer includes—autoworker, painter, leather worker, metal worker, aniline dye worker, paper manufacturer, dental technician, textile workers, tyre and cable workers, petrol workers, hairdressers, truck drivers, drill press operators, and sewage workers.

◆ *Cigarette smoking*: There is fourfold increase in risk of bladder cancer in smokers. Nitrosamines and 2-naphthylamine excretion are increased in smokers.

◆ *Chronic irritation*: Chronic cystitis associated with prolonged indwelling catheter or bladder calculi is associated with increased risk for squamous cell carcinoma of bladder.

Schistosoma hematobium cystitis is also associated with increased risk of squamous cell carcinoma of bladder.

◆ *Pelvic irradiation*: Women treated with radiotherapy for carcinoma uterus or cervix has increased risk of bladder cancer.

◆ *Cyclophosphamide therapy*: Patient treated with cyclophosphamide has up to ninefold increase in risk of bladder cancer. The latent period of development of such cancer is 6–13 years.

◆ *Chronic arsenic poisoning* is associated with increased risk of bladder cancer.

◆ *Genetic factors*: Some genetic factors have been implicated in bladder cancer. Overexpression of c-erbB2 and ras oncogene is associated with increased risk of bladder cancer.

Inactivation of tumor suppressor gene such as p53 and p16 is similarly associated with increased risk of bladder cancers.

Q. What are the histological types of bladder cancer?

Ans.

◆ *Transitional cell carcinoma*: More than 90% bladder cancers are transitional cell carcinoma. There are various grades of differentiation.

◆ *Squamous cell carcinoma*: Found in association with chronic irritation due to bladder calculi, long-term indwelling catheter or schistosoma cystitis.

◆ *Adenocarcinoma*: Most commonly arises from the urachal remnant near the fundus of the bladder. Vesical adenocarcinoma may also arise from the bladder epithelium associated with exstrophy of bladder. Adenocarcinoma in bladder may be due to secondary invasion from adenocarcinoma of rectum, sigmoid, uterus, breast, prostate, and ovary.

Q. What are the different grades of transitional cell tumors of bladder?

Ans.

◆ *Grade 0—papilloma*: This is a papillary lesion with a fine fibrovascular core covered by normal bladder mucosa. This behaves in a benign fashion and does not recur after excision.

◆ *Grade I—well-differentiated tumors*: The thickened urothelium contains more than seven layers of cells with slight atypia and pleomorphism and rare mitotic figures. When confined to mucosa, this is called papillary urothelial tumors of low malignant potential.

◆ *Grade II—moderately differentiated tumor*: There is a wide fibrovascular core. The cells show more pleomorphism, nuclear cytoplasmic ratio is higher, nucleoli are prominent and mitotic figures are more frequent.

◆ *Grade III—poorly differentiated tumors*: The cells do not differentiate as they progress from the basement membrane to the surface. The cells are markedly pleomorphic and mitotic figures are more frequent.

Q. What are the characteristics of in situ carcinoma of bladder?

Ans. The normal urothelium is replaced by irregularly arranged cells showing pleomorphism, large nuclei, and mitotic figures.

* *Primary carcinoma in situ*: This is the only lesion seen without any other tumor in the bladder.
* *Concomitant carcinoma in situ*: When carcinoma in situ is found in association with invasive cancer elsewhere in the bladder.
* *Secondary carcinoma in situ*: Carcinoma in situ found in a patient who already had a tumor.

Q. What do you mean by superficial bladder cancer?

Ans.
* Nonmuscle invasive bladder cancers are called superficial bladder cancer.
* Trigone and lateral walls of the bladder are the common sites of involvement.
* These are usually papillary tumors, single or multiple, which grow in exophytic fashion toward the bladder lumen with a narrow stalk, attached to the bladder wall.
* The adjacent mucosa may show dilated vessels and appears edematous and there may be carcinoma in situ change (concomitant carcinoma in situ).
* These includes:
  – *pTa tumors*—tumors not involving the lamina propria.
  – *pT1 tumors*—tumors involving the lamina propria but not the muscle coat.

Q. What are the characteristics of muscle invasive bladder cancers?

Ans.
* These are usually solid tumors with a low-tufted surface.
* These are often large and broad based with a surface ulceration.
* The chances of local invasion, lymphatic, and blood spread are high.
* Prognosis is also very poor.
* These include:
  – T2—invaded up to the muscle coat
  – T3—involved the full thickness of the bowel wall but no paravesical extension
  – T4—invaded the paravesical tissues, pelvic wall, or the adjacent organs.

Q. How does the bladder carcinoma spread?

Ans.
* *Direct spread*: The mucosal lesion invades the muscle and then spreads to extravesical tissue may involve the adjacent organs and the pelvic wall.
* *Lymphatic spread*: The growth may spread to the pelvic lymph nodes—paravesical nodes, obturator, external iliac, internal iliac, and common iliac nodes.
* *Blood spread*: May spread to the distant site via the bloodstream once the tumor invades the muscle coat. Hematogenous spread may occur to the liver, lungs, bone, adrenal glands, and intestine.
* *Implantation*: Spread by implantation may occur in the denuded urothelium, resected prostatic fossa, or traumatized urethra. Implantation occurs commonly in poorly differentiated tumors.

Q. What is TNM staging for carcinoma of urinary bladder (Tables 18.1 and 18.2)?

Table 18.1: Tumor, nodes, and metastasis (TNM) staging for carcinoma of urinary bladder	
1. Primary tumor (T)	
TX	Primary tumor cannot be assessed
T0	No evidence of primary tumor
Ta	Noninvasive papillary carcinoma
Tis	Carcinoma in situ: "flat tumor"
T1	Tumor invades subepithelial connective tissue
T2	Tumor invades muscularis propria
pT2a	Tumor invades superficial muscularis propria (inner half)
pT2b	Tumor invades deep muscularis propria (outer half)
T3	Tumor invades perivesical tissue
pT3a	Microscopically
pT3b	Macroscopically (extravesical mass)
T4	Tumor invades any of the following: prostatic stroma, seminal vesicles, uterus, vagina, pelvic wall, abdominal wall
T4a	Tumor invades prostatic stroma, uterus, vagina
T4b	Tumor invades pelvic wall, abdominal wall
2. Regional lymph nodes (N)	
Regional lymph nodes include both primary and secondary drainage regions. All other nodes above the aortic bifurcation are considered distant lymph nodes.	
NX	Lymph nodes cannot be assessed
N0	No lymph node metastasis
N1	Single regional lymph node metastasis in the true pelvis (hypogastric, obturator, external iliac, or presacral lymph node)
N2	Multiple regional lymph node metastasis in the true pelvis (hypogastric, obturator, external iliac, or presacral lymph node metastasis)
N3	Lymph node metastasis to the common iliac lymph nodes
3. Distant metastasis (M)	
M0	No distant metastasis
M1	Distant metastasis

Table 18.2: Anatomic stage/prognostic groups
Primary tumor (T):
T0—no evidence of primary tumor
TIS—carcinoma in situ
Ta—noninvasive papillary carcinoma
T1—tumor invading subepithelial connective tissue
T2—tumor invading the muscle coat
T3—tumor invading the full thickness of bladder wall
T4—tumor invading the perivesical tissue or into the prostate, uterus, vagina or rectum.

Contd...

Contd...

Lymph nodes (N):

N0—no regional lymph node metastasis
N1—metastasis to a single lymph node 2 cm or less in greatest dimension
N2—metastasis to single lymph nodes more than 2 cm but not more than 5 cm or multiple lymph nodes none more than 5 cm
N3—metastasis to lymph node more than 5 cm in greatest dimension.

Distant metastasis (M):

M0—no distant metastasis
M1—distant metastasis present.

Stage	T	N	M
Stage 0a	Ta	N0	M0
Stage 0is	Tis	N0	M0
Stage I	T1	N0	M0
Stage II	T2a	N0	M0
	T2b	N0	M0
Stage III	T3a	N0	M0
	T3b	N0	M0
	T4a	N0	M0
	T4b	N0	M0
Stage IV	Any T	N1-3	M0
	Any T	Any N	M1

(T: tumor; N: node; M: metastasis)

Q. How patients with bladder cancer usually present?

Ans.

◆ Painless hematuria is the most common mode of presentation. May be gross or microscopic. Usually intermittent hematuria.
◆ Recurrent attacks of cystitis are common—pain hypogastrium, frequency, and dysuria are common.
◆ Retention of urine—A pedunculated tumor or clot may cause retention of urine.
◆ Flank pain due to ureteric obstruction.
◆ Constant pelvic pain usually suggests extravesical spread of the tumor.

Q. Which investigations may help in diagnosis of bladder cancer?

Ans.

◆ Cystourethroscopy
◆ Urine for malignant cell
◆ Intravenous urography
◆ OEG seen.

Q. How will you treat superficial bladder cancer?

Ans.

◆ TURBT (transurethral resection of bladder tumor) and histopathological examination of resected specimen.

- *Adjuvant therapy*:
  - Single well-differentiated or moderately differentiated pTa tumor—no adjuvant therapy. Regular follow-up cystoscopy initially at 3 monthly interval for 2 years. Afterwards, yearly cystoscopy.
  - Multiple pTa tumors well differentiated or moderately differentiated—6 weeks course of intravesical chemotherapy with mitomycin-C, or Adriamycin.
  - pT1 tumors—single tumor—TURBT followed by intravesical chemotherapy with bacillus Calmette–Guerin (BCG).
- *Multiple tumors*—TURBT followed by intravesical chemotherapy with BCG or immediate radical cystectomy.

Q. How will you treat invasive bladder cancers?

Ans. Results of treatment are not encouraging and 5-year survival with different modalities of treatment is around 40%. The options for treatment are:
- *Surgery*:
  - *Partial cystectomy*—for small adenocarcinoma of the bladder, partial cystectomy may be considered.
  - Radical cystectomy with pelvic lymphadenectomy. Now standard treatment for pT2 and pT3 tumors.
  - Radical cystectomy is not feasible in patients with pT4 tumors.
- Radical radiotherapy
- Systemic chemotherapy with a combination of agents using cisplatinum, methotrexate, Adriamycin, and vinblastine.

■ BENIGN ENLARGEMENT OF PROSTATE (FIG. 18.21)

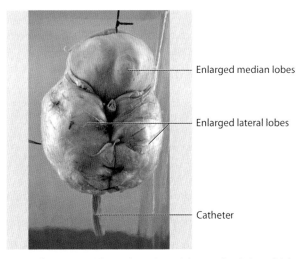

Enlarged median lobes

Enlarged lateral lobes

Catheter

Fig. 18.21: This is a specimen of prostate with two laterals and the median lobe, which are enlarged in size. The prostatic urethra is delineated by a catheter inside the specimen. The area of anterior commissure is sutured with silk. This is a specimen of benign enlargement of prostate

Q. What are the etiological factors for benign prostatic hyperplasia (BPH)?

Ans. Benign prostatic hyperplasia occurs in men over the age of 50 years.

♦ *Hormonal theory*:
  – Although androgens do not cause BPH, the development of BPH requires the presence of testicular androgens. The enzyme 5-alpha reductase converts testosterone to 5-dihydrotestosterone (5-DHT), which promotes prostatic growth.
  – The role of estrogen in BPH is not well established. Serum estrogen level increases in men with age and there are increased intraprostatic levels of estrogens in men with BPH.
  – BPH occurs due to imbalance of testosterone and estrogen in aging men. A relatively higher estrogenic influence in the aging of men is responsible for development of BPH. Estrogen sensitizes the prostatic tissues to 5-DHT, which promote prostatic growth.
  – A number of intermediate peptide growth factors like epidermal growth factor (EGF) and insulin-like growth factor also induce prostatic growth.

♦ *Neoplastic theory*: BPH is due to a benign neoplastic lesion—fibromyoadenoma.

Q. What are the parts of prostate?

Ans. In relation to the urethra and the ejaculatory ducts, the prostate is divided into five lobes:
1. *Anterior or commissural lobe*: Thin part lying anterior to the urethra.
2. *Two lateral lobes*: Part of the prostate lying on either side lateral to the urethra.
3. *Middle lobe*: The triangular wedge of tissue lying between urethra and the two ejaculatory ducts is the middle lobe.
4. *Posterior lobe*: Portion of the prostate lying behind the ejaculatory ducts and the urethra is called the posterior lobe.

Q. What are the different zones in the prostate?

Ans. The prostate is divided into three zones:
1. *Peripheral zone*: This area lies mostly posteriorly and is the area from where most carcinomas arise.
2. *Central zone*: This area lies posterior to the urethra and above the ejaculatory duct.
3. *Periurethral transitional zone*: This area lies laterally to the urethra.

Q. What are the capsules of prostate?

Ans.

♦ *False capsule*: As the BPH develops, the peripheral zone of the prostate gets compressed and forms the false capsule.

♦ *Anatomical or true capsule*: Fibrous sheath outside the compressed peripheral zone forms the anatomical or true capsule.

♦ *Periprostatic sheath*: This is the condensation of the endopelvic fascia around the true capsule. The prostatic venous plexus lies in-between the true capsule and the periprostatic sheath.

Q. What are the pathological changes in benign hyperplasia of prostate?

Ans.

♦ BPH starts in the periurethral transitional zone.

♦ There is hyperplasia of the connective tissue stroma and the glands.

♦ The overgrowth of the fibrous tissue and the plain muscles may form fibromyomatous nodules.

◆ There may be variations in stromal and epithelial proliferation. Majority of the early nodules are stromal in character. Later, the glandular proliferation predominates.
◆ The glands are lined by tall columnar epithelium with formation of papillary processes. The glandular lumen may contain eosinophilic proteinous material known as corpora amylacea.

Q. What are the effects of benign prostatic hyperplasia?

Ans.
◆ *Effects on the urethra*: As the prostate enlarges upwards, the prostatic urethra gets elongated and curved. Due to enlargement of both lateral lobes, there may be compression of the prostatic urethra. This results in narrowing of stream during micturition.
 – Median lobe enlargement causes a ball valve like action at the internal urethral
 – Meatus resulting in obstruction to the flow.
◆ *Effects on bladder:* The base of the bladder is elevated.
 – Due to obstruction in the neck, the bladder wall hypertrophies resulting in trabeculation and formation of diverticula in the bladder.
 – Due to elevation of bladder neck, there is formation of a postprostatic pouch, which results in stagnation of urine in the postprostatic pouch and cystitis.
 – Because of stagnation of urine and infection, there is increased incidence of stone formation.
 – Congestion of veins in the bladder may result in formation of vesical piles, which may rupture resulting in hematuria.
◆ *Effects on kidney and ureter*:
 – Due to backpressure, there is dilatation of ureters and there may be vesicoureteric reflux
 – Bilateral hydronephrosis
 – Ascending infection—pyelonephritis
 – Chronic renal failure.

Q. How patients with BPH usually present?

Ans.
◆ *Irritative symptoms due to BPH (prostatism)*:
 – Frequency of micturition, particularly nocturnal frequency
 – Urgency of micturition and urge incontinence
 – Nocturnal enuresis.
◆ *Obstructive symptoms due to BPH (hesitancy)*:
 – Delay in initiation of the act of micturition
 – Narrowing of stream and poor flow unimproved by straining
 – Dribbling
 – Impaired bladder emptying with large volume of residual urine
 – Chronic retention of urine
 – Acute retention of urine.
◆ *Other symptoms*:
 – Hematuria
 – Urinary infection
 – Chronic renal failure.

Q. How will you evaluate a patient of BPH?

Ans.

◆ Clinical history and examination
◆ *Rectal examination*: Assess degree of enlargement, consistency, and any mucosal fixity
◆ Blood urea and creatinine
◆ Ultrasonography of kidney ureter and bladder region
◆ Transrectal ultrasonography
◆ Uroflowmetry
◆ FNAC in suspected cases of carcinoma prostate
◆ Blood for prostate-specific antigen (PSA)
◆ Cystourethroscopy.

Q. What is the medical treatment for BPH?

Ans.

◆ *Indications*: Patient presenting with mild symptoms may benefit with conservative treatment.
◆ *Drugs*:
  – *Alpha-adrenergic drugs*: Finasteride inhibits smooth muscle contraction.
  – *5-alpha reductase inhibitors*: Terazosin blocks the enzyme 5-alpha reductase preventing conversion of testosterone to 5-DHT.
  These drugs given over a period of 1 year may help a good number of patients.

Q. What are the indications of operative treatment of BPH?

Ans.

◆ Severe symptoms of prostatism
◆ *Uroflowmetry*—maximum flow rate less than 10 mL/s and an increased residual urine volume
◆ Chronic retention of urine
◆ Acute retention of urine
◆ Hemorrhage
◆ Associated with stone formation
◆ Deterioration of renal function.

Q. What are the different options of surgical treatment?

Ans.

◆ Transurethral resection of prostate (TURP)
◆ Transurethral vaporization of prostate (TUVP)
◆ Transurethral laser ablation of prostate
◆ *Open surgery*:
  – Transvesical prostatectomy (Freyers)
  – Retropubic prostatectomy (Millins).

■ TESTICULAR TUMORS (FIGS 18.22A AND B)

Q. What are the cells of origin of seminoma testis?

Ans. The seminoma arises from the germinal epithelium of the secretory tubules of the testis.

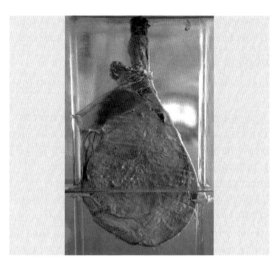

Fig. 18.22A: This is a specimen of testis along with part of the spermatic cord. The testis is cut open showing a tumor involving the whole of the testis. The tumor appears gelatinous, uniform in appearance appears lobulated. There is no evidence of extension of the tumor outside the testicular capsule. So, this is a specimen of seminoma of testis

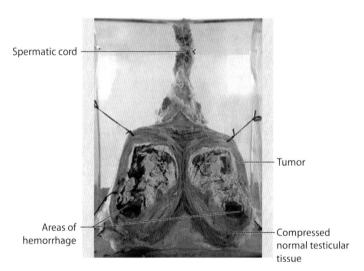

Fig. 18.22B: This is a specimen of testis and part of the spermatic cord. The testis is cut open showing a mass inside the testis, and tumor has a variegated appearance. There are areas of necrosis and hemorrhages and there are islands of solid tissues within the tumor. An area of compressed normal testicular tissue is seen near the lower pole. The tumor has not invaded outside the testicular capsule. So, this is a specimen of teratoma of testis

Q. What are the histological characteristics of seminoma testis?

Ans. These tumors contain varied types of cells. In some, the cells are large with clear cytoplasm and resemble the spermatocytes of the testicular tubules. In others, the cells are smaller with darkly staining nuclei with much less cytoplasm. The tumor cells are often markedly eosinophilic. The cells are arranged in sheets or bands and mitotic figures may be numerous.

Q. What are the histological types of seminomas?

Ans. Seminomas are subclassified depending on the histopathological characteristics and metastatic potential:

* *Typical seminoma:* Most common variety occurs in men between 30 years and 40 years.
  – Histologically, it contains islands or sheets of large cells with clear cytoplasm and dense staining nucleus. Syncytiotrophoblastic elements occur in 10–15% cases and related to beta-human chorionic gonadotropin (β-hCG) production.
* *Spermatocytic seminoma*: Occurs in men older than 50 years.
  – Histologically, consists of cells that vary in size containing deeply pigmented cytoplasm and a large nucleus and resembles cells in different phases of maturing spermatogonia. The metastatic potential of spermatocytic seminoma is extremely low.
* *Anaplastic seminoma*: This is a more aggressive and lethal variant of typical seminoma.
  – Histologically, the cells have greater mitotic activity, cellular anaplasia, and nuclear pleomorphism.
  There is higher incidence of local invasion and metastatic potential is also high.

Q. What are the cells of origin of teratoma?

Ans. The teratoma arises from the totipotent cells in the rete testis and may contain different types of cells in varying combinations.

Q. What are the different histological types of teratoma?

Ans. Depending on the degree of differentiation, the teratomas may be subclassified as:

* *Teratoma differentiated*:
  – There is no recognizable malignant component.
  – Dermoid cyst containing mature ectodermal, mesodermal, and endodermal component is a typical example.
* *Malignant teratoma intermediate (teratocarcinoma)*:
  – Contains incompletely differentiated cells.
  – In type A, there may be some mature tissues.
  – In type B, there are no mature tissues.
* *Malignant teratoma anaplastic (embryonal carcinoma)*: This is an embryonal carcinoma derived from yolk sac and composed of anaplastic cells.
  – These cells secrete alpha fetoprotein.
* *Malignant teratoma trophoblastic (choriocarcinoma)*: Microscopically contains both syncytiotrophoblastic and cytotrophoblastic cell components.
  – Very aggressive tumors and spread early to the distant site.
  – This cell often produces hCG.

Q. What are the nongerm cell tumors of testis?

Ans. The nongerm cell tumor includes:

* *Leydig cell tumor*:
  – Prepubertal interstitial cell tumor
  – These cells elaborate testosterone and result in sexual precocity and muscular development.

* *Sertoli cell tumor*:
  - Postpubertal interstitial cell tumor
  - These cells elaborate feminizing hormones and result in gynecomastia, loss of libido, and aspermia.

Q. What are the etiological factors for development of testicular tumors?

* *Cryptorchidism*: A number of factors are responsible for increased incidence of testicular tumors in undescended testis—abnormal germ cell morphology, elevated temperature, interference with blood supply, endocrine dysfunction, and gonadal dysgenesis.
* *Trauma*: Trauma is an event that prompts medical attention rather than a causative factor.
* *Hormones*: Fluctuation of hormones has been held responsible for development of testicular tumors. Sons of women exposed to diethylstilbestrol have increased risk of testicular tumors.
* *Testicular atrophy*: Nonspecific or mumps-associated atrophy of the testis has been suggested as a potential causative factor for development of testicular tumors.
* *Patients with Klinefelter's syndrome* or *testicular dysgenesis* have increased incidence of testicular tumors.

Q. How does the testicular tumor spread?

Ans.
* *Direct spread*: Local spread is late, as the tumor is confined by the tough tunica albuginea. May spread to the epididymis and the spermatic cord. Scrotal involvement is rare.
* *Lymphatic spread*: Spread by lymphatics is common. The first echelon of lymph nodes are situated in the paraaortic lymph nodes at the level of renal vessels. There is free crossover of the lymphatics from the right to the left. The mediastinal lymph nodes may be involved later. The Virchow's gland may also be involved. The seminomas more commonly spread by lymphatics.
* *Blood spread*: Teratomas particularly embryonal carcinomas and choriocarcinomas more commonly spread by bloodstream. Metastasis may occur to the lungs, liver, brain, and bones.

Q. What is the TNM staging for testicular tumors?

Ans. *See* Surgical Short Cases Section, Page No. 672, Chapter 15.

Q. What are the implications of serum markers?

Ans.
* Serum markers alpha-fetoprotein (AFP) and beta-hCG are elevated in patients with nonseminomatous germ cell tumors. Both markers may be elevated in 40% of patients and one of the markers may be elevated in 90% patients.
* hCG may be elevated in some cases of seminomas. Elevation of AFP always indicates the presence of a teratomatous element.
* Serum markers are also useful for follow up. Rising concentration of these serum markers in follow up indicates active metastases, long before the disease becomes obvious on clinical and radiological examination.

Q. How patients with testicular tumor present?

Ans.
* Painless testicular swelling. There may be an associated secondary hydrocele.

- Abdominal mass due to metastasis in the lymph nodes.
- Enlargement of Virchow's lymph nodes (left supraclavicular node).
- Chest pain, cough, or hemoptysis due to chest metastasis.
- Low back pain or bone pain due to skeletal metastasis.
- Gynecomastia due to systemic endocrine disturbance.
- General symptoms like anorexia, and weight loss due to metastatic disease.

Q. Management of testicular tumors.

Ans. *See* Surgical Short Cases Section, Page No. 670, 671, Chapter 15.

■ CARCINOMA PENIS (FIG. 18.23)

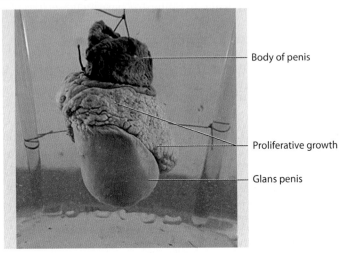

Fig. 18.23: This is a specimen of partial amputation of penis showing a proliferative mass involving the region of corona glandis. The resection margin is about 3 cm proximal to the tumor. So, this is a specimen of carcinoma penis

Q. What are the premalignant lesions of penis?

Ans.
- *Cutaneous horn:* Develops over a pre-existing skin lesion like wart, nevus, or traumatic abrasion. Characterized by overgrowth and cornification of overlying epithelium. Microscopically show hyperkeratosis, dyskeratosis, and acanthosis.
- *Balanitis xerotica obliterans:* This is a genital variation of lichen sclerosis and presents as a whitish patch on the prepuce or glans. The glans may appear white, indurated, and edematous. Microscopically, the lesion show atrophic epidermis with loss of rete pegs and there is infiltration of lymphocytes and histiocytes.
- *Leukoplakia:* These lesions present as solitary or multiple whitish plaques that often involves the prepuce and the glans. Microscopically, there are hyperkeratosis, parakeratosis, hypertrophy of the rete pegs, dermal edema, and lymphocytic infiltration.
- *Phimosis* and *chronic balanoposthitis.*
- *Genital wart or condyloma acuminata*: This is caused by human papilloma virus. The lesion consists of soft friable papillary masses in the prepuce, glans, or the shaft of the penis.

Microscopically consists of outer layer of keratinized tissue covering papillary fronds. The epithelium consists of well-ordered rows of squamous cells.

* *Buschke–Lowenstein tumor (verrucous carcinoma)*: This is a locally invasive papillary lesion. Microscopically, the tumor forms a luxuriant mass composed of broad, rounded rete pegs consisting of well-differentiated squamous cells.
* *Erythroplasia de Queyrat or Paget's disease of the penis*: The lesion consists of a red and velvety marginated lesion of glans or prepuce. Microscopically, the normal mucosa is replaced by atypical hyperplastic cells, containing hyperchromatic nuclei and mitotic figures. This is actually a carcinoma in situ.

Q. What are the macroscopic types of carcinoma penis?

Ans. Grossly, carcinoma penis may be:

* Flat or infiltrating type
* Proliferative type
* Ulcerative type.

Q. What are the microscopic types of carcinoma penis?

Ans.

* *Squamous cell carcinoma*: This is the most common type of carcinoma penis. This consists of epithelial pearls, cells showing hyperchromatic nuclei, and varying degrees of mitotic activity. Depending on the degree of differentiation, there may be four grades of squamous cell carcinoma of the penis.
* *Adenocarcinoma*: Rarely, adenocarcinoma may arise from the smegma-secreting glands.
* *Malignant melanoma*.
* *Basal cell carcinoma*.

Q. How does the carcinoma penis spread?

Ans.

* *Direct spread*: The lesion grows slowly. Buck's fascia acts as a temporary natural barrier for invasion of the growth into the corpora cavernosa. Once the Buck's fascia is invaded, there is rapid extension of the growth into the corporal body and there is chance of vascular dissemination. Involvement of the urethra is very rare.
* *Lymphatic spread*: Metastasis occurs to the inguinal (superficial and deep) and iliac lymph nodes. Metastatic enlargement of the regional lymph nodes leads to skin necrosis, infection, death from inanition, or massive hemorrhage due to invasion of femoral vessels.
* *Blood spread*—is extremely rare.

Q. How do the lymphatics of the penis drain?

Ans. The lymphatics from the prepuce and the skin of the shaft of the penis drain into the superficial inguinal lymph nodes.

The lymphatics from the glans and the lymphatics from the corporal body form a plexus at the base of the penis. The lymphatics from this plexus drain into the superficial inguinal lymph nodes on either side. There are crossover of the lymphatic channels on either side. Some lymphatics drain directly into the deep inguinal lymph nodes.

Efferent channels from the superficial inguinal lymph nodes drain into the deep inguinal lymph nodes and thence to the iliac lymph nodes (external iliac, internal iliac, and obturator nodes).

Q. What is Jackson's staging for carcinoma penis?

Ans. *See* Surgical Short Cases Section, Page No. 658, Chapter 15.

Q. What is TNM staging for carcinoma penis?

Ans. *See* Surgical Short Cases Section, Page No. 657, Chapter 15.

Q. Clinical presentation and management.

Ans. *See* Surgical Short Cases Section, Page No. 651–660, Chapter 15.

■ CARCINOMA OF BREAST (FIGS 18.24A TO D)

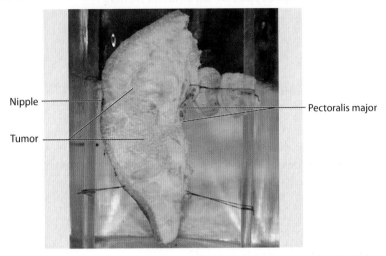

Fig. 18.24A: This is a specimen of a slice of breast showing an irregular mass within the breast parenchyma. There is no definite capsule around the tumor. The tumor appears to have infiltrated the skin. The nipple appears retracted. Few fibers of pectoralis major are seen at the deeper line of resection. Two enlarged lymph

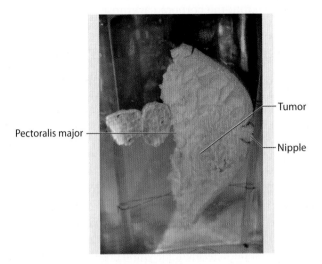

Fig. 18.24B: This is the other side of the slice of breast showing the same tumor

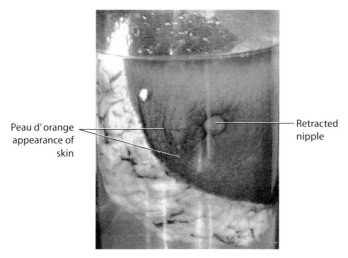

Fig. 18.24C: This is a mastectomy specimen showing a retracted nipple and areola, peau d'orange change in the skin. The other side is to be seen to comment about the tumor

nodes are also seen with the specimen. So, this is a specimen of carcinoma of breast

Q. What are the cells of origin of carcinoma breast?

Ans.
- *Ductal carcinoma*: The malignant tumor arises from the epithelial cells lining the mammary ducts.
- *Lobular carcinoma*: The malignant tumors arise from the cells lining the breast lobules or the acini.

Q. What are the pathological types of carcinoma breast?

Ans.
- *Carcinoma in situ*: This is a preinvasive cancer wherein the malignant cells have not breached the basement membrane.
- *Infiltrating carcinoma*: The malignant cells penetrate the basement membrane and invade the surrounding connective tissue. Once they infiltrate, the cells no longer give rise to tubular or acini formation and grow as solid masses of cells.
- *Scirrhous carcinoma*:
  – This occurs in a small breast with diminished vascularity.
  – The tumor is usually small but is uncapsulated and invades the breast in all directions.
  – The tumor is fibrous and light gray in color, the cut surface appears concave and it cuts with a gritty sensation.
  – Microscopically, the tumor is composed of spheroidal epithelial cells in a fibrous stroma.

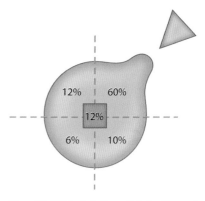

Fig. 18.24D: Relative distribution of breast cancers in different quadrant of the breast

The cells derived from the ductal epithelium exhibit no glandular arrangement and lies in solid masses or finger-like columns. The stroma consists of abundant fibrous stroma. The elastic lamina of the ducts shows striking overgrowth. Toward the periphery of the tumor, the stroma is less dense and the epithelial cells are present in greatest numbers.

- *Medullary or encephaloid carcinoma*:
  - This occurs usually in young women with well-developed breast.
  - This tumor is usually bulky and softer than the scirrhous variety.
  - Microscopically, the cells are either spheroidal or columnar and grow in columns of solid masses showing mitotic figures. The stroma is scanty and there is lymphocytic infiltration.
- *Colloid carcinoma*:
  - These are usually bulky and soft in consistency.
  - Microscopically, the cells contain abundant mucin. The mucoid material is the product of the malignant epithelial cell. At first, this lies within the cell and cell gets distended with mucin giving it an appearance of signet ring cells. Later, the mucoid material is set free in the intercellular stroma.
- *Inflammatory carcinoma of breast*:
  - This usually occurs in patients during pregnancy or in lactation period wherein the breast is very vascular.
  - This is a highly aggressive type of cancer, which grows rapidly to large size and prognosis is poor.
  - The breast becomes diffusely swollen, warm, and painful; and dilated veins appear under the skin, which becomes edematous due to lymphatic invasion of the tumor cells.
  - On cross-section, the tumors appear as a soft, hemorrhagic, and infiltrating mass with large areas of necrosis.
  - Microscopically, the epithelial cells show every sign of extreme malignancy. The cells show abundant mitotic figures and the cells vary greatly in size and shape. There is invasion of growth into the vessels and subdermal lymphatics.
- *Paget's disease of nipple*:
  - This is a superficial manifestation of an underlying breast carcinoma.
  - There is an eczema-like lesion involving the nipple and areola. There is eventual destruction of nipple and areola.
  - Subsequently, an underlying mass will appear in the breast.
  - Microscopically, the lesion contains characteristic cells, which are large, ovoid with abundant, clear, and pale-staining cytoplasm and are situated in the Malpighian layer of the epidermis.

Q. What are the different skin changes in carcinoma breast?

Ans.

- *Peau d' orange*: The skin of the breast becomes tense, thickened, and edematous—not due to direct cancer invasion to the skin but from obstruction of the subdermal lymphatic channels by the malignant growth. The attachment of the hair follicles and the sweat ducts results in depression in the lymphoedematous skin giving the appearance of an orange peel.
- *Tethering of skin*: There is infiltration of the Cooper's ligament by the malignant cells. Because

of attachment of the Cooper's ligament to the skin, it gets tethered to the mass. Appearance of skin dimples on pushing the lump suggests skin tethering.

* *Direct invasion of the skin by the tumor*: As the tumor grows, the subdermal emboli of neoplastic cells fill the endolymphatic spaces and ultimately involve the corium of the skin. The tumor cells in the corium of the skin continue to grow and result in exfoliation and ulceration.
* *Skin nodules*: Multiple skin nodules may appear around the primary tumors or following excision of the tumor, the nodule may appear around the scar. The nodules result from invasion of the skin from below by cells derived from the growing edge of the tumor.
* *Carcinoma en cuirasse*: This occurs in advanced stage of the disease. The skin over the growth becomes fixed and indurated and the induration spreads progressively and involves whole of the breast and adjacent skin. There may be secondary cancerous nodules over this thickened skin. This results from direct infiltration of the skin by the growth. Some regard it as secondary to edema of lymphatic obstruction.

Q. What is the relative distribution of breast cancers in different quadrant of the breast?

Ans.
* Upper outer quadrant—60%
* Upper inner quadrant—12%
* Lower outer quadrant—10%
* Lower inner quadrant—6%
* Central quadrant—12%.

Q. What are the important risk factors for development of carcinoma breast?

Ans.
* *Old age*: The risk of breast cancer increases with increasing age.
* *Sex*: *Common in females*: Incidence in male is only 1%.
* *High-socioeconomic status*: Incidence is little higher in patient of higher socioeconomic status.
* *Dietary factors*: Diet high in fat is associated with increased risk of breast cancer.
* *Smoking and alcohol*: Associated with slightly increased risk.
* *Early menarche, delayed menopause*, and *late first pregnancy* are associated with increased estrogenic effect and pose an increased risk of breast cancer.
* *Hormone replacement therapy:* There is slight increase in relative risk particularly in high-risk patients—benign breast disease and patients with family history of breast cancer.
* *Radiation exposure*: Exposure to ionizing radiation is associated with increased risk of breast cancer.
* *Family history of breast cancer*: There is threefold to fourfold increase in risk of breast cancer in patients with family history of breast cancer.
* *Genetic factors*: Patients with positive *BRCA1* or *BRCA2* gene are associated with increased risk of breast cancer.
* *Prior breast cancer* increases the risk of opposite breast cancer.

Q. What are the modes of spread of carcinoma breast?

Ans.
* *Direct spread*: The tumor grows and involves the adjacent quadrant of the breast. The tumor

grows toward the chest wall and invades the pectoral muscles, serratus anterior, and the bony chest wall. The tumor grows superficially and invades the overlying skin.

- *Lymphatic spread*: Occurs both by permeation and embolization. Lymphatic spread occurs to the axillary lymph nodes and to the internal mammary nodes. In advanced disease, lymphatic spread may occur to the supraclavicular nodes, opposite breast, and the opposite axillary nodes.

The disease may spread by lymphatic channel to the peritoneal cavity and tumor cell may implant on the ovaries giving rise to Krukenberg's tumor.

- *Spread by bloodstream:* Blood-borne metastasis occurs most commonly to bones—in lumbar vertebra, femur, thoracic vertebra, ribs, and skull. Metastasis may also occur in the liver, lungs, brain, adrenals, and ovaries.

Q. What is TNM staging of cancer breast?

Ans. *See* Surgical Long Cases Section, Page No. 260–262, Chapter 5.

Q. What is Manchester staging of breast cancer?

Ans.
- *Stage I*: Tumor confined to breast without chest wall fixity. No axillary lymph node metastasis. If skin is involved less than the size of the lump.
- *Stage II*: Same as stage I + axillary lymph node metastasis, mobile.
- *Stage III*: Tumor confined to breast—skin involvement more than the area of the palpable tumor but confined to the breast. Lump may be fixed to the pectoral muscle but not to the chest wall, fixed axillary lymph nodes, and of the arm.
- *Stage IV*: Lump fixed to the chest wall—skin involvement beyond the area of the breast. Metastasis to the opposite breast, axilla, or distant metastasis.

Q. What is Columbia clinical classification of breast cancer?

Ans.
- *Stage A*: Tumor confined to breast. No skin or chest wall fixity. No axillary lymph node metastasis.
- *Stage B*: Same as stage A + axillary lymph node metastasis, mobile, less than 2.5 cm in dimension.
- *Stage C*: Tumor confined to the breast, with skin fixity, or chest wall fixity. Axillary lymph node metastasis, fixed or more than 2.5 cm in greatest dimension.
- *Stage D*: Distant metastasis present. Extensive skin involvement with satellite nodules, edema of the arm, supraclavicular and internal thoracic lymph node metastasis and metastasis to lungs, brain, bone, and liver.

Preoperative Preparations

Chapter

19

■ INTRODUCTION

Once the diagnosis is reached and surgery is contemplated, a preoperative evaluation is required taking into account both the underlying disease for which specific surgery is to be performed as well as any preexisting/coexisting medical conditions which have a bearing on operative management. This is important to identify significant abnormalities which might influence the outcome of surgery. Preoperative preparation includes:
- General assessment for fitness for the surgery and anesthesia
- Correction of the underlying coexisting medical disease
- Informed consent explaining the operative risk
- General preparation for major surgery
- Prophylactic measures against some postoperative complications.

PREOPERATIVE PREPARATION FOR AN ELECTIVE MAJOR SURGERY

In addition to diagnostic workup for the underlying disease the general assessment for fitness for surgery and anesthesia is done by:
- **Detail history:** The objective is to find out any coexisting medical disease and any risk factors:
  - Any history of respiratory disease—cough, hemoptysis, breathlessness, any history of chronic bronchial asthma
  - Any history of cardiac disease—chest pain, breathlessness, any history of ischemic heart disease or hypertension
  - Any history of diabetes—duration, controlled with diet, oral hypoglycemic agents or insulin
  - Any history of bleeding diathesis and whether on any treatment
  - Any other systemic disease pertaining to gastrointestinal system, urinary system or nervous system
  - Any history of drug and alcohol intake
  - Any previous history of general anesthesia and any adverse reactions like intractable vomiting, apnea or malignant hyperpyrexia (due to succinylcholine).

- **Detail physical examination:**
  - *General survey*—mental state/nutrition/hydration status/any abnormalities of jaw and neck/any skin infection
  - *Systemic examination:*
    - Cardiovascular system
    - Respiratory system
    - Nervous system
    - Gastrointestinal system
    - Musculoskeletal system.
- **Investigations:**
  - *Baseline investigations*
    - Complete hemogram: Hb%, red blood cell (RBC) count, packed cell volume (PCV), total leukocyte count (TLC), differential leukocyte count (DLC), platelet count
    - Blood biochemistry: Blood sugar, urea and creatinine
    - Urine for routine and microscopic examination
    - Chest skiagram, posteroanterior (PA) view
    - Electrocardiography (ECG), particularly in patients over 40 years and in patients with cardiac disease and hypertension.
  - *Special investigations:* Based on the suspected coexisting disease:
    - In patients with respiratory disease [chronic obstructive pulmonary disease (COPD)]:
      » Pulmonary function test— forced expiratory volume-1 (FEV1) and forced vital capacity (FVC) are good indicators of obstructive and restrictive lung disease
      » Sputum culture and sensitivity
      » Arterial blood gas analysis.
    - In patients with cardiovascular disease:
      » Echocardiography
      » Treadmill test
      » Coronary arteriography in patients with significant ischemic heart disease
    - In patients with bleeding diathesis:
      » Bleeding time, clotting time, prothrombin time (PT), partial thromboplastin time— Kaolin activated (PTTK) and platelet count
    - In patients with jaundice:
      » Liver function test
      » Tests for viral markers— hepatitis B surface antigen (HBsAg), hepatitis B e-antigen (HbeAg), hepatitis B core antigen (HBcAg), hepatitis B virus (HBV) antibody and hepatitis B core (HBc) antibody.
- **Correction of the underlying coexisting medical disease:**
  - Treatment of the underlying respiratory disease. Antibiotics for respiratory infection, bronchodilator for obstructive airway disease, chest physiotherapy
  - Treatment of hypertension and ischemic heart disease. Treatment of hypertension with antihypertensive drugs. Significant coronary artery disease requires angioplasty or coronary artery bypass graft before major elective surgery
  - Control of diabetes mellitus
  - Correction of malnutrition: By enteral or parenteral nutrition
  - Correction of anemia by blood transfusion
  - Prophylaxis against tetanus infection.

* **Informed consent:** Patient and the responsible relatives should be explained about the disease and the planned surgical treatment, its risks and possible consequences in understandable terms and this should be recorded in a chart. Patient should also be explained about other surgical and medical treatment for the presenting problem and their advantage and disadvantages. The patient or the responsible relative should sign this informed consent in advance. A good preoperative counseling particularly in situations requiring amputation and creation of temporary or permanent stoma will allay the fears and anxiety of the patient.
* **General preparation:** On the day before surgery final preoperative orders are written.
  – *Skin preparation:* Shaving is commonly used for removal of hair. However, shaving may cause tiny wounds in the skin and may be associated with increased incidence of skin infection. Alternatively depilatory creams may be used for hair removal. Depilatory creams may sometimes cause allergic reaction. The hairs may also be removed by clipping. Clipping is now regarded as a better way of hair removal. A preoperative shower with an antiseptic solution on the day before surgery and on the morning of the day of surgery has been claimed to reduce the incidence of skin infection.
  – *Diet:* Omit solid food 12 hours before surgery and liquids 6–8 hours before surgery.
  – *Purgatives and enemas:* Patient with well-regulated bowel habits does not require preoperative purgative or enemas except in colorectal surgery or in abdominal operations likely to be associated with delayed bowel recovery.
  – *Premedications:* Benzodiazepines are commonly used as premedications. They act both as anxiolytic and hypnotic. Diazepam, lorazepam, oxazepam or nitrazepam may be used as a premedication. They are effective within 1 hour of oral administration and action lasts for 2–4 hours.
  – *Nasogastric tube:* Routine use of nasogastric tube is not required particularly for operations like cholecystectomy. If the patient has gastric outlet obstruction or intestinal obstruction a nasogastric tube is to be inserted preoperatively for decompression of the stomach.
  – *Catheterization:* Preoperative catheterization is required for pelvic operations and in situations where monitoring of urine output is required during operation and in the postoperative period.
  – *Blood transfusion:* In operations where there is anticipation of blood loss, adequate units of blood should be kept reserved with proper grouping and cross matching so as to make the blood available during surgery.
  – *Preoperative volume correction*: If the patient is thought to have volume deficit before operation adequate replacement should be done to correct the fluid and electrolyte deficit before operation.
  – *Continuing medications:* Patient receiving corticosteroid, antihypertensive, digoxin and L-thyroxine should continue all these drugs in the perioperative period. Oral anticoagulants, aspirin and antiplatelet drugs should be withdrawn 5–7 days before surgery to prevent excessive bleeding during surgery.
  – *Prophylaxis against surgical infections:* Meticulous surgical technique and strict aseptic precautions are required to prevent surgical infections. Prophylactic antibiotics are not required in clean operations. Prophylactic antibiotics are however required in clean contaminated and contaminated operations. In grossly contaminated operations the antibiotics should be continued in the postoperative period for 5–7 days. Prophylactic antibiotics should be administered at induction of anesthesia. Antibiotics administered

1–2 hours after contamination is not effective. Depending on length of operation antibiotics dose may need to be repeated.

Therapeutic concentration of the antibiotic should be achieved in the blood before skin incision. The antibiotics administered should be bactericidal in nature and the choice of antibiotics should depend on the common pathogen most likely to be encountered in a given situation.

- *Prophylaxis against tetanus infection:* Past history of immunization is important to plan immunization for tetanus prophylaxis.

- **Immunization history unknown or not immunized:**
  - Active immunization by three doses of adsorbed tetanus toxoid intramuscularly at 1 month interval. Afterwards a booster dose may be given 5 years after the primary course and again after 10 years.
  - For tetanus prone wounds patient should also be given a dose of human tetanus immunoglobulin 250 IU intramuscularly for passive immunization.

- **Fully immunized in childhood:**
  - For minor or non-tetanus prone wound no vaccine is required if patient has received the last dose within 10 years. If last dose was taken earlier than 10 years, one dose of tetanus toxoid is to be given.
  - For tetanus prone wound no vaccine is required if the last dose was taken within 5 years. If last dose was taken earlier than 5 years one dose of tetanus toxoid is to be given.
  - Tetanus immunoglobulin is not required if the patient is fully immunized earlier.

- **Prophylaxis against deep vein thrombosis:** A number of factors influence development of deep venous thrombosis in postoperative period. These include age of the patient, nature and duration of surgery, presence of jaundice, malignant disease, cardiac disease, past history of deep venous thrombosis. Depending on these risk factors the patient has been stratified into high-risk, intermediate-risk and low-risk group.
  - *In low-risk group,* anticoagulants are not required for deep vein thrombosis prophylaxis. Graduated elastic stockinette and early ambulation following surgery are required to prevent development of deep venous thrombosis.
  - *In intermediate-risk and high-risk group,* prophylaxis against deep venous thrombosis may be achieved with the use of:
    - Unfractionated heparin
    - Low molecular weight heparin
    - Graduated elastic stockinette.

Q. What is ASA (American Society of Anesthesiologist) grading for assessment of risk for major surgery and anesthesia?

Ans.

- *Class 1:* Normal healthy individual. No coexisting morbid condition.
- *Class 2:* Mild to moderate systemic disease, e.g. controlled diabetes and hypertension.
- *Class 3:* Severe systemic disease which is not incapacitating, e.g. uncontrolled diabetes, hypertension and heart disease with limited exercise tolerance.
- *Class 4:* Incapacitating systemic disease which is life threatening, e.g. severe and persistent angina.
- *Class 5:* A moribund patient who is not expected to live and surgery performed as a last resort. *E*: Surgery performed as emergency.

PREOPERATIVE PREPARATION IN A CASE OF TOXIC GOITER

General preparation is same as described earlier: History, physical examination and routine investigations. The special investigations depend on the presence of any comorbid condition. Specific preparation for patients with thyrotoxicosis.

- Special investigations
  - Thyroid profile: T3, T4 and thyroid stimulating hormone (TSH)
    - Ultrasonography of thyroid gland
    - Radionuclide thyroid scan in selected cases
    - The aim is to ensure that the patient is as near euthyroid as possible before surgery.
- Treatment is started with antithyroid drugs:
  - *Neomercazole* (5 mg tablets): 10 mg, 8 hourly or 6 hourly. 30–40 mg/day for 8–12 weeks
    - When patient reaches the euthyroid status reduce the dose to 5 mg TDS
    - If the patient shows signs of hypothyroidism or the gland shows signs of increase l-thyroxine may be started in low dose (50–100 µg).
- *Beta-blocker:* Propranolol 40 mg TDS or nadolol 80 mg OD gives rapid symptomatic relief and should be continued for 7 days postoperatively
- *Anxiolytic drug:* May be given
- *Assessment of response:*
  - Sleeping pulse rate
  - Repeat thyroid profile.
- *Lugol's iodine:* 10 drops TDS for 10–14 days before surgery:
  - Reduces vascularity of the thyroid gland
  - Blocks release of thyroid hormones during surgery.
  An alternative to Lugol's iodine is potassium iodide tablets, 60 mg TDS.

Q. If the patient has reaction to the antithyroid drugs, how will you prepare him for surgery?

Ans. If the patient develops reaction to antithyroid drugs, the alternative way of preparation would be by:

- *Use of beta-blocker:* Propranolol—start with 40 mg thrice daily. Dose may be increased to 80 mg thrice daily. Alternatively nadolol may be used 80–160 mg once daily.
- *Use of Lugol's iodine* or potassium iodide tablets 10–14 days before surgery. This regime provides a rapid way for preparation of thyrotoxic patient for surgery.

PREOPERATIVE BOWEL PREPARATION FOR COLORECTAL SURGERY

Good preoperative bowel preparation is required before colorectal surgery to reduce the incidence of wound infection and anastomotic leakage.

In addition to general preparation, the specific preparation for colorectal surgery includes:

- **Mechanical preparation of bowel:**
  - *Diet:*
    - Low residue diet 48–72 hours before surgery
    - On day before surgery only clear liquid is allowed
    - No feed on the day of surgery.

– *Bowel wash:* Balanced electrolyte solution with polyethylene glycol—available as a powder (peglec) is to be dissolved in 1 liter of water and taken on the day before surgery. This is an effective way of bowel preparation. This brings about osmotic catharsis and may render the whole gut empty.

– *Antibiotic preparation:* Mechanical wash of the colon does not sterilize the gut.

Bacterial count in the colon may be reduced by administration of luminal antibiotics like neomycin 1 gram + erythromycin base 1 gram, on the day before operation at 1 PM, 3 PM and 11 PM when surgery is planned at 9 AM next day.

A systemic antibiotic is also administered (e.g. ceftriaxone + metronidazole) before induction of anesthesia and after 6 hours and 16 hours in postoperative period.

If there is contamination during surgery, the antibiotics may be continued for 2–3 days.

Q. What are the other methods of mechanical bowel preparation?

Ans.

◆ Total or whole gut irrigation: A Ryle's tube is passed beyond the duodenojejunal flexure.

◆ With the patient sitting on a comode/couch, normal saline is passed through the Ryle's tube at the rate of 2–3 liters/hour. This clears the whole gut. When clear saline passes per rectum, the bowel is clean. Once clear fluid passes per rectum the wash should be continued for a further period of 1 hour. About 8–9 liters of saline are required. This procedure is contraindicated in persons with cardiovascular disorders, as sodium overload may precipitate heart failure.

◆ Osmotic catharsis: Administration of oral mannitol induces osmotic catharsis and empties the colon of its contents.

◆ Elemental diet for 3–5 days before surgery. Elemental diet is a predigested food which gets absorbed by the terminal ileum and leaves no residue thereby rendering an empty colon.

◆ On-table-lavage: In cases with stenotic lesion presenting with subacute obstruction. Done at the time of emergency surgery. The procedure involves:

– Isolate colon—appendectomy is done—a purse-string suture is applied at the base of appendix and a tube is passed into the colon. Another purse-string is applied in the colon proximal to the site of obstruction and a tube is passed into the colon by making a nick and the purse-string suture is tied around the tube. Normal saline is run into the colon through the proximal tube and the fluid drained out through the distal tube. The whole colon may be washed off well by on table colonic lavage.

PREOPERATIVE PREPARATION IN A CASE OF GASTRIC OUTLET OBSTRUCTION

Q. What are the electrolyte changes in patients with gastric outlet obstruction?

Ans. These patients are chronically dehydrated due to vomiting and have electrolyte abnormalities. Initially due to vomiting, the major loss is fluid rich in hydrogen and chloride ion resulting in hypochloremic metabolic alkalosis. At this stage serum sodium and potassium is usually normal. To compensate for this metabolic alkalosis the kidney excretes low chloride and more bicarbonate. While losing bicarbonate the kidney also loses sodium. The reaction of urine is alkaline.

When the gastric losses continue the patient becomes progressively more dehydrated and hyponatremic. In an attempt to conserve the circulating volume and to conserve sodium the kidney absorbs sodium preferentially and excretes hydrogen ion and potassium ions. The reaction of urine becomes acidic due to loss of hydrogen ion in urine.

At this stage in spite of metabolic alkalosis the kidney excretes acidic urine. This is called paradoxical aciduria. Hence, the alkalosis becomes more severe and the hyponatremia and hypokalemia becomes more marked.

Secondary to the metabolic alkalosis plasma ionized calcium may fall and may result in tetany and disturbances of conscious level.

In addition to general preparation, patient with gastric outlet obstruction needs some specific preparation.

The preparation includes:
- *Correction of dehydration:* Either by oral fluid or by intravenous (IV) normal saline infusion.
- Adequate urine output suggests proper hydration.
- *Correction of electrolyte imbalance:* By IV infusion of normal saline.
- Once adequate urine output is established potassium should be supplemented to correct hypokalemia.
- *Correction of anemia:* By blood transfusion.
- *Correction of hypoproteinemia:* Either by oral high protein diet or by amino acid, fresh frozen plasma or human albumin transfusion.
- *Gastric lavage:* Gastric lavage is done before each feed 4–5 days prior to surgery. Gastric lavage removes the food residue, decreases the mucosal edema and also brings back the gastric tonicity.
- *Correction of hypocalcemia:* IV calcium gluconate will correct associated hypocalcemia.

PREOPERATIVE PREPARATION IN A CASE WITH OBSTRUCTIVE JAUNDICE

- **Detail history and physical examination:** To establish the cause of jaundice.
  - In addition enquire about systemic symptoms and a detail systemic examination to ascertain any coexisting medical disease
  - The cause of obstructive jaundice may be ascertained by taking history (dark eyes and urine, pruritus and pale stool), general examination, biochemical investigations and radiological investigations.
- **Investigations:**
  - *Routine:* See earlier preparation for major elective surgery
  - *Special:*
    - Complete liver function test: Serum bilirubin (total, conjugated and unconjugated bilirubin), serum protein (total protein, albumin and globulin and albumin globulin ratio), serum enzymes [serum glutamic oxaloacetic transaminase (SGOT), serum glutamic pyruvic transaminase (SGPT)], alkaline phosphatase. The latter is especially elevated in biliary obstruction]
    - Prothrombin time expressed as INR (international normalized ratio)
    - Imaging:
      » Ultrasonography
      » Magnetic resonance cholangiopancreatography (MRCP)
      » Endoscopic retrograde cholangiopancreatography (ERCP)
      » CT scan of abdomen.

Metabolic problems in a patient with obstructive jaundice:

- *Malnutrition with hypoproteinemia*
- *Increased incidence of infection*
- *Bleeding tendency due to deficit of vitamin K*
- *Renal problems:* Increased chance of renal failure in postoperative period (hepatorenal syndrome). The causes of renal failure is multifactorial:
  - Most common cause of renal failure in patients with obstructive jaundice is gram-negative endotoxemia
  - Decreased intravascular volume
  - Kidneys are more sensitive to ischemia
  - Bile salt deposition in the renal tubules
  - Anemia
  - Diminished carbohydrate reserve
  - Dehydration.

Preoperative preparation involves correction of the above metabolic abnormalities to reduce the development of postoperative complications.

- **Correction of malnutrition and hypoproteinemia:**
  - Increased dietary protein
  - Transfusion of fresh frozen plasma
  - Transfusion of amino acid or human albumin.
- **Prevention and control of infection:** For prophylaxis, broad-spectrum antibiotics are started 24 hours before surgery. Combination of broad-spectrum antibiotics like:
  - Ampicillin + gentamicin + metronidazole or cefuroxime + metronidazole or ceftriaxone + metronidazole.
- **Control of bleeding tendency***:* A prothrombin time index of more than 80% is required before surgery. Vitamin K deficiency is corrected by administration of vitamin K 10 mg intramuscularly once daily until prothrombin time comes within normal range. A 5–7 days course is usually adequate.
- **Maintenance of renal function:** The patient is to be kept well-hydrated. Plenty of fluids by mouth. On day of operation, IV fluid is to be started from morning. In case of inadequate urine output (1 mL/kg/hr) frusemide or mannitol may be administered. Earlier injection mannitol was used routinely in preoperative, intraoperative and postoperative period to prevent renal failure. However, it is not routinely used nowadays. Avoid nephrotoxic drugs.
- **Correction of anemia:** By blood transfusion.
- **Building up of hepatic glycogen stores***:* By plenty of oral glucose and carbohydrate, and IV dextrose infusion.

PREOPERATIVE PREPARATION OF A PATIENT WITH DIABETES MELLITUS

Q. What are the problems in patients with diabetes mellitus?

Ans. Long-standing diabetes mellitus leads to complications which may involve all the systems.

- *Vascular changes:*
  - Microvascular changes:
    - Nephropathy

  - Neuropathy: Motor/sensory/autonomic
  - Ocular
 – Macrovascular changes:
  - Coronary vascular disease
  - Peripheral vascular disease
  - Cerebrovascular disease
* *Nonvascular changes:*
 – Gastroparesis
 – Sexual dysfunction
* *Increased incidence of infection.*

Q. What are the problems in patients with diabetes coming for surgery?

Ans.
* Increased incidence of infective complications
* Perioperative hypoglycemia or hyperglycemia
* Diabetic ketoacidosis or hyperosmolar states:
 – Impairment of wound healing due to decreased phagocytic activity, impaired proliferation of fibroblasts and associated microangiopathy
 – Increased incidence of cardiac complications like acute myocardial infarction or fatal arrhythmias
 – Associated autonomic neuropathy may cause vomiting, abdominal distension, bladder disturbances.

Q. What are the preoperative investigations for a diabetic patient due for elective major surgery?

Ans. Preoperative evaluation of diabetic patient should include:
* A good history and clinical evaluation to assess any underlying comorbid conditions
* Complete hemogram
* Blood urea, creatinine and serum electrolytes
* Urinary albumin and creatinine ratio
* Electrocardiography and echocardiography
* Assessment for retinopathy (fundus examination).

Q. What are the goals of perioperative management in patient with diabetes mellitus?

Ans. Perioperative management of glucose levels revolves around several key objectives:
* Reduction of overall patient morbidity and mortality
* Avoidance of severe hyperglycemia or hypoglycemia
* Maintenance of physiological electrolyte and fluid balance
* Prevention of ketoacidosis
* Establishment of certain glycemic target levels less than 180 mg/dL in critical patients and less than 140 mg/dL in stable patients.

Management of diabetic patient in the perioperative period depends on:
* Nature of surgical trauma
* Duration of perioperative fasting
* Blood sugar controlled by what measure—diet, oral hypoglycemic or insulin?

Management of patients controlled on insulin:

- The optimum blood sugar level in the perioperative period is 100–200 mg%. If blood sugar is less than 100 mg% chance of hypoglycemia is more, whereas if blood sugar is more than 200 mg%, the incidence of infective complications are increased
- Patient should be admitted 2–3 days before surgery
- Long-acting insulin should be stopped and soluble insulin started
- Patient should be the first case in the operating list in morning. The aim is to prevent perioperative hyperglycemia and hypoglycemia. Maintenance of strict normoglycemia is not advocated. 1 unit of soluble insulin neutralizes 2 g of dextrose.
  - For minor surgery:
    - Omit morning dose of insulin
    - Start previous diet and insulin regimen after surgery
  - For major surgery:
    - *Intraoperative management:*
      » On the day of surgery omit the morning dose of insulin
      » Check fasting blood sugar
      » Start glucose potassium insulin (GKI) infusion—10% dextrose charged with 15 units of insulin and 10 mmol of potassium chloride (KCl) to run 100 mL/hr
      » If fasting blood sugar is less than 100 mg%, charge 10 units of insulin and if fasting blood sugar is more than 200 mg%, charge 20 units of insulin in the 10% dextrose bottle
      » If the duration of surgery is more than 1 hour, blood sugar should be checked hourly during the operation. If within acceptable range, no extra insulin required. If blood sugar is high, give additional insulin subcutaneously.
    - *Postoperative management:*
      » Postoperatively patients are usually managed by GKI regimen (glucose potassium and insulin infusion also known as Alberti regimen)
      » 10% dextrose solution charged with 15 units of soluble insulin and 10 mmol of potassium is infused at the rate of 100 mL/hr
      » Blood sugar is checked hourly:
        ▷ Blood sugar should be maintained in the range of 100–200 mg%
        ▷ If blood sugar is outside the target range the infusion bottle is to be changed.
        ▷ If blood sugar <100 mg%—add 10 units insulin to 10% dextrose
        ▷ If blood sugar >200 mg%—add 20 units insulin to 10 % dextrose
        ▷ If blood sugar is >400 mg% in the postoperative period glucose infusion is to be stopped. Start on normal saline drip and hourly IV insulin till blood sugar comes down to 200–250 mg%. Then start GKI infusion.
- As soon as the patient is able to tolerate oral feeding—IV fluid is withdrawn and oral feeding and subcutaneous insulin is restarted. The IV insulin should be withdrawn after about 1 hour of subcutaneous insulin injection.
- The insulin requirement increases over the baseline requirements on the day of surgery and first two postoperative days and usually comes down to normal by the 3rd postoperative day following an uncomplicated surgery. The mean insulin requirement increases 66% on the day of surgery and 23% and 15% on 1st and 2nd postoperative days.

Q. What is the alternative insulin regimen for perioperative management?

Ans. Alternatively insulin injection may be administered by an infusion pump using a sliding scale. 10% dextrose with 10 mmol of potassium chloride is run at the rate of 100 mL/hr. 0.5 mL (50 units) of injection insulin is taken in a syringe containing 49.5 mL of normal saline and placed in a syringe driver. Blood sugar is checked hourly. The rate of insulin infusion is adjusted depending on the blood sugar level is given in Table 19.1.

Table 19.1: Rate of insulin infusion depending on the blood sugar level

Blood glucose (mg%)	Insulin infusion units (hour)
<100	None
100–140	1
140–200	2
200–400	3

Management of patients controlled on oral hypoglycemic agents (OHA)

- *For minor surgery:*
  - Omit morning dose of OHA
  - Operate early in the morning. The diabetic patient should be the first case on the day's list
  - Postoperatively: Start on previous diet + OHA
- *For major surgery:*
  - *If well-controlled*
    - Omit morning dose of OHA. Sulfonylurea drugs should be stopped on the day before the operation
    - Check blood sugar on morning of operation
    - If well-controlled, start glucose-potassium-insulin (10% dextrose solution charged with 15 units of insulin and 10 mmol of potassium chloride—GKI) drip to run intraoperatively 100 mL/hr. If duration of operation is more than 1 hour, intraoperative blood sugar is to be checked and additional insulin administered if blood sugar is above the acceptable range
    - Postoperatively, manage with GKI infusion or glucose potassium infusion and insulin by a sliding scale (see earlier).
    - Omit IV fluids as soon as possible and start oral diet and previous dose of oral hypoglycemic agent
  - *If not well-controlled on oral hypoglycemics*
    - Stop oral hypoglycemic agents and start short acting human insulin, administered twice or thrice daily
    - Subsequent management is same as patients controlled on insulin (see earlier).

Management of patients controlled by diet restrictions

- *For minor surgery:*
  - No special preparation is required
  - Patient resumes usual diabetic diet immediately after operation.
- *For major surgery:*
  - Monitor blood glucose immediately before operation, during operation (if duration of operation is >1 hour) and hourly after operation
  - Restrict glucose infusion in the perioperative period. Each 5% dextrose bottle should be neutralized with 8 units of insulin

– If control is good, i.e. blood glucose is in the range of 100–200 mg%, no additional insulin is required
– If at any time the blood sugar is above 200 mg%, then IV insulin should be administered either by GKI regime or by the sliding scale.

PREPARATION OF PATIENT WITH ASSOCIATED HEART DISEASE FOR SURGERY

The risk of surgery and anesthesia is increased in patients with coexisting heart disease, which may be apparent or undiagnosed. Cardiac disease may be exacerbated by the stress of surgery and anesthesia due to changes in heart rate, blood pressure, blood volume and increased catecholamine release.

Q. What is Goldman's cardiac risk index?

Ans. Goldman's cardiac risk index is a scoring system for predicting cardiac complications. This includes:

◆ Third heart sound/increased jugular venous pressure (JVP)	11
◆ Recent myocardial infarction	10
◆ Nonsinus rhythm or premature atrial contraction	7
◆ > premature ventricular contraction	7
◆ Age >70 years	5
◆ Emergency operation	4
◆ Poor general condition	3
◆ Intrathoracic/intraperitoneal/aortic surgery	3
◆ Important valvular stenosis	3

Depending on the score cardiac complication rate may be predicted:

Score	Complication rate
0–5	1%
6–12	7%
13–25	14%
>26	78%

Q. What are Eagle's criteria for cardiac risk stratification?

Ans. The Eagle's criteria include:

◆ Age >70 years	1
◆ Diabetes mellitus	1
◆ Angina	1
◆ Q wave in ECG	1
◆ Ventricular ectopics	1

Score:

- ◆ <1: low risk. No further tests required
- ◆ 1–2: Needs noninvasive tests
- ◆ >3: Needs angiography

Q. What are American Heart Association (AHA) criteria to stratify patient with cardiac risk factor for surgery?

Ans. The American Heart Association (AHA) criteria to stratify patient with cardiac risk factor for surgery are given in Table 19.2.

Table 19.2: American Heart Association (AHA) criteria to stratify patient with cardiac risk factor for surgery

Clinical predictors of increased perioperative cardiovascular risk

Major
- Unstable coronary syndromes
  - Acute or recent myocardial infarction (MI)
  - Unstable or severe angina
- Decompensated heart failure
- Significant arrhythmias
  - High-grade atrioventricular block
  - Symptomatic ventricular arrhythmias in the presence of underlying heart disease
  - Supraventricular arrhythmias with uncontrolled ventricular rate
- Severe valvular disease

Intermediate
- Mild angina pectoris (Canadian class I or II)
- Previous MI by history or pathologic Q waves
- Compensated or prior heart failure
- Diabetes mellitus (particularly insulin-dependent)
- Renal insufficiency

Minor
- Advanced age (>75 years)
- Abnormal electrocardiography results (e.g. LVH, LBBB, ST-T abnormalities)
- Rhythm other than sinus (e.g. atrial fibrillation)
- Low functional capacity (e.g. inability to climb one flight of stairs with a bag of groceries)
- History of stroke
- Uncontrolled systemic hypertension

(LVH: left ventricular hypertrophy; LBBB: left bundle branch block)

A preoperative cardiac evaluation will include:
- *A detail history:* Enquire about breathlessness, palpitation, exercise intolerance, chest pain or chest discomfort, any radiation of pain, any history of syncopal attack, history of hypertension, swelling of the legs. Any history of diabetes and hyperlipidemia (increases the risk of cardiac disease).
- *A detail cardiovascular system examination:* Pulse—any irregularity, blood pressure, apex beat (heart enlargement), heart sounds, any added sound, any heart murmur, mitral valve prolapse.

Investigations suggested are:
- ECG—may reveal any rhythm disturbances; left ventricular hypertrophy. Any evidence of ischemic heart disease or myocardial infarction (Q wave, ST changes, T wave abnormalities)
- Echocardiography

- Chest X-ray
- Treadmill test, thallium scintigraphy for evaluation of ischemic heart disease
- 24 hours Holter monitoring
- Cardiac catheterization and coronary angiography in patients with valvular heart disease and coronary artery disease.

Q. What should be the timing for surgery in patient with cardiac disease?

- Patient who had recent myocardial infarction within 6 months—elective surgery should be delayed by 6 months
- Patient who has history of myocardial infarction more than 6 months ago and effort—angina is not unfit for elective surgery
- Patient who underwent coronary artery bypass graft can safely undergo elective surgery
- Patient underwent percutaneous transluminal coronary angioplasty (PTCA)—elective surgery after 4–6 weeks.

Specific measures:

- Hypertension should be well-controlled before elective major surgery
- If there is evidence of ischemic heart disease appropriate treatment:
  - If there is gross coronary artery disease elective major surgery should be preceded by coronary artery bypass graft or coronary balloon angioplasty
  - In presence of mild disease—medical treatment is continued and patient may undergo elective surgery under intensive cardiac monitoring.
- Patient with valvular heart disease are at increased risk for developing infective endocarditis after any invasive procedure
- In upper GI procedure beta hemolytic streptococci is the principal organism
  - Antibiotics—amoxicillin, ampicillin/clindamycin
- In lower GI and GU procedure—entercocci are principal organisms
- Antibiotics—ampicillin/aminoglycosides/vancomycin
- Atrial fibrillation, atrial flutter and sustained ventricular tachycardia—require pacemaker implantation before surgery.

PREPARATION OF PATIENT WITH CHRONIC RESPIRATORY DISEASE FOR ELECTIVE MAJOR SURGERY

Patient with chronic obstructive airway disease has increased incidence of respiratory failure in the postoperative period. Postoperative respiratory failure is aggravated by restriction of respiratory movement due to postoperative pain.

Q. Which factors increase the risk of postoperative pulmonary complications?

Ans.

- Increasing age >60 years
- Low serum albumin
- Obesity
- Associated comorbid conditions:
  - Previous stroke

- Congestive cardiac failure (CCF)
- Acute renal failure (ARF)
- Chronic steroid therapy
- Blood transfusion
- Chronic obstructive pulmonary disease (COPD)
- Pneumonia
- Obstructed sleep apnea.

Preoperative evaluation will include:

- *Detail history:* Cough, breathlessness, chest pain, hemoptysis. History of chronic bronchial asthma.
- *Clinical examination:* Clubbing, cyanosis, respiratory rate, position of trachea. Shape and movement of chest. Percussion note any dullness or hyperresonance on either side of the chest. Auscultation—breath sounds. Any added sounds crepts and rhonci.
- *Relevant investigations:*
  - Chest X-ray
  - Baseline arterial blood gas analysis
  - If there is chronic obstructive airway disease: Pulmonary function test, measurement of peak expiratory flow rate (PEFR), vital capacity (VC) and forced expiratory volume in one second (FEV 1) allow objective assessment of obstructive or restrictive pulmonary diseases.

Measures to be taken in the perioperative period:

- *Chest physiotherapy*
- *Stop smoking at least 10–15 days before operation*: Following stoppage of smoking there may be initially reactive bronchorrhea which may block the respiratory passage.
- *Antibiotics:* Patients with active respiratory tract infection should receive appropriate antibiotics, chest physiotherapy and oxygen supplementation. Elective surgery should be delayed till chest infection is adequately treated.
- *Prophylactic antibiotics* are required to prevent respiratory tract infection.
- *Analgesia:* Adequate postoperative pain relief. Avoid nonsteroidal anti-inflammatory drugs (Diclofenac or rofecoxib) and narcotics. Continuous epidural anesthesia with sensoricaine may be tried.
- *Bronchodilators:* In patient with chronic obstructive pulmonary disease bronchodilators as inhaler helps to overcome the bronchospasm.
- *Steroids as inhaler* are also very effective.
- *Oxygen inhalation:* Patient with gross respiratory diseases should receive perioperative oxygen supplementation depending on the blood gas analysis.
  Patient who developed respiratory failure will need ventilatory support.

PREOPERATIVE PREPARATION OF PATIENT WITH CHRONIC RENAL DISEASE

Renal dysfunction can cause multiple organ system dysfunction and may cause morbidity and mortality in surgical patients.

Evaluation of patient with renal disease will include:

- Detail history and clinical examination
- Investigations:
  - Complete hemogram
  - Blood urea and creatinine
  - Serum electrolytes Na, K, Cl, Ca, Mg
  - Arterial blood gas
  - Chest X-ray.

Q. What are the problems in patient with renal disease?

Ans. Advanced renal disease is associated with:

- Anemia
- Platelet dysfunction
- Leukocyte dysfunction and immunosuppression
- Hyperkalemia
- Hypocalcemia
- Hyperphosphatemia
- Hyponatremia
- Metabolic acidosis
- Catabolic state.

Management:

- *Anemia*—treated with erythropoietin
- *Platelet dysfunction*—platelet transfusion
- *Hypocalcemia*—administer calcium
- *Hyperphosphatemia*—administer phosphate binding antacids
- *Hyperkalemia*—may need dialysis
- *Hyponatremia*—volume restriction or dialysis
- *Metabolic acidosis*—sodium bicarbonate when serum bicarbonate level <15 mmol/L
- *End-stage renal disease*—patient needs dialysis before surgery and also in postoperative period.

Indications of hemodialysis:

- Blood urea nitrogen: >80 mEq/L
- Serum K: >5.5 mEq/L
- Persistent acidosis
- Acute volume overload
- Uremic symptoms.

Avoid secondary renal insult by:

- Avoid nephrotoxic drugs
- Maintain intravascular volume
- Adjustment of some drug dosage depending on creatinine clearance.

Minor Surgical Procedures

INSERTION OF A NASOGASTRIC TUBE

Q. What are the indications for inserting a nasogastric tube?

Ans.

- Decompression of the stomach during upper abdominal surgery
- To empty stomach in intestinal obstruction
- To decompress the stomach postoperatively
- For gastric lavage for preparation of patients of gastric outlet obstruction for operation
- To monitor gastric bleeding
- For feeding.

Q. How will you insert the nasogastric tube?

Ans.

- Explain the patient that a tube needs to be inserted through his nose. Patient has to swallow the tube. There may be some cough during insertion of the tube.
- Lubricate the Ryle's tube (usually No. 16 Fr or 14 Fr) with 2% xylocaine jelly.
- Choose the nostril, which has the wider channel.
- Pass the Ryle's tube horizontally through the nose. As the Ryle's tube touches the posterior pharyngeal wall, the patient will gag.
- Patient may be given a little water to sip. The tube is then slowly advanced as the patient is asked to swallow the tube. During swallowing, the cricopharyngeus muscle will relax and the tube will enter into the esophagus. The tube is further advanced till the second ring in the tube lies at the level of nostril when the tip will lie in the stomach.
- The tube is secured to the nose with an adhesive tape. The tube is then connected to a plastic drainage bag to siphon out the stomach contents. If required, the stomach content may be sucked out hourly.

Q. How to confirm that the tube is in stomach?

Ans.

- Aspirate the tube with a syringe—aspiration of greenish-gray fluid confirms that the tube is in stomach.

◆ Inject about 50 mL of air through the tube and listen with a stethoscope over the epigastrium—audible gurgling sound in the epigastrium will confirm that the tube is in stomach.

◆ Listen to the end of the tube—the sound of moving air will indicate that the tube is in trachea and not in stomach.

Q. What are the characteristics of a Ryle's tube?

Ans.

◆ Usually, 1-meter long made of transparent plastic tubing.

◆ There are a few lead shots near the rounded tip of the tube. These lead shots are radiopaque and make the tip heavier for easy introduction.

◆ There are number of side holes in the tube near the tip.

◆ There are number of markings in the body of the tube.

◆ The first circular marking with a single line is at 40 cm from the tip of the Ryle's tube and when inserted up to this mark, the tip is lying at gastroesophageal junction.

◆ The second circular marking with two lines is situated at 50 cm from the tip of the tube and when inserted up to this mark, the tip lies in the body of the stomach.

◆ The third circular marking with three lines is situated at 60 cm from the tip of the tube and when inserted up to this mark, the tip of the Ryle's tube lies at the pyloric region of the stomach.

◆ The fourth circular marking with four lines is situated at 70 cm from the tip of the tube and when inserted up to this mark, the tip of the Ryle's tube lies at the duodenum.

STARTING AN INTRAVENOUS LINE

Patient is to be explained that an intravenous (IV) line is to be set up for which a needle is required to be punctured through his skin into the vein.

Requirements

An appropriate size IV cannula (18 G or 20 G for adults and 22 G for infants), a tourniquet, sterile gloves, alcohol swab, and dressing for the cannula.

Procedure

◆ Wash hands and wear sterile gloves.

◆ Apply a tourniquet above the elbow and ask the patient to close and open the first a few times to make the veins visible.

◆ The selected site is cleaned with an alcohol swab.

◆ The cannula is opened from the sterile pack and held with two wings together with the bevel of the needle pointing upward.

◆ The vein to be punctured is steadied and the skin is punctured with the cannula keeping the cannula at about 15° to the skin.

◆ The needle with the cannula is advanced through the subcutaneous tissue into the vein. As the cannula enters, the vein blood will be seen flushed into the distal end of the cannula.

◆ The needle is further advanced a few millimeters inside the vein.

* The cannula is held steady. The needle is withdrawn slightly and the plastic cannula is advanced into the vein over the metal needle. The metal needle and the tourniquet are removed.
* The open end of the cannula is connected to the tubing of an IV line.
* The cannula is secured in place by a sterile dressing and adhesive tape.

Color Code and Cannula Size

* Blue—22 G
* Pink—20 G
* Green—18 G
* Gray—16 G
* Brown—14 G.

ARTERIAL BLOOD GAS

Q. How will you collect blood for arterial blood gas (ABG) analysis?

Ans. Arterial blood gas analysis provides information about oxygen, carbon dioxide level in the blood, and overall metabolic status of the body.
* Patient is explained that a blood sample is required to be drawn for blood gas analysis.
* *Site of puncture*: Radial, brachial, and femoral artery are the usual sites for collecting a blood sample for ABG analysis.
* *For a radial arterial stab*: The forearm is kept supinated and the area cleaned with an alcohol swab and the radial artery is palpated.
* 0.1 mL of heparin is drawn into a 2-mL syringe.
* The radial pulse is felt with the index and the middle fingers. In-between the index and the middle fingers, the radial artery is punctured by a vertically held 23 G needle on a 2-mL syringe. The puncture of the artery may be appreciated by a feel. Withdraw 1.5 mL of blood. The needle is withdrawn and firm pressure is applied over the puncture site for about 3 minutes and a dressing is applied over the puncture site.
* Any air bubble aspirated is immediately expelled from the syringe.
* Seal the syringe with a plastic cap. Place it on ice and the sample is sent to the laboratory immediately.

Q. What may be the problem, if sample is analyzed after a long time?

Ans. If the sample is left in room temperature for long time, unimpeded white blood cell metabolism consumes oxygen and increases the carbon dioxide level, so the result will be fallacious.

Q. What will happen, if some air bubble is left in the syringe?

Ans. If some air bubble is left with the sample, it may falsely show high-oxygen level in the sample.

Q. If the sample contains more heparin, what may be the problem?

Ans. Excessive dilution with heparin will falsely reduce the pH of the sample.

ESTABLISHING A CENTRAL VENOUS LINE BY SUBCLAVIAN VEIN PUNCTURE

Indications of Central Venous Cannulation

- Measurement of central venous pressure and pulmonary capillary wedge pressure.
- For parenteral nutrition.
- For rapid administration of IV fluid in cases of shock.
- For insertion of temporary pacemaker electrode.

Requirements

Sterile gloves, alcohol swab, 1% lignocaine injection, 10 mL syringe, scalpel and blade, 20-G needle with a syringe, catheter and a guidewire, suture, and sterile dressings.

Procedure

- Patient is explained the procedure.
- Wash hands and wear sterile gloves.
- Patient lies supine with head tilted down by 5° to avoid air embolism. A sand bag is laid longitudinally between the shoulder blades (Fig. 20.1).
- Clean the skin around the right clavicle with an antiseptic solution and the area is draped.
- Infiltrate the skin below the midpoint of the right clavicle with 1% lignocaine.
- Make 3-mm nick with a scalpel to allow easy entry of the needle.
- Introduce a 20-G needle on a 10-mL syringe beneath clavicle and above the first rib and the needle is pushed deeper in the direction of the suprasternal notch. The entry into the subclavian vein is appreciated by a typical feel, as the needle pierces the vein wall (Fig. 20.2).
- If the needle is in the vein, blood will be drawn easily into the syringe. The syringe is withdrawn keeping the needle inside the subclavian vein.
- A guidewire is introduced through the needle into the subclavian vein.
- The needle is removed keeping the guidewire inside the vein.

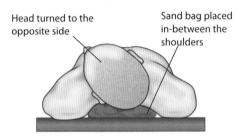

Fig. 20.1: Central venous cannulation. A sandbag is placed between the shoulders and the patient's chin is turned to the left

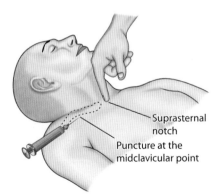

Fig. 20.2: Establishing a central venous access by subclavian vein puncture

- The catheter is passed over the guidewire and the tip of the catheter is introduced up to the upper part of the superior vena cava (Fig. 20.3).
- The guidewire is removed and the cannula is secured in place by a suture. The catheter is then connected to an IV line. A sterile dressing is applied over the puncture site.
- The position of the catheter tip may be confirmed by a chest X-ray. This will also exclude pneumothorax.

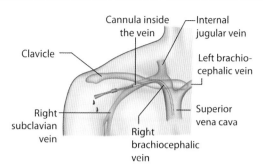

Fig. 20.3: Cannula placed in superior vena cava

Complications of Subclavian Vein Cannulation

- *Subclavian artery puncture*: Blood comes in the syringe under pressure. The needle should be immediately withdrawn and entry wound firmly pressed for a few minutes.
- Pneumothorax
- Air embolism
- Venous thrombosis
- Catheter-related sepsis
- Chylothorax.

INTERNAL JUGULAR VEIN CANNULATION

Procedure

- The patient should be explained about the procedure.
- Patient is placed supine with head tilted down 5° to distend the neck veins (Fig. 20.4).
- Clean the neck with antiseptic solution.
- Inject 1% lignocaine at the apex of the triangle formed by the two heads of sternocleidomastoid and the clavicle.
- At the apex of the triangle, make a 3-mm incision with a scalpel to allow easy insertion of the needle and the cannula.

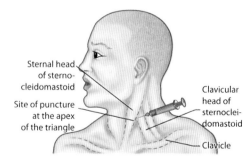

Fig. 20.4: Internal jugular vein cannulation

- Through the puncture in the skin, introduce a 20-gauge needle fitted with a syringe and direct it laterally downward and backward till the internal jugular vein is punctured just beneath the skin and the clavicular head of sternocleidomastoid. The placement of the needle inside the vein is confirmed by aspirating blood. The syringe is disconnected and a guidewire is introduced through the needle into the vein and the needle is withdrawn.

- Introduce a venous catheter over the guidewire into the vein and the guidewire is withdrawn. The end of the cannula is then connected to an IV line.
- The catheter is secured to the skin with a suture and dressing applied.
- A postprocedure chest X-ray will confirm the position of the tip of the catheter and will also exclude pneumothorax.

CATHETERIZATION FOR RETENTION OF URINE

Requirements

Sterile gloves, Foley's catheter, 2% xylocaine jelly, povidone–iodine solution, 10-mL syringe, distilled water, Urobag, sterile dressing, and sterile draping sheet.

Procedure

- Explain to the patient that a catheter will be introduced through his urethral orifice. Reassure that it will be a painless procedure.
- Scrub and put on sterile gloves.
- Patient supine with legs apart.
- Clean the genitalia with an antiseptic solution and drape the area.
- The uncircumcised foreskin is retracted, and the glans penis and the corona are exposed.
- The glans penis is cleaned with antiseptic solution.
- Take 20 mL of 2% xylocaine in the syringe and introduce it through the external urethral meatus into the urethra and press the external urethral meatus to prevent the jelly spilling out and massage the undersurface of the penis to allow the jelly to go further down.
- Wait for 5 minutes.
- The penis is held vertically upwards to straighten the penile urethra by encircling a sterile gauge around the penis.
- The lubricated Foley's catheter is then pushed gently through the external urethral meatus and gradually advanced till it reaches the bladder when urine will be seen coming through the catheter.
- The catheter is advanced a little further.
- About 15–20 mL of water is introduced through the side channel of the catheter to inflate the balloon.
- After the balloon is inflated, the catheter is pulled outward to confirm that the balloon is properly inflated.
- The catheter is then connected to an Urobag. The preputial skin is brought back over the glans penis to prevent development of paraphimosis.
- In case of chronic retention, the bladder should be emptied slowly.

Q. What may be the causes of failure to introduce the catheter?

Ans.
- Catheter may be too large.

- Inadequate anesthesia—if patient resists insertion of catheter.
- Stricture of urethra.
- Prostatic enlargement.
- Bladder neck stricture.
- Tight phimosis.
- Meatal stenosis.

Q. If you cannot pass a Foley's catheter, what other catheter may be tried?

Ans. A stiff catheter—Gibbon's catheter or a stiff rubber catheter may be tried.

Q. What are the complications of catheterization?

Ans.
- Bleeding
- False passage
- Infection.

ABSCESSES

Q. What is an abscess?

Ans. Abscess is localized collection of pus. Patient complains of throbbing pain. The area is swollen, tender, and fluctuant. Overlying skin is red and shiny. If the abscess is large, there may be fever and toxemia.

Q. In which abscesses, the fluctuation is not demonstrable?

Ans.
- Ischiorectal abscess
- Parotid abscess
- Infection in palmar space
- Breast abscess
- Iliac abscess
- Thigh abscess.

Q. What is Hilton's method for drainage of abscess?

Ans. When the abscess is situated in an important site containing major vessels and nerves then there is possibility of injury of underlying structures during drainage of abscess. To avoid this, the abscess drainage in important site is done by Hilton's method.

The skin and subcutaneous tissues are incised with a knife. The point of a hemostat or a sinus forceps is pushed through the most prominent part of the swelling and the blades are then opened. The opening is thus enlarged and pus drained. A finger may be introduced into the abscess cavity and all the loculi broken.

■ DRAINAGE OF PERITONSILLAR ABSCESS

Procedure

- *Anesthesia*: Local anesthesia by spraying 4% xylocaine into the pharynx or general anesthesia with endotracheal intubation (Fig. 20.5).
- *Incision*:
  - Using a No. 11 knife, incise the mucosa over the abscess. A sinus forceps is then thrushed into the abscess and its blades are opened. Suck the pus quickly.
  - If there is bleeding, the abscess cavity may be packed.

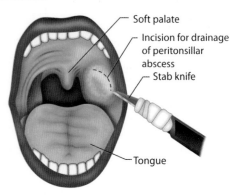

Soft palate

Incision for drainage of peritonsillar abscess

Stab knife

Tongue

Fig. 20.5: Drainage of peritonsillar abscess

■ LUDWIG'S ANGINA

Q. What is Ludwig's angina?

Ans. This is a severe bilateral brawny cellulitis of the sublingual and submandibular region. If neglected, this may cause respiratory obstruction due to edema of the glottis or by pushing the tongue against the roof of the mouth.

Q. How infection occurs in this area?

Ans. This may be secondary to:
- Suppuration in a lymph node.
- Suppuration may arise from a septic focus in the gums or teeth.

Q. What antibiotic?

Ans. Penicillin (10–15 million units) per 4–6 hours with metronidazole.

Procedure

- *Anesthesia*: General anesthesia is preferable.
- *Incision*:
  - A generous incision is made below the lower border of the mandible in the neck skin crease. There will be inflammatory edema in the deeper tissues (Fig. 20.6).
  - Cut through the skin and deep fascia.

Thrush a sinus forceps into the abscess cavity and open it up. All the pus is drained. A corrugated rubber sheet drain is inserted into the abscess cavity.

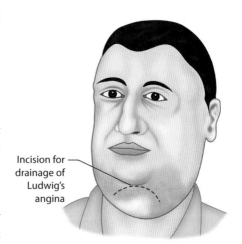

Incision for drainage of Ludwig's angina

Fig. 20.6: Ludwig's angina

■ PAROTID ABSCESS

Predisposing Factors

- Poor oral hygiene
- Debilitated patient
- Postoperative period when no proper mouth care is given
- Dehydration.

Procedure

- *Anesthesia*: General anesthesia (Figs 20.7A and B).
- *Incision*:
  - Start incision anterior to the tragus and go around the ear lobule to the mastoid and then take the incision downward along the anterior border of sternocleidomastoid in the upper part of the neck. The skin and subcutaneous tissue are incised and the skin flap is raised.
  - The parotid gland is exposed. Multiple incisions are made parallel to the branches of facial nerve. A sinus forceps is thrushed in through these incisions and the pus drained. A corrugated rubber sheet drain is kept and the skin incision closed with interrupted monofilament sutures.

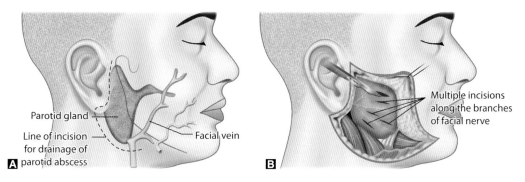

Parotid gland

Line of incision
for drainage of
A parotid abscess

Facial vein

Multiple incisions
along the branches
of facial nerve

B

Figs 20.7A and B: Parotid abscess

■ AXILLARY ABSCESS

Procedure

- *Anesthesia*: General anesthesia.
- *Incision*:
  - Make a 3–5-cm incision just behind the fold of pectoralis major muscle. The skin and subcutaneous tissue is incised (Fig. 20.8).
  - The pus is then drained by Hilton's method. A sinus forceps is thrushed into the abscess

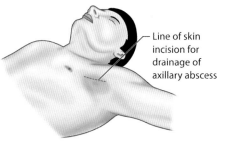

Line of skin
incision for
drainage of
axillary abscess

Fig. 20.8: Axillary abscess

cavity and the blades are opened parallel to the direction of axillary vessels to avoid injury to these structures and the pus drained. A corrugated rubber sheet drain is kept in the abscess cavity.

■ PERINEPHRIC ABSCESS

Perinephric abscess may occur secondary to a cortical abscess in the kidney or may arise due to hematogenous spread of infection.

Position of Patient

♦ Kidney position.

Procedure

♦ *Anesthesia*: General anesthesia.
♦ *Incision*:
  – A 15–20-cm long incision starting posteriorly from the lateral border of erector spinae and then along the bed of the 12th rib (Figs 20.9A to D).
  – Cut-down on the rib and the periosteum of the rib is deflected. The distal two-thirds of the 12th rib is excised. The perinephric space containing the abscess is exposed. A sinus forceps is thrushed into the abscess cavity and the blades are opened and the pus drained out. A corrugated drain is kept in the abscess cavity and the wound may be closed in layers.

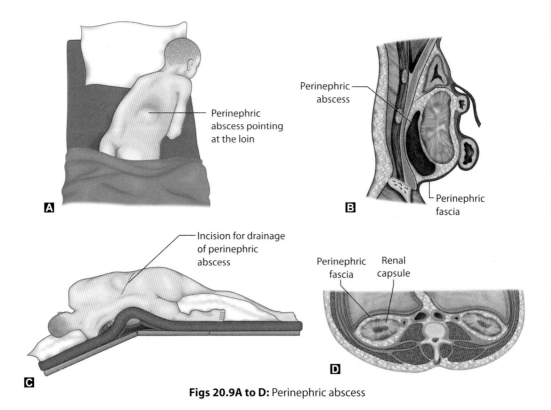

Figs 20.9A to D: Perinephric abscess

■ ANORECTAL ABSCESSES

Q. How does suppuration in perianal region start?

Ans. The infection starts in the anal glands, which mainly lie posteriorly. The infection from these glands may track:

* Downward to form a perianal abscess.
* Upward above the levator ani to form a pelvirectal abscess.
* Laterally to form an ischiorectal abscess. This may spread to the opposite side to form a horseshoe abscess.
* May spread in a submucous plane to form a submucous abscess.

Q. What are the usual organisms?

Ans.

* *Escherichia coli*
* *Staphylococcus aureus*
* *Proteus*
* *Bacteroides*
* *Streptococcus.*

Q. What are the different types of anorectal abscess?

Ans.

* Perianal
* Ischiorectal
* Submucous
* Pelvirectal (Fig. 20.10).

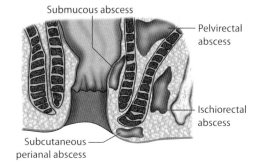

Fig. 20.10: Different types of anorectal abscess.

Q. How will you diagnose perianal suppuration?

Ans.

* *Perianal abscess*: Presents with perianal pain and swelling. There may be fever and toxemia.

  On rectal examination—there is a tense, tender swelling in the perianal region. Fluctuation is usually not demonstrable.
* *Ischiorectal abscess*: The presentation is usually the same but the toxemia may be more.

  On rectal examination—the swelling is usually more lateral; and on rectal examination, there may be a bulge in the lateral wall of the anal canal.
* *Submucous abscess*: Patient presents with rectal pain but no swelling.

  On rectal examination—reveals a soft, diffuse tender swelling bulging into the mucosa.
* *Pelvirectal abscess*: Patient may have general symptoms of fever but no rectal pain or swelling.

  On rectal examination—it may reveal a tender swelling in the lateral rectal wall above the anorectal sling. If the abscess points below into the ischiorectal fossa, a tender swelling may be palpable laterally in the perianal region.

Q. How will you drain perianal or ischiorectal abscess?

Ans.

+ *Anesthesia*: Preferably drained under general anesthesia.
+ *Position of the patient*: Patient in lithotomy position.
+ *Procedure*: A liberal cruciate incision is made over the most fluctuant part of the swelling (Fig. 20.11A). The incision is deepened and as the abscess cavity is entered, the pus will be drained. One finger is introduced through the incision into the abscess cavity and all the loculi are broken (Fig. 20.11B). The corners of the skin flaps are excised to deroot the abscess cavity (Fig. 20.11C).
+ Do a rectal examination and see if there is an associated fistula or not.
+ *If a fistula is not present*: The wound is lightly packed and a T bandage is applied.
+ *If a fistula is present*: The fistulous tract may be laid open and the cavity is lightly packed.
+ *Postoperative*: Daily sitz bath and dressing.

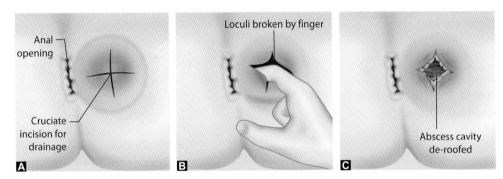

Figs 20.11A to C: Drainage of ischiorectal abscess

■ BREAST ABSCESS

Organisms

+ Most common organism is *Staphylococcus aureus*.

Drainage of Breast Abscess

+ Usually done under general anesthesia.
+ The breast is cleaned with an antiseptic solution—povidone–iodine and draped.
+ The abscess is first aspirated to confirm that pus is present.
+ A para-areolar incision is made over the affected segment of the breast over the most fluctuant part.
+ The incision is deepened to the subcutaneous tissue.
+ A sinus forceps is then inserted into the abscess cavity and the blades are opened and the pus is drained.
+ A finger is then introduced into the abscess cavity and all the loculi within the abscess cavity are broken.
+ The abscess cavity is lightly packed with a gauze or a drain is inserted into the abscess cavity for dependent drainage (Figs 20.12A to E).

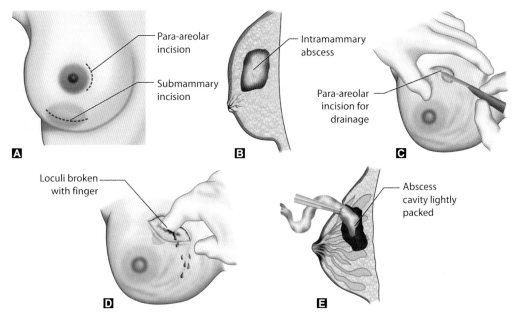

Figs 20.12A to E: Breast abscess

■ HAND INFECTIONS

Acute Paronychia

Q. What is paronychia?

Ans. Paronychia is an infection around the nail.

Q. How will you drain paronychia?

Ans.

* If the pus is present under one corner of the nail:
  – Digital block with a local anesthetic.
  – An incision is made at the angle of the nail. The skin flaps are raised and the corner of the nail is excised (Figs 20.13A to C).
  – If the pus has gone around the nail to the other side.
  – Incision at both corners of the nail. The skin flaps are raised and both corners of the nail are excised. The wound is packed with gauge.

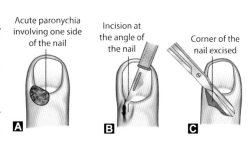

Acute paronychia involving one side of the nail

Incision at the angle of the nail

Corner of the nail excised

Figs 20.13A to C: Drainage of paronychia

■ DRAINAGE OF PULP SPACE INFECTION OF FINGER

Q. What is the anatomical peculiarity of pulp space infection of the finger?

Ans. The pulp of the finger is divided into many small fatty compartments by strands of fibrous tissue running from the skin to the periosteum of the terminal phalanx. A strand of fibrous tissue runs from the distal flexor crease to the periosteum of the terminal phalanx and separates the pulp space from the rest of the finger.

Because of this anatomical peculiarity, infection of the pulp space causes severe throbbing pain, as there is very little space for the pus to expand the pulp space.

Q. How to drain the pulp space infection?

Ans.
- Digital block with 1% injection lignocaine.
- *If the abscess is already pointing to the skin*: An incision is made over the pointing site removing a circular or an elliptical segment of skin. All the loculi are broken and the wound packed with a gauge (Figs 20.14A to D).
- *If the abscess is deep seated and not pointing to the skin*: A J-shaped lateral incision is made close to the free margin of the nail. The pus is drained and the wound is packed with gauze (Fig. 20.14E).

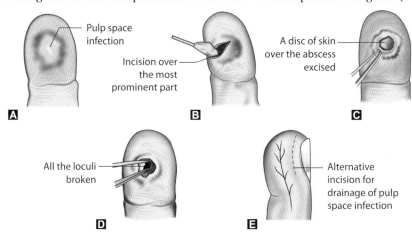

Figs 20.14A to E: Drainage of pulp space infection of finger

Q. How will you drain apical pulp space infection of finger?

Ans.
- Apical pulp space is the area between the distal part of the nail and the distal phalanx.
- Infection in this space causes pain at the tip of the finger with very little swelling and tenderness just under the free edge of the nail.
- *Incision*:
  - Digital block with 1% lignocaine injection.
  - A V-shaped incision at the tip of the finger taking a wedge of the nail (Figs 20.15A and B).

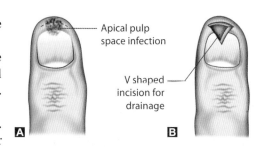

Figs 20.15A and B: Apical pulp space infection

■ VOLAR SPACE INFECTION

The pus may collect in the volar space deep to the epidermis, and deep to the deep fascia or in the tendon sheath. The proximal volar space communicates with the web space.

Collection of pus in the volar space is diagnosed by a swollen and tender finger, which is kept in semiflexion and attempt to straighten the finger causes severe pain.

Q. How to drain?

Ans.

◆ Digital block.
◆ The pus is drained by a transverse incision over the point of greatest tenderness (Fig. 20.16). The tendon sheath is not opened, if it is not infected. Avoid injury to the digital vessels and nerves.

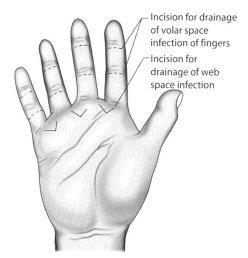

Incision for drainage of volar space infection of fingers

Incision for drainage of web space infection

Fig. 20.16: Incision for drainage of volar space and web space infection

■ WEB SPACE INFECTION

Anatomy of the Web Space

The web spaces lie between the bases of the fingers in the distal part of the palm and are filled with loose fat.

Diagnosis

Severe pain and swelling and the adjacent finger may become separated due to accumulation of good amount of pus.

From the web space, the pus may track to the dorsum of the hand, to the midpalmar space, and to the adjacent web space or to the volar space of the fingers.

Q. How to drain?

Ans.

◆ Median or ulnar nerve block depending on the site of infection (*See* Figs 20.35 and 20.36, Page No. 982, 983).
◆ *Incision*: A V-shaped incision is made on the dorsal aspect in-between the fingers. A sinus forceps is thrushed in and the pus is drained. The wound is lightly packed with gauge (Fig. 20.17).
◆ If the pus is pointing to the palmar aspect, a second V-shaped incision is made on the palmar aspect and the pus is drained (Fig. 20.16).

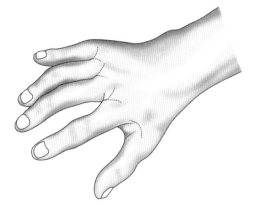

Fig. 20.17: Incision for drainage of web space infection

■ INFECTION OF MIDDLE PALMAR SPACE

Anatomy of Midpalmar Space

The midpalmar space lies between the flexor tendons and the lumbricals anteriorly and the fascia covering the interossei and the metacarpal posteriorly. It is separated from the thenar space by fibrous septa.

Diagnosis

The hand is grossly swollen. The normal hollow of the palm is obliterated and the dorsum of the hand is also swollen. The movement of the middle and ring fingers may be painful.

The infection from the midpalmar space may spread to the space of Parona, and pus tracking up deep to the flexor tendon.

Q. How to drain?

Ans.

- Median nerve block or general anesthesia.
- A transverse incision is made over the middle third of the proximal or distal palmar crease or over the site of maximal fluctuation. The abscess is drained by Hilton's method.

The incision is deepened up to the palmar fascia, which is not incised. A sinus forceps is thrushed in through the palmar fascia parallel to the flexor tendons and the blades are then opened to drain the pus. Avoid injury to the digital vessels, nerves, flexor tendons, or the lumbrical muscles [Fig. 20.18(A)].

■ THENAR SPACE INFECTION

Anatomy of Thenar Space

The thenar space is bounded anteriorly by the palmar fascia, and posteriorly by the transverse head of adductor pollicis. This space is separated from the midpalmar space by a fibrous septum.

Diagnosis

- There is a painful swelling on the thenar eminence and the thumb is abducted.

Q. How to drain?

Ans.

- Median nerve block.
- The thenar space is drained by an incision along the thenar crease. Insert a sinus forceps through the incision into the thenar space and the blades are opened to drain the pus [Fig. 20.18(B)].
- The thenar space may also be entered by an incision in the web between the thumb and the index finger on the dorsal side of the hand.

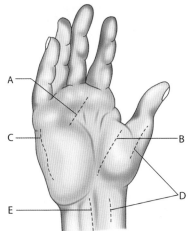

Fig. 20.18: Incisions for drainage of hand infection: A—incision for drainage of midpalmar space infection; B—incision for drainage of thenar space infection; C—incision for drainage of infection of ulnar bursa; D—incisions for drainage of radial bursa; and E—incision for drainage of infection at space of Parona

■ INFECTION OF ULNAR BURSA OF THE HAND

Anatomy

The ulnar bursa is the synovial sheath enclosing the flexor tendon of all the fingers. The flexor tendon sheath of the little finger may continue up to the ulnar bursa. The radial bursa may communicate with the ulnar bursa (Fig. 20.19).

Diagnosis of Infection of Ulnar Bursa

Painful swelling in the palm. There may be a fullness above the flexor retinaculum and edema in the dorsum of hand. The fingers are kept flexed and attempts of extension cause pain, which is most marked in case of little finger. The infection may spread to the radial bursa and there may be pain and swelling along the thumb. Thumb is held in flexion and attempts of extension cause pain.

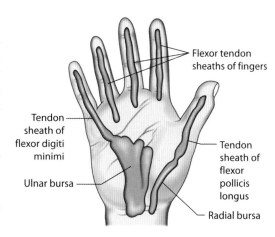

Fig. 20.19: Ulnar bursa, radial bursa, and flexor tendon sheaths of hand

Q. How to drain?

Ans.

* Ulnar nerve block or general anesthesia.
* Skin and deep fascia are incised over the anteromedial aspect of the fifth metacarpal bone [Fig. 20.18(C)]. Retract the abductor digiti minimi and flexor digiti minimi. Divide the attachment of the opponens digiti minimi to the flexor retinaculum. The ulnar bursa is seen bulging. The ulnar bursa is incised and pus drained out. A catheter is introduced into the bursa and the bursa irrigated with normal saline to wash out the pus.
* If there is infection of the flexor tendon sheath of the little finger—a transverse incision on the palmar aspect of the pulp space and volar space is made and deepened to open the flexor tendon sheath. The tendon sheath is then irrigated with normal saline.

Infection of the Radial Bursa

The radial bursa is the continuation of the tendon sheath of the flexor pollicis longus. Infection of a radial bursa results in painful swelling of the thumb and there may be swelling above the flexor retinaculum on the radial side. The thumb is held in flexion and attempt at extension causes pain. If treatment is delayed, the infection may spread to the ulnar bursa and the tendon of flexor pollicis longus may slough.

Q. How to drain?

Ans. A vertical incision along the radial aspect of the proximal phalanx of the thumb. The tendon sheath of the flexor pollicis longus is incised. A probe is passed up through the sheath and a proximal incision is made along the radial side of the wrist. A catheter is introduced into the tendon sheath and irrigated with saline. The wound is not closed and is lightly packed with gauze [Fig. 20.18(D)].

DRAINAGE OF INFECTION IN SPACE OF PARONA

The space of Parona is drained through a longitudinal incision on the side of palmaris longus tendon. The incision is deepened to the deep fascia and then a sinus forceps is thrushed behind the flexor tendons to enter the space of Parona [Fig. 20.18(E)].

INFECTION OF FLEXOR TENDON SHEATHS

The flexor tendon sheaths of the fingers may be infected by a pin prick or by spread of infection from the pulp or from the radial or ulnar bursa.

In flexor tendon sheath infection—there is painful swelling of the finger. The swelling may extend to the distal palm. In case of little finger and the thumb, the swelling may reach above the flexor retinaculum. The finger is partly flexed and extension will cause pain.

Q. How to drain?

Ans. Transverse incision over the flexion crease is made and the incision deepened up to the tendon sheath, which is opened and the pus is drained. If the infection reaches the distal palm additional transverse incision is made over the distal palm and the tendon sheath is opened. A catheter is introduced into the tendon sheath and irrigated with saline. The wound is lightly packed (Fig. 20.20).

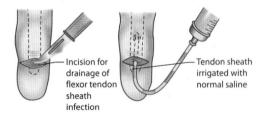

Incision for drainage of flexor tendon sheath infection

Tendon sheath irrigated with normal saline

Fig. 20.20: Infection of flexor tendon sheaths

Q. What may be the sequelae of tendon sheath infection?

Ans.
+ The tendon sheath infection may cause—adhesion of the tendon to the tendon sheath resulting in a stiff finger.
+ If there is collection of pus under tension, it may cause impairment of vascular supply of the tendon and results in ischemic necrosis of the flexor tendons.

ASPIRATION OF PLEURAL FLUID (THORACOCENTESIS)

Q. What are the indications of thoracocentesis?

Ans.
+ Aspiration of pleural fluid, pus or blood for diagnostic and therapeutic purposes.
+ Administration of some drugs intrapleurally.

Requirements

Sterile gloves, povidone–iodine solution, aspiration needle, three-way stop cock, one 5-mL and one 50-mL syringes, a receiver and injection lignocaine, and sterile dressing.

Site of Aspiration

Eighth intercostal space in the midaxillary line or 10th intercostal space in the posterior axillary line. This is usually the dullest area on percussion.

Procedure

* Patient is to be explained about the procedure and reassured that it will be painless.
* Patient sits in a bed with his arms folded and leaning over a bed table.
* Sterilize the skin over the aspiration site with an antiseptic solution like povidone–iodine.
* Infiltrate the skin and subcutaneous tissue and the parietal pleura over the chosen space at the upper border of the rib.
* Insert the needle with the stop cock in closed position piercing the skin, subcutaneous tissue and the pleura (Fig. 20.21). A 50-mL syringe is connected to the end of the stop cock and by turning the stop cock to on position, fluid is aspirated gently with the syringe. The stop cock is turned on to the side channel and the fluid is pushed out from the syringe to the reservoir via the side channel. The process of aspiration is then repeated by turning the stop cock to on position.
* The needle is then removed and the site is sealed with a sterile dressing.
* If the paracentesis is done for only diagnostic purpose 40–50 mL fluid is sufficient for examination.
* For therapeutic aspiration up to 1 L may be aspirated.

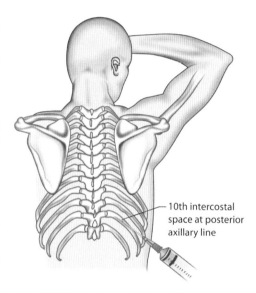

Fig. 20.21: Aspiration of pleural fluid through 10th intercostal space at posterior axillary line

10th intercostal space at posterior axillary line

INSERTION OF A CHEST DRAIN

Indications

* Traumatic hemothorax
* Traumatic pneumothorax
* Drainage of empyema
* Following thoracotomy.

Requirements

Sterile sheets, gloves and gown, antiseptic solution, swabs, injection 1% lignocaine, 5-mL and 50-mL syringe, needle, scalpel blade and suture, needle holder, dissecting forceps, scissors, silastic chest drainage tube and underwater seal drainage bag containing about 200-mL sterile water, one straight clamp, one curved clamp, and dressing and adhesive tape.

Selection of Site

- *For hemothorax*: The chest tube drain is inserted in the midaxillary line or posterior axillary line in the 8th intercostal space.
- *For pneumothorax*: The chest tube drain is inserted in the 2nd intercostal space anteriorly 3–5 cm from the lateral edge of the sternum. The drain may also be inserted in the triangle of safety, which is bounded by the anterior border of the latissimus dorsi, the posterior border of the pectoralis major and the superior border of the fifth rib. In case of pneumothorax, the tube is inserted in an upward direction toward the apex of the lung.

Procedure

- Patient lies comfortably in bed with the backrest lifted to about 45°. Wash hands and put on sterile gloves and gown. Clean the area with an antiseptic solution and drape. The skin, subcutaneous tissue, and the parietal pleura are infiltrated with 1% injection lignocaine.
- A short-skin incision is made with a No. 1 knife at the level of the upper border of the rib at the selected site. Using the curved clamp, the intercostal muscles are separated and reached up to the parietal pleura. The blunt dissection is completed with the index finger down up to the pleura. The chest tube held by a hemostatic forceps is thrushed through the pleura, puncturing it, and the tube is inserted into the pleural cavity.
- Alternatively, the tube may be inserted by using a stilette or a trocar to puncture the pleura.
- The tube is clamped with a hemostatic forceps and the closed end is cut off and the tube is connected to a water seal drainage bag, so that the tube inside the bag remains under the level of the water.
- The drain is fixed to the skin by inserting a stitch through the skin but not piercing the drain.
- Insert a stitch in circular fashion through the skin around the tube and kept untied (which will be tied after removal of the tube).
- A sterile dressing is applied at the exit of the tube.

Q. What are the complications of chest tube insertion?

Ans.
- Hemorrhage
- Damage to intercostal vessels and nerves
- Lung and mediastinal injury
- Infection.

PERICARDIOCENTESIS

Pericardiocentesis is aspiration of fluid from the pericardial cavity. Fluid, pus, or blood may accumulate in the pericardial cavity and may cause pericardial tamponade.

Q. What are the signs of collection of fluid in the pericardial cavity?

Ans.
- Distended neck veins with increased jugular venous pressure
- Pulsus paradoxus—reduction of pulse pressure on inspiration
- Pulsus alternans—QRS complex of alternately varying voltage
- A large cardiac shadow seen in chest X-ray.

Site of Aspiration

- In the epigastrium immediately to the left of xiphisternal junction.

Procedure

- The procedure should be done under electrocardiography (ECG) monitoring.
- The selected site is infiltrated with a local anesthetic solution (1% injection lignocaine).
- The needle fitted with a three-way stop cock is inserted immediately to the left of xiphias junction at an angle of 45° to the horizontal and 10° toward the left arm and pericardium is punctured. By turning the stop cock to the on position, the fluid is aspirated with a 50-mL syringe (Fig. 20.22).

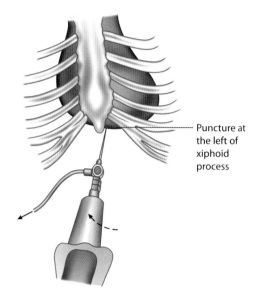

Puncture at the left of xiphoid process

Fig. 20.22: Pericardiocentesis

Q. What may be the complications?

Ans.

- Bleeding due to puncture of the heart by the needle.
- Ventricular fibrillation due to tip of the needle lying in the ventricular wall.

■ PERITONEAL FLUID TAP

Indications

- For aspiration of fluid for diagnostic purpose.
- To relieve respiratory distress due to massive accumulation of peritoneal fluid.

Site of Aspiration

- Usually aspirated at the flank or at the spinoumbilical line lateral to the rectus abdominis muscle.

Method of Aspiration

- Patient is to be explained about the procedure.
- Patient is asked to empty the bladder. Patient lies supine. The abdomen is percussed and the dull area in the flank is marked out.
- Wash hands and wear sterile gloves.
- Clean the skin with antiseptic solution (povidone–iodine) and drape the area with sterile towels.
- Infiltrate the area with 1% injection lignocaine.

◆ Insert a 20-G cannula through the skin and abdominal wall into the peritoneal cavity. The needle is withdrawn. Attach a three-way stop cock at the end of the cannula and the peritoneal fluid is aspirated with a 50-mL syringe (Fig. 20.23).

◆ After aspiration, the cannula is removed and the puncture site is sealed with a sterile dressing and adhesive tape.

◆ For diagnostic purpose, about 50 mL of fluid is enough.

◆ For symptomatic relief about 1,500 mL may be aspirated in one sitting. Aspiration of larger volumes may precipitate hypotension and promotes accumulation of further peritoneal fluid.

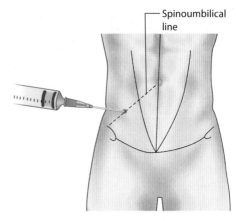

Fig. 20.23: Peritoneal fluid tap

Complications of Peritoneal Fluid Tap

◆ Bleeding
◆ Infection
◆ Injury to intra-abdominal viscera.

CRICOTHYROTOMY

This is an emergency measure to relieve upper airway obstruction where proper resuscitative facilities are not at hand.

The patient is placed supine or propped up against a convenient support. The cricothyroid membrane is marked by sliding a finger down from the thyroid cartilage into the gap between the thyroid and the cricoid cartilage (Fig. 20.24).

A skin puncture is made with a No. 11 knife at the level of the cricothyroid membrane. A large-bore cannula (12 or 14 G) is introduced through the cricothyroid membrane in a

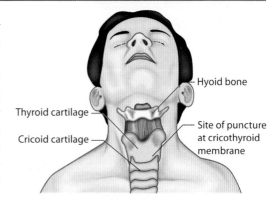

Fig. 20.24: Cricothyrotomy

downward direction. Once the cricothyroid membrane is punctured, the stylet is withdrawn and the cannula is passed down into the trachea.

Once the airway is secured, oxygen can be given through the cannula and the patient is shifted to a hospital.

In dire emergency, simply putting a wide-bore needle through the cricothyroid membrane may save life.

SCLEROTHERAPY FOR PILES

Indications of Sclerotherapy

First-degree and early second-degree piles may be treated by sclerotherapy.

Drugs for Sclerotherapy

- 5% phenol in almond oil
- Sodium tetradecyl sulfate
- Ethanolamine oleate
- Polidocanol.

Procedure

- Patient is explained about the procedure.
- Patient lies in a left lateral position.
- A per rectal examination is done to ensure that the rectum is empty.
- A proctoscope is introduced into the rectum and as the instrument is withdrawn, the pile masses are seen prolapsing into the proctoscope. The primary piles are situated at 3, 7, and 11 o'clock position.
- 2 mL of sodium tetradecyl sulfate is injected into the pedicle of each pile mass. The injection has to be done in the submucous plane at the pedicles of the pile mass (Fig. 20.25). Too superficial an injection will cause blanching of the mucosa and this will cause superficial necrosis.
- Patient should be given high-roughage diet and a stool softener.
- Patient may be reviewed after 6 weeks and further injections may be given, if necessary.

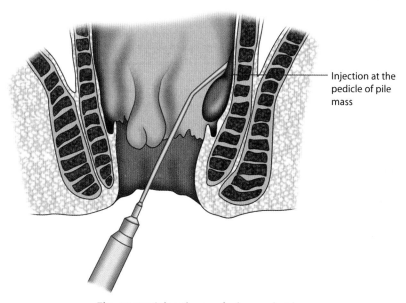

Injection at the pedicle of pile mass

Fig. 20.25: Sclerotherapy for hemorrhoids

SCLEROTHERAPY FOR GANGLION

* Ganglion is a cystic lesion arising from the synovium of a joint capsule or a tendon sheath.
* The fluid is thick and difficult to aspirate.
* The area is cleaned with antiseptic solution. The content of the ganglion is aspirated with 21-G needle and 10-mL syringe. About 2 mL of sclerosant (sodium tetradecyl sulfate) is injected into the ganglion and pressure bandage is applied with a crepe bandage.
* The bandage is maintained for 2 weeks.

LYMPH NODE BIOPSY

* The lymph node biopsy for a superficial node in the neck, axilla, or groin can be done under local anesthesia.
* The area is cleaned with antiseptic solution and draped.
* A local infiltration anesthesia is done by injecting 1% injection lignocaine. The injection is done all around the lymph node to achieve a ring block.
* The skin incision is made along the skin crease and length of the incision should be twice the size of the lymph node to be biopsied. The superficial fascia is incised in the same line.
* If the lymph node is lying deep to the deep fascia, the deep fascia is incised in the same line. The loose tissues around the lymph node are dissected. The lymph node has a small blood vessel, which is ligated and divided and the lymph node is excised.
* The wound is closed in layers.
* The lymph node capsule should not be grasped, as it may distort the histological feature.
* The material is sent to the laboratory in formalin solution.

EXCISION OF SEBACEOUS CYST

* The operation is usually done under local anesthesia.
* The area is cleaned with antiseptic solution and draped.
* Local anesthetic block using 1% lignocaine and ring block all around the cyst. Wait for 5 minutes for local anesthetic effect.
* An elliptical skin incision is made over the cyst centering the punctum (Fig. 20.26A). The skin incision is deepened taking care not to puncture the cyst wall (Fig. 20.26B). The skin flaps are raised and a plane is reached between the subcutaneous tissue and the cyst wall. Once this plane is reached, the cyst is dissected all around with a scissor and the cyst is excised completely (Fig. 20.26C). While dissecting at the depth, care should be taken to avoid any injury to the underlying vessels or nerves. The skin incision is closed with interrupted nonabsorbable sutures (Figs 20.26D and E).

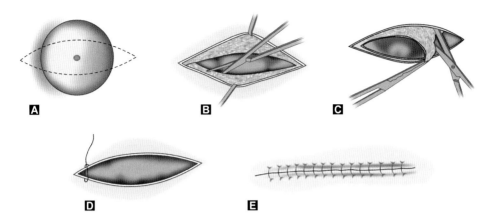

Figs 20.26A to E: Excision of sebaceous cyst

EXCISION OF LIPOMA

Small lipomas may be operated under local anesthesia. The lipomas may lie in different planes—subcutaneous, subfascial, intramuscular, subperiosteal, etc.

Excision of a Subcutaneous Lipoma

- Antiseptic cleaning, draping, and local anesthetic block as in sebaceous cyst.
- A linear skin incision is made over the swelling and the incision is deepened.
- The fat lobules of the lipoma are larger than the subcutaneous fat. There is a thin capsule lining the lipoma. Once the plane between the lipoma and the subcutaneous tissue is reached, the lipoma is shelled out by blunt dissection all around using a finger or a hemostatic forceps. The small vessels supplying the lipoma may be ligated and divided. Hemostasis is secured and the skin incision closed with a nonabsorbable suture taking care to avoid a dead space. The skin incision may be made slightly smaller than the lipoma, as the lipoma may be shelled out from one side by finger dissection and the remaining part dissected similarly.

MANAGEMENT OF INGROWING TOE NAIL

Ingrowing Toe Nail involving One Side of the Nail

- Ingrowing toe nail is a condition of nail margin digging into the nail wall resulting in inflammation of the tissues around the nail. Unilateral ingrowing toe nail is treated with segmental nail bed excision.
- The operation is done under digital nerve block.
- The great toe and the first web space are cleaned with an antiseptic solution.
- The digital nerve block is achieved by injecting 1% injection lignocaine at the base of the great toe on either side. A rubber tourniquet is applied at the base of the great toe.

- One-fifth segment of nail on the ingrown side is to be removed.
- An oblique 1-cm incision is made at the nail-fold angle, extending proximally to the transverse skin crease just distal to the interphalangeal joint.
- The skin flaps are raised proximally and the germinal epithelium of the nail is exposed.
- Following the line of the nail excision the germinal epithelium is excised.
- The skin flaps are replaced and sutured with 3-0 nonabsorbable sutures.
- A paraffin gauze, gauze, and crepe dressing are applied and the tourniquet is removed.

Double Edge Ingrowing Toe Nail

- *Zadek's operation*: Involves radical excision of the germinal epithelium of the whole nail.
- Alternatively, segmental excision of the germinal epithelium of the nail may be done on both sides leaving behind a central nail plate.

DORSAL SLIT OF PREPUCE

- This is indicated in patients with secondary phimosis with a growth underneath the prepuce to take a biopsy from the penile growth or prior to catheterization in patients with phimosis.
- The penis is cleaned with antiseptic solution and draped. Local anesthetic block.
- Two mosquito forceps are lightly applied to the preputial skin without crushing the skin.
- One blade of a pair of scissors is passed under the dorsal prepuce and a dorsal midline cut is made stopping a few millimeters from the corona.
- The bleeding points are tied with 3-0 chromic catgut sutures.
- Interrupted sutures are then used to appose the outer and the inner edges of the cut prepuce.

SCLEROTHERAPY FOR VARICOSE VEINS

Indications of Sclerotherapy for Varicose Veins

- Minor varicosities confined below the knee.
- Residual and recurrent varicosities following operations.

Contraindications of Sclerotherapy

- Saphenofemoral or saphenopopliteal incompetence
- Recurrent phlebothrombosis
- Persistent leg edema
- If associated with underlying deep-venous thrombosis.

Sclerosants Used

- *Sodium tetradecyl sulfate*—3% solution for larger veins and 0.5% for spider or thread veins.
- *Ethanolamine oleate*—5% solution.

The sclerosant causes sterile inflammation of the intima. The resultant fibrosis and the compression bandaging result in permanent occlusion of the dilated segment of the vein.

Procedure

See Surgical Long Cases Section, Page No. 321–344, Chapter 7.

EXPOSURE AND LIGATURE OF EXTERNAL CAROTID ARTERY

Indications

- In severe maxillofacial injury causing uncontrolled bleeding.
- Bleeding from malignant tumors in head and neck region may be controlled with external carotid artery ligation.
- To control bleeding during meningioma excision.

Anatomy of External Carotid Artery

The common carotid artery divides at the level of the upper border of the thyroid cartilage to form the internal and external carotid arteries. The external carotid artery lies deep to the posterior belly of digastric and ascends upward behind the neck of the mandible and ends by dividing into superficial temporal artery and maxillary artery.

Branches of External Carotid Artery

- Ascending pharyngeal artery
- Superior thyroid artery
- Lingual artery
- Facial artery
- Occipital artery
- Posterior auricular artery
- Maxillary artery
- Superficial temporal artery.

Steps of Exposure

- *Anesthesia*: Local anesthesia or general anesthesia.
- *Position of the patient*: Supine with head end elevated by 10° and head turned to the opposite side and the neck is extended slightly.
- *Incision*: An oblique incision is made in the skin from in front of the mastoid process to the level of the upper border of the thyroid cartilage (Fig. 20.27A). The platysma is incised in the same line. The upper and lower skin flans are raised.
- *Exposure of the carotid sheath*: The anterior border of the sternocleidomastoid is freed by incising the investing layer of the deep cervical fascia. The common facial vein, which comes on the way, is ligated and divided.
- *Exposure of the common carotid artery*: The carotid sheath is opened and the internal jugular vein is retracted and the common carotid artery is seen dividing into the internal and external carotid artery (Fig. 20.27B).

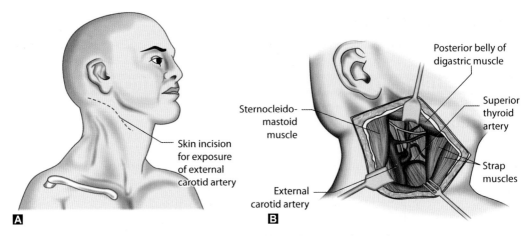

Figs 20.27A and B: Exposure and lying the external carotid artery

The external carotid artery is identified by branches arising from it in the neck. Internal carotid artery has no branch in the neck. The external carotid artery is dissected free and a ligature is passed around the external carotid artery by using an aneurysm needle or a right-angle forceps. The ligature is then tied. The artery needs not be divided.

Q. What may be the problems?

Ans.
- Injury to the hypoglossal nerve, which crosses the bifurcation of the common carotid artery.
- Irritation of the carotid sinus during dissection may cause bradycardia.
- Difficulty in identifying the external carotid artery.

EXPOSURE OF SUBCLAVIAN ARTERY IN THE NECK

Anatomy of Aubclavian Artery

The right subclavian artery arises from the brachiocephalic trunk and the left subclavian artery arises from the arch of the aorta.

The subclavian artery crosses the root of the neck and passes over the first rib behind the scalenus anterior muscle, which divides this artery into three parts:
1. *First part*—part of the artery lying medial to the medial border of the scalenus anterior muscle.
2. *Second part*—part of the artery lying behind the scalenus anterior muscle.
3. *Third part*—part of the artery lying laterally to the scalenus anterior muscle.

Exposure of the Third Part of the Subclavian Artery

Indication

In fracture of the neck of the humerus, there may be injury to axillary artery. Before exploring the hematoma, the proximal control is achieved by exposing the subclavian artery in the neck.

Position of the Patient

Patient supine, head-end elevated by 10°, and head turned to the opposite side. Keep the hands by the side of the patient and draw it downward to depress the shoulder.

Anesthesia

◆ Local anesthesia or general anesthesia.

Incision

A transverse incision is made in the supraclavicular fossa 2 cm above the clavicle from the sternal border of the sternocleidomastoid to the anterior border of the trapezius (Fig. 20.28A).

Procedure

◆ The subcutaneous tissue, platysma, and the deep fascia are incised in the same line. If external jugular comes on the way, it may be ligated and divided (Fig. 20.28B).
◆ The omohyoid muscle is retracted upward and the third part of the subclavian artery is exposed.
◆ The trunk of the brachial plexus lies laterally to the artery and the subclavian vein lies in front of the artery and below it.
◆ The third part of the subclavian artery is dissected and a ligature is passed around the artery by aneurysm needle or a right-angle forceps.

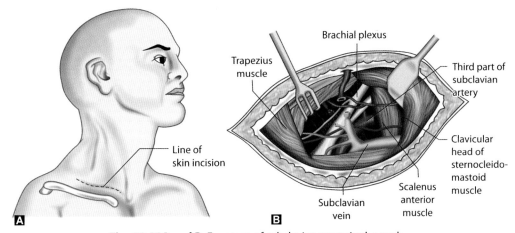

Figs 20.28A and B: Exposure of subclavian artery in the neck

EXPOSURE AND LIGATURE OF THE INTERNAL ILIAC ARTERY

Indications of Internal Iliac Artery Ligation

◆ Severe and continuing uterine hemorrhage following delivery or cesarean section or following abortion is one of the most common indications for unilateral or bilateral internal iliac artery ligation.
◆ Rupture uterus or uterine trauma causing uncontrolled bleeding.

Anesthesia

Regional anesthesia (spinal or epidural) or general anesthesia.

Position of the Patient

Supine.

Incision

Lower midline incision.

Procedure

- Identify the ureter crossing the pelvic brim.
- The ureter crosses the pelvic brim at the level of the bifurcation of the common iliac artery into the external iliac and the internal iliac artery (Fig. 20.29A).
- The peritoneum is incised at this level and the ureter is retracted (Figs 20.29B and C).
- The bifurcation of the common iliac artery is exposed and the internal iliac artery is dissected all around and a ligature is passed around the internal iliac artery by using an aneurysm needle or a right-angle forceps (Figs 20.29D to F).

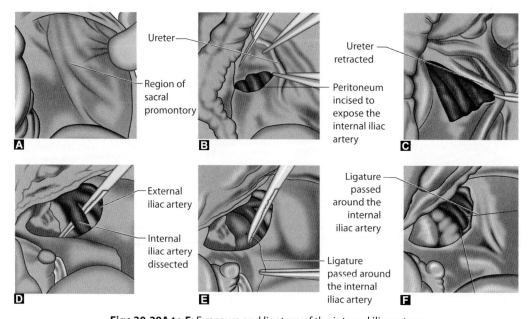

Figs 20.29A to F: Exposure and ligature of the internal iliac artery

EXPOSURE OF THE EXTERNAL ILIAC ARTERY

Anatomy

The external iliac artery arises at the pelvic brim from the common iliac artery and runs to the midinguinal point and courses behind the inguinal ligament and continues as femoral artery in the thigh. The external iliac vein lies medial to it and the psoas muscle lies behind the artery and the femoral nerve lies 1 cm lateral to the artery with genitofemoral nerve running in-between.

Two branches arise from the external iliac artery:

1. Inferior epigastric artery running into the rectus sheath.
2. Deep circumflex iliac artery runs laterally along the inguinal ligament.

Position of the Patient

Supine with moderate Tendelenburg tilt.

Incision

An inguinal incision just above the inguinal ligament (Fig. 20.30A).

Procedure

◆ The skin and subcutaneous tissues are incised. The external oblique aponeurosis is incised along its fibers and the inguinal canal is exposed.
◆ The muscular fibers of the internal oblique are divided. The spermatic cord is retracted upward and medially.
◆ The fascia transversalis is divided and the peritoneum is stripped off medially and the external iliac vessels are exposed.
◆ The external iliac artery is dissected carefully from the external iliac vein and a ligature is passed around the external iliac artery by using an aneurysm needle or a right-angle forceps and the artery may be tied (Fig. 20.30B).

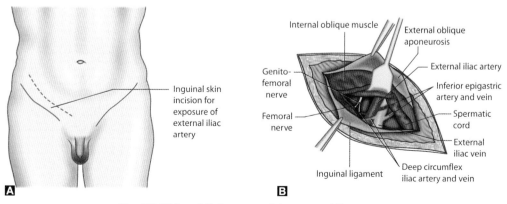

Figs 20.30A and B: Exposure of the external iliac artery

EXPOSURE OF THE FEMORAL ARTERY IN THE THIGH (IN ADDUCTOR CANAL)

Anatomy

The femoral artery starts at the midinguinal point, as the continuation of external iliac artery. It courses in the thigh obliquely first across the femoral triangle and then underneath the sartorius muscle. It ends at the junction of middle and lower third of the thigh by going through a hole in the adductor magnus muscle and continues as the popliteal artery in back of knee joint. In the femoral triangle, the femoral vein lies medially and the femoral nerve lies laterally.

Branches of Femoral Artery

Superficial circumflex iliac, superficial epigastric, superficial and deep external pudendal arteries arise near the origin of the femoral artery. The profunda femoris artery arises 3 cm below the inguinal ligament.

Indication

Penetrating wound in the thigh may require femoral artery ligation. Femoral artery ligation should be done below the origin of the profunda femoris artery to maintain collateral circulation in the leg.

Position of the Patient

Patient supine and the thigh flexed slightly and rotated laterally.

Incision

- A line joining the midinguinal point and the adductor tubercle. The middle third of this line is the femoral artery in the adductor canal.
- Make skin incision over the middle third of the above line (Fig. 20.31A).

Procedure

- The subcutaneous tissue and the deep fascia are incised.
- The sartorius muscle is retracted medially. The fibrous sheath forming the roof of the subartorial canal is incised. The femoral artery is exposed. The femoral artery is carefully dissected from the vein. A ligature may then be passed around the femoral artery using an aneurysm needle or a right-angle forceps (Fig. 20.31B).

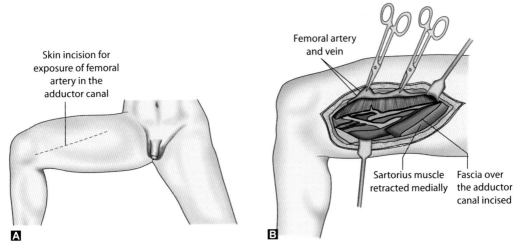

Skin incision for exposure of femoral artery in the adductor canal

Femoral artery and vein

Sartorius muscle retracted medially

Fascia over the adductor canal incised

A   **B**

Figs 20.31A and B: Exposure of the femoral artery in the thigh (in adductor canal)

EXPOSURE OF THE POPLITEAL ARTERY

Anatomy

Popliteal artery begins as a continuation of the femoral artery at an opening in the medial aspect of the adductor magnus. It courses downward in the popliteal fossa and at the lower border of popliteus muscle, it trifurcates into—anterior tibial, posterior tibial, and the peroneal arteries.

Position of the Patient

Patient lies prone. General anesthesia with endotracheal intubation or regional anesthesia.

Incision

Make 15-cm long lazy "S" incision over the center of the popliteal fossa (Fig. 20.32A).

Procedure

- The skin and the subcutaneous tissues are incised. The sural nerve is retracted.
- The deep fascia over the roof of the popliteal fossa is incised in the same line. The hamstring muscle and two heads of the gastrocnemius muscles are then retracted.
- The popliteal artery is carefully dissected from the popliteal vein, which accompanies the artery. The branches arising from the artery are to be preserved to maintain the collateral circulation.

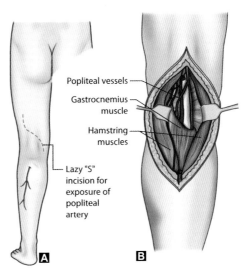

Popliteal vessels

Gastrocnemius muscle

Hamstring muscles

Lazy "S" incision for exposure of popliteal artery

A   **B**

Figs 20.32A and B: Exposure of the popliteal artery

◆ A ligature is passed around the popliteal artery by passing an aneurysm needle or a right-angle forceps around the artery (Fig. 20.32B).

PERIPHERAL NERVE BLOCKS

■ DIGITAL NERVE BLOCK

Procedure

◆ 1% lignocaine hydrochloride without adrenaline is used for digital nerve block (Fig. 20.33).
◆ 5-mL lignocaine is drawn into the syringe and the needle (25 G) is inserted through the dorsal aspect of the interdigital web, 0.5 mL of lignocaine is injected at the point of entry of the needle to block the dorsal digital nerve. The needle is then advanced ventrally and 1 mL of lignocaine is injected to block the palmar digital nerve.
◆ The procedure is repeated on other side of the digit.

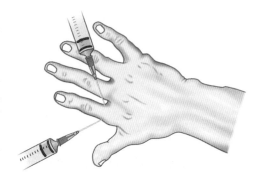

Fig. 20.33: Digital nerve block

■ MEDIAN NERVE BLOCK

Procedure

◆ The median nerve lies at the midline in the wrist immediately below the tendon of palmaris longus (Fig. 20.34).
◆ The forearm is kept supine and the needle is inserted on the ulnar border of the palmaris longus tendon, 2 cm proximal to the distal wrist crease, and 3–5 mL of 1% lignocaine is injected to achieve median nerve block.

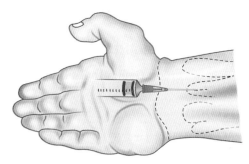

Fig. 20.34: Median nerve block

■ ULNAR NERVE BLOCK

With the forearm supinated the needle is inserted to the radial side of the flexor carpi ulnaris tendon and 3 cm proximal to the distal wrist crease 3–5 mL of 1% lignocaine is injected to achieve ulnar nerve block (Fig. 20.35). The dorsal branch of the ulnar nerve is blocked by subcutaneous injection of 1% lignocaine between the proximal edge of the pisiform bone and the middle of the dorsum of the wrist.

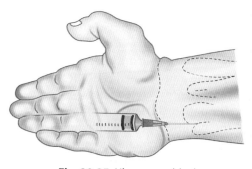

Fig. 20.35: Ulnar nerve block

■ POSTERIOR TIBIAL NERVE BLOCK

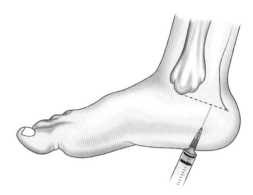

Fig. 20.36: Posterior tibial nerve block

Posterior tibial nerve is blocked by injecting 3–5 mL of 1% lignocaine by inserting needle just anterior to the Achilles tendon at the level of medial malleolus (Fig. 20.36).

Instruments

■ INTRODUCTION

In examination, proper identification of instrument is very important. Mention the complete name of the instrument, e.g. medium-sized curved hemostatic forceps. In next part of the examination it is usually asked, where have you used/seen to have been used this instrument. Try to name some operations where a particular instrument is used and at what step of the operation. Then mention about what are the other uses of this instrument.

Sterilization of the instrument is usually asked. There are various methods for sterilization of instruments. Mention about one method of sterilization best for the particular instrument. If examiner asks about other methods of sterilization then mention about other methods of sterilization.

Q. What is sterilization?

Ans. Sterilization is a process by which all microorganisms like bacteria, fungi, viruses, and the bacterial spores are killed.

Q. What is disinfection?

Ans. Disinfection is the process by which microorganisms are killed or removed excepting the bacterial spores. Disinfection may be:
- *Low level disinfection*: Decreases the overall number of microorganisms. The tubercle bacilli and bacterial spores are not killed.
- *Intermediate level of disinfection*: Kills tubercle bacilli and other microorganism, most viruses and fungi.
- *High level disinfection*: Kills almost all microorganisms but does not kill the bacterial spores.

Q. What are the different techniques of disinfection of instruments?

Ans.
- *Boiling*: Boiling at 100°C for 5 minutes at normal pressure.
- *Formaldehyde vapor*: Instruments kept in formaldehyde vaporizer at 50°C.
- *Glutaraldehyde solution*: Instruments kept dipped in 2% glutaraldehyde solution for 15–20 minutes.
- *Low temperature steam*: Exposure to dry saturated steam at a temperature of 73°C for 20 minutes at subatmospheric pressure.

■ STERILIZATION OF INSTRUMENTS

There are various techniques for sterilization of instruments:

- *Autoclaving*: Autoclaving is a method of sterilization using steam under high pressure.
  - *Standard autoclaving*: involves sterilization at a temperature of 121°C at 15 lb/sq inch pressure for 30 minutes for metallic instruments and 15 minutes for rubber goods (Catheters, gloves, drains, etc.)
  - *High pressure autoclaving*: In central sterilization unit for bulk sterilization high pressure autoclaving is suitable. This involves sterilization at a temperature of 134°C at a pressure of 30 lb/sq inch for 3 minutes.
- *Boiling*: Boiling for half an hour kills all the bacteria and its spores. Boiling of the instruments should be continued for half an hour after water achieves a temperature of 100°C.
- This is not suitable for sharp instruments as there is loss of sharpness due to boiling and there is formation of crust over the instruments
- *Chemical sterilization*: A number of chemicals are used for sterilization of instruments. Sharp instruments are particularly sterilized by keeping them dipped in chemicals.
  - *2% Glutaraldehyde solution (Cidex)*: For sterilization, the instruments should be kept immersed in glutaraldehyde solution for 4 hours.
  - However, for disinfection of instruments, dipping for a period of 15–20 minutes is adequate. Fiber-optic instruments like laparoscope, laparoscopic hand instruments, and cystoscopes are sterilized by keeping them in glutaraldehyde solution. In between cases a period of 15–20 minutes of dipping is adequate for disinfection.
  - *Lysol*: This is used for sterilization of sharp instruments. Dipping in concentrated lysol for 1 hour is adequate for sterilization. If dilute lysol is used, the instrument should be kept immersed for 24 hours.
  - *70% alcohol*: Needles, unused sutures may be kept immersed in 70% alcohol for 12 hours for subsequent use.
  - *Sterilization by peracetic acid (Steris)*: This is effective against all microorganisms including the bacterial spores. The method involves immersion of the instrument in the chemical peracetic acid at a *temperature of 50–56°C* for 12 minutes.
- *Gas sterilization*:
  - *Ethylene oxide gas*: A special ethylene oxide gas chamber is required for sterilization of instruments using ethylene oxide gas. Instruments are kept in the chamber exposed to ethylene oxide for 12 hours, i.e. overnight
    Large ethylene oxide gas chambers are also used for industrial sterilization.
  - *Formaldehyde gas*: Formalin tablets placed in a formalin vaporizer lead to formation of formaldehyde gas. Optical instruments like cystoscope, laparoscope may be sterilized by keeping them in formalin vaporizer for 1 hour.
- *Plasma sterilization*
- *Others*:
  - *Gamma irradiation*: This is not applicable for sterilization of instruments in operative theater setup but is useful for large scale industrial sterilization.
  - *Direct flaming*: In case of urgency when an instrument has fallen down from the operation table and is urgently required, it may be sterilized by direct flaming. The instrument is kept in a bowl and some amount of rectified spirit is poured and flamed. Direct flaming may

achieve a temperature as high as 1,400°C. However, direct flaming is damaging for sharp instruments.

- *Hot air oven*: Ward articles like glass syringes, test tubes may be sterilized in a hot air oven. Keeping the instruments in hot air oven at a temperature of 160°C for 2 hours is adequate for sterilization by this technique.

All the metal instruments are sterilized by autoclaving. All the rubber articles like gloves and catheters are sterilized by autoclaving for 15 minutes instead of 30 minutes required for metal instruments.

Sharp instruments like scissors, needles, and scalpel blades are kept dipped in lysol or glutaraldehyde solution for sterilization.

Parts of an instrument (Fig. 21.1A): A typical surgical instrument consists of:

- Two finger bows for holding the instrument
- A pair of shaft or body of the instrument
- A catch or a ratchet: Once the ratchets are pressed the blades are kept in a closed position
- Blades: A pair of blades constitutes the terminal part of the instrument
- Joint: The two parts of the shaft and the blades are kept attached by a joint. This joint may be either a box joint or a pivot joint.
  - In box joint there is a slot in one shaft and the other shaft is passed through this slot (Fig. 21.1B).
  - In pivot joint the two shafts are attached at one point by a screw (Fig. 21.1C).

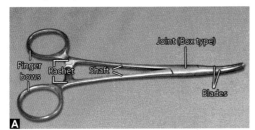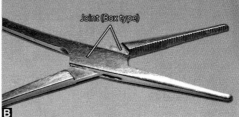

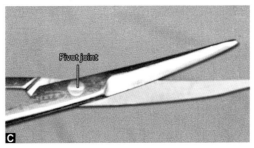

Figs 21.1A to C: Parts of an instrument

▉ RAMPLEY'S SWAB HOLDING FORCEPS

This is a long instrument (average 9.5" in length). The instrument is provided with finger bows and a pair of long shaft. The shaft has a ratchet, a joint, and a pair of blades. The blades are oval, fenestrated and provided with serrations on the inner aspect. This instrument may be straight or curved (Figs 21.2A to C).

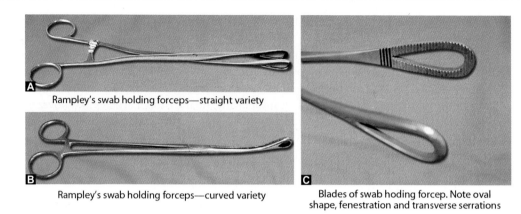

A   Rampley's swab holding forceps—straight variety

B   Rampley's swab holding forceps—curved variety

C   Blades of swab hoding forcep. Note oval shape, fenestration and transverse serrations

Figs 21.2A to C: Swab holding forceps

Uses

- It is used for cleansing the skin with swab dipped in antiseptic solution during all operations
- It is used for holding a swab which is used to clean the blood during dissection of Calot's triangle during cholecystectomy
- The swab held up in the forceps is also used for cleaning the blood in the suture line during gastrojejunostomy, small and large gut anastomosis
- The swab held up in the forceps is also used to strip off the peritoneum from the fascia transversalis while approaching the retroperitoneum for kidney exposure or during lumbar sympathectomy
- It is used for removing the laminated membrane and the daughter cysts during operation of hydatid cyst
- This may be used to hold the fundus and Hartmann's pouch of the gallbladder during cholecystectomy
- This may be used as ovum forceps
- This may be used to swab an abscess cavity
- This may be used as a tongue holding forceps.

Sterilization

It is done by autoclaving.

Q. Why is the instrument long?

Ans.
- The instrument is made longer to enable the surgeon to apply the antiseptic solution to the skin without touching the unsterile field of operation (Figs 21.2A to C)
- The swab held up in between the blades may be used for swabbing at a depth.

Q. How will you remove hair from the skin?

Ans. The skin hair may be removed by shaving or application of epilation cream. Shaving is not a good procedure as it may cause microscopic cuts in the skin where bacterial proliferation may occur overnight. If shaving is to be done at all it should be done in the morning of day of operation. Application of epilating cream is a better choice.

Q. How will you do antiseptic cleansing of skin before operation?

Ans. During all operations the skin needs to be cleansed with antiseptic solution. For abdominal operation the skin from midchest to midthigh should be cleaned. Various antiseptic solutions are used for skin preparation:

- Application of 2–3 layers of povidone iodine which is 2% iodine in polyvinylpyrrolidone. Povidone iodine releases iodine slowly and provides longer duration of antiseptic effect. It is effective against both bacteria and fungus
- Cleansing with spirit, tincture iodine and spirit
- Cleansing with Savlon (Cetrimide solution) and spirit.

Q. What area should you clean for an abdominal operation?

Ans. An area from midchest to midthigh is to be cleaned with antiseptic solution for abdominal operation.

■ TOWEL CLIPS

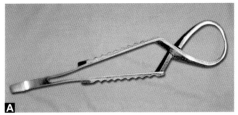

A

Doyens' cross action type towel clip

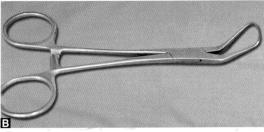

B

Backhaus' towel (corner) clip

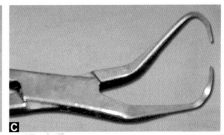

C

Blades of towel clip. Note the curved pointed tip

Figs 21.3A to C: Towel clips

Doyens' Cross Action Type Towel Clip

This is a pincer-like instrument, on pressing the shaft the instrument opens up and on releasing the shaft the instrument closes and the two clips meet each other and provide the pinching action (Fig. 21.3A).

Backhaus' Towel (Corner) Clip

This instrument is provided with finger bows, a ratchet, a pair of shaft, and two sharp hooks. On closing the ratchet the two clips are apposed and on releasing the ratchet the clips open up (Fig. 21.3B).

Uses

- It is used for fixing the draping sheets
- It is used for fixing the diathermy cables, suction tubes, laparoscopic camera cables, and fiber-optic light cables to the draping sheets taking care not to pierce any of these with the towel clip
- It may be used as a tongue holding forceps
- It may be used as cord holding forceps
- It may be used for holding the ribs while elevating a flail segment of chest.

Sterilization

It is done by autoclaving.

Q. What is draping?

Ans. Draping is suitable placement of sheets to isolate the area of operation from the rest of the body. Draping of the operative site reduces the contamination from the adjacent skin areas.

▎BARD-PARKER'S HANDLES

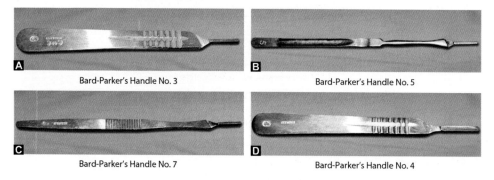

Bard-Parker's Handle No. 3

Bard-Parker's Handle No. 5

Bard-Parker's Handle No. 7

Bard-Parker's Handle No. 4

Figs 21.4A to D: Bard-Parker's handle

Bard–Parker's (BP) handle is a flat stainless steel instrument with one end narrower with a slot on either side for attaching the scalpel blade. A number is written on the handle. The numbers may be 3, 5, 7, and 4 (Figs 21.4A to C).

In scalpel handle No. 4 (Fig. 21.4D) the site for attachment of the blade is little wider than the handle number 3, 5, and 7 where it is little narrower.

Sterilization

It is done by autoclaving.

▎SURGICAL BLADES

Blades number 10, 11, 12, and 15 fit in BP handle number 3, 5, and 7 (Fig. 21.5A).

Blades number 18, 19, 20, 21, 22, 23, and 24 fit in BP handle number 4 (Fig. 21.5B).

The blades are detachable and a new blade is used for every patient, so there is no problem with sharpness of the blade.

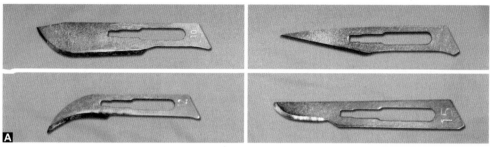

Blades No. 10, 11, 12, 13 and 15 for BP Handle No. 3, 5 and 7

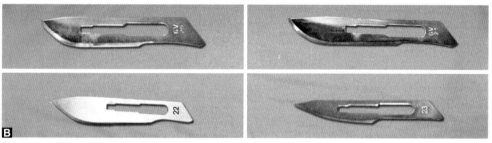

Blades No. 18, 19, 20, 21, 22, 23 and 24 for BP Handle No. 4

Figs 21.5A and B: Surgical blades

Sterilization

Sterilization is supplied in presterilized pack.

Q. What are the uses of BP handle and blade?

Ans.
* It is used to make skin incisions for any operation. The blade numbers 20, 21, 22, 23, and 24 have wide shaft and are used for larger incisions and dissections
* The blade number 15 has a narrow shaft and is used for smaller incisions, while excising a sebaceous cyst or during venesection
* It is used for incision and drainage of an abscess. The blade number 11 is also known as stab knife and is used to incise the skin for drainage of an abscess
* It is used to incise the skin for inserting drains.

Q. Apart from making skin incisions where else is the scalpel used?

Ans.
* The scalpel is also used for sharp dissection to raise skin flaps during mastectomy, incisional hernia repair, during thyroidectomy, and radical neck dissection
* The scalpel is also used to divide the cystic duct and artery during cholecystectomy after these are ligated

- The renal and splenic pedicle may also be divided by a scalpel after ligature during nephrectomy and splenectomy.
- Blade number 11 is used for incision and drainage of abscess.

Q. What are the different abdominal incisions?

Ans. The different abdominal incisions are (Fig. 21.6):

- *Midline incision*:
  - Upper (above the umbilicus)
  - Lower (below the umbilicus)
  - Mid-midline (midline incision centering the umbilicus).

  Indicated in emergency exploratory laparotomy, gastric operations, colonic resection, abdominoperineal resection and anterior resection.

- *Paramedian incision*:
  - Right paramedian incision—vertical incision 2.5 cm to the right of midline. Indicated in gallbladder surgery and right hemicolectomy
  - Left paramedian incision—same incision to the left of midline

  Indicated in gastric operations, left hemicolectomy, and splenectomy.

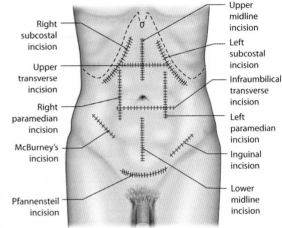

Fig. 21.6: Abdominal incisions

- *Mayo Robson's incision:* Right upper paramedian incision extended like a hockey stick to the midline. Indicated in cholecystectomy.
- *Subcostal incision*:
  - *Right subcostal incision (Kocher's subcostal incision)*—oblique incision 2 cm below and parallel to the right costal margin, extending from midline to beyond the tip of the costal cartilage. Indicated in cholecystectomy, common bile duct exploration, and biliary enteric bypass
  - *Left subcostal incision*—same incision on the left subcostal region. Indicated for splenectomy
  - *Roof top or chevron incision*—bilateral subcostal incision joined in the midline. For pancreatic surgery—Whipple's operation, pancreaticojejunostomy and for liver resection.
- *Transverse incision*:
  - Upper abdominal transverse incision. Indicated for gallbladder surgery and gastric operations
  - Infraumbilical transverse incision. Indicated for exploratory laparotomy in children
  - Suprapubic transverse incision (Pfannenstiel incision). For pelvic operations and prostatectomy.
- *McBurneys' Gridiron incision*: Indicated for appendicectomy.
- *Lanz incision*: It is used for appendicectomy.
- *Inguinal incision:* Incision at the inguinal canal running parallel to the inguinal ligament. It is used for hernia operations.

- *Loin incision or lumbar incision*: Incision from the lateral border of erector spinae downward and forward midway between the 12th rib and the iliac crest up to the lateral border of rectus abdominis. It is used for operations in kidney.
- *Mercedes Benz incision*: Bilateral subcostal incision with vertical incision extending from center of the ∧-shaped cut to the xiphoid process.

■ HEMOSTATIC FORCEPS

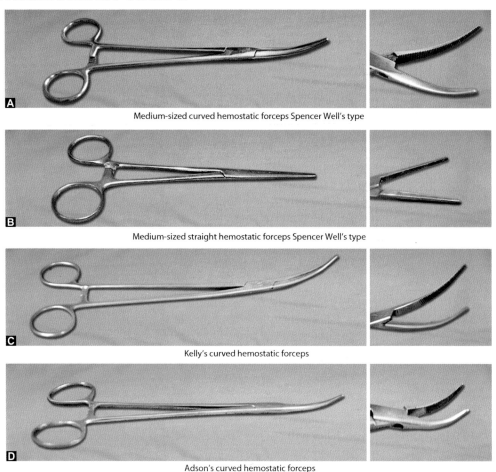

Medium-sized curved hemostatic forceps Spencer Well's type

Medium-sized straight hemostatic forceps Spencer Well's type

Kelly's curved hemostatic forceps

Adson's curved hemostatic forceps

Figs 21.7A to D: Hemostatic forceps. In Spencer Well's variety note the transverse serrations in the whole length of the blade. In Kelly and Adson's variety the transverse serrations are in distal part of the blade

- *Spencer Well's hemostatic forceps* are provided with finger bows, ratchet, a pair of shaft, and a pair of blades. The blades are usually half the length of the shaft. The full length of the blades is provided with transverse serrations. The tips are conical and nontoothed. When the ratchet is closed the blades are apposed (Figs 21.7A and B).
- *Kelly's hemostatic forceps* are longer. The blades are long and the transverse serrations are not present along the whole length of the blades (Fig. 21.7C).

- *Adson hemostatic forceps*: The blades are smaller in comparison to the shaft. The transverse serration is present in the terminal part of the blades (Fig. 21.7D).

Q. How will you differentiate it from a needle holder?

Ans. The hemostatic forceps are lighter instrument. The blades are longer and there are transverse serrations in the blades.

The needle holder is a relatively heavier instrument. The blades are smaller and there are criss-cross serrations in the blade and there may be a groove in the center of each blade.

Uses of Hemostatic Forceps

- It is used during all operations. It is used to hold bleeding vessels while cutting through different layers of tissues
- While making abdominal incisions and during the closure of the incision the hemostatic forceps is used to hold the cut margins of the rectus sheath, linea alba, external oblique aponeurosis, and the surgical peritoneum
- During appendicectomy through McBurney's Gridiron incision the hemostatic forceps may be used to split the internal oblique and transversus abdominis muscle. It may be used to crush the base of appendix during appendicectomy
- While doing intestinal resection and anastomosis, the mesenteric vessels are held in between hemostatic forceps and the desired line of mesentery is divided
- It may be used to dissect the vein while doing venesection in the arm (basilic or cephalic vein) or in the leg (great saphenous vein)
- It may be used for blunt dissection while doing lymph node biopsy, excision of lipoma sebaceous cyst
- It may be used to open an abscess by Hilton's method
- It may be used to hold the end of a ligature while suturing
- It may be used to tie a knot after suturing
- It may be used as a dressing forceps.

Sterilization

It is done by autoclaving.

Q. While making incisions how will you control bleeding?

Ans. Bleeding from the incision site may be controlled with:
- *Simple pressure*: Fine capillary bleeding may be simply controlled by pressure with a mop.
- *Crushing*: The bleeding may be controlled by simply crushing the bleeding point with a hemostatic forceps. Crushing causes curling of tunica media and intima inward and causes occlusion of the lumen of the vessel.
- *Electrocautery*: The bleeding point held by a hemostatic forceps may be coagulated with diathermy.
- *Ligature*: The bleeding point held by a hemostatic forceps may be ligated with chromic catgut sutures.

Q. What is primary hemorrhage?

Ans. Bleeding during operation or at the time of injury.

Q. What is reactionary hemorrhage?

Ans. Reactionary hemorrhage occurs within 24 hours following operation or injury after the primary hemorrhage is controlled.

This may be due to slippage of a ligature or dislodgment of a clot. Resuscitation from shock may increase the blood pressure and may cause reactionary hemorrhage.

Q. What is secondary hemorrhage?

Ans. Secondary hemorrhage usually occurs 7–14 days following the operation or injury. This is usually due to infection and sloughing of vessels.

The secondary hemorrhage is often preceded by "warning hemorrhage" which are bright red stains of hemorrhage from the wound followed by sudden and severe hemorrhage.

Q. What are the characteristics of arterial, venous, and capillary bleeding?

Ans.

* *Arterial bleeding*: Bright red bleeding in spurts which rise and fall with the pulse wave.
* *Venous bleeding*: Dark red bleeding occurring steadily and if large veins are injured flow may be copious.
* *Capillary bleeding*: Bright red, continuous, often rapid ooze.

Q. What is the approximate blood volume in an adult and an infant?

Ans. In adult, normal blood volume is approximately 7% of body weight. So, a 70 kg adult has a blood volume of 5 L.

The blood volume in a child is approximately 8–9% of body weight (80–90 mU/kg of body weight).

Q. What are the different grades of hemorrhage?

Ans.

* *Class I hemorrhage*: Blood volume loss up to 15%.
  In uncomplicated situation:
  - Slight tachycardia, no change of blood pressure or pulse pressure
  - No fluid replacement is required
  - Transcapillary refilling and other compensatory mechanisms restore the blood volume in 24 hours.
* *Class II hemorrhage*: Blood volume loss of 15–30%
  - Tachycardia (heart rate above 100 in an adult), hypotension and decrease in pulse pressure. Decrease in pulse pressure is due to increase in peripheral resistance due to the circulating catecholamines causing an increase of diastolic pressure. Systolic blood pressure may not change initially
  - Urinary output is mildly affected (20–30 mU/hr in an adult).
  These patients may be initially managed with crystalloid infusion but some of these patients may require blood transfusion.

- *Class III hemorrhage:* Blood volume loss of 30–40% (approximate loss of about 2,000 mL of blood in an adult).
  Classic signs of inadequate perfusion:
  - Marked tachycardia and tachypnea
  - Measurable fall of systolic blood pressure
  - Changes in mental state and oliguria.
  In addition to crystalloid infusion these patients will always require blood transfusion.
- *Class IV hemorrhage:* Blood volume loss more than 40%.
  - Life-threatening hemorrhage
  - Marked tachycardia and severe hypotension
  - Urinary output is negligible or anuria
  - Mental state is markedly depressed
  - Cold and pale skin.

Q. How will you treat hemorrhage?

Ans. The basic principles for treatment of hemorrhage are:
- Stop hemorrhage
- Replace the volume lost.

Replacement of blood loss: Initial fluid bolus is administered as rapidly as possible. The initial usual dose is 1–2 L of crystalloid solution in an adult and 20 mL/kg in child.

Patient with class I hemorrhage may not require any fluid replacement. Patient with class III and class IV hemorrhage requires blood transfusion in addition to initial fluid therapy. Patient with class II hemorrhage may be managed only with crystalloid solution infusion but some may require blood transfusion.

Q. What is 3 for 1 rule?

Ans. This is a rough guideline for replacement of crystalloid for blood loss. 3 mL of crystalloid solution replacement is required for loss of each mL of blood.

Q. What is the possible response to the initial fluid therapy?

Ans. The potential response to initial fluid therapy may be:
- *Rapid response:*
  - Patient becomes hemodynamically normal following initial fluid administration and when the fluid administration is slowed to maintenance level
  - No blood transfusion or further fluid bolus is required.
- *Transient response:*
  - Patients respond to initial fluid therapy
  - Starts showing deterioration as the initial fluid administration is slowed down
  - Most of these patients have class II or III hemorrhage
  - These patients have continuing hemorrhage and require blood transfusion and may require surgical intervention.
- *No response or minimal response:*
  - Failure of response to adequate fluid or blood replacement indicate exsanguinating hemorrhage

- Most cases require immediate surgical intervention to control hemorrhage
- Rarely failure of response may be due to pump failure due to cardiogenic shock or cardiac tamponade.

KOCHER'S HEMOSTATIC FORCEPS

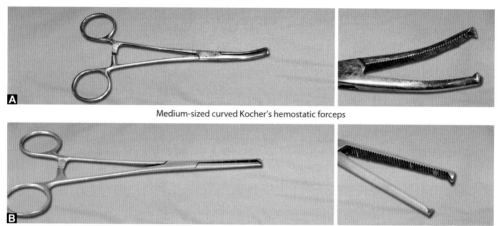

Medium-sized curved Kocher's hemostatic forceps

Medium-sized straight Kocher's hemostatic forceps

Figs 21.8A and B: Kocher's hemostatic forceps. Note the transverse serration and tooth and groove in the terminal part of the blade

Kocher's hemostatic forceps are more or less similar to a Spencer Wells' hemostatic forceps except (Figs 21.8A and B):
- The blades are slightly longer than in a Spencer Well's type of hemostatic forceps
- At the tip of the blades there is a tooth in one blade and a groove in the other blade where the tooth fits when the ratchet is closed. This type of forceps is suitable for holding vessels in tough structures like palm, soles, and the scalp where the vessels tend to retract in the deep fascia. The teeth at the tip of blades help to hold the retracting vessels securely.

Uses

- These are used during appendicectomy operation to crush the base of appendix
- These are used to hold perforating vessels during mastectomy
- These are used to hold the meniscus during meniscectomy
- During subtotal thyroidectomy a series of Kocher's hemostatic forceps are applied around the margin of thyroid gland lobe before excision of the enlarged thyroid lobe
- These are used for holding vessels in the scalp while raising a skin flap for craniotomy
- These are used to hold bleeding vessels while operating on palm and sole
- These are used in obstetrics for artificial rupture of membrane.

Sterilization

It is done by autoclaving.

▮ MOSQUITO HEMOSTATIC FORCEPS

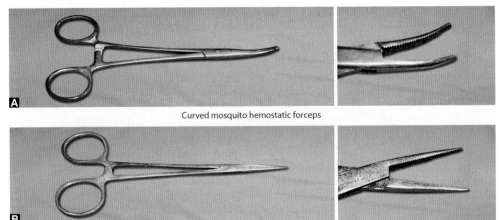

Curved mosquito hemostatic forceps

Straight mosquito hemostatic forceps

Figs 21.9A and B: Mosquito hemostatic forceps. Note the serrations in the whole length of the blade

This instrument is very light, small, and delicate. The blades are smaller in comparison to Spencer Well's type of hemostatic forceps and there are fine transverse serrations in the blades. The tip of the blades is conical and is nontoothed. This instrument is used to hold the small bleeding vessels (Figs 21.9A and B).

Uses

- It is used to hold fine bleeding vessels during cleft lip operation.
- While doing appendicectomy the mesoappendix is punctured at an avascular site by a mosquito forceps and a ligature passed around the mesoappendix and tied before division of the mesoappendix
- While inverting the base of the appendix by a purse string suture the stump of the appendix is held by a mosquito forceps and pushed inward as the purse string suture is tied.
- It is used as hemostatic forceps for operations in infants and children where the vessels are delicate
- It is used during circumcision. Three pairs of mosquito forceps are applied one pair on either side of the preputial orifice and one at the midline raphe where frenulum is attached. The prepuce is then divided starting in the dorsal midline. The skin over the shaft of the penis is retracted and the small vessels on the shaft of the penis are held by mosquito forceps and ligated.

Sterilization

It is done by autoclaving.

MAYO'S PEDICLE CLAMP

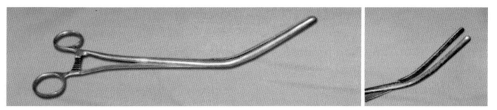

Fig. 21.10: Mayo's pedicle clamp. Note the curved blade and vertical serrations

This is a stout and large forceps. The blades are long and angled to provide a good view at a depth. There are vertical serrations in the blades (Fig. 21.10).

Uses

- It is used during nephrectomy to hold the renal pedicles before division
- It may be used during splenectomy to hold the splenic pedicle.

Sterilization

It is done by autoclaving.

LISTER'S SINUS FORCEPS

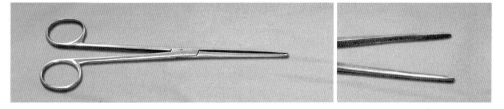

Fig. 21.11: Lister's sinus forceps. Note no ratchet and transverse serrations in terminal part of the blade

This is a long slender instrument with a pair of small blades with transverse serrations. There is no ratchet in the handle (Fig. 21.11).

Uses

- For incision and drainage of abscess by Hilton's method
- It may be used to hold a gauge swab to clean the abscess cavity.

Sterilization

It is done by autoclaving.

Q. What is an abscess? What are the different techniques for abscess drainage?

Ans. Abscess at different locations and management—*See* Minor Surgical Procedure, Page No. 955, 956, Chapter 20.

Q. What is Hilton's method for drainage of abscess?

Ans. During drainage of abscess situated in important areas like axilla and groin, there is chance of injury to the underlying major vessels and nerves if adequate care is not taken. In drainage of abscess in such location the skin and the subcutaneous tissues are incised with a knife. The deep fascia is not incised with a sharp knife but is pierced by thrushing a sinus forceps through the deep fascia and the sinus forceps is then opened up to enlarge the opening in the deep fascia for easy drainage of pus. This is Hilton's method of drainage of abscess.

■ ALLIS TISSUE FORCEPS

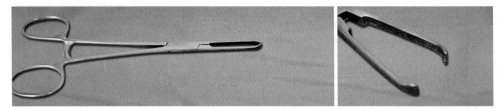

Fig. 21.12: Allis tissue forceps. Note the teeth and grove in the terminal part of the blade

This is a light instrument. The blades are longer and there is a gap between the blades which can accommodate some amount of tissue. The tip of the blades is provided with sharp teeth with grooves in between. When the ratchet is closed the teeth of the one blade fit in the groove of the other blade and vice versa (Fig. 21.12).

Uses

- During laparotomy through midline incision, skin margins may be retracted by applying Allis tissue forceps to the skin margin while linea alba is incised. The linea alba may be lifted up by applying Allis tissue forceps while incising the peritoneum
- While closing the midline incision the linea alba may be held up by Allis tissue forceps during suturing
- It is used to hold the skin margins during incisional hernia operations to raise the skin flaps. It may be used to hold the margins of the fascial gap while dissecting the hernial sac
- It is used during thyroid operations, neck dissection to hold the margins of the skin while raising skin flaps
- It is used to hold the cut margins of the bladder during transvesical prostatectomy or suprapubic cystolithotomy
- It is used to hold the neck of the bladder during bladder neck resection
- It is used to hold the galea aponeurotica while raising a skin flap during craniotomy
- It is used to hold the skin flaps while excising a lipoma, sebaceous cyst or lymph node.

Sterilization

It is done by autoclaving.

■ BABCOCK'S TISSUE FORCEPS

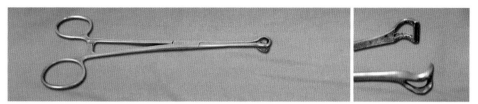

Fig. 21.13: Medium-sized Babcock's tissue forceps. Note the curved fenestrated blade with ridge in one blade and grove in other blade

This is a light instrument. The terminal part of the blades is curved and fenestrated. The tip is provided with a ridge in one blade and groove in the other. When the ratchet is closed the ridge of one blade fits into the groove of the other blade. As there are no teeth this is a nontraumatic forceps. The fenestration in the blade allows some soft tissue to be accommodated in the hollow while holding it (Fig. 21.13).

Uses

- It is used during appendicectomy. Usually three pairs of Babcock's forceps are required during appendicectomy. One pair holds the appendix near its tip, one pair holds the body of the appendix, and the third pair holds the base of the appendix
- It is used during gastrectomy, gastrojejunostomy to hold the margins of the stomach while applying an occlusion clamp
- It is used during small and large intestine resection anastomosis to hold the margins of the gut before applying an intestinal occlusion clamp. In open method of resection anastomosis, intestinal occlusion clamps are not applied. The cut margins of the gut are held up with Babcock's tissue forceps and sutured
- It is used during gastrostomy or jejunostomy to hold the gut while applying purse string suture.
- It is used during choledochoduodenostomy to hold the duodenum before making an incision in the first part of the duodenum
- It is used to hold the cut margins of the bladder during transvesical prostatectomy or suprapubic cystolithotomy.

Sterilization

It is done by autoclaving.

■ LANES' TISSUE FORCEPS

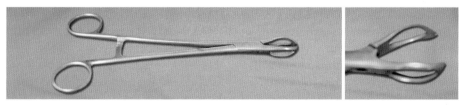

Fig. 21.14: Lanes' tissue forceps. Note the curved stout blade with fenestration and heavy tooth in terminal part of the blade

This is a thick and heavy instrument. The terminal part of the blades is curved and fenestrated. At the tip there is a heavy tooth in one blade with groove in the other blade and with the ratchet in closed position, the tooth and the groove in the blade fits in. Because of stout teeth at the tip this holds tissues firmly but it is traumatizing (Fig. 21.14).

Uses

- It is used during submandibular or parotid gland excision to hold the gland during dissection from the adjacent structures
- During mastectomy it may be used to hold the breast while dissecting it off from the pectoral fascia
- It may be used to fix the draping sheets and also to fix the suction tube and the diathermy cable to the draping sheets as an alternative to towel clip.

Sterilization

It is done by autoclaving.

■ PLAIN DISSECTING FORCEPS

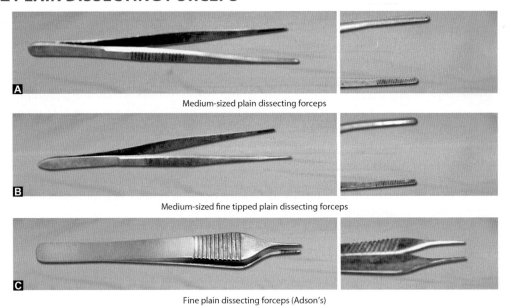

A

Medium-sized plain dissecting forceps

B

Medium-sized fine tipped plain dissecting forceps

C

Fine plain dissecting forceps (Adson's)

Figs 21.15A to C: Plain dissecting forceps. Note transverse serrations and no tooth in the blade

There are grooves on the shaft of the instrument which allows easy gripping. The two limbs of the shaft are so designed that it provides a spring action and the blades are kept apart. Pressing the two limbs of the shaft of the instruments brings the two blades closer and helps in gripping the tissues.

There are transverse serrations at the tip of the blades which help in lifting the tissues and the needle during suturing. There is no tooth at the tip (Figs 21.15A to C).

The plain dissecting forceps are also available as small and long plain dissecting forceps.

Uses

+ It is used during almost all operations to hold delicate structures like peritoneum, vessels, nerves, and muscles during dissection and suturing
+ It is used during appendicectomy to bring out the cecum and to deliver the appendix when it is held by the Babcock's tissue forceps
+ It is used during gastrojejunostomy, gut resection anastomosis to hold the gut margin during suturing
+ It is used to hold blood vessels and nerves during dissection
+ It is used to hold the peritoneum during closure of midline or paramedian abdominal incision.
+ It is used during hernia operation to hold the hernial sac during dissection of the sac from the cord structures
+ Fine tipped forceps is used during nerve repair and vascular anastomosis
+ It is used in pediatric patient to hold the delicate structures during suturing.

Sterilization

It is done by autoclaving.

■ TOOTHED DISSECTING FORCEPS

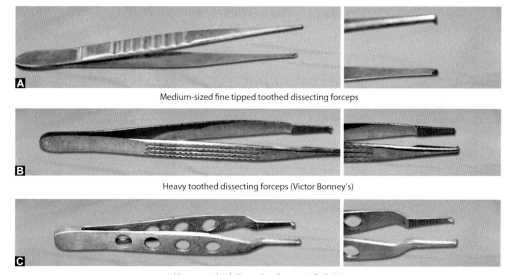

A

Medium-sized fine tipped toothed dissecting forceps

B

Heavy toothed dissecting forceps (Victor Bonney's)

C

Heavy toothed dissecting forceps (Galie's)

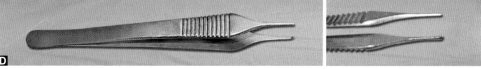

D

Fine tipped toothed dissecting forceps (Adson's toothed dissecting forceps)

Figs 21.16A to D: Toothed dissecting forceps. Note the transverse serrations and tooth in the blade

The design is same as the plain dissecting forceps but there is a tooth at the tip of one blade and a groove at the tip of the other blade. When the blades are approximated the toothed tip fits into the groove. Because of the presence of the tooth, the tissues may be better gripped and there is less chance of slipping (Figs 21.16A to D).

Uses

* It is used during almost all operations to hold tough structures like skin, fascia, and aponeurosis
* It is used to hold the cut skin margins during suturing
* It is used to hold the linea alba or the rectus sheath during closure of abdominal incision
* It is used to hold the scalp during closure of scalp incision
* Fine tipped toothed dissecting forceps is used to hold the cut margins of the prepuce for suturing during circumcision.

Sterilization

It is done by autoclaving.

▉ NEEDLE HOLDERS (FIGS 21.17A TO F)

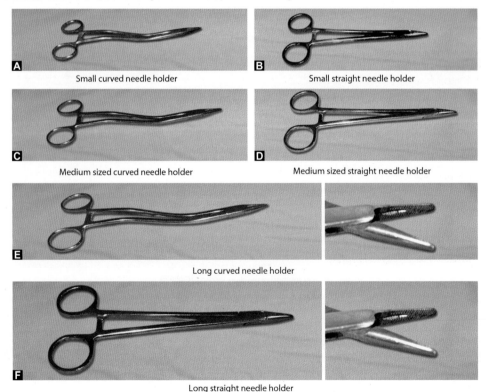

|A| Small curved needle holder
|B| Small straight needle holder
|C| Medium sized curved needle holder
|D| Medium sized straight needle holder
|E| Long curved needle holder
|F| Long straight needle holder

Figs 21.17A to F: Needle holders. Note the criss-cross serrations and groove in the blades

The blades of the needle holder are smaller in comparison to the shaft of the instrument.

There are criss-cross serrations in the blade and there is a longitudinal groove in the center of the criss-cross serration which allows firm gripping of the needle. However, the groove may not be there in all needle holders. The blades of the needle holders may be fine or heavy.

The needle holders with fine blades are used to hold finer needles (2/0, 3/0, 4/0 atraumatic catgut, vicryl, and mersilk).

The small-sized needle holders are used for suturing on the surface.

The long needle holders are used for suturing at the depth inside the abdomen, pelvis or chest.

The curved needle holders are used for suturing in a cavity or at a depth for better visualization.

Uses

These are used to hold the needle for suturing. The needle holders are used in all operations for suturing.

Sterilization

It is done by autoclaving.

Q. Where do you hold the needle with the needle holders for suturing?

Ans. Ideally, the needle should be held by the needle holder at the junction of the anterior two-thirds and the posterior one-third for ease of suturing.

Q. What other instruments will be required for suturing a skin wound?

Ans. Apart from a needle holder following instruments will be required:
- A swab holding forceps for antiseptic cleaning
- A toothed dissecting forceps
- A curved cutting needle
- Suture material—silk or nylon
- A scissor for cutting the ligatures.

■ NEEDLES

Needles are made of stainless steel. There is a sharp pointed tip at one end and an eye at the other end for threading a suture. Atraumatic needles are eyeless. The needles may be curved or straight. Depending on the type of sharp end the needles may be (Figs 21.18 to 21.23):
- Round bodied (Fig. 21.18A)

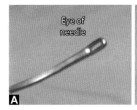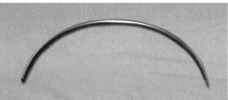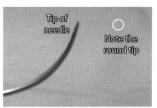

Curved round bodied needle

Fig. 21.18A

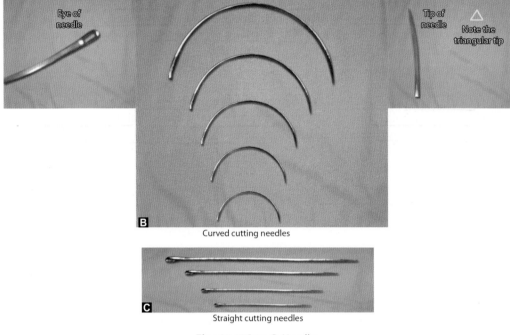

B Curved cutting needles

C Straight cutting needles

Figs 21.18A to C: Needles

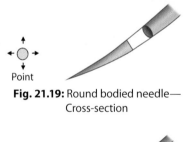

Point

Fig. 21.19: Round bodied needle—
Cross-section

Fig. 21.20: Conventional cutting
needle—Cross-section

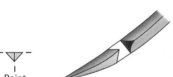

Point

Fig. 21.21: Reverse cutting needle

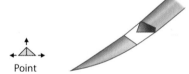

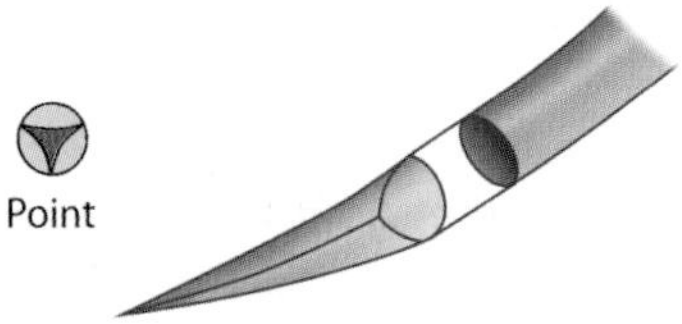

Point

Fig. 21.22: Tapper cut needle

- Cutting (Fig. 21.18B)
- Reverse cutting (Fig. 21.21)
- Taper cut or (Fig. 21.22)
- Blunt (Fig. 21.23).

Q. What are the characteristics of a round bodied needle?

Ans. In round bodied needle, the needle is uniformly round on cross section with a tapering tip. Round

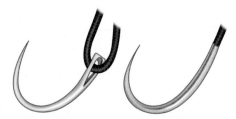

Fig. 21.23: Eyed and eyeless needles

bodied needles are designed to separate tissue fibers rather than cut them as it passes through the tissues and are suitable for suturing soft tissues where easy splitting of tissue fibers are possible, e.g. muscles, intestines, and vessels. After the needle passes, the tissue closes tightly around the suture material thereby forming a leak proof suture line (Figs 21.18A and 21.19).

Q. What are the characteristics of cutting needle?

Ans. Cutting needles are required for penetration of tough structures like fascia, aponeurosis, linea alba, and skin.

The sharp end of conventional cutting needle has a triangular cross-section with the apex on the inside of the needle curvature. The effective cutting edges are restricted to the front section of the needle and runs into a triangulated body which constitutes for half of the length of the needle (Fig. 21.20).

The reverse cutting needle is also triangular in cross-section having the apex of the cutting edge on the outer surface of the needle curvature. This improves the strength of the needle and particularly increases the resistance to bending (Fig. 21.21).

Q. What are taper cut needles?

Ans. This needle combines the initial penetration of a reverse cutting needle with the minimized trauma of a round bodied needle. The cutting tip is limited to the point of the needle, which then tapers out to merge smoothly into a round cross section. These needles are used mostly in vascular surgery (Fig. 21.22).

Q. What are the characteristics of an atraumatic or eyeless needle?

Ans. The eye of the needle with two layers of sutures causes trauma to the tissues through which it passes (Fig. 21.23A).

A needle without an eye is called an atraumatic or eyeless needle. The suture is inserted at the end of the needle by a special technique, so that a single layer of suture is attached at the end of the needle (Fig. 21.23B). This technique of imbrication of the suture at the end of the needle was first devised by Mr George Merson of England and in his memory most of these sutures are called Mersutures.

Q. What are the advantages of using an eyeless needle?

Ans.
- As the needle is eyeless it causes minimal trauma to the tissues.
- This is a disposable needle—so there is no problem with loss of sharpness.
- This is supplied in a presterilized pack—so sterilization before use is not required.
- Faster, more efficient surgery.

Q. What are intestinal needles?

Ans. These are smooth, delicate eyeless needles and allow easy penetration through the soft tissues like stomach, intestines, ureter, and peritoneum.

Q. What are blunt pointed needles?

Ans. These needles with a blunt tip are designed for suturing friable vascular tissues like, liver, spleen, and kidneys (Fig. 21.24).

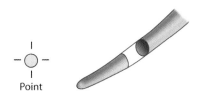

Point

Fig. 21.24: Blunt pointed needle—cross-section

Q. What are the parts of a surgical needle?

Ans.

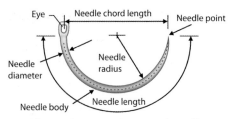

Fig. 21.25: Parts of a surgical needle

* Needle point or sharp apex of the needle (Fig. 21.25)
* *Body*: Which may be straight or curved
* *Eye*: For threading a suture. In atraumatic needles there are no eyes
* *Needle length*: It is the circumferential length of the needle
* *Needle chord length*: This is the linear distance between the pointed tip and the end of the needle.

Q. What do you mean by a 1/4, 3/8, 1/2, and 5/8th circle of a needle?

Ans. This indicates the type of curvature of the needle. One-fourth circle needle means the needle is curved like one-fourth circumference of a circle. Three-eighth circle needle means curvature is more wide and equals three-eighth circumference of a circle. Half circle means the needle is curved like half the circumference of a circle. Five-eighth circle needle means curvature is more wide and equals five-eighth circumference of a circle (Fig. 21.26).

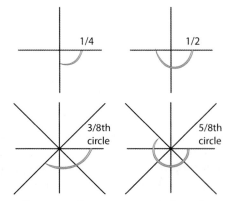

Fig. 21.26: Shapes curvatures of needles

Q. What is the weakest part of the needle?

Ans. The part of the needle near the eye is the weakest part of the needle.

Uses

* The curved round bodied needles are used to suture muscle, peritoneum, and other delicate structures
* The curved cutting needles are used to suture skin and other tough structures like linea alba, anterior rectus sheath, external oblique aponeurosis
* The straight cutting needles are used for suturing skin and other tough structures on the surface
* The atraumatic needles (eyeless needle) with the sutures imbricated at one end is used for suturing during intestinal resection anastomosis, gastrojejunostomy, bilioenteric, pancreaticojejunal anastomosis, and for vascular and nerve anastomosis.

Sterilization

Needles are sterilized by keeping them dipped in concentrated lysol for 1 hour or in dilute lysol for 24 hours. Boiling or autoclaving damages the sharpness of the needle.

■ SKIN CLOSURE CLIPS AND ACCESSORIES

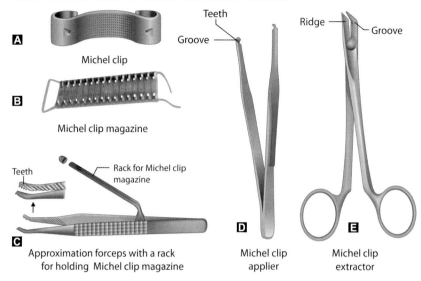

Figs 21.27A to E: Skin closure clips and accessories

- Michel clips are provided with sharp-pointed spike at either end (Fig. 21.27A)
- The Michel clips are supplied in a Michel clip magazine (Fig. 21.27B). Michel clip magazine is loaded into a rack which is attached to a toothed dissecting forceps used to hold the skin margins during application of the clips (Fig. 21.27C)
- The Michel clip applicator resembles a dissecting forceps and there is a groove on either blades near its tip (Fig. 21.27D). The Michel clip is held in this groove and one clip is removed from the magazine holding the clips. Once the Michel clip applier is pressed the shaft of the clips gets bent in the middle and the spike on either side pierces the skin and keeps the skin margins apposed
- With availability of preloaded skin staplers these clips are no longer used.

Sterilization

It is done by autoclaving.

Q. How will you apply these clips?

Ans.
- Michel clips are used for skin closure
- The skin margins are properly apposed and lifted up by holding with the toothed dissecting forceps. One clip is taken from the magazine with the Michel clip applier and the clip is applied to the skin margin by pressing the Michel clip applier. The clip gets bent in the middle and the spike pierces the skin margin on either side keeping the skin margins apposed
- While applying the clips the skin margins have to be apposed properly taking care so that the skin margins do not get inverted.

Q. Where do you apply these clips?

Ans. These clips may be applied for skin incision closure in the neck, abdomen or other sites.

Skin closure with clips is cosmetically better and time required for closure is less. However, these are costly and if not applied properly may cause inversion of skin margins.

Q. How will you remove these clips?

Ans. These clips are removed by Michel clip extractor. Michel clip extractor is an instrument without any ratchet. The blades are curved. In the lower blade there is a groove and in the upper blade there is a ridge (Fig. 21.27E).

For extraction of the Michel clip the lower blade is passed below the middle of the shaft of the applied clip and the instrument is closed. As the upper blade is pressed the clip gets bent outward and the spikes come out of the skin and the clip is thus removed.

■ SKIN STAPLERS

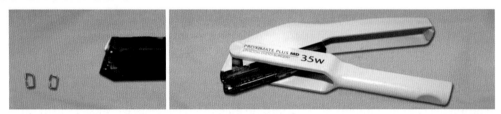

Fig. 21.28: This is a proximate plus skin stapler containing 35 skin staples

Different skin staplers containing preloaded skin staples are available. These staplers contain preloaded staples and are available in presterilized pack (Fig. 21.28).

Uses

These staplers are used for skin approximation in different skin incisions.

■ MAYO'S SCISSORS (FIGS 21.29A TO D)

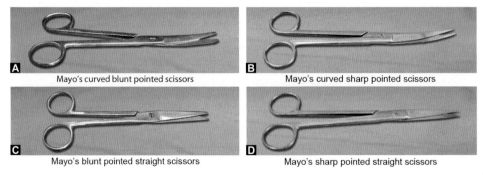

A — Mayo's curved blunt pointed scissors

B — Mayo's curved sharp pointed scissors

C — Mayo's blunt pointed straight scissors

D — Mayo's sharp pointed straight scissors

Figs 21.29A to D: Mayo's scissors. Mayo's scissors are usually long and stout scissors

Mayo scissors may be made from stainless steel or titanium. They may also be available in standard or extra-long scissors, and typically measure between 6 inches (150 mm) and 6 ¾ inches (170 mm) in length.

Uses

+ These are used for cutting sutures
+ These are used during appendicectomy to split the internal oblique and transversus abdominis muscle. After incising the external oblique aponeurosis, the scissors is thrushed through the internal oblique and transversus abdominis muscle with the blades in closed position and then the blades are opened up and the muscles are thus split up
+ These are used to cut tough structures like linea alba, external oblique aponeurosis, anterior and posterior rectus sheath during entry into the abdomen by a midline, paramedian or subcostal incision
+ These may be used to cut dressings
+ These may be used to cut a corrugated rubber sheet drain.

■ MCINDOE SCISSORS

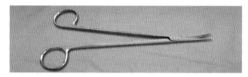

Fig. 21.30: McIndoe scissors. Note the fine, delicate, sharp, and small blades

These are fine scissors. The blades are delicate and smaller than in Mayo's scissors and are used for tissue dissection and cutting delicate structures (Fig. 21.30). In Metzenbaum scissors, the blades are long in comparison to the shaft.

Uses

+ These are used during appendicectomy to cut the external oblique aponeurosis and peritoneum. The mesoappendix is cut after being ligated
+ These are used during herniorrhaphy:
  - To cut the external oblique aponeurosis to expose the inguinal canal
  - To dissect the hernial sac from the cord structures and to open the fundus of the hernial sac.
+ These are used during thyroidectomy:
  - To raise the upper and lower skin flaps by sharp dissection. The upper skin flap is raised up to the upper border of the thyroid cartilage and the lower skin flap raised up to the suprasternal notch
  - To cut the investing layer of the deep cervical fascia in the midline
  - To cut the pretracheal layer of the deep cervical fascia investing the thyroid gland
  - To divide the thyroid vessels (middle thyroid vein, superior thyroid vessels, and the inferior thyroid artery and vein) after their ligature.
+ These are used during mastectomy and incisional hernia operation to raise the skin flap by sharp dissection
+ These are used during radical neck dissection to raise skin flaps by sharp dissection
+ These are used during splenectomy and nephrectomy to cut the pedicles after ligature
+ These are used during cholecystectomy to cut the cystic duct and the artery after they are ligated.

■ METZENBAUM SCISSORS

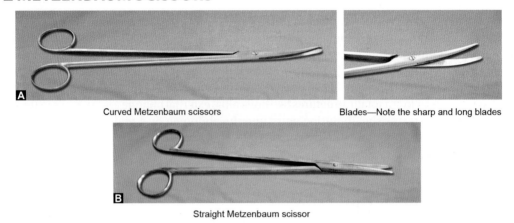

Curved Metzenbaum scissors
Blades—Note the sharp and long blades

Straight Metzenbaum scissor

Figs 21.31A and B: Metzenbaum scissors

This is a long fine scissors with long blades in comparison to the shaft of the instrument. This instrument may be straight or curved (Figs 21.31A and B).

Uses

- The Metzenbaum scissors are used for dissection at the depth. These may be used in above situations as an alternative to McIndoe scissors
- These are used during vagotomy to divide the nerves after ligature
- These are used during cholecystectomy to divide the cystic duct and artery after ligature

■ HEATH'S SUTURE CUTTING SCISSORS

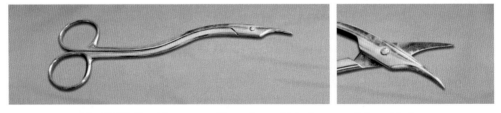

Fig. 21.32: Heath's suture cutting scissors. Note the curved sharp blades

These are the fine scissors curved on angle type. The blades are small, sharp, and at the tip there are serrations. The serrations at the tip allow gripping of the suture material (Fig. 21.32).

Uses

This is used to cut the sutures on the skin or mucosal surface. The suture is held up by a dissecting forceps and one blade of the stitch cutting scissors is inserted into the loop of the suture. The suture is cut close to the entrance of the suture into the skin and then the suture is pulled outside. The exposed part of the suture does not pass through the depth of the wound during removal of the suture.

The serration at the tip of the blade helps in holding of the suture during removal.

Sterilization

Heath's suture cutting scissors are sterilized by keeping them dipped in concentrated lysol for 1 hour or in dilute lysol for 24 hours. Boiling or autoclaving damages the sharpness of the instrument.

LANGENBACH'S RETRACTOR

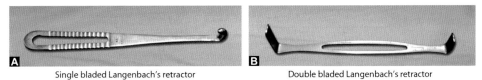

Single bladed Langenbach's retractor   Double bladed Langenbach's retractor

Figs 21.33A and B: Langenbach's retractor

The single bladed Langenbach's retractor has a handle, a long shaft and a flat solid blade. The blade is curved at right angle to the shaft. The tip of the blade is curved at right angle for better retraction of the tissues (Fig. 21.33A).

In double-bladed retractor, there is another flat solid blade at the other end of the shaft (Fig. 21.33B).

Retractors placed suitably help in better visualization of the operative field. The tissue handling may also be minimized. Bleeding may be better seen and controlled with placement of retractors.

CZERNY'S RETRACTOR

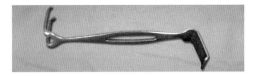

Fig. 21.34: Czerny's retractor

In Czerny's retractor at one end there is a flat blade at right angle to the shaft with the tip curved at right angle while the other end has a biflanged hook (Fig. 21.34).

MORRIS' RETRACTOR

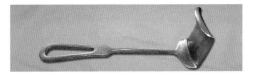

Fig. 21.35: Morris' retractor

The design is like L. The handle is wider and the blade is also wider and the lower end of the blade is curved inward at right angle (Fig. 21.35).

Uses

- These retractors are used for tissue retraction during different operations
- These are used during appendicectomy to retract the layers of the abdominal wall while making the incision. After incising the peritoneum the abdominal wall is retracted with this retractor to visualize the cecum and delivers the cecum and appendix out
- These are used while making and closing different abdominal incisions for ease of working in deeper layers of the abdominal wall
- These are used during thyroidectomy to retract the strap muscles and the sternomastoid for dissection and ligation of the thyroid vessels
- These are used during modified radical mastectomy for retraction of pectoralis major muscle for better visualization during axillary dissection
- These are used during inguinal hernia operation for retraction of different layers for proper visualization during repair of the posterior wall of the inguinal canal
- These are used during radical neck dissection for retraction of skin flaps and sternocleido-mastoid muscle for better visualization at depth.

Sterilization

These retractors are sterilized by autoclaving.

▮ HOOK RETRACTORS

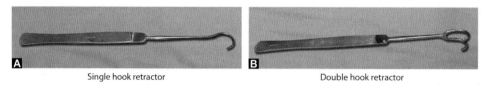

Single hook retractor   Double hook retractor

Figs 21.36A and B: Hook retractor

There is a shaft with handle. There is a single (Fig. 21.36A) or double hook (Fig. 21.36B) at the tip. The tip of the hook may be sharp or blunt.

Uses

- These are used for operation at the surface—for retraction of skin flap and for excision of sebaceous cyst and lipoma
- These are used during venesection for retraction of skin
- These are used during tracheostomy for retraction of skin and thyroid isthmus.

Sterilization

These retractors are sterilized by autoclaving.

CAT'S PAW OR VOLKMAN'S RETRACTOR

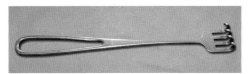

Fig. 21.37: Cat's paw or Volkman's retractor

There are multiple hooks with pointed edges (Fig. 21.37). The pointed edges are helpful for firm retraction. This is used for retraction of skin flaps or fascia for operation at the surface, e.g. excisions of sebaceous cyst, lipoma, dermoid, etc.

Sterilization

These retractors are sterilized by autoclaving.

FISCH NERVE HOOK

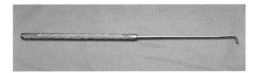

Fig. 21.38: Fisch nerve hook

This is a delicate instrument with a blunt hook at the tip of the shaft (Fig. 21.38).
- This is used for retraction of the nerve during dissection
- Ilioinguinal nerve may be retracted during inguinal hernia operation
- Spinal accessory, hypoglossal, and ansa cervicalis nerve may be retracted during radical neck node dissection.

Sterilization

Sterilization is done by autoclaving.

DEAVER'S RETRACTOR

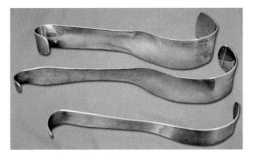

Fig. 21.39: Deaver's retractor

A large curved retractor which is shaped like "S". It is available in different sizes depending on its width (Fig. 21.39).

Uses

* It is used during cholecystectomy for retraction of right lobe of liver
* It is used during truncal vagotomy for retraction of left lobe of liver
* It is used during gastrectomy for retraction of liver
* It is used during pancreaticojejunostomy for retraction of stomach
* It is used during right or left hemicolectomy to retract the abdominal wall while mobilizing the colon from the paracolic gutter
* It is used during kidney operation to retract the abdominal wall
* It is used during anterior resection of rectum or abdominoperineal resection to retract the urinary bladder in male or uterus in female during dissection in the pelvis.

Sterilization

Sterilization is done by autoclaving.

▌SELF-RETAINING ABDOMINAL RETRACTOR (BALFOUR'S TYPE) WITH PROVISION FOR ATTACHMENT FOR THIRD BLADE

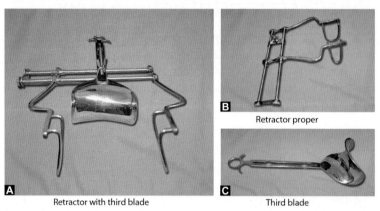

A Retractor with third blade

B Retractor proper

C Third blade

Figs 21.40A to C: Self-retaining abdominal retractor (Balfour's type) with provision for attachment of third blade

There is a horizontal bar on which one of the two blades of the retractor slides. The sliding retractor can be fixed to the horizontal bar by means of a screw. There is another screw in-between the blades which keeps the third blade in position (Figs 21.40A to C).

While applying, the two blades are kept closer and after the abdominal incision is made up to the peritoneum the blades are inserted into the abdomen and blades are separated to retract the abdominal wall. Fixation of the screw in the sliding blade keeps the retractor self-retaining.

The third blade is usually used to retract the costal margin or is used toward the pelvis during pelvic operations.

While a self-retaining retractor is used assistant's hands become free as he does not need to hold the retractor in his hands.

Uses

- It is used to retract the abdominal wall during a number of operations requiring good retraction of the abdominal wall for proper exposure
- It is used in gastric operations (Vagotomy and gastrojejunostomy, gastrectomy)
- It is used in operations on pancreas (Whipple's pancreaticoduodenectomy and pancreaticojejunostomy)
- It is used in intestinal operations (small gut resection and anastomosis, hemicolectomy, abdominoperineal resection, and anterior resection)
- It is used in liver operations (hepatic resection and excision of hydatid cyst)
- It is used in operations on adrenal—adrenalectomy
- It is used in excision of intraperitoneal cysts or sarcomas.

Sterilization

It is done by autoclaving.

■ MILLIN'S SELF-RETAINING BLADDER RETRACTOR WITH A PROVISION FOR ATTACHMENT OF THIRD BLADE

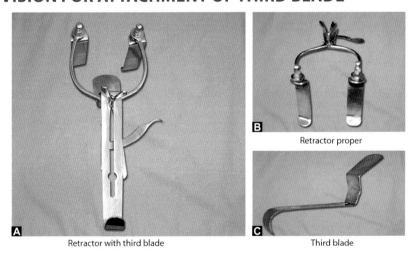

Retractor proper

A Retractor with third blade   **C** Third blade

Figs 21.41A to C: Millin's self-retraining bladder retractor with a provision for attachment of third blade

Two blades are fitted on horizontal bars which can slide and may be fixed by screws.

In-between these two blades there is another screw which may attach the third blade when required. When finger bows are separated the blades are lying closer. When finger bows are approximated the blades are separated (Figs 21.41A to C).

This retractor is used during transvesical prostatectomy. After prostate gland is enucleated, the prostate cavity is packed with roller gauge. Before removal of the pack the self-retaining retractor is inserted into the bladder and the retractor is opened. The third blade retracts the fundus of the bladder. This keeps the bladder wide open and allows proper inspection of the prostate cavity and hemostasis under vision.

Sterilization

Sterilization is done by autoclaving.

■ JOLL'S THYROID RETRACTOR

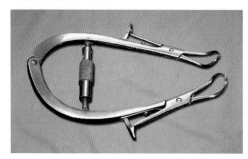

Fig. 21.42: Joll's thyroid retractor

There are two towel clip like forceps at either end. The two flanges can be adjusted by means of a screw mechanism (Fig. 21.42).

This is also a self-retaining retractor used during thyroid operations to retract the skin flaps. After the skin incision is made, the platysma is incised in the same line. The upper and lower skin flaps are dissected and raised. The upper skin flap is raised up to the upper border of the thyroid cartilage and the lower skin flap is raised up to the suprasternal notch. Once the skin flaps are raised the upper and the lower skin flaps are held by the towel clip like forceps attached to the retractor and the retractor is opened by the screw mechanism attached to the retractor.

Sterilization

Joll's thyroid retractor is sterilized by autoclaving.

■ KOCHER'S THYROID DISSECTOR

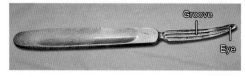

Fig. 21.43: Kocher's thyroid dissector. Note the vertical groove and the eye

The instrument has got a handle and a blade. There are grooves on the handle for firm gripping. The sides of the blade are blunt and there are longitudinal grooves on the upper surface of the blade. There is an eye near the tip of the blade which is meant for passing a ligature (Fig. 21.43).

Uses

◆ This instrument is used during thyroid operations. The dissector may be used to dissect the superior thyroid pedicle and the dissector is passed around the superior thyroid pedicle close to the gland. A ligature is passed through the eye in the blade of the dissector and as the dissector is withdrawn the suture is passed around the thyroid pedicle. Three sutures are passed around the superior thyroid pedicle and tied. The superior pedicle is divided keeping two ligatures toward the upper pole.

◆ The inferior thyroid veins may also be tackled similarly.

Sterilization

It is done by autoclaving.

▮ CORD HOLDING FORCEPS

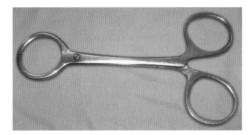

Fig. 21.44: Cord holding forceps

In addition to finger bows and shaft there are two semicircular blades and when the ratchet is closed the blades are apposed and make a circular opening in the blade (Fig. 21.44).

Uses

It is used during hernia operation to hold the spermatic cord so that the cord can be retracted during repair of the posterior wall of the inguinal canal.

Sterilization

It is done by autoclaving.

Q. What is hernia?

Q. What are the different types of hernia?

Q. What is the boundary of inguinal canal?

Q. What is Fruchaud's myopectineal orifice?

Q. What are the parts of a hernia?

Q. What are the coverings of a complete indirect inguinal hernia?

Q. What do you mean by incomplete and complete inguinal hernia?

Q. What is sliding hernia?

Q. What is bubonocele?

Q. What is funicular hernia?

Q. What is herniotomy?

Q. What is herniorrhaphy?

Q. What is hernioplasty?

Q. What is Bassini's technique of herniorrhaphy?

Ans. For answers to these question. *See* Long Cases Section, Page No, 38–68, Chapter 2.

■ MALLEABLE OLIVE POINTED PROBE

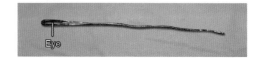

Fig. 21.45: Malleable olive pointed probe with an eye

This is a metallic probe with an olive at the tip and the probe is malleable and there is an eye at the other end (Fig. 21.45).

The instrument is malleable so it can be bent in different ways. The olive point minimizes trauma and reduces the chance of false passage. The eye is meant for passing a ligature which may be passed around a high fistula tract.

Uses

- It is used during fistulectomy operations. The probe is passed from the external opening to emerge from the internal opening. The probe is then bent and an incision around the probe helps in complete excision of the fistulous tract around the probe
- It may be used to pass a ligature through a high fistula in ano for Seton treatment. The malleable probe is passed through the external opening of the fistula and the olive tip emerges from the internal opening. A No. 1 or No. 2 polypropylene suture is passed through the eye of the probe and the probe along with the suture is brought out through the internal opening. By this technique the suture goes through the fistula tract and the two ends of the thread are tied which cuts through the fistula tract gradually and allows healing of the high fistula
- It may be used during fistulotomy or opening a sinus tract. The probe is introduced into the fistula or the sinus tract and the sinus or the fistula is laid open over this probe
- It may be used in assessing the penetrating trauma abdomen to ascertain the depth of the wound and whether it has penetrated the peritoneum or not
- It may be used to assess the length and depth of a sinus tract
- It may be used to sound a sinus tract to ascertain presence of any foreign body.

Sterilization

It is done by autoclaving.

Fistula

Q. What is a fistula?

Ans. Fistula is a tract, usually lined by granulation tissues with openings at both ends of the tract. A fistula in ano is a tract lined by granulation tissue and has an external opening at the perianal skin and internal opening at the anal canal or rectum.

Q. What do you mean by low anal fistula?

Ans. When the internal opening of the fistula lies below the anorectal ring then it is called a low anal fistula. If this fistulous tract is laid open there is no chance of anal incontinence.

Q. What do you mean by high anal fistula?

Ans. When the internal opening of the fistula lies at or above the anorectal ring then it is called a high fistula. Fistulectomy or fistulotomy in such cases may result in incontinence due to division of anorectal ring.

Q. What are the different types of anal fistula?

Ans. The different types of anal fistula include (Fig. 21.46A):

*   *Subcutaneous fistula*: External opening at the perianal skin and the internal opening at the skin lined part of the anal canal.
*   *Submucous fistula*: This is more like a sinus than a fistula. The internal opening is at the anal canal and the tract traverses up to the submucous coat.
*   *Low anal fistula*: The external opening is at the perianal skin and the internal opening lies at the anal canal below the anorectal sling.
*   *High anal fistula*: When the internal opening of the fistula lies at or above the anorectal sling.
*   *Pelvirectal fistula*: In this case the fistulous tract traverses through the levator ani muscle and the internal opening of the fistula is at the rectum.

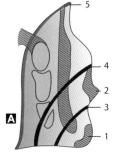

1. Subcutaneous fistula
2. Submucous fistula
3. Low anal fistula
4. High anal fistula
5. Pelvirectal fistula

1. Intersphincteric fistula (low and high)
2. Transsphincteric fistula (low and high)
3. Supralevator fistula

Figs 21.46A and B: Different types of anal fistula

Q. What is Park's classification for perianal fistula?

Ans.

*   *Intersphincteric fistula*: The fistulous tract runs between the internal and the external sphincter.
*   Depending on the internal opening it may be high or low intersphincteric fistula (Fig. 21.46B).
*   *Transsphincteric fistula*: From the external opening at the perianal skin the fistulous tract traverses through both the external and the internal anal sphincter. Depending

on the position of the internal opening at the anal canal this may also be low or high transsphincteric fistula.

◆ *Supralevator fistula*: The fistulous tract traverses through the levator ani muscle and the internal opening is into the rectum.

Q. How perianal fistula develops?

Ans. Perianal fistula develops secondary to:
◆ Perianal abscess (most common cause) which has ruptured spontaneously or is incised late
◆ Associated with specific diseases like tuberculosis or Crohn's disease.

Q. What is Goodsall's rule?

Ans. When the external opening of the fistula lies in the anterior half of the anal opening, then the fistulous tract tends to be straight.

When the external opening of the fistula lies in the posterior half of the anal opening, then the fistulous tract is usually curved and the internal orifice usually lies in the posterior midline. There may be multiple external openings but the internal opening is usually single (Fig. 21.47).

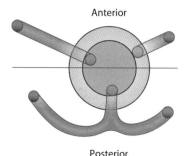
Fig. 21.47: Goodsall's rule

Q. What investigations may help to map out course of perianal fistula?

Ans.
◆ Transrectal ultrasonography (TRUS) or MRI may be helpful in delineation of a complex fistula
◆ Fistulogram is not very helpful for delineation of perianal fistulous tract.

Q. What is watercan perineum?

Ans. Perianal fistula with multiple external openings is called watercan perineum. There may be discharge of pus from multiple openings.

Q. What are the important causes of multiple perianal fistula?

Ans.
◆ Multiple perianal fistula is often associated with tuberculosis, Crohn's disease or lymphogranuloma inguinale
◆ Hidradenitis suppurativa may be associated with multiple perianal sinuses.

Q. What is the treatment for low anal fistula?

Ans. Fistulectomy or fistulotomy is the standard surgical treatment for low anal fistula.

Q. Why fistulectomy and fistulotomy are not suitable for high fistula?

Ans. This will result in anal incontinence.
A staged procedure is advisable in such situation.
◆ Colostomy for fecal diversion
◆ Fistulectomy and repair of sphincter
◆ Colostomy closure after 8 weeks.

Alternatively, Seton treatment may allow healing of the fistula. Under anesthesia a nylon, prolene or silk is threaded on to the eye of the malleable probe is passed through the fistula tract and is tied. At regular intervals the thread is tightened as it cuts through the fistulous tract.

OLIVE POINTED FISTULA DIRECTOR WITH FRENUM SLIT

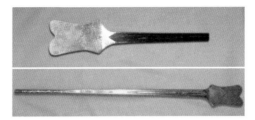

Fig. 21.48: Olive pointed fistula director with frenum slit

This is a metallic probe with an olive at the tip. On the upper aspect there is a groove. The base is broad and flat and there is a slit in the middle (Fig. 21.48).

Uses

* It is used during fistulotomy. The fistula director is passed through the fistula tract from the external to the internal opening and the fistulous tract is incised over the groove in the probe
* In stricture urethra operation the strictured segment may be slit over this probe
* It may be used during tongue tie operation to release the frenulum.

Sterilization

It is done by autoclaving.

PILES HOLDING FORCEPS

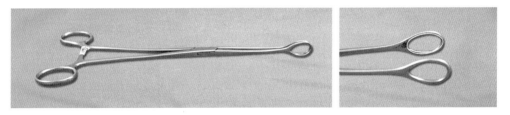

Fig. 21.49: Piles holding forceps. Note the oval blade with fenestration and groove in the terminal part of the blade

The instrument has finger bows, a catch, and a pair of shaft with a pair of blades. The blades are oval with a central fenestration. There is a complete groove on the inner aspect of each blade (Fig. 21.49).

Uses

This instrument is used during piles operation to hold the pile mass.

Sterilization

Sterilization is done by autoclaving.

Q. How will you differentiate it from a swab holding forceps?

Ans. The swab holding forceps is longer and the blades are provided with transverse serrations.

Piles

Q. What are piles?

Ans. Piles are condition of dilated veins occurring in relation to the internal venous plexuses of anal canal with an enlarged and displaced anal cushion.

Q. What are the different types of piles?

Ans. Depending on the location the piles may be:
* *Internal piles*: When the pile mass is lined by the anal mucous membrane and lies internal to the anal orifice.
* *External piles*: When the pile mass is lined by the skin of the anal canal and lies external to the anal orifice.
* *Internoexternal piles*: Combination of internal and external piles.

  Depending on the etiology the piles may be:
* *Primary piles*: When no obvious cause could be found for development of piles
* *Secondary or symptomatic piles*: When the piles develops secondary to some other causes.

Q. What are the important causes of secondary piles?

Ans.
* *During pregnancy*: The important factors for development of piles in pregnancy include:
  – Compression of superior rectal veins by the gravid uterus
  – Relaxing effect of progesterone on the vein walls
  – Increased pelvic circulatory volume.
* *Benign prostate hyperplasis (BPH) or stricture urethra*: Increased straining at micturition
* *Carcinoma of rectum*: Compression of superior rectal vein may give rise to secondary piles
* Chronic constipation with increased straining at defecation.

Q. What are anal cushions?

Ans. The anal cushions are mucosal lining which are gathered predominantly at three places in relation to the three terminal branches of superior rectal artery. The anal cushions are necessary for full continence. Straining at stool leads to downward descent of these anal cushions. Once these anal cushions descend beyond the anal sphincters there is compression of these anal cushions by the anal sphincters resulting in engorgement of the veins of the internal rectal venous plexus leading to formation of internal piles.

Q. What are the primary and secondary sites of piles?

Ans. The primary sites of internal hemorrhoids are at 3, 7, and 11 o'clock position. In-between these primary hemorrhoids there may be smaller secondary hemorrhoids (Fig. 21.50).

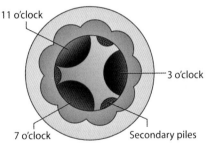

Fig. 21.50: Sites of primary and secondary piles

Q. What are the different grades of piles?

Ans. Depending on size and prolapse of the piles it may be:
- *First degree piles*: Piles that bleed but do not prolapse outside the anal orifice.
- *Second degree piles*: Piles that prolapse outside the anal orifice during defecation and reduce spontaneously or have to be manually replaced and then stay reduced.
- *Third degree piles*: Piles that remain permanently prolapsed outside the anal orifice.

Q. What are the usual presentations of patients with piles?

Ans.
- Painless bleeding per rectum
- Prolapse of the piles mass outside the anal orifice
- Mucus discharge
- Anemia
- May present with complications.

Q. What are the complications of piles?

Ans.
- Strangulation
- Thrombosis
- Ulceration and gangrene
- Portal pyemia and septicemia
- Fibrosis.

Q. What are the nonoperative treatments of piles?

Ans.
- *Injection sclerotherapy*: Indicated in first degree and early second degree piles.
  - Sclerosants used: About 5% phenol in almond or olive oil, sodium tetradecyl sulfate or ethanolamine oleate.
  - Injection is done at the submucosa of the pedicle of the pile mass (*See* Minor Surgical Procedures, Page No. 971, Chapter 20).
- *Barron's banding*: Same indication as above.
- The pile mass is brought into the hollow of the band applicator and on firing the instrument the band is slipped into the pedicle of the pile mass. The band causes ischemic necrosis of the pile mass which sloughs off in a few days.
- *Cryosurgery*: Application of liquid nitrogen (temperature—196°C) causes coagulative necrosis of the pile mass.
- *Photocoagulation*: Application of infrared rays may also cause regression of the pile mass.

Q. What are the indications of surgery for piles?

Ans.

+ Third degree piles
+ Internoexternal piles with a large external piles
+ Failure of nonoperative treatment
+ Thrombosed piles.

Q. What is Milligan-Morgan technique of hemorrhoidectomy?

Ans. This is also called open hemorrhoidectomy. The pile mass is ligated and excised. The cut margins of the anal mucosa and anal skin is left open to heal by granulation.

Q. What is closed hemorrhoidectomy?

Ans. In this technique after ligation and excision of the pile mass the cut margins of the anal mucous membrane and the skin are sutured to close the resulting wound.

■ RIGHT ANGLED FORCEPS (LAHEY'S FORCEPS)

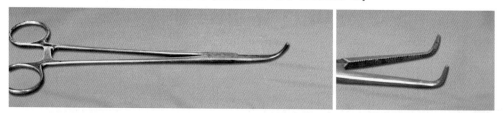

Fig. 21.51: Right angled forceps (Lahey's forceps). Note the 90° angulation and transverse serrations in the blade

Like a hemostatic forceps, this instrument has finger bows, a catch, a pair of shaft, and a pair of blades. The terminal part of blades is bent at right angles to the shaft of the instrument and there are transverse serrations in the blade (Fig. 21.51).

Uses

+ This is usually used to dissect pedicles of important organs and a ligature may be passed around the dissected vessels. This may also be used as a hemostatic forceps to hold a bleeding vessel at a depth
+ This is used during cholecystectomy to dissect the cystic duct and the artery and to pass a ligature around these structures
+ This is used during gastrectomies to dissect and pass ligatures around the left gastric artery, right gastric artery, gastroepiploic vessels before their divisions
+ This is used during vagotomy to dissect the anterior and posterior vagus nerves and pass ligatures around these structures before their division
+ This is used during splenectomy to dissect the splenic artery and the vein and to pass ligature around them
+ This is used during nephrectomy to dissect the renal vessels and to pass ligature around them
+ This is used during thyroidectomy to dissect the middle thyroid vein, superior thyroid pedicle and the inferior thyroid vessels and to pass ligature around them.

Sterilization

It is done by autoclaving.

■ CHOLECYSTECTOMY FORCEPS

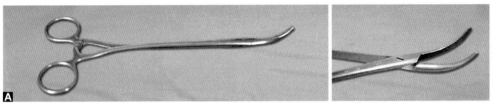

Moynihan's cholecystectomy forceps. Note the heavy blades with transverse serrations

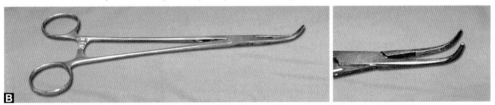

Henry Gray's cholecystectomy forceps. Note the angulation and vertical serrations in the blade

Figs 21.52A and B: Cholecystectomy forceps

These are stout and heavy instruments. In addition to the finger bows and catch there is a pair of long shafts with a pair of relatively small blades with blunt tips. The long instrument helps working at a depth.

In Moynihan's forceps, the blade is slightly angled to the shaft and there are transverse serrations in the blade (Fig. 21.52A).

In Henry Gray's forceps, the blade is longer than in a Moynihan's forceps which is angled at almost right angle to the shaft and there are critical serrations in the blade (Fig. 21.52B).

Uses

- These are used during cholecystectomy. One pair of forceps is used to hold the fundus of the gallbladder and one pair to hold near the Hartmann's pouch. If the gallbladder is long, a third pair of forceps may be used to hold the body of the gallbladder
- The cystic duct and artery may be dissected by Moynihan's forceps. But usually a right angled forceps (Lahey's forceps) is preferred for dissection of the cystic pedicle.

Sterilization

Sterilization is done by autoclaving.

Q. What are the complications of cholecystectomy?

Ans.
- *Immediate complications*:
  - *Anesthetic complications*: Respiratory and cardiac complications

- *Complications due to the procedure:*
  - Bleeding
  - Bile leakage:
    - » Acute biliary peritonitis (Waltman Walters syndrome)
    - » Biloma (localized bile collection)
  - Bile duct injury:
    - » Lateral tear
    - » Complete transection
    - » Partial ligature
    - » Complete ligature
    - » Slippage of cystic duct stump ligature.
- *Delayed complications*:
  - Biliary stricture.

Discussion on Gallstone Disease

See Surguical Long Cases, Page No. 138–144, Chapter 3.

■ DESJARDIN'S CHOLEDOCHOLITHOTOMY FORCEPS

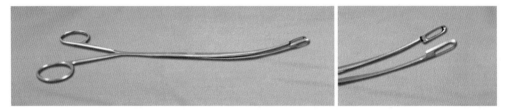

Fig. 21.53: Desjardin's choledocholithotomy forceps. Note no ratchet. Blades having fenestration with groove in the terminal part

This is a long and slender instrument. There are finger bows but no catch. The shafts are curved, in some it is a gentle curve and in other varieties there are different degrees of curvature. The blades are small and fenestrated centrally. There are no serrations in the blade (Fig. 21.53).

Uses

- This is used during choledocholithotomy. The common bile duct is identified by aspirating bile from the bile duct. Two stay sutures are applied in the bile duct by a 3-0 atraumatic catgut suture and a choledochotomy is made in-between the stay sutures. The Desjardin's forceps is then introduced into the bile duct and the stones are removed by holding the stones in the fenestrated blade
- This is used during laparoscopic cholecystectomy. While extracting the gallbladder through the epigastric or umbilical port, as the gallbladder is partially delivered through the port wound, it usually gets stuck if there are large stones in the gallbladder or there are multiple small stones in the gallbladder. The gallbladder is partially delivered through the wound.

The gallbladder is opened and the stone removed from the gallbladder by the Desjardin's choledocholithotomy forceps
* It may also be used during removal of kidney, ureteric or bladder stone.

Sterilization

Sterilization is done by autoclaving.

Q. Why there is no catch in this instrument?

Ans. As this instrument is used for holding stones during its removal, it is not provided with catch. Otherwise stone would be crushed during removal.

■ KEHR'S T-TUBE

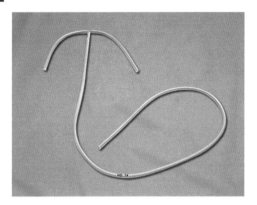

Fig. 21.54: No. 14 Polyvinyl chloride (PVC) Kehr's T-tube

No. 14 PVC (polyvinyl chloride) Kehr's T-tube is available (No. 12, 16, and 18 are also available). Silastic and latex T-tube are also available (Fig. 21.54).

There is a short horizontal limb which is inserted into the bile duct and a long vertical limb which is brought outside.

Uses

* Following choledochotomy, the bile duct is closed over a T-tube, as primary closure of bile duct is associated with higher incidence of leakage
* This is used to drain the bile duct following repair of bile duct injury. The T-tube acts as a stent and is usually kept for about 4–6 weeks
* This may also be used to stent a choledochojejunostomy or choledochoduodenostomy anastomosis
* This may be used as a stent following repair of ureteric injury.

Sterilization

It is done by autoclaving.

T-tube Cholangiography

See X-rays Section, Page No. 813–815, Chapter 17.

Management of Bile Duct Stones

See Surgical Long Cases, Page No. 166–171, Chapter 3.

Q. How T-tube is inserted?

Ans. The short limb is cut to a desired length. The limb passing toward the lower end of the bile duct is kept about 3–4 cm and the limb passing toward the hepatic duct is kept about 2–3 cm. A slit is made in the short limb so that the two openings are connected by the slit and a rim of tube is cut away along the slit made.

The short limb is then inserted into the bile duct. The choledochotomy is then closed with interrupted sutures so that the T-tube fits snugly in the bile duct taking care not to take any bite of the suture in the T-tube.

The long vertical limb of the T-tube is brought out through a stab wound in the skin in lateral abdominal wall and is fixed to the skin by a stitch.

Q. How will you take care of T-tube?

Ans.
- The T-tube is connected to a closed system of drain into a urobag
- The bile is collected in the urobag, measured and evacuated every morning
- A T-tube cholangiogram is done on 8th postoperative day
- If T-tube cholangiogram is normal, the T-tube is clamped overnight and if patient has no problem, on next morning the T-tube is removed by a smart pull. There may be slight leakage of bile for 1–2 days and the tract closes spontaneously.

■ GASTRIC OCCLUSION CLAMPS

- *Moynihan's gastric occlusion clamp:* This is a long instrument with finger bows, a ratchet, and a pair of long shaft provided with a pair of long stout blades. There are transverse serrations in the blade with a linear fenestration along the center of each blade extending near the tip of the blade. The fenestration makes the blade lighter and prevents crushing of tissues. This instrument may be curved (Fig. 21.55A) or straight (Fig. 21.55B).
- *Kocher's gastric occlusion clamp:* Kocher's gastric occlusion clamp is also a long instrument with finger bows, a ratchet, a pair of shaft, and a pair of long blades. The blades are provided with vertical serrations and there are no fenestrations in the blades. This instrument may be straight (Fig. 21.55C) or curved.

Uses

- These are used during gastrojejunostomy to clamp the stomach side for gastrojejunal anastomosis
- These are used during gastrectomy. The line of resection is decided. Two pairs of gastric occlusion clamps are applied along the proximal line of resection and the stomach is divided

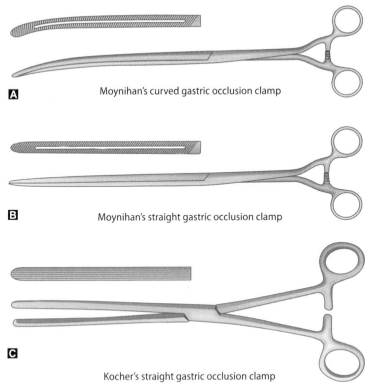

A — Moynihan's curved gastric occlusion clamp

B — Moynihan's straight gastric occlusion clamp

C — Kocher's straight gastric occlusion clamp

Figs 21.55A to C: Gastric occlusion clamps

in-between the two gastric occlusion clamps. Two pairs of intestinal occlusion clamps are applied toward the duodenal end and the stomach is divided in-between.

Sterilization

Sterilization is done by autoclaving.

Q. What are the advantages of using an occlusion clamp?

Ans.
* *Prevents spillage*: When the clamps are applied during gastrointestinal anastomosis, it occludes the lumen of the gut and prevents the spillage of gut contents.
* *Prevents bleeding*: Properly applied clamp also occludes the blood vessels and prevents bleeding during anastomosis.
* *Easier anastomosis*: The applied clamps on either side of anastomosis can be held together and the cut margins are kept closer for easier anastomosis.

Q. What do you mean by closed and open gastrointestinal anastomosis?

Ans. When anastomos is performed by occluding the lumen of the gut by using an occlusion clamp then it is called a closed type of anastomosis.

In open anastomosis, no clamps are applied. The corners of the cut margins are kept steadied by holding with Babcock's tissue forceps or stay sutures and anastomosis is done.

LANE'S PAIRED GASTROJEJUNOSTOMY CLAMPS

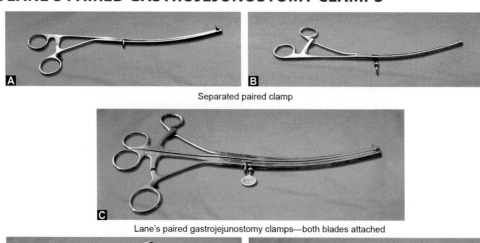

Separated paired clamp

Lane's paired gastrojejunostomy clamps—both blades attached

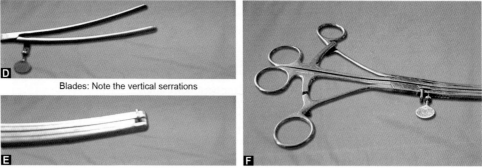

Blades: Note the vertical serrations

Tip of the blades: Note the hook in one blade   Jointing screw for attaching two blades

Figs 21.56A to F: Lane's paired gastrojejunostomy clamps

This is a paired instrument. Each instrument is provided with finger bows, a catch, a pair of shaft, and a pair of long blades provided with longitudinal serrations. Near the tip of one instrument there is a hook which fits the other blade and there is an arrangement of screw in the other blade which fixes the adjacent blade. When properly applied the two instruments are kept side by side keeping the stomach and jejunum apposed. This instrument may be curved (Fig. 21.56A) or straight (Fig. 21.56B).

Uses

This instrument is used during gastrojejunostomy. One pair of clamp is applied to the stomach and one pair is applied to the jejunum. As the two instruments are kept side by side and the screw is tightened the stomach and the jejunum is kept steadied and anastomosis is done easily.

Sterilization

It is done by autoclaving.

Q. What are the indications of gastrojejunostomy?

Ans. Gastrojejunostomy is anastomosis of stomach to the jejunum either by using a loop of jejunum or by using a Roux-en-Y loop of jejunum. The anastomosis may be done to the anterior wall of stomach (Anterior GJ) or to the posterior wall of stomach (posterior GJ). The jejunal loop may be brought up either anterior to the colon (antecolic GJ) or posterior to the colon (retrocolic GJ). The indications are:

* Treatment of peptic ulcer:
  - Gastrojejunostomy is done as a drainage procedure along with truncal vagotomy for treatment of peptic ulcer disease
  - Gastrojejunostomy may be done as a sole procedure in patients with peptic ulcer disease with very poor general condition
  - Pyloric stenosis due to corrosive acid poisoning causing gastric burn and subsequent fibrosis leading to pyloric stricture
  - Carcinoma of stomach:
    - Following lower radical gastrectomy, continuity is maintained by gastrojejunostomy
    - In inoperable carcinoma of stomach causing gastric outlet obstruction
  - Chronic pancreatitis causing gastric outlet obstruction
  - Following Whipple's pancreaticoduodenectomy for periampullary carcinoma or carcinoma of head of pancreas, gastric continuity is maintained by gastrojejunostomy.

Q. What is an ideal gastrojejunostomy?

Ans. A retrocolic, short or no loop, no tension, isoperistaltic gastrojejunostomy with a vertical stoma is considered as an ideal gastrojejunostomy.

A Roux-en-Y gastrojejunostomy has been claimed to be superior as there is no chance of bile reflux gastritis which is common with *loop gastrojejunostomy*.

Q. Describe the steps of truncal vagotomy and gastrojejunostomy.

Ans. *See* Page No. 1097, 1098, Chapter 22.

▌INTESTINAL OCCLUSION CLAMPS

* *Doyen's intestinal occlusion clamps*: These instruments have finger bows, a pair of shaft with a pair of long blades. The blades are lighter and there are vertical serrations in the blade. There is a ratchet, which when closed bring the blades in apposition. These instruments may be curved (Fig. 21.57A) or straight (Fig. 21.57B).
* *Carwardine's twin intestinal occlusion clamps*: These are paired instrument. These are smaller, lighter instrument than Doyen's intestinal occlusion clamps. In addition to finger bows, ratchet, and a pair of shaft and blades, there is a slot on the side of one shaft of one instrument and a screw on the shaft of the other instrument. When applied properly the slot and the screw fit and this keeps this instrument side by side, so that the intestinal loops are kept side by side during anastomosis (Figs 21.58A and B).

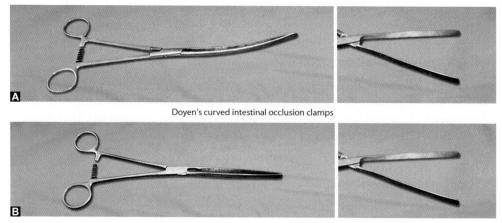

Figs 21.57A and B: Doyen's intestinal occlusion clamps. Note the delicate long blades with vertical serrations

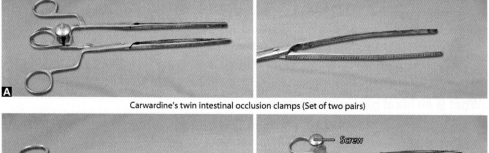

Figs 21.58A and B: Carwardine's twin intestinal clamp. Note the screw, slot, and the delicate blades with vertical serrations

Uses

These instruments are used for gut resection and anastomosis.

Sterilization

It is done by autoclaving.

Q. What are the indications of intestinal resection and anastomosis?

Ans. The important indications are:
- Strangulated hernia with devitalization of gut

- Intestinal obstruction with strangulation causing devitalization of a segment of gut
- Intestinal trauma causing intestinal laceration or devitalization of a segment of a gut due to mesenteric tear
- Intussusception which is irreducible or has caused strangulation of a segment of gut
- Intestinal neoplasm
- Meckel's diverticulum requires excision with a wedge of ileum
- Crohn's disease with stricture or fistula
- Ulcerative colitis not responding to medical treatment
- Intestinal tuberculosis with stricture formation
- Neoplastic lesion in gut either benign or malignant.

Q. What are the different types of intestinal anastomosis?

Ans. Intestinal continuity may be maintained by:
- End-to-end anastomosis
- End-to-side anastomosis
- Side-to-side anastomosis.

Q. What are the different techniques of intestinal anastomosis?

Ans.
- *Standard two layer anastomosis*: Consisting of:
  - Inner layer of suture taking the full thickness of the bowel wall—posterior and anterior through and through layers
  - Outer seromuscular layer—posterior and anterior seromuscular layers
- *Single layer anastomosis*: There are different techniques of applying single layer suture:
  - Simple interrupted suture through the full thickness of the intestine with knot placed toward the mucosal aspect
  - Gambee stitch—suture passed through all layers of the intestine with a loop on mucosa on each side of the anastomosis for better mucosal inversion
  - A single layer extramucosal stitch—suture passed from the serosal aspect and emerges through the submucosa and making a loop on submucosa on each side of the anastomosis.

Q. Which suture material will you prefer for intestinal anastomosis?

Ans.
- *In two layer anastomosis*: Posterior through and through and anterior through and through with absorbable suture—polyglactin (vicryl), polydioxanone (PDS), polyglecaprone (Monocryl) or catgut.
- Posterior seromuscular and anterior seromuscular with mersilk, polyglactin or polydioxanone suture.
- In single layer anastomosis either mersilk or polyglactin sutures are used.
- The size of the suture material for gut anastomosis is 2-0 or 3-0.

Small Gut Resection Anastomosis

Technique of Small Gut Resection Anastomosis

Following laparotomy, the area of gut to be resected is selected. The vessels supplying this segment of the gut are to be ligated and divided. A V-shaped area in the mesentery is marked with the apex pointing toward the root of the mesentery. The vessels supplying the segment of the gut is held by a series of hemostatic forceps and the mesenteric vessels divided in-between the hemostatic forceps.

Two pairs of intestinal occlusion clamps are applied on each side of the intestine which is to be resected. A gauge swab is placed behind the gut and the intestine is divided in-between the occlusion clamps on either side. The escaping gut contents are sucked and swabbed off with the gauge piece. The loop of the intestine is now removed with two pairs of intestinal occlusion clamps still attached to the intestine.

Anastomosis: The occlusion clamps with cut ends of the intestine are approximated so that the cut ends of the bowel lies in close apposition. The anastomosis is done in two layers—a layer of seromuscular sutures and a layer of through and through sutures.

Posterior seromuscular suture is started at the antimesenteric border with 2-0 polyglactin sutures taking bites through the seromuscular layers and continued up to the mesenteric border of the gut and the suture is tied at this end, the suture is kept for continuation of this suture as anterior seromuscular layer.

The posterior through and through suture with 2-0 polyglactin is started at the antimesenteric border and continued around the circumference of the bowel to come back to the starting point as anterior through and through layers. The running sutures should be interlocked at intervals to prevent purse string effect. The suture line is inspected for any bleeding and if necessary additional stitches may be applied.

The anterior seromuscular suture is now continued inverting the through and through layer (Lambert suture).

The gap in the mesentery is apposed with interrupted sutures taking care not to take any bite through the mesenteric vessels.

Drains are not indicated routinely. If there had been perforation of the gut causing peritoneal contamination, then a drain may be inserted.

■ PAYRS' CRUSHING CLAMPS

Payrs' Gastric Crushing Clamps

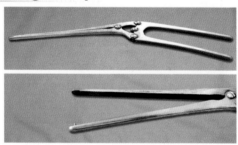

Fig. 21.59: Payrs' gastric crushing clamps. Note the long heavy blades with vertical serrations

These are heavy instruments. The handles are stout and there is a double lever arrangement. The blades are long and heavy and there are vertical serrations in the blade (Fig. 21.59).

The lever arrangement magnifies the pressure of the handle closure to the blades so that it produces a crushing effect, whereby the mucosa is crushed and it curls up.

Uses

These are used during partial gastrectomies. However, most of the surgeons do not use these crushing clamps during gastrectomies. If at all these clamps are used, these clamps are used toward the side of the stomach that is to be resected and the proximal stomach is held up by a gastric occlusion clamp.

Sterilization

It is done by autoclaving.

Q. What are the indications of partial gastrectomy?

Ans.
* Chronic gastric or duodenal ulcer
* Anastomotic ulcer following gastrojejunostomy
* Gastric carcinoma
* Gastrointestinal stromal tumors
* Along with Whipple's pancreaticoduodenectomy, distal stomach is removed. However, in pylorus preserving pancreaticoduodenectomy distal stomach is not removed.

Q. What are the indications of total gastrectomy?

Ans. Total gastrectomy involves resection of whole of the stomach with Roux-en-Y esophagojejunostomy. The important indications are:
* Proximal gastric cancer involving the fundus and cardia
* Cancer involving the midbody of the stomach
* Generalized linitis plastica
* Corrosive stricture involving the whole of stomach
* Zollinger–Ellison syndrome.

Q. How does the crushing clamps functions?

Ans. When the crushing clamp is applied it crushes the muscle and the mucous coat which curls inward and blocks the lumen. The sutures are placed well over the crushed muscle.

Crushing clamps are used at sites where the stump is to be closed, e.g. duodenal stump during gastrectomy and appendix stump during appendicectomy. Crushing clamps should not be used where anastomosis is to be done.

Payrs' Intestinal Crushing Clamps

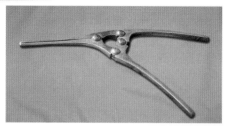

Fig. 21.60: Payrs' intestinal crushing clamps

These instruments resemble gastric crushing clamps, but the blades are smaller and the instrument is little lighter (Fig. 21.60).

Payrs' Appendix Crushing Clamps

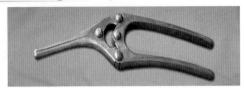

Fig. 21.61: Payrs' appendix crushing clamps

These instruments resemble gastric crushing clamps, but the blades are much smaller and the instrument is little lighter (Fig. 21.61).

Uses of Intestinal and Appendix Crushing Clamps

◆ These may be used to crush the base of the appendix during appendicectomy. However, the base of the appendix is usually crushed with a hemostatic forceps
◆ These may be used to crush the duodenal stump during gastrectomy
◆ These may be used during right hemicolectomy.
  The crushing clamp may be used to crush the ends of ileum and the transverse colon. The ends are then oversewn with sutures and a side to side anastomosis is done.
◆ For intestinal resection anastomosis, two pairs of intestinal occlusion clamps are used and crushing clamps are not used usually.

Sterilization

Sterilization is done by autoclaving.

■ PYELOLITHOTOMY FORCEPS

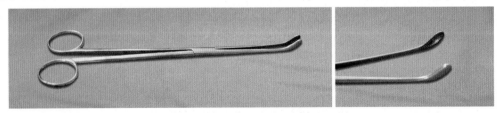

Fig. 21.62: Pyelolithotomy forceps. Note the curved blades with groove and transverse serrations

This is a long instrument, consists of finger bows, a pair of shaft and a pair of blades. The blades are small and oval with transverse serration on the inner side of the blades with a central groove. There is no ratchet in the shaft (Fig. 21.62).

Uses

This instrument is used to hold the stone during nephrolithotomy, pyelolithotomy or ureterolithotomy.

Sterilization

Sterilization is done by autoclaving.

■ SUPRAPUBIC CYSTOLITHOTOMY FORCEPS

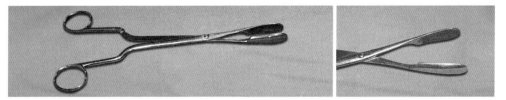

Fig. 21.63: Suprapubic cystolithotomy forceps. Note the long blades with grooves and elevations in the blades

This forceps consists of finger bows—a pair of shaft and a pair of blades. The blades are longer and the inner surface of the blades is provided with fine knobs which help in better gripping of the stones. There are no ratchets in this instrument (Fig. 21.63).

Uses

It is used for suprapubic cystolithotomy. After the bladder is opened by a suprapubic cystotomy the instrument is inserted into the bladder and the stone is removed.

Sterilization

It is done by autoclaving.

Discussion on Renal Calculi

See X-rays Section, Page No. 975–798, Chapter 17.

■ SIMPLE RUBBER CATHETER NO. 10

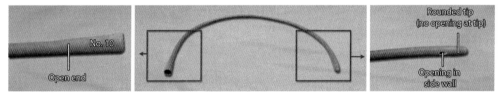

Fig. 21.64: Simple rubber catheter No. 10

This catheter is made of India rubber. The tip is smooth and rounded and there is an opening at the side near the tip. There is an opening at the other end. It comes in variety of sizes—6, 8, 10, etc. (Fig. 21.64).

Q. What does number 10 indicates?

Ans. This is an English scale regarding the diameter of the catheter.
    The diameter is expressed in mm as—Number of catheter/2 + 1.

Q. What are the uses of a simple rubber catheter?

Ans. *Urological use*:
- To differentiate anuria and retention of urine by catheterization of bladder
- To relieve retention of urine by catheterization

- To assess the amount of residual urine after micturition. This, however, can also be done by ultrasonography
- To collect a specimen of urine in an unconscious patient
- *For performing cystography*: The catheter is introduced into the bladder and the dye diluted with normal saline is introduced into the bladder through the catheter
- *For diagnosis of urinary tract injuries*: Catheterization of bladder if revealed hematuria indicates presence of urinary tract injury
- In case of urethral rupture the catheter cannot be negotiated into the bladder
- For administration of intravesical chemotherapy or BCG vaccine for treatment of bladder carcinoma.

Nonurological use:
- *For diagnosis of esophageal atresia in a newborn*: The catheter cannot be passed into the stomach
- It may be used as an oxygen catheter
- It is used during choledocholithotomy for flushing the bile duct with normal saline to remove the sludge and small stones
- It may be used during vagotomy. A catheter is passed around the esophagus to give traction to the esophagus and to identify the vagus nerve
- It may be used to irrigate an abscess cavity.

Q. How will you catheterize a patient presenting with acute retention of urine? What are the complications of catheterization?

Ans. *See* Minor Surgical Procedures, Page No. 954, 955, Chapter 20.

■ FOLEY'S BALLOON CATHETER

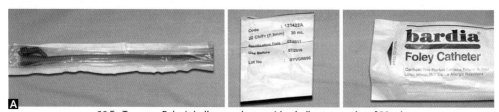

A

22 Fr. Two way Foley's balloon catheter with a balloon capacity of 30 mL

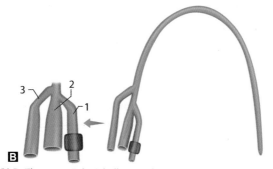

B

B—22 Fr. Three way Foley's balloon catheter with a balloon capacity of 30–50 mL

Figs 21.65A and B: Foley's balloon catheter. 1. Side channel for inflating the balloon; 2. Main channel for drainage; 3. Third channel for drainage or irrigation

This is a variety of self-retaining catheter.
* In two ways Foley's balloon catheter, the side channel is used to inflate the balloon so that it is kept indwelling. There is a valve in the side channel. The main channel is for drainage of urine. The catheter number (No. 16 Fr.) and the balloon capacity (30–50 mL) are mentioned on the main or side channel (Fig. 21.65A)
* In three ways Foley's balloon catheter, there is an additional third channel for either irrigation or drainage (Fig. 21.65B).

Uses

* For relief of retention of urine by urethral catheterization
* It may be used for suprapubic cystostomy
* It may be used for tube nephrostomy
* It may be used for urethral catheterization following urethroplasty
* It may be used for urethral catheterization following open prostatectomy for drainage of bladder. The three way catheter is favored as there is a side channel for irrigation of bladder
* It may be used for drainage of bladder to monitor urine output in critically ill patient or following major operation or major trauma
* It may be used for gastrostomy or jejunostomy
* It may be used for tube cecostomy
* It may be used for cholecystostomy
* For tube thoracostomy for drainage of empyema or hemothorax or for pneumothorax.

Sterilization

Supplied in a presterilized pack and is usually sterilized by gamma irradiation.

Q. What do you mean by a 16 Fr. catheter?

Ans. This is a French scale of measurement. This indicates the circumference of the catheter in millimeter. Diameter of the catheter in mm is calculated by:
   No. of catheter in French scale/3

■ MALECOT'S CATHETER NO. 30 FR

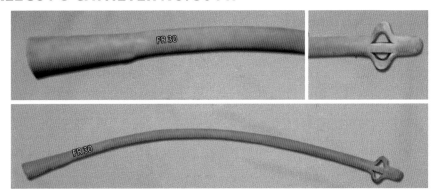

Fig. 21.66: Malecot's catheter No. 30 Fr

This is a type of self-retaining catheter and it is retained after its introduction by its dilated winged end (Fig. 21.66). The dilated winged end may be made straight by introducing a Malecot catheter introducer or by inserting a hemostatic forceps into the dilated end and straightening it over the introducer or hemostatic forceps.

Uses

Like Foley's catheter—except that it is never used for urethral catheterization.

Sterilization

Sterilization is done by autoclaving.

Q. How will you change a suprapubic Malecot catheter?

Ans. Suprapubic cystostomy catheter needs to be changed every 3–4 weeks.
* Local area is cleaned with antiseptic solution
* The catheter is removed by a smart pull
* Another catheter is introduced through the same tract by stretching the tip of the catheter over a catheter introducer.

■ DE PEZZER'S CATHETER NO. 24 FR

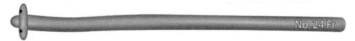

Fig. 21.67: de Pezzer's catheter No. 24 Fr

This is also a self-retaining catheter and it is kept in place after introduction due to its dilated bulbous end (Fig. 21.67).

Uses

Like Foley's catheter—except that it is never used for urethral catheterization.

Sterilization

Sterilization is done by autoclaving.

Q. How are these self-retaining catheters removed?

Ans. Foley's catheter is removed after withdrawing the water from the balloon.
    The Malecot catheter and the de Pezzer catheter are removed by a smart pull.

■ CATHETER INTRODUCER

This is a long metal rod curved like a dilator with a groove in the body with a rounded tip (Fig. 21.68).

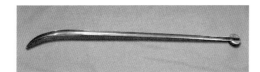

Fig. 21.68: Catheter introducer. Note the groove and curvature of the instrument

Uses

◆ It is used to introduce a Foley's catheter through the urethra when the catheter cannot be introduced in the usual way either due to stricture urethra or prostatic enlargement. But there is risk of false passage in this technique
◆ It may be used to introduce a Malecot or de Pezzer's catheter. The introducer is passed through the catheter and is brought near the tip. The catheter is stretched at the tip over the introducer thereby straightening the tip so that the catheter is introduced through a small opening.

Sterilization

It is done by autoclaving.

▌METALLIC BOUGIE

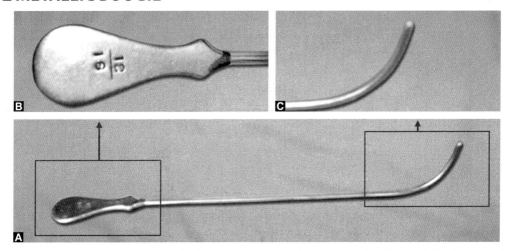

Figs 21.69A to C: (A) Clutton's metallic bougie No. 12/16; (B) Note the handle which is violin shaped and number difference of 4 and (C) terminal part of the blade which curved and having a rounded tip

Characteristics

◆ *Clutton's metallic bougie*: This is a solid, cylindrical metallic instrument. The handle is violin shaped with a long shaft and the terminal end has a smooth curve with a blunt tip. The number written on the handle has a difference of 4. The denominator number denotes the circumference in mm at the base and the numerator denotes the circumference in mm at the tip. This is available in a set of 12 and the different numbers are 6/10, 8/12, 10/14, 12/16 .... 28/32 (Figs 21.69A to C).

♦ *Lister's metallic bougie*: This is identical to a Clutton's metallic bougie. The differences are:
  − The handle is rounded and the tip is olive pointed
  − The number written has a difference of 3 and has same implication as in Clutton's metallic bougie
  − This is also available in a set of 12 (Fig. 21.70).

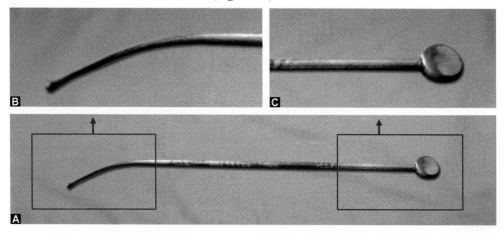

Figs 21.70A to C: (A) Lister's metallic bougie No. 11/14; (B) Note the handle which is round and having a number difference of 3; (C) Note tip which is curved and olive pointed

Uses

♦ Metallic bougie is used for dilatation of urethra in urethral stricture
♦ It is used for dilatation of urethra prior to introduction of cystoscope
♦ It is used during repair of rupture urethra by rail road technique
♦ It is used during choledocholithotomy. This is used as a sound to ascertain presence of bile duct stones. This may be passed through the ampulla of Vater to ascertain the patency of ampulla.

Sterilization

Sterilization is done by autoclaving.

Q. How will you do urethral dilatation?

Ans. Patient lies supine. The external genitalia are cleaned with antiseptic solution (Savlon). 20 mL of 2% xylocaine jelly is introduced through the external urethral meatus into the penile urethra. Wait for 5 minutes.

Stand on the left side of the patient. The penis is held by the left hand. Start dilatation with a 10/14 dilator. The dilator is introduced through the external urethral meatus keeping it parallel to the left inguinal ligament. The dilator is allowed to pass by its own weight. As the dilator goes in bring it to the midline of the abdomen in an anticlockwise direction and as it goes further down bring the dilator down in between the two thighs. Once the dilator goes into the bladder, it can be rotated easily. There should be no pain or bleeding during the procedure.

Q. How will you know if there is any false passage?

Ans.
* There is continuous sense of resistance while introducing the instrument
* The handle cannot be pressed between the two thighs
* The instrument cannot be moved freely from side to side
* Patient may complain of severe pain
* Bleeding per urethra.

Q. For stricture urethra what should be the frequency of dilatation?

Ans. For passable stricture urethra, dilatation at regular interval is the treatment of choice.
* Initially dilatation is to be done once a week for a month. Then:
* Once in a month for a year
* Once every 6 months for 3 years
* Afterwards once a year for lifelong (birthday dilatation).

Q. What are the complications of urethral dilatation?

Ans.
* False passage
* Bleeding
* Fistula formation
* Infection
* Restricture.

Q. When do you consider that a stricture is impassable?

Ans. An impassable stricture is one where a smallest size filiform bougie (1 Fr.) cannot be negotiated through it.

Q. What are the indications of surgical treatment for urethral stricture?

Ans.
* Impassable stricture
* Failure of repeated dilatation
* When dilatation is required at more frequent interval.

▮ FEMALE METALLIC CATHETER

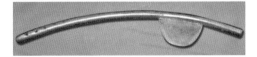

Fig. 21.71: Female metallic catheter

This is a short metallic catheter. The tip is rounded and there are multiple side holes near the tip (Fig. 21.71).

Uses

- It is used during pelvic operations to empty the bladder before the operation to prevent injury to the bladder. Bladder needs to be emptied while doing laparotomy through a lower midline incision
- It may be used to relieve retention if a rubber catheter cannot be passed.

Sterilization

It is done by autoclaving.

■ MALE METALLIC CATHETER

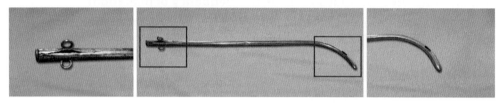

Fig. 21.72: Male metallic catheter. Note the handle with two rings for better grip. Note the tip with curved and rounded end with a side hole

This is a long metallic catheter. Like a dilator the terminal part of the catheter is curved. The tip is rounded and there are side holes in the catheter near the tip. There are two rings near the base for holding the catheter (Fig. 21.72).

Uses

This catheter is used for relief of retention when a simple rubber, Foley's or Gibbon's catheter cannot be passed through the urethra.

Sterilization

It is done by autoclaving.

Q. How will you pass the metallic catheter?

Ans. The patient lies supine and the surgeon stands on the left side of the patient. The external genitalia are cleaned with an antiseptic solution. 20 mL of 2% xylocaine jelly is introduced through the external urethral meatus into the penile urethra and the glans penis is kept pressed for 5 minutes for adequate anesthesia. The metal catheter is lubricated with the xylocaine jelly. Penis is lifted up and steadied with the left hand and the catheter tip is placed at the external urethral meatus keeping it parallel to the left inguinal ligament. Instrument is allowed to go in by its own weight and the handle of the instrument is gradually brought toward the midline over the abdomen. As the catheter goes further, the handle of the instrument is now brought down between the two thighs.

Q. How do you know the catheter has gone into the bladder?

Ans. As the catheter goes into the bladder, there is loss of resistance, the handle can be depressed between the thighs and the instrument can be rotated freely on either side. No bleeding through the urethra and urine will drain through the catheter.

■ VOLKMAN'S SPOON OR SCOOP

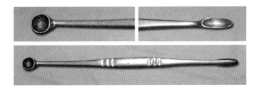

Fig. 21.73: Volkman's spoon or scoop

This is a long metallic instrument with a spoon like ends with sharp edges larger in size on one side and small in size at the other end. The sharp edges allow easy curettage (Fig. 21.73).

Uses

- It is used to curette a chronic abscess cavity either in bone or in soft tissue.
- It may be used to curette a sinus or a fistulous tract.
- It may be used to curette an aneurysmal bone cyst.

Sterilization

It is done by autoclaving.

■ KELLY'S RECTAL SPECULUM (PROCTOSCOPE)

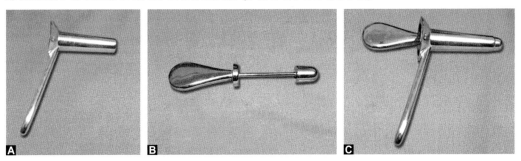

Figs 21.74A to C: (A) Kelly's rectal speculum (proctoscope); (B) Speculum proper; (C) Obturator

The instrument is about 3 inches long.

There is a hollow outer sheath where a handle is attached. The terminal end of the sheath is either round or obliquely cut. The inner rod is called the obturator and its terminal part is smooth and rounded and fits well with the outer sheath. In some instrument, there is arrangement for attachment of a light (Figs 21.74A to C).

Uses

The proctoscope may be used for diagnostic or therapeutic purposes.
- *Diagnostic use*: By proctoscopic examination, it is possible to diagnose following conditions—
  - Diagnosis of piles: the pile mass protrudes into the lumen of the proctoscope
  - An anal or a rectal polyp may be seen protruding into the lumen of the proctoscope
  - Carcinoma of anal canal or rectum may appear as a proliferative mass or an ulcerating lesion
  - Diagnosis of ulcerative colitis: Associated proctitis may appear as red, congested mucosa which bleeds to touch and in some cases pseudopolyps may be seen
  - The internal opening of a perianal fistula may be seen
  - The apex of an intussusception may be seen in the anal canal through the proctoscope.
- *Therapeutic uses*:
  - Used during injection sclerotherapy of piles. The injection is made at the base of the pile mass visualized through the proctoscope
  - Used during polypectomy
  - Used while taking a biopsy from a rectal or an anal growth.

Q. How will you do a proctoscopic examination?

Ans. Patient is explained the procedure and a consent is taken for a digital rectal examination and proctoscopic examination.

Patient is asked to lie in left lateral position. The left leg is kept straight and the right leg is flexed at knee and hip and is drawn toward the abdomen. Patient is asked to relax the buttock and take deep breathing.

The perineal area is inspected to look for any swelling, fistula, sentinel skin tag or any tear in the skin lined part of anal canal.

A digital rectal examination is done first to exclude any painful condition like anal fissure or abscess.

The proctoscope is lubricated with 2% xylocaine jelly and is then introduced into the anal canal at first directed upwards and forward toward the umbilicus and then pushed upward and backward toward the sacrum. The obturator is withdrawn and a light is thrown inside from a torchlight and the interior of the rectum is inspected. The sheath is then gradually withdrawn and rest of the examination is completed.

■ FLATUS TUBE (FIG. 21.75)

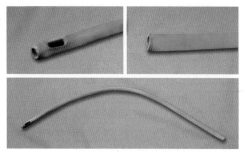

Fig. 21.75: Flatus tube

This is a thick rubber tube. There is an opening at the tip and the tip is rounded and smooth. In addition there are two side openings. The other end is conical.

Uses

* It is used during nonoperative decompression of sigmoid volvulus.
* It may be used to relieve gaseous distension of large gut due to paralytic ileus.

Sterilization

Sterilization is done by autoclaving.

Q. How is the flatus tube inserted?

Ans. Patient is explained the procedure. Patient lies in left lateral position or in lithotomy position.

The flatus tube is lubricated with 2% xylocaine jelly. A digital rectal examination is done before introduction of the tube to exclude any painful anal condition. The flatus tube is then gently passed into the anal canal and then pushed further up. While inserting, in a case of volvulus, there will be resistance in passage of the tube further up. The tube is pushed further up with manipulation and once it goes beyond the point of twist, lots of flatus and feces will come out and there will be deflation of the dilated sigmoid colon. The other end of the tube is kept immersed in a kidney dish containing water.

■ DOYEN'S MOUTH GAG

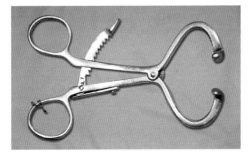

Fig. 21.76: Doyen's mouth gag

In addition to finger bows there is a ratchet lock mechanism in the shaft. The two blades are semicircular in shape and bent in the terminal part. When the finger bows are kept apart the blades are in closed position. When the finger bows are approximated the blades are separated. The instrument is kept self-retaining, once the ratchet is locked (Fig. 21.76).

Uses

This is used to open the mouth during intraoral operations like:
* Glossectomy
* Cleft palate operation

- Removal of calculus from submandibular duct
- Excision of an intraoral ranula
- Taking biopsy from an intraoral or pharyngeal lesion
- Repair of intraoral injuries.

Sterilization

It is done by autoclaving.

■ AIRWAY TUBES

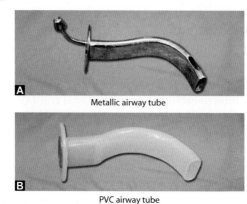

Metallic airway tube

PVC airway tube

Figs 21.77A and B: Airway tubes (PVC: polyvinyl chloride)

- *Metallic airway tube*: Metallic airway tube is a curved stainless steel tube with both ends open. At one end, there are multiple side holes. At the other end, there is flange. The flange is kept outside the teeth (Fig. 21.77A).
- *Rubber/PVC airway tube*: In rubber airway tube, at the proximal end, there is a stainless steel tube fitted inside the rubber tube. This part is kept in-between the teeth (Fig. 21.77B).

Uses

- Pharyngeal airway tube is used to prevent tongue falling back in an unconscious patient. This also prevents tongue bite.
- During anesthesia, airway tube is inserted to prevent falling back of tongue while ventilating with a face mask.
- During post-anesthetic recovery, airway tube may be inserted to prevent falling back of tongue. Oxygen may be administered through the side tube.

Sterilization

It is done by autoclaving.

■ FULLER'S BIVALVED METALLIC TRACHEOSTOMY TUBE

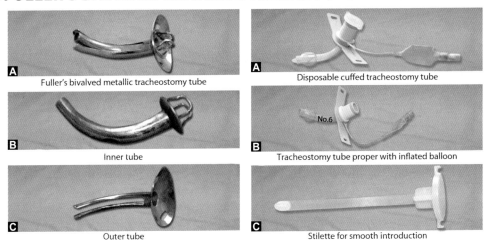

A Fuller's bivalved metallic tracheostomy tube

B Inner tube

C Outer tube

Figs 21.78A to C: Fuller's bivalve metallic tracheostomy tube

A Disposable cuffed tracheostomy tube

B Tracheostomy tube proper with inflated balloon

C Stilette for smooth introduction

Figs 21.79A to C: Disposable cuffed tracheostomy tube No. 6

Fuller's metallic tracheostomy tube comprises:
* An inner tube which is a hollow metallic tube with a terminal rounded opening and an additional opening in the upper wall of the tube. The proximal open end of the tube is provided with a shield which is attached to two metallic rings. They are used to hold the tube during insertion and removal (Fig. 21.78A). The inner tube is longer than the outer tube and when inserted into the outer tube it projects beyond the outer tube (Fig. 21.78B).
* An outer tube which is wider than the inner tube, the outer tube is biflanged. The proximal end of the outer tube is provided with a shield in which there is one opening on either side which is used to pass a tape to fix the tracheostomy tube around the neck (Fig. 21.78C).

The other varieties of tracheostomy tubes are:
* *Cuffed tracheostomy tube usually supplied in a presterilized pack*: This tracheostomy tube may be kept indwelling by inflating the cuff with air. Cuffed tracheostomy is specifically required in unconscious patient who requires assisted ventilation (Figs 21.79A to C).
* *Noncuffed tracheostomy tube*: This is a curved rubber tube with openings at the either end. At the proximal end there is a flap with side openings through which tapes are passed to fix the tracheostomy tube around the neck.

Q. What are the indications of tracheostomy?

Ans. The important indications for tracheostomy are:
* *Mechanical obstruction to upper airway*:
  – Laryngeal diphtheria
  – Foreign body impacted in larynx
  – Acute laryngeal edema
  – Ludwig's angina causing laryngeal obstruction
  – Neck, mouth, and jaw injuries

- Cut throat wound with laryngeal or tracheal injury
- Carcinoma of thyroid
- Bilateral recurrent laryngeal nerve palsy
- Laryngeal tumors.

♦ *In respiratory paralysis*: In respiratory paralysis due to poliomyelitis, Guillain–Barrè syndrome, bulbar palsy, tetanus, and flail chest, patient may require mechanical ventilation for prolonged period.

Tracheostomy is required in such situation for effective tracheobronchial toilet.

♦ *Following some radical surgery*:
- Laryngectomy
- Laryngopharyngectomy
- Following total thyroidectomy if there is associated tracheomalacia.

♦ *For reduction of dead space*: Patient with chronic obstructive or restrictive airway disease with inadequate ventilation may benefit by a 30% reduction of dead space following tracheostomy.

♦ *For aspiration of retained secretions*:
- When the excessive tracheobronchial secretions in unconscious patient
- In patient with major chest or cervical injury
- When tracheobronchial secretion cannot be cleared by simple suction.

Q. Where do you insert the tracheostomy tube?

Ans. Depending on the level of insertion of the tube into the trachea, tracheostomy may be:

♦ *High tracheostomy*: Tracheostomy done above the level of isthmus of thyroid gland.
♦ *Mid tracheostomy*: Tracheostomy done at the level of isthmus of thyroid gland.
♦ *Low tracheostomy*: Tracheostomy done below the level of the isthmus of thyroid gland.
The thyroid isthmus lies at the level of 2nd, 3rd and 4th tracheal rings.

Q. Describe the steps of tracheostomy.

Ans.

♦ Patient is kept supine. Neck is extended by placing a sand bag in-between the two shoulders and head is supported on a head ring.

♦ Antiseptic cleaning and draping. The area is infiltrated with 2% injection of xylocaine.

♦ About 4 cm. transverse skin incision is made in the neck crease 2 cm above the suprasternal notch. The platysma is incised in the same line. The upper and lower skin flaps are raised. The deep fascia is incised in the midline and the strap muscles are retracted laterally.

♦ The thyroid isthmus is dissected by incising the pretracheal fascia and lifted up with a blunt hook. The thyroid isthmus may be divided between clamps and ligated thereby exposing the trachea. 0.5 mL of 2% xylocaine is injected into the trachea to minimize the coughing while introducing the tracheostomy tube. The trachea is steadied by holding the cricoid cartilage with a sharp hook and trachea is incised over the 2nd and 3rd tracheal ring. The opening is dilated by inserting a tracheal dilator and the tracheostomy tube is inserted. An anterior flap of trachea over the 2nd and 3rd tracheal ring may be excised for ease of introduction of tracheostomy tube.

◆ The deep fascia and the skin are closed. A tape is passed through the rim of the tracheostomy tube and tied around the neck.

Q. How will you take care of the tracheostomy tube?

Ans.
◆ Regular suction of the tracheostomy tube maintaining strict asepsis
◆ Inspired air should be adequately humidified
◆ Regular chest physiotherapy
◆ If a metallic tracheostomy is used initially it should be replaced by PVC or rubber tracheostomy tube after 24–48 hours
◆ A spare tracheostomy tube should be kept ready to replace the tracheostomy tube in case it gets blocked by viscid secretion.

Q. What are the complications of tracheostomy?

Ans.
◆ Bleeding due to injury to anterior jugular vein, thyroid isthmus, inferior thyroid vein or arteria thyroidea ima
◆ Tracheal stenosis: Particularly when patient is using cuffed tracheostomy tube for a prolonged period
◆ Surgical emphysema in the neck
◆ Mediastinal emphysema
◆ Blockage of tracheostomy tube and respiratory obstruction
◆ Infection.

■ SINGLE-BLADED BLUNT HOOK

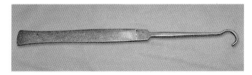

Fig. 21.80: Single-bladed blunt hook

This is used during tracheostomy to retract the strap muscles of the neck and to retract the isthmus of the thyroid gland (Fig. 21.80).

■ SINGLE-BLADED SHARP HOOK

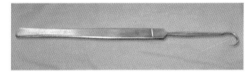

Fig. 21.81: Single-bladed sharp hook

This is used during tracheostomy to steady the trachea by holding the cricoid cartilage with the sharp hook (Fig. 21.81).

■ TRACHEAL DILATOR

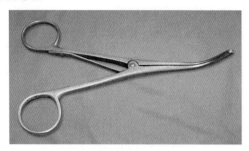

Fig. 21.82: Tracheal dilator

This instrument has finger bows, a pair of shaft, and two blades. The tip of the blades is olive pointed. When the finger bows are kept apart, the blades lie in closed position. When the finger bows are pressed and apposed the blades get separated (Fig. 21.82).

Uses

This instrument is used during tracheostomy. After a stab incision is made over the trachea, the tracheal dilator is introduced into the trachea in closed position. The tracheal dilator is then opened up by pressing the finger bows and the stab wound in the trachea opens up and the tracheostomy tube is then inserted through the gap. The tracheal dilator is then closed by releasing the finger bows and the instrument is withdrawn.

Sterilization

It is done by autoclaving.

■ CORRUGATED RUBBER SHEET DRAIN

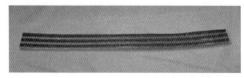

Fig. 21.83: Corrugated rubber sheet drain

This is a corrugated rubber sheet which may be cut to a desired size before use as a drain (Fig. 21.83).

Uses

- It is used to drain blood, pus or bile following some operations.
- It is used following cholecystectomy. The drain is placed in the subhepatic space and in the hepatorenal pouch of Morrison.
- It is used following repair of peptic perforation.
- The drain is kept in the hepatorenal pouch of Morrison.

* It is used following drainage of subphrenic abscess and pelvic abscess. The drain is placed in the subphrenic space or in the pelvis.
* It is used following pancreaticojejunostomy or pancreatic resection. The corrugated rubber sheet drain is placed in the lesser sac as a prophylactic drain which may drain pancreatic juice if there is formation of a postoperative pancreatic fistula.
* It may be used following small or large gut resection anastomosis. The drain is placed in the hepatorenal pouch of Morrison or in the pelvis.
* It may be used following mastectomy. The drain is kept in the axilla and under the breast flap.
* It may be used during repair of incisional hernia. One drain is kept in the preperitoneal space and another drain is kept deep to the skin.
* It is used in hydrocele operation following eversion of sac. A small corrugated rubber sheet drain is placed in the scrotum deep to the dartos muscle.

Sterilization

Sterilization is done by autoclaving.

■ ANEURYSM NEEDLE

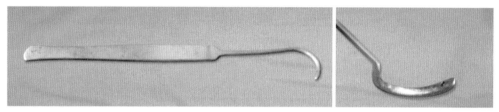

Fig. 21.84: Aneurysm needle. Note the curved blade with groove in inner aspect and eye at tip of the blade

This instrument has got a handle, shaft, and a blade. The terminal part of the blade is blunt, bent at about right angle and there is an eye with groove on the undersurface. The eye is meant for threading a suture (Fig. 21.84).

Uses

* It is used during venesection to pass ligature around the vein. One ligature is passed around the vein to ligate the distal end of the vein. Another ligature is passed around the vein in the proximal part and is tied after venotomy and introduction of the cannula through the vein.
* It may be used during thyroidectomy to pass a ligature around the superior thyroid vessels close to the upper pole of the gland.
* It may be used during nephrectomy to pass a ligature around the renal vessels.
* It may be used during splenectomy to pass a ligature around the splenic vessels.
* It may be used to pass a ligature around an aneurysm at the proximal and distal end of the aneurysm. It was in fact originally used for this purpose.
* It may be used during cholecystectomy to pass ligatures around the cystic duct and the cystic artery.

Sterilization

It is done by autoclaving.

Aneurysm

Q. What is an aneurysm?

Ans. Localized dilatation of a segment of an artery is called aneurysm.

Q. What are true and false aneurysms?

Ans. In true aneurysm, the aneurysm sac wall is lined by all the layers of the arterial wall.

In false aneurysm, the aneurysm sac wall is lined by a single layer of fibrous tissue and the layers of the arterial wall do not cover the aneurysm. The aneurysmal sac communicates with the arterial lumen through a rent in the wall of the artery.

Q. What are the different types of aneurysm?

Ans. Depending on the shape, aneurysm may be:
* *Fusiform*: Dilatation of the whole circumference of the segment of the arterial wall.
* *Saccular*: A part of the circumference of the arterial wall projecting as a bulbous mass.
* *Dissecting*: There is a breach in the tunica intima and the blood forces in between the tunica intima and the tunica media leading to occlusion of the lumen of the artery.

Q. What are the important causes of aneurysm?

Ans.
* Atherosclerosis is the most common cause of aneurysm
* Traumatic
* Collagen vascular disease
* Syphilitic
* Mycotic: Due to bacterial infection.

Q. Which vessels may be affected by aneurysm?

Ans. Aneurysm may affect both large and small-sized vessels:
* *Aorta*: Arch of the aorta, descending thoracic aorta or abdominal aorta
* Carotid, subclavian, axillary, femoral, and popliteal arteries
* Smaller vessels like cerebral, mesenteric, splenic, and renal arteries.

Q. What are the usual presentations of patient with abdominal aortic aneurysm?

Ans.
* *Asymptomatic*: No symptom pertaining to the aneurysm. Diagnosed incidentally by clinical or radiological investigation.
* *Symptomatic*:
  - Low backache or upper abdominal pain
  - Pain in the groin or thigh due to nerve compression. Lower limb swelling due to venous compression

- Emboli may cause distal ischemia and gangrene of the lower limbs. Pulsatile mass in abdomen—showing expansile pulsation
- May present with symptoms and signs of rupture.

Q. How will you diagnose rupture of abdominal aortic aneurysm?

Ans. Abdominal aortic aneurysm may expand gradually leading to rupture. The rupture may occur into the peritoneal cavity (anterior rupture) or into the retroperitoneum (posterior rupture).

- Anterior rupture results in massive bleeding into the peritoneal cavity and very few of these patients survive to reach the hospital.
- Severe abdominal pain.
- Severe hypovolemic shock: Rapid feeble pulse, hypotension, cold clammy extremities, and oliguria
- Posterior rupture results in an expanding retroperitoneal hematoma. Severe abdominal pain or severe backache. Moderate to severe hypotension
- The pulsatile mass is palpable in the abdomen.

Q. What are the important intrinsic features of aneurysm?

Ans.
- There is a swelling along the course of the artery
- The swelling shows expansile pulsation
- On compressing the artery proximal to the swelling, the swelling diminishes in size and the pulsation disappears
- A thrill may be palpable over the swelling
- A bruit may be audible on auscultation over the swelling.

Q. What are the complications of aneurysm?

Ans.
- *Thrombosis*: There may be thrombotic occlusion of the aneurysmal sac leading to distal ischemia.
- *Peripheral embolism*: There may be release of emboli from the thrombus in the aneurysm leading to distal ischemia.
- *Rupture of aneurysm*: Symptoms and signs will depend on the site of involvement.
- *Pressure symptoms:*
  - Venous compression: Distal edema
  - Nerve compression: Tingling, numbness or motor paralysis
  - Pressure on esophagus may cause dysphagia
  - Pressure on trachea may cause dyspnea
  - Pressure on the bones may cause bony erosion, bone pain and pathological fracture.

Q. What investigations may help in diagnosis?

Ans.
- *Ultrasonography of abdomen*: The aneurysm may be diagnosed and the diameter of the aneurysm may be assessed.

- *Aortography*: It may delineate the proximal and distal extent of the aneurysm. If there is a circumferential thrombus in the aneurysm the aortography may not be reliable for assessing the exact diameter of the aneurysm.
- Contrast CT scan of abdomen or MRI of abdomen for better delineation of the aneurysm.

Q. What is the treatment for unruptured abdominal aortic aneurysm?

Ans.
- Symptomatic aneurysm needs treatment
- Aneurysm more than 5 cm in diameter needs treatment.

Q. What is the ideal treatment for abdominal aortic aneurysm?

Ans.
- Aortic bypass graft is the ideal procedure
- The abdominal aorta above and below the aneurysm is dissected. The iliac arteries are also dissected
- Vascular clamps are applied proximal and distal to the site of aneurysm. The aneurysm sac is opened and the thrombus is removed. A dacron or PTFE (polytetrafluoroethylene) graft is anastomosed to the proximal normal aorta and distally anastomosed to the iliac arteries or distal aorta depending on the extent of the aneurysm.

Q. What are the postoperative complications?

Ans.
- Hemorrhage is the most common complication
- Respiratory complications: Collapse, consolidation, and shock lung
- Postoperative renal failure
- Aortoduodenal fistula
- Spinal cord ischemia
- Sexual dysfunction
- Infection.

∎ SUTURE MATERIALS

Types of Suture Materials

Depending on the behavior of the suture material in the tissues, the sutures may be:
- *Absorbable sutures*: These sutures get absorbed in the tissues either by enzymatic digestion or by phagocytosis. Depending on the source, these sutures may be:
  - Natural absorbable sutures:
    - Plain and chromic catgut
  - Synthetic absorbable sutures:
    - Polyglycolic acid (Dexon)
    - Polyglactin 910 (Vicryl)
    - Polyglactin 910 Rapide (Vicryl Rapide)
    - Polydioxanone suture (PDS)
    - Poliglecaprone 25 (Monocryl).
- *Nonabsorbable sutures*: These sutures remain in the tissues for indefinite period. Depending on the source, these sutures may be:

♦ Natural nonabsorbable sutures:
  – Linen thread
  – Silk.
♦ Synthetic nonabsorbable sutures:
  – Polypropylene (Prolene)
  – Monofilament polyamide (Ethilon)
  – Polyester (Ethibond)
  – Nylon.

Depending on the number of strands in the suture materials, sutures may be:
♦ *Monofilament sutures*:
  – Sutures consisting of a single strand of fiber are called monofilament sutures
  – These sutures are smooth and strong
  – Chance of bacterial contamination is less
  – The disadvantage is that knot tied may become loose
  – Polypropylene, Polyamide, Catgut, Monocryl, Polydioxanone, Polyglactin finer sizes 6/0-9/0.
♦ *Polyfilament sutures*:
  – Sutures consisting of multiple strands braided together are called polyfilament sutures
  – They are easier to handle and the knot tied does not slip
  – The disadvantage is that the bacteria may lodge in the crevices of the sutures so these sutures are not suitable in presence of infection, e.g. silk, linen, polyglycolic acid, polyglactin 910, braided polyamide, and braided polyester.

Q. What are the criteria of an ideal suture material?

Ans.
♦ Should have adequate tensile strength
♦ Should incite minimal tissue reaction
♦ Should have easy handling property
♦ Should have good knotting quality
♦ Should be nonallergenic and noncarcinogenic
♦ Should be easily available and cheap.

Descriptions of Different Labelings in a Foil Pack

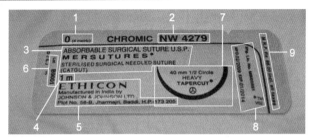

Fig. 21.85: Different labeling in a foil pack. 1. Thickness of the sutures; 2. Code number; 3. Type of suture; 4. Length of the suture; 5. Name of manufacturer; 6. Lot number/batch number; 7. Description of the needle; 8. Manufacturing license number, manufacturing date and expiry date; 9. Price of the foil pack

Different surgical sutures are supplied in a sterile pack. The different labelings in the foil pack indicate (Fig. 21.85):

- The number indicates the thickness of the suture. Depending on the thickness of the sutures, the number may be 2, 1, 1–0, 2–0, 3–0, 4–0, etc. Higher the number, thicker is the suture. 0 prefixed by higher numbers are finer sutures, e.g. 3–0 is thinner than 2–0 sutures.
- Company's code number for a particular suture. NW4226 means No. 1 atraumatic chromic catgut suture on 3/8th circle needle with a needle length of 45 mm and suture length of 76 cm. For different specification of suture materials the code number is different.
- The type of suture contained in the foil pack—absorbable or nonabsorbable, chemical name of the suture and brand name of the suture. The brand name of the suture will vary depending on the manufacturer.
- The length of the suture material contained in the pack. Sutures are available in different sizes—45 cm, 76 cm, 90 cm, 152 cm, etc.
- The name of the manufacturer. This pack is manufactured by ETHICON (Division of Johnson & Johnson). The other manufacturer of suture materials are—Suture India, Futura, Centennial, US Surgical, Aesculap, etc.
- The lot number or batch number of the suture.
- The description of the needle. The needles may be of different sizes—16 mm, 22 mm, 30 mm, 40 mm, 45 mm, etc. The needle may be of different curvatures half circle, 3/5th circle, etc. The needle may be straight or curved.
- Manufacturing License No., manufacturing date and expiry date of the suture material.
- Price of the pack.

Most of the sutures are supplied in a sterilized pack. In examination, mention the following points:

- No. of suture—1/0, 2/0, etc.
- Natural or synthetic
- Absorbable or nonabsorbable
- Type of suture—catgut, polyglycolic acid, polyglactin, etc.
- Whether provided with a needle or not—if there is a needle, description of the needle—length, curvature, round bodied or cutting.
- Length of the suture—45 cm, 70 cm, 90 cm, etc.

■ NATURAL ABSORBABLE SUTURE: CATGUT

The natural absorbable surgical suture derived from the submucosa of the sheep is known as catgut. This is the brand name of this suture manufactured by Ethicon division of Johnson and Johnson. The similar sutures manufactured by other companies include Trugut, Pro Gut, etc. (Figs 21.86A to D).

Characteristics of Catgut

- Derived from the submucosa of sheep's intestine or serosa of cattle's intestine. It is 99% collagen.
- This is absorbed by a process of enzymatic digestion by proteolytic enzymes contained in the polymorphs and macrophages.
- Catgut is easy to handle and knots well.

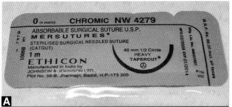

A

This is a sterile pack containing natural absorbable suture, No. 0, chromic catgut on an atraumatic half circle heavy tapercut needle with a needle length of 40 mm and suture length of 1 m

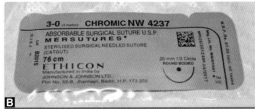

B

This is a sterile pack containing natural absorbable suture, No. 3-0, chromic catgut on an atraumatic half circle round bodied needle with needle length of 20 mm and suture length of 76 cm

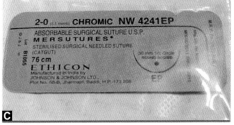

C

This is a sterile pack containing natural absorbable suture, No. 2-0, chromic catgut on an atraumatic half circle round bodied needle with needle length of 30 mm and suture length of 76 cm

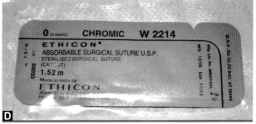

D

This is a sterile pack containing natural absorbable suture, No. 0 chromic catgut with a suture length of 1.52 cm

Figs 21.86A to D: Catgut sutures

- Absorption rate depends on the size of the catgut and whether it is plain or chromicized.
- Plain catgut loses 50% tensile strength in tissues in 3 days and loses all tensile strength in 15 days (Fig. 21.87).
- Plain catgut gets absorbed in tissues within 60 days (Fig. 21.88)
- The chromic catgut loses 50% tensile strength in 7 days and loses all its tensile strength in 28 days (Fig. 21.87).
- The chromic catgut gets absorbed in tissues in 90–100 days (Fig. 21.88).
- In presence of infection the catgut gets absorbed earlier.

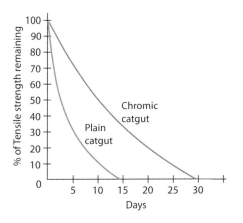

Fig. 21.87: Catgut—in vivo loss of tensile strength

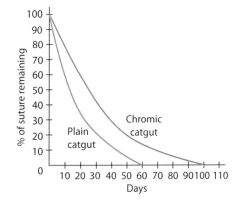

Fig. 21.88: Catgut—in vivo loss of mass: Absorption in tissues

Uses

- *Plain catgut*:
  - Plain catgut is used to tie small subcutaneous vessels
  - Used to approximate subcutaneous tissues during closure of an incision
  - Used during circumcision to suture the cut margins of the prepuce
  - Used in repair of wounds of lip or oral cavity.
- *Chromic catgut*:
  - Used to suture muscles, bowel anastomosis, and closure of peritoneum.
  - Used during appendicectomy. The mesoappendix is tied with 1-0 chromic catgut suture. The base of the appendix is tied with a 1-0 or 2-0 chromic catgut suture. The stump of the appendix may be inverted with a Z or a purse string suture applied with a 2-0 atraumatic catgut suture. The peritoneum, muscles, and the external oblique aponeurosis are apposed by 2-0 chromic catgut sutures.
  - Used during small gut resection anastomosis. In two layer anastomosis, the posterior and anterior through and through layers are applied with 2-0 atraumatic catgut sutures. The seromuscular (anterior and posterior) layer is usually applied with Mersilk. Alternatively all layers may be sutured with 2-0 polyglactin or polyglycolic acid suture.
  - Used during gastrojejunostomy for posterior and anterior through and through layers using a 2-0 atraumatic catgut suture.
  - Used during cholecystectomy. Bleeding from the gallbladder bed may be controlled by suturing the gallbladder bed using 1-0 atraumatic catgut suture mounted on a 45 mm round bodied needle.
- May be used during closure of a subcostal incision—posterior rectus sheath, anterior rectus sheath and external oblique aponeurosis and muscle may be apposed with 1-0 chromic catgut sutures.
- Synthetic absorbable sutures, polyglycolic acid and polyglactin, are replacing catgut suture for most of the uses of catgut.

Q. What do you mean by an atraumatic suture?

Ans. When a suture is attached to an eyeless needle, it is called an atraumatic suture. This concept was first introduced by George Merson of Edinburgh by devising a technique of imbrication of the suture at the end of an eyeless needle. In his memory, these sutures are also known as "Mersutures".

Q. How catgut is prepared?

Ans. This is synthesized from the submucosa of sheep's intestine or serosa of beefs intestine.

The layers of the intestine are scrapped off leaving only the submucosa. This is treated with a fat solvent to wash off the fat. The strips of submucosa are then dried off. The thread so obtained is then cut into different diameters and length. This is plain catgut.

The plain catgut if treated with 20% chromic acid produces chromicized catgut. Treatment with chromic acid alters its property and it stays longer in tissues maintaining tensile strength for a longer time.

Catgut is sterilized by gamma irradiation and is supplied in a sterilized pack containing isopropyl alcohol.

SYNTHETIC ABSORBABLE SUTURES

■ COMMON FEATURES

- Synthesized in laboratory
- These may be monofilament (monocryl, polydioxanone, and finer sizes vicryl) or polyfilament (vicryl and vicryl rapide)
- They can be of natural color or can be colored green (Dexon) or violet (vicryl)
- They are twice as strong as compared to natural absorbable suture
- They are absorbed by a simple process of hydrolysis and evoke minimal tissue reaction
- They have excellent handling properties. Once tied the knots are secure
- These are sterilized by ethylene oxide
- They are available in different sizes, different lengths, swaged into different types of needles
- They maintain tensile strength in tissues for a longer time and absorbed in tissues after a variable time.

■ POLYGLYCOLIC ACID SUTURE (DEXON)

Characteristics

- This is a synthetic delayed absorbable polyfilament suture (Figs 21.89A and B)
- This is a polymer of glycolic acid
- Dexon may be dyed green and may be uncoated or coated with a lubricant to reduce the coefficient of friction
- Polyglycolic acid maintains tensile strength in tissues for about 30 days and gets absorbed in 80–90 days (Figs 21.90 and 21.91).
- Polyglycolic acid suture manufactured by US Surgical is known as Dexon. The polyglycolic acid sutures manufactured by other companies are available as Petcryl and Maxon.

■ POLYGLACTIN SUTURES (VICRYL)

Polyglactin are synthetic absorbable sutures (Figs 21.92A to C). These sutures are available in different sizes like 1, 1-0, 2-0, 4-0, 5-0, 6-0, 7-0, 8-0, and 9-0. The needle may be of different types

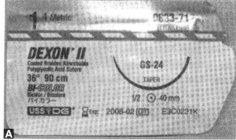

A This is a sterile pack containing synthetic absorbable suture, No. 1, polyglycolic acid (Dexon) on a half circle tapper cut needle with a needle length of 40 mm and suture length of 90 cm

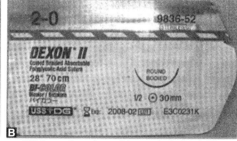

B This is a sterile pack containing synthetic absorbable suture, No. 2-0, polyglycolic acid (Dexon) with a half circle round bodied needle with a needle length of 30 mm and suture length of 70 cm

Figs 21.89A and B: Polyglycolic acid suture

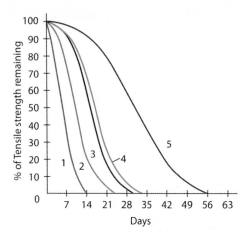

1- Polyglactin 910 rapide (vicryl rapide); 2-Polyglecaprone (monocryl); 3-Polyglycolic acid (dexon); 4-Polyglactin 910 (vicryl); 5-Polydioxanone (PDS II)

Fig. 21.90: Synthetic absorbable sutures—in vivo loss of tensile strength

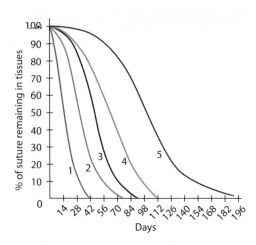

1-Polyglactin 910 rapide (vicrly rapide); 2-Polyglycolic acid (dexon); 3-Polyglactin 910 (vicryl); 4-Polyglecaprone (monocryl); 5-Polydioxanone (PDS II)

Fig. 21.91: Synthetic absorbable sutures—in vivo loss of mass absorption in tissues

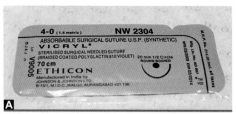

This is a sterile pack, containing No. 4-0, synthetic absorbable suture polyglactin 910 (vicryl), coated, dyed violet, on an atraumatic half circle rounded bodied needle with a needle length of 20 mm and suture length of 70 cm

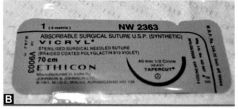

This is a sterile pack, containing No. 1 synthetic absorbable suture polyglactin 910 (vicryl), coated, dyed violet on a 1/2 circle 4 mm heavy tapercut needle with a suture length of 70 cm

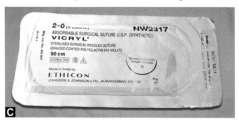

This is a sterile pack, containing No. 2-0 synthetic absorbable suture, polyglactin 910 (vicryl), coated, dyed violet, on an atraumatic half circle rounded bodied needle with a needle length of 30 mm and suture length of 90 cm

Figs 21.92A to C: Polyglactin 910 sutures

40 mm, 30 mm, 22 mm, 16 mm, etc. The suture length may be 90 cm, 70 cm or 45 cm. The needles may be round bodied, cutting or taper cut. These sutures may also be available as undyed vicryl and as coated vicryl. These features will be mentioned in the foil pack. Vicryl is the trade name of the polyglactin 910 suture made by Ethicon (Johnson and Johnson). The brand names of the polyglactin sutures made by other companies are—Truglyde, Centicryl, Safil, etc.

Characteristics

+ Polyglactin 910 are synthetic absorbable polyfilament sutures. The finer polyglactin sutures 5-0, 6-0 are available as monofilament sutures and are used in vascular surgery.
+ Polyglactin (Vicryl) is a copolymer of lactide and glycolide (in a ratio of 90% glycolide and 10% lactide).
+ These sutures are digested by hydrolysis and not by enzymatic digestion, hence incite less tissue reaction.
+ These sutures maintain tensile strength in the tissues for about 28–30 days and get absorbed in 80–90 days (Figs 21.90 and 21.91).

Uses of Polyglycolic Acid and Polyglactin Sutures

+ Indicated in all situations where catgut are used (see above).
+ No. 1 or 1-0 suture may be used for closure of subcostal, paramedian, Pfannenstiel or McBurney's incision.
+ 3-0 or 4-0 sutures on atraumatic needles are used in biliary enteric anastomosis—choledochoduodenostomy, choledochojejunostomy, and hepaticodochojejunostomy.
+ 3-0 or 4-0 sutures are also used in pancreaticojejunal anastomosis—Puestow's lateral pancreaticojejunostomy or pancreaticojejunal anastomosis following Whipple's operation.
+ In small gut resection anastomosis—seromuscular (anterior and posterior) and through (posterior and anterior) layers may be sutured with 2-0 polyglactin or polyglycolic acid sutures.
+ Single-layered anastomosis in large gut may be done with 2-0 polyglactin or polyglycolic acid suture.

■ POLYGLACTIN RAPIDE (VICRYL RAPIDE) SUTURE

Characteristics

+ This is a variety of polyglactin 910 suture (Fig. 21.93). The rapid absorption characteristics of vicryl rapide are achieved by exposure of coated vicryl to gamma irradiation. This results in material with low molecular weight than coated vicryl.
+ This is undyed.
+ Vicryl rapide maintains tensile strength for 10–12 days and gets absorbed in tissues in 42 days (Figs 21.90 and 21.91).

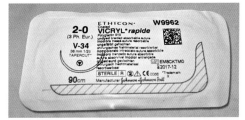

This is a sterile pack containing 2-0 synthetic absorbable suture, polyglactin 910 (vicryl rapide) on an atraumatic half circle tapercut needle with needle length of 36 mm and suture length of 90 cm

Fig. 21.93: Vicryl rapide suture

Uses

+ It may be used for subcuticular sutures.
+ It may be used for skin or mucosal closure.
+ It needs not to be removed, gets spontaneously absorbed.
+ It may be used for circumcision for approximation of cut margins of the prepuce.

Polyglecaprone (Monocryl Suture) (Figs 21.94A and B)

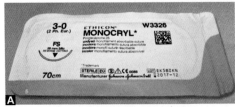
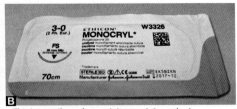

This is a sterile pack containing no. 3-0 synthetic absorbable polyglecaprone (monocryl) suture on an atraumatic 3/8th circle reverse cutting needle with a needle length of 26 mm and suture length of 70 cm

This is a sterile pack containing no. 3-0, synthetic absorbable polyglecaprone (monocryl) suture on an atraumatic half circle visi-black, tapercut needle with a needle length of 26 mm and suture length of 70 cm

Figs 21.94A and B: Polyglecaprone (monocryl sutures)

Characteristics

- This is a synthetic absorbable monofilament suture.
- This is composed of a copolymer of 75% glycolide and 25% caprolactone.
- This is available as an undyed suture or may be dyed violet.
- This has double the strength of chromic catgut.
- It has excellent handling properties, has got very smooth surface, and passes through the tissues with greater ease.
- This suture maintains tensile strength in tissue for 21 days (Fig. 21.90).
- Monocryl is absorbed by hydrolysis in about 90–120 days (Fig. 21.91).
- Monocryl is sterilized by ethylene oxide.

Uses

- Monocryl may be used in situations where catgut sutures are used.
- Used for intestinal anastomosis as an alternative to catgut or polyglactin suture.
- Used for closure of peritoneum.
- Subcutaneous tissue apposition.
- Used in urological procedures—pyeloplasty, ureter repair.

■ POLYDIOXANONE SUTURE (PDS-II) (FIGS 21.95A TO C)

Characteristics

- This is a synthetic, delayed absorbable, monofilament suture formed by polymerizing the monomer "paradioxanone".
- This is dyed violet. PDS II sutures are an improved version of initial PDS suture.
- The soft, pliable and smooth PDS II suture allows easy passage through the tissues and the knotting characteristics of this material is the best among the synthetic absorbable sutures.
- Like polyglactin, it is also available in different sizes-1, 1-0, 2-0, 3-0, 4-0, etc. with different types of needle and different suture lengths.

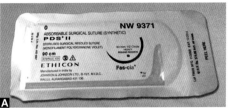

A

This is a sterile pack, containing no. 0, synthetic absorbable polydioxanone (PDS II) suture on an atraumatic half circle heavy round bodied needle with a needle length of 40 mm and suture length of 90 cm

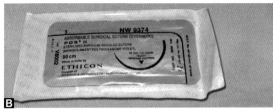

B

This is a sterile pack, containing no. 1, synthetic absorbable polydioxanone (PDS II) suture on an atraumatic half circle heavy reverse cutting needle with a needle length of 40 mm and suture length of 90 cm

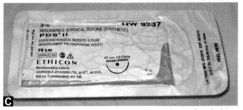

C

This is a sterile pack, containing no. 3-0, synthetic absorbable polydioxanone (PDS II) suture on an atraumatic half circle round bodied needle with a needle length of 20 mm and suture length of 70 cm

Figs 21.95A to C: Polydioxanone suture (PDS-II)

♦ Tensile strength: It maintains tensile strength for a longer period for about 56 days (Figs 21.90 and 21.96).
  – At 2 weeks—70% tensile strength is maintained
  – At 4 weeks—50% tensile strength is maintained
  – At 6 weeks—25% tensile strength is maintained
  – At 8 weeks—loses all tensile strength.
  The suture is absorbed by hydrolysis and complete absorption occurs in about 180–210 days (6–7 months) (Fig. 21.91).

Uses

♦ These sutures are used in all situations where catgut, polyglycolic acid, and polyglactin sutures are used.
♦ No. 1 or 1-0 suture may be used for closure of paramedian or midline and other abdominal incisions.
♦ 3-0 and 4-0 sutures are used for intestinal or biliary enteric anastomosis.

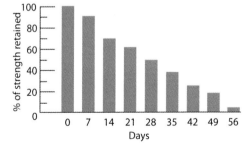

Fig. 21.96: Polydioxanone suture (PDS-II)—in vivo tensile strength retention

■ NATURAL NONABSORBABLE SUTURES: SILK

Silk are natural nonabsorbable sutures.

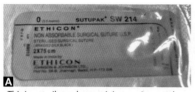 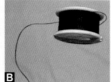 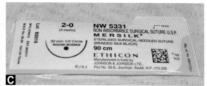

A	B	C
This is a sterile pack, containing no. 0, natural nonabsorbable suture, black braided silk (sutupak), with 2 pieces of suture each with a length of 75 cm	This is a reel containing natural nonabsorbable suture, black braided silk, no. 1-0	This is a sterile pack, containing no. 2-0 natural nonabsorbable suture (black braided silk), Mersilk on a half circle, round bodied, curved, atraumatic needle with a needle length of 30 mm and suture length of 76 cm

Figs 21.97A to C: Black braided silk

Silk may be supplied in sterile pack (sutupak) containing black braided silk which are precut into different sizes and suture thickness may be 6-0 to 3 (Fig. 21.97A). Silk may also be supplied as silk reels which are nonsterile and are available in sizes from No. 6-0 to 4 (Fig. 21.97B) and is sterilized by autoclaving.

Black braided silk mounted on atraumatic needles are available as Mersilk. Mersilk are available in different sizes No. 7-0 to 1, different lengths (45 cm, 76 cm and 90 cm) and with different types of needles, curvature 1/2 circle, 3/8th circle, and needle size of 16 mm, 22 mm, 30 mm, and 40 mm (Fig. 21.97C).

Characteristics

- This is a natural nonabsorbable suture.
- The silk is derived from the cocoon of silk worm larvae.
- This is basically a protein covered initially by an albuminous layer. The albuminous layer is removed by a process called degumming during manufacturing of these sutures. The suture is braided round a core and coated with wax to reduce the capillary action.
- Handling property is best and it knots securely.
- This is sterilized by gamma irradiation.
- The silk for surgical use is dyed black.
- Tensile strength: Silk maintains tensile strength for a longer time and the tensile strength is lost in 2 years' time (Fig. 21.98).

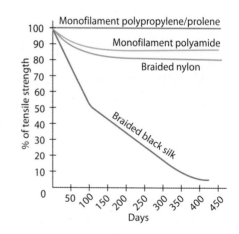

Fig. 21.98: Nonabsorbable suture—in vivo loss of tensile strength

- Once placed in the tissues it incites a polymorphonuclear reaction and a fibrous capsule is formed around the silk in 14–21 days.

Uses

- No. 1 or 1-0 silk sutures are used as ligature.
- It is used during cholecystectomy to ligate the cystic duct and cystic artery.
- It is used during small and large gut resection to ligate the mesenteric vessels.
- It is used to ligate the pedicles during nephrectomy and splenectomy.

- It is used during truncal vagotomy to ligate the anterior and posterior vagus nerve before their division. Two ligatures are applied and the nerve is divided in-between.
- It is used for skin closure either with interrupted or continuous suture.

Uses of Mersilk:

- 2-0 and 3-0 Mersilk is used for anterior and posterior seromuscular sutures in small gut anastomosis and in gastrojejunostomy.
- It may be used to repair the posterior wall of inguinal canal in herniorrhaphy.
- 3-0 Mersilk may be used for pancreaticojejunal anastomosis.
- 4-0 Mersilk may be used for nerve suture.

Q. What are the characteristics of linen sutures?

Ans.

- This is a natural nonabsorbable suture made from flax and the material is cellulose.
- This is twisted to form a polyfilament suture.
- Tissue reaction is similar to silk.
- It has excellent knotting properties.
- It gains 10% tensile strength when wet
- It is used for tying of pedicles and as ligatures.

■ SYNTHETIC NONABSORBABLE SUTURES

Polypropylene Suture

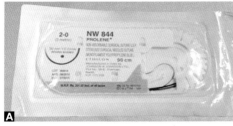
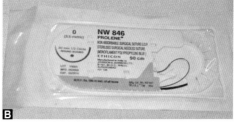

A. This is a sterile pack, containing No. 2-0 synthetic nonabsorbable suture, polypropylene (prolene) on a half circle round bodied atraumatic needle with a needle length of 30 mm and suture length of 90 cm

B. This is a sterile pack, containing No. 0 synthetic nonabsorbable suture, polypropylene (prolene) on a half circle round bodied needle with a needle length of 30 mm and suture length of 90 cm

Figs 21.99A and B: Polypropylene suture

Characteristics

- This is a synthetic, monofilament, nonabsorbable suture (Figs 21.99A and B).
- Polypropylene has structural similarity to protocollagen which is a precursor of collagen.
- This suture is inert and has extremely low tissue reactivity and is nonbiodegradable.
- It has low coefficient of friction and slides through the tissues readily.
- It has a peculiar property. The suture may extend up to 30% before breaking and hence is useful in situations where postoperatively some-elasticity is required on the part of the suture to accommodate postoperative swelling and thereby helps to prevent tissue strangulation.

- Handling is good and knotting is very secured since the material deforms on knotting and allows the knot to bed down on itself.
- It is extremely smooth and does not saw through the tissues.
- Polypropylene sutures are available in a variety of eyeless needles in various sizes from 8-0 to 1. Polypropylene material is also used in polypropylene mesh, which are used for hernia repair and in rectopexy for rectal prolapse.
- Maintains tensile strength for indefinite period.

Uses

- No. 1-0 or no. 1 suture is used for herniorrhaphy for repair of the posterior wall of inguinal canal by different techniques.
- It is used for closure of midline abdominal incision.
- It is used for repair of incisional hernia.
- 2-0 or 3-0 sutures are used for repair of tendon injuries.
- Finer sutures, 4-0 and 5-0, are used for vascular anastomosis and for repair of nerve injury.

Monofilament Polyamide Sutures

Characteristics

- This is a synthetic monofilament nonabsorbable suture and is a variety of nylon (Fig. 21.98).
- This has a very low coefficient of friction and readily passes through the tissues.
- This is an inert suture and incites minimal tissue reaction.
- Maintains tensile strength for a long time. Tensile strength loss after 1 year of implantation is 25% (Fig. 21.100).
- Monofilament polyamide suture has a memory and knot security is poor so 4-5 throws are required for proper knotting.
- Available in different sizes.

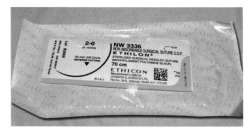

This is a sterile pack containing No. 2-0 synthetic monofilament polyamide suture (ethilon) on a 3/8th circle atraumatic, curved, reverse cutting needle with a needle length of 45 mm and suture length of 70 cm

Fig. 21.100: Monofilament polyamide sutures

Uses

- For closure of skin incision
- For closure of abdominal wall incision
- For herniorrhaphy
- Monofilament polyamide sutures are also available as finer sutures 3–0, 4–0, 5–0 up to 10–0
- The finer sutures are used in vascular surgery.

Nylon Sutures

This is a synthetic nonabsorbable suture, monofilament, white in color. It has high tensile strength and maintains its tensile strength for indefinite period.

Uses

Same as monofilament polyamide sutures.

◼ STAINLESS STEEL WIRE

Stainless steel wire is unique suture material of having very high tensile strength and extreme inertness (Fig. 21.101). Suturing with stainless steel requires perfect technique and poor technique may jeopardize the very purpose of suturing. Too tight a suture may cause tissue necrosis and steel wire can pull or tear out of tissues. Barbs on the end of the steel can traumatize the surrounding tissues. Kinks in the wire can render it practically useless.

This is available in different sizes from No. 5-0 to 6.

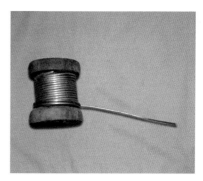

Fig. 21.101: Stainless steel wire

Uses

- In orthopedic operations for suturing bones, e.g. in fracture patella and fracture olecranon
- Closure of midline sternotomy incision
- Interdental wiring for fracture mandible
- Earlier used for herniorrhaphy
- Earlier used for Thiersch's operation.

Sterilization

It is done by autoclaving.

◼ INSTRUMENTS FOR LAPAROSCOPIC SURGERY
LAPAROSCOPIC INSTRUMENTS

Telescope (Figs 21.102A and B)

Telescope is one of the viewing instruments for laparoscopic surgery. These are available as:
- Diameter: 1.9 to 10 mm.
- Lens angulation: 0° and 30 or 45°.

Q. How will you identify 0° and 30° telescopes?

Ans. In 0° telescope, the terminal end of the telescope is rounded and the lens is at the terminal part. This is a forward viewing telescope.

In 30° telescope, the terminal end of the telescope is oblique and the lens is located on the undersurface. This is an oblique viewing telescope.

Q. What is the lens system in the telescope?

Ans. This is a rod lens system incorporated in the rigid metallic tube. This is devised by John Hopkin.

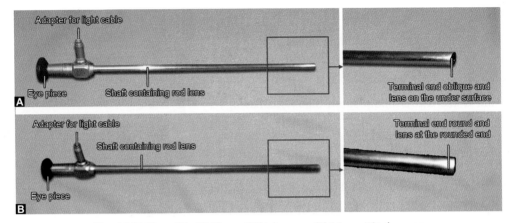

Figs 21.102A and B: (A) 10 mm 30° telescope; (B) 10 mm 0° telescope

Sterilization

There are various ways for sterilization of optical instruments:

* *Chemical sterilization*:
    - 2% glutaraldehyde solution for 4 hours for sterilization and 20 minutes for disinfection
    - Peracetic acid: Dipping for 12 minutes provides high level of disinfection.
* *Gas sterilization*:
    - Ethylene oxide: Keeping in ETO chamber for 12 hours
    - Plasma sterilization.
* *Autoclaving*: The newer generation telescopes are autoclavable and may be sterilized by standard method of autoclaving.

Veress Needle (Figs 21.103A to D)

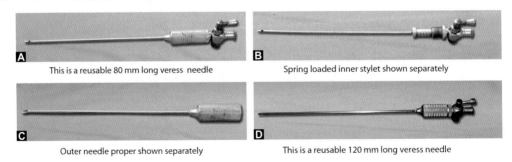

| This is a reusable 80 mm long veress needle | Spring loaded inner stylet shown separately |

| Outer needle proper shown separately | This is a reusable 120 mm long veress needle |

Figs 21.103A to D: Veress needle

Q. What are the parts of this needle?

Ans. This is a spring loaded needle. The outer needle has a sharp end and there is a rounded stylet inside which projects beyond the sharp tip of the needle by spring action.

Q. What is the use of this needle?

Ans. This is used for induction of pneumoperitoneum during laparoscopic surgery.

Q. How will you hold the needle?

Ans. The needle is held in-between the thumb and the index and middle finger. The ring finger is placed to act as a guard to prevent excessive entry of needle into the peritoneal cavity.

Q. How will you insert the needle?

Ans. A subumbilical 10 mm incision is made. The Veress needle is held in-between fingers and placed in the subumbilical incision site at 45° angle directed toward the pelvis and the needle is inserted. Two clicks will be felt once after entry through the linea alba and next as the surgical peritoneum is penetrated. Too much entry should be prevented once the needle enters into the peritoneal cavity appreciated by loss of resistance.

Q. What gas is used for creation of pneumoperitoneum?

Ans. Carbon dioxide gas is ideal for creation and maintenance of pneumoperitoneum during laparoscopic surgery.

Q. What other gases may be used for pneumoperitoneum?

Ans. Earlier different gases were used for pneumoperitoneum like N_2O, oxygen, and air. In view of distinct advantages of carbon dioxide these gases are not used.

Q. What are the advantages of carbon dioxide for use during laparoscopic surgery?

Ans.
- Carbon dioxide is an inert, noncombustible gas.
- Electrocautery may be safely used as CO_2 does not support combustion.
- Carbon dioxide is a highly diffusible and soluble gas. As the carbon dioxide is absorbed from the peritoneal surface, it remains in soluble form in blood as carbonic acid.
- In the lung the carbonic acid splits into water and CO_2 and the CO_2 gas from the alveoli may be removed by hyperventilating by the anesthetist.

Q. What is closed technique of induction of pneumoperitoneum?

Ans. The closed technique of induction of pneumoperitoneum involves blind puncture by using a Veress needle. A 1 cm (5 mm if a 5 mm telescope is to be used) smiling subumbilical incision is made and the Veress needle is inserted at 45° angle pointing toward the pelvis. Alternatively, the needle may be inserted at a right angle to the abdominal wall.

Q. How will you confirm the correct position of the needle in the peritoneal cavity?

Ans. The needle tip should lie free in the peritoneal cavity. The position may be ascertained by:
- Free movement of the needle both side to side and anteroposteriorly.
- Aspirate the needle with a 10 mL syringe. Nothing should come out. If the needle is wrongly placed inside the lumen of gut or urinary bladder, intestinal contents or urine will come on aspiration.
- Introduce about 10 ml of saline through the needle and after injection try to aspirate back. If the needle is in peritoneal cavity the saline would flow freely and no saline could be aspirated back. If the needle tip lies in rectus sheath, the saline may be pushed easily but some amount may be aspirated back.
- *Drop test*: Place a drop of saline at the needle adapter. If the needle is in the peritoneal cavity the drop will be sucked into the peritoneal cavity.

- *Recording the intra-abdominal pressure*: Once the end of the needle is connected to the automatic electronic insufflator the actual intra-abdominal pressure will be seen in the machine. If the needle is in the peritoneal cavity the intra-abdominal pressure will be shown as 0–6 mm Hg. If the machine shows very high pressure there will be no gas flow and the interpretation is either the needle tip is blocked or the needle is not in the peritoneal cavity.

Q. What are the drawbacks of closed technique of pneumoperitoneum?

Ans. Although safe in experienced hand and quick to perform, this is a blind technique and there are higher incidences of injuries due to blind introduction of the Veress needle or the first trocar insertion. There may be bladder, bowel or vascular injury.

Q. What is open technique of induction of pneumoperitoneum?

Ans. This is a safer technique for creation of pneumoperitoneum. The technique involves making a 1 cm subumbilical incision and the underlying linea alba is exposed. The linea alba is picked up by two pairs of Allis tissue forceps and incised under vision. The underlying surgical peritoneum is incised under vision and Hasson cannula is introduced into the peritoneal cavity. The trocar of the Hasson cannula is rounded and does not cause injury to the underlying structures. The cannula is fixed to the skin by two sutures.

Two sutures are applied on either side of the midline over the rectus sheath. The linea alba along with underlying blended parietal peritoneum is incised and the peritoneal cavity is entered. This can be confirmed by inserting a finger. Blunt-tipped Hasson trocar and cannula are inserted under direct vision. The blunt trocar is removed and the cannula is kept in place by fixing with the sutures already placed.

This open technique for creation of pneumoperitoneum is safer as there is least chance of injury to the underlying viscous or vessels.

Trocar and Cannula (Figs 21.104 and 21.105)

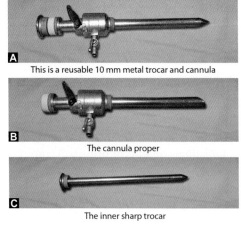

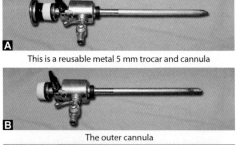

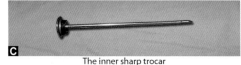

A This is a reusable 10 mm metal trocar and cannula

B The cannula proper

C The inner sharp trocar

Figs 21.104A to C: 10 mm metal trocar and cannula

A This is a reusable metal 5 mm trocar and cannula

B The outer cannula

C The inner sharp trocar

Figs 21.105A to C: 5 mm trocar and cannula

Q. How will you introduce the trocar?

Ans. The top of the trocar rests on the palm and the trocar and cannula is held in between fingers. Utmost care is required during placement of first trocar by blind technique. The trocar is gradually inserted by rotatory movement till loss of resistance is felt. After the telescope attached to the camera is inserted the subsequent trocars are inserted under vision.

Q. What are the uses of trocar and cannula?

Ans. The cannulas are the channels for introduction of the laparoscopic instruments. The inner sharp trocar is required for smooth introduction of the cannula. In the cannula, there is a valve which prevents leakage CO_2 gas so that pneumoperitoneum is maintained well.

The diameter of the cannula should be 1 mm more than the diameter of the instrument that is to be introduced.

Q. How many trocar and cannula you will need for lap chole operation?

Ans. Two 10 mm and two 5 mm cannula are required for lap cholecystectomy operation.

One 10 mm subumbilical port for telescope attached to the camera.

This is cannula part one 10 mm epigastric port inserted to the right of falciform ligament just below the xiphoid. This is surgeon's right hand working port.

One 5 mm right midclavicular port inserted below the right costal margin at the right midclavicular line. This is surgeon's left hand working port.

One 5 mm right anterior axillary port inserted at the level of umbilicus at the right anterior axillary line. This is the assistant port for holding the fundus of the gallbladder.

Maryland Dissector (Fig. 21.106)

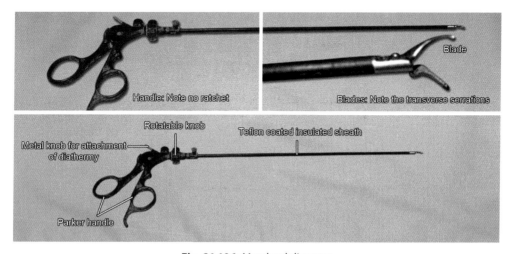

Fig. 21.106: Maryland dissector

Uses

- It is used during laparoscopic cholecystectomy to dissect the cystic pedicle.
- It is used to make a tunnel around the cystic duct and artery for application of clips.
- It is used during other laparoscopic operation for dissections.

Endograsping Forceps: Toothed (Fig. 21.107)

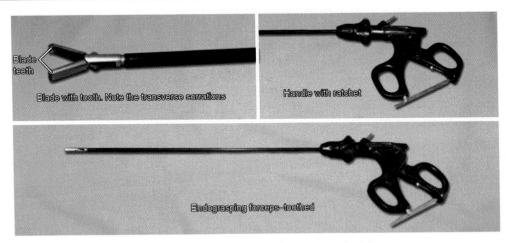

Fig. 21.107: Endograsping forceps—toothed.

Toothed grasper is traumatic. This may be used during Cholecystectomy to hold the funds or the Hartmann pouch, if the gallbladder wall is very thick. May be used during ventral hernia repair to hold the touch structures like the margin of the linea alba for suturing.

Endograsping Forceps: Nontoothed (Fig. 21.108)

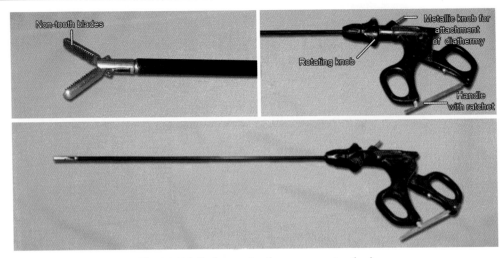

Fig. 21.108: Endograsping forceps—nontoothed

Uses

- It is used to hold tissues.
- In laparoscopic cholecystectomy one grasper hold the fundus and another grasper hold the Hartman's pouch.

Endoscissors: Curved Bladed/Straight Bladed (Fig. 21.109)

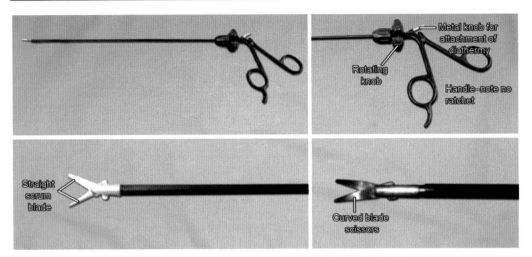

Fig. 21.109: Endoscissors—curved bladed/straight bladed

Uses

- It is used for cutting structures during endoscopic procedures.
- It is used to cut cystic duct and artery after clipping during laparoscopic cholecystectomy.

Suction Irrigation Cannula (Fig. 21.110)

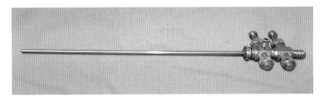

Fig. 21.110: Suction irrigation cannula. Note the two knobs and two channels, one for suction and one for irrigation

Uses

- It is used for suction of blood, fluid, pus during laparoscopic procedure.
- Through irrigation channel fluid can be used for irrigation of the operative area.

Endoscopic Clip Applicator (Fig. 21.111)

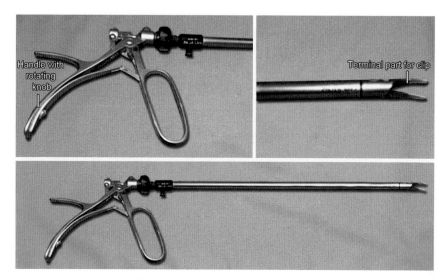

Fig. 21.111: Endoscopic clip applicator

Uses

- It is used for applying titanium clips during laparoscopic procedure.
- It is used to clip the cystic duct and artery before dissection.

Endoscopic Crocodile Forceps (Fig. 21.112)

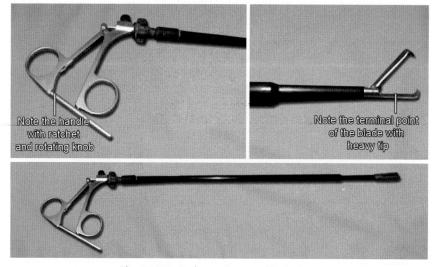

Fig. 21.112: Endoscopic crocodile forceps

Endoscopic Spoon Forceps (Fig. 21.113)

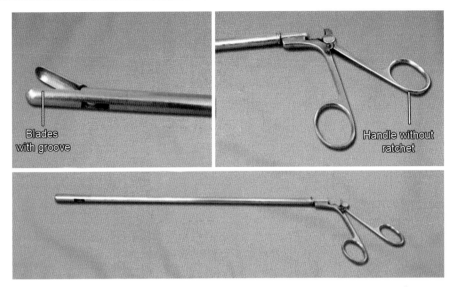

Fig. 21.113: Endoscopic spoon forceps

Uses

It is used during laparoscopic cholecystectomy for picking up spilled out stones.

Endoscopic Diathermy Hook (Fig. 21.114)

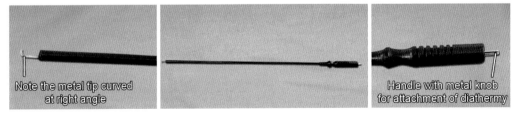

Fig. 21.114: Endoscopic diathermy hook

Uses

- It is used for diathermy dissection during laparoscopic procedure.
- It is used to dissect the gallbladder from the liver bed.

Endoscopic Diathermy Spatula (Fig. 21.115)

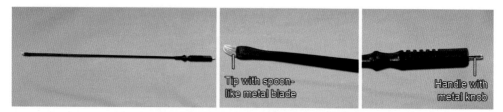

Fig. 21.115: Endoscopic diathermy spatula

Uses

Same as endoscopic hook.

Endo Needle Holder (Fig. 21.116)

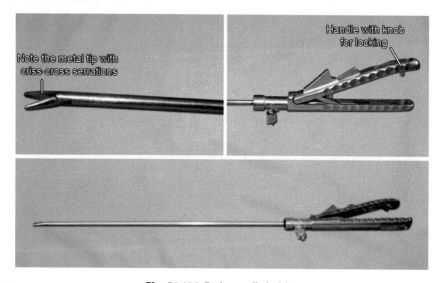

Fig. 21.116: Endo needle holder

Uses

It is used in laparoscopic procedure requiring suturings, e.g. during laparoscopic gastrojejunostomy, choledochoduodenostomy, and gut resection and anastomosis.

Ligaclip—LT 300 (Fig. 21.117)

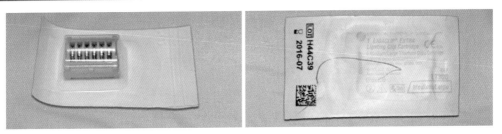

Fig. 21.117: Ligaclip—LT 300

Ligaclip—LT 400 (Fig. 21.118)

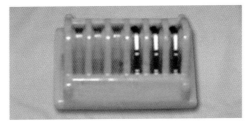

Fig. 21.118: Ligaclip—LT 400

Uses

These are titanium clips used during laparoscopic procedure. These are used to clip a vessel before division. The cystic duct is clipped with this titanium clip before division.

Chapter

Operative Surgery

22

■ STEPS OF LICHTENSTEIN HERNIOPLASTY

Q. Describe the steps of Lichtenstein hernioplasty.

Ans.

- *Anesthesia*: Spinal anesthesia.
- *Position of the patient*: Supine.
- Antiseptic cleaning and draping.
- *Incision*: Inguinal incision. Starting medially at the pubic tubercle and laterally extending beyond the deep inguinal ring 2 cm above and parallel to the inguinal ligament.

  The two layers of subcutaneous tissue (superficial fatty layer—fascia of Camper and the deeper membranous layer—fascia of Scarpa) are incised in the same line as skin by using diathermy. While incising the subcutaneous tissue the superficial epigastric vessels are coagulated and cut. Medially, superficial external pudendal vessels and laterally superficial circumflex iliac vessels may come in the field and needs coagulation and division.
- *Exposure of the inguinal canal*: The external oblique aponeurosis is exposed deep to the subcutaneous tissue. A nick is made in the external oblique aponeurosis. The cut margins are picked up in between two pairs of hemostatic forceps and external oblique aponeurosis is incised medially dividing the superficial inguinal ring and laterally the external oblique aponeurosis is incised beyond the deep inguinal ring.

  The upper flap of external oblique aponeurosis is dissected upward and the conjoint tendon is exposed. The lower flap of external oblique aponeurosis is dissected downward to expose the shining inguinal ligament from pubic tubercle medially to laterally beyond the deep inguinal ring.
- *Dissection of hernial sac*: The spermatic cord along with the hernial sac is dissected in between fingers using a gauze piece and lifted up from the fascia transversalis.

  In case of indirect inguinal hernia the hernial sac lies anterolateral to the cord covered by the cremasteric muscle and the internal spermatic fascia. In case of direct inguinal hernia, the hernial sac lies posteromedial to the cord structures covered by the internal spermatic fascia.

  The cremasteric muscle and fascia is incised and deep to this internal spermatic fascia is incised. The cord structures are splayed in-between fingers and the hernial sac is identified by shiny white margin. The margin of the hernial sac is picked up by a pair of hemostatic forceps and the hernial sac is dissected by sharp dissection from the cord structures taking care not to damage the vas deferens and the testicular vessels.

The hernial sac is dissected from the fundus to the neck of the sac. The neck of the sac is identified by:
- Most constricted part of the sac
- There is a collar of fat pad around the neck
- Inferior epigastric vessels are seen medial to the neck of the sac

+ *Opening of hernial sac and reduction of contents*: The hernial sac is opened at the fundus and the interior of the sac is inspected to exclude a sliding component.

(In case of complete inguinal hernia when the fundus of the hernial sac lies at the bottom of the scrotum, the whole sac need not be dissected. The sac is dissected from the cord structures in the inguinal canal and transected at the middle and the distal part of the sac is left as such. The proximal part of the sac is then dissected up to the neck of the sac). The contents of the hernia are reduced into the peritoneal cavity.

+ *Herniotomy*: The hernial sac is twisted and the neck of the sac is transfixed and the distal sac is excised.

+ *Reinforcement of the posterior wall by placement of a polypropylene mesh*: A standard 15 cm × 7.5 cm sized mesh is required for inguinal hernia. The lateral end of the mesh is split at the lower one-third and upper two-thirds junction to accommodate the spermatic cord. The lower margin of the mesh is fixed to the inguinal ligament starting medially at the fascia over the pubic tubercle extending laterally along the inguinal ligament beyond the deep inguinal ring using 2-0 polypropylene suture. The mesh is medially sutured to the lateral border of the rectus sheath. The mesh is fixed above to the conjoint tendon using 2-0 polypropylene sutures. The split lateral end of the mesh is resutured beyond the spermatic cord to create a neodeep ring.

+ *Closure of external oblique aponeurosis*: The external oblique aponeurosis is sutured using running 1-0 polypropylene suture creating a new superficial inguinal ring.

+ *Closure of subcutaneous tissue and skin*: The skin and subcutaneous tissue is apposed using interrupted sutures with monofilament polyamide. Alternatively, the skin and subcutaneous tissue may be apposed using subcuticular sutures with 3-0 polyglactin.

▐ STEPS OF HERNIOTOMY FOR CONGENITAL HERNIA

Q. Describe the steps of herniotomy for congenital hernia.

Ans. Simple herniotomy is required in infants and children.

+ *Anesthesia*: Operation is usually done under general anesthesia.
+ *Position of patient*: Supine.
+ Antiseptic cleaning and draping.
+ *Skin incision*: A transverse skin incision is made over the groin overlying the deep inguinal ring parallel to the inguinal ligament. The skin and superficial fascia are incised (Fig. 22.1A).
+ *Incising the external oblique aponeurosis*: The external oblique aponeurosis is incised in the same line (Figs 22.1B and C).
+ *Dissection of hernial sac*: The cord with its covering and the hernial sac is isolated and dissected free from the fascia transversalis. The coverings of the cord—external spermatic fascia, the cremaster and internal spermatic fascia are gently teased open just distal to superficial inguinal ring to dissect the hernial sac. The sac is dissected from cord structures (Figs 22.1D and E).

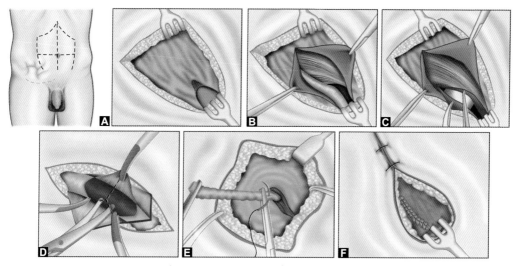

Figs 22.1A to F: Steps of herniotomy

◆ *Opening of sac and reduction of the contents of sac*: The sac is opened and contents of the sac are milked into the peritoneal cavity.
◆ *Transection of the sac*: The sac is transected distal to the deep inguinal ring and the distal part of the sac is left open as such ensuring that there is no bleeding from the distal stump of the sac.
◆ *Ligation of the neck of the sac*: The proximal stump of the sac is held up by a hemostatic forcep and dissected proximally up to the internal inguinal ring. By rotating the clamp, the sac is twisted and ligated by transfixation at the neck and the redundant sac excised (Fig. 22.1F).
◆ *Closure*: The cord structures are covered by closing the covering of the sac.

The external oblique aponeurosis closed with absorbable suture and skin apposed by subcuticular suture (Fig. 22.1F).

Q. What is the difference in technique in older children?

Ans. In child more than 2 years of age, the external and internal rings become widely separated so that direct dissection is no longer possible.

In these cases, skin incision is made slightly laterally over the internal inguinal ring. The skin and superficial fascia is incised. The external oblique aponeurosis is incised and inguinal canal exposed—the external ring is not opened.

The cremasteric fascia and internal spermatic fascia is incised and sac dissected free from the cord structures. The sac is clamped across and the distal part of the sac transected and kept open. The proximal part of the sac is dissected up to the deep ring and tackled as described above.

■ STEPS OF TRANSABDOMINAL PREPERITONEAL OPERATION

Q. Describe the steps of transabdominal preperitoneal (TAPP) operation (Fig. 22.2).

Ans.
◆ *Anesthesia*: General anesthesia with endotracheal intubation.

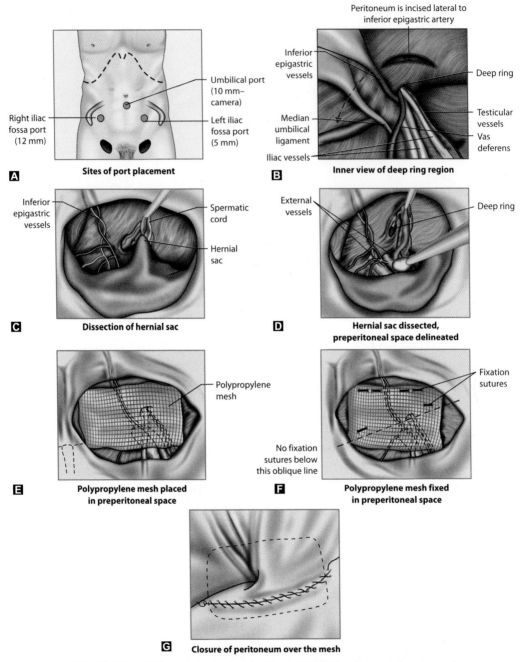

A Sites of port placement

Umbilical port (10 mm–camera)
Right iliac fossa port (12 mm)
Left iliac fossa port (5 mm)

B Inner view of deep ring region

Peritoneum is incised lateral to inferior epigastric artery
Inferior epigastric vessels
Median umbilical ligament
Iliac vessels
Deep ring
Testicular vessels
Vas deferens

C Dissection of hernial sac

Inferior epigastric vessels
Spermatic cord
Hernial sac

D Hernial sac dissected, preperitoneal space delineated

External vessels
Deep ring

E Polypropylene mesh placed in preperitoneal space

Polypropylene mesh

F Polypropylene mesh fixed in preperitoneal space

Fixation sutures
No fixation sutures below this oblique line

G Closure of peritoneum over the mesh

Figs 22.2A to G: Transabdominal preperitoneal (TAPP) laparoscopic hernia repair

- *Position of the patient*: Initially supine. After creation of pneumoperitoneum patient turned to Trendelenburg position with slight elevation of the side to be operated. Monitor kept at the leg end toward the side of hernia. Surgeon stands on the contralateral side. Assistant stands opposite to the surgeon. Bilateral hernia can be operated from either side. Patient's hand kept by the side of trunk and patient well strapped to the table.

Patient should be catheterized.

- *Creation of pneumoperitoneum*: A 10-mm subumbilical incision is made. And a Veress needle inserted into the peritoneal cavity. After confirming the position of the Veress needle in the peritoneal cavity the Veress needle is connected to the automatic electronic insufflator set to 12 mm Hg intra-abdominal pressure and initial flow rate to 1 L/min. Pneumoperitoneum achieved with insufflation of carbon dioxide.
- *Placement of subumbilical ports*: A 10-mm subumbilical port is inserted with gentle rocking movement taking care not to injure the intra-abdominal organ or vessels.
- *Placement of subsequent ports*: Two more 5 mm port is inserted in right and left lower quadrant of the abdomen slightly below the umbilicus lateral to the rectus abdominis taking care not to injure the inferior epigastric vessels.
- *Inspection of pelvic anatomy*: Inspect the bladder, median umbilical fold (containing the obliterated urachus), medial umbilical fold (containing the obliterated umbilical artery), lateral umbilical fold (containing the inferior epigastric artery).
  The indirect hernial sac descends through the deep inguinal ring which is lateral to the lateral umbilical fold. The direct hernial sac descends through the Hesselbach's triangle, which lies medial to the lateral umbilical fold. The triangle of Doom is the area bounded.
  - Laterally by the testicular vessels
  - Medially by the vas deferens
  - Above by the line joining the vas deferens and the testicular vessels.
  The external iliac vessels lie in this triangle.
- *Division of peritoneum*: The hernial contents are reduced. The peritoneum is picked up by a grasper about 2 cm medial to the anterior superior iliac spine about 3–4 cm above the inguinal ligament. The peritoneum is incised at this level by an endoscissor. This incision is then carried medially above the hernial defect up to the medial umbilical fold.
- *Downward reflection of peritoneum and dissection of preperitoneal space*: The incised peritoneum is reflected downward by sharp and blunt dissection and the preperitoneal space is delineated. Medially the dissection is done up to the symphysis pubis. Below the dissection is done up to the obturator foramen. Laterally the dissection is done up to the iliopsoas muscle. Following the Cooper's ligament the deep, inguinal ring is identified.
- *Dissection of hernial sac*: In case of direct hernia, the hernial sac is dissected while lifting the peritoneal flap. In case of indirect inguinal hernia the hernial sac lies anterior to the cord structure. Using two grasping forceps the hernial sac is dissected off from the cord structures taking care not to injure the cord structures. The hernial sac is dissected up to the fundus distally and the proximal limit of dissection is up to the point where the vas deferens and the testicular vessels diverge. If the hernial sac is complete, the hernial sac is transected at the middle and the distal sac kept laid open.
- *Placement and fixation of mesh in preperitoneal space*: A polypropylene mesh size of 12 cm × 15 cm is ideal for inguinal hernia. The mesh is rolled and a suture is placed in the middle of the rolled mesh which helps in better placement and unrolling. The rolled mesh is inserted

into the peritoneal cavity through the 10-mm trocar. The mesh is placed in the preperitoneal space. Medially the mesh is placed up to the symphysis pubis and laterally 2 cm medial to the anterior superior iliac spine. Below the mesh is placed along the Cooper's ligament and lateral to the deep ring along the inguinal ligament. The mesh is unrolled and spread to cover the deep inguinal ring and the Hesselbach's triangle. The mesh is fixed by tacker to the Cooper's ligament medially, above to the anterior abdominal wall. Care is taken not to place any tacker over the triangle Doom and the triangle of pain (lateral to the testicular vessels).

◆ *Repositioning of peritoneal flap and closure of peritoneal defect*: The peritoneal edge is grasped and returned to its normal position. The peritoneal defect is apposed by intracorporeal suturing or by using tackers to avoid contact of mesh with the intra-abdominal viscera.

◆ *Closure of port sites*: 10 mm port site—linea alba apposed by 1-0 polyglactin sutures. Skin apposed with monofilament polyamide sutures.

∎ STEPS OF TOTAL EXTRAPERITONEAL OPERATION FOR INGUINAL HERNIA

Q. Describe the steps of total extraperitoneal (TEP) operation for inguinal hernia.

Ans.

◆ *Anesthesia*: General anesthesia with endotracheal intubation.

◆ *Position of patient*: Same as TAPP operation.

◆ *Placement of subumbilical port*: An infraumbilical 1.5 cm incision is made. The subcutaneous tissue is dissected and the anterior rectus sheath is exposed. The anterior rectus sheath is incised horizontally. The rectus muscle is dissected from the linea alba and retracted laterally.

– *Creation of preperitoneal space*: A balloon trocar is inserted into the space between the rectus abdominis muscle anteriorly and the posterior rectus sheath posteriorly. The baloon is inflated by air and the preperitoneal space is created.

– *Insertion of 10-mm trocar*: The balloon trocar is removed and a 10-mm trocar is introduced into the preperitoneal space thus created and CO_2 gas is insufflated through the cannula and the preperitoneal space is created further.

◆ *Insertion of telescope*: A 10-mm telescope attached to the light source and camera is introduced through the subumbilical cannula. Further creation of the preperitoneal space may be achieved by blunt dissection using the telescope.

◆ *Placement of subsequent ports*: Placement of two more 5-mm ports is required. One 5-mm port is inserted in the midline under direct vision about 1 cm above the symphysis pubis. Another 5 mm port is inserted in the midline midway between the suprapubic and subumbilical trocar. Patient is placed in the Trendelenburg position with the side of the hernia being tilted up.

◆ *Dissection of hernial sac*: The Cooper's ligament is identified lateral to the symphysis pubis and cleared of any preperitoneal fat.

If direct hernia is present, the sac will be readily identified during this dissection and reduced.

◆ *Dissection of indirect hernial sac*: The lateral dissection is done by using a Maryland grasper. The indirect hernial sac lies lateral to the inferior epigastric vessels and anterolateral to the cord structures. The hernial sac is dissected off from the cord structures taking care not to injure the testicular vessels and the vas deferens.

- *Parietalization of the cord structures*: For ease of placement of the mesh, the cord structures are dissected from the preperitoneal loose areolar tissue till the point of divergence of the vas deferens and the testicular vessels.

  During dissection of the preperitoneal space, if the peritoneum is opened inadvertently there will be loss of preperitoneal space due to creation of pneumoperitoneum.

  In this situation the option will be to:
  – Close the peritoneal rent
  – Insert a Veress needle into the peritoneal cavity for deflation or
  – Convert this to a TAPP procedure.
- *Placement and fixation of the mesh*—same as TAPP procedure.

  Desufflation of the peritoneal space by a slow and controlled manner and the trocars are removed.
- *Closure at 10-mm port site* anterior rectus sheath apposed by 2-0 Vicryl suture and skin with monofilament polyamide suture.

■ ANATOMY OF ABDOMINAL INCISIONS

Q. What is the technique of an upper midline abdominal incision?

Ans. Midline incision allows rapid access with minimal blood loss and is an ideal incision for emergency exploratory laparotomy.

- *Skin and subcutaneous tissue*: The skin and subcutaneous tissue is incised in the same line extending from below the xiphoid to just above the umbilicus. If required the incision may be extended below around the umbilicus.
- *Incising linea alba*: Once the skin and subcutaneous tissues are incised the linea alba is exposed. The linea alba is identified by the interdigitating fibers. The linea alba is incised with a knife in the same line for the full length of the skin incision.
- *Incising surgical peritoneum*: Pick up the peritoneum between two pairs of hemostatic forceps and confirm by palpation that no bowel is adherent. Nick the peritoneum in between the hemostatic forceps. Hold the cut margins of the peritoneum with hemostatic forceps. Insert two fingers beneath the cut margin of the peritoneum and divide the peritoneum with scissors up to the full length of the skin incision while incising above cut on one side of the falciform ligament. Care must be taken to look for any adherent viscera to avoid injury while incising the peritoneum.

  In lower midline incision, the linea alba is more wide. Care must be taken while incising the peritoneum toward the lower end to avoid injury to the urinary bladder.

Closure of midline incision: The peritoneum and the linea alba is apposed in single layer with running 0 or 1 polypropylene suture. The bites should be taken at 1 cm interval and 1 cm from the edge of the cut margin.

Skin is closed with interrupted monofilament polyamide suture or silk sutures.

Q. Why linea alba and peritoneum are closed in one layer?

Ans. Mass closure of peritoneum and linea alba is as effective as a layered closure and it is quicker.

Q. What is the length of suture material required for closing an incision?

Ans. The stitches should be applied at 1 cm interval and 1 cm from the edge of the cut margin.
Using this technique, the suture required is 4 times the length of the incision. This is called
Jenkins' rule.

Q. What is the anatomy of paramedian incision?

Ans.

- *Skin and subcutaneous tissue*: Skin incision about 2.5 cm from the midline. Subcutaneous
  tissue incised in the same line.
- *Anterior rectus sheath*: Once the skin and subcutaneous tissues are incised the anterior rectus
  sheath is exposed. Incise the anterior rectus sheath in the same line as skin incision.
- *Separating the rectus abdominis muscle*: A number of hemostatic forceps are applied on the
  medial cut margins of the anterior rectus sheath and lifted up. The rectus abdominis muscle
  is adherent to the anterior rectus sheath at the tendinous intersections. With sharp dissection
  with knife, these tendinous intersections are separated from the medial cut margin of the
  anterior rectus sheath.
- *Retraction of the rectus abdominis muscle*: Once the tendinous intersections are separated
  from the medial cut margins of the rectus sheath the rectus abdominis muscle is retracted
  laterally and the posterior rectus sheath is exposed.
- *Incising the posterior rectus sheath*: The posterior rectus sheath is a composite layer comprising
  of posterior lamella of the internal oblique aponeurosis, transversus abdominis (muscular
  fibers at the upper third and the aponeurotic fibers at the middle third), fascia transversalis,
  extraperitoneal fatty tissue and the parietal peritoneum. In the lower third, the posterior
  rectus sheath is deficient.

  The posterior rectus sheath is lifted up by two pairs of hemostatic forceps and the lifted up
  posterior rectus sheath is palpated in between fingers to confirm that no gut is lifted up. A nick
  is made in the peritoneum. The cut margins of the peritoneum are held by hemostatic forceps
  and the peritoneum incision extended up and down up to the full length of the skin incision.

Closure of paramedian incision: Closure is done in three layers:

1. The peritoneum with posterior rectus sheath is closed with running sutures of 0 or polyglactin
   or polydioxanone.
2. The anterior rectus sheath with running sutures of 0 or 1 polyglactin or polydioxanone.
3. Skin closed with interrupted monofilament polyamide suture.

Q. What is the anatomy of McBurney's gridiron incision?

Ans.

- *Skin incision*: An oblique skin incision of about 5–7 cm length at right angle to the right
  spinoumbilical line passing through the McBurneys' point as the center point.
     (McBurneys' point lies at the junction of medial two-thirds and lateral one third of the right
  spinoumbilical line). The subcutaneous tissue (fascia of Camper and fascia of Scarpa) are
  incised in the same line.
- *External oblique aponeurosis*: A nick is made in the external oblique aponeurosis and the
  external oblique aponeurosis is incised in the same line along the direction of its fibers.

- *Internal oblique and transversus abdominis muscle*: Both internal oblique and transversus abdominis muscle is split along the direction of their fibers. The closed end of a Mayo's scissors is thrushed through both internal oblique and transversus abdominis muscle and the blades are opened. The split is then widened by stretching it between two fore fingers. Two Langenbach's retractors are then inserted to retract the muscles medially and laterally.
- *Peritoneum*: The surgical peritoneum comprising of fascia transversalis, extraperitoneal fatty tissue and the parietal peritoneum is then picked up by two pairs of hemostatic forceps. Palpate the peritoneum to exclude that nothing else is picked up. A nick is made in the peritoneum and the two incised ends are picked up with hemostatic forceps and the peritoneum incision extended up and down up to the full length of the skin incision.

Closure: Closure is done in four layers.

- Surgical peritoneum closed with 1-0 or 2-0 polyglactin suture.
- Internal oblique and transversus abdominis muscles are approximated with interrupted 2-0 polyglactin sutures.
- External oblique aponeurosis apposed with running 2-0 polyglactin sutures.
- Skin approximated with interrupted monofilament polyamide sutures.

Q. What is Lanz incision?

Ans. The Lanz incision is identical to McBurney's incision but here the skin incision is transverse running along the McBurney's point.

Apart from the skin incision, the rest of the approach is like McBurney's incision.

Q. What is the anatomy of Kocher's subcostal incision?

Ans.

- *Skin incision*: About 15 cm long incision begins in the midline below the xiphoid process and runs downward and laterally 2.5 cm below and parallel to the right costal margin. The subcutaneous tissue is incised in the same line.
- *Anterior rectus sheath and the external oblique aponeurosis and muscle*: Once the subcutaneous tissues are incised the anterior rectus is exposed on the medial half of the incision and on the lateral half of the incision, the external oblique aponeurosis and the muscle are exposed. The anterior rectus sheath and the external oblique aponeurosis and the muscle are incised in the same line.
- *Rectus abdominis muscle and the internal oblique muscle*: After incising the anterior rectus sheath and the external oblique, the rectus abdominis muscle is exposed on the medial half of the incision and the internal oblique aponeurosis and the muscle is exposed on the lateral half of the incision. The rectus abdominis muscle is divided across the direction of its fibers. The internal oblique aponeurosis and the muscle are divided along the direction of its fibers.
- *Posterior rectus sheath*: The posterior rectus sheath, comprising of posterior lamella of internal oblique, transversus abdominis muscular fibers, fascia transversalis, extraperitoneal fatty tissue and the parietal peritoneum is exposed next. The posterior rectus sheath is picked up by two pairs of hemostatic forceps and a nick is made in the sheath. The cut margins are then held up by hemostatic forceps and the incision on the posterior rectus sheath is extended medially up to the midline and laterally divides the transverses abdominis muscle and the surgical peritoneum up to the lateral extent of the skin incision.

The 8th, 9th, and 10th intercostal nerves are seen running between the internal oblique and the transversus abdominis muscle.

Closure: Closure is done in three layers.

1. The peritoneum with the posterior rectus sheath is apposed with running 1-0 polyglactin sutures. Laterally, this layer also takes the internal oblique and the transversus abdominis muscle.
2. Next the anterior rectus sheath and the external oblique aponeurosis and the muscle is approximated with running 1-0 polyglactin sutures.
3. Skin approximated with interrupted monofilament polyamide sutures.

Q. What is the anatomy of transverse abdominal incision?

Ans.
+ *Skin*: The skin and the subcutaneous tissue are incised transversely at the desired level.
+ *Anterior rectus sheath*: The anterior rectus sheath is incised in the same line as the skin.
+ *Rectus abdominis muscle*: There are two ways of approach through the rectus abdominis muscle.
+ *Transverse division of transversus abdominis muscle*: Both the rectus abdominis muscles are divided transversely and the posterior rectus sheath is exposed. This is suitable in upper abdominal incision, where there are tendinous intersections where the recti are adherent to the anterior rectus sheath. The recti muscles do not retract.
+ *Vertical separation of the recti*: This is suitable in lower abdominal incision where the recti do not have tendinous intersections. The anterior rectus sheath is dissected upward and downward from the rectus abdominis muscle by sharp dissection. The two recti muscles are then widely separated by blunt dissection and stretching in between the fingers.
+ *Posterior rectus sheath or the peritoneum*: In upper abdominal incision, the posterior rectus sheath is exposed and incised transversely.

In lower abdominal incision after vertical separation of the recti the surgical peritoneum (comprising of parietal peritoneum, extraperitoneal fatty tissue with the fascia transversalis) are exposed and are incised vertically.

Closure of transverse incision: Closure is done in layers.

+ Posterior rectus sheath or peritoneum, extraperitoneal fatty tissue with fascia transversalis— approximated with running 1-0 polyglactin sutures. The divided recti muscles do not require any suture.
+ *Anterior rectus sheath*: Approximated with running 1-0 polyglactin sutures.
+ Skin approximated with interrupted stitches with monofilament polyamide sutures.

■ STEPS OF D2 GASTRECTOMY FOR GASTRIC CANCER

Q. Describe the steps of D2 gastrectomy for gastric cancer.

Ans.
+ *Anesthesia*: General anesthesia with endotracheal intubation.
+ *Position of the patient*: Supine.
+ Antiseptic dressing and draping.

- *Incision*: Midline incision starting below the xiphisternal junction to halfway between the umbilicus and the symphysis pubis. The skin and subcutaneous tissue are incised in the same line.
- *Division of linea alba*: The linea alba is incised in the same line.
- *Division of surgical peritoneum*: The fascia transversalis, extraperitoneal fatty tissue and the parietal peritoneum are lifted up in between two pairs of hemostatic forceps and a nick is made in the peritoneum and the opening in the peritoneum is then extended in the same line.
- *Exploration of the abdomen*: Assess for distant spread liver metastasis, peritoneal deposits, omental deposits, pelvic deposits and presence of ascites. In presence of distant metastasis, curative resection is not attempted. If resectable, resection of the primary growth offers best palliation.
- *Assessment of lymph node status*: Assess the site of involvement and number of lymph nodes involved whether mobile or fixed. Gross lymph node involvement also precludes a curative resection.
- *Assessment for resectability*: Assess the local growth, the location, size and depth of invasion, involvement of adjacent structures. Gross invasion to adjacent structures precludes a curative resection. Involvement of transverse mesocolon and tail of pancreas may be managed with resection of a segment of colon and tail of pancreas.
- *Division of greater omentum and anterior layer of transverse mesocolon*: The procedure begins with division of greater omentum from the transverse colon by sharp dissection through a bloodless plane. Some small blood vessels may be controlled with diathermy.
  The greater omentum is cleared from the whole of transverse colon. The anterior layer of transverse mesocolon is incised and stripped-up up to the anterior surface of the pancreas.
- *Division of right gastroepiploic vessels*: As the greater curvature is lifted up along with the greater omentum the right gastroepiploic vessels are seen entering the pyloric end of greater curvature. The right gastroepiploic vessels are divided in between ligatures.
- *Division of left gastroepiploic vessels*: The proximal line of gastric resection is decided, which is 6 cm proximal to the proximal margin of the growth. The left gastroepiploic vessel is ligated and divided along the greater curvature. If more proximal division is required, the short gastric vessels may require ligature and division.
- *Division of lesser omentum (gastrohepatic ligament)*: The gastrohepatic omentum is dissected and divided close to the porta hepatis and the right gastric artery is ligated and divided close to its origin from the hepatic artery. The omentum to the right of ascending part (1st part) of the duodenum is divided and the duodenum is kocherized.
- *Division of duodenum*: Once the right gastric artery and right gastroepiploic arteries are tied the first part of the duodenum is dissected all around. Two pairs of soft clamps are then applied and the stomach divided just beyond the pylorus.
  The subpyloric and the suprapyloric lymph nodes are also included with the specimen.
- *Closure of duodenal stump*: The duodenal stump is closed in 2 layers—first layer with through and through continuous 3-0 polyglactin sutures and a second layer of inverting suture with 3-0 Mersilk.
- Alternatively, the duodenum may be divided with a linear cutter which cuts the duodenum and staples both the cut ends.
  The duodenal stump may also be closed with a linear stapler.

- *Dissection of lymph nodes*: The divided stomach is lifted up and the lymph nodes in the gastric bed are dissected. The lymph nodes along the hepatic artery are dissected up to their origin. The lymph nodes along the splenic artery are dissected up to the hilum of spleen. The left gastric artery is divided at its origin from the celiac trunk and the lymph nodes around the left gastric artery and celiac trunk are resected en bloc.
- *Resection of the stomach*: Two pairs of gastric occlusion clamps are applied obliquely.

  On the lesser curvature side the line of resection is just below the cardia. On the greater curvature side the line of resection is just below the last short gastric vessels. It should be at least 6 cm proximal to the proximal margin of the tumor. The stomach is then transected between the two pairs of occlusion clamps.

  Alternatively, the stomach may be divided by using GIA linear cutter.
- *Gastrojejunal anastomosis*: The proximal loop of the jejunum is brought up through a rent in the transverse mesocolon and placed alongside the transected stomach. Afferent loop may be brought to the lesser curvature and efferent loop to the greater curvature side. Two pairs of Babcock's tissue forceps are applied to the jejunal loop and a light intestinal occlusion clamp is applied to the jejunum and holding the two clamps together, the stomach and jejunum are kept side by side.

  Alternatively a Roux-en-Y gastrojejunal anastomosis may be done.

  A continuous seromuscular suture is applied between the stomach and the jejunum with 3-0 Mersilk.

  To create a valvular anastomosis the upper part of the cut end of the stomach is closed with through and through sutures using 3-0 polyglactin sutures leaving 5 cm area open. The jejunum is incised for 5 cm and is anastomosed with the remaining cut end of the stomach. The posterior through and through and anterior through sutures are applied with continuous 3-0 polyglactin suture. The anterior seromuscular layer is applied with continuous 3-0 Mersilk suture.
- *Fixation of stomach to the mesocolon rent*: The anastomosis is brought down through the rent in the mesocolon. The margins of the mesocolon rent are sutured to the stomach wall by interrupted stitches.
- *Placement of drain*: A 26 Fr tube abdominal drain is kept in hepatorenal pouch of Morrison close to the duodenal stump.
- *Closure*: Peritoneum and linea alba closed in single layer with continuous No. 1 polypropylene suture.

  Skin closed with interrupted monofilament polyamide suture.

■ STEPS OF TOTAL GASTRECTOMY

Q. What are the indications of total gastrectomy?

Ans.
- Adenocarcinoma of stomach.
- GIST involving large portion of stomach.
- Zollinger-Ellison syndrome.
- Life threatening gastric hemorrhage.

Steps of total gastrectomy:

- *Anesthesia:* General anesthesia with endotracheal intubation.
- *Position of patient:* Supine.
- Antiseptic cleaning and draping.
- *Incision:* A long midline incision from xiphisternum to 8 cm below the umbilicus.

   If the lower esophagus in invaded and needs resection, a left thoracoabdominal incision gives adequate exposure.

Exploration of abdomen:

Assess the local tumor as to whether it is resectable or not. Invasion to aorta, IVC or celiac axis indicates non-resectability.

   Invasion to left lobe of liver, body or tail of pancreas and colon is not a contraindication for resection as the involved organ can be resected en bloc provided there is no distant metastasis.

   Presence of moderate metastasis is not a contraindication for palliative resection of tumour.

- *Omentectomy:* The entire greater omentum is separated from the transverse colon by sharp dissection along the embryonic fusion plane. Also resect the superior layer of the transverse mesocolon avoiding injury to middle colic vessels.
- *Division of right gastroepiploic vessels (RGEV):* Division of gastrocolic omentum and superior layer of transverse mesocolon exposes the anterior surface of the pancreas and duodenum alongwith the RGEV. The right gastroepiploic vessels are ligated and divided close to their origin and the lymph nodes are swept towards the specimen.
- *Resection of lesser omentum:* The gastrohepatic omentum is incised close to the liver and swapt towards the specimen. The right gastric artery arising from the hepatic artery is ligated and divided.
- *Division of duodenum:* Mobilise the duodenum by Kocher maneuver. Dissect the 1st part of the duodenum free from the anterior surface of the pancreas.
- *Transection by linear cutter:* A 55 mm linear cutter may be used to staple and transect the duodenum 2.5 cm beyond the pylorus.
- *Hand sewn closure:* Two pairs of intestinal occlusion clamps are applied 2.5 cm beyond the pylorus and the duodenum is transected using a cutting diathermy. The duodenal stump is closed in 2 layers using 2-0 PDS suture.

The proximal cut end of the duodenum may be ligated by No. 1 silk suture.

- *Celiac axis dissection and ligation of left gastric artery:* The divided stomach is lifted up and towards the left and the LGA is seen emerging from the celiac trunk. The left gastric artery is dissected using a right angled forceps and divided The loose areolar tissue and the lymph nodes are taken with the specimen side.
- *Division of left gastroepiploic vessels (LGEV) and gastrosplenic ligament containing short gastric vessels:* The left gastroepiploic vessels arising from the splenic artery is dissected, ligated and divided. The gastrosplenic ligament containing the short gastric vessels are ligated and divided completely.
- *Dissection of lymph nodes around the hepatic artery:* The peritoneum overlying the hepatic artery is incised and all the lymph nodes around the common hepatic artery upto the origin of gastroduodenal artery is taken down with the specimen.
- *Dissection of lymph nodes around the splenic artery and splenic hilum:* Nodes in the subpyloric region and lymph nodes around the splenic artery along the upper border of the pancreas upto the splenic hilum is dissected and taken along with the specimen.

- *Dissection of esophagogastric junction:* The avascular left triangular ligament is divided and the left lobe of the liver is retracted towards the right. Incise the peritoneum over the abdominal part of the esophagus. The esophagus is dissected free from the crura of the diaphragm. The esophagus is encircled with fingers. Both the anterior and posterior vagal trunks are divided. The most cephalad part of the gastrohepatic omentum is divided. There may be an accessory hepatic branch from the left gastric artery which needs to be ligated and divided. The esophagophrenic ligament is divided and the incision is carried around the fundus to divide the avascular gastrophrenic ligament. The whole stomach is now free.

  An intestinal occlusion clamp is applied around the esophagus and the esophagus is transected at the proposed level. The transection of the esophagus is done 5 cm -6 cm proximal to the proximal margin of the growth.

- *Preparation of a Roux en Y loop of jejunum:* A Roux en Y loop of jejunum is fashioned 15-20 cm from the duodenojejunal flexure (Attachment of ligament of Treitz). Make an incision at the mesentery after ligating and dividing the marginal vessels. Further vessels of the arcade are divided taking care to maintain the vascularity at the transected end of the jejunum. A linear cutter of 55 mm will transect and staple the ends of the jejunum.

  The distal limb of the jejunum is brought up to the end of transected esophagus through a rent in the transverse mesocolon to the left of middle colic artery.

Esophagojejunal Anastomosis (End-to-Side): Hand sewn end-to-side esophagojejunostomy: The anticipated site of the esophageal transaction is 5–6 cm proximal to the proximal margin of the growth. If the diaphragmatic hiatus is excessively large, narrow it by applying 1-2 interrupted suture using 2–0 polypropylene suture.

The Roux loop of jejeunum is fixed to the undersurface of the diaphragm by few interrupted suture to prevent tension on the suture line of esophagojejunostomy.

A jejunostomy is made on the antimesenteric border of the side of jejunum.

two layered anastomosis is made: Interrupted sutures with 4-0 polyglactin

- Posterior seromuscular sutures
- Posterior through and through sutures
- Anterior through and through sutures
- Anterior seromuscular sutures.

End-to-side Stapled Esophagojejunostomy:

Apply stay sutures at the transected end of the esophagus at two corners and middle of anterior and posterior cut ends. Pass a sizer into the cut end of the esophagus and assess which size stapler will be suitable. For esophagojejunal anastomosis a 28 or 31 mm circular stapler is suitable. A purse string suture is applied at the cut end of the esophagus using a 2–0 polypropylene suture. The anvil of the circular stapler is inserted into the esophagus and the purse string suture is tied snugly around the rod of the anvil.

The Roux en Y loop of jejunum is brought up through a rent in the transverse mesocolon. The lubricated end of the cartridge of the circular stapler is inserted into the jejunum through the cut end of the jejunum. By opening the stapler the rod of the cartridge is punctured through the antimesenteric border of the jejunum.

Reattach the anvil rod to the rod of the cartridge properly and ensure that the attachment is tight. Tighten the screw (clockwise) at the base of the circular stapler and see that the anvil is brought in close contact with the cartridge. When the approximation is completed, fire the device by pulling the trigger. Then turn the wing nut anticlockwise one and half turn, rotate the device and deliver the anvil from the esophagus. The index finger should easily pass through the anastomosis.

The end of the jejunum is closed by firing a 55mm (3.5 mm staple height) linear stapler about 1–2 cm beyond the esophagojejunal anastomosis.

End-to-side Jejunojejunostomy

An end-to-side jejunojejunostomy is done 45–50 cm distal to the esophagojejunostomy. A single layer interrupted suture with 3-0 polyglactin suture is ideal.

Placement of Drain

A wide bore tube drain is placed at the heaptorenal pouch of Morrison.

Closure of Abdomen

Single layer continuous suture closure with No.1 loop PDS suture. Skin apposed with interrupted monofilament polyamide suture.

◼ STEPS OF TRUNCAL VAGOTOMY AND GASTROJEJUNOSTOMY

Q. Describe the steps of truncal vagotomy and gastrojejunostomy.

Ans.

- *Anesthesia*: General anesthesia with endotracheal intubation.
- *Position of the patient*: Supine.
- Antiseptic cleaning and draping.
- *Incision*: An upper midline incision extending from xiphoid to the umbilicus. The skin subcutaneous tissue, linea alba and the surgical peritoneum incised in the same line.
- *Exploration of abdomen*: A thorough exploration of abdomen to identify any associated disease. The site of the ulcer is palpated.
- *Exposure of the abdominal part of the esophagus*: A self-retaining retractor is placed to retract the abdominal wall on either side. The left triangular ligament of liver is incised and the left lobe of liver is retracted toward the right to expose the abdominal part of the esophagus. The peritoneum reflecting from the esophagus is incised transversely for about 3–4 cm on either side.
- *Division of the anterior vagus nerve*: The stomach is held by the assistant pulling it downard and outward. The anterior vagus now stands out in front of the abdominal part of the esophagus and gastroesophageal junction is well seen. The anterior vagus nerve is dissected with a right angled forceps. The nerve trunk is held by two pairs of hemostatic forceps both above and below and the intervening 1 cm of the nerve trunk is excised. The proximal and distal cut ends are ligated with silk sutures.
- *Division of posterior vagus nerve trunk*: The gastrohepatic omentum is divided close to the cardioesophageal junction and lesser sac is entered. The stomach is held by the assistant upward and outward and the posterior vagal nerve trunk is identified by finger dissection in the groove between posterior wall of esophagus and the aorta. The thick nerve trunk is dissected using a right angled forceps, held by two pairs of hemostatic forceps at upper and lower dissected end and the intervening 1 cm of segment is excised. The cut ends are ligated with black silk.

- *Drainage procedure*: Truncal vagotomy should be combined with a drainage procedure. This may be achieved either with pyloroplasty or gastrojejunostomy.
- *Roux-en-Y gastrojejunal anastomosis*: Earlier a loop gastrojejunostomy was usual practice. But a nowadays a Roux-en-Y gastrojejunal anastomosis is preferred.
- *Fashioning of a Roux loop of jejunum*: The Roux loop is fashioned about 15 cm from duodenojejunal flexure. The jejunal loop is held up by the assistant and the mesentery is illuminated. The vessels in the mesentery are well seen. At the point of proposed jejunal transection, the mesentery is divided after the mesenteric vessels are dissected, ligated and divided taking care to maintain adequate blood supply to both the proximal and distal limb of the loop after division. The jejunum is transected at the point of division of the mesentery. The distal loop may be lengthened by dividing the intermediate branches joining the arcade, taking care to maintain the blood supply via the adjacent arcade.
- *Closure of the end of distal jejunal limb*: The end of the distal jejunal limb is closed in two layers using inner through and through (all coat) layers using 3-0 polyglactin sutures and outer seromuscular layer using same suture.
- *Gastrojejunal anastomosis*: A posterior gastrojejunostomy is preferred. An incision is made in the transverse mesocolon to the right of middle colic vessels (space of Riolan). The posterior wall of the stomach is held up by two pairs of Babcock's tissue forceps and delivered through the rent in the transverse mesocolon. A pair of gastric occlusion clamp is applied keeping an adequate length of the stomach beyond the clamp. The distal limb of the Roux-en-Y loop is brought close to the stomach keeping the closed end toward the left. An intestinal occlusion clamp is applied to the jejunum and the stomach and jejunum kept side by side. The anastomosis is done in following layers:
  - A continuous posterior seromuscular suture apposing the stomach to the jejunum with 3-0 polydioxanone suture (PDS suture).
  - About 5 cm gastrotomy and jejunotomy is made using diathermy knife parallel to the seromuscular suture applied.
  - The next layer is posterior through and through taking all layers of stomach and jejunum using 3-0 polyglactin suture.
  - Once posterior through and through layer is completed the same suture is continued as continuous anterior through and through layer taking all coats of the stomach and jejunum. The occlusion clamps are removed and check for any bleeding.
  - The anastomosis is completed by applying continuous anterior seromuscular layer using 3-0 PDS.
- *Closure of the mesocolon rent*: The stomach wall is anchored to the mesocolon rent by applying few interrupted 3-0 Mersilk suture to prevent internal herniation through the mesocolon rent.
- *Jejunojejunal anastomosis*: The jejunal continuity is maintained by jejunojejunal anastomosis about 35 cm distal to the gastrojejunal anastomosis. The proximal jejunum is kept by the side of distal jejunum at the site of proposed anastomosis. A jejunotomy is made at the antimesenteric border of the distal jejunum matching the lumen of the proximal jejunal limb. The anastomosis is done by single layer interrupted all coat stitches using 3-0 PDS suture.
- *Approximation of the cut margin of jejunal mesentery*: The cut margin of the proximal jejunal mesentery is apposed to the distal jejunal mesentery by interrupted 3-0 Mersilk suture to prevent internal herniation. Care should be taken so that jejunal vessels are not punctured while taking these stitches.

- *Closure*: The surgical peritoneum and the linea alba is closed in single layer by a continuous suture using No. 1 loop PDS suture. Skin is apposed by interrupted 2-0 monofilament polyamide suture.

STEPS OF REPAIR OF PEPTIC PERFORATION

Q. Describe the steps of repair of peptic perforation.

Ans.
- General anesthesia with endotracheal intubation and assisted ventilation.
- *Position of patient*: Supine.
- Antiseptic dressing and draping.
- Abdomen opened by an upper midline incision. Skin and subcutaneous tissues are incised. The linea alba is incised in the same line. The surgical peritoneum is lifted up in-between two pairs of hemostatic forceps and incised in-between the pairs of hemostatic forceps. The peritoneum incision is then extended up and down. As soon as the peritoneum is incised, gas and bile stained peritoneal fluid escape.
- The peritoneal fluid is aspirated and the site of perforation is localized. The liver is retracted by a Deaver's retractor and the stomach is drawn downward by the assistant using a moist sponge (Fig. 22.3A). The distal stomach and the duodenum are inspected.
- Simple closure of the perforation is the preferred surgical treatment.
- Three or four interrupted polyglactin (Vicryl) or polyglycolic acid (Dexon) sutures are inserted along the axis of the gut. The central stitch traverses through the center of the perforation (Fig. 22.3B).
- The corner sutures are tied first and the central stitch is tied last. The suture line may be reinforced by placing a tag of omentum over the site of perforation and the sutures are tied over the omentum (Fig. 22.3C).
- After closure of the perforation the meticulous peritoneal toilet is done. The subphrenic paces, paracolic gutters and the pelvis are cleared of all turbid fluid and these areas are irrigated with normal saline and the lavage fluid aspirated back.

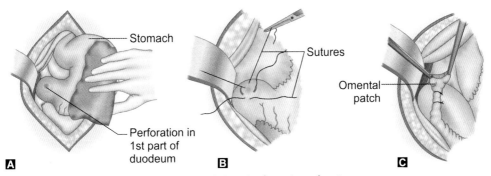

Stomach

Sutures

Omental patch

Perforation in 1st part of duodeum

A **B** **C**

Figs 22.3A to C: Repair of peptic perforation

- A drain is placed in the hepatorenal pouch of Morrison and abdomen is closed. However, the use of drain is not always essential.
- The peritoneum and the linea alba is closed with a continuous No. 1 polypropylene sutures. The skin is closed by interrupted sutures using monofilament polyamide sutures.

Postoperative management:

- Nasogastric aspiration is to be continued.
- Intravenous fluid to maintain fluid and electrolyte balance.
- Antibiotics:
  - Injection: Cefotaxime 1 g IV twice daily.
  - Injection: Amikacin 500 mg IV twice daily.
  - Injection: Metronidazole 500 mg IV thrice daily.
- Intravenous ranitidine or omeprazole.
- Monitoring of pulse, blood pressure, respiration, temperature, and urine output.
- Once bowel sounds return and the patient passes flatus, oral fluid is started and by 3–5 days patient is given semisolid diet.

■ STEPS OF LAPAROSCOPIC CHOLECYSTECTOMY

Q. Describe the steps of laparoscopic cholecystectomy.

Ans.

- *Anesthesia:* The operation is done under general anesthesia with endotracheal intubation.
- *Antiseptic cleaning and draping:* From midchest to midthigh.
- *Position of the patient:* Initially patient is supine. The position is changed after induction of pneumoperitoneum. Patient is placed in reverse Trendelenburg position with right side up position.
  - *Establishment of pneumoperitoneum:* Intra-abdominal pressure is preset to 12–14 mm Hg in automatic insufflator. An 1 cm size smiling incision is made below the umbilicus. A Veress needle is inserted into the abdomen at right angle taking care not to injure the underlying abdominal organs or big vessel. The position of the needle inside the peritoneal cavity is confirmed by injecting about 5 mL of saline and reaspirating it. If the needle is in correct place the saline could be pushed easily and on aspiration nothing will come. This can also be confirmed by drop test. A drop of saline is placed at the back of needle and abdominal wall is lifted up. The needle is in correct place, the saline drop will be sucked in. Once the needle is confirmed to be in the peritoneal cavity, it is connected to an automatic carbon dioxide insufflator by the insufflation tube. The carbon dioxide flow is started at slow rate (1–2 L/min). Afterward the flow rate is increased. Once the abdomen is inflated to a sufficient level the Veress needle is withdrawn.
  - *First trocar entry:* The first trocar is placed blindly and there is risk of injury to the underlyin viscera or vessels. A 10-mm trocar and cannula is inserted into the abdomen below the umbilicus and trocar is removed keeping the cannula in place.
  - *Introduction of the telescope attached to a video camera and light cable:* The video camera light cable attached to 30°, 10 mm telescope is inserted into the peritoneal cavity through the infraumbilical trocar.

– *Inspection of the peritoneal cavity*: The picture of the abdominal cavity is now displayed in the video screen.

  The pelvis is inspected first and then attention is drawn toward the gallbladder.

– *Introduction of 2nd, 3rd, and 4th port (Fig. 22.4A)*: The next three ports are made under direct vision.

  The second 10 mm port is made at the epigastrium below the xiphoid just to the right of midline so that the trocar goes into the abdomen to the right of falciform ligament.

  One 5 mm port is made in the right midclavicular line just below the right costal margin and a second 5 mm port is made in the right anterior axillary line at the level of the umbilicus.

  One toothed grasper is introduced through the anterior axillary port and this grasps the fundus of the gallbladder and pushes it up toward the diaphragm thereby exposing the site of Calot's triangle. One more grasper is introduced through the midclavicular port to hold the Hartmann's pouch of the gallbladder. Through the epigastric port is inserted a Maryland dissector attached to a diathermy.

– *Dissection of cystic pedicle and the Calot's triangle (Fig. 22.4B)*: The patient is positioned reversed Trendelenburg's position with the right side up to allow the intestine to fall away from the right hypochondriac region. With the Maryland dissector the anterior leaf and the posterior leaf of the cystic pedicle is teased off and the cystic duct and artery is dissected clearly. Posterior dissection of the Calot's triangle is the most important initial step. Anterior dissection of the Calot's triangle is complementary and should be done after the posterior dissection is done. A large window is created between the cystic duct and the artery so that the clips may be applied easily.

– *Application of clips and division of cystic duct and artery (Fig. 22.4C)*: Once the cystic duct and artery is cleared off they are clipped with titanium clips applied by a 10-mm clip applier inserted through the epigastric port. Three clips are applied in the cystic duct and three in the cystic artery and the duct and artery is divided by an endoscissors keeping two clips in the cystic duct and artery toward the bile duct side.

– *Dissection of the gallbladder from gallbladder bed of liver (Figs 22.4D and E)*: Once the cystic duct and the artery are divided the gallbladder is now dissected by using a unipolar diathermy hook from the liver bed.

– *Irrigation and suction*: Once the gallbladder is free, the gallbladder bed is irrigated with normal saline and check for any bleeding which may be controlled by diathermy coagulation.

– *Extraction of gallbladder*: The separated gallbladder is then held up by a crocodile forceps and removed through the epigastric port.

– *Placement of drain*: Placement of a drain is optional. If there is slight oozing or if the surgery is difficult then a tube drain may be placed in the hepatorenal pouch of Morrison for 24–48 hours.

– *Closure of the incision*: The cannulas are withdrawn and the incisions are closed. The sheath in the 10 mm port areas are closed with Vicryl sutures.

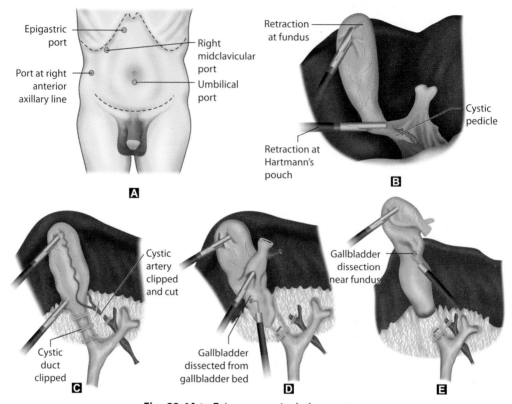

Figs 22.4A to E: Laparoscopic cholecystectomy

Q. Why do you prefer laparoscopic cholecystectomy?

Ans.

- Laparoscopic cholecystectomy has been established as a gold standard for the treatment of gallstone diseases.
- Surgery is safe in the hands of a trained surgeon.
- Less pain, less hospital stay
- Cosmetic
- Early return to work is possible
- More acceptance by the patient.

Q. While you take consent for laparoscopic cholecystectomy what should you tell the patient?

Ans. Laparoscopic cholecystectomy sometimes need conversion to open procedure if there is gross adhesion and the anatomy in the area of Calot's triangle is not clear and there is excessive bleeding. So an informed consent is to be taken from the patient that if laparoscopic procedure is not safe, it may need conversion to open cholecystectomy.

■ OPEN CHOLECYSTECTOMY

Q. What are the indications of cholecystectomy?

Ans.

- Gallstone disease
- Chronic cholecystitis
- Acute cholecystitis
- Mucocele of gallbladder
- Empyema of gallbladder
- Cholesterolosis of gallbladder
- Porcelain gallbladder
- Carcinoma of gallbladder
- Gallbladder polyp
- Acalculous cholecystitis
- Traumatic rupture of gallbladder
- Along with Whipples' operation.

Steps of open cholecystectomy:

- *Anesthesia:* General anesthesia with endotracheal intubation.
- *Position of the patient:* Supine. If intraoperative cholangiogram is required then patient should be placed on a special operation table with transparent top. There should be provision for insertion of a Bucky grid for placement of an X-ray plate for exposure.
- *Antiseptic cleaning and draping:* Antiseptic cleaning by application of povidone-iodine solution from midchest to midthigh.
- *Incision:* Right subcostal incision (Kocher's incision).
- *The structures incised in Kocher's subcostal incision.*
- *Preliminary exploration:* The stomach, duodenum, colon, pancreas and liver are examined first. The gallbladder is examined, look for color, any adhesions, palpated for any calculi. The supraduodenal part of the common bile duct is palpated at the free margin of the lesser omentum with index finger in the epiploic foramen and thumb in front to exclude presence of any calculi. The retroduodenal part of the common bile duct is palpated by keeping the finger tips along the lateral border of the second part of the duodenum and by placing the thumb anteriorly in the groove between the duodenum and the pancreas.
- *Placement of mops:* The next step is good exposure. Three mops are placed. The first mop is placed in the hepatorenal pouch to retract the right colic flexure downward. The second mop is placed in the lower part of the wound to retract the duodenum, transverse colon and the small intestine. The third mop is placed more medially to retract the stomach.
- *Retraction and exposure:* Deep retractors are placed and held by the assistants for good exposure. One Deaver's retractor retracts the right lobe of the liver upward and another Deaver's retractor retracts the lower part of the wound.
- *Dissection of the cystic pedicle:* The fundus of the gallbladder is held by a Moynihan's cholecystectomy forceps. Another Moynihan's cholecystectomy forceps is applied at the Hartmann's pouch and the gallbladder is retracted downward and to the right. The anterior layer of the peritoneum covering the cystic duct and artery is snipped off with a scissors and

the cystic duct and artery dissected by blunt dissection using a peanut swab. The cystic artery often runs anterior to the cystic duct.

◆ *Ligation of cystic artery and duct*: The cystic artery is dissected by using a right angle forceps and two ligatures of No. 1-0 silk suture are passed around the cystic artery. These are then tied and the cystic artery is divided in-between the ligatures. Similarly the cystic duct is dissected by using the right angle forceps and two ligatures are passed around the cystic duct. These ligatures are tied and the cystic duct divided in-between the ligatures. For safety one additional ligature may be applied in the cystic artery and the duct.

◆ *Dissection of gallbladder from liver*: The gallbladder is retracted by using the Moynihan's cholecystectomy forceps and a finger is insinuated between the gallbladder and the liver and the gallbladder is gently dissected from its bed. As the gallbladder is lifted from its bed, fine fringes stand out. These are divided with diathermy or ligated and divided, as fine vessels are present in these strands. As the gallbladder is dissected, the peritoneal reflection from the gallbladder to the liver is divided with scissors or diathermy knife. A fringe of peritoneum is kept on either side of the gallbladder bed. While lifting the gallbladder from gallbladder bed in liver, look for any cholecystohepatic duct.

◆ *Hemostasis*: The gallbladder bed is checked for bleeding. Bleeding points are either ligated or coagulated with diathermy. A hot moist pack may also control minor bleeding in the gallbladder bed. The margins of the raw area of the gallbladder bed may be apposed with interrupted or continuous sutures of chromic catgut.

◆ *Drainage*: A drainage tube is kept in the subhepatic space.

◆ *Closure*: Closure is done in layers (see abdominal incisions).

Q. What is retrograde cholecystectomy?

Ans. The usual technique of cholecystectomy described above—ligation of cystic duct and artery and dissection of gallbladder from its bed starting from the neck to the fundus is called retrograde cholecystectomy.

Q. What is fundus first cholecystectomy?

Ans. If there is dense adhesion at the Calot's triangle area and the anatomy is not discernible, then attempt at dissection of cystic duct and artery may result in excessive bleeding or inadvertent injury to the bile duct. In such situation it is safer to start dissection of the gallbladder fundus from the gallbladder bed in the liver and dissection carried toward the neck of the gallbladder and the cystic duct and artery ligated and divided. This is called fundus first cholecystectomy.

Excessive traction of the mobilized gallbladder may cause kinking of the bile duct and may result in bile duct injury.

If dense adhesion prevents isolation of cystic artery and cystic duct clearly, it is better to keep a part of the gallbladder neck. The gallbladder is transected at the neck and the cut margins are suture ligated.

■ STEPS OF CHOLEDOCHOLITHOTOMY

Q. Describe the steps of choledocholithotomy (Figs 22.5 to 22.8).

Ans. If operated for gallstones and common bile duct stones—Kocher's subcostal or right paramedian or midline incisions.

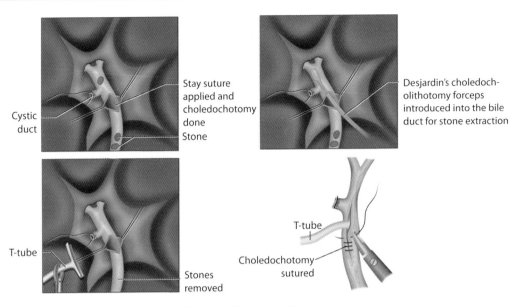

Cystic duct

Stay suture applied and choledochotomy done

Stone

Desjardin's choledoch-olithotomy forceps introduced into the bile duct for stone extraction

T-tube

T-tube

Stones removed

Choledochotomy sutured

Fig. 22.5: Choledocholithotomy

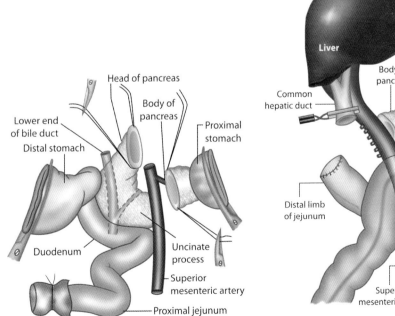

Head of pancreas

Body of pancreas

Lower end of bile duct

Distal stomach

Duodenum

Proximal stomach

Uncinate process

Superior mesenteric artery

Proximal jejunum

Fig. 22.6: Structures that are to be removed in Whipple's operation are shown to the right of superior mesenteric artery

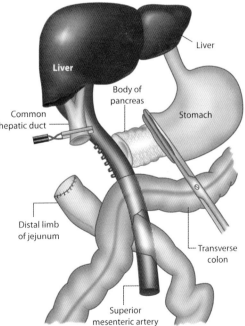

Liver

Liver

Body of pancreas

Common hepatic duct

Stomach

Distal limb of jejunum

Transverse colon

Superior mesenteric artery

Fig. 22.7: Structures as seen before anastomosis

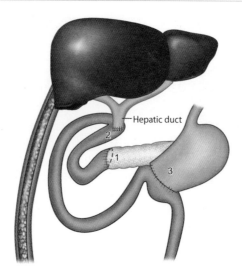

Fig. 22.8: Reconstruction after pancreaticoduode-nectomy. (1) Choledochojejunostomy; (2) Pancre-atojejunostomy; (3) Gastrojejunostomy

A laparotomy is done and presence of gallbladder and common bile duct stone confirmed by palpation. The gallbladder is held by Moynihan's cholecystectomy forceps and the peritoneum of the cystic pedicle is dissected and the cystic duct and artery is dissected. Cystic artery ligated and divided. A suture is passed around the cystic duct for ease of lateral retraction.

- *Identifying the bile duct*: The bile duct is dissected by lifting and incising the peritoneum from its anterior aspect. Bile duct identified by aspirating bile.
- *Application of stay sutures*: Two stay sutures are applied on either side of the supraduodenal part of the bile duct using 3-0 atraumatic chromic catgut suture.
- *Making a choledochotomy*: Choledochotomy is done in supraduodenal part of common bile duct in between the stay sutures and the incision extended for about 2 cm.
- *Removal of CBD stones*: A Desjardin's choledocholithotomy forceps is introduced into the bile duct and the stones removed. This may be aided by introduction of a choledochoscope through the choledochotomy and stone may be extracted by a Dormia basket catheter introduced through the choledochoscope.

    The bile duct is then irrigated with normal saline to flush off the small fragments of stone or debris.

    An intraoperative cholangiogram is done to ascertain complete clearance of the bile duct stones.

- *Introduction of tube*: A T tube is fashioned for placement in the bile duct. The horizontal limb is deroofed and proximal end kept for about 2–5 cm and distal end kept for about 4 cm. The choledochotomy is closed keeping a T tube in the bile duct.

    Alternatively a *choledochoduodenostomy* may be done.

■ STEPS OF CHOLEDOCHODUODENOSTOMY

Q. Describe the steps of choledochoduodenostomy.

Ans. This is usually done following choledocholithotomy.

+ *Anesthesia*: General anesthesia with endotracheal intubation.
+ *Position of patient*: Supine
+ Antiseptic cleaning and draping.
+ *Incision*: Approach is as in open cholecystectomy, through Kocher's subcostal incision.
+ *Cholecystectomy*: Mops are placed to expose the area of Calot's triangle.
+ Gallbladder is held by Moynihan's cholecystectomy forceps at the fundus and the Hartmann's pouch and the cystic pedicle is dissected, ligated and divided.
+ *Choledocholithotomy*: The cystic duct stump is retracted to reach the bile duct.
+ The peritoneum in front of the bile duct is incised and the bile duct is exposed. Bile duct is confirmed by aspiration of bile.
+ Two stay sutures are applied on either side of the midline in the anterior wall of bile duct using 3-0 chromic catgut suture.
+ A choledochotomy is done and the stones are removed from the bile duct using Desjardin's choledocholithotomy forceps. The bile duct is irrigated with saline to clear off any residual stone or debris.
+ Choledochoduodenostomy
+ *Mobilization of the first part of duodenum*: The first part of the duodenum is mobilized by dividing the hepatoduodenal ligament. The right gastric artery is ligated and divided. This allows first part of the duodenum to be brought up for choledochoduodenostomy without tension.
+ *Incision on duodenum*: Choledochotomy is already made for removal of bile duct stones. A similar incision is made in the anterior wall of duodenum along its axis.
+ *Anastomosis*: Anastomosis is done with interrupted suture using 4-0 polyglactin or polydioxanone.
+ Take bite from the angle of the duodenotomy to the middle of the choledochotomy on either side. Interrupted suture at 3 mm interval is taken between the duodenum and the bile duct forming the posterior wall. All the sutures in the posterior wall are then tied.
+ The anterior layer of sutures are then taken between the duodenum and the bile duct and tied at the end.
+ *Closure*: Check for hemostasis. A drain is kept in the hepatorenal pouch of Morrison.
+ Incision is closed in layers.

■ STEPS OF WHIPPLE'S PANCREATICODUODENECTOMY

Q. Describe the steps of Whipple's pancreaticoduodenectomy.

Ans.

+ *Anesthesia*: General anesthesia with endotracheal intubation.
+ *Position of the patient*: Supine.

- Antiseptic cleaning and draping.
- *Incision*: A long midline incision extending from xiphoid to well below the umbilicus. The subcutaneous tissue is incised in the same line. The linea alba and the surgical peritoneum is incised in the same line and the peritoneal cavity entered (in obsese patient with wide costal, margin a roof top incision provides better exposure).
- *Exploration of abdomen*: Assess for distant metastasis—presence of ascites, liver, omentum, and pelvis is examined for presence of any nodules. Presence of distant metastasis is a contraindication for resection. Mobile lymph nodes within the area of resection are not a contraindication for resection. However, presence of fixed nodes is a contraindication for resection.
- *Assessment for resectability*: This involves a number of steps to decide about the resectability.
- *Exposure of the duodenum and the head of the pancreas*: The peritoneum lateral to the right colic flexure is incised and the colic flexure is dissected down to expose the duodenum and the head of the pancreas. While doing so the right gastroepiploic vein draining into the superior mesenteric vein needs ligature and division.
- *Kocherization of duodenum*: The peritoneal attachment at the lateral border of second part of duodenum is incised and the duodenum kocherized lifting it up from the inferior vena cava, aorta and the retroperitoneum. Any infiltration of the tumor into the inferior vena cava or aorta is a contraindication for resection. The first part of the duodenum is also mobilized by incising the peritoneum from the superior border of the duodenum up to the foramen of Winslow.
- *Exposure of the pancreas*: The greater omentum is divided in between ligature and the head, neck, and body of the pancreas is exposed well. Small vessels in front of the head pancreas need ligature and division for proper exposure of the head of the pancreas.
- *Exposure and dissection of superior mesenteric vessels*: The Kocher's maneuver is extended to the third part of the duodenum. The third part of the duodenum is mobilized and the superior mesenteric vessels are identified crossing the third part of the duodenum, superior mesenteric artery (SMA) to the left and superior mesenteric vein (SMV) to the right. Small vessels joining the middle colic vein, SMV from the pancreaticoduodenal vein needs ligature and division. An attempt is made to create a tunnel between the superior mesenteric vein and the neck of the pancreas. A judgment is made at this stage regarding tumor invasion into the SMV or portal vein. Any invasion indicates inoperability.

  However, nowadays if expertise is available, it is possible to resect a segment of portal vein with the tumor followed by reconstruction with a prosthetic graft.
- *Dissection of hepatoduodenal ligament and portal structures*: The hepatoduodenal ligament is divided close to the liver and the peritoneum and the loose areolar tissue over the bile duct, hepatic artery and the portal vein are dissected along with the pericholedochal lymph nodes. The bile duct is dissected all around. The gastroduodenal artery arising from the hepatic artery is dissected, ligated and divided. This gives a good exposure of the portal vein. An attempt is now made to complete the tunnel between the neck of the pancreas and the portal vein. If there is no invasion into the portal vein the resection can proceed.
- *Cholecystectomy and division of bile duct*: The cystic artery is dissected and ligated. The gallbladder is dissected off from the liver bed starting with the fundus and dissected up to the bile duct. The already dissected bile duct is divided above the cystic duct insertion.

◆ *Division of gastrohepatic omentum and lymph nodes*: The lesser omentum is incised close to the liver and the peritoneum over the common hepatic artery (CHA) is incised. The lymph nodes around the CHA is dissected and swept down toward the specimen. The lymph nodes around the common bile duct and the portal vein are also swept down toward the specimen.

◆ *Distal gastrectomy*: While dissecting the hepatic artery, the right gastric artery is dissected, ligated and divided close to the pylorus. The distal third of the stomach needs resection in Whipple's operation. The right gastroepiploic artery is dissected, ligated and divided near the lower border of the pylorus. The left gastric arcade along the lesser curvature is dissected, ligated and divided at the site of proposed gastric resection. The left gastroepiploic arcade is also dissected, ligated and divided at the greater curvature at the site of proposed gastric resection. Two pairs of intestinal occlusion clamps are applied and the stomach divided in-between.

◆ *Division of the neck of the pancreas*: Two pairs of stay sutures are applied along the upper and lower border of the junction of body and neck of the pancreas to minimize bleeding. A soft clamp may be applied to the specimen side and the neck of the pancreas is transected using cutting diathermy. While doing so the portal vein lying behind the neck of the pancreas is safeguarded by placing a dissector in-between the neck of the pancreas and the portal vein.

◆ *Division of the jejunum*: The duodenojejunal flexure is identified at the infracolic compartment. The ligament of Treitz is identified and incised taking care not to injure the inferior mesenteric vein. Two pairs of intestinal occlusion clamps are applied about 10 cm from the D-J flexure and the jejunum is transected. The mesentery of the proximal jejunum is incised close to the jejunal wall taking care not to injure the superior mesenteric artery or vein. A double row of short vessels runs from the fourth part of duodenum to the uncinate processes. These vessels are dissected, ligated and divided.

Once these vessels are divided, the divided jejunum may now be brought to the right behind the superior mesenteric vessels.

◆ *Division of uncinate process*: At this stage the only attachment of the specimen is between the uncinate process and the superior mesenteric vessels. There are multiple short vessels running between the uncinate process and the superior mesenteric vessels. These vessels are dissected in small bits, ligated and divided, taking care not to injure the superior mesenteric vessels.

◆ *Removal of specimen*: Once the uncinate process is cleared off from the superior mesenteric vessels, the specimen consisting of gallbladder, common bile duct, distal third of the stomach, head, neck, and uncinate process of the pancreas, whole of duodenum, proximal 10 cm of jejunum along with regional lymph nodes are now free to be removed.

◆ *Reconstruction*: Once resection is complete reconstruction is to be done to maintain pancreatic, biliary, and gastric continuity.

◆ *Pancreaticojejunal anastomosis*: The jejunal loop is lengthened by dividing the vascular arcade in the mesentery taking care to maintain the vascularity at the cut end of the jejunum. The cut end of the jejunum is closed by 2 layers of sutures, inner through and through layers taking all coats of jejunum with 3-0 polyglactin sutures. Outer seromuscular layer with 3-0 interrupted Mersilk sutures. The jejunal limb is brought up through a rent in the transverse mesocolon in an avascular area to the right of middle colic vessels.

- An end to side pancreaticojejunal anastomosis is done in 2 layers. Interrupted 4–0 PDS sutures are applied between the posterior pancreatic capsule with the posterior seromuscular coat of jejunum.
  - A jejunotomy is made at the level of pancreatic duct. Using 4–0 PDS suture the pancreatic duct mucosa is sutured to the all coats of the jejunum first applied posteriorly and then anteriorly.
  - The anastomosis is completed by interrupted sutures using 4-0 PDS apposing the anterior pancreatic capsule with anterior seromuscular coat of jejunum.
- *Hepaticodochojejunostomy*: About 15 cm distal to the pancreaticojejunal anastomosis an end to side hepaticodochojejunostomy is done. A jejunotomy is made in the jejunum matching the hepatic duct diameter. A single layer anastomosis is done by taking all coats of jejunum and the hepatic duct with interrupted 4-0 PDS sutures.
- *Gastrojejunal anastomosis*: About 15 cm distal to the hepaticodochojejunostomy an end to side gastrojejunal anastomosis is done in 2 layers. The posterior seromuscular suture is applied first by a running 4-0 PDS suture. The gastrotomy is partially closed by all coats running suture with 4-0 PDS, leaving about 5 cm for anastomosis. The posterior through and the anterior through suture is applied by running 4-0 PDS sutures taking all coats bite of the stomach and jejunum. The anastomosis is completed by applying running anterior seromuscular layer with 4-0 PDS.
- *Closure of transverse mesocolon rent*: The rent in the transverse mesocolon is sutured to the seromuscular coat of the jejunum with interrupted 3-0 Mersilk to prevent internal herniation through the mesocolon rent.
- *Feeding jejunostomy*: A feeding jejunostomy is done 15 cm distal to the gastrojejunal anastomosis. A No. 20 Fr Foleys catheter is used for creating a feeding jejunostomy and the catheter brought out through a stab wound. This is useful for maintaining nutrition in postoperative period in situation of delayed gastric emptying or development of pancreatic fistula.
- *Placement of drain*: A wide bore drain is placed in the hepatorenal pouch of Morrison close to the pancreaticojejunal anastomosis.
- *Closure of abdomen*: Surgical peritoneum with linea alba in single layer with running suture using 1 polypropylene or 1 PDS suture. Skin apposed with interrupted 2-0 monofilament polyamide sutures.
  The jejunostomy tube and the drainage tube are fixed to the skin.

▮ STEPS OF LATERAL PANCREATICOJEJUNOSTOMY

Q. Describe the steps of lateral pancreaticojejunostomy.

Ans.

- *Anesthesia*: General anesthesia with endotracheal intubation.
- *Position of the patient*: Supine.
- Antiseptic cleaning with povidone-iodine and draping by placement sterile sheets.
- *Incision*: A roof top or chevron incision gives very good exposure. In patient with narrow costal margin a long upper midline incision extending from below the xiphoid to about 4 cm below the umbilicus also gives adequate exposure.

+ *Preliminary exploration of abdomen*: On opening the peritoneum, the abdomen is explored for diagnosis of any unforeseen pathology. Pancreas is palpated for confirmation of diagnosis.
+ *Exposure of pancreas*: The gastrocolic omentum is divided in between ligature and the body and tail of pancreas is exposed. The head of pancreas is exposed by dividing the duodenocolic ligament and reflecting the right colic flexure downward. While doing so the right gastroepiploic vein needs dissection and division after ligature. The small branches of gastroduodenal artery also need division for exposure of the entire head of the pancreas.
+ *Kocherization of duodenum*: An incision is made in the posterior parietal peritoneum at the lateral border of second part of duodenum and the duodenum kocherized lifting it up from the inferior vena cava and posterior abdominal wall. The head of the pancreas can now be palpated properly.
+ *Exposure of body and tail of pancreas*: The gastrocolic ligament is divided in between ligature and the body and tail of pancreas is exposed.
+ *Identification and opening of pancreatic duct*: A grossly dilated duct with calculi in lumen can be easily palpated. If the duct is not palpable a hypodermic needle is inserted into the pancreatic parenchyma lateral to the neck of the pancreas at the upper one-third and lower two-thirds junction. As the needle reaches the pancreatic duct pancreatic juice will start flowing out. The needle is kept in that position. Following the shaft of the needle the pancreatic parenchyma is incised with a diathermy knife and the pancreatic duct is opened up. A metal dilator is inserted through the opened duct toward the body and tail of the pancreas and the duct is opened by incising the pancreatic parenchyma using a diathermy knife to minimize bleeding. The dilator is then inserted toward the head of the pancreas and the duct is opened similarly keeping 1 cm margin from the medial border of the duodenum to prevent injury to the vessels lying in the pancreaticoduodenal groove.
+ *Removal of ductal calculi*: Using Desjardin's choledocholithotomy forceps all the stones and debris are cleared from the pancreatic duct. Some stones and debris may be cleared by irrigating the duct lumen with saline.
+ *Pancreatic head coring*: For adequate pain relief a proper head coring is also required. The thickened pancreatic parenchymal tissue of the head of pancreas is excised in piecemeal using electrocautery keeping a 1 cm rim of tissue around the medial border of the duodenum.
+ *Creation of a Roux-en-Y loop of jejunum*: A Roux-en-Y limb of jejunum is created about 15 cm distal to the duodenojejunal flexure. The vessels in the mesentery are divided in such a fashion so that blood supply to both the proximal and distal limb is well maintained. The jejunum is divided and the cut end of the distal jejunal limb is closed by 3-0 PDS in two layers (inner through and through layers and outer interrupted seromuscular layers).
+ *Pancreaticojejunal anastomosis*: The distal limb of the Roux-en-Y loop is brought up behind the transverse colon through an avascular area in the mesocolon to the right of middle colic vessels (space of Riolan).

The jejunum is placed by the side of the opened pancreatic duct. A longitudinal jejunotomy is made along the antimesenteric border matching the opening in the pancreatic duct. A single layer pancreaticojejunal anastomosis is done by interrupted through and through stitches taking bites in all layers of jejunum and the pancreatic parenchyma and the duct mucosa using 4-0 PDS suture.

(Alternatively a two-layer anastomosis may be done. A outer layer of continuous suture taking seromuscular coat of jejunum and the pancreatic parenchyma using 4-0 Mersilk. An inner layer of interrupted suture taking jejunal mucosa and the pancreatic duct mucosa using 4-0 PDS suture.

- *Closure of mesocolon rent*: The mesocolon rent is closed by taking interrupted suture between the margin of the mesocolon rent and the jejunal serosa.
- *Jejunojejunal anastomosis*: The intestinal continuity is maintained by doing a jejunojejunal anastomosis about 35 cm distal to the pancreaticojejunal anastomosis. Single layer jejunojejunal anastomosis is done with interrupted all coats stitch using 4-0 PDS sutures.
- *Closure of jejunal mesenteric gap*: The mesenteric gap between the proximal and the distal jejunum loop is apposed by interrupted sutures using 3-0 Mersilk
- *Placement of drain*: Check for hemostasis and a wide bore abdominal drain (No. 32 Fr) is placed in the hepatorenal pouch of Morrison.
- *Closure*: Closure in layers. The internal oblique, transversus abdominis and the surgical peritoneum laterally and the posterior rectus sheath medially is apposed by continuous suture using No.1 PDS suture.

The external oblique muscle and aponeurosis laterally and the anterior rectus sheath medially is apposed by a continuous suture using 1 PDS suture.

The skin is approximated by interrupted 2-0 monofilament polyamide sutures.

■ STEPS OF RIGHT HEMICOLECTOMY

Q. Describe the steps of right hemicolectomy.

Ans. (For growth in cacum and ascending colon a standard right hemicolectomy involves resection of terminal 10 cm of ileum, cecum, ascending colon and right two-thirds of transverse colon along with whole of greater omentum and the regional lymph nodes epicolic, paracolic, intermediate and the central lymph nodes).

- *Anesthesia*: General anesthesia with endotracheal intubation.
- *Position of patient*: Supine.
- Antiseptic cleaning with povidone-iodine and draping.
- *Incision*: A long midline incision from midepigastrium to about 5 cm below the umbilicus. Skin subcutaneous tissue, linea alba and surgical peritoneum incised in the same line.
- *Exploration of abdomen*: Assessment for metastasis, presence of ascites, any distant spread to liver, omentum, peritoneum and pelvis. Palpate for involvement of regional lymph nodes— epicolic, paracolic, intermediate, and central lymph nodes (lymph nodes around the origin of superior mesenteric vessels).

  Assessment of the local growth to decide about the resectability. Assess whether the growth has invaded the posterior abdominal wall, ureter, gonadal vessels and duodenum and pancreas. Any adherence of small gut to the growth.
- *Exteriorization of small gut*: For ease of dissection the whole of small gut is exteriorized and wrapped in a moist towel taking care not to twist the mesentery.
- *Division of greater omentum*: The greater omentum is ligated and divided close to the greater curvature of stomach preserving the gastroepiploic arcade.

- *Mobilization of right colon*: The cecum and the ascending colon are retracted medially and the peritoneum is incised using diathermy along the white line of Toldt at the right paracolic gutter. The right colon along with the terminal ileum is reflected toward the left to expose the vessels supplying the right colon—ileocolic, right colic, and the middle colic vessels. While doing so, care is taken to prevent injury to the structures lying deep to the right colon—gonadal vessels, right ureter, and the duodenum. Small bleeding in the retroperitoneum may be controlled by placement of a moist mop.
- *Divisions of vessels of right colon*: The vessels supplying the terminal 10 cm of ileum are dissected, ligated and divided. The ileocolic vessels and the right colic vessels are ligated as high as possible. The right branch of the middle colic vessels are ligated close to its origin from the trunk of middle colic artery. The mesentery in-between these vessels are divided and taken with the specimen.
- *Dissection of lymph nodes*: While dissecting and ligating the vessels all the lymph nodes along these vessels are dissected and taken along with the specimen. The lymph nodes around the trunk and origin of the superior mesenteric trunk is also dissected and removed along with the specimen.
- *Division of terminal ileum and the transverse colon*: Two pairs of intestinal occlusion clamps are applied at the site of proposed ileal resection and the ileum is resected using cutting diathermy.
- *Division of transverse colon*: Two pairs of intestinal occlusion clamps are applied at the site of proposed transverse colon resection and the colon is divided using cutting diathermy. Care is taken to preserve the blood supply to the end of ileum and the transverse colon.
- *Ileocolic anastomosis*: A two layer anastomosis is done. The anastomosis may be done either as end-to-end, or the cut ends may be closed and a side-to-side anastomosis (functional end-to-end anastomosis) may be done.
  - The posterior seromuscular suture is applied by interrupted suture using 3-0 Mersilk sutures.
  - The posterior through and through and anterior through layer is applied by running suture using 3-0 polydioxanone (PDS).
    The anterior seromuscular suture is completed by interrupted 3-0 Mersilk sutures.
    (Alternatively a single layer anastomosis may be done by interrupted suture using 3-0 PDS suture).
- *Closure of mesenteric gap*: The gap between the mesentery of ileum and transverse mesocolon is closed by interrupted suture using 3-0 Mersilk.
- *Placement of drain*: Hemostasis is checked and a tube drain is placed at hepatorenal pouch of Morrison by making a stab incision at the right lumbar region.
- *Closure of abdomen*: The surgical peritoneum and the linea alba is closed by running suture using No. 1 loop PDS suture.
  Skin is apposed by interrupted 2-0 monofilament polyamide sutures. The drain tube is fixed to the skin.

■ STEPS OF LOW ANTERIOR RESECTION

Q. Describe the steps of anterior resection (or low anterior resection).

Ans.

- *Anesthesia*: General anesthesia with endotracheal intubation.
- *Position of patient*: Growth in upper rectum if hand sewn anastomosis is contemplated patient should be in supine.

  For growth in midrectum or lower rectum, if the decision might change to abdominoperineal resection (APR) during operation or anastomosis is contemplated with a circular stapler patient should be in modified lithotomy position.
- *Incision*: A lower midline incision from just above the symphysis pubis to about 5 cm above the umbilicus. The skin subcutaneous tissue, linea alba and surgical peritoneum is incised in the same line.
- *Exploration of abdomen*:
  - Assessment for presence of ascites, any distant spread to liver, omentum, peritoneum and pelvis. Palpate for involvement of regional lymph nodes—pararectal lymph nodes and central lymph nodes (lymph nodes around the origin of inferior mesenteric artery).
  - Assessment of the local growth to decide about the resectability. Assess whether the growth has invaded the posterior or lateral pelvic wall and ureter.
- *Exteriorization of small gut*: The whole small gut is delivered outside and kept wrapped in moist towel taking care not to twist the mesentery.
- *Mobilization of sigmoid and descending colon*: The mobilization starts on the left side of the pelvic brim. The left leaf of mesosigmoid is incised close to the pelvic brim in an avascular area. This incision is taken upward toward the splenic flexure. The avascular plane between the mesosigmoid and the posterior pelvic wall is being entered by sharp dissection and the rectosigmoid junction along with superior rectal vessels are lifted up. The left ureter crossing the apex of the mesosigmoid is safeguarded during this dissection. The right leaf of the mesosigmoid is then incised going upward up to the bifurcation of aorta and going down up to the point in lateral pelvic wall where the mesosigmoid reaches the lateral pelvic wall peritoneum. During this dissection the right ureter is safeguarded.
- *Mobilization of splenic flexure and descending colon*: The lateral peritoneum along the line of Toldt is incised taking this incision upward up to the splenic flexure. The leinocolic and the renocolic ligaments are then divided and the splenic flexure brought down to ensure a tension-free colorectal anastomosis.

  Ligation of inferior mesenteric vessels and lymphatic dissection. The inferior mesenteric artery is dissected close to its origin at the aorta and the lymph nodes around are dissected toward the colon. The inferior mesenteric artery is dissected beyond the origin of the left colic artery, ligated and divided. The inferior mesenteric vein is dissected near the duodenojejunal flexure, ligated and divided close to the lower border of the pancreas and the lymphatic tissue around this is taken down with the colon.

  The lymphatic tissue around the bifurcation of the aorta and the common iliac vessels are taken down toward the specimen. The intervening mesentery is divided.

  Mobilization of the mesorectum and the rectum: This is the most important step in anterior resection.

- *Posterior or presacral dissection*: The mobilized sigmoid colon is drawn upward and forward which opens up the presacral space. The avascular areolar tissue which surrounds the mesorectum is identified and divided by sharp dissection. This dissection is initially carried downward in the midline along the curve of the sacrum up to the coccyx. Beyond this the dissection carried forward in front of the anococcygeal raphe dividing the Waldeyer's fascia. This dissection has to be done in proper plane preserving the presacral vessels and nerves.
- *Lateral dissection*: The dissection from the posterior midline is carried around the lateral wall of the mesorectum and sharp dissection is done along the lateral pelvic wall. The dissection is first done on the left side and the lateral ligament is put on stretch by retracting the rectum toward the right. A right angled forceps is used to dissect the lateral ligament and the right angled forceps is passed around the lateral ligament, which is divided by using diathermy. Sometimes the middle rectal vessels running along the lateral ligament needs ligature and division. With similar maneuver the right lateral ligament is divided. While dividing the lateral ligament the ureter and the hypogastric nerves are taken care of to prevent injury to these structures.
- *Anterior dissection*: The anterior dissection is different in male and female patients.
  - *In male patient*: The bladder is retracted anteriorly by a Lloyd–Davis retractor or a Deavers retractor and the peritoneum lining the rectovesical pouch is incised. This peritoneal incision is extended laterally to the lateral pelvic wall. The posterior leaf of the incised peritoneum along with the Denonvilliers' fascia is picked up with a long hemostatic forceps and retracted in an upward and posterior direction. By sharp dissection (using diathermy or a Metzenbaum scissor), the rectum along with the mesorectum is separated from the seminal vesicle and the prostate. Few bleeding vessels during this dissection may be controlled by diathermy.
  - *In female*: Then uterus is retracted anteriorly and the peritoneum of the rectouterine pouch (pouch of Douglas) is incised and the incision is carried on either side to the lateral pelvic wall. The posterior leaf of the incised peritoneum along with Denonvilliers' fascia is picked up by a long hemostatic forceps and retracted in a posterior and cephalad direction and the rectum along with mesorectum is separated from the cervix and the posterior vaginal wall, small bleeding during this dissection may be controlled by using diathermy.
- *Division of proximal colon*: (The extent of colonic resection for anterior resection is 7 cm proximal to the proximal margin of the growth. The distal margin for anterior resection is 5 cm from the distal margin of the growth. For low anterior resection this margin may be as low as 2 cm. In ultralow anterior resection even a 1 cm distal margin is acceptable).
  At the point of proposed resection of proximal colon, the marginal artery is dissected, ligated and divided. Two pairs of intestinal occlusion clamps are applied at the site of proposed resection of colon and the proximal colon is divided by cutting diathermy in-between the intestinal occlusion clamps.
- *Division of rectum*: At the point of proposed rectal resection, the superior rectal artery is dissected and ligated close to the rectal wall. A C-shaped occlusion clamp is applied around the rectum distally and an intestinal occlusion clamp is applied proximally and the rectum is divided in-between using cutting diathermy. The specimen is removed.
- Colorectal anastomosis

- *Hand-sewn anastomosis*: A single layer colorectal anastomosis is done with interrupted suture using 4-0 polydioxanone or Mersilk suture either by full thickness suture or extramucosal suture.
- *Stapler anastomosis*: In low or ultralow anterior resection a stapler anastomosis is preferable. This is done by using a circular stapler. The rectal stump is closed by applying a purse string suture using 1-0 polypropylene suture. The anvil of the circular stapler is passed into the proximal cut end of the colon and the end of colon closed around the anvil by a purse string suture. The handle of the circular stapler is passed through the anal canal and delivered through the rectal stump by a sharp puncture. The anvil is fitted into the handle of the circular stapler. The stapler knob is gradually closed whereby the colonic end is brought closer to the rectal stump. Once the indicator in the stapler shows that is in the firing range. The stapler is unlocked and fired. This will create colorectal anastomosis. Once the anastomosis is done the stapler is opened up by turning the knob one and half turn and the stapler is delivered out through the anal canal.
- *Checking the donuts*: The anvil is opened up and the donut is examined. Two complete donut indicates that a proper anastomosis has been done.
- *Testing the anastomosis*: An intestinal occlusion clamp is applied to the colon proximal to the anastomosis. Pour normal saline into the pelvis so that the site of anastomosis remains under the saline. Using a 50 mL syringe air is pushed into the rectum through the anal canal. Look for any air bubble escaping through the anastomosis. In perfect anastomosis there should be no leakage of air through the anastomosis.
- *Proximal diversion colostomy or ileostomy*: When there is any doubt regarding the colorectal anastomosis, a proximal diversion transverse colostomy or ileostomy is preferable to safeguard the anastomosis.
- *Placement of drain*: Hemostasis is checked and a tube drain is placed inside the pelvis.
- *Closure of abdomen*: The surgical peritoneum and linea alba in single layer using No. 1 loop PDS. Skin closed with interrupted suture using monofilament polyamide sutures.

■ STEPS OF ABDOMINOPERINEAL RESECTION

Q. Describe the steps of abdominoperineal resection.

Ans.

- *Anesthesia*: General anesthesia with endotracheal intubation.
- *Position of patient*: Patient is placed in a modified lithotomy Trendelenburg position. The operating surgeon stands on the left side of the patient. Operation is simultaneously done by two teams of surgeons.
- Antiseptic cleaning and draping of both abdomen and perineal area with povidone-iodine and draping done to expose the abdomen and perianal area.
- *Incision*: A midline incision is made starting just above the symphysis taking the incision up to the right of umbilicus to about 5 cm above the umbilicus. The subcutaneous tissue, linea alba and the surgical peritoneum is incised in the same line.
- *Exploration of abdomen*: A self-retaining retractor is applied for better exposure. General exploration of abdomen to assess for any ascites, omentum, peritoneal surface, pelvis, and liver for any metastasis. Assess the regional lymph nodes for any enlargements. Palpate the rest of the large gut for any evidence of synchronous growth.

Assess the rectal growth for deciding about resectability. If the tumor is fixed to the prostate, seminal vesicle or the growth is fixed to the sacrum posteriorly, it is not wise to proceed with resection.

- *Mobilization of sigmoid colon*: The sigmoid colon is lifted up and toward the right. The left leaf of the mesosigmoid is incised at its apex and the incision is carried upward up to the sigmoid colon and descending colon junction and carried distally up to the base of the bladder in male (in female up to the lateral margin of posterior vaginal wall). During this dissection, the left ureter crossing the sigmoid mesocolon is taken care of. The sigmoid colon is lifted up from the posterior pelvic wall by sharp dissection. The sigmoid colon is then retracted up and toward the left and the right leaf of the mesosigmoid is incised. This incision is carried-up up to the bifurcation of the aorta and carried below around the lateral pelvic wall up to the base of the bladder in male (in female up to the lateral margin of posterior vaginal wall).While doing so the right ureter is taken care of. The peritoneal incision is joined anteriorly across the base of the bladder in male and in female around the posterior vaginal wall.

- *Ligation of inferior mesenteric vessels and lymphatic dissection*: The inferior mesenteric artery is dissected close to its origin at the aorta and the lymph nodes around are dissected toward the colon. The inferior mesenteric artery is dissected beyond the origin of the left colic artery, ligated and divided. The inferior mesenteric vein is dissected near the duodenojejunal flexure, ligated and divided close to the lower border of the pancreas.

  The lymphatic tissue around the origin of inferior mesenteric artery and lymph nodes around the bifurcation of the aorta and the common iliac vessels are taken down toward the specimen. The intervening mesentery is divided.

  – *Mobilization of the mesorectum and the rectum*: This is the most important step in APR.

  – *Posterior or presacral dissection*: The mobilized sigmoid colon is drawn upward and forward which opens up the presacral space. The avascular areolar tissue which surrounds the mesorectum is identified and divided by sharp dissection. This dissection is initially carried downward in the midline along the curve of the sacrum up to the coccyx. Beyond this, the dissection carried forward in front of the anococcygeal raphe dividing the Waldeyer's fascia. This dissection has to be done in proper plane preserving the presacral vessels and nerves.

  – *Lateral dissection*: The dissection from the posterior midline is carried around the lateral wall of the mesorectum and sharp dissection is done along the lateral pelvic wall. The dissection is first done on the left side and the lateral ligament is put on stretch by retracting the rectum toward the right. A right angled forceps is used to dissect the lateral ligament and the right angled forceps is passed around the lateral ligament which is divided by using diathermy. Sometimes the middle rectal vessels running along the lateral ligament needs ligature and division. With similar maneuver the right lateral ligament is divided. While dividing the lateral ligament the ureter and the hypogastric nerves are taken care of to prevent injury to these structures.

  – *Anterior dissection*: The anterior dissection is different in male and female patients.

    - *In male patient*: The bladder is retracted anteriorly by a Lloyd–Davis retractor or a Deavers retractor and the peritoneum lining the rectovesical pouch is incised. This peritoneal incision is extended laterally to the lateral pelvic wall. The posterior leaf of the incised peritoneum along with the Denonvilliers' fascia is picked up a long hemostatic forceps and retracted in an upward and posterior direction. By sharp dissection (using diathermy or a Metzenbaum scissor), the rectum along with the mesorectum is separated from the seminal vesicle and the prostate. Few bleeding vessels during this dissection may be controlled by diathermy.

- *In female*: Then uterus is retracted anteriorly and the peritoneum of the rectouterine pouch (pouch of Douglas) is incised and the incision is carried on either side to the lateral pelvic wall. The posterior leaf of the incised peritoneum along with Denonvilliers' fascia is picked up by a long hemostatic forceps and retracted in a posterior and cephalad direction and the rectum along with mesorectum is separated from the cervix and the posterior vaginal wall. Small bleeding during this dissection may be controlled by using diathermy.

♦ *Division of sigmoid colon*: The point of division of sigmoid colon is 7 cm proximal to the proximal margin of the growth. Adequate length of sigmoid (about 5 cm) is required to create an end sigmoid colostomy. At the proposed site of sigmoid transection, the marginal artery is dissected, ligated and divided. Two pairs of intestinal occlusion clamps are applied and the sigmoid colon divided in-between using cutting diathermy.

♦ *Perineal dissection*: The perineal dissection ideally starts when the abdominal surgeon has decided about the resectability of the tumor and the abdominal and perineal dissection should proceed simultaneously.

A purse string suture is applied around the anal orifice.

♦ *Perineal incision*: An elliptical incision is made around the anal orifice and the incision is extended anteriorly 3–4 cm from the anal verge and posteriorly the incision is extended up to the tip of the coccyx.

♦ *Lateral dissection*: The medial leaf of the incised skin margin is lifted up and medially by using a pair of Allis tissue forceps and the lateral skin leaf is retracted laterally by using a skin hook. The incision is deepened into the perirectal fat up to the pelvic diaphragm (levator ani). The anterior and posterior branches of inferior hemorrhoidal vessels which run in the ischiorectal fossa below the levator ani are coagulated and divided. This dissection is done on either side.

♦ *Posterior dissection*: The posterior leaf of the skin margin is lifted up posteriorly and the incision is deepened down. The anococcygeal ligament is divided using diathermy. A dense layer of fascia (Waldeyer's fascia attaches the posterior rectum and mesorectum to the presacral and precoccygeal area. The anal canal is lifted and the Waldeyer's fascia is divided using electrocautery and this dissection is continued upward in the presacral space till the perineal surgeon reaches the area reached by the abdominal surgeon.

♦ *Division of levator ani*: The index finger is inserted through the presacral area and the finger is swept across the superior aspect of the levator ani muscle on each side of the pelvis and levator ani muscle is divided on either side of the lateral pelvic wall. The puborectalis muscle is also divided.

♦ *Anterior dissection*: The anterior incision is deepened along a plane at the posterior border of deep transverse perineal muscle. The rectourethralis muscle is divided.

- *In male*: The attachment of anterior mesorectum to the prostate and seminal vesicle has already been divided by the abdominal surgeon. The remaining attachment of the anterior mesorectum to the neck of the prostate is dissected from the perineal side. Once the mesorectum is dissected all around the specimen is now free to be removed from the perineal side.

- *In female*: The attachment of the anterior mesorectum to the posterior vaginal wall is divided till the area reached by the abdominal surgeon is met. Once the mesorectum is dissected all around the specimen is removed from the perineal side.

- *Closure of the perineal incision*: The perineal wound is irrigated. A suction drainage tube is placed in the perineal wound which is brought out through the posterior aspect of the perineal wound. The muscles of the pelvic floor do not require to be sutured in the midline. The ischiorectal fat pad and subcutaneous tissue of the pelvis is apposed with 2-0 polyglactin sutures.

  Skin is apposed with interrupted 2-0 monofilament polyamide suture. The skin may also be apposed by subcuticular suture (if there is gross contamination, the perineal wound may be kept open by placement of a gauze pack).

- *Construction of end sigmoid colostomy*: The ideal site of colostomy should be marked before the operation starts. The colostomy should be located in left lower quadrant of the abdomen. The colostomy should be placed at the junction of medial one-third and lateral two-thirds junction of left spinoumbilical line. At the site of proposed colostomy, the skin is picked up by a pair of Allis tissue forceps and a circle of skin is excised appropriate to the diameter of colon. The subcutaneous tissue is incised.

- A cruciate incision is made over the anterior rectus sheath. The rectum abdominis muscle is split by using a straight hemostatic forceps.

- The posterior rectus sheath is picked up by two pairs of hemostatic forceps and the posterior rectus sheath along with peritoneum is incised.

- The cut end of the sigmoid colon is brought out through this wound by using a Babcock's tissue forceps, taking care so that there is no rotation of the end of the sigmoid colon. The colon is fixed to the anterior rectus sheath using interrupted 2-0 polyglactin sutures. The colostomy is constructed by taking interrupted suture with 3-0 polyglactin suture, taking all coats of the sigmoid colon and the subcutaneous tissue.

- *Closure of lateral space*: The lateral space between the exteriorized sigmoid colon is obliterated by taking few interrupted suture between the seromuscular coat of the sigmoid colon and the posterior parietal peritoneum. This prevents development of internal herniation in postoperative period.

- *Abdominal closure*: The pelvic cavity is irrigated with normal saline. The pelvic peritoneum is apposed by suturing with 2-0 polyglactin sutures.

  The surgical peritoneum and linea alba are apposed by suturing with No. 1 polypropylene or No. 1 PDS suture. The skin is apposed with interrupted monofilament polyamide sutures.

■ STEPS OF TRANSVERSE COLOSTOMY

Q. Describe the steps of transverse colostomy.

Ans.

- Indications of transverse colostomy:
  - To relieve left colonic obstruction
  - For fecal diversion to safeguard against leakage following low anterior resection or left colonic anastomosis
  - Fecal diversion in patient with rectovaginal fistula or Hirschsprung's disease.

- *Anesthesia*: General anesthesia. It may also be done under regional or local anesthesia.
- *Position of patient*: Supine.
- Antiseptic cleaning and draping.
- *Skin incision*: The site of the colostomy should be planned well before the operation. The ideal site of right transverse colostomy is at the right upper quadrant of the abdomen at a point midway between the right subcostal margin and the umbilicus over the rectus abdominis muscle.

  A transverse incision is made at a point midway between the right costal margin and the umbilicus. The incision extends medially 2 cm to the right of midline and laterally extending just beyond the lateral border of the rectus sheath. The subcutaneous tissue is incised in the same line.
- *Incising the anterior and posterior rectus sheath and the peritoneum*: A cruciate incision is made over the anterior rectus sheath. The rectus abdominis muscle is exposed. The rectus abdominis muscle is split by inserting a Kelly hemostatic forceps and the posterior rectus sheath is exposed. The posterior rectus is lifted up by two pairs of hemostatic forceps and incised in-between. The peritoneal opening is stretched by inserting two fingers.
- *Delivery of the transverse colon*: The transverse colon is identified by looking at taenia coli, haustration and attachment of the greater omentum and transverse mesocolon. The greater omentum attached to the transverse colon is divided close to the colon for about 6–7 cm and the transverse mesocolon is identified. The antimesenteric border of the transverse colon is held up by a pair of Babcock forceps and delivered out in the wound. The loop of colon should remain out of the wound without any tension.
- *Insertion of a colostomy device through the transverse mesocolon*: The transverse colon is pulled up and a rent is made in the transverse mesocolon in an avascular area close to the mesenteric border of the colon and a plastic colostomy device is passed through the rent to keep the colon in place so that it does not retract.
- *Fixation of the colon*: The projecting colon is fixed to the anterior rectus sheath by few interrupted suture using 2-0 polyglactin sutures.
- *Construction of colostomy*: A 5-cm long incision is made in the colon along the taenia coli. The edges of the colon are turned back and the cut margin of the colon is sutured to the subcutaneous tissue by interrupted 3-0 polyglactin sutures.

  A colostomy bag may be applied to the skin around the colostomy so that the opening in the bag snugly fits around the opened up colon.
  - *Skin closure*: The remaining skin incision site is apposed by interrupted monofilament polyamide suture.

◼ STEPS OF CLOSURE OF COLOSTOMY

Q. Describe the steps of closure of colostomy.

Ans. Before closure of colostomy the primary cause has to be treated.

The distal colon should be assessed by either colonoscopy or radiographic examination with barium (distal cologram) to assess patency of the distal colon up to the rectum.
- *Anesthesia*: Regional anesthesia.
- Antiseptic cleaning and draping.

◆ *Mobilization of the colostomy*: 6–8 interrupted 3-0 Mersilk sutures are inserted around the mucocutaneous junction of colostomy. These sutures are kept long and held up by a number of hemostatic forceps for traction. An incision is made around the edge of the colostomy taking about 2 mm fringe of skin around the colostomy. If required, the incision may be extended on either side in a transverse plane.

Traction is applied in the sutures already placed around the colostomy, and the colon is dissected all around up to the rectus sheath. The dissection is done further up to the peritoneum and the peritoneum is opened all round and the colon is mobilized well.

◆ *Freshening the margin of colostomy*: The fringe of skin around the colostomy is excised up to the margin of mucosa and the mucosa of the colon is freed all around.

◆ *Closure of colon*: The incision in the colon is closed with interrupted sutures taking all coats with 3-0 PDS. The apposition may also be done with interrupted sutures taking the seromuscular coats (extramucosal stitch).

◆ *Closure of abdominal wound*: Single layer closure of posterior and anterior rectus sheath with running No. 1 PDS suture.

Skin apposed with interrupted monofilament polyamide sutures.

■ STEP OF APPENDICECTOMY

Q. Describe the steps of appendicectomy.

Ans.

◆ General anesthesia with endotracheal intubation (appendicectomy may also be done under regional anesthesia—spinal or epidural).

◆ Position of the patient: Supine.

◆ Antiseptic cleaning and draping.

◆ *Incision*: McBurneys' Gridiron incision. An oblique skin incision of about 3 inches (1 inch above and 2 inches below the spinoumbilical line) is made at right angle to the right spinoumbilical line passing through the McBurneys' point (Fig. 22.9A). The skin and subcutaneous tissues are incised in the same line.

◆ *Division of external oblique aponeurosis*: A nick is made in the external oblique aponeurosis and the external oblique aponeurosis is incised along the direction of its fibers (Fig. 22.9B).

◆ *Splitting internal oblique and transversus abdominis muscle*: The internal oblique muscle is exposed and deep to it lies the transversus abdominis muscle. A Mayo's scissor is thrushed with the blades closed through the internal oblique and the transversus abdominis muscle and the blades are opened up to split both these muscles along the direction of their fibers (Fig. 22.9C).

◆ *Incising the peritoneum*: Two Langenbachs' retractors are inserted deep to these muscles and the peritoneum is exposed. The peritoneum is lifted by two pairs of hemostatic forceps and a nick is made in the peritoneum and the peritoneal incision is then extended along the line of skin incision (Fig. 22.9D).

◆ *Identifying the cecum*: As soon as peritoneum is opened turbid or clear fluid may escape from the peritoneal cavity (this fluid may be due to peritoneal reaction to local inflammation). The cecum is identified by its pale color, presence of taenia coli and absence of mesentery.

◆ *Delivering the cecum and the appendix*: The cecum is delivered into the wound by holding it with a plain dissecting forceps. The cecum is grasped with a moist sponge and is delivered

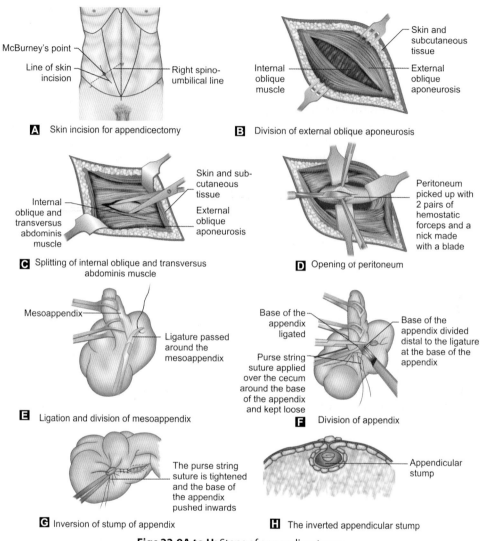

McBurney's point
Line of skin incision
Right spino-umbilical line

A   Skin incision for appendicectomy

Skin and subcutaneous tissue
Internal oblique muscle
External oblique aponeurosis

B   Division of external oblique aponeurosis

Internal oblique and transversus abdominis muscle
Skin and sub-cutaneous tissue
External oblique aponeurosis

C   Splitting of internal oblique and transversus abdominis muscle

Peritoneum picked up with 2 pairs of hemostatic forceps and a nick made with a blade

D   Opening of peritoneum

Mesoappendix
Ligature passed around the mesoappendix

E   Ligation and division of mesoappendix

Base of the appendix ligated
Purse string suture applied over the cecum around the base of the appendix and kept loose
Base of the appendix divided distal to the ligature at the base of the appendix

F   Division of appendix

The purse string suture is tightened and the base of the appendix pushed inwards

G   Inversion of stump of appendix

Appendicular stump

H   The inverted appendicular stump

Figs 22.9A to H: Steps of appendicectomy

into the wound further when the appendix will come into view. If appendix is not visible, follow the anterior taenia coli in the cecum which will guide into the base of the appendix.

♦ *Division of the mesoappendix*: The appendix is held by Babcock's tissue forceps—one applied near the tip, one applied at the body of the appendix and another Babcock's tissue forceps applied at the base of the appendix. The mesoappendix is clamped with one or more pair of hemostatic forceps and divided and ligated. Alternatively, a mosquito hemostatic forceps is thrushed through an avascular area in the mesoappendix near its base and a ligature passed around the mesoappendix and ligated. The mesoappendix attached toward the appendix is then divided (Fig. 22.9E).

♦ *Division of the base of appendix*: The base of the appendix is crushed by applying a hemostatic forceps. A ligature of 1-0 chromic catgut is then passed around the base of the appendix at the crushed area and the base of the appendix is ligated. A hemostatic forceps is applied at the appendix about 5 mm distal to the site of ligature at the base of appendix. The appendix is divided with a knife close to the forceps and the stump of the appendix is swabbed with povidone-iodine lotion (Fig. 22.9F).

The appendix, swab, knife with the hemostatic forceps which are contaminated are kept in a bowl and removed from the operation field.

* *Burying the base of appendix*: Most surgeons do not invert the base of appendix routinely. If the stump of the appendix is to be inverted, a purse string suture is applied on the cecal wall around the base of the appendix. The stump of the appendix is held by a dissecting forceps and the purse string suture is tightened and the stump of the appendix is inverted as the purse string suture is tied (Figs 22.9G and H).
* *Check for hemostasis*: The mesoappendix stump is checked for bleeding.
* *Look for Meckel's diverticulum*: Bring out the terminal ileum and look up to two feet from the ileocecal junction to exclude any associated Meckel's diverticulum.
* *Closure*: The wound is closed in layer.

Q. What is retrograde appendicectomy?

Ans. When the appendix is retrocecal, the tip may not be accessible easily. If the base is easily accessible a retrograde appendicectomy is preferred in such situation.

The base of the appendix is dissected by passing a hemostatic forceps through the mesoappendix. The base of the appendix is crushed by a hemostatic forceps applied around the base of the appendix. The crushed base of the appendix is then ligated with 1-0 chromic catgut sutures. A hemostatic forceps is applied 5 mm distal to the ligature at the base of the appendix and the appendix is divided in-between. The mesoappendix is then held between the hemostatic forceps and divided and ligated from the base up to the tip. Once whole of the mesoappendix is ligated the appendix becomes free and is removed.

Q. When you should not crush the base of appendix during appendicectomy?

Ans.
* If the appendix is gangrenous.
* If there is perforation at the base of the appendix.
* If the base of appendix and the cecum is edematous.

Q. How many ports are required for laparoscopic appendicectomy?

Ans. Three ports are required:
* Infraumbilical 10 mm port—for telescope and the camera.
* One 5 mm port in the right iliac fossa.
* One 10/5 mm port in left iliac fossa or suprapubic area.

■ SPLENECTOMY

Q. What are the indications of splenectomy?

Ans.
* *Splenic trauma*: Severe degree of splenic injury requires splenectomy. Mild splenic trauma may be managed with splenic conserving surgery.

- Chronic hemolytic diseases like hereditary spherocytosis, thalassemia, and sickle cell anemia.
- Idiopathic thrombocytopenic purpura.
- Hypersplenism causing pancytopenia due to portal hypertension, lymphomatous infiltration or in leukemias.
- Splenic cysts, splenic abscess or tumors.
- Incidental splenectomy in association with radical gastrectomy or shunt surgery for portal hypertension.

Steps of splenectomy:

- *Anesthesia*: General anesthesia with endotracheal intubation.
- *Position of the patient*: Supine with a sand bag placed under the left side of the chest.
- *Incision*: Approach is either by a long midline or left subcostal incision (see abdominal incision).
- *Exploration*: The spleen is examined. The liver, gallbladder and the bile duct are examined.
    In hemolytic anemias there may be stones in the gallbladder or in the common bile duct. Thorough exploration of the abdomen is to be done for presence of any splenunculi or lymphadenopathy.
- *Mobilization of the spleen*: The left hand is passed between the spleen and the diaphragm and the spleen is drawn toward the abdominal incision. This maneuver brings the lienorenal ligament in view. The posterior leaf of the lienorenal ligament is incised with the scissors and the spleen is mobilized and delivered into the abdominal wound.
- *Division of splenic vessels*: As the spleen is mobilized into the wound, the posterior surface of the hilum of the spleen is dissected. The splenic vein and artery come into view. The splenic artery is seen running along the upper border of the pancreas. The splenic artery is dissected using a right angle forceps and three ligatures of No. 1 silk are passed around the artery and are ligated. The splenic artery is divided in-between the ligatures keeping two ligatures toward the proximal side. The splenic vein is dissected carefully taking care not to injure the pancreatic tail. Three ligatures are passed around the splenic vein and the ligatures are tied. The splenic vein is divided keeping two ligatures toward the portal vein side.
- *Division of short gastric vessels*: The short gastric vessels run in the gastrosplenic ligament.
    The gastrosplenic ligament is divided in-between series of hemostatic forceps and ligated with No. 1-0 silk.
- *Division of anterior leaf of lienorenal ligament*: Once the gastrosplenic ligament, splenic vessels are divided and the pancreatic tail is dissected from the splenic hilum, the anterior leaf of the lienorenal ligament is exposed. This is usually avascular and may be divided with the scissors.
    The spleen is now free to be removed.
- *Placement of drain and closure*: A suction drain is kept in the splenic bed and the abdomen is closed in layers.

Postoperative management:

- Intravenous fluid to maintain hydration. IV fluid is continued till bowel sounds return. This usually takes about 48–72 hours.
- Nasogastric aspiration.
- Prophylactic antibiotics.
- Vaccination against pneumococcal and *Haemophilus influenzae* infection.

◼ NEPHRECTOMY

Q. What are the indications of nephrectomy?

Ans.

- Carcinoma of kidney
- Severe renal injury with avulsion of renal pedicle
- Hydronephrosis with nonfunctional kidney
- Renal calculus with gross destruction of kidney
- Chronic pyelonephritis
- Pyonephrosis of kidney
- Donor nephrectomy for transplantation.

Nephrectomy through a loin incision:

- *Anesthesia*: General anesthesia with endotracheal intubation.
- *Position of the patient*: For approach to the right kidney, patient lies in left lateral position.
  The upper arm is supported on an arm rest and is used for venous cannulation and blood pressure measurements. The left lower limb is kept flexed at the hip and knee to 90° and the right lower limb is kept extended supported on a pillow kept between the two legs. The area between the right costal margin and the iliac crest is opened by lifting the kidney bridge and breaking off the table toward the leg end. The position is maintained by a leather strap or a broad band of adhesive strap fixing the iliac crest and the greater trochanter to the operation table. The right shoulder is also anchored to the operation table by adhesive strap.
- Antiseptic dressing and draping
- *Skin incision*: The skin incision starts from the angle between the 12th rib and the lateral border of the erector spinae muscles and passes downward and forward about 1 cm below the 12th rib to a point about 2 cm above and anterior to the anterior superior iliac spine up to the lateral border of the rectus sheath.
  The subcutaneous tissue is incised in the same line.
- *Division of superficial muscles*: In the posterior part of the wound, the latissimus dorsi muscle is incised. In the anterior part of the wound, the external oblique muscle and the aponeurosis is incised.
  In the posterior part of the wound once the latissimus dorsi is incised the serratus posterior inferior muscle is exposed. The serratus posterior inferior muscle is also incised. At the anterior part of the incision, the internal oblique muscle and aponeurosis is incised in the same line.
- *Division of thoracolumbar fascia*: An incision is made in the thoracolumbar fascia taking care not to injure the subcostal nerve. The incision is carried backward up to the lateral border of the erector spinae muscle. Using a Gallies swab, with blunt dissection the parietal peritoneum is stripped off from the transversus abdominis muscle.
  The transversus abdominis muscle is divided by carrying forward the incision in the thoracolumbar fascia. Hemostasis is secured.
- *Exposure of perinephric space*: The cut margins of the thoracolumbar fascia are retracted and the parietal peritoneum is further stripped off medially and the perinephric space is exposed.
- *Incision of perirenal fascia*: The perirenal fascia (fascia of Gerota) is lifted at the lateral aspect with two pairs of hemostatic forceps and incised with a knife in-between the hemostatic forceps. The incision in the perirenal fascia is then extended with a scissors.

- *Exposure of the kidney*: Once the perirenal fascia is incised the pale yellow perinephric fat is exposed and deep to this fat lies the kidney.
- *Mobilization of kidney*: By blunt finger dissection, the kidney is mobilized. The lower pole, posterior surface and the anterior surface of the kidney are mobilized. There may be an accessory artery and vein at the lower pole while mobilizing. These vessels should be clamped and divided.
- *Division of the ureter*: The upper ureter is identified, dissected and divided in-between clamps and the cut ends are ligated. The proximal ureter is followed up to the hilum.
- *Division of the renal vessels*: The renal artery lies posterior to the renal vein and approach from the posterior aspect will allow better tackling of the artery. The artery should be ligated before the vein to avoid congestion of blood in the kidney. A right angle forceps is used to dissect and pass ligatures around the artery. Three ligatures are passed and the vessel is triply ligated. The renal artery is divided keeping two ligatures toward the proximal side.
  The renal vein is similarly dissected, triply ligated and divided keeping two ligatures toward the inferior vena cava side.
- *Mobilization of the upper pole of the kidney*: After the renal vessels are ligated and divided, the upper pole is mobilized separating the adrenal from the upper pole of the kidney by blunt dissection taking care to avoid injury to the adrenal gland.
- *Check for hemostasis*: After the kidney is removed, the renal fossa is exposed well and inspected carefully to look for any bleeding which may be controlled with diathermy or ligature. A tube drain is kept in the renal fossa.
- *Closure of the incision*:
  - *Closure is done in layers*:
    - Transversus abdominis muscle with running 0 chromic catgut or Vicryl sutures
    - Internal oblique and serratus posterior inferior with running 0 chromic catgut or Vicryl sutures
    - External oblique and latissimus dorsi with running 0 chromic catgut or Vicryl sutures
    - Skin closed with interrupted monofilament polyamide sutures.

■ STEPS OF MODIFIED RADICAL MASTECTOMY

Q. Describe the steps of modified radical mastectomy (Patey).

Ans.
- General anesthesia with endotracheal intubation.
- Patient is placed supine with the arm on the operated side supported on an arm table.
- Antiseptic cleansing and draping.
- The position of the lump is delineated.
- *Skill incision (Fig. 22.10A)*: A transverse elliptical skin incision is made encircling the nipple and areola and encompassing 5 cm of skin margin around the mass.
- *Raising of skin flaps (Figs 22.10B and C)*: The skin flaps are raised by sharp dissection with scalpel or scissor in the plane between the subcutaneous fat and the mammary fat. The upper skin flap is raised up to the clavicle and the lower skin flap is raised up to the upper quadrant of the rectus sheath. The bleeding points are coagulated with diathermy taking care to avoid burn of the skin.
- *Raising the breast (Fig. 22.10D)*: The uppermost part of the breast is dissected off from the fascia covering the pectoralis major. A cleavage is created between the breast tissue and the

fascia covering the pectoralis major and the whole breast is lifted off from the pectoralis major fascia. The perforating vessels on the medial side are controlled with diathermy or are ligated. The breast is lifted above from the level of the clavicle, below up to the upper quadrant of the rectus sheath, medially up to the midline and laterally up to latissimus dorsi. The breast is allowed to hang laterally keeping the axillary tail of the breast in continuity with the axillary lymph nodes.

◆ *Axillary dissection (Fig. 22.10E)*: The lateral border of the pectoralis major is cleared of the loose areolar tissue and all the loose areolar tissue and level I lymph nodes in the axilla are cleared taking care not to injure the axillary vessels and the nerves. The pectoralis minor muscle is dissected and it is divided from its insertion into the coracoid process. The level II and III lymph nodes are then dissected off from the axilla. The lateral dissection is carried up to the anterior border of the latissimus dorsi. The clearance of the lymphatics and the loose areolar tissue is kept confined to the anterior and inferior aspect of the axillary vein and no attempt is made to clear the structures above the vein. The structures so separated are dissected away from the chest wall by dissection using a peanut swab. The nerve to serratus anterior is identified along the lateral chest wall and preserved. Nerves to latissimus dorsi is identified running along the subscapular vessels and preserved. The intercostobrachial nerve is dissected and preserved.

Hemostasis is secured.

◆ *Closure (Fig. 22.10F)*: A suction drain is inserted—one tube kept in the axilla and another tube kept underneath the breast flap. The skin incision may be closed with a subcuticular sutures or interrupted silk or nylon sutures. After skin closure the vacuum drain is activated and fluid is squeezed out from beneath the skin flaps and the skin flaps adheres to the chest wall.

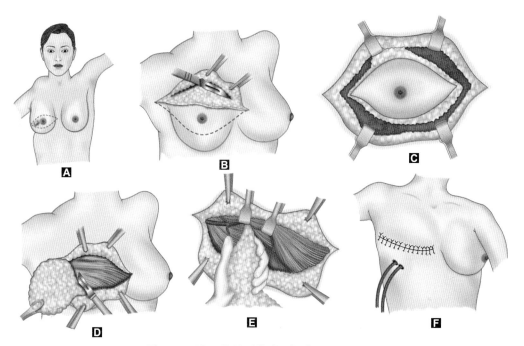

Figs 22.10A to F: Modified radical mastectomy

Q. What structures are to be preserved during modified radical mastectomy?

Ans.

+ Long thoracic nerve (supplies serratus anterior).
+ Thoracodorsal nerve (supplies latissimus dorsi).
+ Cephalic vein.
+ Axillary vein.

■ STEPS OF LUMBAR SYMPATHECTOMY

Q. Describe the steps of lumbar sympathectomy.

Ans.

+ *Anesthesia*: General anesthesia with endotracheal intubation.
+ *Position of patient*: Supine with slight tilting by placing a pillow behind the loin on the side of operation.
+ Antiseptic dressing and draping.
+ *Incision*: An oblique lumbar incision starting from the lateral border of the erector spinae and then extended medially up to the lateral border of the rectus abdominis. The skin and the subcutaneous tissues are incised in the same line.
+ *Division of abdominal flat muscles and aponeurosis*: The external oblique muscle and aponeurosis are incised in the same line as skin incision.
  The internal oblique and the transversus abdominis muscles are cut in the same line.
+ *Stripping of the peritoneum*: Once the flat muscles are divided, the extraperitoneal fatty tissue and the peritoneum are exposed. This layer is stripped off medially by dissecting with a swab taking care not to open the peritoneum. If the peritoneum is opened inadvertently, it should be sutured with 1-0 chromic catgut sutures.
+ *Identification of the sympathetic chain*: The sympathetic chain is situated in the lateral side of the body of the lumbar vertebrae medial to the medial margin of the psoas muscle. On the right side, this is overlapped by the inferior vena cava and on the left side this is overlapped by aorta.
  The sympathetic chain is identified by the presence of ganglia and the rami communicantes passing from the ganglia. The first lumbar ganglion is situated high up under cover of the crus of the diaphragm and contains both *gray* and *white rami* communicantes. The *white rami* communicans carries the preganglionic fibers and the *gray rami* communicantes carries the postganglionic fibers.
  For complete sympathetic denervation of the lower limb the lst, 2nd, 3rd, and 4th lumbar ganglia are to be removed. If bilateral sympathectomy is contemplated, the 1st lumbar ganglion on one side is to be preserved. Bilateral division of 1st lumbar ganglion will result in sterility due to paralysis of the ejaculatory mechanism.
+ *Dissection of the sympathetic chain*: The first lumbar ganglion is identified and dissected by using a right angled forceps and divided in-between ligatures. The sympathetic trunk is then dissected downward up to the 4th lumbar ganglia lying behind the common iliac vessels and divided in-between ligatures at this point. While dissecting the sympathetic chain some lumbar vessels might need ligature and division.
+ Closure of incision in layers.

STEPS OF TOTAL THYROIDECTOMY

Q. Describe the steps of total thyroidectomy.

Ans.

- *Anesthesia*: General anesthesia with endotracheal intubation.
- *Position of patient*: Patient is supine, neck extended by placing a pillow in-between the shoulder blades and head resting on a ring.
- *Dressing and draping*: Povidone-iodine painting done from the level of the chin to the upper chest. Three towel draping done for the head and operative area isolated by further placement of draping.
- *Incision*: The approach is through a cervical collar incision made 2 cm above the suprasternal notch extending from posterior border of one sternocleidomastoid to the posterior border of opposite sternocleidomastoid. The skin incision is marked by pressing with a thread on the skin (Garrotte mark). The collar incision is made, the skin, superficial fascia, and platysma are cut. The platysma is incised at a little higher level than the skin (Fig. 22.11A).
- *Raising the skin flaps*: The upper skin flap, superficial fascia and the platysma are dissected and the upper flap is raised up to the upper border of the thyroid cartilage. The lower flap of skin, superficial fascia and the platysma are raised up to the suprasternal notch (Fig. 22.11B).
- *Incision of deep cervical fascia*: The investing layer of the deep cervical fascia is incised in the midline. If the anterior jugular veins come on the way, these may be ligated and divided (Fig. 22.11C).
- *Raising the fascial and strap muscles flap*: The investing layer of the deep cervical fascia along with the strap muscles are lifted up from the thyroid gland to expose the lateral lobes of the gland covered by the pretracheal fascia (Fig. 22.11D). The pretracheal fascia is incised and the finger passed around the plane between the pretracheal fascia and the thyroid gland. If the enlarged lobes are large, the strap muscles may be divided at an upper level as the nerves enters the strap muscles from below.
- *Division of the middle thyroid vein*: The thyroid lobe is mobilized medially and the middle thyroid vein is identified passing from the middle of the lateral lobe to the internal jugular vein (IJV). The middle thyroid vein is dissected and divided in between ligatures (Fig. 22.11E).
- *Division of superior thyroid vessels*: The muscles are retracted upward and laterally and the superior pole of lateral lobe of thyroid is exposed. The superior thyroid vessels are dissected close to the upper pole of the lobe. The superior thyroid artery and vein should be ligated separately. Three ligatures are passed around the superior thyroid artery, ligated and divided keeping two ligatures toward the proximal side. The superior thyroid vein is ligated and divided similarly. Care should be taken to avoid damage to external laryngeal nerve (Fig. 22.11F).
- *Division of inferior thyroid artery*: The gland is retracted medially and the branches of the inferior thyroid artery are identified entering the lower pole of the thyroid lobe. At this stage the recurrent laryngeal nerve is identified running vertically up along the tracheoesophageal groove. The parathyroid glands are identified and preserved. The individual branches of the inferior thyroid artery are identified and divided in between ligatures (Fig. 22.11G).
- *Division of inferior thyroid veins*: The inferior thyroid veins emerge from the lower pole of the lateral lobe. These veins are dissected and divided in between ligatures.

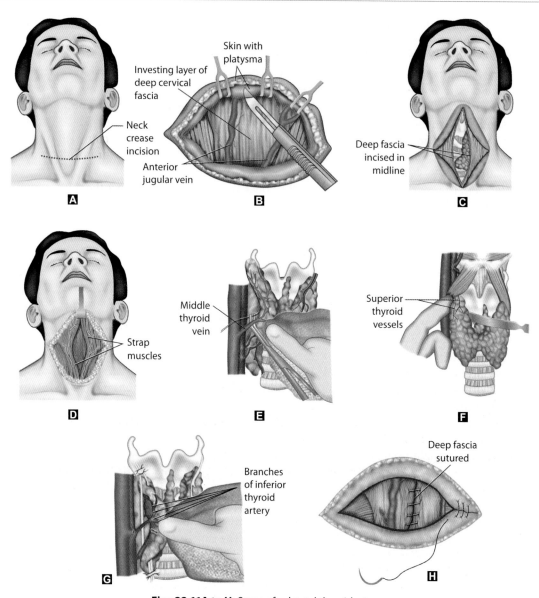

Figs 22.11A to H: Steps of subtotal thyroidectomy

The dissection on the other side now divides the middle thyroid vein, superior thyroid vessels, inferior thyroid artery branches and the inferior thyroid veins in the same way as done above.

* *Dissection of the thyroid isthmus*: The thyroid isthmus is dissected free from the trachea by using a thyroid dissector. Arteria thyroidea ima if present should be dissected, ligated and divided.

Once these vessels are ligated and divided, thyroid lobes and isthmus are attached to the larynx and trachea by pretracheal fascia and Berry's ligament. The small vessels from tracheal

and esophageal branches are cauterized and divided. The pretracheal fascia and Berry's ligament is then divided taking care not to injure the recurrent laryngeal nerve.
- *Control of bleeding and placement of drain*: All bleeding points are checked and bleeding controlled with ligatures or diathermy coagulation. Two suction drainage tubes are kept one each at the sites of resected lobe.
- *Closure*: The investing layer of the deep fascia is apposed with interrupted 3-0 polyglactin sutures. The platysma is apposed with 3-0 polyglactin sutures. The skin is apposed with interrupted monofilament sutures or by subcuticular sutures.

STEPS OF LEFT HEMITHYROIDECTOMY

Q. Describe the steps of left hemithyroidectomy.

Ans.
- *Anesthesia*: General anesthesia with endotracheal intubation.
- *Position of the patient*: Patient supine with neck extended by placing a sand bag in-between the shoulder blades, head resting on head ring. The head end is elevated by about 15° to reduce the venous congestion.
- *Antiseptic dressing and draping*: Antiseptic cleaning with povidone-iodine from chin to midchest. Three towel draping for head area. A Mayo's table is placed over the chest area and draping done by placement of jaconate and sterile sheets.
- *Incision*: Cervical collar incision along the skin crease 2 cm above the suprasternal notch and extending from posterior border of one sternocleidomastoid to the posterior border of opposite sternocleidomastoid. The skin incision is marked by pressing the line of incision with a black silk thread (Garrotte mark).

  The skin and subcutaneous tissue is incised and the platysma muscle is incised at little higher level along the same line of skin incision.
- *Raising of skin flaps*: Both the upper and lower skin flaps is to be raised.

  The upper skin flap is lifted up by applying a pair of sharp skin hook and dissection is carried out in subplatysmal plane and the upper skin flap is lifted up up to the upper border of thyroid cartilage.

  The lower skin flap is lifted up similarly and the dissection done in subplatysmal level up to the suprasternal notch. Small bleeding vessels may be controlled with electrocautery.
- *Incising the investing layer of deep cervical fascia*: Once the skin flaps are raised these are held up by applying a pair of Joll's thyroid retractor and the skin flaps are retracted by opening the Joll's thyroid retractor. A nick is made in the investing layer of deep cervical fascia in the midline. The cut margins are picked up by two pairs of hemostatic forceps and the incision extended above up to the upper border of thyroid cartilage and below up to the suprasternal notch. If the anterior jugular vein comes in the way, this may be ligated and divided.
- *Exposure of the thyroid lobe*: The investing layer of deep cervical fascia is picked up by a number of hemostatic forceps and the strap muscles (superficial—sternohyoid, omohyoid and the deeper sternothyroid) are lifted up from the thyroid lobe by blunt dissection. Once this is done, the thyroid lobe covered by pretracheal fascia is exposed.

  If the thyroid lobe is hugely enlarged, for proper exposure the strap muscles may be divided transversely at a higher level (as the nerve supply comes from below).

- *Incising the pretracheal fascia*: The pretracheal fascia covering the thyroid lobe is picked up by hemostatic forceps and incised. A plane is created between the pretracheal fascia and the thyroid lobe on the side to be operated.
- *Division of middle thyroid vein*: This is the first vessel to be tackled in thyroidectomy as it is a slender vessel and is a direct tributary of IJV. The thyroid lobe is retracted medially and the middle thyroid vein is identified emerging from the middle of the thyroid lobe running transversely into the IJV. The vein is dissected by a right angled forceps and two ligatures are passed around the vein, ligated and the vein is divided in between two ligatures.
- *Division of superior thyroid vessels*: The strap muscles are retracted laterally and the thyroid lobe is retracted downward and medially to expose the superior pole of the lateral lobe of the gland. The superior thyroid vessels are dissected close to the upper pole of the gland taking care not to injure the external laryngeal nerve. The superior thyroid artery and vein should be ligated separately. Three ligatures are passed around the superior thyroid artery, ligated and divided keeping two ligatures toward the proximal side. The superior thyroid vein is ligated and divided similarly.
- *Division of inferior thyroid artery*: The earlier concept was to tie the inferior thyroid artery away from the gland to avoid injury to the recurrent laryngeal nerve. However, this is associated with higher incidence of parathyroid infarction.
  - The recent concept is to ligate the individual branches of the inferior thyroid artery close to the gland. The thyroid lobe is retracted further medially and the parathyroid gland and the recurrent laryngeal nerve are identified running in the tracheoesophageal groove. The individual branches of the inferior thyroid artery is dissected using a right angled forceps, ligated and divided in-between ligature, taking care not to injure the recurrent laryngeal nerve.
- *Division of inferior thyroid vein*: The inferior thyroid vein emerges from the lower pole of the lateral lobe of the gland. The inferior thyroid veins are dissected with right angled forceps, ligated and divided in between ligature.
- *Dissection of thyroid isthmus*: The thyroid lobe is dissected from the trachea and esophagus by dividing the pretracheal fascia and the Berry's ligament (thickening of pretracheal fascia attached to the cricoid cartilage).
  - The thyroid lobe is lifted up and medially. Lower pole of the isthmus is dissected from the trachea and if an arteria thyroidea ima is present, this is to be dissected, ligated and divided. The isthmus is dissected from the anterior surface of trachea. A pair of hemostatic forceps is applied at the junction of the isthmus with opposite lobe and the isthmus is divided with a knife, taking care not to injure the underlying trachea. The cut margin of the isthmus is overrun with 3-0 polyglactin sutures.
- *Closure*: Check for hemostasis. Any bleeding needs to be controlled with diathermy or ligature.
- *Placement of drain*: A suction drain is placed in the neck at the site of resected lobe.
- *Closure*: The investing layer of deep cervical fascia is approximated with interrupted 3-0 polyglactin sutures. The platysma is apposed by a running 3-0 polyglactin suture. The skin is apposed by subcuticular suture using 3-0 polyglactin.

▮ STEPS OF SUPERFICIAL PAROTIDECTOMY

Q. Describe the steps of superficial parotidectomy.

♦ General anesthesia with endotracheal intubation.

♦ *Position of patient*: Supine with neck extended by placing a sand bag below the shoulder blade. Head resting on a head ring and turned to the opposite side of operation. Head end elevated by 15° to reduce venous congestion. Eyes covered with an eye pad.

♦ Antiseptic cleaning and draping.

♦ *Incision*: An S-shaped cervicomastoidfacial incision is made. The incision starts below the zygomatic arch taken in front of the tragus turns around the ear lobule bending backward to the mastoid process and then curves downward transversely in the skin crease of the neck.

♦ *Raising of skin flaps*: The cervical, part of the incision is deepened first then the mastoid and finally the facial part of the incision. The incision is deepened down to the subcutaneous tissue and the platysma. The anterior skin flap is picked up by a sharp skin hook and the anterior skin flap is raised by sharp dissection below the platysma up to the anterior border of the parotid gland. Superiorly the skin flap is raised up to the zygomatic arch. The posterior skin flap along with the ear lobule is lifted up to some extent to expose the sternocleidomastoid muscle (SCM) and the mastoid process, and cartilaginous part of the external auditory canal.

♦ *Exposure and dissection of the posterior margin of the parotid gland*: The external jugular vein is dissected ligated and divided at the lower pole of the gland. The great auricular nerve exposed may be divided if required for ease of subsequent dissection. The dissection is done between the anterior border of SCM and the posterior border of the parotid gland upward to reach up to the mastoid process. Small bleeding vessels along the anterior border of SCM need control with electrocautery. The SCM is retracted laterally to expose the posterior belly of digastric and the stylohyoid muscle.

♦ *Identification of facial nerve*: There is a dense layer of temporoparotid fascia which extends from tympanomastoid fissure to the posterior border of parotid gland. This fascia is incised and deep dissection is done along the anterior border of mastoid process. The assistant retract the parotid gland medially. As the dissection is deepened there appears multiple small branches of posterior auricular artery which needs electrocautery and division. The deep dissection is done further to reach the junction of cartilaginous and bony part of the external auditory canal. The facial nerve is identified emerging from the stylomastoid foramen lying in front of the styloid process and at the junction of cartilaginous and bony part of the external auditory canal. The nerve runs transversely or obliquely for about 1–2 cm and divides into temporofacial (upper) and cervicofacial (lower) division and enters into the faciovenous plane of the parotid gland dividing the gland into superficial and deep lobe.

    Small bleeding vessels may be controlled with pressure packing or by use of bipolar diathermy.

♦ *Dissection of facial nerve branches*: All the facial nerve branches are traced from the point of entry of the nerve into the gland up to its exit from the anterior border of the gland. A curved mosquito forceps with concavity upward is pushed between the nerve branch and the parotid tissue of the superficial lobe in front in small bits and the overlying parotid tissue divided using scissors or bipolar cautery. This is continued up to the anterior border of the gland. All the nerve branches are dissected in the same way. The zygomatic branch is traced up toward the zygomatic arch at the upper pole of the gland and the cervical branch is traced at the lower pole toward the neck. The other branches are traced to the anterior border of the gland.

- *Removal of superficial part of the gland*: As all the nerve branches are dissected and the overlying parotid tissue divided the whole of superficial part of the gland now lies free with attachment of the parotid duct at the anterior border of the gland. The parotid duct is ligated at the anterior border of masseter muscle and the superficial part of the gland is removed.

    A suction drain is placed at the parotid fossa, brought out through a stab wound in the anterior skin flap in the neck.

- *Closure*: Closure is done in single layer with interrupted 3-0 monofilament polyamide suture. Alternatively the platysma may be apposed by 3-0 polyglactin suture and the skin apposed by subcuticular suture using 3-0 polyglactin.

■ STEPS OF SUBMANDIBULAR SIALOADENECTOMY

Q. Describe the steps of submandibular sialoadenectomy.

Ans.

- *Anesthesia*: General anesthesia with endotracheal intubation.
- *Position of patient*: Patient supine, neck extended by placing a sand bag in-between shoulder blades, head resting on head ring and chin turned to the opposite side. Head end elevated by 15° to reduce venous congestion.
- Antiseptic cleaning with povidone-iodine and draping. Head area draped with three towel technique.
- *Incision*: A transverse neck crease skin incision is made 3–4 cm below the lower border of the mandible medially extending up to 2 cm lateral to midline and laterally extending up to the point below the angle of lower jaw.
- *Raising of skin flaps*: The skin incision is deepened to incise the subcutaneous tissue, platysma and the investing layer of deep cervical fascia. The upper skin flap is reflected up toward the lower border of the mandible, taking the deep cervical fascia along with the skin flap to prevent injury to the marginal mandibular branch of facial nerve. The lower skin flap is similarly raised to expose the superficial lobe of the submandibular gland. While raising the skin flaps the superficial vein including the anterior facial vein needs to be ligated and divided.
- *Mobilization of superficial lobe of submandibular gland*: The superficial lobe of the submandibular gland is retracted superiorly and then lower pole of the gland is dissected toward the posterior end. Toward the posterior end of the lower pole, the trunk of facial, artery and vein are identified, dissected, ligated and divided. The superficial lobe of the gland is mobilized by combination of sharp and blunt dissection. At the upper pole of the superficial lobe of the gland, the facial artery and vein are again encountered, dissected ligated and divided close to the gland.
- *Mobilization of the deep part of the gland*: As the superficial lobe of the gland is mobilized the posterior border of the mylohyoid muscle is identified and the mylohyoid muscle is retracted to expose the deep part of the gland which lies between the mylohyoid and the hyoglossus muscle. Multiple small vessels lying between mylohyoid and hyoglossus muscle needs division with electrocautery.

◆ *Identification of lingual nerve*: The deep part of the submandibular gland is retracted downward to identify the lingual nerve as a broad band of white tissue running above the submandibular duct.
  – The lingual nerve runs forward over the hyoglossus initially above the submandibular duct and then crosses the superficial aspect of the duct and winds round the lower border of the duct to cross its medial aspect from below upward.
◆ *Dissection and division of submandibular duct*: The submandibular duct emerges from the anterior end of the deep part of the gland and runs on the hyoglossus muscle in close relation to the lingual nerve. The submandibular duct is dissected up to, the floor of the mouth taking care not to injure the lingual nerve and the hypoglossal nerve. The submandibular duct is ligated with 2-0 polyglactin suture and divided close to the floor of the mouth. The lingual nerve runs first above the submandibular duct then winds round it from lateral to medial side.
◆ *Removal of deep part of the gland*: The deep part of the gland is mobilized and dissected off from the hyoglossus muscle taking care not to injure the hypoglossal nerve which lies deep to the deep part of the gland on the hyoglossus.
◆ *Closure*: Hemostasis secured. A suction drain is placed at the submandibular fossa. The subcutaneous tissue with the platysma is apposed with running 3-0 polyglactin suture. Skin apposed with 3-0 polyglactin subcuticular suture or with interrupted suture using 3-0 monofilament polyamide suture.

■ STEPS OF TYPE I MODIFIED RADICAL NECK DISSECTION

Q. Describe the steps of type I modified radical neck dissection.

Ans. There are three types of modified radical neck dissection:
◆ *Type I*: Radical neck dissection with preservation of spinal accessory nerve (SAN).
◆ *Type II*: Radical neck dissection with preservation of SAN and the IJV.
◆ *Type III*: Radical neck dissection with preservation of all three structures—(1) SAN, (2) IJV and (3) the SCM.
◆ *Anesthesia*: General anesthesia with endotracheal intubation.
◆ *Position of the patient*: Patient supine, arms on the sides of the body. Head turned to the opposite side resting on a head ring and the head end elevated by about 15° to reduce the venous congestion.
◆ *Antiseptic dressing and draping*: The antiseptic cleaning with povidone-iodine from chin to the midchest. Three towel draping for the head and draping of the remaining area by placement of sterile sheets to expose the site of the operation.
◆ *Incision*: For unilateral dissection a Y-shaped incision is made. The horizontal limb of the Y starts from the point below the chin and taken downward toward the hyoid bone and then curves upward toward the mastoid process. The vertical limb of the incision starts from the middle of the horizontal limb and then continue downward in an S-shaped manner and ends just above the clavicle. The skin incision is deepened to incise subcutaneous fat and the platysma.
◆ *Raising of skin flaps*: The posterior skin flap is raised first. The skin flap with subcutaneous tissue and platysma is lifted up by two skin hooks and the skin flap is lifted up by sharp dissection from the underlying soft tissue till the anterior border of trapezius. While lifting the posterior skin flap the SAN entering the anterior border of trapezius should be preserved.

- While raising the upper skin flap two branches of facial nerve cervical branch and the marginal mandibular branch has to be preserved. To do so, the deep fascia is incised at the level of hyoid bone and extending up to the fascia covering the submandibular salivary gland. The upper skin flap along with the deep fascia attached to the upper flap is lifted up by sharp dissection up to the lower border of mandible taking care not to injure the branches of facial nerve.
- The medial or anterior skin flap is lifted up by skin hooks and lifted in a subplatysmal plane by sharp dissection just beyond the midline medially and below up to the clavicle exposing the supraclavicular fossa.

- *Early division of SCM and IJV*: The lower end of the SCM at its origin from the sternum and clavicle is dissected and divided by diathermy knife. The SCM is lifted up to expose the carotid sheath.
  - The fascia covering the carotid sheath is incised and the lower end of the IJV is dissected by using a right angled forceps and 3 silk ligatures are passed around the IJV and IJV is ligated and divided keeping two ligatures distally. The lower cut end of the IJV may be transfixed with 3-0 Mersilk. While dissecting the IJV the vagus nerve should be taken care of.

- *Supraclavicular dissection*: The posterior triangle of the neck is divided by the inferior belly of omohyoid into the upper occipital and lower supraclavicular triangle. The fascia over the fat pad lateral to IJV is incised and the fat pad with the lymph nodes isdissected up. While doing so the phrenic nerve running over the scalenus anterior muscle is preserved. All the fat pad along with supraclavicular lymph nodes are dissected off from the supraclavicular triangle taking care not to breach the prevertebral fascial layer covering the brachial plexus. While dissecting the supraclavicular triangle the external jugular vein needs to be dissected ligated and divided. The transverse cervical vessels also need ligature and division. The inferior belly of omohyoid is dissected close to its origin from the upper border of scapula and divided by diathermy.

- *Dissection of Chaissaignac's triangle*: This is the area between the medial border of scalenus anterior muscle, IJV and the common carotid artery. The loose areolar tissue and the lymph nodes are cleared from this area by sharp and blunt dissection. Important structures like thyrocervical trunk, vertebral vein, and thoracic duct on the left side and jugular lymphatic trunk on the right side lies in this area. These structures are to be preserved carefully.

- *Dissection of occipital triangle*: Before starting dissection of occipital triangle the SAN needs to be dissected and safeguarded. The SAN is identified at the posterior border of SCM at the junction of upper one-third and lower two-thirds. This is about 1 cm above the Erb's point where the great auricular nerve turns around the posterior border of SCM. Once the nerve is identified the SAN nerve is dissected along the posterior triangle up to the anterior border of trapezius at its lower third. The nerve may also be identified using a nerve stimulator.

  Once the SAN is safeguarded, the dissection proceeds along the anterior border of trapezius up to the mastoid process and all loose areolar tissue and the lymph nodes in the occipital triangle are cleared of the ascending branch of transverse cervical artery running along the anterior border of trapezius needs ligature and division.

- *Division of upper end of SCM*: Taking care of the SAN, the SCM is lifted up up to its insertion into the mastoid process. The upper end of SCM is dissected free and divided close to its insertion. The IJV is exposed.

- *Division of upper end of IJV and carotid dissection*: As the SCM and IJV are lifted up, the level III and level IV lymph nodes are cleared off along with the IJV. The upper end of IJV is dissected and 3 silk ligatures are passed around and ligated. The upper end of the IJV is now divided keeping 2 ligatures toward the proximal side. Near the termination of IJV the posterior belly of digastric muscle may be lifted up to clear the level II lymph nodes. While dissecting the level II, III, and IV nodes, the vagus nerve and common carotid artery is to be taken care of.
- *Dissection of level I lymph nodes*: The fat in the submental area is incised and cleared. The anterior belly of the digastric muscle is exposed. The superficial lobe of the submandibular gland is exposed. The upper border of the submandibular gland is freed by dissecting and dividing the facial vein and artery in between ligature at the lower border of the mandible. The lower border of the superficial lobe is similarly freed by dissecting, ligating and dividing the facial artery and the vein at lower pole of the gland. The mylohyoid muscle is retracted in a forward direction to identify the deep part of the submandibular gland. The lingual nerve is identified as a broad band along the upper pole and the branches from the lingual nerve to the submandibular ganglion is ligated and divided. The lingual nerve crosses around the submandibular duct. The submandibular duct is dissected up to the floor of the mouth, ligated and divided. The hypoglossal nerve running in between the deep part of the submandibular gland and the hyoglossus muscle is also preserved. All the loose areolar tissue and the lymph nodes from submental triangle and submandibular triangle are cleared off by sharp and blunt dissection. The small vessels that come on the way are controlled by electrocoagulation. The lower pole of parotid gland is excised and overrun with 3-0 Vicryl sutures.
- *Check for hemostasis*: Hemostasis is checked and any bleeding is controlled by electrocautery. The wound is irrigated with normal saline.
- *Placement of drain*: Two 12 Fr tube drain is placed through the posterior flap and connected to a vacuum drainage bag.
- *Closure*: The subcutaneous tissue and the platysma are apposed by 3-0 polyglactin sutures. Skin is approximated by interrupted 3-0 monofilament polyamide suture. Alternatively, skin may be apposed by subcuticular suture or skin staplers.

■ VENOUS CUT DOWN (VENESECTION)

This involves exposure of a vein, venotomy and introduction of a wide bore cannula inside the vein under direct vision.

A long cannula may be passed down the vein up to the superior vena cava and central venous pressure (CVP) may be measured.

Indications of Venesection

- For intravenous access in shocked patient requiring rapid infusion of fluid
- For prolonged period of intravenous fluid therapy
- For parenteral nutrition
- For measurement of central venous pressure.

Sites

- Great saphenous vein at the ankle or at the groin
- Basilic vein at the arm
- Cephalic vein at the deltopectoral groove.

Q. Describe the steps of venous cut down?

Ans.

Procedure:

- Wash hands and wear sterile gloves
- The area is cleaned with an antiseptic solution (povidone-iodine) and draped with towel
- Inject 1% lignocaine at the site transversely across the vein to be cannulated (Fig. 22.12A).
- A small transverse incision is made across the selected vein. The incision is deepened up to the subcutaneous tissue.
- The subcutaneous tissue is incised (Fig. 22.12B).
- The vein is isolated by blunt dissection (Fig. 22.12C).

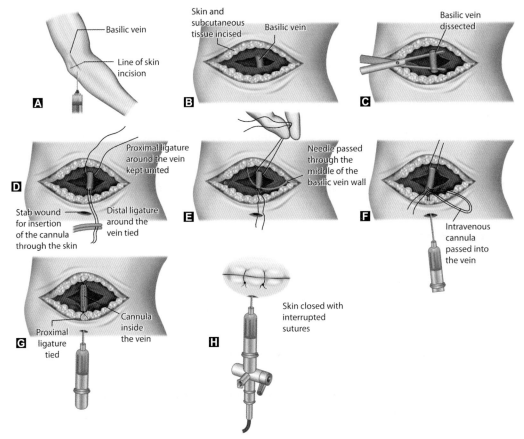

Figs 22.12A to H: Steps of venesection

- Two ligatures are passed around the vein. The distal one is tied and held by a hemostatic forceps (Fig. 22.12D).
- A curved needle is passed through the middle of the basilic vein wall and the vein wall in front of the needle is incised (Fig. 22.12E).
- A No. 6 or 9 sterile infant feeding tube is introduced through the venotomy and the cannula is advanced proximally so that its tip lies in the superior vena cava. The proximal ligature is tied to fix the cannula within the vein (Figs 22.12F and G).
- The end of the cannula is connected to an intravenous fluid channel.
- The skin incision is closed with interrupted skin sutures (Fig. 22.12H).
- The cannula is fixed to the skin by a suture passed around the cannula.
- Sterile dressing is applied.

▌TRACHEOSTOMY

Q. What are the indications of tracheostomy?

Ans. *See* Instruments Section. Page No. 1051–1053, Chapter 21

Q. Describe the steps of tracheostomy.

Ans.
- *Position of patient:* Patient supine with neck extended by placing a sand bag in—between the shoulder blades and head supported with a ring.
- *Anesthesia:* Usually done under local anesthesia by injecting 1% lignocaine hydrochloride.
- *Incision:* For elective tracheostomy a transverse neck crease incision is made midway between cricoid cartilage and the suprasternal notch. In emergency a vertical incision from the lower border of the thyroid cartilage to the suprasternal notch may be used.
- *Procedure*:
  - The skin, subcutaneous tissue and the platysma is incised in the same line. The investing layer of the deep cervical fascia is incised in the midline and the strap muscles are retracted on either side.
  - The thyroid isthmus is exposed. This isthmus is divided in the midline in between forceps and the trachea is exposed. The trachea is held fixed by a single hook retractor. A 1–2 cm vertical incision is made on the trachea centering 3rd or 4th tracheal ring using a No. 11 knife. A tracheal dilator is inserted into the trachea with the blades in closed position. The blades are opened and a cuffed tracheostomy tube is inserted into the trachea through the tracheotomy. The tracheostomy tube is fixed by a strap tied around the neck. The bleeding from the cut ends of the thyroid isthmus is controlled. The skin is closed with interrupted silk stitches.

Q. What are the complications of tracheostomy?

Ans.
- Bleeding from the thyroid isthmus or brachiocephalic vein and inferior thyroid veins
- Blockage of tracheostomy tube—may result even in death.
- Tracheal stenosis.

■ GASTROSTOMY

Indications

- *For feeding in patients with esophageal obstruction*: Corrosive stricture or carcinoma of esophagus.
- For gastric decompression in a postoperative patient when passage of a nasogastric tube is not feasible
- *In cases of duodenal fistula*: Two tubes may be inserted through the gastrostomy. One kept in the duodenum proximal to the site of leakage for aspiration and another tube passed beyond the duodenum 25–30 cm beyond the fistula for feeding.

Q. Describe the steps of gastrostomy.

Ans.

- *Anesthesia*: General anesthesia or local anesthesia. For local anesthesia inject 20 mL 0.5% of injection lignocaine in the skin and subcutaneous tissue. After incising the skin and subcutaneous tissue, another 20 mL is injected along the linea alba and the parietal peritoneum.
- *Incision*: About 5 cm midline vertical incision starting from just below the xiphoid.
- *Procedure*:
  - Skin and subcutaneous tissues are incised along the line of incision (Fig. 22.13A).
  - The linea alba is incised in the midline.
  - The peritoneum is lifted in between the hemostatic forceps and a nick is made in the parietal peritoneum and the incision in the peritoneum is extended.
  - The wound margin is retracted and the stomach is identified (Figs 22.13B and C).
  - The skin below the left costal margin is infiltrated with injection lignocaine and an incision is made lateral to the outer border of rectus abdominis (Fig. 22.13D).
  - The gastrostomy tube (22 Fr Foley's or Malaecot's catheter) is brought into the abdomen through this stab wound (Fig. 22.13E).
  - The stomach is held by two pairs of Babcock's tissue forceps. A stab wound is made in the anterior wall of the stomach high up in the body between the greater and lesser curvature of the stomach (Fig. 22.13F). The gastrostomy tube is introduced through the stab wound with the tip directed toward the pylorus
  - A purse string suture is applied around the stab wound and is tightened around the tube. Insert two more purse string suture around each 0.5 cm apart inverting the previous layers (Fig. 22.13G).
  - The stomach wall is fixed to the parietal peritoneum by 2 or 3 interrupted chromic catgut sutures (Fig. 22.13H).
  - The incision is closed in layers. The gastrostomy tube is fixed to the skin.

Q. What is Witzel gastrostomy?

Ans. In Witzel gastrostomy instead of series of purse string suture, the gastrostomy tube is buried in the stomach wall by creating a tunnel in the stomach wall. The wall of the stomach on either side of the gastrostomy tube is sutured to create the tunnel.

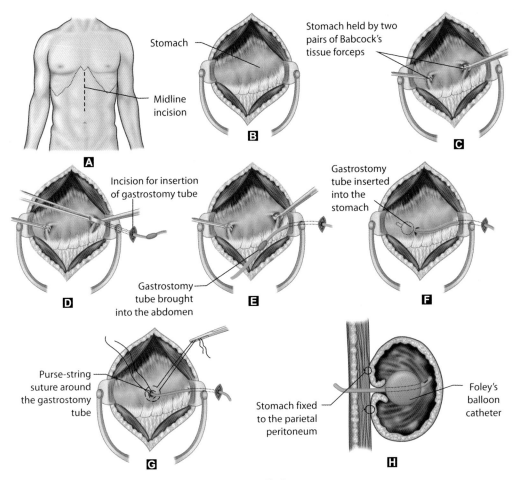

Figs 22.13A to H: Gastrostomy

Q. What is Deepage Janeway gastrostomy?

Ans. This is a technique of permanent gastrostomy. A flap is raised from the anterior wall of the stomach and is formed into a tube. The stomach tube is brought out and sutured to the skin to create a permanent gastrostomy.

Q. What are the other techniques of gastrostomy?

Ans.
* Laparoscopic gastrostomy
* Percutaneous endoscopic gastrostomy.

Q. Why it is not desirable to do a gastrostomy in a patient with inoperable carcinoma of esophagus?

Ans. In inoperable carcinoma of esophagus patient has problems of swallowing of food and saliva. Gastrostomy allows feeding but does not provide any relief for the distressing problems of swallowing of the saliva. So it is not desirable to do gastrostomy. Some form of esophageal stenting is preferable.

■ STEPS OF EVERSION OF SAC

Q. What are the steps of eversion of sac (Fig. 22.14)?

Ans.

♦ Antiseptic dressing and draping.

♦ *Anesthesia*: Operation is done under local anesthesia. The spermatic cord is infiltrated with 2% lignocaine hydrochloride. The scrotal skin along the line of incision is also infiltrated with lignocaine hydrochloride.

♦ *Skin incision*: A vertical incision is made parallel to the median raphe of the scrotum.

♦ *Incising the layers of scrotum*: The incision is deepened to cut the dartos muscle the scrotal fascia and the hydrocele sac lined by the parietal layer of the tunica vaginalis is exposed.

♦ *Incising the parietal layer of tunica vaginalis*: The tunica vaginalis sac is separated from the dartos muscle layer by finger dissection and a space created between the tunica vaginalis and the dartos.

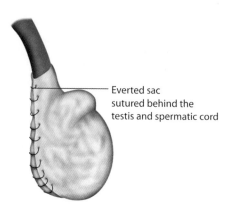

Everted sac sutured behind the testis and spermatic cord

– An incision is made over the tunica vaginalis in an avascular area anteriorly away from the testis, epididymis and cord structures and fluid drained.

Fig. 22.14: Eversion of sac

– The tunica vaginalis incision is then extended and testis delivered out of the tunica vaginalis sac.

♦ *Eversion of sac*: The cut margin of the tunica vaginalis sac is everted around the testis.

♦ *Suturing the cut margins of tunica vaginalis*: The cut margin is stitched behind the testis with 1-0 chromic catgut sutures.

♦ *Repositioning of testis into the scrotum*: The testis with the everted hydrocele sac is reinserted into the scrotal sac taking care so that there is no rotation of the testis. This is ascertained by keeping the head of the epididymis superiorly and sinus of the epididymis laterally.

♦ *Check for hemostasis*: If there is oozing, a corrugated rubber sheet drain may be placed into the scrotum.

♦ *Closure*: The internal spermatic fascia, cremasteric fascia, external spermatic fascia and the dartos muscle are apposed by a continuous 2-0 chromic catgut sutures. Skin is apposed by interrupted monofilament polyamide suture. A coconut bandage is applied.

■ CIRCUMCISION

Indications

♦ Religious: Muslims and Jews
♦ Phimosis
♦ Paraphimosis.

Q. Describe the steps of circumcision (Figs 12.15A to F).

Ans.

- In adults this is usually done under local anesthesia and in children usually done under general anesthesia.
- The penis is cleaned with an antiseptic solution (povidone-iodine) and draped with a sterile sheet.
- Infiltration anesthesia using 1% lignocaine injection (without adrenaline). The local anesthetic is injected all around the base of the penis. Wait for 5 minutes.
- The tip of the prepuce is grasped with two pairs of mosquito forceps and the adhesion between the prepuce and the glans penis is separated (Fig. 22.15A).
- A dorsal cut is made in the prepuce with scissors extending proximally up to 5 mm of the corona glandis (Fig. 22.15B). The cut is then taken around the penis to the ventral aspect toward the frenulum and the preputial skin is excised (Figs 22.15B to D).

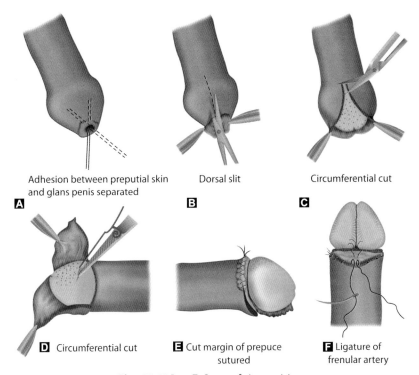

Adhesion between preputial skin and glans penis separated

A

Dorsal slit

B

Circumferential cut

C

D Circumferential cut

E Cut margin of prepuce sutured

F Ligature of frenular artery

Figs 22.15A to F: Steps of circumcision

- Once the prepuce is excised there are bleeding from a number of points. The skin is retracted over the penis and the bleeding points are held up by mosquito forceps and ligated with 3-0 catgut sutures.
- The skin edges are then sutured with 3-0 chromic catgut sutures. The dorsal and ventral midline sutures are applied first and the remaining cut edges of the prepuce is sutured with interrupted 3-0 chromic catgut sutures (Fig. 22.15E). A figure of eight stitch in ventral midline controls the frenular artery (Fig. 22.15F).
- A light dressing is applied.

Chapter

Surgical Anatomy

23

■ INTRODUCTION

Surgical anatomy is one component of oral and practical examination.

This section contains surgical anatomy related to discussion of long and short cases.

The relevant anatomy discussed along with illustrations. For more details students may refer to any standard book on Surgical Anatomy.

■ INGUINAL CANAL

Q. What are the boundaries of inguinal canal (Fig. 23.1)?

Ans. Inguinal canal is an oblique canal with a length of about 3.8 cm, situated at the lower part of anterior abdominal wall and extends from the deep-inguinal ring to the superficial inguinal ring.

This canal is bounded:

◆ *Anteriorly*: By the external aponeurosis along its whole length and reinforced laterally by the muscular fibers of the internal oblique.
◆ *Posteriorly*: By the fascia transversalis throughout and reinforced medially by the conjoint tendon.
◆ *Medially*: By the lateral border of the rectus sheath.

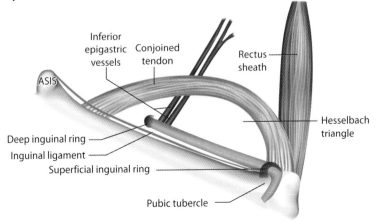

Fig. 23.1: Surgical anatomy of inguinal canal

- *Roof*: Formed by the conjoined tendon and arched fibers of internal oblique and transversus abdominis.
- *Floor*: Formed by the lacunar ligament medially and the inguinal ligament laterally.

Q. What is Hesselbach's triangle?

Ans. The medial part of the inguinal canal is Hesselbach's triangle being bounded:
- Laterally by the inferior epigastric vessels.
- Medially by the lateral border of the rectus sheath.
- Base is formed by the upper concave surface of the medial part of the inguinal ligament and the lacunar ligament.

Q. What are the contents of inguinal canal?

Ans. The inguinal canal contains:
- Spermatic cord in male and round ligament of uterus in female.
- In addition, the ilioinguinal nerve traverses through the inguinal canal.
- The nerve does not come through the deep ring enters the inguinal canal by piercing the internal oblique muscle and emerges out through the superficial inguinal ring.

Q. What are the constituents of spermatic cord?

Ans. The spermatic cord comprises of:
- Vas deferens
- Testicular artery
- Artery to the vas
- Artery to the cremaster
- Pampiniform plexus of veins
- Testicular lymphatic vessels
- Testicular sympathetic plexus
- Genital branch of genitofemoral nerve.

Q. What are the coverings of spermatic cord?

Ans. The coverings of spermatic cord are outside inwards:
- *External spermatic fascia*: Derived from the external oblique aponeurosis and covers the cord beyond the superficial inguinal ring.
- *Cremasteric muscle and fascia*: Derived from the internal oblique aponeurosis.
- *Internal spermatic fascia*: Derived from the fascia transversalis.

Q. What is Fruchaud's myopectineal orifice (Fig. 23.2)?

Ans. This is osseo-musculoaponeurotic hiatus in the lower abdomen through which all groin hernia occurs.

This is bounded:
- *Laterally* by the iliopsoas muscle

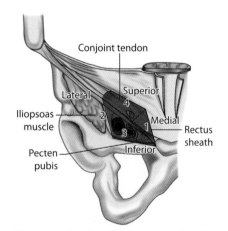

Fig. 23.2: Fruchaud myopectineal orifice is bound—by (1) lateral border of rectus sheath, (2) iliopsoas muscle, (3) pecten pubis, and (4) conjoint tendon

* *Medially* by the lateral border of the rectus sheath
* *Below* by the pecten pubis
* *Above* by the arched fibers of internal oblique and transversus abdominis.

Q. What is the anatomy of deep-inguinal ring?

Ans. The deep-inguinal ring lies 1.25 cm above the inguinal ligament at the midinguinal point (a point midway between the symphysis pubis and anterior superior iliac spine). This is actually not an opening but the mouth of a prolongation of fascia transversalis dragged down by the gubernaculum. The inferior epigastric vessels lie medial to the deep-inguinal ring.

   The spermatic cord in male and round ligament in female emerge through the deep-inguinal ring.

Q. What is the anatomy of superficial inguinal ring (Fig. 23.3)?

Ans. The superficial inguinal ring is formed by splitting of external oblique aponeurosis at its insertion medially. Base is 1.25 cm and the height is 2.5 cm.

The boundary of superficial inguinal ring is:

* *Base*: Formed by the pubic crest.
* *Medially*: Superomedial crus of external oblique aponeurosis.
* *Laterally*: Inferolateral crus of external oblique aponeurosis:
    - The two crura are joined by intercrural fibers.

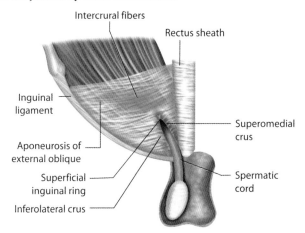

Fig. 23.3: Schematic diagram of superficial inguinal ring

Q. What structures emerge through the superficial inguinal ring?

Ans. In addition to spermatic cord in male and round ligament of uterus in female, the ilioinguinal nerve emerges through the superficial inguinal ring.

Q. What are the different ligaments in relation to external oblique aponeurosis?

Ans. The different ligaments in relation to external oblique aponeurosis are:
* *Inguinal ligament (Poupart ligament)*:
    - This is a condensation of the lower part of the aponeurosis of the external oblique aponeurosis. This is usually 10 cm in length and is attached laterally to the anterior superior iliac spine and medially to the pubic tubercle.

- The lateral part of the inguinal ligament is thick, rounded, and cord like. The medial part of the inguinal ligament is flat and bent upon itself, so that it has an upper concave surface. This concave upper surface of the ligament forms the floor of the inguinal canal.
- *Lacunar ligament*:
  - This is one of the extensions of inguinal ligament. This is triangular in shape. The apex is attached to the pubic tubercle. The base is free, concave, and forms the medial boundary of the femoral ring. The lower surface is convex and the upper surface is concave and forms the floor of the inguinal canal medially.
- *Cooper's ligament or pectineal ligament*:
  - This is the continuation of the lacunar ligament along the pecten pubis of the pubic ramus and may extend up to the iliopubic eminence.
  - The femoral vessels run in-between the inguinal ligament and the Cooper's ligament and are enclosed by the femoral sheath.
- *Reflected part of the inguinal ligament*:
  - This starts from the lateral crus of the superficial inguinal ring and passes behind the superficial inguinal ring, and in front of the conjoint tendon to get blended with the linea alba.

Q. Which structures pass deep to the inguinal ligament (Fig. 23.4)?

Ans. The following structures pass deep to the inguinal ligament from lateral to medial side:
- Iliacus muscle
- The lateral femoral cutaneous nerve passing in front of the iliacus muscle
- Femoral nerve lies in the groove between the iliacus and the psoas major muscle. Nerve to pectineus arises from the femoral nerve passes behind the inguinal ligament and supplies the lateral part of the pectineus muscle.
- Psoas major muscle
- Pectineus muscle
- In-between the inguinal ligament and the pectineus and psoas major lies the femoral sheath with its contents (femoral artery, femoral vein, and lymphatics).

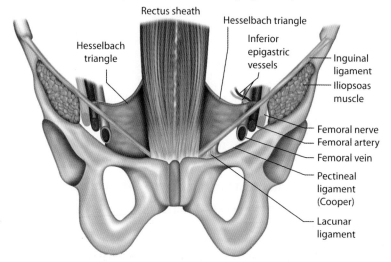

Fig. 23.4: Schematic diagram of inguinal ligament

Q. What is conjoint tendon?

Ans. The conjoint tendon or falx inguinalis is formed by the fusion of lower fibers of internal oblique and transversus abdominis. The conjoint tendon arches behind the superficial inguinal ring and medial part of the inguinal canal (forming the posterior wall of the medial part of the inguinal canal) and is inserted into the pubic crest and the pectineal line of the pecten pubis.

Q. What is femoral sheath?

Ans.
* This is a fascial sheath presents in the groin enclosing the femoral vessels.
* Femoral sheath is funnel-shaped with wide mouth upwards.
* Formed by the prolongation of the fascia of the abdomen.
  - The anterior layer of femoral sheath is formed by the prolongation of fascia transversalis behind the inguinal ligament descending to about 4 cm below the inguinal ligament.
  - The posterior layer of the femoral sheath is formed by the prolongation of the fascia iliaca.
  - The medial and lateral wall is formed by the blending of the two layers.

Q. What are the different compartments of femoral sheath (Fig. 23.5)?

Ans. The femoral sheath is divided into three compartments by two septa:
* *Lateral or arterial compartment*: Contains the proximal part of the femoral artery with its branches. The femoral branch of genitofemoral nerve lies at first anterior and then lateral to the artery.
* *Intermediate or the venous compartment*: This contains the femoral vein. The great saphenous terminates into the femoral vein at saphenous opening.
* *Medial or lymphatic compartment*: This is also called femoral canal. This contains loose areolar tissue, one deep-inguinal lymph node (lymph node of Cloquet), and lymphatic vessels.
* *The opening of the femoral canal* proximally is known as femoral ring, which is covered by femoral septum, which is formed by condensation of extraperitoneal fatty tissue.

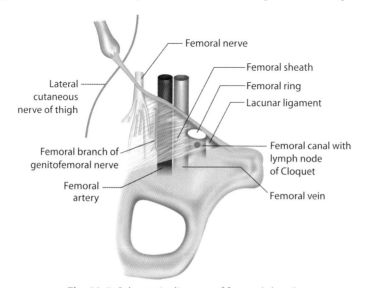

Fig. 23.5: Schematic diagram of femoral sheath

Q. What is the boundary of femoral ring (Fig. 23.5)?

Ans.

- *Anteriorly*: Inguinal ligament
- *Posteriorly*: Fascia covering pectineus and Cooper's ligament
- *Medially*: Concave margin of lacunar ligament
- *Laterally*: Septum separating the femoral vein.

Q. Which factors normally prevent development of hernia in the groin?

Ans. The following factors are important in preventing development of hernia at the groin:

- *Obliquity of the inguinal canal*: Provides a flap valve like action preventing descent of abdominal contents through the inguinal canal.
- *Shutter mechanism*: When there is increase of intra-abdominal pressure, the anterior wall of the canal contracts and presses against the deep-inguinal ring thereby shutting the deep-inguinal ring thereby preventing escape of abdominal contents through the deep-inguinal ring.
  - In the medial part of the inguinal canal, the conjoint tendon forming the posterior wall comes forward and shuts the medial part of the inguinal canal thereby preventing any escape of abdominal contents through the inguinal canal.
  - The arched fibers of the internal oblique and the transversus abdominis forming the roof of the canal also contract and descend down thereby decreasing the height of the inguinal canal from above.
  - *Ball valve mechanism*: Contraction of cremaster muscle draws up the spermatic cord toward the superficial ring thereby occluding the superficial inguinal ring.
  - *Slit valve mechanism*: Contraction of external oblique aponeurosis results in approximation of two crura of the superficial inguinal ring, preventing herniation through the superficial inguinal ring.

Q. What is processus vaginalis and what is its fate?

Ans. This is a pouch of peritoneum dragged down during the descent of gubernaculum of testis or ovary. This extends from the deep-inguinal ring and emerges through the superficial inguinal ring to the bottom of scrotum in male and labia majora in females.

- *Fate of processus vaginalis*: Normally the part of the processus vaginalis from the deep-inguinal ring to the upper pole of testis disappears and the distal part in the scrotum persists as tunica vaginalis of testis.

Q. What are the abnormalities of processus vaginalis?

Ans. There may be some abnormalities in relation to persistence of processus vaginalis:

- Whole of processus vaginalis may persist leading to congenital hydrocele or hernia.
- The processus vaginalis may persist from just beyond the deep-inguinal ring to the upper pole of testis, leading to a funicular type of hydrocele.
- The intermediate part of the processus vaginalis may persist and may lead to formation of encysted hydrocele of the cord.
- The processus vaginalis may persist from beyond the deep ring to the bottom of the scrotum leading to infantile hydrocele.

Q. What is the boundary of femoral triangle?

Ans.
* *Above (base)*: Inguinal ligament
* *Laterally*: Medial border of sartorius
* *Medially*: Medial border of adductor longus
* *Apex*: By meeting of medial border of adductor longus and medial border of sartorius
* *Roof*: Skin, superficial fascia, and deep fascia of thigh
* *Floor*: Medial to lateral—adductor longus, pectineus, iliacus, and psoas muscles.

Q. What are the contents of femoral triangle?

Ans. The contents of femoral triangle are:
* *Femoral artery and its branches*:
  - *Three superficial branches*—superficial external pudendal, superficial epigastric, and superficial circumflex iliac.
  - *Three deep branches*—deep external pudendal, profunda femoris, and muscular branches.
* *Femoral vein*—lies medial to the artery and the tributaries corresponds to the arterial branches.
* *Nerves*—femoral nerve lies lateral to the femoral artery, nerve to pectineus, femoral branch of genitofemoral nerve, and lateral cutaneous nerve of thigh.
* *Inguinal lymph nodes*—superficial and deep-inguinal lymph nodes.

■ ANATOMICAL CONCEPT IN VIEW OF LAPAROSCOPIC REPAIR OF HERNIA

Q. What is preperitoneal space?

Ans. This is a potential space lying in-between the fascia transversalis and the parietal peritoneum. In laparoscopic hernia repair, the mesh is placed in this space.

Q. What is space of Retzius?

Ans. The potential area deep to the fascia transversalis and lying behind the symphysis pubis and the anterior wall of the bladder is the space of Retzius. This space traced laterally is described as the space of Bogros. This space lies between the fascia transversalis and the peritoneum.

Q. What are the different umbilical ligaments and folds?

Ans. When the groin area is viewed from within the peritoneal cavity following structures are seen (Fig. 23.6):
* *Median umbilical ligament and median umbilical fold:* The midline peritoneal fold lifted by the obliterated urachus is known as median umbilical fold. The obliterated urachus is the median umbilical ligament.
* *The peritoneal fold raised by the obliterated umbilical artery is the medial umbilical fold* and the obliterated umbilical artery is the medial umbilical ligament.
* *The peritoneal fold* raised by the inferior epigastric vessels is the lateral umbilical fold.

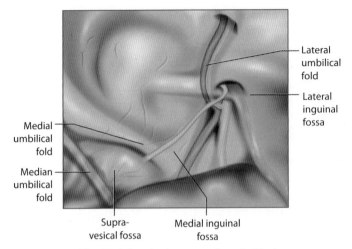

Fig. 23.6: Inguinal anatomy from behind

Q. What are supravesical fossa and the inguinal fossa?

Ans.
- *Supravesical fossa*: The space between the median umbilical fold and the medial umbilical fold.
- *Medial inguinal fossa*: The space between the medial umbilical fold and the lateral umbilical fold site of direct inguinal hernia.
- *Lateral inguinal fossa*: The space lying lateral to the lateral umbilical fold (Fig. 23.6). Site of indirect inguinal hernia.

■ ANTERIOR ABDOMINAL WALL

Rectus Sheath

Q. How is rectus sheath formed (Figs 23.7A to D)?

Ans. Rectus sheath is a musculoaponeurotic sheath enclosing the rectus abdominis and the pyramidalis muscle. The rectus sheath is formed by the aponeurosis of external oblique, internal oblique, and the muscular fibers and aponeurosis of transversus abdominis. The anterior and posterior wall of the rectus sheath varies at different levels and is formed as follows:
- *Rectus sheath above the lower costal margin*:
  - The anterior wall of the sheath is formed only by the external oblique aponeurosis.
  - The posterior wall of the sheath is deficient here and the rectus abdominis muscle is attached to the lower costal cartilages and the xiphoid process (Fig. 23.7A).
- *Rectus sheath from the costal margin up to midway between the umbilicus and xiphoid process*:
  - The anterior wall of the rectus sheath at this level is formed by the external oblique aponeurosis and the anterior lamella of the internal oblique aponeurosis.
  - The posterior wall of the sheath is formed by the posterior lamella of the internal oblique aponeurosis, muscular fibers of the transversus abdominis, fascia transversalis, extraperitoneal fatty tissue, and the parietal peritoneum. All these layers are blended to form the posterior rectus sheath (Fig. 23.7B).

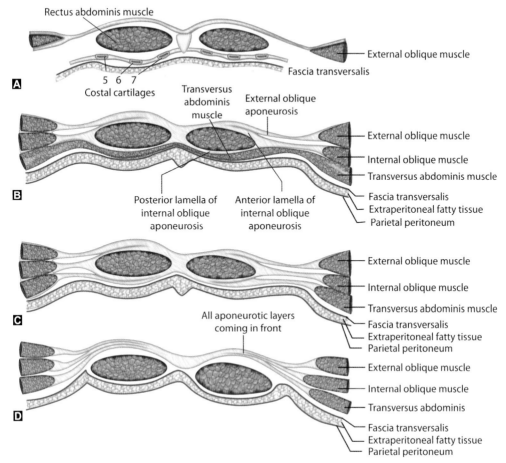

Figs 23.7A to D: Formation of rectus sheath at three levels. (A) Above the level of costal margin; (B) Between costal margin and a point midway between umbilicus and symphysis pubis; (C) Below the point midway between umbilicus and symphysis pubis; (D) Above the symphysis pubis

- *Rectus sheath from the above level to midway between the umbilicus and the symphysis pubis.*
  - The anterior wall of the sheath is formed by the external oblique aponeurosis and anterior lamella of the internal oblique aponeurosis.
  - The posterior wall is formed by the same layers as in level II except that the transversus abdominis is aponeurotic at this level (Fig. 23.7C).
- *Rectus sheath from the above level up to the symphysis pubis:*
  - The anterior wall of the sheath at this level is formed by the aponeurosis of all three muscles—(1) external oblique, (2) internal oblique, and (3) the transversus abdominis.
  - The posterior wall of the rectus sheath is deficient at this level and the rectus abdominis muscle lies on the fascia transversalis (Fig. 23.7D).

Q. What are the contents of rectus sheath?

Ans. The contents of the rectus sheath include:
- Rectus abdominis muscle
- Pyramidalis muscle

* Inferior epigastric artery and vein
* Superior epigastric artery and vein
* Terminal parts of 7th to 12th (subcostal) nerves along with their collateral branches.

These nerves run in-between the transversus abdominis and internal oblique muscle and enter the rectus sheath by piercing the posterior lamella of the internal oblique, supply the rectus abdominis muscle by entering into the muscle from its lateral side. The nerve comes out as anterior cutaneous nerve by piercing the anterior rectus sheath.

Q. What is linea alba?

Ans. This is the median raphe formed by the interlacing fibers of the anterior rectus sheath.

Above the umbilicus, the linea alba is wide (about 1.25 cm) and below the umbilicus, it becomes linear.

Above it is attached to the xiphoid process. Below it splits into two layers—(1) superficial and (2) deep. The superficial fibers are attached to the anterior surface of the symphysis pubis. The deep fibers are attached to the posterior surface of the pubic crest.

Q. What is the fascial disposition in anterior abdominal wall?

Ans. Deep to the skin, there are two layers of superficial fascia in the abdomen. There is no deep fascia in the abdomen.

Disposition of superficial fascia of abdomen:

The superficial fascia of abdomen consists of:

* An outer fatty layer (fascia of Camper)
* An inner membranous layer (fascia of Scarpa).

The two layers of the superficial fascia are distinctly discernible below the level of umbilicus.

Q. What are the prolongations of fascia of Scarpa?

Ans.

* The fascia extends to the thigh below the inguinal ligament to about 1.25 cm and blends with the deep fascia (fascia lata) of the thigh.
* Medial to the pubic tubercle the fascia extends over the penis as fascia of the penis and over the scrotum as dartos muscle. This fascia extends into the perineum as fascia Colles. The fascia Colles covers transversus perinei superficialis muscle and is attached to the perineal membrane.
* In the midline, the fascia of Scarpa is attached to the linea alba and is prolonged downward to form the two ligaments of the penis.
* The fundiform ligament is attached to the linea alba above and splits to enclose the penis and is attached to the median raphe of the scrotum.

The suspensory ligament of the penis is attached to the front of the symphysis pubis and the fascia of the shaft of the penis.

Q. What is the disposition of fascia transversalis in abdomen?

Ans. Fascia transversalis is a tough fibrous membrane covering the deep surface of transversus abdominis muscle.

Extent:

* Anteriorly, the fascia is blended at the linea alba and becomes continuous with the opposite side.

- Posteriorly, it is continuous with the anterior layer of thoracolumbar fascia and at the lateral border of the kidney becomes continuous with the fascia of Gerota (renal fascia).
- Below, it is attached to the inner lip of the ventral segment of the iliac crest, inguinal ligament, pubic crest, and the pecten pubis and becomes continuous with the fascia iliaca.
- Above, it is continuous with the diaphragmatic fascia.

Q. What are the prolongations of fascia transversalis?

Ans. The fascia transversalis has prolongations outside the abdominal wall as:
- Prolongation through the deep-inguinal ring around the spermatic cord as internal spermatic fascia.
- Prolongation over the femoral vessels deep to the inguinal ligament as anterior layer of femoral sheath.

Q. What are the coverings of kidney (Fig. 23.8)?

Ans. The coverings of kidney are:
- *The fibrous capsule*: Thin membrane closely investing the kidney.
- *Perinephric fat*: This is a layer of adipose tissue lying between the fibrous capsule and the renal fascia.
- *Renal fascia or fascia of Gerota*: This is a fibroareolar sheath investing the kidney.
- *Paranephric fat*: This is a layer of adipose tissue lying outside the renal fascia. This also fills the paravertebral gutter posterior to the kidney.

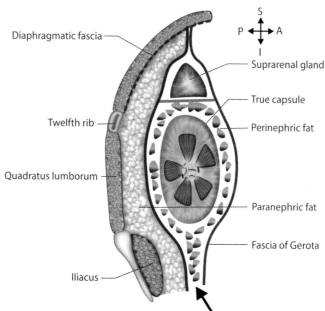

Fig. 23.8: Coverings of kidney. Note that fascial capsule is open inferiorly as shown by the arrow

Q. What is the disposition of renal fascia?

Ans. The renal fascia consists of:
- Anterior layer or fascia of Toldt
- Posterior layer or fascia of Zuckerkandl.

A number of trabeculae connect the renal fascia to the fibrous capsule across the perinephric fat.

♦ Traced above the two layers meet at the upper pole of the kidney and then split to enclose the suprarenal gland and meet again at the upper pole of the suprarenal gland and becomes continuous with the fascia covering the diaphragm.

♦ Traced below the two layers remain separate and enclose the ureter. The anterior layer fuses with the extraperitoneal fatty tissue at right iliac fossa and the posterior layer gets blended with the fascia iliaca.

♦ Laterally, the two layers fuse together and become continuous with the fascia transversalis.

♦ Medially, the anterior layer passes in front of the renal vessels and becomes continuous with the fascial covering of the abdominal aorta and inferior vena cava. The posterior layer becomes continuous with the fascia covering the quadratus lumborum and the psoas major muscle.

At the medial border of the kidney, there is a septum between the two layers of the fascia. The renal vessels pierce this septum and enter into the hilum of the kidney.

■ ESOPHAGUS

Q. What is the extent of esophagus?

Ans.

♦ In an adult of average height, the length of the esophagus is about 25 cm.

♦ Begins at the lower border of the cricoid cartilage at the level of 6th cervical vertebra.

♦ Terminates at the gastroesophageal junction at the level of T11 vertebra.

♦ Distance from incisor teeth to beginning of esophagus—15 cm.

♦ Distance from incisor teeth to gastroesophageal junction—40 cm.

Q. What are the esophageal sphincters?

Ans. There are sphincters at the commencement and termination of the esophagus.

♦ *Upper esophageal sphincter:* This is an anatomical sphincter formed by the inferior constrictor muscle of the pharynx. This muscle consists of two parts:

  1. *An upper oblique fibers (thyropharyngeus)* arising from the cricoid and the thyroid cartilage and encircle the hypopharynx and are inserted into the median raphe.

  2. *The lower horizontal fibers (cricopharyngeus)* arising from the cricoid cartilage and pass horizontally backward round the pharynx and are inserted into the median raphe at the back.

     During swallowing, the upper oblique fibers contract and propel the food downwards and the lower horizontal fibers relax to allow the food to pass into the esophagus.

♦ *Lower esophageal sphincter:* There is no anatomical lower esophageal sphincter. The esophagogastric junction acts as a physiological sphincter.

  The esophageal hiatus is surrounded by the left limb of the right crus. The median arcuate ligament is a tough, 1–3 mm wide fibrous condensation of the medial fibrous borders of the two crura of the diaphragm. This does not contribute to the competence of esophagogastric junction. This is used to anchor the fundus of the stomach during fundoplication operation.

Q. How pharyngeal diverticulum is formed?

Ans. Incoordination of action of thyropharyngeus and the cricopharyngeus, with failure of cricopharyngeus to relax, results in increased intrapharyngeal pressure and leads to formation of a pharyngeal diverticulum.

Q. What are the sites of normal constriction of esophagus?

Ans. There are four sites of normal constriction in the esophagus:
1. At the commencements, at the pharyngoesophageal junctions, at the lower border of the cricoid cartilage, and lying at a distance of 15 cm from the incisor teeth.
2. At the point of crossing by the aorta—about 22.5 cm from the incisor teeth.
3. At the point, where it is crossed by the left root of the lung—about 27.5 cm from the incisor teeth.
4. At the esophageal opening in the diaphragm—about 37.5 cm from the incisor teeth.

Q. What is the arterial supply of the esophagus?

Ans.
* *Above*: By branches of inferior thyroid artery and esophageal branches of the aorta.
* *Below*: By the branches from left gastric and inferior phrenic arteries.

Q. What is the venous drainage of esophagus?

Ans.
* The cervical esophagus drains into the inferior thyroid veins and thence into the brachiocephalic veins.
* The left half of the thoracic esophagus drains into the hemiazygos vein and thence into the brachiocephalic vein.
* The right half of the thoracic esophagus drains into the azygos system of veins and thence intro the superior vena cava.
* The cardioesophageal junction and the abdominal esophagus drain into the coronary, splenic, and retroperitoneal and inferior phrenic veins. There is free communication between the portal and systemic veins. In portal hypertension, these veins may become engorged and form esophageal varices.

Q. How the lymphatics from esophagus are drained (Fig. 23.9)?

Ans. Lymph nodes draining the esophagus are divided into:
* *Paraesophageal lymph nodes*: These lymph nodes lie on the wall of the esophagus. These include cervical, upper, middle, and lower thoracic paraesophageal nodes and paracardiac nodes.
* *Periesophageal lymph nodes*: They are located on the structures lying adjacent to the esophagus. These include cervical, scalene, paratracheal, subcarinal, posterior mediastinal, diaphragmatic, left gastric, lesser curvature, and celiac nodes.
* *Lateral esophageal nodes*: These are located lateral to the esophagus and receive efferent lymphatics from the para- and periesophageal nodes. These include posterior triangle nodes, hilar, suprapyloric, common hepatic, and greater curvature lymph nodes.

The lymphatic vessels arising from the mucous membrane form a submucous plexus. The lymphatic vessels in the submucosa run up and down and penetrate the muscular layer and form a plexus in the adventitial coat. These adventitial lymphatics drain into the adjacent lymph nodes.

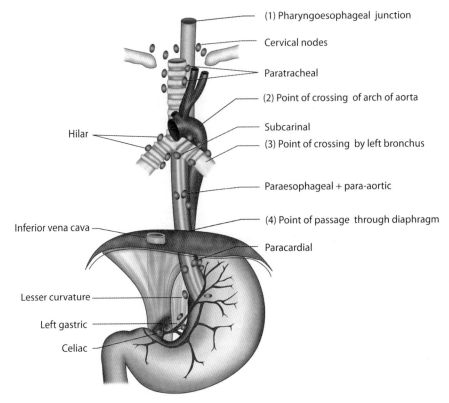

(1) Pharyngoesophageal junction

Cervical nodes

Paratracheal

(2) Point of crossing of arch of aorta

Subcarinal

(3) Point of crossing by left bronchus

Hilar

Paraesophageal + para-aortic

(4) Point of passage through diaphragm

Inferior vena cava

Paracardial

Lesser curvature

Left gastric

Celiac

1, 2, 3, 4—Sites of normal constrictions

Fig. 23.9: Sites of normal constriction of esophagus (1, 2, 3, 4) and groups of lymph nodes draining the esophagus

Q. What is the nerve supply of esophagus?

Ans.
* *Cervical esophagus*: Recurrent laryngeal nerve and branches from the middle and inferior cervical ganglia.
* *Thoracic esophagus*: By branches from the esophageal plexus, from the thoracic splanchnic nerves, and branches from the sympathetic nerve trunk.
* *Abdominal esophagus*: By branches from the anterior and posterior gastric nerves, which arise from the esophageal plexus.

■ STOMACH

Q. What are the parts of stomach (Fig. 23.10)?

Ans. Anatomically, the stomach is divided into:
* *Fundus*: This is the part of the stomach lying above a horizontal plane from the cardiac notch to the greater curvature.
* *Body of the stomach*: This is the part of the stomach lying between the fundus and the pyloric part of the stomach, being demarcated from the pyloric part of the stomach by a plane drawn from the incisura angularis to the greater curvature.

* *The pyloric portion of the stomach*: This extends from the distal part of the body to the pyloric constriction. This is further subdivided into:
  – *Pyloric antrum*: Extends from the incisura angularis to another plane drawn from the right end of the bulging of the greater curvature.
  – *Pyloric canal*: The narrowed part of the distal stomach extending from the end of the pyloric antrum to the pyloric orifice.

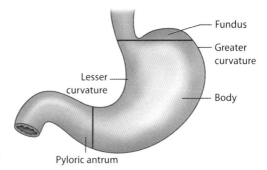

Fig. 23.10: Parts of stomach

* *Lesser curvature of the stomach*: This is the concave border of the stomach and is continuous with the right free border of the esophagus.
* *Greater curvature of the stomach*: This is the convex border of the stomach and starts at the left border of the esophagus, where it joins the stomach.

Q. What are the different gastric glands?

Ans. Histologically, there are three different types of gastric glands in different parts of the stomach:
1. *Cardiac glands*: These are mucous-secreting glands and situated in a small area of the stomach around the esophagogastric junction.
2. *Body or fundic glands*: These glands are situated in the fundus and body of the stomach. The mucosa contains two varieties of cells—(1) the zymogenic cells secrete pepsin and (2) the oxyntic cells secrete hydrochloric acid.
3. *Pyloric glands*: The pyloric glands are mucous-secreting glands. These glands also secrete gastrin.

Q. How lymphatic drainage of stomach occurs?

Ans. *Intrinsic lymphatics of stomach*:
Lymphatics of stomach start in the subepithelial layer and form a plexus around the gastric glands (periglandular plexus). Lymphatic vessels from the periglandular plexus pierce the muscularis mucosae and form a submucous plexus. Lymphatic vessels from the submucous plexus pierce the circular and the oblique muscle coat and form an intramural plexus. Lymphatics from the intramural plexus pierce the longitudinal muscle coat and the serous coat to drain into the adjacent lymph nodes.

For lymph node stations for drainage of gastric lymphatics (*See* Surgical Long Case Section, Page No. 110, Chapter 3).

Q. What is the arterial supply of stomach (Fig. 23.11)?

Ans. There are major and minor arteries supplying the stomach. These include:
* *Vessels along the lesser curvature*:
  – *Left gastric artery*—branch of celiac trunk
  – *Right gastric artery*—branch of hepatic artery.
  These two arteries anastomose along the lesser curvature and divide into anterior and posterior branches and supply the body and pyloric part of the stomach.

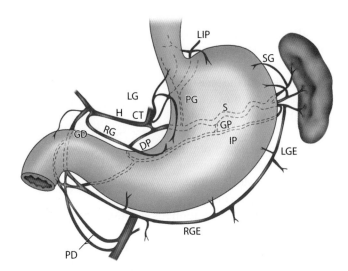

Fig. 23.11: Arterial supply to the stomach. (LIP: left inferior phrenic artery; SG: short gastric artery; LGE: left gastroepiploic artery; RGE: right gastroepiploic artery; S: splenic artery; GP: great pancreatic artery; IP: inferior pancreatic artery; PD: pancreaticoduodenal artery; DP: dorsal pancreatic artery; GD: gastroduodenal artery; RG: right gastric artery; H: hepatic artery; CT: celiac trunk; LG: left gastric artery)

- *Vessels along the greater curvature*:
  - *Right gastroepiploic artery*—a branch of gastroduodenal artery.
  - *Left gastroepiploic artery*—a branch of splenic artery.
  These two arteries anastomose along the greater curvature and give off branches, which supply the body and pyloric part of the stomach.
- *Short gastric arteries*, which are branches of splenic artery, run along the gastrosplenic ligament and supply the fundus of the stomach.
  Some branches from gastroduodenal artery supply the pyloric part of the stomach.

Q. What is the venous drainage of stomach?

Ans. The veins follow the arteries along the lesser and greater curvature:
- *Veins along the lesser curvature*:
  - Right gastric vein drains into the portal vein.
  - Left gastric vein drains into the portal vein.
- *Veins along the greater curvature*:
  - Right gastroepiploic vein drains into the superior mesenteric vein.
  - Left gastroepiploic vein drains into the splenic vein.
  - Short gastric vein drains into the splenic vein.
  Prepyloric vein of Mayo runs anterior to the pylorus of the stomach and connects the right gastric vein with the right gastroepiploic vein.

Q. What is the distribution of vagal trunk in stomach (Fig. 23.12)?

Ans. The right and left vagus nerves enter into the abdomen through the abdomen through the esophageal opening in the diaphragm and continue as anterior and posterior vagus nerve, respectively.

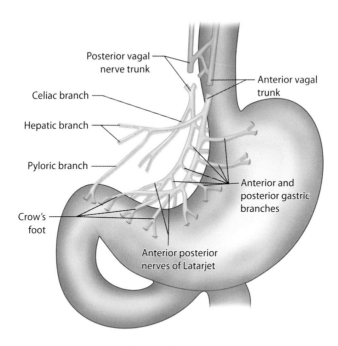

Fig. 23.12: Distribution of vagus nerve in stomach

The anterior vagus nerve gives off the hepatic branch and continues along the lesser curvature and gives off branches to the anterior wall of the fundus and body of the stomach. The anterior vagal trunk then continues as anterior nerve of Latarjet and ends like a crows feet supplying the pyloric region of the stomach.

The posterior vagus nerve gives off celiac branch and then continues along the lesser curvature of the stomach giving off branches supplying the posterior wall of the fundus and the body of stomach and then continues as posterior nerve of Latarjet and supplies the pyloric region of the stomach.

Q. What is the arterial supply of colon (Fig. 23.13)?

Ans. The colon is supplied with branches from superior and inferior mesenteric arteries.

- *Cecum*: Supplied by anterior and posterior cecal arteries, which are branches of inferior division of ileocolic artery.
- *Ascending colon*: Supplied by right colic artery, which is a branch of superior mesenteric artery. The right colic artery divides into ascending and descending branches. The ascending branch joins with the right branch of middle colic artery and the descending branch joins with the superior branch of ileocolic artery.
- *Right colic flexure*: This is supplied by the ascending branch of right colic artery and the right branch of middle colic artery.
- *Transverse colon*: Right two-thirds of transverse colon develops from the midgut, hence it is supplied by the middle colic branch of superior mesenteric artery and the left one-third develops from the hind gut and is supplied by the inferior mesenteric artery. The middle colic artery divides into right and left branch. The right branch joins with the ascending branch

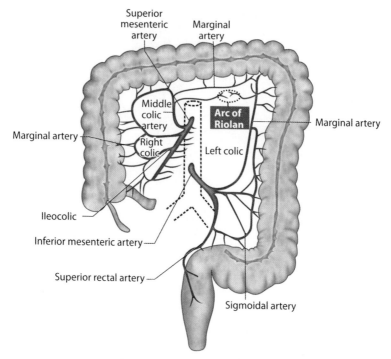

Fig. 23.13: Arterial supply of colon

of right colic artery and the left branch joins with ascending branch of left colic artery. The end arteries vasa recta arise from the marginal artery running along the mesenteric border of the colon.

* *Descending colon*: Supplied by the left colic branch of the inferior mesenteric artery.
* *Sigmoid colon*: Supplied by the sigmoid branches of the inferior mesenteric artery.

Q. What is the lymphatic drainage of colon (Fig. 23.14)?

Ans. Lymphatic of the colon starts at the submucosa and emerges through the serous coat and drains into the following groups of lymph nodes:

* *Epicolic lymph nodes*: These lymph nodes lie on the wall of the colon.
* *Pericolic lymph nodes*: These lymph nodes lie along the terminal vessels (vasa recta) entering the wall of the colon.
* *Intermediate lymph nodes*: These lymph nodes lie along the main branches of the vessels supplying the colon (ileocolic, right colic, middle colic, left colic, and sigmoid branches).
* *Principal lymph nodes*: These are preaortic lymph nodes, which lie along the origin of the superior and inferior mesenteric arteries for the aorta.

The terminal lymphatics from the cecum, ascending colon, and the right half of the transverse colon drain into the superior mesenteric lymph nodes. The terminal lymphatics for the left half of the transverse colon, descending colon, and the sigmoid colon drain into the inferior mesenteric lymph nodes.

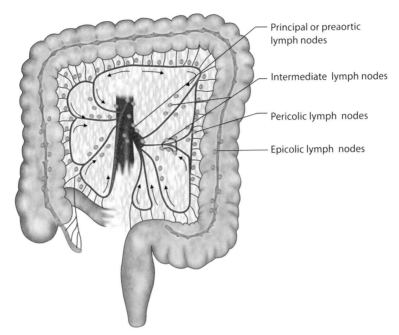

Fig. 23.14: Lymphatic drainage of colon

Labels on figure:
- Principal or preaortic lymph nodes
- Intermediate lymph nodes
- Pericolic lymph nodes
- Epicolic lymph nodes

Q. What is the blood supply of rectum and anal canal (Fig. 23.15)?

Ans. The rectum and anal canal are supplied by the following arteries:

- *Superior rectal artery*: This is the continuation of inferior mesenteric artery. This divides into right and left branches and near the middle of the rectum, it divides into further branches and pierces the muscle of the rectum and descends in the submucous coat up to the level of sphincter ani internus and anastomose with the branches of middle and inferior rectal arteries.
- *Middle rectal artery*: This is branch of anterior division of the internal iliac artery. It runs along the lateral ligaments of the rectum and pierces the muscle coat of the rectum and anastomoses with the branches of the superior and inferior rectal arteries.
- *Inferior rectal artery*: This is a branch of internal pudendal artery. This traverses the ischiorectal fossa and divides into a number of branches, which pierce the anal canal and anastomose with the superior and middle rectal arteries.
- *Median sacral artery*: Arises from the posterior surface of the bifurcation of aorta and supplies branches to the lower rectum and anal canal.

Q. What is the venous drainage of rectum and anal canal (Fig. 23.16)?

Ans. The veins start in the anal valves, as columns of veins at the following sites:

- At 11 o'clock position (anterior and right)
- At 3 o'clock position (anterior and left)
- At 7 o'clock position (posterior and right).

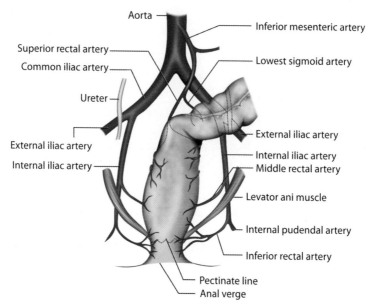

Fig. 23.15: Arterial supply to the rectum and anus

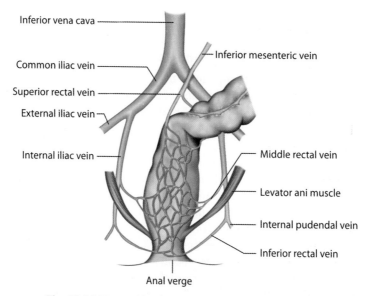

Fig. 23.16: Venous drainage of the rectum and anal canal

In addition, there are columns of veins:
* At 1 o'clock position (anterior and left)
* At 5 o'clock position (posterior and left).

(Dilatation of veins at 11, 3, and 7 o'clock position forms primary piles. The dilatation of veins at 1 and 5 o'clock position forms secondary piles).

These columns of veins ascend in the submucous coat of the rectum and form a plexus in lower part of the rectum—internal rectal venous plexus. From this venous plexus, the drainage occurs as:

◆ *Veins* from the upper part of the plexus pierce the circular and longitudinal muscle coat of rectum and form a venous plexus in the pararectal tissue—external rectal venous plexus. The veins from this plexus drains as:
  – *From the upper part* of the external venous plexus, 6–7 veins emerge on either side, which ascend up joins to form a single vein known as superior rectal vein, which ascends behind the rectum and continues as the inferior mesenteric vein in the pelvic mesocolon. The inferior mesenteric vein ends at the splenic vein and receives sigmoid vein and left colic vein as tributaries.
  – *From the lower part* of the external rectal venous plexus, 6–8 veins emerge on either side, which join to form middle rectal vein, one on either side, which drains into the internal iliac vein.
◆ *There is a plexus of veins* in the skin lined part of the anal canal, which communicates above with the internal rectal venous plexus. These veins drain via the inferior rectal veins into the internal pudendal vein.

Q. How the lymphatics from rectum and anal canal are drained (Figs 23.17 and 23.18)?

Ans. *Intrinsic lymphatics of the rectum*: Lymphatics of the rectum start in the mucous membrane and form a plexus in the submucous coat. Lymphatics from the submucous plexus pierce the circular muscle and form an intramural plexus in-between the circular and the longitudinal muscle coat of the rectum. Lymphatics from the intramural plexus pierce the longitudinal muscle coat of the rectum and form an extramural plexus.

Lymphatic drainage:

◆ From the upper part of the extramural plexus, the lymphatic vessels drain into the pararectal lymph nodes lying in the

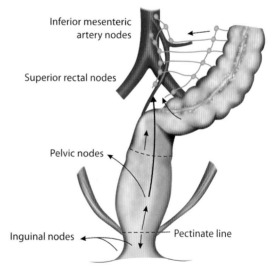

Inferior mesenteric artery nodes

Superior rectal nodes

Pelvic nodes

Inguinal nodes

Pectinate line

Fig. 23.17: Lymphatic drainage of the rectum and anal canal

pararectal tissue. The efferent lymphatics from the pararectal lymph nodes drains as:
  – Efferents from the upper pararectal lymph nodes ascend along the superior rectal vessels and then along the inferior mesenteric vessels and drain into the preaortic lymph nodes lying along the origin of the inferior mesenteric artery.
  – Efferents from the other pararectal lymph nodes drain into the common iliac and internal iliac lymph nodes.
◆ From the lower part of the extramural lymphatic plexus, the lymphatics run laterally and form another plexus on the levator ani and drain ultimately into the internal iliac lymph nodes.

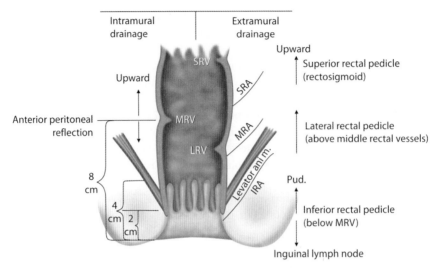

Fig. 23.18: Lymphatic drainage of the rectum and anal canal. (SRV: Superior rectal valve; MRV; middle rectal valve; LRV: lower rectal valve; SRA: superior rectal artery; MRA: middle rectal artery; IRA: inferior rectal artery)

Lymphatics of the anal canal:

* Lymphatics of anal canal above the pectinate line:
  - Lymphatics run with the rectal lymphatics and join the plexus on the levator ani. From this, the lymphatics drain into the internal iliac lymph nodes.
* Lymphatics of anal canal below the pectinate line:
  The lymphatics from the skin lined part of the anal canal drain into the medial group of superficial inguinal lymph nodes.

■ ANATOMY OF LIVER AND EXTRAHEPATIC BILIARY SYSTEM

Q. What is the average weight of liver?

Ans.
* The liver is the largest organ of the body
* In adult male—1.4 kg–1.8 kg
* In adult female—1.2 kg–1.4 kg.

Q. What are anatomical lobes of liver (Fig. 23.19)?

Ans. The liver is demarcated into right and left lobes anatomically by the attachment of falciform ligament in front and above and below and behind by the fissure for ligamentum teres and ligamentum venosum. The right lobe constitutes 5/6th and the left constitutes 1/6th of the liver.

Q. What are physiological or surgical right and left lobes of liver (Fig. 23.20)?

Ans. The physiological right and left lobe of liver is demarcated by an imaginary plane called cholecysto-caval plane, which passes through the floor of gallbladder fossa and inferior vena cava. These lobes are supplied by the right and left branches of the hepatic artery and portal vein and the bile drains into the corresponding right and left hepatic ducts. The caudate lobe

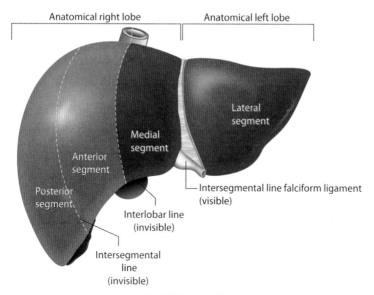

Fig. 23.19: Lobes of liver

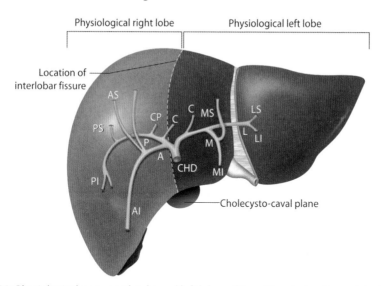

Fig. 23.20: Physiological or surgical right and left lobes of liver. (A: anterior; C: caudate; I: inferior; L: lateral; M: medial; P: posterior; S: superior; CHD: common hepatic duct; CP: caudate process)

belongs to the physiological left lobe of the liver. However, it receives supply from both the right and left branches of hepatic artery and portal vein.

Q. What are the segments of liver (Fig. 23.21)?

Ans. French anatomist, Couinaud, described eight segments in the liver depending on the distribution of branch of hepatic artery, portal vein, and bile duct. The segments are functional units of the liver being supplied by a branch of hepatic artery, portal vein, hepatic duct, and drained by a tributary of hepatic vein.

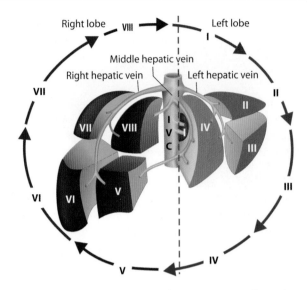

Fig. 23.21: Segments of liver. Arrows indicate positions of hepatic segments according to clockwise order I to VIII

There are eight segments in the liver—segments I–IV in left lobe of liver and segments V–VIII in right lobe of the liver.

- Segment I is the anatomical caudate lobe of the liver.
- Segment II is located in the lateral end of the left lobe.
- Segment III is the medial end of the anatomical left lobe.
- Segment IV is between the ligament of teres and the segment III.
- Segments V and VI in anterior aspect of right lobe.
- Segments VII and VIII in posterior aspect of right lobe.

Q. What are ligaments in relation to the liver (Fig. 23.22)?

Ans. The following ligaments are attached to the liver:

- *Falciform ligament*: A sickle-shaped peritoneal fold connects the liver to the undersurface of diaphragm and anterior abdominal wall up to the umbilicus. It consists of two layers of peritoneum and at the free margin contains ligamentum teres.
- *Coronary ligament*: It consists of upper layer reflected from the liver to the diaphragm and lower layer reflected from the liver to the kidney (hepatorenal ligament).
- *Right triangular ligament* connects right lateral surface of the liver to the diaphragm.

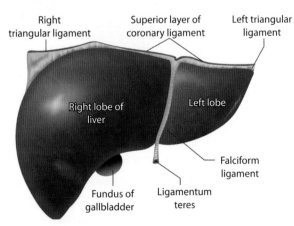

Fig. 23.22: Ligaments in relation to the liver

◆ *Left triangular ligament*: It connects the upper surface of the left lobe to the diaphragm.
◆ *Lesser omentum*: It consists of two layers of peritoneum and connects the lesser curvature of the stomach and proximal 2.5 cm of duodenum to the liver.

Q. What is portal fissure (Fig. 23.23)?

Ans. This is a nonperitoneal H-shaped fissure located in posterior and inferior surface of the liver. The right limb of the fissure consists of groove for inferior vena cava and fossa for gallbladder. The left limb of the fissure consists of fissure for ligamentum teres and ligamentum venosum. The horizontal limb of the fissure is formed by the porta hepatis.

Q. What is porta hepatis (Fig. 23.23)?

Ans. This is a nonperitoneal transverse fissure on the under surface of the liver through which the hepatic artery (right and left branches) and the portal vein (right and left branches) enter into the liver and the hepatic ducts (right and left branches) and lymphatics exit from the liver.

The relation of structures at the porta hepatis from before backwards is:

◆ Hepatic ducts in the front
◆ Branches of hepatic artery
◆ Branches of portal vein.

Q. What is ligamentum teres?

Ans. Ligamentum teres is the remnant of left umbilical vein and runs from the umbilicus to the fissure for ligamentum teres and ends in left branch of portal vein in the inferior surface of liver. This runs in the free margin of the falciform ligament.

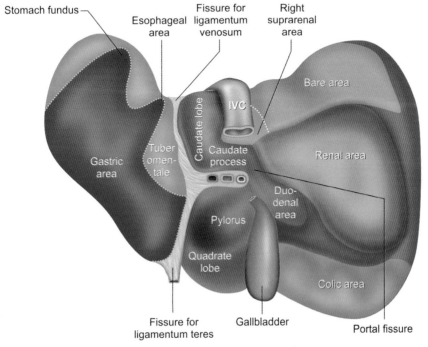

Fig. 23.23: Schematic diagram of porta hepatis

Q. What is ligamentum venosum?

Ans. This is remnant of ductus venosus, which in fetal life connects the left branch of portal vein with the left hepatic vein or the inferior vena cava. This lies in the fissure for ligamentum venosum in the inferior surface of liver.

Q. What constitutes extrahepatic biliary system (Fig. 23.24)?

Ans. The extrahepatic biliary tree consists of:
- Right and left hepatic ducts
- Common hepatic duct
- Gallbladder and cystic ducts
- Common bile duct
- Ampulla of Vater.

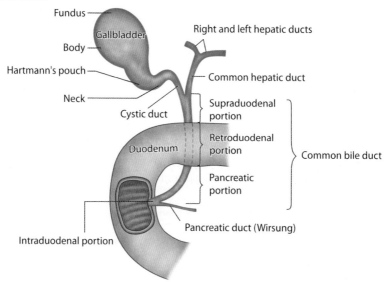

Fig. 23.24: Anatomy of extrahepatic biliary system

Q. What are the parts of gallbladder?

Ans. The gallbladder lies in the gallbladder fossa on the undersurface of the liver. This is a pear-shaped structure with an average length of 7–12 cm and capacity of 30–50 mL. The gallbladder consists of:
- *Fundus*: Part of the gallbladder projecting beyond the inferior border of the liver.
- *Body*: Part of the gallbladder extending from the end of the fundus to the neck of gallbladder.
- *Neck*: The neck of the gallbladder forms an S-shaped curve and connects the body of the gallbladder to a narrow infundibulum, which is continued as cystic duct. From the neck, a small diverticulum may project toward the duodenum. This is known as Hartmann's pouch. The portion of the neck giving attachment to the Hartmann's pouch is known as isthmus of gallbladder.

Q. What is the peculiarity in structure of gallbladder?

Ans. The gallbladder consists of three coats—(1) mucous, (2) fibromuscular, and (2) serous coat. There is no submucous coat in gallbladder.

The mucous membrane is thrown into innumerable folds, which sink into the muscle coat. These are called crypts of Luschka.

The muscle fibers are arranged in a criss-cross fashion and are well developed near the neck of the gallbladder.

The serous coat covers the gallbladder on all sides except part of the gallbladder in contact with the gallbladder bed in liver.

Q. What is the disposition of hepatic ducts, cystic duct, and common bile duct (Fig. 23.24)?

Ans. The right and left hepatic ducts emerge at the porta hepatis. The left hepatic duct purses a longer course than the right hepatic duct. These two ducts join at the confluence to form the common hepatic duct.

The common hepatic duct is 3 cm in length and runs in the free margin of the lesser omentum.

The cystic duct emerges from the neck of the gallbladder is 3 cm long and joins the right margin of the common hepatic duct (CHD) to form the common bile duct.

The common bile duct is 7.5 cm long and is divided into four parts:

1. *Supraduodenal part*: 2.5 cm long runs in the free margin of lesser omentum lying to the right of hepatic artery and in front of portal vein.
2. *Retroduodenal part*: Lying behind the first part of the duodenum.
3. *Infraduodenal part* lies in the groove or in a tunnel in the posterior surface of the head of pancreas.
4. *Intraduodenal part*: Runs obliquely through the wall of the second part of the duodenum, dilates to form the ampulla of Vater and joined by the pancreatic duct opens at the posteromedial wall of the duodenum at the major duodenal papilla.

Q. What are the sphincters around the bile duct (Fig. 23.25)?

Ans.

* *Sphincter choledochus (sphincter of Boyden)*: Sphincter around the terminal part of the bile duct.
* *Sphincter pancreaticus*: This is the sphincter muscle around the terminal part of the pancreatic duct.
* *Sphincter of Oddi*: Sphincter around the ampulla of Vater.

Q. What is the blood supply of gallbladder and biliary tree (Figs 23.26A and B)?

Ans. The gallbladder is supplied by the cystic artery, which is usually a branch of right hepatic artery. The cystic artery arises behind the common hepatic duct, crosses behind, and enters the gallbladder (Fig. 23.26A).

An accessory cystic artery arising from the gastroduodenal artery may also supply the gallbladder (Fig. 23.26B).

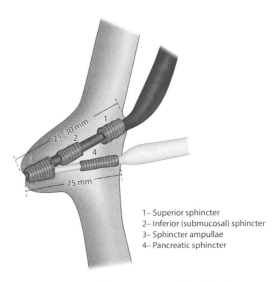

1– Superior sphincter
2– Inferior (submucosal) sphincter
3– Sphincter ampullae
4– Pancreatic sphincter

Fig. 23.25: Sphincters around the bile duct

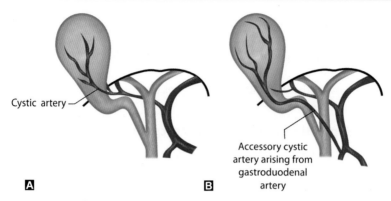

Cystic artery

Accessory cystic
artery arising from
gastroduodenal
artery

A   **B**

Figs 23.26A and B: Arterial supply of gallbladder

The bile duct is supplied by two vertical arteries arising from the hepatic artery running along the bile duct at 3 and 9 O'clock position and giving off circumferential arteries anteriorly and posteriorly.

Q. What is Moynihan's hump (Fig. 23.27)?

Ans. This is one of the anomalies in relation to the course of hepatic artery. The hepatic artery makes a tortuous course in front of the bile duct near the entry of cystic duct. The cystic artery arising from this hump or the hump of right hepatic artery is usually short. This is a dangerous anomaly, as hepatic artery may be confused with cystic artery and may be clipped during cholecystectomy.

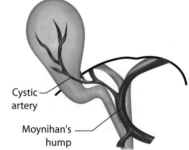

Cystic
artery

Moynihan's
hump

Fig. 23.27: Moynihan's hump

Q. How venous drainage of gallbladder occurs?

Ans. The cystic veins draining the gallbladder do not accompany the cystic artery. These veins pierce the fossa for the gallbladder and drain into the intrahepatic part of portal vein. Rarely, cystic vein drains into the right branch of portal vein.

Q. What is the lymphatic drainage of biliary tree (Fig. 23.28)?

Ans. The lymphatics of gallbladder drain into the cystic lymph node of Lund. The cystic lymph node lies at the junction of cystic duct and common hepatic duct. The efferent from the cystic lymph nodes drains into the pericholedochal lymph nodes and lymph nodes at the porta hepatis and superior and posterior pancreaticoduodenal lymph nodes. These lymphatics then pass into the celiac lymph nodes.

Q. What is the boundary of Calot's triangle (Fig. 23.29)?

Ans. The Calot's triangle is bounded:
- Above by the inferior surface of liver
- Below by the cystic duct
- Medially by the common hepatic duct.

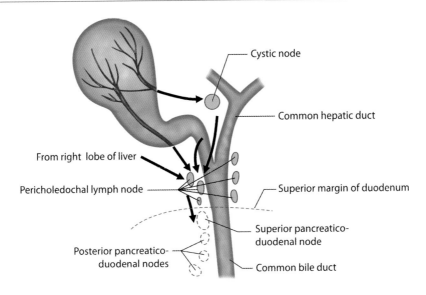

Fig. 23.28: Lymphatic drainage of biliary tree

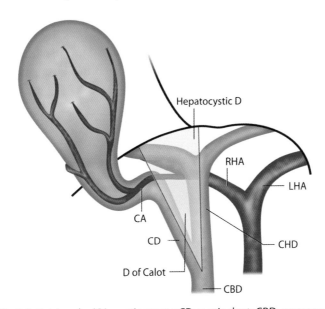

Fig. 23.29: Calot's triangle. (CA: cystic artery; CD: cystic duct; CBD: common bile duct; RHA: right hepatic artery; LHA: left hepatic artery; CHD: common hepatic duct)

Q. What are the functions of gallbladder?

Ans. Gallbladder performs a number of functions:
- *Storage of bile*: Gallbladder stores the bile during fasting. In fasting state, the bile secreted by the liver is diverted into the gallbladder via the cystic duct, as the sphincter of Oddi remains in spasm.

- *Concentration of bile*: Gallbladder concentrates the bile by active absorption of water, sodium bicarbonate, and sodium chloride. The gallbladder is 5–10 times concentrated than the liver bile.
- *Emptying of bile*: In response to feeding, the gallbladder contracts and the sphincter of Oddi relaxes, and resulting in emptying of bile into the duodenum. This is mediated by the hormone cholecystokinin.
- *Secretion mucous*: Gallbladder has the capacity of secretion of mucous. About 20 mL of mucous is secreted by the gallbladder mucosa per day. If the cystic duct is obstructed due to any reason, the bile cannot enter into the gallbladder and the mucous secreted by the gallbladder remains pent-up in the gallbladder resulting in mucocele of gallbladder.

Q. What are the location and parts of pancreas (Fig. 23.30)?

Ans. Pancreas (Greek word—"Pan" means all and "kreas" means flesh) weighs approximately 80–90 g and is located in the retroperitoneum behind the stomach and from the concavity of the duodenum to the hilum of the spleen.

The pancreas consists of following parts:

- *Head*: Lies within the concavity of the duodenum. Constitutes about 30% of the mass of pancreas.
- *Neck*: The junctional area between the head and body of the pancreas. The neck of the pancreas overlies the superior mesenteric vein and the formation of portal vein.
- *Body*: Extends from the left margin of the portal groove to the tail of the pancreas.
- *Tail*: The extreme left portion of pancreas lying between two layers of lienorenal ligament extending up to the hilum of the spleen.
- *Uncinate process*: This is a triangular projection from the lower and left portion of the head of pancreas, which passes upwards and medially behind the superior mesenteric vessels.

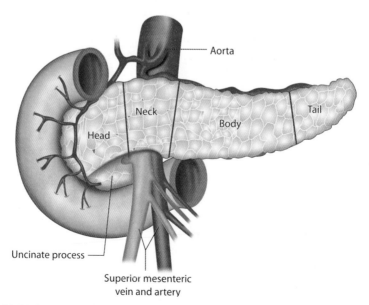

Fig. 23.30: Five parts of pancreas. The line between the body and the tail is arbitrary

Q. What is the disposition of pancreatic duct (Fig. 23.31)?

Ans. The main pancreatic duct (duct of Wirsung) drains the tail, body, and ventral part of the head of the pancreas and joins the common bile duct to form the ampulla of Vater and opens in the posteromedial wall of the second part of the duodenum over the major duodenal papilla.

The minor pancreatic duct (of Santorini) draining the part of the head of the pancreas into the posteromedial wall of the second part of the duodenum above the opening of ampulla of Vater over the minor duodenal papilla.

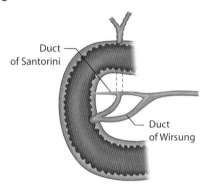

Fig. 23.31: Disposition of pancreatic duct.

Q. How does the pancreas develop?

Ans. The pancreas develops from the dorsal and ventral pancreatic bud.

The dorsal and pancreatic bud arises from the dorsal side of the duodenum and forms the body and tail of pancreas. The duct arising from the dorsal bud and draining the body, and tail opens in the minor papilla.

The ventral pancreatic bud arises from the base of the hepatic diverticulum and forms the head, neck, and uncinate process of the pancreas. The duct draining the head and neck area opens into the major duodenal papilla distal to the opening of dorsal duct. Fusion occurs between the two buds and the ducts also fuses.

The ventral duct and the distal portion of the dorsal duct fuse and form the main pancreatic duct (duct of Wirsung).

The proximal portion of the dorsal duct forms the minor pancreatic duct (duct of Santorini).

Q. What is pancreas divisum (Fig. 23.32)?

Ans. Pancreas divisum is a congenital anomaly, where there is failure of fusion of dorsal and the ventral pancreatic duct.

In this condition, the dorsal pancreatic duct draining the body and tail of the pancreas opens into the minor duodenal papilla.

The ventral pancreatic duct draining the head and neck of the pancreas opens into the major duodenal papilla.

This may result in functional obstruction of the minor duodenal papilla draining the major part of the pancreas resulting in recurrent pancreatitis.

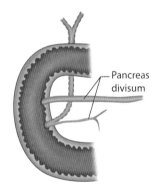

Fig. 23.32: Schematic diagram of pancreas divisum

Q. What is the islet of Langerhans?

Ans. These are endocrine cells in the pancreas and constitutes about 10–20% of pancreatic mass. This consists of:

* Beta cells (70%)—secretes insulin.
* Alpha cells (20%)—secretes glucagon.
* Delta cells—secretes somatostatin.
* Pancreatic polypeptide cells—secretes pancreatic polypeptide.
* Vasoactive intestinal polypeptide (VIP) cells—secretes vasoactive intestinal polypeptide.

Q. What is the arterial supply of pancreas (Fig. 23.33)?

Ans.

◆ *Head and neck*: Supplied by superior and inferior pancreaticoduodenal arteries. Superior pancreaticoduodenal artery is the branch of gastroduodenal artery, and inferior pancreaticoduodenal artery is the branch of superior mesenteric artery. Each of these arteries gives off dorsal and ventral branches and an anastomotic network is formed on the ventral and dorsal aspect of the head of pancreas.

◆ *Body and tail*: Supplied by the pancreatic branches of splenic artery. One of these branches is large and accompanies the main pancreatic duct and is known as arteria pancreatica magna. Occasionally, a dorsal pancreatic branch arising from splenic artery or celiac trunk may supply the dorsal surface of the pancreas.

  A capillary plexus supplies the islet cells and the acini.

◆ *Venous drainage*: The veins follow the arteries and drain into the superior mesenteric vein, splenic vein, and the portal vein.

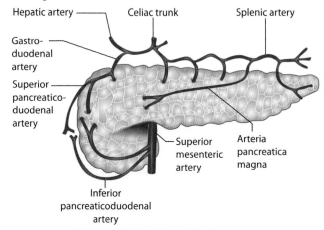

Fig. 23.33: Arterial supply of pancreas

Q. What is the effect of secretin and pancreozymin on pancreatic secretion?

Ans. In response to a meal pancreas secretes juice-containing enzymes and bicarbonates.

  The hormone secretin released by the duodenal mucosa stimulates pancreas to secrete pancreatic juice rich in bicarbonate.

  The hormone pancreozymin (cholecystokinin) released by the duodenal mucosa in response to food stimulates pancreas to secrete a juice rich in enzymes.

  Vagal stimulation increases volume of pancreatic secretion.

■ APPENDIX

Q. What is the length of appendix?

Ans. The length of appendix is highly variable and ranges between 2 cm and 20 cm.

Q. What are the parts of appendix?

Ans. The appendix has a base, body, and tip. The mesentery attached to the appendix is known as mesoappendix.

Q. Where the base of appendix is located (Fig. 23.34)?

Ans. The base of the appendix is attached to the posteromedial wall of the cecum 2 cm below the ileocecal junction.

If the teniae coli in the cecum are traced downwards all the three teniae coli converge to the base of the appendix and continue as the longitudinal muscle coat of the appendix.

On the surface, the base of the appendix lies at McBurney's point, which is located at the right spinoumbilical line (line joining between the anterior superior iliac spine and the umbilicus) at the junction of medial two-thirds and lateral one-third.

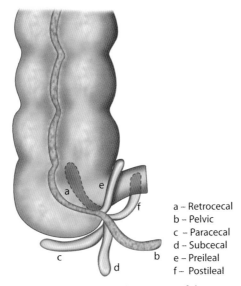

a – Retrocecal
b – Pelvic
c – Paracecal
d – Subcecal
e – Preileal
f – Postileal

Fig. 23.34: Different anatomical positions of the appendix

Q. What is mesoappendix?

Ans. This is the mesentery of the appendix attached to the mesenteric border of the appendix. The mesoappendix contains the appendicular vessels. The mesoappendix does not extend up to the tip of the appendix and the appendicular vessels stop just before the tip of the appendix. The tip of the appendix is the least vascular area, and in obstructive type of appendicitis, the most common site of gangrene is the tip of the appendix.

Q. Which vessels supply the appendix?

Ans. The appendix is supplied by appendicular artery, which is a branch of inferior division of ileocolic artery. The appendicular artery is an end artery.

Sometimes an accessory appendicular artery may arise from the posterior cecal artery and may supply the appendix in addition to appendicular artery.

Q. Why appendix is known as abdominal tonsil?

Ans. The submucous coat of appendix contains lots of lymphoid follicles. The presence of lymphoid follicles is one important etiological factor for development of appendicitis.

Q. What are the different locations of appendix (*see* **Fig. 23.34**)?

Ans. The base of the appendix is usually located at the McBurney's point. The body and the tip of the appendix may lie at different locations and hence named according to the location as:
* *Retrocecal* (60–70%): Most common location and lies behind the cecum.
* *Pelvic* (20–30%): Second most common location lies toward the pelvis.
* *Paracecal* (1–2%): Lies along the side of the cecum.
* *Subcecal* (1%): Lies below the cecum.
* *Splenic* (1–2%): Lies toward the terminal ileum. May be:
  - *Preileal*: Runs in front of the terminal ileum
  - *Postileal*: Runs behind the terminal ileum.

Ectopic appendix: Due to malrotation of the gut, the appendix along with cecum may be located in left iliac fossa or in the right subhepatic region.

Q. What is the extent and branches of abdominal aorta (Fig. 23.35)?

Ans.
* *Extent of abdominal aorta*: The descending thoracic aorta is continued as abdominal aorta at the lower border of the T12 vertebra passing through the aortic hiatus of the diaphragm behind the median arcuate ligament. It runs in front of the vertebral body of L1 to L4 lying little to the left side of the midline. At the level of the body of L4 vertebra, it terminates by dividing into two common iliac arteries.

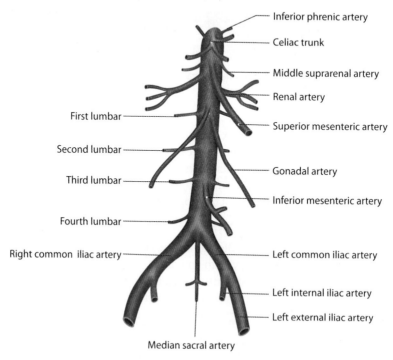

Fig. 23.35: Branches of abdominal aorta

Branches: The branches of abdominal aorta include:

- *Ventral branches*: Three unpaired ventral branches supply the gastrointestinal tract.
  - *Celiac trunk*: Divides into left gastric, hepatic, and splenic arteries.
  - *Superior mesenteric artery*: Gives off inferior pancreaticoduodenal, jejunal, and ileal branches, middle colic, right colic, and terminates as ileocolic artery.
  - *Inferior mesenteric artery*: Gives off left colic, sigmoid branches, and terminates as superior rectal artery.
- *Lateral branches*: These are paired branches.
  - *Inferior phrenic arteries*: First branch of abdominal aorta arise at the level of T12 vertebra
  - *Middle suprarenal arteries*
  - *Renal arteries*
  - *Testicular* or ovarian arteries.
- *Dorsal branches:* These are:
  - *Lumbar arteries*—four pairs
  - *Unpaired median* sacral arteries.

Q. What are the branches of celiac trunk (Fig. 23.36)?

Ans. This is the first ventral branch of abdominal aorta. This subdivides into:

- *Left gastric*: Runs along the lesser curvature and anastomoses with the right gastric artery. Gives off branches to esophagus, fundus of stomach, body, and cardiac end of stomach.
- *Hepatic artery*: The hepatic artery runs in the gastrohepatic omentum. Part of the hepatic artery from its origin to the origin of gastroduodenal artery is called the common hepatic artery. Part of the hepatic artery from the origin of gastroduodenal artery to its bifurcation is called the hepatic artery proper. The branches of hepatic artery includes:
  - Gastroduodenal, which divides into superior pancreaticoduodenal and right gastroepiploic artery.
  - Right gastric

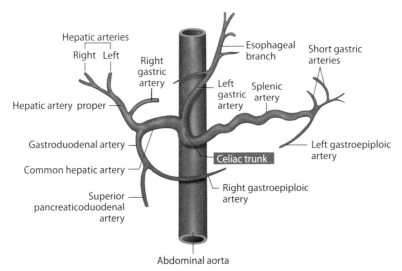

Fig. 23.36: Branches of celiac trunk

- *Branches to bile duct*: Arteries to the bile duct run at 3 O'clock and 9 O'clock position.
- Cystic artery arises from the right branch of the hepatic artery.
- *Two terminal branches*: Right and left hepatic branches supplying the corresponding lobes of the liver.
- An accessory hepatic artery may arise from the superior mesenteric artery or left gastric artery.
- *Splenic artery*: Runs along the upper border of pancreas and reaches the splenic hilum. The branches of splenic artery are:
  - Short gastric branches
  - Left gastroepiploic artery.

Q. What are the branches of superior mesenteric artery (Fig. 23.37)?

Ans. The superior mesenteric artery is a ventral branch of abdominal aorta and arises at the level of L1 vertebra. The branches include:
- *Inferior pancreaticoduodenal*: Runs in the pancreaticoduodenal groove and anastomoses with the superior pancreaticoduodenal artery.
- Middle colic
- Right colic
- Ileocolic
- Jejunal and ileal branches.

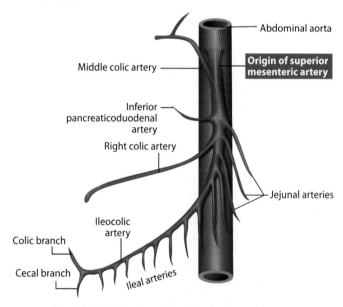

Fig. 23.37: Branches of superior mesenteric artery

Q. What are the branches of inferior mesenteric artery (Fig. 23.38)?

Ans. Inferior mesenteric artery is a ventral branch of the aorta at the level of L3 vertebra. The branches include:
- Left colic artery
- *Sigmoid artery*: May be more than one in number
- *Superior rectal artery*: Inferior mesenteric artery continues as the superior rectal artery.

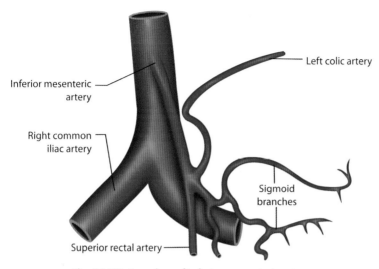

Fig. 23.38: Branches of inferior mesenteric artery

Q. What are the extent and tributaries of inferior vena cava (Fig. 23.39)?

Ans.

- *Origin:* The inferior vena cava is formed by the union of right and left common iliac vein at the level of the 5th lumbar vertebra about 2.5 cm to the right of midline.
- *Termination:* The inferior vena cava opens at the lower and posterior part of right atrium. This opening is guarded by the valve of the inferior vena cava.
- *Tributaries of inferior vena cava:*
  - Right and left common iliac veins, which join to form the inferior vena cava

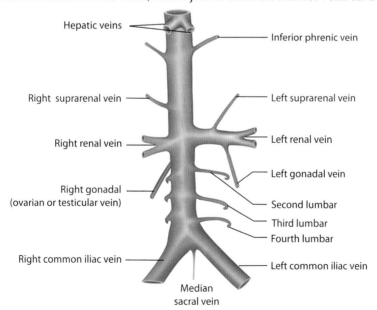

Fig. 23.39: Tributaries of inferior vena cava

   – Median sacral vein
   – Lumbar veins
   – Lumbar azygos vein
   – Right testicular or ovarian vein (the left gonadal vein drains into left renal vein)
   – Right and left renal veins
   – Right suprarenal vein (left suprarenal vein drains into left renal vein)
   – Right inferior phrenic vein (left inferior phrenic vein drains into left suprarenal vein)
   – Hepatic veins (right, middle, and left hepatic veins).

Q. Describe anatomy of portal vein (Fig. 23.40).

Ans. The portal system of veins carries blood from the abdominal part of the gastrointestinal system, spleen, pancreas, and gallbladder to the liver.

The blood in the portal system traverses through two sets of capillaries:

- First set of capillary in the wall of the gut
- Second set of capillary at the liver, where the blood drains into the sinusoids and from there the blood is returned via the hepatic veins and the inferior vena cava.
- *Origin of portal vein*: This is formed by the union of superior mesenteric vein and the splenic vein behind the neck of the pancreas.
- *Course of portal vein*:
  The portal vein ascends behind the neck of the pancreas and the pyloric part of the stomach and runs in the free margin of the lesser omentum running in-between and behind the bile duct and the hepatic artery. The bile duct lies in the right free margin and the hepatic artery lies to the left of the duct. As the vein reaches to the porta hepatis, it divides into the right and left branches and enters into the liver.

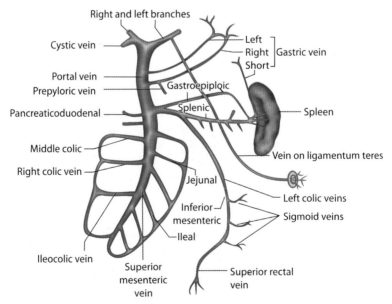

Fig. 23.40: Anatomy of portal vein

Tributaries of portal vein:

- Superior mesenteric vein
- Splenic vein (inferior mesenteric vein drains into the splenic vein)
- Right gastric vein
- Left gastric vein (coronary vein)
- Cystic vein
- Sometimes, prepyloric vein
- Superior pancreaticoduodenal vein
- Paraumbilical vein drains into left branch of portal vein.

Q. What are the sites of portacaval anastomosis (Fig. 23.41)?

Ans.

- *At the abdominal part of the esophagus*:
  - *Portal*: Esophageal tributaries of left gastric vein
  - *Systemic*: Esophageal tributaries of azygos and accessory hemiazygos vein.
- *At the dentate line of anal canal*:
  - *Portal*: Superior rectal vein
  - *Systemic*: Middle and inferior rectal veins.
- *Around the umbilicus*:
  - *Portal*: Paraumbilical vein
  - *Systemic*: Thoracoepigastric and superficial epigastric.
- In portal hypertension, these veins form a bunch of dilated veins around the umbilicus (caput medusae).
- *In the bare area of liver*:
  - *Portal*: Veins from the liver
  - *Systemic*: Diaphragmatic veins.

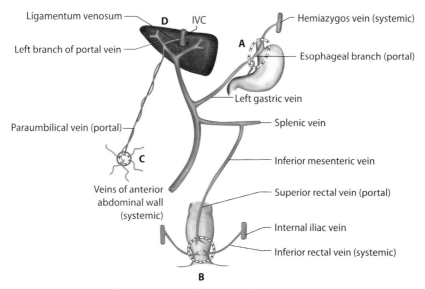

Fig. 23.41: Sites of portacaval anastomosis

◆ *In the retroperitoneum*:
  – *Portal*: Veins of colon and duodenum
  – *Systemic*: retroperitoneal veins and veins from kidney.
◆ *If, due to developmental error*, the ductus venosus remains patent then there is direct communication between the left branch of portal vein and the inferior vena cava providing a portacaval anastomosis.

Q. Describe anatomy of renal vein (Fig. 23.42).

Ans. *Formation of renal vein*: The interlobular vein carries blood from the cortex and medulla and drains into the venous arcades lying along the base of the medullary pyramids. These arcades drain into the interlobar veins, which join to form lobar veins. These lobar veins join to from 5–6 tributaries, which ultimately form the renal vein.

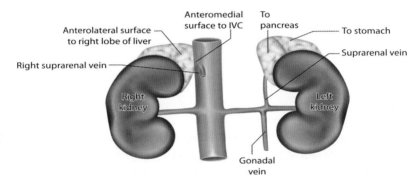

Fig. 23.42: Anatomy of renal vein

Termination of renal vein:

The right renal vein is short and drains into the inferior vena cava. There are no tributaries of right renal vein.

The left renal vein is long (about 7.5 cm), and passes anterior to the abdominal aorta and drains into the inferior vena cava at a little higher level than the right renal vein. The left renal vein receives following tributaries:
◆ Left adrenal vein
◆ Left gonadal vein (testicular or ovarian)
◆ Sometimes left inferior phrenic vein.

▌AUTONOMIC NERVOUS SYSTEM

Q. What constitutes the autonomic nervous system?

Ans. The autonomic nervous system consists of:
◆ Sympathetic nervous system
◆ Parasympathetic nervous system.

Q. What constitutes the sympathetic nervous system?

Ans. The sympathetic nervous system consists of:
* *Preganglionic sympathetic fibers*: These are axons of the nerve cells located at the lateral horn cells of the spinal cord at all the thoracic and upper two lumbar segments (T1–L2. thoracolumbar outflow).
* Sympathetic trunk with the sympathetic ganglia and other paravertebral ganglia.
* Postganglionic sympathetic fibers.

Q. What constitutes the parasympathetic nervous system?

Ans. The parasympathetic nervous system consists of:
* Preganglionic fibers arising from the brain and the sacral segments of the spinal cord (craniosacral outflow).

The preganglionic cranial fibers arise from:
* Edinger–Westphal nucleus (runs along IIIrd nerve)
* Superior and inferior salivary nucleus (runs along VIIth and IXth nerve)
* Dorsal motor nucleus (runs along Xth nerve).

The sacral fibers arise in the gray matter of the spinal cord from second to fourth sacral segments.
* Peripheral parasympathetic ganglia
* Postganglionic parasympathetic fibers.
    The peripheral autonomic nervous system is under the control of central autonomic centers in the brainstem, hypothalamus, and the cerebral cortex.
    The preganglionic sympathetic fibers are short synapses with many postganglionic neurons and these result in an enhanced effect following a sympathetic discharge.
    The preganglionic parasympathetic fibers are long and synapse with only few postganglionic neurons, so the parasympathetic discharge results in a more limited effect.

Q. What are the important neurotransmitters in autonomic nervous system?

Ans.
* *Preganglionic sympathetic fibers*: Acetylcholine
* *Postganglionic sympathetic fibers*: Noradrenaline, except postganglionic fibers to the sweat glands where the neurotransmitter is acetylcholine
* *Preganglionic parasympathetic fibers*: Acetylcholine
* *Postganglionic parasympathetic fibers*: Acetylcholine.

Q. What are white rami communicantes?

Ans. The white rami communicantes carry the preganglionic sympathetic fibers from the spinal nerves into the sympathetic trunk.
    The preganglionic fibers of the sympathetic system arise from the lateral horn cells of the spinal cord from T1 to L2 segments. These fibers exit from the spinal cord along the anterior nerve roots of the spinal nerve and then run a short course along the mixed spinal nerve and exit from the mixed spinal nerve via a white rami communicantes to enter into the sympathetic trunk. So the white rami communicantes are present from T1 to L2 spinal nerves to the corresponding sympathetic ganglia. The postganglionic fibers pass through the gray rami communicantes to the spinal nerve and runs along the vessels.

Q. What constitutes the sympathetic nervous system?

Ans. The gray rami communicantes carry postganglionic sympathetic fibers from the sympathetic ganglia to the corresponding spinal nerves. The gray rami communicantes are present from the cervical to the sacral segments of the sympathetic trunk to the corresponding spinal nerves.

Q. What are the characteristics of sympathetic trunks?

Ans. Sympathetic trunks situated one on either side of the vertebral body consist of ganglia joined by nerve fibers. The sympathetic trunks extend above to the base of the skull and end below in front of the coccyx as ganglion impar.

There are following sympathetic ganglia along the sympathetic trunks:
- *Three cervical ganglia*: Superior, middle, and inferior cervical ganglia
- Eleven thoracic ganglia
- Four lumbar ganglia
- Four sacral ganglia.

Developmentally, each spinal nerve segment had one ganglion. Due to subsequent fusion, the numbers of ganglia are reduced.

The ganglia from T1 to L2 communicantes with the corresponding spinal nerves via the white rami communicantes. The gray rami communicantes are, however, present in all the sympathetic ganglia connecting the ganglia to the corresponding spinal nerves.

Q. What is the distribution of postganglionic sympathetic fibers?

Ans. The postganglionic sympathetic fibers are distributed as:
- *Somatic fibers*:
  The preganglionic sympathetic fibers enter into the sympathetic trunk via the white rami communicantes to synapse with the ganglia corresponding spinal segment or in a ganglia higher or lower in the sympathetic trunk. The postganglionic fibers exit through the gray rami communicantes to the corresponding spinal nerves. These postganglionic fibers are distributed via the spinal nerves as:
  - Vasomotor fibers to the cutaneous blood vessels
  - Sudomotor fibers to the sweat glands
  - Pilomotor fibers to the arrectores pilorum.
- *Visceral fibers*:
  - Thoracic viscera are supplied by the postganglionic fibers arising from the cervical and upper thoracic ganglia via the cardiac, esophageal, and pulmonary plexuses.
  - Abdominal viscera are supplied by the fibers, which exit from the sympathetic trunk without synapsing and run along the greater, lesser, and the lowest splanchnic nerves and synapse in the ganglia of one of the prevertebral plexuses.
  - Fibers to the adrenal medulla run through the sympathetic trunk without synapsing and run through the greater splanchnic nerve and celiac plexus into the adrenal medulla where they synapse with the ganglion cells, which have same embryologic origin as the sympathetic ganglia.
- Postganglionic fibers to the cranial structures like salivary glands, and dilator pupillae are carried via the gray rami communicantes, which accompany the carotid vessels.

Q. What are the characteristics of lumbar sympathetic trunk?

Ans. The lumbar sympathetic trunk lies retroperitoneally on the anterolateral surface of the bodies of lumbar vertebrae. The sympathetic trunk lies medial to the psoas muscle. On the right side, it is partially overlapped by the inferior vena cava and the left side it is partially overlapped by the abdominal aorta.

There are four lumbar sympathetic ganglia. The L2 and L3 lumbar sympathetic ganglia usually fuse to form a single ganglion. The branches of lumbar sympathetic trunk include:

- The ventral rami of L1 and L2 spinal nerve give off white rami communicantes to the corresponding lumbar ganglia. These white rami communicantes carries preganglionic fibers to the sympathetic trunk.
- Gray rami communicantes to all lumbar spinal nerves.
- Splanchnic nerves arising from the lumbar ganglia join the celiac, intermesentcric, and superior hypogastric plexus.

▌BREAST

Q. What are the quadrants of breast (Fig. 23.43)?

Ans. One vertical and one horizontal line are drawn through the nipple. The area of the breast corresponding to the nipple areolar complex is the central quadrant. The outer quadrant is:

- Upper outer quadrant
- Upper inner quadrant
- Lower outer quadrant
- Lower inner quadrant.

Q. What is the extent of normal breast (Fig. 23.43)?

Ans. The extent of the normal breast varies in nulliparous and multiparous women.
In nulliparous women the breast extends:

- Above, up to the second rib
- Below, up to the sixth rib
- Medially, up to the lateral border of sternum
- Laterally, up to the anterior axillary line.

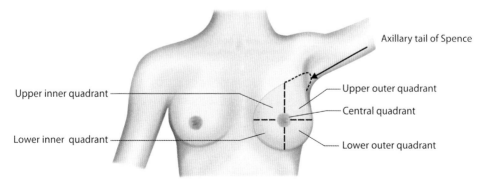

Fig. 23.43: Quadrants of breast and tail of Spence

In multiparous women the breast extends:

- Above, up to the clavicle
- Below up to the eighth rib
- Medially, up to the midline
- Laterally, up to the posterior axillary line.

The axillary tail of breast is a prolongation of a part of the breast toward the axilla.

Q. What are breast lobules?

Ans. The lobules are the structural units of breast. This consists of acini lined by cuboidal or columnar cells. Each lobule is drained by a ductule and 10–100 ductules join to form a lactiferous duct.

There are 15–20 lactiferous ducts in each breast. These ducts run circumferentially and open into the nipple. These lactiferous ducts are lined by specialized myoepithelial cells. At the terminal part of the lactiferous ducts, there is an ampulla, which stores milk before discharge.

Q. What is the ligament of Cooper?

Ans. These are fibrous strands extending from the breast parenchyma to the skin of the breast. When cancers cells spread along these fibrous strands there appear dimpling of the skin due to attachments of the ligaments to the skin.

Q. What are the boundaries of axilla (Fig. 23.44)?

Ans. Axilla is a pyramidal-shaped space between the upper part of the arm and lateral side of the upper chest wall. The axilla has four walls, an apex, and a base.

- *Apex is bounded*:
    - Anteriorly by the clavicle
    - Posteriorly by the upper border of the scapula
    - Medially by the upper border of the first rib
    - Laterally by the coracoid process.

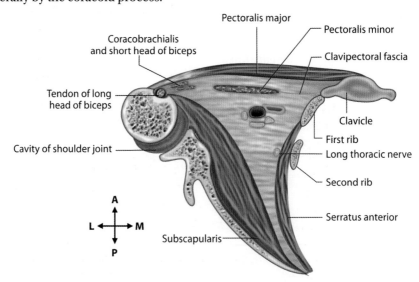

Fig. 23.44: Cross-section of axilla to show its wall

- Base of the axilla is formed by the axillary fascia stretching between the pectoralis major and latissimus dorsi.
- Anterior wall of the axilla is fleshy and is formed by the pectoralis major muscle throughout and behind this by the pectoralis minor and subclavius muscle enclosed within the clavipectoral fascia. Anterior axillary fold is formed by the lateral border of the pectoralis major muscle.
- Posterior wall of the axilla is formed by the subscapularis, latissimus dorsi, and teres major muscle.
  The posterior axillary fold is formed by the subscapularis latissimus dorsi and the teres major muscle.
- The medial wall of the axilla is formed by the upper four or five digitations of the serratus anterior muscles and second to sixth ribs with the intercostal muscles being covered by the serratus anterior muscle.
- Lateral wall of the axilla is formed by upper part of the shaft of the humerus and the conjoint origin of the coracobrachialis and the short head of biceps brachii.

Q. What are the origins and insertion of pectoralis major muscle?

Ans.

- *Origin*: The pectoralis major muscle arises by two heads:
  1. *Clavicular head*: Arises from anterior aspect of the clavicle
  2. *Sternal head*: Arises from the anterior surface of the body of the sternum meeting in the midline with opposite muscle and above extends up to the sternoclavicular joint blending with the clavicular head.
- *Insertion:* The pectoralis major muscle is inserted by a trilaminar aponeurosis into the lateral lip of the bicipital groove of the humerus. The fibers of the clavicular head are inserted by anterior lamina and blend with the middle lamina lying behind it. The sternal fibers get folded upon themself and are inserted by middle and posterior lamina. The upper sternal fibers pass onto the middle lamina and the lower sternal fibers pass onto the posterior lamina. The lowest fibers of origin become the highest fibers of insertion.

Q. What are the actions of pectoralis major muscle?

Ans. The pectoralis major muscle helps in adduction and medial rotation of the shoulder.

The clavicular head of the muscle helps in flexion of the shoulder by raising the humerus during pushing.

The sternal head of the muscle helps in extension of the shoulder joint by bringing the flexed humerus downward and backward to the side.

Q. What is the nerve supply of the muscle?

Ans. It is supplied by both the medial and lateral pectoral nerves arising from the medial and lateral cord of the brachial plexus. The medial pectoral nerve pierces the pectoralis minor muscle and supplies both the muscles.

Q. What are the origins of the pectoralis minor muscle?

Ans.

- *Origin*: This arises from the anterior surfaces of the second to sixth rib and the adjacent costal cartilages.
- *Insertion*: This is inserted by an aponeurosis into the coracoid process near its tip.

Q. What is nerve supply of the pectoralis major and minor muscle?

Ans. It is supplied by medial and lateral pectoral nerves.

Q. What is the disposition of clavipectoral fascia?

Ans. This is a fascial condensation lying between the pectoralis minor and the clavicle.

Attachment of clavipectoral fascia:

- *Above,* it splits to enclose the subclavius. The superficial layer is attached to anterior margin of the subclavian groove on the inferior aspect of clavicle. The deep layer is attached to the posterior margin of the subclavian groove and is continued into the neck with deep cervical fascia covering the inferior belly of omohyoid.
- *Below,* it splits to enclose the pectoralis minor muscle and at the lower border of pectoralis minor, it is continued as the suspensory ligament of axilla.
- *Laterally,* it is attached to the coracoid process and the coracoclavicular ligament.
- *Medially,* it is attached to the first rib and blends with the fascia covering the first and second intercostal space.

Q. Which structures pierce the clavipectoral fascia?

Ans. The following structures pierce the clavipectoral fascia:
- Cephalic vessels
- *Lateral pectoral nerve*—a branch of lateral cord supplies the pectoralis major muscle
- Acromiothoracic vessels
- Lymphatic vessels.

Q. What are the parts of axillary artery?

Ans. Axillary is the continuation of the subclavian artery and extends from the outer border of the first rib and the outer border of the teres major muscle, wherein it is continued as the brachial artery.

Axillary artery is divided into three parts in relation to the pectoralis minor muscle.
- *First part:*
  - Part of the artery lying between the outer border of the first rib and the upper border of pectoralis minor.
- *Second part:*
  - Part of the artery lying behind the pectoralis minor muscle.
- *Third part:*
  - Part of the artery lying between the lower border of the pectoralis minor and the lower border of teres major muscle.

Q. What are the branches of axillary artery (Fig. 23.45)?

Ans. One branch from first part, two branches from second part, and three branches from third part of axillary artery are as follows:
- *First part:* (One branch) superior thoracic artery.
- *Second part:* (Two branches)
  1. *Thoracoacromial:* Arises at upper border of pectoralis minor, and pierces pectoralis minor divides into four branches—(1) clavicular, (2) pectoral, (3) acromial, and (4) deltoid branches.
  2. *Lateral thoracic:* Runs along the lower border of the pectoralis minor to the chest wall.

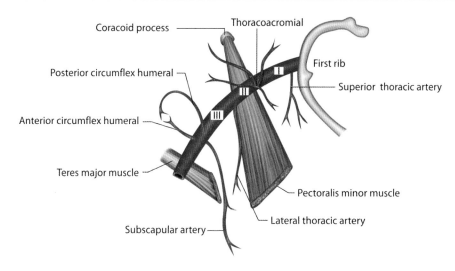

Fig. 23.45: Branches of axillary artery

- *Third part:* (Three branches)
  1. *Subscapular:* Largest branch runs along the posterior wall of the axilla. Gives off circumflex scapular artery, which forms a plexus on the dorsum of scapula.
  2. Posterior circumflex humeral
  3. Anterior circumflex humeral. The circumflex arteries encircle the surgical neck of the humerus. The posterior circumflex humeral accompanies the axillary nerve.

Q. What are the different groups of axillary lymph nodes?

Ans. *See* Surgical Long Cases Section, Page No. 237, Chapter 5.

Q. What are the contents of the axilla?

Ans. The contents of the axilla are:
- Vessels of the upper limbs
- Nerves of the upper limbs
- Two heads of the biceps brachii
- Origin of the coracobrachialis
- Loose areolar tissue and the lymph nodes.

Q. What are the origins and insertion of serratus anterior muscle?

Ans.
- *Origin:* The serratus anterior muscle arises by fleshy digitations from the outer surfaces of the upper eight ribs. The fibers arising from the upper four ribs lie deep to the pectoralis minor muscle and the fibers arising from the next four ribs interdigitate with the fibers of external oblique muscle of the abdomen.
- *Insertion:* This is inserted on the costal aspect of the medial border of the scapula and by a larger triangular insertion at the costal surface of the inferior angle of the scapula and a smaller triangular area at the costal surface of the upper angle of the scapula.

◆ *Action*: The serratus anterior helps in pulling the scapula forward while the arm is raised either in front of the body or away to the side. If paralyzed the medial border and the inferior angle of the scapula will project from the back during the above movement, this is known as winging of the scapula.

◆ *Nerve supply*: By long thoracic nerve.

Q. What are the layers of scalp (Fig. 23.46)?

Ans. The scalp is the soft tissue covering of the skull and consists of:

◆ *S*: Skin
◆ *C*: Subcutaneous tissue
◆ *A*: Galea aponeurotica and occipitofrontalis
◆ *L*: Loose connective tissue
◆ *P*: Pericranium.

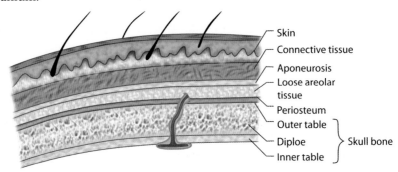

Fig. 23.46: Schematic diagram of layer of scalp

Q. What is the peculiarity of subcutaneous tissue of scalp?

Ans. The subcutaneous tissue of scalp consists of a close network of fibrofatty tissues and is attached firmly to the overlying skin and the underlying galea aponeurotica. Numerous vessels are found in this layer. The walls of the blood vessels are densely adherent to the fibrous tissue.

In case of scalp injury, these vessels remain open in the network of fibrous tissue resulting in profuse bleeding. The bleeding can be controlled by pressure over the injured scalp against the bone.

Q. What is the disposition of galea aponeurotica?

Ans. The galeal or the epicranial aponeurosis is a thin tendinous sheet, which unites the occipital and frontal bellies of occipitofrontalis muscle.

Behind, it extends between the two bellies of occipitofrontalis muscle and is attached to the external occipital protuberance and highest nuchal line. In front, it sends a narrow slip between the two bellies of frontalis muscle and blends with the subcutaneous tissues at the root of nose. Laterally, it blends with the temporal fascia.

Q. What are the peculiarities of loose areolar layer of the scalp?

Ans. The loose areolar tissue lies deep to the aponeurotic layer. The loose areolar tissue contains few small arteries and some important emissary veins. The emissary veins are valveless and connect the superficial veins of the scalp with the diploic veins of the skull bones and intracranial venous sinuses.

An infection in this layer may rapidly spread to intracranial venous sinuses, so this layer of the scalp is also known as danger area of the scalp.

Collection of blood or pus in this layer produces generalized swelling of the scalp posteriorly extending up to the highest nuchal line and anteriorly extends up to the upper eyelid as there is no bony attachment of the frontalis muscle.

Q. What is the blood supply of the scalp (Fig. 23.47)?

Ans. The scalp has a rich blood supply and a small cut may cause profuse bleeding. The following arteries supply the scalp:
+ Supratrochlear and supraorbital arteries, branches of ophthalmic artery run along the corresponding nerves.
+ Superficial temporal artery, the smaller terminal branch of the external carotid artery runs up in front of the tragus along with auriculotemporal nerve.
+ Posterior auricular artery, a branch of external carotid artery ascends behind the pinna.
+ Occipital artery, a branch of external carotid artery runs up in occipital region along with greater occipital nerve.

The venous drainage occurs through:
+ Supratrochlear and supraorbital veins, which join at the medial angle of the orbit to form the facial vein.
+ Superficial temporal vein, which joins with the maxillary veins in the substance of the parotid gland to form the retromandibular vein.
+ Posterior auricular vein, which joins with the posterior division of the retromandibular vein to form the external jugular vein.
+ Occipital vein, which drains into the occipital venous plexus. The occipital venous drains into both the vertebral vein and internal jugular vein.

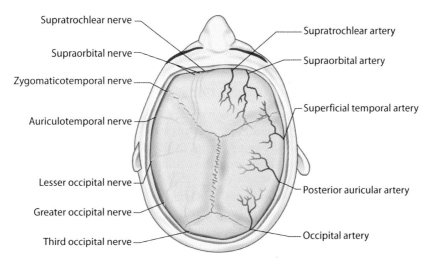

Fig. 23.47: Scalp—arterial supply shown on right and nerve distribution shown on left.
Veins are not shown, but follow the arteries

The veins of the scalp freely anastomose with each other and are connected to the diploic veins of the skull bone. These veins also communicate with the intracranial venous sinuses through the valveless emissary veins.

Q. What is the nerve supply of the scalp (Fig. 23.48)?

Ans. The nerves supply of the Scalp are as follows:
- Supratrochlear and supraorbital nerves, which are branches of ophthalmic nerve.
- Zygomaticotemporal nerve, a branch of maxillary division of trigeminal nerve.
- Temporal branch of facial nerve supplies the frontal belly of occipitofrontalis.
- Auriculotemporal nerve, a branch of mandibular division of trigeminal nerve.
- Posterior branch of greater auricular nerve.
- Posterior auricular branch of facial nerve supplies occipital belly of occipitofrontalis muscle.
- Lesser occipital nerve from C1 nerve of cervical plexus.
- Greater occipital nerve from C2 of cervical plexus.
- The third occipital nerve from dorsal ramus of C3 nerve.

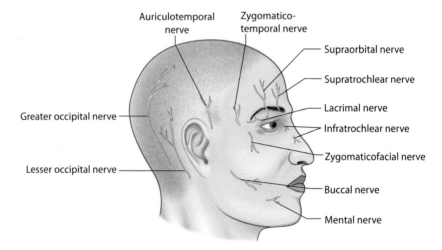

Fig. 23.48: Nerve supply of the scalp

Q. What are the veins of the face (Fig. 23.49)?

Ans. The nerves supply of the Scalp are as follows:
- *Facial vein*: The facial vein begins as the angular vein at the inner angle of the orbit by joining of supratrochlear and supraorbital veins. In the neck, the facial vein is joined by anterior division of retromandibular vein and forms the common facial vein, which drains into the internal jugular vein.
- *Retromandibular vein*: The retromandibular vein is formed within the substance of the parotid gland by joining of superficial temporal and maxillary vein. At the lower pole of the parotid gland, the retromandibular vein divides into anterior and posterior division.
  The anterior division joins the facial vein to form the common facial vein. The posterior division joins with posterior auricular vein to form the external jugular vein.

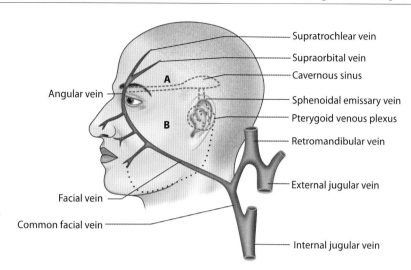

Fig. 23.49: Veins of the face

- *External jugular vein*: The external jugular vein is formed by joining of posterior division of retromandibular vein and the posterior auricular vein. The external jugular vein drains into the subclavian vein.
- The occipital vein joins the suboccipital venous plexus, which drains either into the internal jugular vein or into the vertebral vein.
- *Anterior jugular vein*: The anterior jugular vein is formed below the chin by union of small veins from the submandibular region and descends downwards in the neck on either side of the midline.

Q. What is the sensory nerve supply of the face (Fig. 23.50)?

Ans. The face is supplied by sensory branches of three divisions of the trigeminal nerve—(1) ophthalmic, (2) maxillary, and (3) mandibular divisions. Three distinct areas in the face are supplied by these nerves:

1. *Ophthalmic zone*: Tip and sides of the nose, forehead, and the upper eyelid.
2. *Maxillary zone*: Upper lip, part of the sides of the nose lower eyelid, malar prominence, and a small portion of temporal region.
3. *Mandibular zone*: Lower lip, chin, skin overlying the mandible excluding the angle, cheek, part of pinna, external acoustic meatus, and most of the temporal region.
   An area near the angle of the mouth is supplied by the greater auricular nerve.

The following nerves supply the different areas of the face:

- *Branches from the ophthalmic division*:
  - *Lacrimal nerve*—supplies the lateral part of the upper eyelid.
  - *Supraorbital nerve*—supplies the forehead and the scalp up to the vertex.
  - *Supratrochlear nerve*—supplies the middle of the forehead and scalp.
  - *Infratrochlear nerve*—supplies the medial part of the upper eyelid and side of the nose.
  - *External nasal nerve*—supplies the tip and ala of the nose.

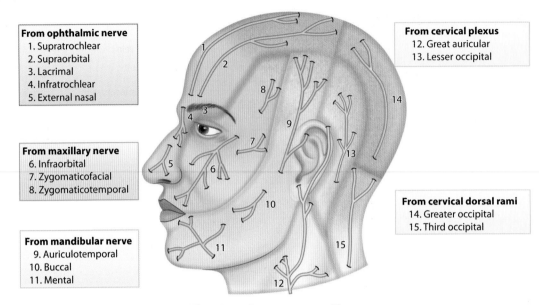

From ophthalmic nerve
1. Supratrochlear
2. Supraorbital
3. Lacrimal
4. Infratrochlear
5. External nasal

From maxillary nerve
6. Infraorbital
7. Zygomaticofacial
8. Zygomaticotemporal

From mandibular nerve
9. Auriculotemporal
10. Buccal
11. Mental

From cervical plexus
12. Great auricular
13. Lesser occipital

From cervical dorsal rami
14. Greater occipital
15. Third occipital

Fig. 23.50: Sensory nerves of face

- *Branches from the maxillary division of trigeminal nerve*:
  - *Infraorbital nerve*: Continuation of maxillary nerve and emerges through the infraorbital foramen and divides into three branches:
    1. Palpebral branch supplies the lower eyelid.
    2. Labial branch supplies the upper lip and cheek.
    3. Nasal branch supplies the sides and ala of the nose.
  - *Zygomaticofacial nerve*—emerges through the zygomatic foramen and supplies the overlying skin.
  - Zygomaticotemporal nerve supplies the temporal region.
- *Branches from the mandibular division of trigeminal nerve*:
  - *Auriculotemporal nerve*: Runs vertically upwards across the posterior root of zygoma and divides into:
    - *Auricular branch*—supplies the pinna and the external acoustic meatus.
    - *Temporal branch*—supplies the skin over the temporal region.
  - *Buccal branch*—supplies skin over the cheek and also the mucous membrane of the cheek after piercing the buccinator muscle.
  - *Mental nerve*—emerges through the mental foramen supplies the skin and mucous membrane of the lower lip.

Q. How do the face and lips develop?

Ans. During the second week of intrauterine life, the face of the embryo is represented by an area bounded cranially by the neural plate caudally by the pericardium and laterally by the mandibular process of the first pharyngeal arch on each side. A depression appears in the center of this area known as stomodeum. The inner lining of the stomodeum is the buccopharyngeal membrane and at 4th week of intrauterine life, the buccopharyngeal membrane disappears and the stomodeum communicates with the foregut.

A number of processes develop around the stomodeum and help in development of face.

■ CERVICAL FASCIA

Q. What is the disposition of cervical fascia?

Ans. Fascial investment of the neck is the cervical fascia. The cervical fascia is broadly divided into:

* Superficial cervical fascia
* Deep cervical fascia.

The superficial cervical fascia is a thin fascial layer, which lies between the *dermal layer of the skin* and the *deep cervical fascia.*

Q. Which structures lies in the superficial cervical fascia?

Ans. The following structures lies in relation to the superficial cervical fascia:

* Fat in obese individual, there is more fat in the superficial fascia.
* Platysma muscle.

The *platysma* muscle is situated on the anterior aspect of the neck and arises by two heads from the fascia covering the *pectoralis major* and *deltoid*. These fibers from the two heads cross the clavicle and meet in the midline, and fusing with the muscles of the face.

The nerve supply of platysma is via the cervical branch of the *facial nerve.*

* Cutaneous nerves
* Superficial blood vessels of the neck
* Superficial lymphatic vessels and superficial cervical lymph nodes.

Q. What is the disposition of deep cervical fascia?

Ans. The deep cervical fascia is located underneath the superficial fascia and invests all the deeper structures of the neck. The different layers of the deep cervical fascia are:

* Investing layer
* Pretracheal layer
* Prevertebral layer.

Q. What is the disposition of investing layer of deep cervical fascia (Fig. 23.51)?

Ans. The investing layer of deep cervical fascia extends as follows:

* Posteriorly attached to the ligamentum nuchae and the spines of cervical vertebrae.
* This fascial layer splits to enclose the trapezius muscle and runs medially to form the roof of the posterior triangle.
* At the lateral border of the sternocleidomastoid, it splits to enclose the sternocleidomastoid muscle and runs medially to form the roof of the anterior triangle of the neck and becomes continuous with investing layer of the deep cervical fascia of the opposite side.
* Superiorly this fascial layer is attached to the:
  - External occipital protuberance
  - Superior nuchal line
  - Mastoid process
  - Base of the mandible.
  This layer splits to enclose the parotid and submandibular salivary glands.

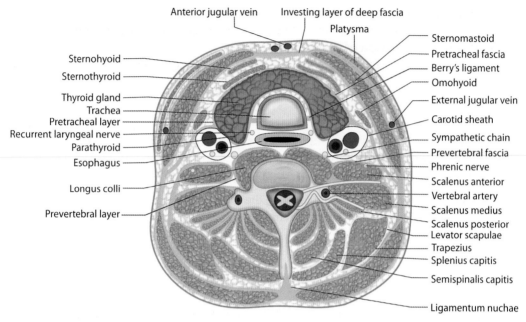

Fig. 23.51: Disposition of layers of cervical fascia

Inferiorly, this fascial layer is attached to the:

- Spine of scapula
- Acromion process
- Clavicle and the upper border of the manubrium sterni.

This fascial layer splits inferiorly to form the suprasternal space of burns and the supraclavicular space.

Anteriorly, this fascial layer is attached to the symphysis menti and hyoid bone above and becomes continuous with the investing layer of the fascia of the opposite side.

Q. What is the disposition of pretracheal layer of the deep cervical fascia?

Ans. Deep to the sternocleidomastoid muscle, a fascial prolongation reaches the thyroid gland where it splits to enclose the thyroid gland and medially this gets blended with the fascial covering of the trachea.

A part of this pretracheal fascia extending between the thyroid gland and the cricoid cartilage is thickened to form the Berry's ligament.

Superiorly, this layer is attached to the hyoid bone, oblique line of thyroid cartilage and the cricoid cartilage.

Inferiorly, this layer invests the thyroid veins run behind the brachiocephalic vein and gets blended with the fascial covering of the arch of the aorta.

Q. What is the disposition of prevertebral layer of the deep cervical fascia?

Ans. This layer invests the prevertebral muscles and forms the floor of the posterior triangle of the neck.

Superiorly, this fascial layer is attached to the base of the skull.

Inferiorly, this fascial layer is attached to the anterior longitudinal ligament and the body of the fourth thoracic vertebra.

Anterior to the prevertebral fascia is the retropharyngeal space containing loose areolar tissue.

Carotid sheaths:

The carotid sheaths are paired fascial sheath, which enclose important vessels and nerves. The carotid sheath extends from the *base of the skull to the thoracic mediastinum. This is of clinical importance as a pathway for the spread of infection. The fascial layers of the carotid sheath are derived from the pretracheal, prevertebral, and investing layers of the deep cervical fascia.*

The contents of the carotid sheath are:

- Common carotid artery (which bifurcates within the sheath into the external and internal carotid arteries).
- Internal jugular vein.
- Vagus nerve.

Q. What is the relevance of these fascial dispositions?

Ans. The cervical fascia forms different compartments in the neck. A superficial skin infection is prevented from spread into the deep neck space by the tough investing layer of the deep fascia.

Infections occurring deep to the deep fascia may spread along the fascial planes.

Infection posterior to the prevertebral fascia: Initially forms a prevertebral abscess. The pus may erode through the prevertebral fascia and reach the retropharyngeal space. Through the retropharyngeal space, the pus may point into the thorax.

Laterally, the pus may point laterally into the posterior triangle of the neck and thence to the axilla.

Infection between the investing layer of the deep cervical fascia and the pretracheal fascia: The pus can track down into the chest in anterior mediastinum.

■ THYROID GLAND

Q. What are the parts of thyroid gland?

Ans. Thyroid gland, weighing about 25 g, is a butterfly-shaped structure located in the front and sides of the lower part of the neck. The gland consists of:
- Right and left lateral lobes
- Isthmus
- Sometimes, a pyramidal lobe may project upwards from the isthmus.

Q. Where is the thyroid gland located?

Ans. The thyroid gland is located in the thyroid region.

Each of the lateral lobes extends above up to the oblique line of the thyroid cartilage and below up to the fourth or fifth tracheal ring.

The isthmus of the thyroid gland lies over the second, third, and fourth tracheal rings.

Q. What are the parts of each lobe of the thyroid gland?

Ans. The thyroid lobe consists of two borders and three surfaces:
- *Borders*:
  - The anterior border is thin and is related to the anterior branch of superior thyroid artery.
  - The posterior border is broad and rounded and is related to the branch of the inferior thyroid arteries and the parathyroid glands.
- *Surfaces*: There are three surfaces:
  1. The anterolateral surface is convex and is covered by sternothyroid, sternohyoid, superior belly of omohyoid, and medial border of sternocleidomastoid.
  2. The medial surface is related to two tubes—(1) trachea and (2) esophagus, two nerves—(1) external laryngeal and (2) recurrent laryngeal, and two muscles—(1) inferior constrictor of pharynx and (2) cricothyroid.
  3. Posterior surface is related to carotid sheath.

Q. What is the disposition of the isthmus of the thyroid gland?

Ans. The isthmus of the thyroid gland joins the two lobes and lies over the second, third, and fourth tracheal rings.

The isthmus has superior and inferior borders and anterior and posterior surfaces. The posterior surface lies over the second, third, and fourth tracheal rings.

Q. What is pyramidal lobe?

Ans. This is described as a third lobe and may be present in some cases extending from the upper border of isthmus and may extend up to the hyoid bone.

Q. What is levator glandulae thyroideae?

Ans. In some cases, a fibrous band may be present extending from the body of the hyoid bone to the isthmus or to the pyramidal lobe.

Q. What are the capsules of the thyroid gland?

Ans. The capsules of the thyroid gland are:
- *True capsule*: Formed by condensation of the connective tissue of the gland.
- *False capsule*: The pretracheal layer of the deep cervical fascia splits to enclose the thyroid gland and forms the false capsule.

A rich venous plexus lies deep to the true capsule of the thyroid gland. So, during thyroidectomy dissection is done between the false and true capsules of the thyroid gland. Dissection deep to the true capsule will result in excessive bleeding.

Q. What is the blood supply of thyroid gland (Fig. 23.52)?

Ans. *Arterial supply*: The arterial supply is by:
- *Superior thyroid artery*: First branch of external carotid artery. Runs in close relation to the external laryngeal nerve at its initial course and at the upper pole divides into an anterior and posterior branch.

- *The anterior branch* runs along the anterior border of the lateral lobe and continues along the upper border of the isthmus to anastomose with the same artery of the opposite side.
- *The posterior branch* runs along the posterior border of the lateral lobe and anastomoses with an ascending branch of inferior thyroid artery.

♦ *Inferior thyroid artery*: A branch of thyrocervical trunk (branch of subclavian artery) runs deep to the carotid sheath and reaches the lower pole of the thyroid gland gives off four to five branches, which supply the thyroid gland. An ascending branch anastomoses with the posterior branch of superior thyroid artery and supplies the parathyroid glands. The recurrent laryngeal nerve is in close relation to the inferior thyroid artery close to the gland.

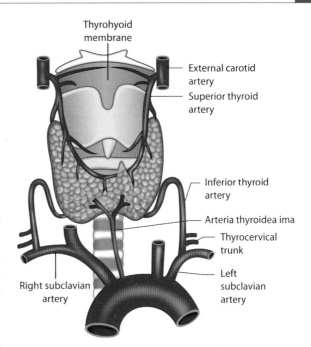

Fig. 23.52: Arterial supply of thyroid gland

♦ *Arteria thyroidea ima*: In about 3% of patients, there may be an additional supply by arteria thyroidea ima, which arises from the brachiocephalic trunk or arch of the aorta and enters into the lower part of the isthmus.

♦ *Tracheal and esophageal branches*: In addition to the above named arteries, the thyroid gland is also supplied by minor branches arising from the tracheal and esophageal branches.

Venous drainage (Fig. 23.53):

The venous drainage is via:

♦ *Superior thyroid vein*: Runs along the superior thyroid artery and drains into the internal jugular vein.

♦ *Middle thyroid vein*: A short and slender vein emerges from the middle of the thyroid lobe and drains into the internal jugular vein.

♦ *Inferior thyroid veins*: Emerges at the lower of the lateral lobes and joins at the lower border of the isthmus and drains into the left brachiocephalic vein.

♦ *A fourth thyroid vein (vein of Kocher)*: May present emerging between the middle and inferior thyroid vein and drains into the internal jugular vein.

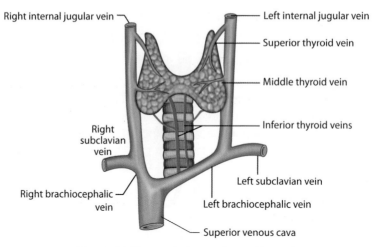

Fig. 23.53: Venous drainage of thyroid gland

Q. What is the lymphatic drainage of thyroid gland (Fig. 23.54)?

Ans. There is a rich lymphatic plexus within the thyroid gland. The lymphatics emerge from the gland and drain as:

- From upper part of the gland—to level II, level III, level V lymph nodes, and prelaryngeal lymph nodes (level VI)
- From lower part of the gland, the lymphatic reaches the level IV, level V, and pretracheal lymph nodes (level VI).

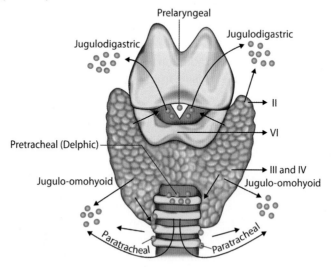

Fig. 23.54: Lymphatic drainage of thyroid gland

Q. How does the thyroid gland develop?

Ans. *See* Surgical Short Cases Section, Page No. 492, Chapter 11.

Q. What are fates of thyroglossal duct?

Ans. *See* Surgical Short Cases Section, Page No. 492, Chapter 11.

Q. What is the location of parathyroid glands?

Ans. There are two pairs of parathyroid glands each weighing about 50 mg. They lie as:

- *Superior parathyroid gland*: Develops from fourth branchial pouch. More constant in position. Lies at the middle of the lateral lobe along the posterior border of the thyroid gland. Lies close to the arterial anastomosis of superior and inferior thyroid artery.
- *Inferior parathyroid gland*: Develops from the third branchial pouch. Their location is variable and may lie:
  - Within the thyroid capsule near the lower pole.
  - Outside the thyroid capsule immediately above the inferior thyroid artery.
  - In superior mediastinum in an ectopic location.

Q. What are the branches of arch of the aorta?

Ans. The branches of the arch of the aorta are:

- *Brachiocephalic trunk*—divides into right subclavian and the right common carotid artery.
- *Left common carotid artery*
- *Left subclavian artery*
- *Arteria thyroidea ima* in some cases.

■ SUBCLAVIAN ARTERY

Q. What are the parts of subclavian artery (Fig. 23.55)?

Ans. The subclavian artery is a branch of brachiocephalic trunk on the right side and branch of arch of the aorta on the left side.

The subclavian artery extends from the sternoclavicular joint to the outer border of the first rib where it is continued as axillary artery.

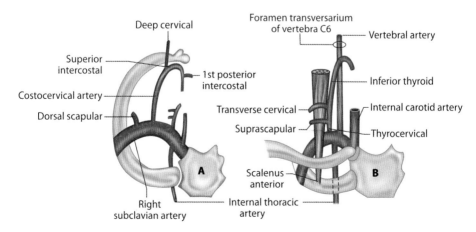

Fig. 23.55: Branches of right subclavian artery

The subclavian artery is crossed by scalenus anterior muscle and is divided into three parts in relation to this muscle.

1. *First part*: Lies medial to the scalenus anterior muscle
2. *Second part*: Lies behind the scalenus anterior muscle
3. *Third part*: Lies lateral to the scalenus anterior muscle.

Q. What are the branches of subclavian artery?

Ans. The branches of subclavian artery are:

- *Vertebral artery*: Arises from the first part of subclavian artery (first and largest branch). Ascends in the foramen transversarium of cervical vertebrae and the skull through foramen magnum and joins with the vertebral artery of the opposite side to form the basilar artery.
- *Internal thoracic artery*: Arises from the inferior aspect of the first part of the subclavian artery. Descends in the thorax lying posterior to the costal cartilages and ends at the level of sixth rib by dividing into superior epigastric and musculophrenic arteries.
- *Thyrocervical trunk*: Arises from the front of the first part of the subclavian artery. This divides into:
  - Inferior thyroid artery
  - Suprascapular
  - Transverse cervical artery.
- *Costocervical trunk*: Arises from the dorsal aspect of the second part of subclavian artery. The costocervical trunk divides into:
  - Deep cervical artery
  - Superior intercostal artery, which divides into first and second posterior intercostal artery.
  - *Dorsal scapular artery*: Occasionally arises from the third part of the subclavian artery.

■ ANATOMY OF COMMON CAROTID ARTERY IN THE NECK (FIG. 23.56)

Common carotid artery on the right is a branch of brachiocephalic trunk and on the left side, this is a branch of arch of the aorta.

In the neck, this artery lies in the carotid sheath lying medial to the internal jugular vein and anteriorly covered by the sternocleidomastoid muscle.

The artery lies in front of the transverse processes of lower four cervical vertebrae and ends at the level of upper border of thyroid cartilage by dividing into external and internal carotid arteries.

Branches: Apart from two terminal branches, there are no other branches in the neck.

Q. What is carotid sinus?

Ans. Carotid sinus is a slight dilatation at the termination of the common carotid artery or at the beginning of internal carotid artery. At the region of the carotid sinus, the tunica media is thin but the tunica adventitia is thick and contains a rich nerve plexus derived from the glossopharyngeal nerve and sympathetic nerve. The carotid sinus acts as a baroreceptor and helps in regulation of blood pressure.

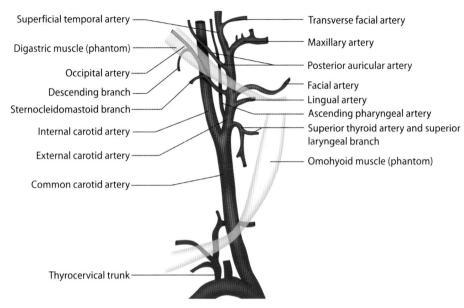

Superficial temporal artery

Digastric muscle (phantom)

Occipital artery

Descending branch

Sternocleidomastoid branch

Internal carotid artery

External carotid artery

Common carotid artery

Thyrocervical trunk

Transverse facial artery

Maxillary artery

Posterior auricular artery

Facial artery

Lingual artery

Ascending pharyngeal artery

Superior thyroid artery and superior laryngeal branch

Omohyoid muscle (phantom)

Fig. 23.56: Branches of external carotid artery

Q. What is carotid body?

Ans. This is a small oval and reddish-brown structure situated behind the bifurcation of common carotid artery. Supplied by a rich nerve plexus derived from glossopharyngeal, vagus, and sympathetic nerves. This acts as a chemoreceptor and responds to changes in oxygen, carbon dioxide, and pH of blood.

Q. What are the branches of external carotid artery (Fig. 23.56)?

Ans. The external carotid artery begins at the level of the upper border of the thyroid cartilage medial to the sternocleidomastoid muscle and anterior to the transverse process of C4 vertebra.

The external carotid artery terminates behind the neck of mandible by dividing into maxillary and superficial temporal artery.

The branches of external carotid artery may be grouped as:

- *Anterior branches*:
  - Superior thyroid artery
  - Lingual artery
  - Facial artery
- *Posterior branches*:
  - Occipital
  - Posterior auricular
- *Medial branch*:
  - Ascending pharyngeal
- *Terminal branch*:
  - Maxillary
  - Superficial temporal.

Q. What are the different triangles in the neck (Fig. 23.57)?

Ans. There are different triangles in the neck. Broadly these are:

- *Anterior triangle*: *Boundary*:
    - – *Anteriorly*: Midline of the neck from chin to the suprasternal notch.
    - – *Posteriorly*: Lateral border of the sternocleidomastoid.
    - – *Base*: Lower border of the mandible and a line joining between the angle of mandible and mastoid process.
    - – *Apex*: Lies at the suprasternal notch.
- *Posterior triangle*: *Boundary*:
    - – Anteriorly, lateral border of sternocleidomastoid.
    - – Posteriorly, medial border of trapezius.
    - – Base is formed by the clavicle.
    - – Apex at the mastoid process where trapezius and the sternocleidomastoid meet.

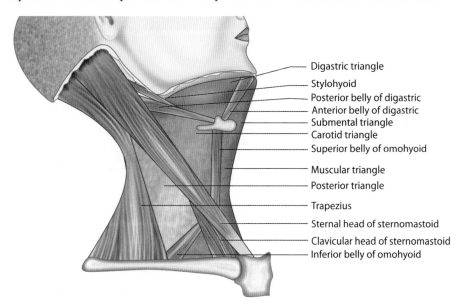

Digastric triangle
Stylohyoid
Posterior belly of digastric
Anterior belly of digastric
Submental triangle
Carotid triangle
Superior belly of omohyoid
Muscular triangle
Posterior triangle
Trapezius
Sternal head of sternomastoid
Clavicular head of sternomastoid
Inferior belly of omohyoid

Fig. 23.57: Triangles of neck

Q. What are the subdivisions of anterior triangle of the neck?

Ans. The anterior triangle is subdivided into number of triangles:

- Submental triangle
- Digastric or submandibular triangle
- Carotid triangle
- Muscular triangle.

Q. What is the boundary of submental triangle?

Ans. Submental triangle is bounded by:

- On either side—anterior belly of digastrics
- Base is formed by the body of the hyoid bone
- Floor formed by the right and left mylohyoid muscles.

Q. What is the boundary of digastric or submandibular triangle?

Ans. Digastric triangle is bounded by:
* Anteroinferiorly—by the anterior belly of digastric muscle
* Posteroinferiorly—by posterior belly of digastric muscle
* Base is formed by the lower border of the mandible and a line joining from the angle of the mandible to the tip of mastoid process
* Floor is formed by the mylohyoid muscle anteriorly and hyoglossus posteriorly and a small part of middle constrictor of the pharynx.

Q. What is the boundary of carotid triangle?

Ans. Carotid triangle is bounded by:
* *Anterosuperiorly*: Posterior belly of digastric muscle and stylohyoid
* *Anteroinferiorly*: Superior belly of omohyoid
* *Posteriorly*: Anterior border of sternocleidomastoid muscle
* Floor is formed by middle constrictor of pharynx, inferior constrictor of pharynx, and thyrohyoid membrane.

Q. What is the boundary of muscular triangle?

* *Anteriorly*: Midline of the neck from body of the hyoid bone to the suprasternal notch.
* *Posterosuperiorly*: Superior belly of omohyoid.
* *Posteroinferiorly*: Anterior border of sternocleidomastoid muscle.

Q. What are infrahyoid muscles?

Ans. There are two layers of infrahyoid muscles:
1. *Superficial layer*: Sternohyoid medially and superior belly of omohyoid
2. *Deeper layer*: Sternothyroid and thyrohyoid muscles.

These muscles are supplied by ventral rami of first, second, and third spinal nerves via ansa cervicalis.

Q. When these muscles need to be divided during thyroidectomy, where will you divide?

Ans. If these muscles need division during thyroidectomy, they are to be divided at a higher level as the nerve supply reaches these muscles from below.

Q. What is ansa cervicalis (Fig. 23.58)?

Ans. This is a loop of nerve lying in front of the carotid sheath and the larynx and supplies the infrahyoid muscles.
* *Formation*:
  - *Superior root*: From the descending branch of hypoglossal nerve. Its fibers are derived from the ventral rami of first cervical nerve.

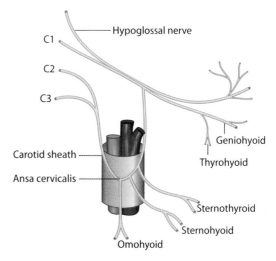

Fig. 23.58: Ansa cervicalis

- Inferior root is formed by the branches from ventral rami of second and third cervical nerve.
  - *Supply*: Branch from the superior root supplies the superior belly of omohyoid.
  - Branch from the ansa supplies the sternohyoid, sternothyroid, and inferior belly of omohyoid.

■ CERVICAL LYMPH NODES

There are large number of lymph nodes in the neck.

Based on relation to deep cervical fascia, the lymph nodes are broadly grouped into:
- *Superficial cervical lymph nodes*—lying superficial to deep cervical fascia
- *Deep cervical lymph nodes*—lying deep to deep cervical fascia.

Based on the anatomical location, they are grouped into:
- *Horizontal chain of lymph nodes*: These include:
  - Occipital
  - Posterior auricular
  - Preauricular
  - Parotid
  - Facial
  - Anterior cervical (superficial and deep) includes infrahyoid, prelaryngeal, paralaryngeal, pretracheal, and paratracheal lymph nodes
  - Submental
  - Submandibular
  - Superficial cervical.
  Vertical chain of deep cervical lymph nodes: These include:
  Lymph nodes along the internal jugular vein deep to the sternocleidomastoid muscle.
- Upper deep cervical (jugulodigastric)
- Lower deep cervical (jugulo-omohyoid)
- Lymph nodes along the posterior border of sternocleidomastoid muscle and anterior border of trapezius and lymph nodes in the supraclavicular fossa (posterior triangle).

Q. What are the different levels of lymph nodes in the neck?

Ans. From surgical point of view, the different groups of cervical lymph nodes are classified into different levels based on their anatomical location.

There are six levels of lymph nodes in the neck (Fig. 23.59):

1. *Level I*: Submental lymph nodes lying in the submental triangle (IA) and submandibular lymph nodes situated in the submandibular triangle (IB).
2. *Level II (upper jugular group)*: Lymph nodes located around the upper third of the internal jugular vein from the level of carotid bifurcation to the base of the skull (from base of the skull to the level of hyoid bone).
3. *Level III (middle jugular group)*: Lymph nodes located around the middle third of the internal jugular vein extending from the carotid bifurcation above to the cricothyroid membrane below (from level of hyoid bone to the cricoid cartilage).

4. *Level IV (lower jugular group)*: Lymph nodes located around the lower third of the internal jugular vein lying between the cricothyroid membrane above and the clavicle below (from the level of cricoid cartilage to the clavicle).
5. *Level V (posterior triangle group)*: Lymph nodes located in the posterior triangle extending laterally up to the anterior border of the trapezius and medially up to the lateral border of sternomastoid. The supraclavicular nodes are also included in this group.
6. *Level VI (anterior compartment group)*: This includes the perilaryngeal, pericricoid and peritracheal nodes lying above up to the hyoid bone, below up to the suprasternal notch, and laterally extend up to the medial border of sternomastoid. (Lymph nodes in the anterior mediastinum are included as level VII nodes).

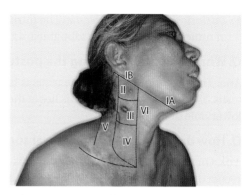

Fig. 23.59: Levels of lymph nodes in the neck

■ SALIVARY GLANDS

Q. What is the boundary of parotid region?

Ans. *See* Surgical Short Cases Section, Page No. 537, Chapter 12.

Q. What is the disposition of parotid fascia?

Ans. *See* Surgical Short Cases Section, Page No. 538, Chapter 12.

Q. What are the parts of parotid gland?

Ans. The parotid gland is divided into superficial and deep parts by faciovenous plane of Patey.

The retromandibular vein is formed within the gland by joining of superficial temporal and maxillary vein, which divides into anterior and posterior division, as it emerges from the gland.

The facial nerve emerges from the stylomastoid foramen and enters into the parotid gland lying superficial to the veins.

■ ANATOMY OF TESTIS, BLOOD SUPPLY AND LYMPHATIC DRAINAGE

Q. What are the coverings of testis?

Ans. The coverings of the testis are the layers of the scrotum and the intrinsic coverings of the testis. These are from outside inwards:

- Skin
- Dartos muscle
- External spermatic fascia
- Cremasteric fascia
- Internal spermatic fascia
- Parietal layer of tunica vaginalis

♦ *Intrinsic coverings of the testis*: The intrinsic coverings of the testis include the visceral layer of tunica vaginalis, tunica albuginea, and tunica vasculosa.

Q. What structure lies along the posterior border of the testis?

Ans. The posterior border of the testis is broad and the epididymis lies along the posterior of testis. The head of the epididymis lies at the upper pole and the tail of the epididymis lies at the lower pole of the testis.

Q. How do you identify the lateral surface of the testis?

Ans. On the lateral surface, the epididymis overhangs the testis and is separated by a semilunar recess of tunica vaginalis sac called sinus of the epididymis. So, the lateral surface of the testis is identified by the presence of sinus of epididymis.

Q. What is the internal structure of testis (Fig. 23.60)?

Ans. The testis is covered by a tough fibrous layer known as tunica albuginea. Near the posterior border, a fibrous vertical partition projects into the interior of testis known as mediastinum of testis.

From the convex anterior surface of the mediastinum testis, numerous fibrous septa project to the anterior border of the testis dividing the testis into 200–300 lobules. Within these lobules, there are 2–3 seminiferous tubules, which are convoluted.

The straight part of the seminiferous tubules ascends in the mediastinum of testis and joins with adjacent tubules and forms a plexiform network known as rete testis.

About 15–20 efferent ductules arise from the upper part of the rete testis and enter the head of the epididymis. These efferent ductules join to form a single duct known as canal of the epididymis and by convolutions form the body and tail of the epididymis. At the tail of the epididymis, this is continued as the vas deferens.

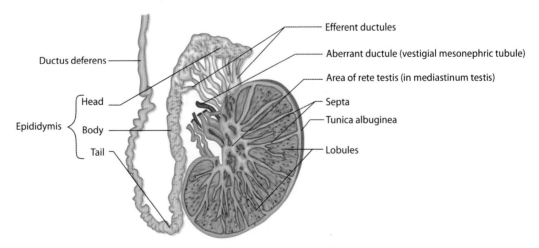

Fig. 23.60: Internal structure of testis

Q. What are the interstitial cells of testis?

Ans. The interstitial cells include:
- *Sertoli cells*: These are polyhedral cells lie along the basement membrane of seminiferous tubules. These cells provide nutrition to the growing spermatogonia and also secrete some estrogen.
- *Leydig cells*: These are polyhedral cells located in the lobules outside the basement membrane of seminiferous tubules. These cells secrete testosterone. These cells are abundant in fetal life, disappear at birth and reappear at puberty, and persist throughout the reproductive period of life.

Q. What is the blood supply of testis (Fig. 23.61)?

Ans.

Arterial supply:

The testis is principally supplied by the testicular artery, which is a lateral branch of abdominal aorta at the level of L1 vertebra.

The testis may also be supplied by the artery to the vas, which is a branch of superior vesical artery.

A minor supply may come from cremasteric artery, which is a branch of inferior epigastric artery.

Venous drainage:

The testis is drained by pampiniform plexus formed by 15–20 veins emerging from the upper pole of the testis. At the level of the superficial inguinal ring, these veins join to form 4–5 veins and at the level of deep-inguinal ring these veins join further to form two veins and at the retroperitoneum, these two veins join to form a single testicular vein. The right testicular veins drain at the inferior vena cava and the left testicular vein drains into the left renal vein.

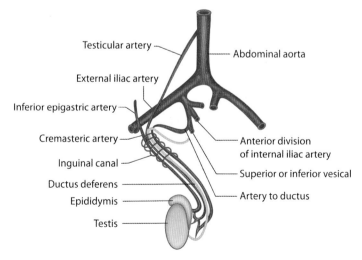

Fig. 23.61: Arterial supply of testis

Q. How does the lymphatic of testis drain (Fig. 23.62)?

Ans. The lymphatics of testis follow the vessels and drain into the para-aortic lymph nodes at the level of L1 vertebra.

Q. How does the testis develop (Fig. 23.62)?

Ans.

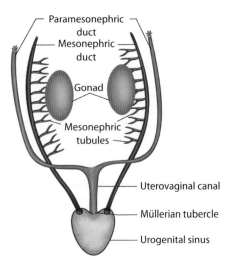

Fig. 23.62: Development of testis

* The testis develops in the retroperitoneum from the genital ridge, which lies medial to the mesonephros at the level of first lumbar vertebra around 4th to 6th week of intrauterine life.
* The cells of the genital ridge proliferate and migrate into the mesoderm of the mesonephros as solid cords known as testis cords.
* The central cells of these cords degenerate and canalization occurs leading to formation of seminiferous tubules and the rete testis.
* This rete testis joins the blind ends of the mesonephric tubules attached to the Wolffian duct and recanalization occurs.
* The mesonephros disappears by 10th week of intrauterine life. The mesonephric duct (Wolffian duct) persists and forms the epididymis and vas deferens.
* The developing testis is attached to the posterior abdominal wall by mesorchium, which transmits the neurovascular bundle of the testis.
* The germ cells are derived from the wall of the primitive yolk sac and migrate into the mesoderm of the mesonephros and get incorporated within the testis cords. These germ cells form spermatogonia, which are the precursors of spermatozoa.
* The interstitial cells of testis are derived from the mesoderm between the testis cords. These cells secrete testosterone, which is required during testicular development and descent.
* The mesoderm of the mesonephros cuts off the connection of the testis cords from the genital ridge and forms the tunica albuginea. This mesoderm also forms the mediastinum testis and septa testis.

Q. What is the chronology of testicular descent? (*See also* Page No. 640, Chapter 15)

Ans. Testes develop in the lumbar region. The descent starts after 2nd month and traverses the following route to reach the scrotum.
* *Lumbar region:* Remains up to the 2nd month.
* *Iliac fossa:* Traverse the retroperitoneum from 2nd to 3rd month and lies at right iliac fossa at the end of 3rd month.
* *Deep-inguinal ring:* Descends from right iliac fossa to the region of deep-inguinal ring during 3rd to 4th month. The testes remain at the region of the deep-inguinal ring from 4th to 7th month.
* *Superficial inguinal ring:* The testis traverses the inguinal canal during 7th to 8th month and lies at the superficial ring at the end of 8th month.

+ *Root of the scrotum*: Runs from superficial inguinal ring to the root of the scrotum during 8th to 9th months and remains at the root of the scrotum at the end of 9th month.
+ *Bottom of the scrotum*: Testes descend to the bottom of the scrotum shortly before birth or after the birth.

Q. What are the systems of veins in lower limbs (Fig. 23.63)?

Ans. The venous drainage of lower limb occurs through following system of veins:

+ *Deep veins*: The deep veins in the legs start in the plantar aspect of the foot and the dorsum of the foot and accompany as venae comitantes of the arteries in the legs, venae comitantes of posterior tibial vein and the anterior tibial vein. The venae comitantes of posterior tibial vein and the venae comitantes of the anterior vein join to form the popliteal vein, which lie alongside the popliteal artery and continued higher up as the femoral vein, which is continued as the external iliac vein.

+ *Superficial system of veins*: Great saphenous vein starts from medial side of dorsal venous arch joined by medial marginal vein of foot runs in front of the medial malleolus ascends along subcutaneous surface of tibia and then passes one hands breadth behind the medial border of the patella and the ascend in the thigh to end at femoral vein at the saphenous opening, which lies 3.5 cm below and lateral to pubic tubercle.

+ The short saphenous vein starts from the lateral side of the dorsal venous arch joined by the lateral marginal vein of the foot and ascends in the leg behind the lateral malleolus and runs in the posterior aspect of the leg running between the two gastrocnemii. This ends at the popliteal vein at a variable distance of 2–15 cm from the knee joint line.

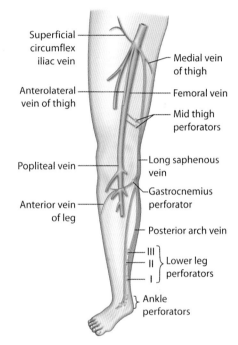

Fig. 23.63: Superficial veins in the lower limb

+ *Communicating vein*: These are superficial veins lying superficial to the deep fascia communicating between the great and short saphenous veins.

+ *Perforating veins*: These are veins, which connect the superficial system of veins to the deep veins. The perforating veins may be:
  – Direct perforators, which join directly between the superficial and deep veins
  – Indirect perforators of the perforating veins from superficial vein join the venous plexus in the muscle and from the venous plexus in the muscle another perforating vein drains into the deep vein thereby indirectly connecting the superficial and deep veins.

Q. What are the common sites of perforating veins?

Ans. In great saphenous system:

* Saphenofemoral junction at saphenous opening—largest perforator
* Adductor canal perforator (Hunterian perforator) at midthigh
* Perforator above the knee
* Perforator below the knee (Boyd's perforators)
* Medial ankle perforator at 5 cm, 10 cm, and 15 cm above the medial side of the leg (Cockett and Dodd perforators)
* Perforators at the level of ankle (May or Kuster perforator)
* Apart from these constant perforators, there are some other inconstant perforators at different level joining the superficial and deep system of veins.

In short saphenous system:

* Saphenopopliteal junction situated at 2 cm below to 15 cm above the knee joint line.

FASCIAL COMPARTMENTS OF THE THIGH

The thigh extends from the groin to the knee. The thigh is divided into three compartments by following fascial attachments (Fig. 23.64):

1. *Medial intermuscular septum*: Fascial extension of deep fascia of the thigh and is attached to the medial lip of the linea aspera. This separates the medial compartment of the thigh from anterior compartment.

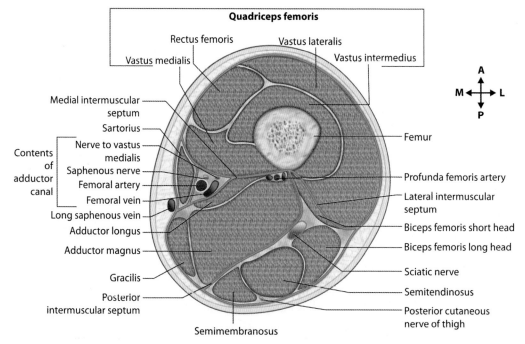

Fig. 23.64: Cross-section at the level of midthigh to depict the osteofascial compartments of thigh with their content

2. *Lateral intermuscular septum*: Fascial extension forms the deep fascia of the thigh and is attached to the lateral lip of the linea aspera. This separates the anterior compartment of the thigh from the posterior compartment.
3. *Posterior intermuscular septum*: This is a thin fascial layer extending deeper from the deep fascia of the thigh and separates the medial compartment from the posterior compartment of the thigh.

Anterior or extensor compartment of the thigh:

- *Muscles*: Two extensors
  - Sartorius
- *Quadriceps femoris*: Vastus medialis, vastus lateralis, vastus intermedius, and rectus femoris
- *Vessels*: Femoral artery and vein
- *Nerves*: Femoral nerve and lateral cutaneous nerve of the thigh.

Medial or adductor compartment:

- *Muscles*:
  - Adductors
  - Adductor longus
  - Adductor magnus
  - Gracilis.
- *Nerves*: Branches of obturator nerve and medial cutaneous nerve of thigh.

Posterior or extensor compartment:

- *Muscles*: Hamstring muscles
- *Biceps femoris*: Short head and long head
  - Semitendinosus
  - Semimembranosus
- *Nerves*: Sciatic nerve. At popliteal fossa divides into common peroneal and posterior tibial nerve
  - Posterior femoral cutaneous nerve
- *Vessels*: Femoral vessels continued as popliteal vessels.

Q. What is the boundary of femoral triangle?

Ans. This is the triangular area in the upper third of the thigh below the inguinal ligament (Figs 23.65A and B).

Boundary of femoral triangle:

- Above—by the inguinal ligament
- Medially—by the medial border of adductor longus muscle
- Laterally—by the medial border of sartorius muscle
- Apex—formed by the meeting point of sartorius and adductor longus muscle
- Roof is formed by the fascia lata pierced by the great saphenous vein ending at the femoral vein at the saphenous opening
- Floor of the femoral triangle is formed by: (Medial to lateral):
  - Adductor longus muscle
  - Pectineus

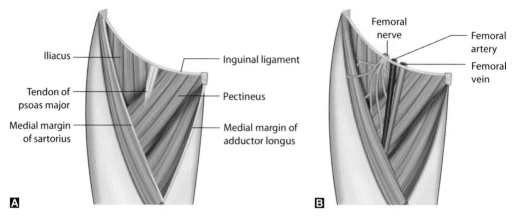

Figs 23.65A and B: (A) Showing boundaries and floor of the femoral triangle; (B) Showing the main content of femoral triangle

- Tendon of psoas muscle
- Iliacus muscle.

Contents of femoral triangle:
- *Femoral sheath with its contents*:
  - Cloquet lymph nodes
  - Femoral vein with its tributaries
  - Femoral artery with its branches in the femoral triangle
- Femoral nerve
- Inguinal lymph nodes
- A part of lateral femoral cutaneous nerve
- Femoral branch of genitofemoral nerve.

Adductor Canal

Q. What are the boundaries of adductor canal?

Ans. The adductor canal is an intermuscular tunnel in the middle third of the thigh. This extends from the apex of the femoral triangle to the adductor hiatus through which the femoral vessels enter into the popliteal fossa.

The adductor canal is bounded:
- Anteromedially—by the sartorius muscle
- Anterolaterally—by the vastus medialis
- Posteriorly—by the adductor longus and adductor magnus
- Roof is formed by the fibrous membrane bridging the gap between the vastus medialis and the adductor muscle.

Q. What are the contents of adductor canal?

Ans. The contents of the adductor canal are:
- Femoral artery

- Femoral vein
- Saphenous nerve
- Nerve to vastus medialis.

Popliteal Fossa

Q. What are the boundaries of popliteal fossa?

Ans. Popliteal fossa is diamond-shaped space at the back of the knee (Figs 23.66 and 23.67).

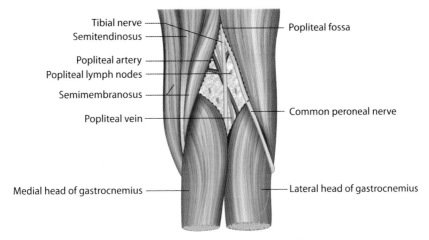

Fig. 23.66: Popliteal fossa—boundaries and contents

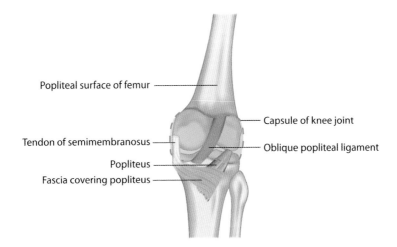

Fig. 23.67: Structures forming the floor of popliteal fossa

The boundaries are:

* Superomedially—by semimembranosus and semitendinosus
* Superolaterally—by the tendon of biceps femoris
* Inferomedially—by the medial head of gastrocnemius
* Inferolaterally—by the tendon of plantaris and lateral head of gastrocnemius
* Roof is formed by the popliteal fascia—pierced by the short saphenous vein, as it terminates into the popliteal vein.
* Floor is formed by:
    - Popliteal surface of the femur
    - Posterior aspect of the knee joint
    - Pectineus muscle attached to the popliteal surface of the tibia.

Q. What are the contents of popliteal fossa?

Ans. The contents of popliteal fossa are:
* Popliteal artery
* Popliteal vein
* Common peroneal and tibial nerves
* Loose areolar tissue
* Popliteal lymph node.

■ FASCIAL COMPARTMENTS IN THE LEG

The leg extends from below the knee joint up to above the ankle joint. There are four osteofascial compartments in the leg (Fig. 23.68).

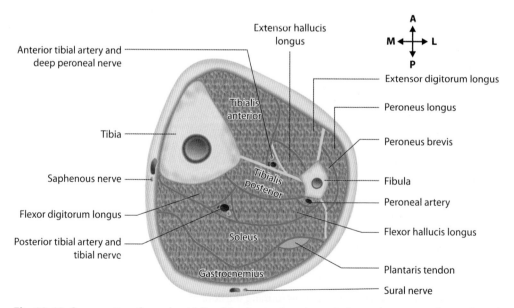

Fig. 23.68: Cross-section through middle of the leg to show boundaries and contents of osteofascial compartments of leg

The medial surface of the tibia is subcutaneous and the deep fascia of the leg is blended with the periosteum of tibia on the medial side.

◆ The interosseous membrane is the fibrous membrane attached to the posterior border of the tibia and the medial border of the fibula.
◆ The intermuscular septa are extensions from the deep fascia of the leg.
◆ The anterior intermuscular septum is attached along the anterior border of the fibula.
◆ The posterior intermuscular septum is attached along the posterior border of the fibula.

The compartments in the leg are:

◆ *Anterior compartment (extensor compartment)*: Area between the anterior border of the tibia and the anterior intermuscular septum attached along the anterior border of the fibula.
  – Muscles in the anterior compartment of the leg:
    - Tibialis anterior
    - Extensor hallucis longus
    - Extensor digitorum longus
    - Peroneus tertius
  – *Nerve*: Deep peroneal nerve
  – *Vessels*: Anterior tibial artery and vein.
◆ *Lateral compartment (peroneal compartment)*: Area between the anterior and posterior intermuscular septa.
  – Muscles in the lateral compartment:-
    - Peroneus longus
    - Peroneus brevis
  – *Nerve*: Branches of deep peroneal nerve
  – *Vessels*: Peroneal artery and the vein.
◆ *Posterior compartment (flexor compartment)*: Area between the posterior intermuscular septum and the medial border of the tibia. The posterior compartment is further subdivided into superficial and deep posterior compartment by a transverse intermuscular septum.
  – *Superficial posterior compartment*:
    - *Muscles*:
      » Medial and lateral heads of gastrocnemius
      » Plantaris
      » Soleus.
    - *Nerve*:
      » Sural nerve.
  – *Deep posterior compartment*:
    - *Muscles*:
      » Tibialis posterior
      » Flexor hallucis longus
      » Flexor digitorum longus
      » Popliteus.
    - *Nerve*:
      » Posterior tibial nerve.
    - *Vessels*:
      » Posterior tibial vessels.

Index

Page numbers followed by *f* refer to figure and *t* refer to table.

A

Abdomen 85, 92, 102, 1154
  burst 748
  CECT scan of 107, 200
  closure of 1097, 1110, 1113, 1116
  computed tomography scan of
    242, 756, 786, 791, 939
  examination of 6, 41, 211, 349,
    401, 683
  exploration of 780, 1093, 1095,
    1097, 1108, 1112, 1114, 1116
  feel of 94
  local examination of 87, 714, 727
  movement of 6
  palpation of 92*f*
  plain X-ray of 738, 781
  preliminary exploration of 1111
  quadrants of 90*f*
  region of 90*t*
  shape of 6
  temperature of 92*f*, 93*f*
  ultrasonography of 596, 700,
    756, 791
  upper part of 776*f*, 803*f*
  X-ray of 781*f*
Abdominal
  aorta, branches of 1178, 1178*f*
  compartment syndrome 74
  distension, stage of 779
  flat muscles, division of 1128
  injury 695
  pain
    chronic 831
    dull upper 178
  wall 73, 79, 94*f*
    anterior 1152
    defects 668
    lower 618
  wound, closure of 1121
Abdominoperineal resection 1116
  steps of 1116
Abductor
  digiti minimi 481
  longus, rupture of 611
  pollicis
    brevis 478, 479*f*, 481
    longus 466, 466*f*, 468

Aberrant renal vessel 907
Aberrant thyroid, lateral 307
Abortion, threatened 558
Abrahamson nylon darn repair 62
Abscess 955, 1000
  anorectal 959
  appendicular 732, 734, 868
  axillary 957, 957*f*
  chronic 238
  drainage of 955, 1000
  formation, stage of 504
  iliac 955
  pancreatic 713, 742
  pelvirectal 959
  perianal 959
  perinephric 958, 958*f*
  prostatic 751
  psoas 611, 730
  submucous 959
  subphrenic 703, 803, 805
Acalculous cholecystitis 145, 146,
    900, 1103
  development of 900
Accessory nerve, spinal root of 3
Achalasia 816, 817
  cardia 816, 817, 820
    diagnosis of 817
  cricopharyngeal 818
Achlorhydria 857
Acid-fast bacilli 756
Acidity 2
Acidosis, metabolic 948
Aciduria, paradoxical 106
Acinic cell
  carcinoma 537
  tumor 543
Acoustic neuroma 456
Acral lentiginous melanoma 406,
  407
Acrocyanosis 449
Acromion, angle of 357*f*
Actinomycosis 830, 869
Adamantinoma 589
Addison's disease 24
Adductor canal 980, 981, 1216
  boundaries of 1216
  contents of 1216
  perforator 328*f*

Adductor longus tendon 52*f*, 327*f*
Adductor pollicis 476, 476*f*, 481
Adenoacanthoma 573, 864
Adenocarcinoma 537, 820, 864,
  903, 915, 927
  metastatic 512
  pancreatic ductal 184
Adenoid cystic carcinoma 537, 543
Adenolymphoma 537, 539, 540
Adenoma 537
  monomorphic 537
  oxyphilic 537
  pleomorphic 537
  trabecular 307
  umbilical 615, 616
Adenomatous
  polyposis coli 862, 878
  polyps, types of 878
Adiposis dolorosa 395
Adrenal gland 222, 794
Adrenalectomy, medical 263
Adrenergic blocking drugs, alpha
  753
Adrenocorticotropic hormone
  263, 317, 413
Adriamycin 120, 248, 516
Adson's test 521, 521*f*
Aerobic gram-negative bacilli 768
Air hunger 189
Airway 679
  management 83
  tubes 1050, 1050*f*
Albendazole 191
Alcohol 736, 986
  intake, chronic 820
Alkaline phosphatase 939
Allantois 617
Allergic reaction 339
Allergy 273
Allis tissue forceps 1000, 1000*f*
Alloderm 724
Alopecia 248
Amebic point 88
Amelanotic melanoma 405
Ameloblastoma 589-591
American Association for Surgery
  708

American College of Radiology 239
American Heart Association 945, 945*t*
American Joint Committee on Cancer System 113
American Society of Anesthesiologists 936
Amikacin 506
Aminosalicylic acid 506
Amoxicillin 374
Ampulla of Vater 1170
Amputation, role of 433
Amyloidosis, secondary 223
Anabolic steroid 598
Anal
  canal 876*f*, 1163, 1164*f*, 1165
    lymphatics of 1166
  cushions 1024
  fistula
    high 1021
    low 1021, 1022
    types of 1021, 1021*f*
Analgesics 743
Anaplastic carcinoma, biopsy report revealed 654
Anderson-Hynes pyeloplasty 218*f*
Anemia 5, 13, 73, 117, 134, 223, 748, 830, 831, 838, 839, 906, 948
  correction of 939, 940
  megaloblastic 137
  mild 14
  moderate 14
  severe 14
Anesthesia 460, 746, 960, 977, 978, 1107
  apinal 53
  epidural 53
  local 53
Aneurysm 1056, 1057
  causes of 1056
  complications of 1057
  false 1056
  needle 1055, 1055*f*
  types of 1056
Angioembolization, role of 707
Angiography 360, 688
  role of 152
Angioma 402
  strawberry 441, 442
Angiosarcoma 308
  malignant 307
Anguli oris, depressor 557
Ankle
  brachial
    blood pressure index 359, 375

joint, movement of 348
  region of 325*f*
Ann Arbor staging system 515*t*
Anomalous pancreaticobiliary duct junction 175, 902, 903
Anorectal
  abscess, types of 959, 959*f*
  anomalies 554
  defects 668
Anorexia 117, 178, 128, 223, 838, 839
Anosmia 847
Ansa cervicalis 1207, 1207*f*
Antibioma 238, 763
Antibiotic 369, 607, 947, 956
  prophylactic 79, 84, 741, 947
  therapy 368, 372, 373
    optimal duration of 372
Anticoagulant therapy 336
Antilymphocyte serum 225
Antireflux surgery, role of 818
Antiseptic cleaning and draping 1103, 1131, 1135
Antithyroid drugs 300, 301, 937
Antitubercular drug 505, 913
  second lines of 506
  treatment 913
Antral stasis 856
Antrectomy 130
Anxiety neurosis 297
Anxiolytic drug 937
Aorta
  abdominal 1178
  dissecting aneurysm of 735
Aortic
  aneurysm, abdominal 1056-1058
  bodies 525
Apendicitis, acute 729, 834, 835, 865, 866*f*, 867, 868
Apert's syndrome 558
Apex beat 7
Aphthous ulcer 572
Apical pulp space infection 962*f*
Appendectomy 730, 731, 736, 836
  indications of 835
  open 835
  techniques of 835
Appendicectomy 1121, 1123
  laparoscopic 1123
  retrograde 1123
  steps of 1121, 1122*f*

Appendicitis
  development of acute 833, 867
  diagnosis of acute 730
  gangrenous 868
  recurrent 139, 833, 835
  retrocecal 834
Appendicular
  abscess, drainage of 734
  lump, conservative treatment of 733
Appendix 61, 1176
  anatomical positions of 1177*f*
  burying base of 1123
  carcinoma of 835
  crushing clamps 1038
  division of base of 1122
  endometriosis of 835
  length of 1176
  locations of 1178
  mucocele of 835, 868
  of testis, cyst of 627
  part of 871*f*, 1176
Appetite 2
  loss of 85
Arch of aorta, branches of 1203
Areola 227, 929*f*
Arnold-Chiari malformation 460, 461
Arrhythmias 302
Arteria dorsalis pedis 348, 355*f*
  pulse 355
Arterial
  blood gas analysis 951
  bypass graft 364
  compartment 1149
  disease
    occlusive 359, 447
    peripheral 339
  hemangioma 441
  insufficiency 367
  ischemia 374
  pulses 323
Arteriovenous fistula 342, 450, 451, 449, 452, 455
  congenital 451
Arteriovenous malformation 336
Artery 520, 521*f*, 659, 1101
  disposition of 538
  lingual 975, 1205
  ovarian 1179
  vertebral 1204
Ascaris lumbricoides 809
  cycle of 809
Ascites 154, 838
  pancreatic 742

Aspergillosis 801, 802
Aspirate catheter 697
Aspiration
    method of 969
    site of 967, 969
Asthenia 117
Astler-Coller's modification 206
    for Dukes staging 840, 882
Atherosclerotic peripheral
    vascular disease 345, 365, 447
Atraumatic needle 1007
Atrophy, subsequent 60
Auricular
    artery, posterior 975
    nerve, great 538, 546
Auriculotemporal nerve 538
Auscultation 6, 7, 27, 41, 89, 213,
    275
Autoimmune diseases 339, 447
Autonomic nervous system 1184,
    1185
Axilla 246, 400
    boundaries of 1188
    contents of 1191
Axillary
    artery
        branches of 1190, 1191f
        parts of 1190
    dissection 1127
    lymph node 229, 235, 236,
        237f, 268f
        dissection 243, 271
        groups of 1191
    nerve 470
    node, anterior group of 235
    pulse 356
        palpation of 357f
    surgery, role of 253, 267
    vein 250, 1128
Axonotmesis 471

B

Babbit hypothesis 184
Babcock's stripper 334
Babcock's tissue forceps 1001,
    1001f, 1032
Bacillus-calmette-guerin vaccine
    919
Backache, low 838
Backhaus' towel clip 989
Bacteria 897
Bacterial
    endocarditis, subacute 755

infection 867
    peritonitis, stage of 779
    proliferation 746
Bacteroides 867, 959
    fragilis 369
Baker's cyst 765
Balanitis
    recurrent 648
    xerotica obliterans 653, 657,
        926
Balanoposthitis
    chronic 657, 926
    recurrent 648
Ball valve mechanism 1150
Ballance's sign 700
Balthazar grading and score 739t
Bard-Parker's handle 990, 990f
Barium enema 775, 836
    double contrast 200, 886
Barium-meal study, role of 107
Barrett's esophagus 820
Barron's banding 1025
Basal acid output 857
Basal cell carcinoma 391, 422,
    422f, 423-425, 573, 927
    sclerosing 425
    site of 425
    type of 424
Basal cell nevus syndrome 428
Basal pneumonia 726, 735
    right side 805
Bassini's repair 55
    lichtenstein modification of 55
    modified 55, 55f, 65
Battle's pararectal incision 73
Beck's triad 693
Beetroot ingestion 755
Bentonite flocculation test 191
Berry's, ligament of 279
Berry's sign 275, 283
Beta-lactamase inhibitor 369
Bethesda system 287
Biceps
    brachii, tendon of 356f
    femoris 1215
Bile duct 140, 148, 171, 807, 809,
    1106
    carcinoma of 184
    common 140, 142, 143, 155,
        167, 709, 806f, 807f, 808,
        810f, 813f, 1170, 1173
    consequences of worm in 809
    distal 172
    division of 1108

intraduodenal part of 183
    obstruction 181
    stones 169, 170, 815
        management of 1030
        recurrent 169
        residual 169
        secondary 169
    stricture 148, 172
    transcystic exploration of 168
Biliary
    colic, classical attack of 144,
        899
    communication 188
    tract disease 139, 904
    tree 143, 1171
        lymphatic drainage of 1172,
            1173f
Billroth gastrectomy 130
Biopsy
    excisional 425
    incisional 242, 425, 431, 535,
        572
    techniques of 425
Bird's beak deformity 791
Bitots spot 12
Black pigment stones 894
Bladder 1047
    cancer 918
        development of 914
        superficial 916, 918
    carcinoma of 751, 754, 916
    closure 668
    exstrophy of 668
    in situ carcinoma of 916
    neck
        fibrosis 751
        muscular hypertrophy 751
        obstruction 219
    outflow obstruction 908
    outlet obstruction, symptoms
        of 909
    pain 215
    region, part of 796f
    stone 751
    USG of 68
Bleeding 120, 133, 134, 334, 666,
    704
    control of 1131
    tendency, control of 940
Bleomycin 120, 516
Blindness 457
Blister formation 368
Blood 42, 107, 221, 298
    disorders 447

dyscrasia 755
loss 996
pressure 5, 22, 679, 680, 722
measurement of 22f
persistent 22
segmental 359, 375
transfusion 935, 947
vessels 439
Bloom-Richardson grading system 259
Blue nevus 415
Blunt abdominal trauma, treatment of 698, 703, 780
Blunt pointed needle 1007, 1007f
Body
carcinoma of 161
mass index 12
temperature, normal 23
Boey's score 743, 743t
Bone
cyst
aneurysmal 589
solitary 589
diseases 134
grafting 563
involvement 433
lengthening, Ilizarov technique of 364
marrow biopsy 514
metastasis 257
pathological fracture of 458
scan 221
Bony
cage, normal 800f
jaw swelling 589
Borderline resectable
disease 154
pancreatic cancer 163, 165
Borrmann's classification 117, 863
Botulinum toxin, role of 818
Bow sign 629
Bowel
circumference of 61
enema, small 829f
injury 60
obstruction
cause of small 783
large 790, 791
sounds 6, 189
Bowen's disease 420, 657
Boyden, sphincter of 1171
Brachial blood pressure index 375
Brachial plexus 469, 469f
cords of 469

injury, complete 482
lesion, causes of 482
root of 470
traction injury of 483
trunks of 469
Brachial pulse 356
palpation of 356f
Brachiocephalic trunk 1203
Brachioradialis 468
muscle 466, 466f
Brachytherapy 434
role of 434
Bradycardia 21, 686
Brain
computed tomography scan of 459
metastasis 257
Brainstem, hemangioblastomas of 910
Branchial arches 497
constituents of 497
sixth 498
Branchial cartilage 501
Branchial cleft 497
Branchial cyst 487, 494-497, 527
development of 497f
Branchial fistula 500, 500f
tract 500
Branchial sinus 499, 499f, 500
excision of 501
Branchiogenic carcinoma 501
Branham's sign 450
Breast 226, 228, 232, 246, 508, 594, 599, 801, 1187
abscess 955, 960, 961f
drainage of 960
advanced carcinoma of 255
architecture of 239f
cancer 243, 246, 248, 253, 254, 256, 264-266, 270, 854, 929f, 931
advanced 252, 253, 271
Columbia clinical classification of 932
development 264, 595
familial 263
hereditary 263
male 596, 854
management 269
Manchester staging of 932
metastatic 255-256
molecular subtypes of 263
sporadic 263
treatment of 266, 271

carcinoma 4, 226, 238, 239, 242, 247, 251, 255, 256, 258, 263, 264, 266-271, 764, 928
metastatic 256, 764
TNM staging for 259
conservation, role of 254
conserving surgery 246, 247, 250, 854
cyst 763
elephantiasis of 646
examination 238f, 764
fibroadenoma of 238, 598, 763
imaging 239
reporting 853
BI-RADS system of reporting of 852
inflammatory carcinoma of 254, 930
lesion 241, 242
malignant 763
nonpalpable 258
lobules 1188
locally advanced carcinoma of 251, 251f, 252, 764
lump 243
malignancy 239, 853
mass 240, 241
normal 1187
parenchyma 928f
quadrants of 231f, 929f, 1187, 1187f
reconstruction 269
tissue 232, 232f, 239
tuberculosis of 238, 763
upper quadrant of 239f
Breath sound 680, 848
Broad-spectrum antibiotics 730, 743, 805
Bronchial carcinoma 598
Bronchodilators 947
Brown pigment stones 894
Bruit 89
Bubonocele 43, 62
Buccal mucosa 583
Buccinator muscle 534, 534f
Buerger's angle of circulatory insufficiency 354
Buerger's disease 345, 349, 349f, 360, 362-365, 447, 759
Buerger's exercise 363
Buerger's test 347
Bulbar sclera, upper 14f
Buphthalmos 442
Burhene technique 170, 815

Burn 721
  chemical 721
  circumferential 725
  deep 721
  depth of 720, 721
  electrical 721
  first-degree 720, 723
  fourth-degree 721, 723
  full thickness 721
  injury 399, 721, 724
    severe 719
  second-degree 720, 723
  shock 399, 722
    causes of 399, 722
    management of 723
  superficial 721
  third-degree 721, 723
  wound 721, 723, 725
Bursa, subcutaneous 453
Bursitis, subhyoid 278
Buschke-Löwenstein tumor 653,
  660, 927

C

Cachexia 838
Calcitonin gene-related peptide
  317
Calcium deficiency 137
Calculi, pancreatic 794
Calculus 755
  anuria 799
Calf muscle 350f
  hematoma 765
Calot's triangle 142, 1101, 1102,
  1104, 1172, 1173
  boundary of 142, 142f, 1172
  dissection of 1101
Camellotte sign 190
Cancer
  breast, TNM staging of 932
  colon 889
  pancreatic 162, 811, 812
Cannonball metastasis 221, 799,
  801f
Cannonball shadows, causes of
  801
Cannula 1074
  uses of 1075
Capillary
  bleeding 995
  blood glucose 157
  filling time 347, 354
  hemangioma 441
    types of 441

refilling, test for 347, 353
wedge pressure, pulmonary
  370
Capreomycin 506
Capsular tear, small 702
Capsule, fibrous 1155
Carbon dioxide, advantages of
  1073
Carcinoembryonic antigen 201,
  317
  role of 841
Carcinogens 175, 427, 902
Carcinoid tumor 830, 837, 864, 869
Carcinoma 134, 159, 219, 306, 308,
  537, 579, 582, 816, 821
  adenosquamous 903
  adrenocortical 598
  anaplastic 315
  breast 248, 253, 404, 764, 930,
    931
    cells of origin of 929
    development of 931
    pathological types of 929
    treatment of 271
  cecum 839
  cheek, types of 583
  colon 204-206, 790, 836
    development of 838
    TNM staging for 840
  descending colon 199
  en cuirasse 931
  esophagus 819, 820
    development of 820
    types of 820
  gallbladder 96, 172-175, 902,
    902f, 903
    development of 175, 903
  head of pancreas, development
    of 158
  in situ 657, 929
    primary 916
    secondary 916
  kidney 221, 223, 225, 844, 845,
    910, 911
    cells of origin of 909
    development of 223
  lip 577, 582
    types of 581, 582
    ultraviolet radiation-
      induced 580
  male breast 594, 595
  metachronous 884
  mucoepidermoid 537
  of colon, Dukes staging for 840,
    882

of gallbladder, TNM for 175,
    904
  of rectum, Dukes staging for
    885
  of stomach, TNM for 865
  of urinary bladder, TNM
    staging for 917
  oral 574t
  pancreas 153
  papillary 307, 308, 314, 493,
    755, 914
  parotid gland 540, 541, 541f
  penis 651, 655-657, 926, 926f,
    927
    gross types of 657
    Jackson staging of 658, 928
    TNM classification of 657
    types of 927
  periampullary 147-149, 152,
    154, 158, 171, 172
  primary 306, 830, 869
  rectal 886
  scirrhous 929
  stomach 104, 107, 108, 115,
    824, 825
    advanced 115
    staging of 825
  synchronous 884
  thyroid 279, 291, 293, 305f, 306,
    309
  tongue 573, 573f, 574, 576-579
    development of 573
    types of 573
  types of 586
Card test 475
Cardiac
  anomalies 554
  disease 946
  glands 1159
  node, right 110
  risk stratification 944
  tamponade 689, 693, 848
  toxicity 248
Cardiovascular failure 770
Cardiovascular system 727, 934
  examination of 7, 41, 349
Carnett's test 102
Carney's triad 120
Caroli's disease 183, 184
Caroticocavernous fistula 847
Carotid
  angiogram 523
  artery 283, 524
    aneurysm 523
    external 976f
    left common 1203
    ligature of external 975

body 525, 1205
    hyperplasia 525
    tumor 522, 523, 523f, 524,
        525
    pulsation 275
    pulse 357
        palpation of 283f, 357f
    sinus 1204
    triangle, boundary of 1207
Carpal tunnel syndrome 521
Cart wheel appearance 186
Carwardine's twin intestinal clamp
        1033, 1034f
Casonis test 191
Cat's paw 1015
    retractor 1015f
Catabolic state 948
Catgut sutures 1061f
Catheter 954
    introducer 1042, 1043f
Causalgia 473
Cavernous sinus thrombosis
    bilateral 296
    unilateral 296
Cavity
    oral 553
    pericardial 968
Cecal volvulus 792, 793
Cecum 790, 1161
    carcinoma of 202
    part of 871f
Celiac axis dissection 1095
Celiac trunk branches of 1179,
        1179f
Cell
    carcinoma, transitional 755,
        915
    nuclear grooving of 308
Cellulitis 765
Central venous cannulation 952f
    indications of 952
Cephalic vein 250, 1128
Cerebellar
    hemangiomata 223
    sign 8
Cerebellum, hemangioblastomas
    of 910
Cerebral
    contusion 686, 687
    edema 687
    hemisphere 442
    laceration 686
Cerebrospinal fluid 460, 682, 847
Cervical
    auricle 501

dermoid 496
    cyst 491
esophagus 1158
fascia 1197
    deep 1131, 1197, 1198
    disposition of 1197
    incision of deep 1129
    layers of 1198f
    superficial 1197
lymph node 5, 19, 404f, 503,
        537, 1208
    bilateral 513f
    deep 1208
    examination of 275
    metastatic 503, 507, 507f,
        511
    superficial 1208
lymphadenitis
    chronic 496, 539
    tubercular 501-503, 503f,
        507
lymphadenopathy 535
    chronic 503
rib 518, 518f, 520-522
    types of 520f
spondylosis 521
Cervicodorsal sympathectomy
        448, 449
    role of 448
Cetrimide solution 192
Chaga's disease 816
Chaissaignac's triangle, dissection
    of 1136
Charcot's triad 169
Cheek, carcinoma of 582, 582f, 584
Chemical
    carcinogens 427
    peritonitis, stage of 778
    sterilization 986, 1072
    sympathectomy 362
Chemoreceptor organs 525f
Chemotherapy 158, 248, 253, 255,
        435, 764, 802
    regimes of 120, 256, 516
    role of 114, 174, 180, 225, 256,
        434, 543, 656
    side effects of 248, 516
    systemic 119
Chenodeoxycholic acid 144, 898
Chest
    computed tomography scan of
        242
    drain, insertion of 967
    examination of 36, 401, 682

injury 689, 690, 847
    metastasis 802
    movement of 7
    pain 3
        exertional 302
    physiotherapy 947
    shape of 7
    trauma, major 848
    tube insertion, complications
        of 968
    wall swelling 31f
    X-ray 42, 140, 200, 205, 298,
        332
Chew-and-spit test 858
Cheyne-Stokes breathing 23
Cholangiocarcinoma 148, 171,
        172, 177-180
    development of 178
    periampullary 180
    TNM classification for 179,
        179t
    types of 178
Cholangiography, intraoperative
    170
Cholangiohepatitis 181
Cholangitis 184, 189
    acute 178, 726
    recurrent 144, 184, 898
    sclerosing 148, 172
Cholecystectomy 142, 142f, 143,
        146, 147, 170, 174, 1102,
        1107, 1108
    complications of 1027
    forceps 1027, 1027f
    indications of 1103
    laparoscopic 141, 1100, 1102,
        1102f
    open 141, 141f, 1103
    radical 173
    retrograde 1104
    simple 174
    steps of open 1103
Cholecystitis 184
    acute 88, 96, 144, 145, 726, 729,
        735, 898, 899, 900, 904, 1103
    chronic 85, 88, 126, 138, 139,
        144, 894f, 898, 899, 1103
Choledochal cyst 175, 181, 183,
        184, 902
    complications of 184
    treatment of 184
    types of 183, 183f
Choledochocoele 183
Choledochoduodenostomy 157,
        1106, 1107
    steps of 1107

Choledochojejunostomy 1106
Choledocholithiasis 148, 149*f*,
　　166-168, 171, 181
Choledocholithotomy 170, 1104,
　　1105*f*, 1107
　　laparoscopic 171
　　open 171
　　steps of 1104
Choledochotomy 1106
Cholelithiasis 181, 894*f*
Cholesterol 144, 897
　　crystals 497
　　gallstones 143, 795, 894
　　solubility 146*f*
　　stone 143, 144, 795, 896
Cholesterolosis, microscopic
　　appearance of 901
Chordee correction 664, 664*f*
Choriocarcinoma 924
Chromaffinomas 456
Chromogranin 317
Chromosomal defect 259
Chylocele 621, 623, 624, 645
Chylothorax 953
Ciliospinal reflex, loss of 483
Cilostazole 448
Cimino's fistula 452
Ciprofloxacin 374, 506
Cirrhosis 184
Cirsoid aneurysm 442, 443, 443*f*
Clammy extremities 700
Claudication, progress of 345
Clavipectoral fascia, disposition
　　of 1190
Claw hand 477
　　deformity 481
Cleft lip 553, 554, 556, 558, 563*f*,
　　565, 567
　　bilateral 555, 557, 561, 562*f*
　　　complete 555*f*, 562, 564*f*
　　　incomplete 561, 562
　　central 555, 555*f*
　　complete 555
　　complicated 556
　　development of 558
　　incomplete 555
　　isolated 561
　　lateral 555
　　repair of 561
　　simple 556
　　unilateral 555, 557, 557*f*, 559
　　　complete 555*f*
　　　incomplete 554*f*, 555*f*
Cleft palate 554, 563, 565-567
　　bilateral complete 564*f*

complete 564
development of 558, 565
incomplete 564
repair of 568*f*
surgery 568
types of 565*f*
Clindamycin, combination of 374
Cloquet's hernia 611
Cloquet's node, enlargement of
　　611
Closed loop obstruction 746, 787
Clostridium
　　novyi 771
　　perfringens 771
　　septicum 771
Clubbing, degrees of 16
Clutton's metallic bougie 1043,
　　1043*f*
Coccidioidomycosis 801, 802
Cock's peculiar tumor 391
Cold
　　abscess 496, 526
　　agglutinins 447
　　nodule 288, 293
Colectomy
　　subtotal 202
　　total 204, 878
　　transverse 839, 1119
Colic artery
　　left 1180
　　middle 110
Colic flexure, right 839, 1161
Collagen disease 64
Collapsed lung, margin of 848
Collar stud abscess, stage of 504
Colloid
　　carcinoma 930
　　goiter 284, 289
　　nodule 285, 291, 293, 294
　　solution 723
Colon 203*f*
　　arterial supply of 1161, 1162*f*
　　ascending 1161
　　carcinoma of 199, 202, 206,
　　　879-883
　　closure of 1121
　　descending 839, 1114, 1162
　　epiploicae 82
　　fixation of 1120
　　lymphatic drainage of 1162,
　　　1163*f*
　　polyposis of 876, 877*f*
　　portion of 203*f*
　　segment of 886*f*
　　transverse 203, 790, 1161

Colonic
　　cancer 205, 841
　　　TNM classification for 206,
　　　　207*t*, 882
　　carcinoma 204, 208, 838, 839,
　　　841, 882, 883
　　development of 881
　　diagnosis of 839
　　obstructing 839, 840
　　types of 206, 838, 879, 880*f*
　　Crohn's disease 833
　　gas shadows 782
　　obstruction 812
　　polyps, types of 206, 876
　　pseudo-obstruction 793
　　surgery 839
　　tuberculosis, left 200
Colonoscopy 886
Colorectal
　　cancer 201
　　carcinoma 206, 881, 881*f*
　　surgery 937
Colostomy
　　closure of 1120
　　construction of 1120
　　device, insertion of 1120
　　freshening margin of 1121
　　mobilization of 1121
Colovesical fistula communication
　　36
Common bile duct, disposition
　　of 1171
Complement fixation test 191, 645
Compression bandaging, role of
　　397
Concomitant carcinoma in situ
　　916
Condyloma acuminata 653, 926
Confusion, transient 339
Congestive cardiac failure 765, 947
Conjoint tendon 1146*f*, 1149
Consanguineous marriage 558
Consciousness, transient loss of 686
Conservative surgery 192
Constipation 784
Constrictor muscle, inferior 528
Contact dissolution 815
Contrast-enhanced computed
　　tomography scan, role of 218,
　　431
Conventional
　　chemotherapy, role of 124
　　cutting needle 1006*f*
Cooper's ligament 57, 62, 63, 66,
　　69, 612, 931, 1087, 1148, 1188

Cope's technique 873
Cord
 encysted hydrocele of 621,
  625-627, 630
 fibrous 615
 holding forceps 1019, 1019*f*
 hydrocele of 33, 44
 lipoma of 44, 627, 630
 lymphangioma of 627
 structures, parietalization of
  1089
Core needle biopsy 239
Corona glandis, region of 926*f*
Coronary ligament 1168
Corrugated rubber sheet drain
  1054, 1054*f*
Corrugator supercilii 533, 534*f*
Cosmetic deformity 454
Costal cartilage, calcification of
  794
Costocervical trunk 1204
Cough 3
Courvoisier's law 96, 149, 149*f*, 167
Cranial fossa fracture
 anterior 847
 middle 847
Cranial nerve palsy 3
Craniostenosis 296
Cranium
 computed tomography scan of
  386
 examination of 8, 41, 349
Cricothyrotomy 970, 970*f*
Crile's method 278, 278*f*
Criminal nerve of Grassi 129, 129*f*
Crohn's disease 11, 790, 830-832,
  837, 869, 871, 881, 1035
 development of 831
 left colonic 200
Crohn's ileitis, acute 729
Cronkhite-Canada syndrome 876,
  879
Crossed leg test 348, 354, 354*f*
Crushing clamps functions 1037
Cryoglobulinemia 447
Cryosurgery, role of 423
Cryptorchidism 675, 925
Crystal clear fluid 628
Curettage, role of 423
Curling's ulcer 725
Cushing's syndrome 24, 223, 296,
  317
 facies of 10*f*
Cutaneous malignancies,
 development of 427

Cutaneous nerve, medial 469, 469*f*
Cyanosis 5, 15, 680, 848
 central 15, 15*f*
 peripheral 15
Cyclophosphamide 120, 248
Cycloserine 506
Cyst 34, 183*f*, 186, 188-190, 386,
  486
 aspiration of 486
 biliary relationship of 186
 chronic 197
 complex 295
 congenital 185, 198
 excision of 188
 false 385
 fluid 497
 intraperitoneal rupture of 189
 large 628
 layers of 892
 location of 186
 neoplastic 199
 number of 186
 parapelvic 216
 pressure of 189
 proliferative 185
 pseudopancreatic 193, 194*f*
 resection of 182
 retention 197, 762
 rupture of 184, 189
 sebaceous 384, 388-391, 393,
  453
 sequestration 198
 size of 186
 small 628
 thyroglossal 37, 278, 487, 490,
  490*f*, 491-493, 497
 traumatic 185
 true 198
 urachal 617
Cystadenocarcinoma 160, 199
Cystadenoma, mucinous 199
Cystectomy technique of 187
Cystic
 artery 1173
  and duct, ligation of 1104
 degeneration 185, 454
 duct 806*f*, 1101, 1170, 1173
  disposition of 1171
  stump 143
 hygroma 33, 484-487, 496, 497
  complications of 487
  fates of 485
 islet cell tumors 199
 lesion 185, 453

 neoplasms 199
 pedicle 142
  dissection of 1101, 1103
 swelling 185
 vein 1183
Cysticercosis 199
Cystine stones 797
Cystitis, acute 755
Cystoenterostomy 182
Cystogastrostomy 194*f*, 195
Cystography 756
Cystojejunostomy 194
Cystolithotomy forceps,
 suprapubic 1039, 1039*f*
Cystopericystectomy 192
Cystosarcoma phyllodes 599, 600,
  600*f*
Cystostomy, suprapubic 753
Cystourethroscopy 918
Cytarabine 120
Cytotoxic chemotherapy 158
Czerny's retractor 1013, 1013*f*

D

Dacarbazine 516
Dacron mesh 77
Dahl Froment's sign 788
Dalrymple's sign 276
Damage control surgery 712
Danazol therapy 617
Dasatinib 124
Daughter cyst 188, 892
De Pezzer's catheter 1042, 1042*f*
Deaver's retractor 1015, 1015*f*
Decubitus 5, 11
Deep cervical fascia, disposition
 of 1197
Deep ring occlusion test 41, 49, 601
Deformity 482, 562
Dehydration 746
 correction of 939
Delaire's technique 561
Dense stellate soft tissue mass 239
Dental cyst 487, 497, 587-589
 contents of 588
Dentigerous cyst 487, 497, 588,
  589
Depressed fracture, open 846
Dercum's disease 395
Dermagraft 724
Dermal
 burn
  deep 720, 723
  superficial 720

flares 344
graft 664
nevus 415
Dermatitis 12
Dermatomyositis 447
Dermoid
    cyst 198, 382, 383, 383f, 384,
        384f, 385, 386, 386f, 387,
        389, 390, 453, 526
    complications of 387
    preauricular 384f
    submental 388f
    types of 386
    postanal 386
    sequestration 385
    subhyoid 489
    teratomatous 386
    type of 385
Deroofing operation, role of 906
Desjardin's choledocholithotomy
    forceps 1028, 1028f
Desmoid tumor 618, 619, 732
    development of 619
Devine and Horton's operation
    651
Dexrabeprazole 128
Dextran solution 723
Diabetes 74, 159, 162
    control of 368
    mellitus 73, 159, 297, 339, 713,
        726, 940, 941
        maternal 558
Diabetic foot 365, 367, 368, 372,
        374, 375
    classification systems of 379
    infection 369-371, 373, 380
        classification schemes 380t
    ulcer 376-378, 378f
        development of 376
Diabetic neuropathy 365
Diaphragm, domes of 780
Diarrhea 134, 137, 159, 304, 830,
        838
    chronic 831
    postvagotomy 138
Dietl's crisis 909
Digastric triangle, boundary of
        1207
Digital mammography 851
Digital nerve block 982, 982f
Digoxin 598
Dipping method 104f
Directly observed therapy short
    course treatment regimen 505
Discoid lupus erythematosus 581

Disinfection 985
    intermediate level of 985
Dissection, anterior 1115, 1117,
        1118
Distant metastasis 111, 154, 160,
        207, 224, 255, 262, 431, 436,
        508, 510, 544, 672
Distension, abdominal 73, 784
Distress, respiratory 759
Diverticulum, appendicular 835
Donor nephrectomy 1125
Doom, triangle of 633, 633f
Dorsal
    interossei 474, 475f
    scapular
        artery 1204
        nerve 470
Dorsalis pedis artery 367
Double duct sign 152
Down's syndrome 558
Doxorubicin 516
Doxycycline 374
Doyen's cross action type towel
    clip 989
Doyen's intestinal occlusion
    clamps 1033, 1034f
Doyen's mouth gag 1049, 1049f
Drain 963, 964, 965, 966
    paronychia 961
    placement of 82, 83, 1094,
        1097, 1101, 1110, 1112,
        1113, 1116, 1124, 1131,
        1132, 1137
Drop test 1073
Drugs 736
Duct
    carcinoma 762, 763
    dilatation 239
    ectasia 762, 763
    fistula 551
    papilloma 762-764
    submandibular 546, 547, 547f,
        551
    thyroglossal 491, 491f, 492,
        492f
Ductal
    calculi, removal of 1111
    carcinoma in situ 241
        high-grade 851
    injury 712
Dukes staging 206
Dumbbell neurofibroma 456
Dumbbell parotid tumor 545
Duodenal
    cap, region of 822f

fistula 134, 713, 1140
hematoma 710
ileus 828
    chronic 828
injury 710, 711
    nonoperative treatment of
        711
    laceration 710
    obstruction 157, 812, 826, 828
    point 88
    stricture 828
    stump 135
        blow out 805
        closure of 1093
    ulcer 804
        chronic 124, 126, 127, 130,
            132, 133t, 133, 139, 822,
            828
        complications of 125
    wall thickening 709
Duodenum 132, 710, 855, 1107
    anterior wall of 780
    barium meal X-ray of 822f,
        823f, 825f, 827f
    division of 1093, 1095
    double contrast barium X-ray
        of 823
    first part of 1107
    Kocherization of 1108, 1111
Dynamic venography 343
Dyselectrolytemia 746
Dysphagia 445
    sideropenic 581

E

Eagle's criteria 944
Ear pain, cause of 576
Eastern cooperative oncology
    group scale 5, 9
Ecchymosis 336
Echinococcosis 191
Echinococcus 889, 890
    antigen 185
    granulosus 188, 889
        adult worm of 890f
        lifecycle of 891f
    multilocularis 188, 889, 892
Ectopia vesicae 666, 667f, 668, 669
Ectopic
    pregnancy 729, 731
    testis 641, 642
        location of 641f
    thyroid gland 388, 491

Eczema 341
Edema 5, 16, 228, 368, 765
    laryngeal 758
    pancreatic 710
Ehlers-Danlos syndrome 64
Elbow 400
Electrocardiography 42, 242, 298, 332, 360, 369
Electrolyte
    imbalance, correction of 939
    serum 107, 372
Electromyography 470
Elephantiasis
    causes of 455
    graecorum 455
    neurofibromatosa 454, 455
Embolic gangrene 759
Embryonal carcinoma 924
Empyema 46, 96, 189
    drainage of 967
    thoracis 726
Encephalocele 46
Encephaloid carcinoma 930
Endo needle holder 1080, 1080f
Endocrine
    deficiency, pancreatic 713
    disorder 135
    factors 639, 663
Endocyst, functions of 188, 892
Endograsping forceps 1076
Endometrial cancer 249
Endometrioma 617
Endoscissors 1077, 1077f
Endoscopic
    biopsy, role of 121
    clip applicator 1078, 1078f
    crocodile forceps 1078, 1078f
    diathermy
        hook 1079, 1079f
        spatula 1080, 1080f
    drainage, problems of 195
    internal urethrotomy 719
    pyelolysis 219
    retrograde
        cholangiopancreatography 167, 707, 806, 807, 807f, 808f, 810, 939
        cholnagiography 806f
    sphincterotomy 171
    spoon forceps 1079, 1079f
    submucosal resection 116
        technique of 116

ultrasonography, role of 153, 163
Endovenous laser
    ablation 335
    surgery 337
Enema, contrast 791
Enophthalmos 483
Enterobacter aerogenes 369
Enterocele 44, 61
Enteroclysis 829f
Enterocutaneous fistula 36
Enterocystoma 615
Enterogenous cyst 198
Enzyme
    deficiency 663
    linked immunosorbent assay 132, 185
    pancreatic 738
Epidermal burns 723
Epidermodysplasia verruciformis 428
Epidermoid carcinoma 799
Epididymal cyst 44, 390, 621, 627, 628, 630
Epididymis 628
    cyst of 627, 628
Epididymo-orchitis 627, 670
Epigastric hernia 608, 608f
    false 608
    true 608
Epigastrium 91
Epilepsy, acute 726
Epispadias 554
Epistaxis 847
Epithelial
    dysplasia, mild-to-moderate 570
    tumors 307, 537
Epithelioid granuloma 504
Epulis 592
    benign 593
    carcinomatous 593
    false 593
    fibrous 592, 593
    malignant 593
    types of 593
Erb-Duchenne paralysis 482
Erectile dysfunction 650
Erythema 368
Erythrocyte sedimentation rate 8, 221, 242, 288, 332, 360, 504
Erythroplakia 570, 573, 581

Erythroplasia of Queyrat 657, 660, 927
Escherichia coli 369, 959
Esomeprazole 128
Esophageal
    carcinoma 821
    dilatation 818
    myotomy, long 818
    nodes, lateral 1157
    obstruction 1140
    resection 821
    spasm, diffuse 818
    sphincter 1156
        lower 1156
        upper 1156
    stenosis, upper 528
Esophagectomy transhiatal 821
Esophagitis, chronic 820
Esophagogastric junction, dissection of 1096
Esophagojejunal anastomosis 1096
Esophagojejunostomy
    end-to-side stapled 1096
    hand sewn end-to-side 1096
Esophagoscopy 527
Esophagus 508, 1156
    abdominal 1158
    part of 1097
    advanced carcinoma of 821
    arterial supply of 1157
    barium swallow X-ray of 816, 816f, 818f, 819f
    carcinoma of 818, 1141
    diffuse spasm of 818
    dilatation of 816f
    lower end of 132, 816f, 821, 856
    nerve supply of 1158
    normal constriction of 1157
    venous drainage of 1157
Essels along lesser curvature 1159
Estrogen 258, 598
Ethambutol 505, 506
Ethanolamine oleate 974
Ethionamide 506
Ethylene oxide gas 986
European Hernia Society Groin Hernia Classification 65t
Everolimus 124
Excessive coffee consumption 223
Excessive salivation, cause of 576
Exertional breathlessness 302
Exocrine insufficiency, pancreatic 713

Exogenous daughter cyst 191
Exomphalos 604
  major 604f, 605
    management of 605
  minor 604
  sac 604
Exophthalmos 276, 280, 280f, 281f, 296, 303
  bilateral 296
  causes of 296
  grades of 296
  malignant 297
  unilateral 296
Exostosis 444
Extensor
  carpi radialis
    brevis 468
    longus 468
  carpi ulnaris 468
  digiti minimi 468
  digitorum longus 468
    muscle 466f
  indicis 468
  muscles
    deep 468f
    superficial 468f
  pollicis
    brevis 467, 467f, 468
    longus 466, 466f, 468
External genitalia, palpation of 213
Extracorporeal shock wave
  lithotripsy, role of 815
Extradural hematoma 687, 847
Extrahepatic
  bile duct 183
  biliary system 1166
    anatomy of 1170f
    constitutes 1170
  biliary tree 183
    dilatation of 183
  cysts, multiple 183
Extraperitoneal operation, steps of
  total 1088
Extremities
  examination of 683
  temperature of 679
  venous disease, lower 331
Extrinsic compression near
  pylorus 105
Eyelids, lower 13f
Eyes
  signs 280
  yellowish discoloration of 85
Eystadenoma 185

F

Face
  sensory nerves of 1196f
  vein of 1194, 1195f
Facial
  acne 10f
  artery 975, 1205
  nerve 545, 1133
    branches of 536, 536f, 1133
    injury 542
    palsy 533, 546
    trunk 535
  vein 1194
Facies 5, 10
Fahrenheit or centigrade scale 23
Falciform ligament 1168
Fallopian tubes 61
Familial adenomatous polyposis
  coli 838, 877, 878
Fascia 61, 1146
  pretracheal 1132
  prevertebral 31f
  transversalis 63, 1155
    disposition of 1154
Fat
  necrosis, traumatic 238, 763
  perinephric 1155
  saponification 710
Fatigue 304
Fecal impaction 790
Fecaliths 794, 833
Fegan's test 323, 329, 329f
Femoral
  aneurysm 611
  artery 1151, 1216
    branches of 980, 1169
    exposure of 980,, 981f
  canal
    boundary of 610
    contents of 610
    opening of 1149
  hernia 44, 50, 51, 52f, 609-612
    incidence of 610
    right-sided 609f
    sac, hydrocele of 611
    strangulated 611
  pulse 355, 356f
  ring, boundary of 610, 1150
  sheath 1149, 1149f, 1216
    boundaries of 610f
    compartments of 1149
  tail 642
  triangle 641, 641f, 1216f

  boundary of 1151, 1215
  contents of 1151, 1216
  floor of 1216f
  vein 1151, 1217
Fetal exposure 675
Fever 2, 3, 85, 145, 189, 368, 786, 830
  continuous 23
  intermittent 23, 831
  remittent 23
  types of 23, 24f
Fibers
  lower horizontal 1156
  postganglionic
    parasympathetic 1185
    sympathetic 1185, 1186
  preganglionic
    parasympathetic 1185
    sympathetic 1185
  somatic 1186
Fibroadenoma 599, 599, 764
  hard 599
  pathological types of 599
Fibroadenosis 762, 764
Fibrocystic disease 198
Fibrolipoma 394
Fibroma 384, 390, 393, 453, 535
Fibrosarcoma 430
Fibrous histiocytoma, malignant
  438
Fibular bone graft 581
Filarial
  epididymo-orchitis 645
  infection 645
  scrotum 643
Filariasis 455, 644, 645
Fine needle aspiration cytology
  121, 221, 241, 285, 404, 504, 511, 512, 524, 654, 870
  role of 432
Fingers
  dorsal aspect of 92f
  dorsum of 352f
Fisch nerve hook 1015f
Fissure, portal 1169
Fistula 36, 499, 1021
  development of 497f
  formation 493
  internal 198
  pancreatic 713
  pelvirectal 1021
  perianal 1021
  subcutaneous 1021
  submucous 1021

thyroglossal 493, 494
transsphincteric 1021
urachal 617, 618
urethrocutaneous 36, 666
vesicovaginal 36
Fistulectomy 1022
Fistulotomy 1022
Fitzpatrick's operation 651
Flail chest 693, 848
central 694
lateral 694
major 694, 849, 850
minor 694, 849, 850
Flail segment 850
fixation of 850
paradoxical movement of 693
Flank pain 911
Flatus tube 1048, 1048*f*, 1049
Flexor
carpi ulnaris 474, 477
compartment 477, 478*f*, 1219
digiti minimi 481
digitorum
profundus 474, 479, 480*f*
superficialis 479, 480*f*
pollicis
brevis 481
longus 478, 478*f*
tendon sheaths 965*f*
infection of 966, 966*f*
Floor of mouth, carcinoma of 584
Fluid 625, 784
and electrolyte
balance 135, 787
retention 249
balance chart 743
collection
acute 739, 742
peripancreatic 710
therapy 722
Fluorodeoxyglucose positron
emission tomography 153
Foam sclerotherapy 335, 338
complications of 339
Foley's balloon catheter 1040,
1040*f*
Foley's catheter 80, 955
Follicular
adenoma 285, 291, 292, 305-
307
carcinoma 292, 307, 308, 310,
314
low-grade 308
neoplasm 293

Foot ulcer 378, 379
Formaldehyde vapor 985
Fossa, supraclavicular 357*f*
Fourth branchial arch 498
Fowler-Stephens procedure 638
Fracture
comminuted 845*f*
depressed 846
pathological 223
Fragment, depressed 846
Frey's syndrome 539
Froment's sign 476, 476*f*
Fruchaud's myopectineal orifice
66, 66*f*, 1146, 1146*f*
Fuchsig's test 354, 354*f*
Fuller's bivalve metallic
tracheostomy tube 1051, 1051*f*
Fulminant sepsis 374
Fundic glands 1159
Fundus 1158
first cholecystectomy 1104
Fungal infection 801, 802
Fungi 897
Funicular direct inguinal hernia 69

G

Gait 5, 8, 11
Galactocele 763
Galea aponeurotica, disposition
of 1192
Gallbladder 88, 96, 96*f*, 139, 145,
148, 149*f*, 167, 170, 178, 183*f*,
894*f*, 895, 895*f*, 1070, 1171
adenomyomatosis of 175, 902
arterial supply of 1172*f*
cancer 176
advanced 174
carcinoma of 144, 146, 148,
171, 172, 174, 175, 177, 184,
898, 902-904, 1103
cholesterolosis of 901, 902,
1103
dissection of 1101, 1104
empyema of 144, 145, 172, 898,
900, 1103
extraction of 1101
functions of 1173
lumen of 895
mucocele of 144, 145, 172,
895*f*, 898, 900, 1103
palpation of 167
parts of 1170
perforation of 805
point 88

polyp 175, 902, 1103
strawberry 146
structure of 1170
traumatic rupture of 1103
venous drainage of 1172
Gallstone 134, 144, 184, 736, 794,
898
asymptomatic 796
composition of 795
development of 144, 898
disease 140, 175, 177, 736, 795,
894, 902, 1028, 1103
formation of 896
ileus 144, 784, 898
large 146
pancreatitis 741
pigment 143, 894
radiopaque 794
silent 146, 796, 901
types of 143, 795, 894
Gamma
glutamyltransferase 707
glutamyltranspeptidase 168
irradiation 986
Ganglioneuromas 456
Gangrene 144,, 347
Gangrenous cholecystitis, acute
896*f*
Gardner's syndrome 877, 879
Gas 784
filled ileal loops 782
gangrene 771
sterilization 986, 1072
Gastrectomy 137
distal 1109
indications of 113, 1037, 1094
partial 131
radical 113
total 113, 1037
Gastric
artery
left 1159
right 1159
short 1160, 1160*f*
biopsy 132
cancer 114-117, 862, 863, 863*f*,
865, 1092
advanced 117, 863
development of 117, 865
diffuse 863
intestinal type 863
proximal 113
TNM classification for 111,
111*t*

carcinoma 114, 825
  advanced 825
  types of 825
distension 79
glands 1159
hemorrhage, life threatening
  1094
lavage 109, 939
lymphoma 117, 120, 131
  Ann Arbor staging of 118
  primary 117-119
  secondary 118-120
  types of 117
occlusion clamps 1030, 1031f
outlet obstruction 11, 103-106,
      124, 125, 157, 826-828,
      938
  cause of 827
  consequences of 827
  palliation of 174
  relief of 158
peristalsis 91f
point 88, 127
resection 114
ulcer 858
  benign 822, 823, 855, 859
  chronic 126, 127, 131-133,
      133t, 139, 823, 824, 856,
      858, 859
  complications of 824
  excision of 131
  types of 133
vein
  left 1183
  right 1183
vessels
  division of short 110, 1124
Gastrinoma 135
Gastritis
  acute 735
  chronic 131
Gastroduodenal artery, branch
  of 1160
Gastroepiploic
  artery
    left 1160, 1160f
    right 1160, 1160f
  vessels 110
    division 1093, 1095
    right 110
Gastroesophage 819f
Gastroesophageal
  junction 819f
  reflux disease 143

Gastrohepatic
  ligament 1093
  omentum, division of 1109
Gastrointestinal
  secretions, volumes of 784
  stromal tumor 105, 120
    TNM classification for 122,
      122t
  system 934
  tract 508, 698, 790
Gastrojejunal anastomosis 1094,
  1098, 1110
Gastrojejunocolic fistula 134
Gastrojejunostomy 125, 130, 131,
      134, 156, 157, 1033, 1097,
      1106f
  indications of 1033
  steps of 1033, 1097
  stoma of 132, 856
Gastrosplenic ligament 1095
Gastrostomy 1140, 1141f
  techniques of 1141
Gatifloxacin 506
Gelbard's operation 651
Genetic testing, role of 264
Genital defects
  female 668
  male 668
Genital wart 926
  long-standing 657
Genitalia 620
  external 6, 88, 89
Genitofemoral nerve, genital
  branch of 60, 1146
Gerota's fascia 222, 1155
Gestational thyrotoxicosis 304
Giant
  cell 593
    granuloma 589
    Langhans type of 504
  fibroadenoma 599
  incisional hernia 79
  mesh placement, bilateral 63
  ventral hernia, repair of 83
Gilbert's classification 64
Gingivoperiosteoplasty 563
Gland
  deep part of 1134, 1135
  fistula 551
  sebaceous 390
  submandibular 547f, 548, 550,
    551
  superficial part of 1134
Glandular hypospadias 666

Glans penis 656
  leukoplakia of 657
Glanuloplasty 664, 666
Glasgow score 740
Glaucoma 442
Globular swelling measurement
  of 29
Glomangioma 444
Glomerulonephritis, acute 755
Glomus
  body 444
  intravagale 525
  jugulare 525
  tumor 402, 444, 444f
Glossitis 12f
  cheilitis 12
  chronic superficial 573
  syphilitic 573
Glutaraldehyde solution 985, 986
Goiter 284
  huge 279
  nodular 308
  retrosternal 279
    prolongation of 279, 279f
  simple multinodular 305
  toxic 937
Goldman's cardiac risk index 944
Gonadotropin-releasing hormone
  638
Goodsall's rule 1022, 1022f
Gorlin syndrome 428
Graham's patch 743, 779
Granulocyte-macrophage colony-
  stimulating factor 376
Granuloma 755
Graves' disease 295, 297, 298, 304
Greater omentum, division of
  1093, 1112
Groin hernia 64, 66
  laparoscopic repair of 57
  recurrent 59
  repair 58
Growing toe nail, double edge in
  974
Gstrointestinal lymphomas,
  primary 118
Gubernaculum testis 640
Guillotine method 649
Gynecomastia 595, 598
  bilateral 596, 597, 597f
  causes of 598
  idiopathic 597

H

Haemophilus influenzae 1124
Hamartomas 443
Hamartomatous lesions 444
Hamper laparoscopic dissection 59
Hand infection 961
  drainage of 964*f*
Hand sewn
  anastomosis 1116
  closure 1095
Hard palate, carcinoma of 586
Hartley Dunhill procedure 290
Hartmann's procedure 792, 833
Harvey's sign 347, 353
Hashimoto's thyroiditis 285, 307, 308
Head
  and neck carcinoma, TNM classification for 508
  coring, pancreatic 1111
  injury 685
  lesion, pancreatic 151
  of pancreas, carcinoma of 96, 147, 158, 161
  rising test 102*f*
Headache 2, 3, 339
Heart rate 680
  normal 21
Heartbeat, irregular 304
Heat sensitivity 304
Heath's suture cutting scissors 1012, 1012*f*
Heel ulcer 377
Heineke-Mikulicz pyloroplasty 130, 130*f*
Heineke-Mikulicz technique 664
Helicobacter pylori 127, 132*f*, 856, 862
  infection 117, 131, 132, 175, 159, 856, 862
Heller's operation 818
Hemagglutination test, indirect 191
Hemangioma 307, 439, 439*f*, 440, 442, 444, 453, 455, 489, 527, 537
  cavernous 441
  complications of 443, 460
  plexiform 441, 442
  types of 441
Hemangiosarcoma 430
Hematemesis 2, 133
Hematocele 621, 623, 624, 626, 670

Hematoma 334, 666, 763
  acute subdural 689
  intracranial 687
  peripancreatic 710
  subcapsular 707
  subdural 688, 847
Hematuria 2, 713, 754, 798, 905, 906, 909
  gross 911
  painless 223
Hemicolectomy, right 839, 1112
Hemimandibulectomy 572, 590, 591
Hemithyroidectomy 290, 310, 1131
Hemoglobin 221, 369, 680
Hemogram, complete 107, 140, 221, 288, 294, 360, 399, 596, 644, 700, 728
Hemoperitoneum 702, 705
Hemoptysis 3, 223
Hemorrhage 60, 198, 302, 341, 387, 394, 443, 758, 759, 923*f*, 968, 996
  grades of 995
  intracystic 190
  intramural 830, 869
  postoperative 759
  primary 995
  reactionary 995
  secondary 713, 995
  subconjunctival 847
Hemorrhagic fluid 904*f*
Hemorrhoidectomy
  closed 1026
  Milligan-Morgan technique of 1026
Hemorrhoids 971*f*
Hemostasis 1104
Hemostatic forceps 993, 993*f*
  uses of 994
Hemothorax 968
  management of 849
  massive 689
  traumatic 691, 849, 967
Hemotympanum 847
Henry Gray's forceps 1027
Heparin, low-molecular weight 703, 766
Hepatic
  adenoma 185
  artery 154, 182, 1095
    common 110
    left 1173
    right 1173
  duct 806*f*, 807*f*, 813*f*, 1169

  common 1167*f*, 1170, 1171, 1173
    disposition of 1171
  dysfunction 911
  flexure 203*f*
  glycogen stores 940
  injury 705
    conservative treatment of 704
  metastasis 257
  resection, role of 707
  trauma 705, 707
Hepaticodochojejunostomy 1110
Hepaticojejunostomy 156*f*
Hepatobiliary iminodiacetic acid scanning 750
Hepatoduodenal ligament
  dissection of 1108
Hepatoma 185
Hernia 38, 43, 59, 66, 67, 594, 790
  bilateral 59, 64
  complete 44
  complications of 66
  congenital 33, 600-602, 1084
  contents of 60, 66
  development of 67
  direct 50, 52
  distal extent of 62
  fundus of 47*f*
  incisional 71, 72*f*, 73, 77
  incomplete 43
  inflamed 66, 67
  irreducible 66
  laparoscopic repair of 1151
  large 64
    incisional 74
  location of 65
  obstructed 40, 59, 66
  operation, open 59
  recurrence of 60, 70
  reduction of 47*f*
  repair 54*f*, 56, 77
  sac
    indirect 56
    posterior wall of 61*f*
  strangulated 59, 66, 67
  swelling 46, 53
  umbilical 602, 603, 606, 603*f*
Hernial sac 60, 61, 61*f*, 626
  dissection of 1083, 1084, 1087, 1088
  hydrocele of 66, 624, 625
  opening of 1084
  parts of 60, 60*f*

Herniography 67
Hernioplasty 60, 62
Herniorrhaphy 60
    indications of 602
Herniotomy 55, 602
    steps of 1084, 1085*f*
Hesselbach's triangle 52, 68, 69, 1146
Hiatus hernia 126, 139, 143
Hilton's method 1000
Hip joint, movement of 348
Histaminase 317
Histoplasmosis 801
Hodgkin's disease, histologic types of 514
Hodgkin's lymphoma 503, 515, 516
Homan's sign 331, 765
Hormonal
    stimulation, defective 640
    theory 920
    therapy, side effects of 639
    treatment, role of 638
Hormone 925
    replacement therapy 265
    therapy 255, 764, 802
        role of 248, 225, 596
    treatment 754
Horner's syndrome 275, 483
Hot
    air oven 987
    nodule 288
Human
    chorionic gonadotropin 304, 638
    low-density lipoprotein 360
Humerus, mid-shaft of 464
Hürthle cell
    carcinoma 316
    neoplasm 316
    tumors 315, 316
Hutchinson's melanotic freckle 414, 415
Hydatid cyst 186-192, 199, 889, 892, 893
    complications of 189, 893
    enlargement of 191
    layers of 893
    sequelae of 189, 893
    treatment of 192
Hydatid disease 188, 190, 191, 801, 889
Hydatid fluid 188, 893
Hydration status 5, 11
Hydrocele 33, 60, 497, 623, 624, 634

bilocular 625
complications of 626
congenital 44, 625
development of 624
fluid 487
funicular 625
infantile 625
infected 623
operation 623
primary 624
relief of 623
secondary 624
tapping of 624
types of 625
Hydrocephalus 459, 460, 462
Hydronephrosis 216, 217, 217*f*, 218, 219, 220, 842, 843, 904, 906, 907*f*, 908, 909, 1125
bilateral 219, 909
causes of
    bilateral 843, 908
    unilateral 843, 906
complications of 220, 909
grades of 843
surgery 219
unilateral 219
Hydronephrotic sac 908
Hydroxydaunomycin 120
Hyoid
    arch 498
    bone 491, 492
Hypercalcemia 223, 911
    transient 249
Hypercalcitoninemia, persistent 319
Hyperchloremic acidosis 669
Hyperemia, zone of 721
Hyperkalemia 948
Hyperkinesia 302
Hypernephroma 909
Hyperparathyroidism 736, 798
    brown tumor of 589
Hyperphosphatemia 948
Hyperplasia
    benign 219
    prostatic 68, 920, 921, 1024
    pseudoepitheliomatous 421
Hyperplastic
    candidiasis, chronic 581
    polyp, hyperplastic 877
Hyperprolactinemia 762
Hyperpyrexia 23
    malignant 751, 933
Hypertension 22, 73, 223, 905, 906, 911

intra-abdominal 84
portal 93, 184, 189, 812
treatment of 906
Hyperthermia 631, 770
Hyperthyroidism 304
    primary 303
    secondary 304, 305
    symptom of 273
    types of 303
Hypertonic saline 723
Hypertrophic pyloric stenosis, adult 105
Hypertrophic scar 395, 397
Hypoalbuminemia 765
Hypocalcemia correction of 939
Hypochondrium
    left 91
    right 91
Hypogastrium 91, 100*f*
Hypoglossal nerve 3
Hypoglycemic attacks 812
Hyponatremia 948
Hypopharynx 508
Hypopigmentation 428
Hypoproteinemia 74, 748, 940
    correction of 939, 940
Hypospadias 554, 660-663
    anterior 662
    development of 663
    distal penile type of 661*f*
    middle 662
    posterior 662
    repair
        complications of 666
        principle of 664
    types of 662, 662*f*
Hypotension 22, 189, 368, 686, 693, 700
Hypothenar muscles 474, 481
Hypothermia 23
Hypothyroidism 762
    symptom of 273
Hypoxia 631

I

Ileocecal valve function 790
Ileostomy 878, 1116
Ileum, part of 871*f*
Iliac artery
    exposure of external 979, 979*f*
    ligature of internal 977, 978*f*
Iliac fossa 96*f*, 1212
    left 91
    right 91, 731, 831

Iliac spine, anterior superior 48f,
49f, 356f
Iliopsoas
bursa 611
muscle 1146f
Imatinib resistant disease 123
Immunity
cell-mediated 769
humoral 769
Immunosuppressive therapy 74,
146
Impalpable testis 635, 641
Incision 977, 1093, 1103, 1107,
1108
abdominal 992, 992f, 1089
closure of 1101, 1126
subcostal 992
transverse 992
type of 749
Incisional hernia
development of 73
laparoscopic repair of 79
mesh repair of 78
midline 74, 75
repair of 76, 78, 79
Infection 190, 198, 387, 391, 394,
443, 454, 460, 736, 905, 906, 968
Infectious Diseases Society of
America 380
Inflammation, stage of 504
Inflammatory polyp 877
Ingrowing toe nail 973
Inguinal canal 64, 601, 1145, 1150
boundaries of 1145
contents of 1146
exposure of 1083
posterior wall of 64
surgical anatomy of 1145f
Inguinal fossa
lateral 1152
medial 1152
Inguinal hernia 42, 43, 51, 51f, 56,
57, 68, 610, 611, 621, 1088
complete 61
direct 44, 50f, 52, 65, 68, 68f, 69
funicular type of 44
indirect 44, 50, 50f, 52, 65, 69
recurrent 70, 70f
repair of 56, 57
right-sided 42f
Rives prosthetic repair of 63
surgery 53
types of 44f, 62
unilateral 59

Inguinal ligament 55f, 356f, 1147,
1148, 1148f
reflected part of 1148
Inguinal lymph node 404, 658,
1151
metastasis, left 652f
Inguinal pouch, superficial 641,
641f, 642
Inguinal ring
deep 640, 1212
superficial 47f, 1147, 1212
Inguinal tail, superficial 642
Inguinoscrotal
regions 39f
swelling 45f
Inhalational injury 721
Initial fluid therapy 996
Injection sclerotherapy 1025
indications of 337
Injury
high-grade 702
level of 473
mechanism of 678
pancreatic 708, 711-713
pancreaticoduodenal 708, 709
penetrating 708
types of 473
Insomnia 302
Insulin test, role of 858
Intensity modulated radiotherapy
434
Intermittent porphyria, acute 726
Intermuscular septum
lateral 1215
medial 1214
Internal inguinal ring, large 64
Interossei muscles 474
Interphalangeal joint, movement
of 348
Intersphincteric fistula 1021
Interstitial cell tumors 671
Intestinal anastomosis
techniques of 1035
types of 1035
Intestinal fluid, sequestration of
746
Intestinal
metaplasia, types of 117, 865
needles 1007
obstruction 134, 746, 786
acute 726, 729, 730, 782,
784, 785, 787, 870
causes of small 783
simple 746

subacute 784, 870
occlusion clamps 1033
perforation 805
Intestine 61, 801
acquired diverticula of 874
Intradermal nevi 414
Intrahepatic biliary radicles 807f,
808f, 813f
Intraoperative cholangiography,
role of 170
Intraperitoneal rupture 190
Intratesticular hyperperfusion
injury 631
Intratumor injection 244
Intravenous fluid 607, 743
Intussusception 871-873
development of 872
diagnosis of 873
Invagination test 46, 47f
Ionizing radiation 265, 427
Iron deficiency anemia 137
Irritation, chronic 573
Ischemic
colitis 790, 837
damage 830, 869
gangrene 518f
stage of 364, 447
limb 376
revascularization of 377
Ischiorectal abscess 955, 959, 960
drainage of 960f
Ishikawa
classification 164f
radiographic criteria 164
Islet of Langerhans 1175
Isoniazid 505
Isoperistaltic gastrojejunostomy
130
Isotope scanning, role of 288
Itching 189

J

Jacksonian epilepsy 442
Japanese classification of early
gastric cancer 863, 863f
Jaundice 2, 5, 14, 15, 74, 184, 189,
748, 838
obstructive 144, 147, 148, 150,
166, 167, 170, 171, 178, 181,
189, 898, 939
painless progressive 159, 161
palliation of 174
relief of 158, 174

Jejunal
    limb, end of distal 1098
    loop 782, 829
    mesenteric gap, closure of
        1112
    mesentery 1098
    stricture 829
Jejunogastric intussusception 134
Jejunojejunal anastomosis 1098,
    1112
Jejunojejunostomy, end-to-side
    1097
Jejunostomy, feeding 1110
Jejunum
    division of 1109
    Roux loop of 1098
Joffroy's sign 276, 281, 281*f*
Joint sensation 8
Joll's thyroid retractor 1018, 1018*f*
Jugular vein
    anterior 1195
    cannulation, internal 953, 953*f*
    external 1195
    internal 19, 19*f*, 20
Jugular venous
    pressure 17, 17*f*
    pulsation 17*f*
    pulse wave 18*f*
Junctional nevus 414, 415
Juvenile polyps 876

K

Kanamycin 506
Kangri cancer 420
Kaposi's sarcoma 402
Karnofsky scale 5, 9
Keetley-Torek technique 638
Kehr's sign 700
Kehr's T-tube 1029, 1029*f*
Kelly's hemostatic forceps 993
Kelly's rectal speculum 1047,
Keloid 395, 396
    complications of 397
    development of 396
    nonprogressive 396
    scar 302
    spontaneous 396
    treatment of 397
Kerley's lines 800
Kidney 88, 98, 214, 222, 801
    ballottability of 214*f*
    carcinoma of 216, 220, 223,
        754, 756, 909, 1125

coverings of 1155, 1155*f*
cut section of 907*f*
exposure of 1126
gross destruction of 1125
hydatid cyst of 216, 221
hydronephrotic 220
lump 200
mass 223
mobilization of 1126
nonfunctional 220, 1125
palpation of 99*f*, 213
pyonephrosis of 1125
simple cyst of 216
stone 794
    radiopaque 794, 796
tuberculosis of 221, 912, 913
upper pole of 1126
USG of 68
Killian's dehiscence 527, 528
Klatskin's tumor 180
Klinefelter's syndrome 595, 598,
    925
Klippel-Trenaunay syndrome 452
KLittre's hernia 61
Klumpke's paralysis 482
Knee 400
    elbow position 102*f*
    joint, movement of 348
Koch's lymphadenitis 388, 523
Koch's postulate regarding
    infection 768
Kocher's clamps 82
Kocher's gastric occlusion clamp
    1030
Kocher's hemostatic forceps 997,
Kocher's incision 141
Kocher's maneuver 1108
Kocher's subcostal incision 992,
    1103
    anatomy of 1091
Kocher's test 275
Kocher's thyroid dissector 1018,
    1018*f*
Kocher's vein of 1201
Krukenberg's tumor 932
Kussmaul's sign 693
Kyphosis 457

L

Labii inferioris, depressor 557
Labiomental muscles 557
Lacrimal nerve 1195
Lactated Ringer's solution 722, 723
Lacunar ligament 1148

Ladd and Gross technique 637
Ladd's band 828
Lahey's forceps 1026, 1026*f*, 1027
Lahshal system 565
Lane's paired gastrojejunostomy
    clamps 1032, 1032*f*
Lanes' tissue forceps 1001, 1001*f*
Langenbach's retractor 1013,
    1013*f*, 1091, 1121
Lanz incision 992, 1091
Laparoscopy 635, 820
    role of 153, 168, 219
Laparotomy, indications of 702
Laryngeal nerve
    nonrecurrent 307
    palsy
        bilateral recurrent 307, 758
        recurrent 302, 759
Laryngocele 46
Larynx 275, 278, 507
Latarjet, nerve of 129
Latissimus dorsi 250, 1128
    myocutaneous flap 269
Laugier's femoral hernia 611
Lauren's classification 116, 862
Lavage fluid 697
Leg
    edema, persistent 974
    rising test 102*f*
    ulcers, causes of 339
Leiomyoma 105
Leiomyosarcomas 105, 438
Lemesurier technique 561
Lens system in telescope 1071
Lentigo 414
Lentigo maligna 415
    melanoma 406
Leprosy 598
    nodular 455
Lesser omentum 1169
Leucovorin 120
Leukemoid reaction 223
Leukocyte
    count
        differential 8, 221, 242, 288,
            332, 360, 485, 779
        total 8, 125, 221, 242, 288,
            332, 360, 485, 684, 779
    dysfunction 948
Leukoplakia 420, 568, 573, 581,
    926
    development of 569
    oral 568
    types of 569

Leukoplakic change 568
Leukoplakic patch 421, 569, 570
  biopsy of 569
  excision of 570
Levator anguli oris 534, 534*f*
Levator ani, division of 1118
Levator glandulae thyroideae 1200
Levator labii superioris 556, 556*f*
  alaeque nasi 556, 556*f*
Levofloxacin 506
Lichen planus, oral 581
Lichtenstein hernioplasty, steps
  of 1083
Lichtenstein mesh
  hernioplasty 55
  repair 54*f*
Lichtenstein tension-free repair
  54, 65
Lieberkuhn, crypts of 880
Lienorenal ligament, division of
  anterior leaf of 1124
Ligament, left triangular 1169
Ligamentum teres 1169
Ligamentum venosum 1170
Limb
  ischemia, chronic 363
  ischemic ulceration of 377
  lower 348
  motor system of lower 348
  temperature of 351
Limy bile 795
Linea alba 1154
  division of 1093
Linen sutures 1069
Linitis plastica 863
Lip
  carcinoma of 579, 579*f*
  develop 557
    lower 558
  muscles of 556*f*
    abnormalities of 557
  surgery 582
Lipodermatosclerosis 341
Lipoma 384, 390, 392, 393, 394,
  453, 535, 539, 611
  complications of 394
  excision of 973
  surface of 393
Lipoprotein
  high-density 761
  low-density 761
  very low-density 761
Liposarcoma 394, 430, 438

Lisch nodules 457
Lister's metallic bougie 1044, 1044*f*
Lister's sinus forceps 1077*f*
Lithogenic bile 146, 901
Littre's hernia 62
Liver 88, 94, 96, 103, 140, 148, 183*f*,
  185, 805
  abscess 726, 735
    rupture of 805
  anatomical lobes of 1166
  anatomy of 1166
  average weight of 1166
  delineate upper border of 95
  disease, chronic 598
  enlargement 186
  function test 140, 150, 167, 172,
    200, 205, 221, 242, 596,
    728
  hydatid cyst of 185, 189, 193
  injury 704
    grades of 703
    minor 705
  lobes of 1167*f*
  metastasis 154, 257
    multiple 154
  metastatic 185
  palpation of 213
  resection 192
    left lobectomy 192
    right lobectomy 192
  segmental resection of 188
  segments of 1167, 1168*f*
  simple cyst of 193
  trauma 707
  wedge resection of 192
Lobular carcinoma 763
Local cyanosis, stage of 364, 447
Local syncope, stage of 446
Lockhart's operation 651
Lockwood, tail of 641, 641*f*
Loin incision 993
Loin pain 223
Lord's operation 623
Lothiessan's repair 57
Lovibond's angle 15, 16, 16*f*
Lower limb, elephantiasis of 646
Ludwig's angina 956, 956*f*
Lumbar
  arteries 1179
  azygos vein 1182
  hernia 613, 613*f*
  incision 993
  region 1212

sympathectomy 361, 362, 1128
  steps of 1128
sympathetic trunk 362, 1187
triangle
  boundary of inferior 613
  superior 613*f*
  veins 1182
Lumbosacral
  meningocele 459, 461
  meningomyelocele 461*f*
  region 460
Lumen of appendix, obstruction
  of 867
Lump 88, 731, 763, 870
  abdominal 185
  appendicular 733, 868, 732
  fixity of 232, 430
  pectoral fixity of 233
  serratus anterior fixity of 234
  skin fixity of 430
Lung 801, 802
  diseases, occupational 802
  injury 968
  metastasis 257
Luteinizing hormone releasing
  hormone 249, 638
Lymph node 18, 19*f*, 20, 20*f*, 110,
  154, 283, 310, 402, 405, 417,
  453, 503, 506, 577, 581, 584,
  585, 654, 672, 676, 794, 856
  apical group of 236, 236*f*
  biopsy 972
  dissection 112, 113, 417, 455,
    550, 1094, 1095, 1113
    elective 403, 403
    radical 542
  division of 1109
  draining esophagus 1158
  enlargement, cause of 417, 577
  epicolic 1162
  examination of regional 27, 36,
    37, 229, 348, 484
  groups of 283
  horizontal chain of 1208
  intermediate 1162
  involvement 266, 411
  levels of 18*f*, 237, 1208, 1209*f*
  local 222
  mass 148, 172, 181
  metastasis 154, 172, 305*f*, 308,
    404, 404*f*, 578
    management of 422
  metastatic 404, 523, 578
  nonpalpable 655

para-aortic 110
paraesophageal 1157
pericolic 1162
periesophageal 1157
prelaryngeal 278
pretracheal 278, 491
principal 1162
regional 111, 160, 207, 224,
    260, 408, 436, 508, 509, 510,
    544, 672
stations of stomach 110*f*
status 1093
submental 388
subpyloric 110
supraclavicular 20*f*
suprapyloric 110
Lymphadenectomy, prophylactic
    655
Lymphadenitis, tubercular 504,
    505
Lymphangioma 444, 455, 537
subhyoid 489
Lymphangiosarcoma 430
Lymphatic
    channels develop 486
    cyst 185, 527
    drainage 1165
    leukemia, chronic 504, 507
    obstruction 455, 645
        causes of 645
    spread 574, 582, 802, 882
    tissues 444
    vessels 362
Lymphedema 239
    causes of 267
Lymphocele 60
Lymphocyte 117
    activated killer cells 225
    depletion 514
    predominance 514
Lymphocytic infiltration 412
Lymphocytic thyroiditis 293
Lymphoid tissue 117
Lymphoma 117, 172, 181, 200,
    308, 507, 514, 515, 515*f*, 671,
    830, 837, 869
    low-grade malignant 308
    malignant 307, 308, 513, 513*f*
    metastasis of 535
    staging of 515*t*
Lynch syndrome 838, 881
Lysol 986
Lytle's repair 64, 64*f*

M

Mafenide acetate 725
Magnetic resonance
    angiography 375
    cholangiopancreatography
        140, 167, 810, 939
Malabsorption syndrome 297
Malaise 159
Malecot's catheter 1041, 1041*f*
    suprapubic 1042
Malignancy
    delayed development of 669
    high-grade 308
Malignant cell 221, 918
Malignant disease 5, 748
Malignant melanoma
    metastatic 412
    TNM staging for 408, 408*t*
Malignant peripheral nerve sheath
    tumor 438
Malleable olive pointed probe
    1020
Malleolus, medial 327*f*
Malnutrition 73, 74, 940
    correction of 940
    infantile 811
Mammogram
    false-negative 854
    false-positive 854
Mammography 239, 239*f*, 851,
    851*f*, 852-854
    malignant lesion in 239, 852
Mandible 590
Mandibular arch 498
Manubrium sterni 275, 395*f*
Marfan syndrome 64
Marginal mandibular resection
    586
Marion's disease 219
Marjolin's ulcer 426, 427
    development of 427
Maryland dissector 1075, 1075*f*
Mass 870
    abdominal 831, 838
    appendicular 734
Masseter muscle 532*f*
Mastectomy 929*f*
    indications of 247
Mastication, muscle of 498
Mastoid process 1197
Maternal estrogens 675
Maxilla, part of 845*f*
Maxillary artery 498, 975

Mayo Robson's incision 141, 992
Mayo's pedicle clamp 999, 999*f*
Mayo's repair, drawbacks of 78
Mayo's scissors 1010, 1010*f*
McBurney's gridiron incision 992,
    994
    anatomy of 1090
McBurney's incision 734
McBurney's point 88, 730, 1090
McBurneys' gridiron incision 1121
McIndoe scissors 1011, 1011*f*
Meatal stenosis 219, 666
    acquired 219
    congenital 219
Meatoplasty 664
Mebendazole 191
Mechlorethamine 120, 516
Meckel's diverticulum 61, 62, 132,
    615-617, 729, 730, 856, 874-
    876, 1035, 1123
Median nerve 470
    block 982, 982*f*
    injury 477
    medial root of 469
    motor supplies of 477
    palsy 478, 481
    sensory supplies of 477, 481,
        481*f*
Median sacral
    artery 1163
    vein 1182
Median umbilical
    fold 1151
    ligament 1151
Mediastinal cyst 386
Mediastinal injury 968
Mediastinal shift 848, 680
Mediastinal syndrome, superior
    514, 517
Mediastinitis 528
Medullary carcinoma 307, 308
Melanocyte 405
    stimulating hormone 413
Melanoma
    benign 414
    development of 405
    malignant 245, 400, 401, 401*f*,
        404, 404*f*, 405, 407, 407*f*,
        408, 410-412, 573, 927
    nodular 406
    subungual 445
    types of 406

Melanuria 411
Melena 133, 838
Memory, transient loss of 686
Menarche, age of 4
Meningitis 460
Meningocele 46, 384, 385, 458-461
Meningomyelocele 458, 461
Menopause, premature 248
Menstruation 265
Mental retardation 442
Mentalis 557
Mercedes Benz incision 993
Mesenteric artery
    branches of
        inferior 1180, 1181f
        superior 1180, 1180f
    inferior 1179
    superior 155f, 1105f, 1179
Mesenteric cyst 193
Mesenteric gap, closure of 1113
Mesenteric vein
    portal vein impingement,
        bilateral superior 154
    superior 1183
Mesenteric vessels, ligation of
    inferior 1117
Mesentery
    root of 110
    twisting of 786
Mesh
    fixation of 1089
    placement of 63
Mesoappendix 866f, 1177
    division of 1122
Mesocolon rent, closure of 1098,
    1112
Metacarpophalangeal joints 466,
    466f
Metallic airway tube 1050
Metallic bougie 1043
Metallic catheter 1046
    female 1045, 1045f
    male 1046, 1046f
Metastasis, pulmonary 223, 802
Metastatic disease 435
Methotrexate 120
Methysergide 447
Metronidazole 369
Metzenbaum scissors 1012, 1012f
Meyer's stripper 334
Microcarcinoma 307
Microcarcinoma, papillary 308
Microdochectomy 764
Microsclerotherapy 338

Micturition
    frequency of 211
    painful 913
Midclavicular plane 90
Midline incision, closure of 1089
Midpalmar space
    anatomy of 964
    infection, drainage of 964f
Midtarsal joint movement 348
Migratory thrombophlebitis 159
Miliary shadows, causes of 801
Miliary tuberculosis 801
Millard's operation 559
Millard's repair 561
Millard's rotation advancement
    operation 560f
    technique 562f
Millin's self-retaining bladder
    retractor 1017, 1017f
Mini-cholecystectomy 142
Miosis 483
Mirault-Blair technique 561
Mitotic rate assessment 409
Mixed stones, composition of 898
Mobile inguinal lymph node 655
Mobile lymph nodal metastasis
    578
Mobilize spleen 702
Möbius sign 276, 281, 282f
Mohs micrographic surgery 421
Moles 414
Molluscum fibrosum 454
Monoblock dissection 403
Monocryl sutures 1066f
Monofilament polyamide sutures
    1070, 1070f
Monostotic fibrous dysplasia 589
Morgagni, cyst of 627
Morris' retractor 1013, 1013f
Moses' sign 331
Mosquito hemostatic forceps 998,
    998f
Motor neuron disease 521
Motor system 7
Mouth
    carcinoma floor of 585
    floor of 488f, 489, 507, 577, 585,
    586
Moxifloxacin 506
Moynihan's cholecystectomy
    forceps 1103
Moynihan's forceps 1027
Moynihan's gastric occlusion
    clamp 1030
Moynihan's hump 1172, 1172f

Moynihan's method 97
Mucocele 96
Mucosal melanoma 510t
Mucous membrane 901f
Muffled heart sounds 693
Muir-Torre syndrome 428
Multinodular goiter 284f, 285,
    288-290, 304
Multiple trauma, severe 677
Mumps orchitis 598
Mupirocin 725
Murphy's kidney punch 215
Murphy's sign 88, 97, 97f, 139
Muscle 30, 477, 556, 566, 1091,
    1215
    abdominal 51, 51f
    bilabial 556, 556f
    cremasteric 61, 1146
    cricopharyngeus 528
    deep 477
    division of superficial 1125
    guard 805
    invasive bladder cancers 916
    nerve supply of 1189
    of forearm, deep 468
    power 463
        grade 359
    superficial 468, 477
    thyropharyngeus 528
    tone, abdominal 51f
    wasting 350, 358
    weakness, proximal 302
Muscular elements 498
Muscular triangle, boundary of
    1207
Muscularis propria 206
Musculocutaneous nerve 470
Musculoskeletal system 934
Myasthenia like syndrome 302
Mycobacterium tuberculosis 870
Myelocele 462
Myelosuppression 248
Mylohyoid 498
Myocardial infarction, acute 726,
    735
Myotomy, cricopharyngeal 527
Myxedema, pretibial 303

N

Naffziger method 280, 280f
Nanocrystalline silver 725
Narath's femoral hernia 611
Nasal
    cavity 507

deformity 557
  correction of 561
nerve, external 1195
Nasogastric
  aspiration 79, 607
  suction 743, 748
  tube 80, 935, 949
    insertion of 949
Nasolabial muscles 556, 556*f*
Nasopharynx 507
National Comprehensive Cancer
  Network 154
National Institute of Clinical
  Excellence 58
Nausea 159, 249
Neck 400
  anterior triangle of 1206
  dissection
    anterior compartment 513
    elective 575
    functional 575
    radical 512, 575
    types of 512
  examination of 530
  lymph node dissection 542
  node
    dissection, classical radical
      512
    metastasis, bilateral 512
  of pancreas, division of 1109
  of sac, ligation of 1085
  prophylactic irradiation of 573
  swellings 484
  triangle of 1206*f*
  veins 5, 693
Necrosis
  pancreatic 739, 742
  score 739
Necrotizing soft tissue infection
  771, 772
Needle 1005, 1006*f*
  aspiration cytology 535
  holders 1004, 1004*f*
  part of 1008
Neoadjuvant chemotherapy, role
  of 115, 435
Neoadjuvant therapy 165, 166
Neomercazole 300, 937
Neoplastic
  lesion 828
    benign 763, 764
  polyp, benign 877
  theory 920

Nephrectomy 716, 1125
  indications of 716, 914, 1125
  radical 222
Nephrolithotomy, percutaneous
  731, 799
Nephron sparing surgery 225
Nephrotic syndrome 223, 911
Nerve 439, 538, 1151, 1215
  apinal 457
  blocks, peripheral 982
  compression 520
  conduction velocity 470
  infraorbital 1196
  infratrochlear 1195
  injury 336, 462, 472
    types of 471
  invasion, recurrent 307
  lateral root of median 470
  lesion 348
  lingual 1135
  peripheral 472
  repair 473
  roots 469
  subscapular 470
  supratrochlear 1195
  type of 473
Nervous system 934, 1184
  dysfunction of 681
  examination of 7, 41, 349, 401
  sympathetic 1185, 1186
Neural tissues 444
Neurilemmoma 537
Neuroblastomas 456
Neurofibroma 384, 390, 393, 444,
  452, 453, 453*f*, 454, 457, 537,
  539
  complications of 454
  painful 454
  solitary 454
  types of 454
Neurofibromatosis
  generalized 454, 456, 457
  plexiform 454, 455, 455*f*
Neurofibrosarcoma 430
Neurolipoma 395
Neuroma 456
  false 456
  true 456
Neuropathy 339, 366, 378
Neuropraxia 471
Neurotmesis 472
Nevin's staging for carcinoma of
  gallbladder 175, 903

Nevolipoma 395
Nevus
  benign 413, 414
  compound 414, 415
  flammeus 441
Nicoladoni's sign 450
Night blindness 12
Nipple 227
  discharge 226
    abnormal 762
  displacement of 231, 231*f*
  reconstruction 269
  retracted 929*f*
  retraction 239
Nitrosamines 175
Nodal metastasis 410
Nodular goiter, complications of
  289
Nodule, toxic 301
Non-Hodgkin's lymphoma 517
  types of 517
Nonneoplastic polyp, benign 876
Nonpolyposis colorectal cancer,
  hereditary 862
Nonsteroidal anti-inflammatory
  drugs 131
Nontoxic multinodular goiter 276,
  284, 285, 288, 289
Nose, root of 460
Nottingham prognostic index 259
Nuchal line, superior 1197
Nuclear pleomorphism 259
Nutrition 5
Nutritional
  deficiency 558
  deficit 134
Nylon sutures 1070

O

Obesity 67, 265
Oblique aponeurosis
  closure of external 1084
  division of external 1121
  external 1090, 1091, 1147
Oblique muscle, internal 1091
Obstruction, biliary 172
Obstructive pulmonary disease,
  chronic 934, 947
Occipital protuberance, external
  1197
Occipital triangle, dissection of
  1136

Occipitofrontalis, frontal belly of 533, 533*f*
Ochsner's clasping test 479, 480*f*
Ochsner-Sherren regime 733
Oddi, sphincter of 1171
Oesch phlebectomy hook 334
Ofloxacin 506
Ogilvie syndrome 790, 793
Olfactory nerve palsy 3
Ombredanne's technique 638
Omentectomy 114, 1095
Omentocoele 61
Omentopexy 188
Omentoplasty 364
    partial 192
Omentum 61, 82
    division of lesser 1093
Omeprazole 128
Oncovin 120, 516
On-table colonic lavage, role of 840
Oophorectomy, surgical 249
Operation, type of 73, 748
Ophthalmic division 1195
Ophthalmoplegia 303
Opponens digiti minimi 481
Opponens pollicis 478, 479*f*, 481
Optic nerve palsy 3
Optical urethrotomy 754
Oral
    aromatase inhibitor 249
    carcinomas, TNM
        classification of 574
        staging grouping for 575
    intake, failure of 746
    pill 264
Orbicularis
    oculi 533, 533*f*
    oris 534, 534*f*, 556, 556*f*
Orbital proptosis 303
Orbital tumor 296
Orchidectomy 638
    high-inguinal 671*f*
Orchidopexy 636, 637*f*, 643
    principle of 636
    steps of 636
Orchiectomy, indications of 71
Organs, palpation of 88
Oropharynx 507
Orthoplasty 664, 664*f*
Osler-Rendu-Weber syndrome 442
Osteoclastoma 589
Osteoma 589

Osteomyelitic sinus 427
Osteomyelitis 37, 370, 373, 374, 591
    long-standing 420
    of mandible, chronic 591
Osteosarcoma 589, 801
Ovarian ablation 257
Ovarian cyst, twisted right 729
Ovary 801
Oxalate stones 797, 798
Oxygen
    inhalation 190, 947
    tension, transcutaneous 375
Oxyuris vermicularis 867

P

Pachydermatocele 454
Packed cell volume 684
Paget's disease 263*f*, 657, 927, 930
Paget's test 33
Pain 25, 38, 127, 210, 226, 334, 354*f*, 368, 518, 908
    abdomen 2, 85, 219, 737, 778
        acute 726
    abdominal 184, 784, 790, 812, 838
    acute 726, 729, 735
    cause of 149, 608
    duration of 25
    epigastric 159
    management 83
    over swelling 25
    palliation of 174
    penile 650
    periodicity of 25, 133
    persistent severe pain 812
    prostatic 215
    radiation of 25, 38
    relief of 158, 174
    sensation 467
    site of 25, 345
Palate
    develop 565
    primary 563
    submucus cleft of 564
Pallor 700
Palmar interossei 475, 475*f*
Palmar space, infection of middle 964
Palmaris brevis 481
Palomo's operation 632, 633
    laparoscopic 633
Palpation
    deep 6
    superficial 6, 88

Palpebral conjunctiva, lower 13*f*
Pampiniform plexus 630, 630*f*, 1146
Pancoast tumor 521
Pancreas 140, 159, 194, 198, 710, 805
    arterial supply of 1176, 1176*f*
    body of 195, 1111
    carcinoma 149, 152, 153, 156, 158, 161-163, 163*t*
    cystadenocarcinoma of 193
    cystadenoma of 193
    develop 1175
    divisum 736, 811, 1175, 1175*f*
    exposure of 1108, 1111
    gallbladder, carcinoma of 149
    head of 1108
    hydatid cyst of 193
    parts of 1174, 1174*f*
    pseudocyst of 185, 193, 194, 198
    tail of 161, 195, 1111
Pancreatectomy
    distal 113, 711, 812
    total 156
Pancreatic artery
    great 1160*f*
    inferior 1160*f*
Pancreatic cancer, TNM
    classification for 159, 160*t*
Pancreatic duct 807, 810
    dilated 810*f*
    disposition of 1175, 1175*f*
    normal dimension of 811
    obstruction 811
    opening of 1111
Pancreatic fluid, reflux of 897
Pancreatic head
    laceration of 712
    massive injury of 712
Pancreatic injury
    causes of 708
    conservative treatment of 711
Pancreatic trauma
    grades of 712
    types of 708
Pancreaticoduodenal
    injury
        combined 712
        treatment of 710
    trauma, complications of 713
    vein, superior 1183
Pancreaticoduodenectomy 156*f*, 161, 163, 1106*f*

Pancreaticojejunal anastomosis
1109, 1111
Pancreaticojejunostomy 156*f*
lateral 1110
Pancreatitis 85, 184, 713, 736
acute 144, 726, 729, 736-739,
739*t*, 740, 741, 898
autoimmune 736, 811
chronic 126, 139, 148, 155, 159,
161, 162, 172, 181, 195, 735,
810-812
complications of acute 742
development of acute 736
hereditary 811
intermediately severe 739
mild acute 738
severe 739
Pancreatojejunostomy 1106*f*
Pancreozymin 1176
Pantaloon hernia 62
Pantoprazole 128
Papillae 308
Papillary tumors, multiple 914*f*
Papilloma 573, 755
Paragangliomas 525
Paralysis
below knee, complete 483
respiratory 1052
Paralytic ileus 134, 746, 786
Paramedian incision
anatomy of 1090
closure of 1090
Paraphimosis 648
reduction of 648*f*
Parasitic infection 801
Parasternal heave, left 7
Parasympathetic nervous system
1184, 1185
Parathyroid
gland 319, 320
blood supplies of 319
interior 319
location of 1203
superior 319
hyperplasia 319
insufficiency 302
Paraumbilical hernia 605, 605*f*,
606, 607
complications of 606
Paraumbilical vein drains 1183
Parenchymal laceration, distal 712
Parenteral nutrition, total 135
Paris staging system 118
Park's classification 1021
Parkland formula, modified 722

Paronychia
acute 961
drainage of 961*f*
Parotid abscess 955, 957, 957*f*
Parotid carcinoma 542, 543
TNM classification of 544, 544*t*
Parotid cyst 539
Parotid duct 532, 532*f*
disposition of 538
orifice 532, 532*f*
Parotid fascia, disposition of 538
Parotid fistula
causes of 551
types of 551
Parotid gland 530, 532, 538, 539
adenolymphoma of 535
carcinoma of 535
deep lobe of 545
deep part of 531, 533
malignant tumors of 541
parts of 537, 1209
posterior margin of 1133
Parotid lymphoma 549
Parotid region, boundary of 537
Parotid swelling 532
Parotid tumor, mixed 531, 531*f*,
532, 536, 537, 539, 540
Parotidectomy 546
superficial 535, 535*f*, 1133
total 542
Patch repair 65
Patey's modified radical
mastectomy 249
Payrs' appendix crushing clamps
1038, 1038*f*
Payrs' gastric crushing clamps
1036, 1036*f*
Payrs' intestinal crushing clamps
1037, 1037*f*
Peau d' orange 234, 235*f*, 267,
929*f*, 930
Pecten pubis 1146*f*
Pectineal ligament 1148
Pectoral nerve
lateral 470
medial 469
Pectoralis major muscle 31*f*, 233*f*,
234*f*, 269, 1189
nerve supply of 1190
origins of 1189
Pelvic
abscess 734, 784
anatomy, inspection of 1087
appendicitis, peculiarities of
834

appendix 734
colon 203
injuries 717
irradiation, previous 59
lymph node dissection 655
mass 342
mesocolon
long 789
narrow attachment of 789
Pelvicalyceal system 844*f*, 904*f*,
907*f*
Pelvis, examination of 683
Pelviureteric junction obstruction
218, 843
Pemberton's sign 276, 280, 280*f*
Penile
curvature, degree of 664
deformity 650
hypospadias, distal 665
prosthesis, role of 651
Penis
anatomical parts of 659, 659*f*
arterial supplies of 659
bulb of 659
carcinoma of 245, 404, 652,
652*f*, 657
drain, lymphatics of 927
edema of 60
elephantiasis of 645
lymphatic drainage of 659*f*
palpation of 213*f*
partial amputation of 926*f*
premalignant lesions of 926
secondary carcinoma of 660
total amputation of 654
Peptic perforation 742, 743, 768,
777, 778
management of 859
repair of 779, 1099, 1099*f*
Peptic ulcer 131, 143, 458, 729,
780, 855, 856
acute 726
benign 856
causes of recurrent 135
chronic 131, 735, 856, 857, 859
complications of 133, 133*t*,
134, 859
disease 126
recurrent 135, 136
site of 132
surgery 134, 138, 862
treatment 128
Peptostreptococcus 369, 371
Peracetic acid 986
Percutaneous
aspiration, role of 192

catheter drainage of
pseudocyst, role of 195
Perforated peptic ulcer, acute 735
Perforating veins, common sites
of 1214
Periampullary region, carcinoma
of 154
Perianal disease 831
Perianal fistula 1022
causes of multiple 1022
Perianal region 959
Perianal suppuration 959
Pericardiocentesis 968, 969*f*
Pericholecystic adhesion, gross
182
Pericystectomy, partial 192
Pericystojejunostomy 192
Perineal dissection 1118
Perineal incision 1118
closure of 1119
Perineal tail 641
Perinephric space, exposure of
1125
Perineum 641, 641*f*
Periostitis 341
Peripheral ischemia, signs of 351,
351*f*
Peripheral nerve, structure of 471
Perirenal fascia, incision of 1125
Peristaltic sound 89
Peritoneal cavity 189, 1073
inspection of 1101
Peritoneal defect, closure of 1088
Peritoneal flap 1088
Peritoneal fluid tap 969, 970*f*
complications of 970
Peritoneal lavage 190, 697
Peritoneal metastasis 154
Peritoneal reaction, stage of 778
Peritoneum 1091, 1092, 1121
division of 1087
downward reflection of 1087
incising surgical 1089
stripping of 1128
Peritonitis 133, 189, 747, 748
biliary 144, 898
development of 778
diffuse 189
Peritonsillar abscess, drainage of
956, 956*f*
Peritumor injection 244
Peroneal compartment 1219
Peroneal nerve injury 483
Perthes' test 331
modified 323, 329

Pethidine 743
Peutz-Jegher's syndrome 24, 24*f*,
876, 879
Peyronie's disease 650, 651
causes of 650
Pfannenstiel incision 68
Pharyngeal
artery, ascending 975
diverticulum 1157
fistula 528
pouch 497, 525-529
Pharyngoplasty 568
Pharynx, constrictor muscles of
529*f*
Phenacetin nephropathy 223
Pheochromocytoma 297, 318, 456,
457, 910
Phimosis 646, 646*f*, 647, 657, 926
complications of 648
secondary 649
Phleboliths 794
Phlebothrombosis, recurrent 974
Phosphate stones 797, 798
Phrenic arteries, inferior 1179
Phyllodes tumor 599
Pierre Robin's syndrome 558
Pigmented nevi 414
Piles 1024-1026
causes of secondary 1024
complications of 1025
external 1024
grades of 1025
holding forceps 1023, 1023*f*
internal 1024
internoexternal 1024
nonoperative treatment of
1025
primary 1024, 1025*f*
sites of 1025
secondary 1024, 1025*f*
sites of 1025
symptomatic 1024
types of 1024
Piperacillin 369
Pizzillo's method 278, 278*f*
Plasma
calcitonin level 319
sterilization 986
Plastibell technique 649
Platelet
derived growth factor 376
dysfunction 948
Platysma 534, 534*f*
Pleural fluid, aspiration of 966
Plug repair 65

Plummer-Vinson syndrome 573
Plunging ranula 488, 488*f*, 489, 496
Pneumonia 947
Pneumoperitoneum 1073, 1100
closed technique of 1074
creation of 1087
induction of 1074
Pneumothorax 953, 968
open 689
traumatic 691, 692, 849, 850,
967
Polyarteritis nodosa 447
Polycystic disease 186, 216
Polycystic kidney 221, 755, 904,
905
complications of 906
disease 905
adult 223, 905
infantile 906
Polycystic liver disease 190
Polycystic renal disease 906
Polycythemia 223, 911
Polydioxanone suture 1066, 1067*f*
Polyglactin
rapide suture 1065
sutures 1065
Polyglecaprone 1066, 1066*f*
Polyglycolic acid 77
mesh 77
suture 1063, 1063*f*
uses of 1065
Polyp 876
hamartomatous 876
Polyposis coli 4
Polypropylene
mesh 77
suture 1069, 1069*f*
Polytetrafluoroethylene
mesh 77
placement of 79
Polytrauma 848
Polyvinyl chloride 1050
Popliteal artery, exposure of 981,
981*f*
Popliteal fossa 1217, 1217*f*
boundaries of 1217
contents of 1218
Popliteal pulse 355
palpation of 356*f*
Popliteal vein, arterialization of
364
Porcelain gallbladder 902, 1103
Porokeratosis 428
Port sites, closure of 1088
Port wine stain 441, 442
Porta hepatis 1169, 1169*f*

Portacaval anastomosis, site of 1183, 1183*f*
Portal vein 154, 182
 anatomy of 1182, 1182*f*
 branches of 1169
 course of 1182
 left branch of 1183
 obstruction 812
 origin of 1182
 tributaries of 1183
Positron emission tomography 674
 role of 431
Postauricular dermoid cyst 383*f*
Postburn
 contracture 397, 398
 scar 427
Postcholecystectomy syndrome 143
Postcibal syndrome 136, 137
Posterior component separation technique 80
Posterior surface, palpation of 277*f*
Postfixed brachial plexus 469
Postileal appendicitis, peculiarities of 834
Postvagotomy diarrhea, causes of 138
Poupart ligament 1147
Povidone iodine 725
Precordium, shape of 7
Prednisolone 516
Prednisone 120, 516
Preperitoneal mesh repair, open 65
Preperitoneal space
 creation of 1088
 dissection of 1087
Prepuce, dorsal slit of 974
Preputial skin, abnormal 662
Preputioplasty 647, 647*f*
Prepyloric vein 1183
Presacral dissection 1115, 1117
Presbyesophagus 818
Pressure, simple 994
Primary bile duct stones 169
Procarbazine 120, 516
Processus vaginalis 639
 abnormalities of 1150
 fate of 1150
Proctocolectomy total 878
Profundoplasty 364
Pronator teres 479, 480*f*
Propranolol 447
Prostaglandin 317
Prostate 755, 801, 920

benign
 enlargement of 752, 919
 hyperplasia of 751, 755, 920
 capsules of 920
 carcinoma of 751, 754, 755
 parts of 920
 transurethral
  laser ablation of 922
  resection of 922
  vaporization of 922
Prostatectomy
 retropubic 922
 transvesical 922
Prostatitis 751
Proteus mirabilis 369, 371
Proton-pump inhibitor 127, 128
Proximal colon, division of 1115
Proximal stomach total gastrectomy 119
Pseudoachalasia 817
Pseudoaneurysm 702
Pseudoarthroses 457
Pseudocyst 193, 196-198
 acute 742
 complication of 198, 812
 endoscopic drainage of 195
 external drainage of 196
 formation, causes of 197
 intervention of 196
 large 195
 pancreatic 713, 739
 postacute 197
 sequelae of 196
 types of 197
Pseudopolyps 886
Pseudoptosis 483
Puberty 657
Pubic symphysis closure 668
Pubic tail 641
Pubic tubercle 51, 51*f*, 52*f*, 327, 327*f*
Pulp space infection 962
 anatomical peculiarity of 962
 drainage of 962*f*
Pulsatile
 bone swelling 223
 movements 87
Pulse 5, 679, 722
 alternans 968
 paradoxus 693, 968
 peripheral 355
 rate 740
 wave
  tension of 21
  tracing 359

Punch biopsy 425
Purulent discharge 368
Pyelography, retrograde 218, 843
Pyelolithotomy forceps 1038, 1038*f*
Pyelolymphatic backflow 908
Pyelonephritis
 acute 730, 731
  right-sided 726
 chronic 139, 1125
 recurrent 669
Pyeloplasty
 dismembered 843
 nondismembered 844
 types of 218
Pyelotubular backflow 908
Pyemia, portal 868
Pyloric
 antrum 1159
 canal 1159
 exclusion procedure 711
 glands 1159
 stenosis 126
Pyloroplasty 126, 130, 131
Pylorus conserving pancreaticoduodenectomy 156
Pyocele 626
Pyogenic
 granuloma 402, 445
 lymphadenitis, chronic 503, 507
Pyonephrosis 909
 tuberculous 216
Pyramidal lobe 1200
Pyramidalis muscle 1153
Pyrazinamide 505, 506
Pyrexia 23, 751
 high-grade 805
Pyriform 39
Pyuria 2

Q

Quadrantectomy 247
Quadriceps femoris 1215
Quadruple ligation 451*f*
Quinolone 369

R

Rabeprazole 128
Radial artery, segment of 22*f*
Radial bursa 965*f*
 drainage of 964*f*
 infection of 965

Radial forearm flap 581
Radial nerve 464, 469, 470
  injury 463, 463*f*, 467*f*
  sensory supply of 467
Radial pulse 355
  palpation of 21*f*, 356*f*
Radiation
  enteritis 830, 837, 869
  exposure 308, 558
  therapy 255
    role of 247
Radical gastrectomy, lower 109,
  110
Radical mastectomy, modified
  250, 253, 268, 764, 1126,
  1127*f*, 1128,
Radical neck dissection, modified
  506, 513, 575, 1135
Radioactive
  iodine uptake test 297
  thyroid scanning 288
Radiofrequency ablation 335, 337
  contraindications of 336
  principle of 335
  treatment, complications of
    336
Radioiodine 301
  scanning 306
  therapy 301
    drawback of 301
    role of 300
Radioisotope scanning, role of 292
Radiolucent bile duct stone 806*f*
Radionuclide
  scanning, role of 493
  thyroid scanning 297
Radiopaque shadows, multiple
  796*f*
Radiotherapy 423, 455, 512, 572,
  764
  administration of 578
  external beam 434
  indications of 250, 578
  limitations of 424
  role of 114, 124, 174, 180, 225,
    256, 421, 424, 427, 433, 576,
    584, 591, 656, 821
  techniques of 434
Radius, segment of 581
Ramhorn penis 643, 643*f*
Rami communicantes 362
Rampley's swab holding forceps
  987
Randall's plaque 798
Ranson criteria 740
Ranula 487-489
  complications of 489

Rapid test 191
Raspberry tumor 615, 616
Raynaud's disease 445-448
Raynaud's phenomenon 346, 363,
  446, 447
Raynaud's syndrome 445, 449
Reactive hyperemia test 357
Rectal artery
  inferior 1163, 1166*f*
  middle 1163, 1166*f*
  superior 1163, 1166*f*, 1180
Rectal cancer
  development of 884
  TNM staging for 885
Rectal incontinence 669
Rectal temperature 740
Rectal valve
  lower 1166*f*
  middle 1166*f*
  superior 1166*f*
Rectum
  abdominoperineal resection of
    884*f*
  carcinoma of 883-886, 1024
  division of 1115
  intrinsic lymphatics of 1165
  lymphatic drainage of 1165*f*,
    1166*f*
  venous drainage of 1163, 1164*f*
Rectus abdominis muscle 1091,
  1092, 1153
  retraction of 1090
  role of 74
Rectus sheath 1152
  anterior 1090-1092
  contents of 1153
  formation of 1153*f*
  lateral border of 1146*f*
  posterior 1090-1092
Red blood cell 13
Reducible hernia 43
Reed-Sternberg giant cells 514
Reflexes 348
  abdominal 8
  deep 8
  esophagitis 126
  superficial 8
Refractory metabolic alkalosis 106
Regional limb perfusion 412
Regional lymphadenectomy, role
  of 433
Renal
  angiography 222
  arteries 1179

arteriography 756
calculi 1039, 1125
  recurrent 458
  right-sided 139
cell carcinoma 225, 909, 910
  development of 910
  papillary 910
  TNM classification of 224
disease 948
  chronic 947
  end-stage 948
failure 765, 770
  acute 947
  chronic 74, 220, 598, 799,
    905, 906, 909
fascia 1155
  disposition of 1155
function, maintenance of 940
infection 798
injury 714, 716
  complications of 716
  grades of 714
  severe 1125
lump 214, 905, 908
pain 905, 913
pelvis 755
stones 797, 798, 799
  complications of 798
  types of 797
transplant 146
trauma 715, 716
  diagnosis of 714
tuberculosis 794, 913, 914
vein
  anatomy of 1184, 1184*f*
  formation of 1184
  termination of 1184
vessels 222
  division of 1126
Renorrhaphy 716
Residual bile duct stones,
  management of 815
Respiration 5, 23
Respiratory
  disease, chronic 846
  distress
    causes of 283
    severe 680, 689, 758, 848
  movements 87
  obstruction 302
  rate 7, 740
  system 934
    examination of 7, 41, 349
Reticular varices 344
Retina 457

Retinal angiomas 910
Retractile testis 642
Retrobulbar tumor 296
Retrocecal appendicitis, acute 726
Retromandibular vein 1194
Retroperitoneal
    adhesions 640
    air 709
    bile staining 710
    cyst 216, 386
    duodenal lymph nodes 110
    lump 102*f*
    lymph node dissection 674
    swelling 732
    tumor 200, 221
Reynold's pentad 169
Rhabdomyoma 393
Rhabdomyosarcoma 430, 535
Rheumatoid
    arthritis 447
    nodules 801
Rhinorrhea 847
Rhonchi 7
Rib
    fracture 690
        first 690
        isolated 691, 849
        lower 690
        multiple 847*f*
    graft 581
Richter's hernia 61, 61*f*, 784
Riedel's thyroiditis 279, 305
Rifampicin 505, 506, 755
Right angled forceps 1026, 1026*f*
Right great toe, dry gangrene of 759
Rigid metal pin stripper 334
Rising test 88
Rives preperitoneal mesh repair 69
Rives Stoppa's technique 78
Road traffic accident 677, 685, 695,
    708, 713, 717
Robson's staging 911
Roof top or Chevron incision 992
Rotter's node 235, 236
Round bodied needle 1006, 1006*f*
Roux-en-Y
    cholecystojejunostomy 157
    cystojejunostomy 188
    gastrojejunal anastomosis
        1098
    loop of jejunum, creation of
        1111
Rubber catheter, simple 1039,
    1039
Rubella infection 558

Rupture 198, 626
Rutherford Morrison incision 734
Ryle's tube 157, 950

S

Sac
    body of 60
    calcification of 626
    contents of 1085
    coverings of 60
    fundus of 60
    ligation of 60
    mouth of 60
    neck of 60
    opening of 1085
    transection of 1085
Saccular diverticulum 183
Sacral region 17*f*
Salivary calculi, composition of
    548
Salivary gland 507, 530, 537, 543,
    547, 1209
    carcinoma, TNM classification
        of 544, 544*t*
    major 509*t*
    malignant lymphoma of 548
    submandibular 547, 547*f*, 550,
        551
    swelling, submandibular 496
Salmon patch 441
Salpingitis, acute 729
Saphena varix 344, 611
Saphenofemoral junction 326,
    332, 333*f*
Saphenous
    nerve 1217
    system 325*f*
    varicosity, short 336
    vein, arterialization of 364
        great 324, 329*f*, 351*f*, 352*f*
        small 338
Sarcoidosis 801
Sarcoma 308
    synovial 430, 438
Saturday night palsy 470
Scalene triangle 520*f*
Scalp 507
    blood supply of 1193
    dermoid 391
    layer of 1192, 1192*f*
    nerve supply of 1194, 1194*f*
    subcutaneous tissue of 1192
Scarpa, fascia of 641, 1154
Schamroth sign 15, 16, 16*f*

Schwannomas 456
Schwartz test 323, 327
Sciatic nerve palsy 483
Scleroderma 445, 447
Sclerosant injection 486
Sclerosis
    nodular 514
    systemic 339
Sclerotherapy 337, 338, 440, 440,
    971, 971*f*, 972, 974
    complications of 338
    contraindications of 974
    indications of 971, 974
    role of 623
Scolicidal
    agents 192
    solution 190
Scoliosis 457
Scorpion bite 736
Scrotal
    sac 641
    sebaceous cyst 392
    swelling 45*f*
    tail 641
    temperature 631
Scrotum 45*f*, 392, 1142
    bottom of 1213
    elephantiasis of 643, 643*f*, 645
    filariasis of 621
    root of 45*f*, 1213
    swelling, root of 45*f*
Sebaceous cyst
    complications of 391
    excision of 972, 973*f*
    infected 391
    multiple 392*f*
Sebaceous horn 391
Self-retaining abdominal retractor
    1016, 1016*f*
Seminoma 671
    anaplastic 924
    mixed 671
    testis 923
    types of 924
    typical 924
Senile keratosis, pigmented 402
Sensation, deep 8
Sensory
    nerve dysfunction 464
    system 7, 348
Sentinel lymph node 243, 243*f*,
    244, 403, 404, 655
    average number of 245
    biopsy 243-245
        advantages of 243, 404

contraindications of 245
role of 243, 433, 655
Sepsis, systemic 368
Septicemia 868
Seroma formation 336
Serotonin 317
Serous cystadenoma 199
Serratus anterior muscle 234f,
1191
Sertoli cell tumor 925
Serum
calcium level 221
glutamic
oxaloacetic transaminase
939
pyruvic transaminase 939
lactate dehydrogenase level
413
tumor markers 672
staging of 673t
Shock 680, 786
anaphylactic 189
hypovolemic 722
psychogenic 722
septicemic 722, 779
wave lithotripsy, extracorporeal
171, 731, 799
Shoelace darn technique 76, 76f
Shouldice repair 56, 65, 69
modified 65
Shouldice technique 54, 54f
Shprintzen syndrome 558
Sialadenitis, chronic 535, 546, 547,
547f
Sialoadenectomy, submandibular
1134
Sickle cell disease 726
Sigmoid artery 1180
Sigmoid colectomy 204
Sigmoid colon 203, 790, 1162
division of 1118
long redundant 789
mobilization of 1117
part of 884f
resection 839
Sigmoid volvulus 788, 790, 791
development of 788
Sigmoidoscopic decompression
792
Silbar procedure 638
Silver
nitrate 192, 725
sulfadiazine 725
Simple melanocytic tumors, types
of 414

Single bladed blunt hook 1053,
1053f
Sinus 36
formation, stage of 504
Sjögren's syndrome 548
Skeletal
defects 668
deformities 457
elements 498
tissues 444
Skin 30, 381, 382, 419, 988, 1089,
1090, 1092
burn 336
cancer, nonmelanoma 405
closure clips 1009, 1009f
direct invasion of 931
fixity 30f, 232
flap 423, 1126, 1129, 1131,
1133-1135
incision 244, 991, 1090, 1091,
1120, 1125
irritations, chronic 420
manifestations 189
nodules 931
over
abdomen 6, 87
breast 228
swelling 274
perfusion pressure 376
pigmentation 338, 339, 341
preparation 935
staplers 1010
temperature 347
tethering of 232, 232f, 930
thinning of 304
ulceration of 338
wound 1005
Skinfold thickness 12f
Skull
bone fracture 845
fracture 687
simple linear fracture of 846
Sleep apnea, obstructed 947
Sliding hernia 61, 61f
Slip sign 393
Slit valve mechanism 1150
Small cysts, multiple 904f
Small gallstones, multiple 146
Small gut, exteriorization of 1112,
1114
Small intestine 790, 869f
part of 825f
segment of 871f
Small polyps, multiple 886f
Smooth tongue 12f

Sodium tetradecyl sulfate 974
Soft fibroadenoma 599
Soft palate 14f
muscles of 566f
Soft tissue
sarcoma 428, 429, 429f, 430,
432-438, 801
development of 437
management of 433
recurrent 437
TNM staging for 436
types of 438
tumor 431
Solar keratosis, treatment of 420
Somatostatin 317
Space of Retzius 58, 82, 1151
Speech, defective 556, 566
Spence, tail of 1187f
Spencer Well's hemostatic forceps
993
Spermatic cord 45f, 213f, 1146
constituents of 1146
coverings of 1146
lymph vessel of 646
palpation of 41
part of 923f
Spermatic fascia
external 61, 1146
internal 1146
Spermatocele 627, 628
Spermatocytic seminoma 924
Sphincter choledochus 1171
Sphincter pancreaticus 1171
Sphygmomanometer 22
Spider nevus 441
Spinal cord
compression 257
hemangioblastomas of 910
Spine, examination of 8, 41, 349
Spironolactone 598
Spleen 88, 97, 103, 148, 805
delayed rupture of 699
hydatid cyst of 193
mobilization of 1124
palpation of 97f, 213
subcapsular hematoma of 701
Splenectomy 1123
complications of 702
indications of 1123
steps of 1124
Splenic artery 110, 1095, 1160f,
1180
branch of 1160
Splenic flexure 203f
mobilization of 1114

Splenic hilum 110, 1095
Splenic injury 699, 702
    grades of 701
    types of 699
Splenic pedicle, avulsion of 702
Splenic rupture
    signs of 700
    symptoms of 700
Splenic trauma 700-702
    major 700
Splenic vein 1183
Splenic vessels, division of 1124
Split thickness skin grafting 423
Splitting internal oblique 1121
Squamous cell carcinoma 67, 339,
        416, 416f, 417, 418, 420, 421,
        537, 573, 820, 864, 903, 915,
        927
    metastatic 511
    recurrence of 421
    types of 421
Squamous papilloma 445, 455
    pigmented 402
Squint 3
Stab injury abdomen 780
Stainless steel wire 1071, 1071f
Staphylococcus aureus 369, 371,
        371f, 372, 959, 960
Staphylococcus epidermidis 371
Stapler anastomosis 1116
Stay sutures, application of 1106
Steatorrhea 137, 159, 717, 870
Steering wheel injury 708
Stellate ganglion 449
Stellwag's sign 276, 282, 282f
Stenosis 133
    congenital 219
Stenotic lesion 837
Sterile pyuria 913
Sterilization 985, 986, 988, 990,
        991, 994, 997-1009, 1013-
        1024, 1027, 1029, 1031,
        1033, 1034, 1037-1050,
        1054-1056, 1071, 1072
Sternocleidomastoid muscle 357f,
        497, 499f
    posterior border of 20f
    right 32f
Sternomastoid tumor 523
Steroid 74, 131
    therapy, chronic 947
Stethoscope, placing bell of 283f
Stickler syndrome 558
Stitch granuloma 302

Stomach 116, 132, 189, 790, 801,
        805, 855, 949, 1158, 1160
    adenocarcinoma of 1094
    anterior wall of 780
    arterial supply of 1159
    barium meal
        series of 824f
        X-ray of 822f, 823f,
            825f-827f
    body of 1158
    carcinoma of 103, 107, 108,
            112, 113, 116, 117, 131,
            138, 860, 862, 862f, 863,
            864
    distal part of 860f, 861f
    double contrast barium X-ray
        of 823
    fixation of 1094
    greater curvature of 105f, 1159
    hour glass 133
    intrinsic lymphatics of 1159
    lesser curvature of 1159
    lymphatic drainage of 110,
        1159
    lymphoma of 105
    musculature of 105
    normal emptying time of 827
    parts of 1158, 1159f
    pyloric
        portion of 1159
        region of 824f
    resection of 1094
    venous drainage of 1160
Stomal obstruction 134
Stomatitis 12
Stones, formation of 909
Stoppa reapir 65
Straight line repair 561
Strangulation
    obstruction 746, 747, 786, 790
    signs of 792
    symptoms of 792
Strap muscles flap 1129
Streptococcus faecalis 768
Streptococcus pyogenes 486, 768,
        771
Streptomycin 506
Stress
    incontinence 215
    ulcers 725
Sturge-Weber syndrome 442
Subclavian artery 1203
    anatomy of 976
    branches of 1203f, 1204

exposure of 976, 977f
    left 1203
    parts of 1203
    puncture 953
    third part of 976
Subclavian pulse, palpation of 357
Subclavian vein
    cannulation, complications of
        953
    puncture 952, 952f
Subcostal incision
    left 992
    right 141, 992
Subcutaneous
    lipoma, excision of 973
    tissue, closure of 1084
Subdermal tissue overlying tumor
        244
Subepithelial connective tissue
        657
Subfascial endoscopic perforator
        surgery 339
Subhyoid bursal cyst 491
Submandibular
    duct
        dissection of 1135
        division of 1135
    gland
        carcinoma of left 549f
        superficial lobe of 1134
    salivary gland
        carcinoma of 549
        left 546
    sialoadenectomy, steps of 1134
Submental dermoid,
    complications of 389
Submental triangle, boundary of
        1206
Subphrenic abscess
    causes of 804
    drainage of 805
Subphrenic pus collection
    signs of 805
    symptoms of 805
Subphrenic spaces 803, 804f
Subscapular lymph node
    palpation 236
Subtotal radical gastrectomy,
    distal 119
Subtotal thyroidectomy, steps of
        1130f
Subumbilical ports, placement
    of 1087
Succinylcholine 933
Succussion splash 104f

Sucking breast milk 556
Suction irrigation cannula 1077, 1077f
Sulfamethoxazole 374
Sunderland's classification 472
Superficial parotidectomy, steps of 1133
Superficial surgical site infection 770
Superficial temporal artery pulse, palpation of 357f
Superficial thrombophlebitis, small region of 338
Superior lumbar triangle, boundary of 614
Superior mesenteric vessels, dissection of 1108
Supraclavicular dissection 1136
Supraclavicular lymph nodes
   examination of 229
   palpation of 237
Supraclavicular nodes 20
Supradiaphragmatic nodes 110
Suprahyoid thyroglossal cyst 388
Supralevator fistula 1022
Supraomohyoid neck dissection 513
Supraorbital nerve 1195
Suprarenal arteries, middle 1179
Suprarenal vein, right 1182
Supravesical fossa 1152
Sural nerve 334
Surgery
   complications of 524
   indications of 705, 731, 1026
   laparoscopic 1073
   radical 192, 542
Surgical blades 990, 991f
Surgical needle, parts of 1008, 1008f
Surgical peritoneum, division of 1093
Suture
   material, type of 749
   synthetic
      absorbable 1063, 1064f
      nonabsorbable 1069
   thickness of 1059f
   type of 1059f
Swab holding forceps 988f, 1024
Swelling 25, 27-30, 186, 210, 226, 281, 304, 382, 400, 453, 458, 489, 530, 540, 621, 686, 700
   abdomen 85
   compressibility of 34f

congenital 381
consistency of 30
examination of 452, 629
face 3
feet 3, 368
fixity of 31, 31f
inspection of 26f
intra-abdominal 732
large 440
malignant 381
margin of 29, 30f
smooth contour of 240
surface of 29f, 35f
Swiss cheese defect 74
Sympathetic chain, dissection of 1128
Sympathetic trunk 362, 1186
Symphysis pubis 48f, 49f, 356f, 1153, 1153f
Syringomyelia 521
Syringomyelocele 462
Systemic lupus erythematosus 339, 447, 755

T

Tabes mesenterica 869
Tachycardia 21, 189, 302, 368, 700
Tamoxifen therapy 249
   side effects of 249
Tanner's slide 55
Taper cut needles 1007
Tapping, complications of 624
Tazobactam 369
Telescope 1071
   insertion of 1088
Teletherapy 579
Temperature
   over breast 232f
   steam, low 985
Temporal artery, superficial 975
Temporal pulse, superficial 357
Tender spots, deep 88t
Tenderness, abdominal 170, 786, 805
Tendon sheath infection 966
   sequelae of 966
Tennison's repair 561
Tension pneumothorax 689, 692, 848
Tensor palate 498
Tensor tympani 498
Teratocarcinoma 924
Teratogenic drugs 558
Teratoma 386, 671

cells of origin of 924
mixed 671
types of 924
Terminal ileum, division of 1113
Terminal phalanx, resorption of 364
Testes, palpation of 213
Testicular
   artery 1146
      injury 634
   atrophy 60, 642, 598
   descent, chronology of 640, 640f, 1212
   enlargement 625
   function 631
   lymphatic vessels 1146
   swelling 60
   sympathetic plexus 1146
   tumors 598, 675, 621, 669, 670, 671, 675, 922, 925
      development of 675, 925
      management of 926
      TNM staging for 672
   vessels, short 640
   volume 632
Testis 508, 624, 639, 801
   anatomy of 1209
   arterial supply of 1211f
   atrophy of 626
   bilateral impalpable 641
   blood supply of 1211
   coverings of 1209
   defective development of 640
   descent of 639
   development of 1212, 1212f
   drain, lymphatic of 1212
   emergent 642
   epididymis, palpation of 41
   internal structure of 1210, 1210f
   interstitial cell of 1211
   lateral surface of 1210
   nongerm cell tumors of 924
   posterior border of 1210
   venous drainage of 633
Tetanus
   infection 936
   prophylaxis 725
Tetany, cause of 106
Thenar muscle 474, 481
Thenar space infection 964
   drainage of 964f
Thenar space, anatomy of 964
Therapeutic embolization, role of 222

Thermography 257
Thigh abscess 955
Thoracic
    artery, internal 1204
    esophagus 1158
    nerve, long 250, 1128
Thoracocentesis, indications of
    966
Thoracodorsal nerve 250, 470,
    1128
Thoracolumbar fascia, division
    of 1125
Thoracoscopy, role of 820
Thoracotomy 967
    indication of 691, 849
Thread veins 344
Thrombectomy, venous 766
Thrombolytic therapy 766
Thrombophilia 767
Thrombophlebitis, superficial
    336, 339
Thrombosis 443
    venous 334, 953
Thyrocervical trunk 1204
Thyroglobulin, role of 314
Thyroglossal cyst
    complications of 493
    locations of 491f
    pathology of 492
Thyroglossal duct, fates of 1203
Thyroglossal fistula, lining
    epithelium of 494
Thyroid 272, 284, 507, 801
    acropachy 303
    anaplastic carcinoma of 315
    antibody 306
    artery
        division of inferior 1129,
            1132
        inferior 1201
        superior 975, 1205
    cancer 308-312, 315
        anaplastic 311, 313
        extrathyroidal extension of
            320
        medullary 313, 317
        TNM staging for 311
    carcinoma 306, 310, 320, 316,
        802
        anaplastic 315
        development of 306
        differentiated 314
        familial medullary 318

TNM staging for 311
    types of 308
cartilage 357f, 523
cyst 285, 291, 293, 295
disease 272
gland 277, 278, 279f, 283, 283f,
    290, 492, 1199, 1200,
    1202
    arterial supply of 1201f
    benign tumor of 285
    blood supply of 1200
    capsules of 1200
    carcinoma of 276, 285, 305
    disposition of isthmus of
        1200
    isthmus of 277, 278f, 491
    lymphatic drainage of 1202,
        1202f
    palpation of 277, 277f, 278,
        278f
    parts of 1199
    venous drainage of 1202f
hormone 285
insufficiency 302
isthmus, dissection of 1130,
    1132
lesions 294
lobe
    exposure of 1131
    posterior surface of 277
medullary carcinoma of 292,
    306, 316
nodule 285, 287, 288, 293, 294
    solitary 285, 291-294, 309,
        318f, 491, 523, 756
profile study 285
region 274f
stimulating hormone 285, 304,
    317, 937
storm 302
swelling 279, 283, 285, 287
tissue 290
    residual 315
tumors
    prognostic classification of
        308
    types of 307
vein
    division of inferior 1129,
        1132
    division of middle 1129,
        1132
    fourth 1201
    inferior 1201

middle 1201
    superior 1201
    vessels, division of superior
        1129, 1132
Thyroidectomy 319, 1207
    complications of 302
    near total 290, 310
    role of total 290
    steps of total 1129
    subtotal 290, 299
    total 290, 318, 319, 758, 1129
Thyroiditis 304
    chronic 285
    granulomatous 305
Thyrotoxic myopathy 303
Thyrotoxicosis 296-300, 302, 303,
    598
    facies of 10f
    neurological manifestations of
        302
    primary 276, 295, 295f, 297
    recurrent 301
    secondary 289
    treatment of 301
Thyroxine binding globulin 298
Tibia, intercondylar area of 356f
Tibial artery pulse, anterior 355
Tibial nerve block, posterior 983,
    983f
Tibial pulse
    anterior 355f
    posterior 355
Tinel's sign 473
TIRADS classification system 286
Tissue
    diagnosis, role of 165
    necrosis 771
    subcutaneous 83, 381, 382,
        1089, 1090
    suture repair 65
Toe
    brachial index 375
    nail, management of ingrowing
        973
Toilet mastectomy 254
Tongue 14f, 507
    carcinoma of 570, 571, 571f
    drains, lymphatics of 576
    excision of 577
    posterior third of 577
    protrusion of 491, 491f
Tonsil, abdominal 866
Toothed dissecting forceps 1003,
    1003f

Towel clips 989, 989*f*
Toxemia 786
Trachea 275, 278
   position of 7
Tracheal
   dilator 1054, 1054*f*
   obstruction 289
Tracheomalacia 758, 759
Tracheostomy 307, 1052, 1139
   complications of 1053, 1139
   high 1052
   indications of 1051, 1139
   low 1052
   mid 1052
   tube 1052, 1053
      cuffed 1051
      disposable cuffed 1051*f*
      noncuffed 1051
Traction test 627, 627*f*
Transabdominal preperitoneal
   operation, steps of 1085
   repair 58, 65
Transcystic bile duct stone
   extraction, limitations of 168
Transcyte 724
Transhepatic
   cholangiography,
   percutaneous 152, 775
   route, percutaneous 171
Transillumination test 622*f*
Transitional cell tumors, grades
   of 915
Transluminal coronary
   angioplasty, percutaneous 946
Transpyloric plane 90
Transverse abdominal incision,
   anatomy of 1092
Transverse colon
   delivery of 1120
   division of 1113
   volvulus of 793
Transverse colostomy, steps of
   1119
Transverse incision, closure of
   1092
Transverse mesocolon 1120
   anterior layer of 1093
   rent, closure of 1110
Transverse nasalis 556, 556*f*
Transverse preputial island flap
   repair 665
Transverse rectus abdominis
   myocutaneous flap 269
Transversus abdominis muscle
   1091, 1092, 1121

Trapezius muscle, anterior border
   of 20*f*
Trauma 339, 624, 626, 675, 736,
   755, 925
   abdominal 698, 710
   pancreaticoduodenal 709
Traumatic arteriovenous fistula
   450, 450*f*
Traumatic ulcer, long-standing
   573
Treacher-Collins syndrome 558
Treitz, ligament of 828
Tremor 282, 304
Trendelenburg's operation 333,
   337
Trendelenburg's test 323, 324
Triceps muscle 464, 464*f*
Trigeminal nerve
   mandibular
      branch of 498
      division of 1196
   maxillary division of 1196
   palsy 3
Triglyceride cholesterol 761
Trimethoprim 374
Triple tube decompression 711
Trocar 1074
   entry, first 1100
   uses of 1075
Troisier's sign 162
Tropical eosinophilia 802
Trousseau's sign 162
Trucut needle biopsy 293, 316
Truncal vagotomy 125, 130, 131,
   1097
   steps of 1033, 1097
Trypanosoma cruzi 816
T-tube 1030
   cholangiogram 775, 813, 813*f*,
      814, 814*f*, 1030
   cholangiography,
      postoperative 170
   removal of 815
Tubercle bacilli 506, 830
Tubercular stricture, pathogenesis
   of 869
Tuberculosis 148, 172, 181, 505,
   653, 755, 830, 837, 869, 870
   abdominal 870
   hyperplastic 830, 870
   ileocecal 729, 829, 830
   intestinal 869, 870
   pulmonary 3, 297, 505
   ulcerative type of 830

Tuberosity, tibial 350*f*
Tubule formation 259
Tubulodermoid 386
Tuchsig's test 348
Tumor 307, 755, 931
   cells 223, 535
      prevent intraluminal spread
         of 204
   characteristics 252
   grade 246, 911
   histologic grade of 259*t*
   histological grade of 258
   inoperable 542
   local excision of 590
   marker 117
      serum levels of 672
      study, role of 165
   mucoepidermoid 543
   multiple 919
   nonepithelial 307
   noninvasive 754
   primary 111, 207, 224, 260, 436,
      508-510, 544, 574, 656, 672
   resectable 154
   size 911
   stage 319
   thickness 408, 412
   type of 642
   ulceration of 412
   vein interface 164
Tunica
   adventitia 363
   albuginea plication 664
   intima 363
   media 363
   vaginalis 1142
      sac 623
      suturing cut margins of
         1142
Turban tumor 425, 456
Turcot's syndrome 877, 879
Turnbull's no touch technique 202
Typhlitis, acute 729
Typhoid carriers, chronic 175, 902
Tyrosine kinase inhibitors 124

U

Ulcer 35, 366, 381
   benign 855, 857, 859
   cancer 226, 857, 862
   chronic 420, 427
   deep 371
   edge of 36*f*

excision of 131
healing of 340
infective 339, 572
local examination of 35
malignant 339
over breast 228
parts of 35f
postradiation 427
recurrent 134
syphilitic 572
traumatic 572
tubercular 572, 870
tuberculous 36
venous 339, 420
Ulceration 391, 443, 460
Ulcerative colitis 11, 881, 886-889
development of 887
extraintestinal manifestation of 888
grades of 888
Ulnar bursa 965f
infection of 964f, 965
Ulnar claw hand 477
Ulnar nerve 469, 470, 474, 481
block 982, 982f
injury 473, 473f, 477, 477f
palsy 473, 481
sensory supply of 474f
Ultrasonography 217, 239, 240, 413, 785
role of 240
transrectal 1022
Umbilical hernia, repair of 604f
Umbilical ligaments 1151
Umbilicus 87, 91, 616, 1152, 1153, 1153f
position of 6
Undescended testis 554, 634, 635, 635f, 638, 640, 642
complications of 642
incidence of 640
University of Texas Health Science Center San Antonio Classification System 379t
Upper paramedian incision, right 141
Ureter 755
division of 1126
removal of 222
USG of 68
Ureteric colic 2, 729, 731
Ureteric stenosis, congenital 907
Ureterocele 907
Ureterosigmoidostomy 669

Urethra 620, 755
develop, normal 663
prostatic 919f
rupture 718
stricture 1024
Urethral
dilatation 754, 1044
complications of 1045
diverticulum 666
injury, grades of 718
meatus, external 662
obstruction 908
rupture
triad of 718
types of 718
stricture 666, 1045
traumatic 719
treatment of 754
valve 618
congenital posterior 219
Urethrography 756
Urethroplasty 664, 665
Asopa's technique of 666
open 754
technique of 665f
Urge incontinence 215
Urinary
bladder 60, 61f, 755, 914f
benign papilloma of 914
carcinoma of 917t
development of 667f
lumen of 914f
palpation of 213
papillary carcinoma of 914
portion of 61
catheterization 79, 607
citrate 798
defects 668
diversion procedure, types of 669
excretion 738
infection 798
output 722
retention 60, 754
stasis 798
tuberculosis 912
Urination, frequency of 913
Urine
acute retention of 751, 1040
exfoliative cytology of 221
retention of 954
Urography, intravenous 217, 221, 756, 775, 842, 842f, 844, 844f, 918

Ursodeoxycholic acid 144, 898
Urticaria 189
Uterus 801

V

Vacuum-assisted closure 376, 377
Vagal trunk 1160
Vaginal hydrocele 33, 620, 621, 625, 630, 670
bilateral 621f
Vagotomy 130, 138
highly selective 129, 129f, 131
Vagus nerve
distribution of 1161f
division of anterior 1097
palsy 3
trunk, division of posterior 1097
Valvular failure 342
Vancomycin 369, 372
Varicella zoster virus 816
Varicocele 44, 627-631, 634
development of primary 631
grades of 632
ligation of 633
management of 633
operation, complications of 634
primary 630
secondary 630
types of 630
unilateral 631
Varicogram 344
Varicose ulcer 339, 341
treatment of 340
Varicose vein 321, 323, 324f, 334, 335, 337, 341, 343, 452, 974
complications of 341
primary 342
radiofrequency ablation
secondary 342
surgery 334
treatment of 335, 336, 339
Vas deferens 60, 1146
develops 639
short 640
Vascular
disease 36
peripheral 345
element 498
endothelial growth factor 364
hamartomas 444
Vasoactive intestinal peptide 317

Vasodilator drugs, role of 448
Vasovagal reaction 339
Vastus medialis 1217
Vatalanib 124
Vein 538, 1160, 1213
   communicating 1213
   deep 342, 1213
   draining penis 659
   empty segment of 353*f*
   plexus of 1165
   short saphenous system of 333
   superficial system of 1213
   systems of 1213
   thrombosis
      acute deep 336
      deep 84, 765-767
      development of deep 767
Vena cava
   inferior 222, 1181, 1181*f*
   injury, inferior 706
   obstruction
      inferior 93
      superior 93, 296
   superior 953*f*
   thrombosis, inferior 342
   tributaries of inferior 1181
Venesection
   indications of 1137
   steps of 1138*f*
Venography 343, 344
   ascending 332
Venous
   cut down 1137, 1138
   obstruction, deep 341
   surgery, role of direct 341
   thrombosis, deep 331, 334,
      336, 338, 339, 341, 342, 765
   ulcer
      long-standing 427
      recurrence of 340
Ventral hernia, repair of 80
Veress needle 1072, 1072*f*
Verrucous carcinoma 583, 927
Vertebral anomalies 554
Vertical incision 73
Vessels 1160, 1215
   of right colon, division of 1113

Vestibulocochlear nerve palsy 3
Vicryl rapide suture 1065*f*
Vinblastine 516
Vincristine 120, 516
Viral orchitis 675
Virchow's gland 18, 503
Virchow's lymph node 18, 19*f*
Visceral fibers 1186
Vision, double 3
Vitamin
   B complex deficiency 12
   C deficiency 12
   deficiency 12, 798
Vitellointestinal duct 615, 874, 875
   abnormalities of 615, 615*f*
   persistent 614, 614*f*
Vocal fremitus 7
Volar space infection 963
Volkman's retractor 1015, 1015*f*
Volkman's spoon or scoop 1047,
   1047*f*
Volvulus 790
   recurrence of 792
Vomiting 2, 85, 133, 159, 248, 249,
   746, 784, 827
   bilious 134
von Graefe's sign 276, 280
von Hippel-Lindau disease 223,
   910
von Recklinghausen's disease 454,
   456-458
Vulva, elephantiasis of 646

W

Wagner's grading system 379
Wardill-Kilner-Veau four flap
   technique 568*f*
Warm nodule 288
Warthin tumor 537
Water Lily sign 186
Water soluble contrast study 793
Watercan perineum 1022
Water-soluble contrast studies 745
Web space
   anatomy of 963
   infection 963, 963*f*

Wedge biopsy, deep 425
Wegener's granulomatosis 801
Weight loss 2, 85, 137, 159, 178,
   223, 830, 831, 838, 839
Whipple's operation 155, 155*f*,
   156, 157, 161, 163, 765, 812,
   1103, 1105*f*
Whipple's
   pancreaticoduodenectomy
      712, 1033, 1107
   steps of 1107
Whipple's procedure 161, 712
White blood cell 380, 770
White rami communicantes 1185
Witzel gastrostomy 1140
Worm infestation 181, 897
Worm, lifecycle of 890
Wound
   complications 84
   dehiscence 460
      abdominal 748
      treatment of 748
   drainage 749
   healing 377
   hematoma 73
   infection 60, 73, 302, 460, 528,
      666, 768, 771, 772
   postoperative 769
Wrist 400
   extensor 465, 465*f*
   flexors 479, 480*f*

X

Xanthine stones 797
Xeroderma pigmentosum 405,
   420, 428
Xerophthalmia 12

Z

Zieman's test 50, 50*f*
Zollinger-Ellison syndrome 855,
   858, 1094
Zygomatic arch 357*f*

Opinions About the Book

"Bedside Clinics in Surgery, a book which is needed by the undergraduate and postgraduate students alike. It forms the logical next step to 'Clinical Surgery' by Dr Das, and may even replace it as the student's companion for clinical cases.

One of the prime difficulties in reading textbooks is the long paragraphs and prose, uninterrupted by photographs, diagrams or color diagrams. The author has successfully overcome this by formatting the text as questions and answers. The inclusion of photographs, especially color pathology slides, is welcome.

Each section starts with an outline for describing a case. This would be extremely useful for the students, as they know which points are to be stressed during presentation. I would further commend the author in pointing out errors usually made by the students, e.g. saying 'nothing significant' in family history."

I have not come across another book, which covers the case, from a clinical point of view so well, e.g. even the doses and side effects of antituberculous drugs are given. Hence, the student does not have to cross-refer to a number of books.

One of the problems, postgraduate students face, is the variety of ways in which a problem can be tackled. This book gives the most widely accepted technique of doing so.

The inclusion of pathology specimens is the first of its kind as far as I know. Description of X-rays and instruments makes it a complete book for the exam-going students.

—AK Attri, JIMA, November 2005 Issue

"The book has an interesting question and answer format, which is exam oriented. I found it to be informative and accurate. The diagrams are clear and simple. The instruments and pathology specimens are clear."

**—Dr Benjamin Perakath, Professor and Head
Department of Surgery Unit V, Christian Medical College, Vellore, India**

"I like it very much. I have recommended it to my students. The clinical examination, eliciting signs, writing a case sheet, common questions that will be asked and answers to the questions, surgical pathology, instruments, operative procedures and totally the presentation of book shows the experience and expertise of the author. I am sure a student who has no knowledge can excel with this book in hand and do well in the examination."

**—Dr B Kanchana, Professor and Head, Department of Surgery
Aarupadai Veddu Medical College and Hospital
Kirumampakkam, Puducherry, India**

"Students from our institute are also looking for an additional book on surgery clinics to do better than others in practical examination."

**—Dr Suneel Kumar Gadikota, Associate Professor of General Surgery
Kamineni Institute of Medical Sciences, Narketpally, Nalgonda, Andhra Pradesh, India**

"The book has great scope for undergraduates, postgraduates and staff as well. It includes all contemporary material. The book is a boon for undergraduates as the text is made very easy to understand and in friendly language with most frequently asked questions in examinations."

—Dr Gurpal Singh Chhabda, Associate Professor of General Surgery
Kamineni Institute of Medical Sciences, Narketpally, Nalgonda, Andhra Pradesh, India

"I have gone through the book titled as *Bedside Clinics in Surgery* by Dr Makhan Lal Saha, which is highly educative and complete in all aspects of the surgery for the students of undergraduate and postgraduate courses. Everything is discussed in a comprehensive manner on long and short cases including traumatic and emergency services. It is also a rare phenomenon to discuss in detail about the X-ray procedures and surgical pathology pertaining to the patients. It has also a practical discussion procedures. No other book discusses in such a great length about the instruments which are quite crucial for exam-appearing students. Though it is not a substitute for textbook of surgery, it gives readymade guidelines for the students appearing for undergraduate and postgraduate examinations."

—Superintendent, Osmania General Hospital, Hyderabad, Andhra Pradesh, India

"The book is good and it will be useful to the undergraduates and postgraduates in surgery."

—Dr BS Gedam, Professor
Department of Surgery, Government Medical College, Nagpur, India

"It has plenty of information for a quick revision before examinations or even before presentations. Highly recommended."

—Dr RCM Kaza, Professor
Department of Surgery, Maulana Azad Medical College, New Delhi, India

"The question and answers given in each chapter are the frequently asked questions in any standard examination by the examiner.
The author should be congratulated for using the clinical photographs from his own collection and colleagues. The book covers not only clinical surgery but also X-rays, surgical pathology, preoperative preparations, minor surgical procedures and instruments."

—Dr N Dorairajan, Professor, Department of Surgery
Madras Medical College, Chennai, Tamil Nadu, India

"Keeping in view the practical and viva-voce of MBBS examinations, the book has been designed in a different style. The content of the book is precise and methodical. Series of common long and short cases with related questions will prove helpful to the students. The author has very well compiled the common operative procedures; details of routine instruments and various common radiographs."

—Prof M Amanullah Khan, Chairman, JN Medical College
Aligarh Muslim University, Aligarh, Uttar Pradesh, India

Dr Saha has done a very good job and the book is a very useful not only for undergraduates but also for postgraduate students as well. The section on short cases in surgery is particularly helpful for the students and gives them relevant information as a question-answer session."

—Dr Navneet Kaur, UCMS and Guru Tegh Bahadur Hospital, Delhi, India

"I have gone through the book and found to be useful for the undergraduate students and I strongly recommend this book for reference to MBBS students."

—Dr AT Kamble, Professor and Head, Department of Surgery
Indira Gandhi Government Medical College, Nagpur, Maharashtra, India

"The book discusses all the probable questions that may be asked in the clinical examination. The author must be a good examiner and also observed the questions asked by other examiners in the clinical examination. The investigations described are relevant to the clinical cases. The surgical pathology, X-rays, surgical procedures and instruments described are adequate and essential for surgical students.

I recommend this book for all MBBS students. Junior teaching faculty members will be benefited by reading this book and will help them in taking bedside clinics."

—Dr D Premkumar, Professor and Head, Department of Surgery
IRT—Perundurai Medical College and Hospital, Tamil Nadu, India

"It is a pleasure to write a prologue for the book *Bedside Clinics in Surgery* authored by Dr Makhan Lal Saha on the eve of publication of the revised second edition. This book has been already an extremely popular entity in the earlier editions. A comprehensive book like this is hardly available in this country to cater the needs of both undergraduate and postgraduate students of surgical mainstream. The clinical part of the book exhaustively deals with examination and diagnosis with suitable explanations along with a comprehensive coverage of the theoretical background. The pictorial inclusion of a variety of surgical cases is an asset of this publication. The addition of Operative Surgery has widened the scope of this book to be a total guide for examination of the subject. The book is well recommended for the students of surgery."

—Dr BP Chakravarty, Professor of Surgery, Ex-Professor and Head, Department of Surgery
RG Kar Medical College and Hospital, Kolkata, West Bengal, India
Bankura Sammilani Medical College, Bankura, West Bengal, India
MGM Medical College and Hospital, Jamshedpur, Jharkhand, India